Essentials of Endodontics

Second Edition

Essentials of Endodontics

Second Edition

Vimal K Sikri

MDS, DOOP(PU), DEME(AIU), FICD

former Professor and Head
Department of Conservative Dentistry and Endodontics, and
Principal, Punjab Government Dental College and Hospital
Amritsar, Punjab
India

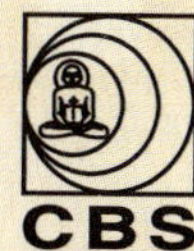

CBS Publishers & Distributors Pvt Ltd

New Delhi • Bengaluru • Chennai • Kochi • Kolkata • Mumbai

Bhopal • Bhubaneswar • Hyderabad • Jharkhand • Nagpur • Patna • Pune • Uttarakhand • Dhaka (Bangladesh)

Disclaimer

Science and technology are constantly changing fields. New research and experience broaden the scope of information and knowledge. The author has tried his best in giving information available to him while preparing the material for this book. Although all efforts have been made to ensure optimum accuracy of the material, yet it is quite possible some errors might have been left uncorrected. The publisher, the printer and the author will not be held responsible for any inadvertent errors, omissions or inaccuracies.

Essentials of
Endodontics
Second Edition

ISBN: 978-93-87964-69-3

Second Edition 2019
First Edition 2012

Published by Satish Kumar Jain and produced by Varun Jain for
CBS Publishers & Distributors Pvt Ltd
4819/XI Prahlad Street, 24 Ansari Road, Daryaganj, New Delhi 110 002
Ph: 23289259, 23266861, 23266867 Fax: 011-23243014 Website: www.cbspd.com
e-mail: delhi@cbspd.com; cbspubs@airtelmail.in

Corporate Office: 204 FIE, Industrial Area, Patparganj, Delhi 110 092
Ph: 4934 4934 Fax: 4934 4935 e-mail: publishing@cbspd.com; publicity@cbspd.com

Branches

- **Bengaluru:** Seema House 2975, 17th Cross, K.R. Road, Banasankari 2nd Stage, Bengaluru 560 070, Karnataka
  Ph: +91-80-26771678/79 Fax: +91-80-26771680 e-mail: bangalore@cbspd.com
- **Chennai:** 7, Subbaraya Street, Shenoy Nagar, Chennai 600 030, Tamil Nadu
  Ph: +91-44-26260666, 26208620 Fax: +91-44-42032115 e-mail: chennai@cbspd.com
- **Kochi:** 42/1325, 1326, Power House Road, Opp KSEB Power House, Ernakulam 682 018, Kochi, Kerala
  Ph: +91-484-4059061-65 Fax: +91-484-4059065 e-mail: kochi@cbspd.com
- **Kolkata:** No. 6/B, Ground Floor, Rameswar Shaw Road, Kolkata-700014 (West Bengal), India
  Ph: +91-33-2289-1126, 2289-1127, 2289-1128 e-mail: kolkata@cbspd.com
- **Mumbai:** 83-C, Dr E Moses Road, Worli, Mumbai-400018, Maharashtra
  Ph: +91-22-24902340/41 Fax: +91-22-24902342 e-mail: mumbai@cbspd.com

Representatives

• Bhopal	0-8319310552	• Bhubaneswar	0-9911037372	• Hyderabad	0-9885175004
• Jharkhand	0-9811541605	• Nagpur	0-9021734563	• Patna	0-9334159340
• Pune	0-9623451994	• Uttarakhand	0-9716462459	• Dhaka (Bangladesh)	01912-003485

Printed at Goyal Offset Printers, GT Karnal Road, Industrial Area, Delhi, India

to

Divine energy of learning and knowledge

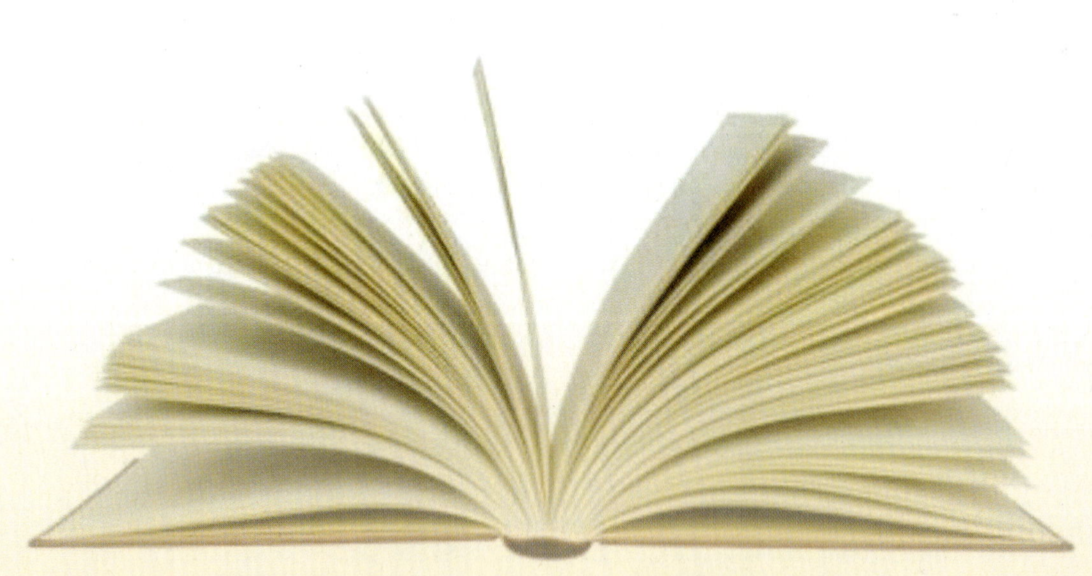

I owe, the Almighty God, gratitude for all His blessing

Contributors

Ankit Sikri
Associate professor
Bhojia Dental College and Hospital
Baddi (Himachal Pradesh) 173205
Email: sikriankit@gmail.com

Annupriya Sikri
Reader
National Dental College and Hospital
Gulabgarh
DeraBassi 140507 (Punjab)
Email: annupriya05@gmail.com

Arathi Ganesh
Professor and Head
Sri Ramachandran Dental College
SRMC and RI (DU)
Porur, Chennai 600116
Email: drarthiganesh@gmail.com

Arpit Sikri
Assistant Professor
Sudha Rustagi College of Dental Sciences and Research
Faridabad 121003
Email: arpitsikri@gmail.com

B Rajkumar
Professor and Had
BBD College of Dental Sciences
BBD University, Faizabad Road
Lucknow 226028
E mail: office@bbdcods.edu.in

Devendra Chopra
Reader
Saraswati Dental College and Hospital
233, Tiwari Ganj, Chinhat
Lucknow (UP) 227105
Email: drdevendra45@gmail.com

Faizal CP
Professor and Head
Kannur Dental College
Anjarakandy PO
Kannur (Kerala) 670612
Email: drfaizalcp@gmail.com

Gomty Mahajan
Associate professor
Department of Microbiology
Punjab Institute of Medical Sciences
Jalandhar, Punjab 144011
Email: drgomty@gmail.com

Jyotsana Sikri
Senior lecturer
Sudha Rustagi College of Dental Sciences and Research
Faridabad 121003
Email: jyotsanasikri@gmail.com

Mahantesh Yeli
Professor and Head
SDM College of Dental Sciences and Hospital
Dharwad 580009
Email: mantuuu@yahoo.com

Mahima Mohit
Professor
SDM College of Dental Science
Sattur, Dharwad 580009
Email: mahima702002@yahoo.co.in

Mamta Kaushik
Professor
Army College of Dental Sciences
ACDS Nagar (Chennapur–CRPF Road)
Jai Jawahar Nagar, Secunderabad 500087
Email: mamkaushik@gmail.com

Puneet Girdhar
Assistant Professor
Punjab Govt. Dental College and Hospital
Amritsar 143001
Email: puneetgirdhar@gmail.com

Rajesh Pillay
Professor and Head
PMS College of Dental Science and Research
Golden Hills, Venkode
Trivandrum 695028
Email: pmscollege@gmail.com

S Balagopal
Vice Principal and Professor and Head of the Department
Tagore Dental College and Hospital
Chennai 600127
Email: sbalagopal@yahoo.com

Shashirekha Govind
Professor
Institute of Dental Sciences
K-8, Kalinga Nagar
Bhubaneswar 751003
Email: shashirekha123@yahoo.com

Vasudev Ballal
Professor
Department of Conservative Dentistry and Endodontics
Manipal College of Dental Sciences
Manipal 576104
Email: drballal@yahoo.com

Viresh Chopra
Faculty of Endodontology
Oman Dental College
PO Box-835, Mina Al Fahal, Postal Code 116
Sultanate of Oman
Email: info@omandentalcollege.org

Foreword

Endodontics is fundamental to the modern clinical practice of dentistry. As evidenced by this timely, authorative book *Essentials of Endodontics* has over the years, grown and expanded to become a multifaceted branch of the art and science of dentistry.

As in all branches of dentistry, successful clinical outcomes are highly dependent on the knowledge, understanding, skill and meticulous attention to detail by the clinician. This book provides the knowledge and through the careful structuring and presentation by Dr Sikri and the many eminent contributors, the opportunity to develop a sound understanding of contemporary endodontics. Given the appropriate application of this knowledge and understanding, those who read and otherwise consult this 'treasure house' of information should be able to look forward to practising highly effective and professionally rewarding endodontics. In this way Dr Sikri and his colleagues will fulfil their mission in sharing their expert knowledge and understanding, enthusiasm and quest for excellence in "principle-based" endodontics.

Dr Sikri and his colleagues who have contributed to this highly commendable book, together with the publishers are to be congratulated on the way in which they have brought together and lucidly presented a considerable mass of important information in respect of modern endodontics in an easy to read, user-friendly and extensively illustrated text. This book is a great credit to all those involved in its preparation and publication.

This book is highly recommended to both students and practitioners wishing to provide their patients with high quality, state-of-the-art endodontics. Endodontics as presented in this book will enhance clinical success in the management of diseased and damaged teeth with a compromised, let alone nonvital pulpodentinal complex.

Nairn HF Wilson DSc (h.c.), PhD, MSc, BDS, FDS, FFD, FGDP (UK), DRD
Dean and Head of King's College London
Dental Institute

Preface to the Second Edition

Any book is considered worth reading if readers' analysis is positively assessed by the author. A good number of students, after analysing the first edition, suggested modifications in text and flow. Endodontics, being a dynamic subject, need upgradation on periodic basis; coupled with incorporating wishes of the readers.

Tremendous changes have occurred since the first edition was published; both in our understanding of the basic biology of the disease process as well as the development of techniques and gadgets used in endodontic therapy. The focus of second edition is primarily to update the text incorporating all the advances in materials, instruments and techniques, which have revolutionized endodontics in the past couple of years; and also add valued knowledge to biological/biocompatible approach in the treatment phase. Recently, advances in microbial dynamics and understanding of nuances of root canal variations have made endodontic prognosis more predictable.

The present edition is thoroughly updated. A few new chapters are added, viz. Drugs used in Endodontics, Endodontic Case Selection: Treatment Planning, Ethics in Endodontics, etc. Another few chapters are bifurcated, expanding text and figures, vis-à-vis the developments in the subject. The important sub-subjects are summarized in boxes for ready reference of the readers. Many line diagrams and clinical photographs are added in every chapter for easy to understanding of the text. The language of the text, as usual, is kept lucid and simple.

Summarily, the book will be an asset for the undergraduate and postgraduate students as well as teachers and practitioners interested in the subject of 'Endodontics'.

I am thankful to Dr Nitin Verma, Assistant Professor, GDC, Amritsar, for updating the chapter on Surgical Endodontics. I am whole heartedly grateful to Dr Vivek Hegde (Pune) and Dr Mahalaxmi (Chennai) for photographs of their endodontic cases. I am thankful to my students, Dr Tejinder, Dr Komal, and Dr Neha for reading the manuscript.

Completing this book would not have been possible without contributions from multitude of academicians and eminent teachers. My wife, Dr Poonam Sikri, my sons, Dr Ankit, Dr Arpit and my daughter-in-laws, Dr Annupriya, Dr Jyotsana whole-heartedly supported me in this adventure.

Last but not the least, I am thankful to all those who helped me directly or indirectly in compiling the manuscript of the book.

I look forward to your suggestions, comments and criticism for future improvement in the book.

Vimal K Sikri

Preface to the First Edition

Over the years in my profession, I have realized that there is no limit to learning much more in the subject you think you know well. In more than three decades of my teaching career, I have always encouraged my students to raise more and more questions. Students' queries have provided me with an enriching experience that has endorsed my belief that learning is a never ending process. The knowledge that gathered in these years, complimented with my long clinical experience is all enshrined in this book *Essentials of Endodontics*.

It has been rightly said that knowledge lies in the accumulation of the facts and wisdom in its simplification. The book in your hand is simple and comprehensive, made to serve as an introductory text for students as well as a useful guide for the practitioners. The concepts presented in the book have been developed over the time under the influence of my teachers and co-operation of my colleagues and students.

Like all sciences, endodontic therapy is also based upon sound principles. Every effort has been invested to make this book authentic, scholarly and self-evident. Color coded key information boxes serve as easy to use navigational aids for the students. While going through the text the readers will find solutions to myriad endodontic challenges. A chapter 'Resinifying therapy in endodontics'—a solution to many endodontic problems has been added for the benefit of clinicians and practitioners.

A loving heart is said to be the beginning of all knowledge. I am sincerely grateful to Almighty God, the constant source of my strength for bestowing upon me that requisite heart. I have had the good fortune of working under a great teacher, Dr SS Dua, whose blessings and continuous patronage have led this book to see the light of the day.

I would like to extend special thanks to all those who have contributed their experiences in the form of text and photographs in this book. I extend my gratitude to my colleagues in the department, Dr Renu Bala Sroa, Professor; Dr Baljeet Sidhu, Demonstrator and Dr Jagan Jyot, Medical Officer whose suggestions have been carefully considered and acted upon. Dr Nitin Verma has been of valuable help in re-organizing the chapter on 'Surgical Endodontics'. I am thankful to Mr Vipul for making beautiful Corel diagrams, to Mr Ashwani Mahajan for his ready-to-help attitude and to Dr Puneet Girdhar and Dr Sachin Dev Mehta for bearing with my over-occupation especially during travelling. I express my heartfelt thanks to Dr Anil Chandra of CSJM Medical University, Lucknow, Dr Deepak Grover and Dr Gurpreet of National Dental College, DeraBassi, Dr Aamir of Govt. Dental College, Srinagar, Dr Isha Narang of BHU, Varanasi and Dr Agam Bhatnagar of SGT Dental College, Gurgaon for contributing in the form of photographs. I eulogize the efforts of my students Dr Gulvinder, Dr Payal, Dr Amrit Preet, Dr Preeti Jain, Dr Meenu Garg, Dr Ruchika Arora, Dr Laxmi Gahlot, Dr Isha Sood, Dr Garima Malhotra, Dr Ibadat Preet Kaur, Dr Shalini Sinha, Dr Mandeep Kaur, Dr Priyanka Setia and Dr Shikha Sharma for organizing manuscript and the photographs.

Last but not the least I am thankful to my wife, Dr Poonam and my dear sons, Dr Ankit and Arpit for their encouragement during preparation of this manuscript and also during countless hours of organizing and editing the text.

A book is a treasure house upon which we can draw again and again and I hope this book proves to be a real one.

Vimal K Sikri

Contents

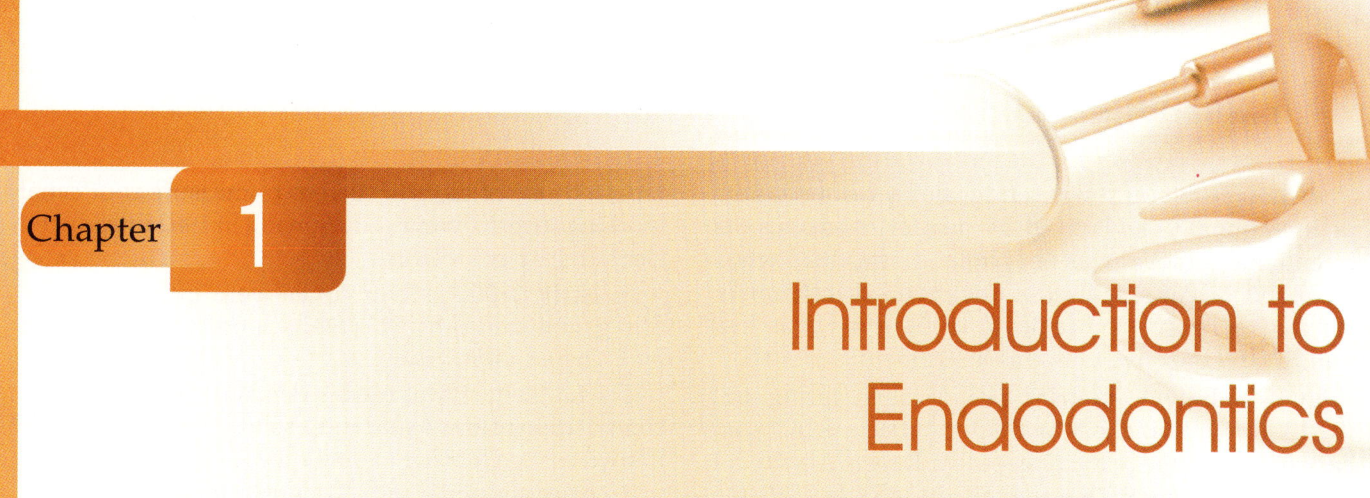

Chapter 1

Introduction to Endodontics

Endodontics, the name derived from 'Endo' means inside, 'Dont' means the tooth and 'ics' means the study; that is, the study of inside of the teeth. The pulp, which is inside the tooth, is a specialized connective tissue encased by dentin. The dentin is further covered by enamel in the coronal part and cementum in the radicular part. The collective study of physiology and pathology of pulpal tissue along with their sequalae is 'Endodontics'.

DEFINITIONS

The science dealing with diseases of pulp and the periapical tissues is endodontics. It is defined as *'the division of dental science that deals with etiology, diagnosis, treatment and prevention of diseases of dental pulp and their sequelae'*.

SCOPE OF ENDODONTICS

Pulpal and periapical diseases are common in dentistry. Untreated cases lead to bone destruction and subsequent extraction of the concerned tooth. Endodontics provides treatment to such cases and the tooth can be saved; protecting stomatognathic system in functions. Endodontics can be beneficial in variety of cases, such as:

- Pulp exposures (complete or partial)
- Periapical abscess
- Root fractures
- Root perforations
- Teeth with incomplete apical root development
- Endodontic implants
- Replants
- Transplants (autotransplants or allotransplant)
- Occlusal trauma causing reversible pulpitis
- Overzealous root planing and curettage, leading to pulpal sensitivity
- Extensive infrabony pocket formation extending beyond the root apex
- Surgical intervention of pulpal problems (apicoectomy, hemisection, etc.)
- Developmental anomalies of pulpal tissue.

EVOLUTION OF ENDODONTICS

The evolution of scientific development in endodontics dates from the third decade of 17th century. Literature on the early history of endodontics is sparse and undocumented as early history of dentistry. The beginning of endodontics is both slow and late. It was further retarded by the focal infection theory. Only in 1956, it attained a degree of acceptability and respect when the American Board of Endodontics was established.

An archaeological excavation by the department of antiquities and museums in northern Negev desert (Israel) recovered the skeletal remains of 25 people buried in a mass grave approximately in 200 BC. Subsequent analysis of the dentition showed one skeleton with a 2.5 mm bronze wire implanted in maxillary right lateral incisor. This is the first archaeological evidence of endodontic procedure performed in ancient Israel, which is documented.

On the radiograph, the root canal appears to have been artificially widened to a depth of 2.5 mm in preparation for insertion of the wire. This implies direct intervention by a skilled dental practitioner rather than a haphazard procedure performed by a layman.

The pulp of an aching tooth was often cauterized either by a red-hot cautery or by means of a chemical or a weak acid. The use of a hot wire has been mentioned by F. Hoffman (1753) in his book *A Treatise on the Teeth; their Disorders and Cure.*

Josiah Flagg of Boston, the first American to practice dentistry exclusively, relieved pain of an abscessed tooth by creating an opening into the crown, leading to the pulp cavity. He named this operation as 'tapping the pulp'.

Although the pulp was left to die by cauterization, or intentionally devitalized by heat or chemicals; its intentional removal was not planned until 1824 when Delmond of Paris devised a fine, hooked instrument for that purpose. The removal of the pulp was less painful and effective with this instrument.

In 1838, Edwin Maynard took a watch spring and filed it down to make a four-sided broach, which can entwine and remove the pulp easily. Robert Arthur cut barbs on broaches with a penknife in 1853. In 1885, the Gates Glidden drill and in 1904, the K-file were introduced. Standardization of instruments was proposed by Trebitsch in 1929 and again by Ingle in 1958 but again meant to be reviewed for rotary Ni-Ti instruments.

Following removal of the entire pulp, radicular space preparation was done by step-back or telescopic technique since 1969 as first described by Clem and Weine. Another major breakthrough for root canal preparation as crown down technique was given by John Pappin and Marshall in 1980, followed by "Balanced force" concept by Roane in 1985.

Philip Pfaff performed the conventional pulp capping of diseased pulp in 1756. In 1874, Adolf Witzed of Germany tried pulp mummification with different materials. In 1836, in "Guide to sound Teeth", Shearjashub Spooner introduced a technique for pulp devitalization of the pulp by arsenic. This technique continued for well over 100 years. Chapin A. Harris of Baltimore, one of the founders of the first dental school, who also used the drug at the same time; however, he warned against its use because of arsenic potential to damage the teeth and soft tissue. About the middle of the 19th century, efforts were made to conserve the pulp with medicaments such as creosote, Canada balsam and alcohol. The agent used was wiped over the exposed pulp and it was capped with metal disk, oiled silk, asbestos, plaster of Paris, lead or tin foil, collodion, etc.

Root canal filling actually preceded removal of the entire pulp. After the removal of the pulp, the canal was filled with some foreign substance often gold foil. Documentary proof of gold foil fillings in 1809 by Edward Hudson of Philadelphia is available. In 1890, Gramm used copper points, which were plated with gold to prevent dissolution.

Guttapercha, an extract of trees of sapodilla family, mixed with lime, quartz and feldspar; was introduced in 1850 and marketed under the name of Hill's stopping. In 1867, GA Bowman of St. Louis used guttapercha points for filling of root canals.

Working length determination was performed by radiographic technique since 1908 as first described by Meyer L. Rhein. In 1918, Custer for the first time reported use of electric current to measure root canal working length. Eventually Sunada in 1962 introduced electronic apex locators.

In early 1930's, silver cones were introduced for filling root canals by H. Trebitsch and later modified by E. Jasper of St. Louis.

The first cement was used in dentistry in 1856. A crude composition of zinc oxide and a solution of zinc chloride known as oxychloride of zinc was popular at that time.

Two outstanding English dentists, John Hunter, who wrote, 'The Natural History of Human Teeth (1778)', and Joseph Fox strongly advocated transplantation of tooth. Hunter used to boil the teeth before transplantation. Since venereal diseases were rampant, boiling of teeth was preferred. However, it was not done for reasons of sterility but rather for removal of the attached soft tissue. Hunter first successfully implanted a human tooth in a cock's comb.

James Gardette, (1950) another Philadelphia dentist, is given credit for intentional replantation of teeth in America.

In 1864, Stanford C. Barnum of New York invented rubber dam for keeping the operative field clear of saliva and soft tissues.

Otto Walkoff in 1891 introduced camphorated monochlorophenol as an intracanal medicament, which he found to be more effective and less irritating.

Wilhelm Konrad Roentgen discovered X-ray in 1895. Two weeks after Roentgen announced his discovery, a pioneer in endodontics, Professor Otto Walkhoff, took radiograph of his own teeth, exposing the plate for 25 minutes.

In 1906, Dr John P Buckley mixed cresol with formalin, which became known as Formocresol, and is still the favoured intracanal medicament among practising endodontists.

Until the late 1850s, ice and heat had been used to determine whether the pulp was dead or alive. In 1867, Magitot of France, suggested the use of an electric current to determine if vitality was present in a tooth. However, Marshall in 1891 popularized it. Focal infection theory promulgated by William Hunter in 1910 was blindly followed in dentistry, particularly in root canal treatment.

Local anesthesia was discovered in 1884, when at the suggestion of Sigmund Freud; Carl Koller, a Viennese ophthalmologist, first used a solution of cocaine as a topical anesthetic for eye surgery. In 1885, William S. Halsted of New York, made the first block injection (a mandibular bone) with the cocaine solution. Myer in 1904 developed 'Myer Dental Obtunder' a high-pressure syringe for anesthetizing the pulp and in 1906 infiltration anesthesia was introduced by Vaughan.

The placement of calcium hydroxide as a sub-base in deep cavities where the removal of all decay would expose the pulp (indirect pulp capping) has been used successfully since its introduction by Walter Hess in 1951.

Numerous agents are being used for smear layer removal from the root canals, like EDTA (15% Ethylenediaminetetraacetate acid) since 1957 by Nygaard-Ostby followed by Fehr in 1963 who introduced EDTAC (15% EDTA + Cetrimide) and Steward 1969 RC Prep (10% urea peroxide + 15% EDTA). Citric acid in 40% concentration was first used by Tidmarsh in 1978 followed by 20% concentration by Wayman (1979) and 10% citric acid by Baugmgartner (1984). Koskinen reported the success of several cases using Tubulicid (38% benzalkonium chloride, EDTA, 50% citric acid) in 1975 followed by Largal Ultra (15% EDTA, Cetrimide, NaOH) in 1980. Salvizol another root canal chelating agent with broad spectrum bactericidal activity (5.0% aminoquinaldinium diacetate) was introduced by Kaufman in 1981. Torabinejad first used MTAD containing citric acid and doxycycline as decalcifying substances in 2003.

The period of dentistry in the early part of 20th century was characterized by the introduction of basic sciences, especially Endodontics. As we go back to 200 years of progress in endodontics, it is almost like comparing the stone age with the present technologies (Table 1.1). Various sciences have contributed to a much better understanding of the physiology and pathology of pulp, enabling us to examine and compare it in health and disease.

Table 1.1	Evolution of Endodontics
200 BC	First evidence of endodontic dentistry with 2.5 mm bronze wire in maxillary right lateral incisor
500 AD	Aetius first recorded endodontic surgical procedure (the incision and drainage of an acute abscess)
1725	Lazare Riviere used clove oil as obtundent, later used oil of cinnamon, camphor or turpentine
1728	Pierre Fauchard in his textbook "Le Chirurgien Dentiste" first described dental pulp
1746	Pierre Fauchard described removal of pulp
1753	F. Hoffman advocated cauterization of pulp with hot wire
1756	Philip Pfaff described pulp capping of diseased pulp
1757	Bourdet described a therapy of extracting carious teeth, followed by filling the canals with gold and re-implanting them
1778	John Hunter advocated re-implantation when crown was partially destroyed due to caries
1783	Woofendale used cautery for destroying the pulp to relieve pain
1809	Edward Hudson plugged root canal with gold foil in anterior teeth only
1820	Leonard Koecker used hot wire for cauterization of exposed pulp and covered with a lead foil for its cooling effect
1824	Delmond devised a fine, hooked instrument for pulp extirpation
1836	Shearjashub Spooner advised pulp devitalization by Arsenic
1838	Edwin Maynard filed an instrument into a four sided broach
1839	World's first dental journal was introduced
1847	Edwin Truman introduced gutta-percha as a filling material
1850	Hill introduced Guttapercha mixed with lime, quartz and feldspar marketed under the name of Hill's stopping
1850	WW Codman confirmed that the aim of pulp capping proposed by Koecker in 1821, was to form a dentin bridge
1853	Robert Arthur introduced barbs and handles on broaches
1864	Stanford C. Barnum introduced rubber dam
1866	Chase introduced pulp mummification
1867	GA Bowman introduced gutta-percha points for root canal filling
1867	Magitot suggested use of electric current to determine vitality of pulp
1879	Witzel introduced phenol
1880	Brophy used heat to check the status of pulp, traced sinus tract
1883	Perry used gutta-percha wrapped around a gold wire
1883	WE Harding differentiated between pulp capping of an accidental and intentional exposure
1884	Carl Koller firstly used topical local anaesthesia with cocaine
1885	Lepkoski advised use of formalin despite of arsenic to 'dry' pulp

(Contd...)

1

Table 1.1	Evolution of Endodontics (*Contd...*)
1885	William S Halsted described first local anesthesia block injection, a mandibular nerve block with a cocaine solution
1890	Gramm introduced copper points for filling root canals, later gold plated them to prevent discoloration
1891	Otto Walkoff introduced camphorated monochlorophenol as intracanal medicament
1900	Price described periapical radiolucencies as 'blind abscesses' and advised use of radiographs for diagnosis of pulpless teeth
1904	Frank Billings directed attention on relationship between oral sepsis and bacterial endocarditis
1904	Myer introduced High Pressure Syringe for anesthetizing the pulp, 'Myer Dental Obtunder'
1906	Vaughan introduced infiltration anaesthesia
1906	John P Buckley introduced formocresol
1908	Meyer L Rhein introduced a technique for determining canal length and level of obturation
1909	EC Rosenow developed the theory of 'focal infection' in a study of bacterial aspects of root canal treatment
1910	William Hunter devised 'focal infection theory'
1918	Custer investigated the electronic method for root length determination
1930	BW Hermann introduced calcium hydroxide
1930	H Trebitsch introduced silver cones for root canal filling
1955	Kuttler defined the apical anatomy of cemento-enamel junction with regard to working length determination
1957	Richman credited with the use of ultrasonics in endodontics
1957	Nygaard-Ostby introduced EDTA (ethylenediaminetetraacetate acid)
1960	Theodore H Maiman introduced LASER
1961	Ostby described role of blood clot in endodontic therapy
1962	Sunada introduced electronic apex locator
1963	Fehr introduced EDTAC (15% EDTA + Cetrimide)
1965	Leon Goldman first use laser on a tooth
1966	Frank described apexification technique
1969	Clem and Weine introduced 'Step-back' or telescopic technique for root canal preparation
1969	Steward introduced RC prep (10% Urea peroxide and 15% EDTA)
1971	Weichman first attempt to use laser in endodontic surgery
1971	Inoue developed electronic apex locator Sonoexplorer (low frequency electronic apex locator)
1974	Schilder described vertical compaction of guttapercha
1977	FS Yee introduced obtura unit for root canal filling
1977	Baumann described the use of operating microscope in endodontics
1978	Ben Johnson introduced Thermafil
1978	Apotheker and Jako: Concept of extreme magnification in the form of operating microscope
1979	McSpadden introduced the Thermomechanical compaction
1979	Detsch described the use of endoscope in endodontic diagnosis
1979	Cox and Cooke first described C shaped canal
1980	John Pappin and Marshall introduced 'Crown-down' preparation for canal preparation
1981	Chayes-Virginia Inc.: Dental operating microscope (named Dentiscope)
1983	Cvek introduced partial pulpotomy
1984	Baumgartner used citric acid (10%) for smear layer removal in root canals
1985	Roane introduced 'Balance Force' concept for canal preparation
1986	Hasegawa introduced Endocater (high frequency electronic apex locator)
1987	Harmeet Walia introduced Nickel-Titanium instruments in endodontics
1989	S Senia introduced light speed instruments

(*Contd...*)

Table 1.1 Evolution of Endodontics (*Contd...*)

1990	Carlsen and Alexandersen described Radix entomolaris
1993	Torabinejad developed mineral trioxide aggregate (MTA)
1993	Lussi, Nussbacher Grosrey described non-instrumentation technique
1993	APIT/Endex (third gen Electronic apex locator) developed by Frank and Torabinejad
1994	Ben Johnson introduced Profile instruments
1995	McSpadden introduced Quantec instruments
1996	Buchanan introduced Hand Greater taper files
1996	Hoshino and Colleagues introduced Triple antibiotic paste
1999	Endox system was introduced by Haffner and colleagues
1999	Bingo 1020 (fourth generation apex locator)
2000	Edward Lynch and Aylin Bayson developed Healozone
2000	Arias introduced electrochemically activated water as irrigation solution
2001	Clifford Ruddle and team developed protaper system in co-operation with Dentsply
2001	Micro-mega developed Hero Shapers
2002	John McSpadden introduced K3 Endo
2003	Jai and Albert introduced Resilon as an obturating material
2003	Torabinejad introduced irrigant MTAD (4.25% citric acid, 3% doxycycline, 0.5% Tween 80)
2004	Dr Goodis introduced V-taper
2005	Zehnder introduced irrigant HEBP (7% 1-Hydroxyethylidene-1,1-bisphosphonate)
2005	Liberator was introduced by Miltex
2006	Protaper Universal system was introduced
2006	Fukumoto introduced intracanal aspiration technique
2006	Koch and Brave introduced Activ GP
2007	Franklin introduced Monobloc concept
2007	Endovac was introduced by Hoafs and D Edson
2007	Tulsa dental specialties Introduced M wire technology
2007	Greater taper series X was introduced by Dr S Buchnan
2008	Dr Richard Mounce introduced Twisted file
2008	Ghassan Yared introduced a concept of canal preparation using only one NiTi rotary instruments
2009	Pierre Machtou, Bob Sharp and Cliff Ruddle introduced endoactivator irrigation system
2009	George Eliades introduced vibringe irrigation system
2009	Endosequence post preparation technique was developed by Dr Ali Nasseh
2010	Redent Nova introduced self adjusting file
2010	Ghasson Yared introduced Reciproc
2011	Dentsply introduced Wave One
2012	FKG Dentaire introduced RaCe
2012	Coltene-Whaledent introduced Hyflex-CM
2012	Micro-Mega introduced Revo-S file
2013	Micro-Mega introduced One shape
2013	Dentsply introduced ProTaper Next
2014	Neolix France introduced NeoNiTi file system
2015	Coltene-Whaledent introduced Canal Pro Cr-2 Endomotor with reverse motion
2015	File retrieval kit by Dr Yoshi Teruachi
2016	Autosyringe introduced by vista dental
2017	Carl Zeiss introduced Civil Zeiss extara 300

OUTCOME OF ENDODONTIC THERAPY

In biology, the term 'outcome' can never be defined. Age old phrase 'body tissues never follow text' is true in all therapies; equally true in endodontics. The 'outcome' is based on several factors, and taking care of each of these factors can minimize failures; however, one factor 'iatrogenic' is beyond the control of all of us. Therefore, the prognosis (the forecast of a disease) may not be definite.

In endodontic therapy, the term 'prognosis' applies to chances of healing; thereby, saving the tooth. The outcome of the treatment is evaluated in terms of clinical normalcy (absence of symptoms) and radiographic normalcy (reduction or disappearance of radiolucency) associated with the tooth. These results are better stated and communicated in terms of healing as follows:

Healed: Follow-up reveals a combined clinical and radiographic normalcy.

Healing: Considering the fact that healing takes considerable time, it is described as a combination of clinical normalcy and reduced radiolucency.

Functional: Follow-up reveals a residual radiolucency combined with clinical normalcy. The residual radiolucency may have been either reduced or remain unchanged in size.

The terms 'healed', 'healing' and 'functional' indicate the outcome of endodontic therapy; routinely used for treatment success.

Factors of Prognosis

There are various preoperative, intraoperative and post-operative factors which influence the outcome of endodontic therapy.

Preoperative Factors

a. *Tooth location*: It has been observed that certain teeth (maxillary canines, maxillary second premolars and mandibular canines) have a better prognosis than other teeth; however, any difference between anterior and posterior teeth has not been documented. Maximum failure rate has been observed in mandibular first premolar.
b. *Symptoms*: Preoperative symptoms may be a reflection of the types and numbers of micro-organisms in root canal system. Nevertheless, the healing rate is comparable for both symptomatic and asymptomatic teeth.
c. *Size of the lesion:* Smaller lesions up to 5.0 mm diameter have shown better prognosis than the larger lesions.
d. *Periodontal condition:* The preoperative periodontal condition of the tooth does not influence prognosis of the endodontic therapy. Periodontal diseases may advance on its own rate, subsequently tooth loss becomes imminent.
e. *Systemic health:* The influence of systemic health has not been established to a great extent; however, it is seen that medically compromised patients are at high risk of developing infections.

Intraoperative Factors

a. *Apical extent of treatment:* Extrusion of filling materials beyond the root end generally results in a poor prognosis. The impaired prognosis may result due to over instrumentation and displacement of infected debris into the periapical area.
b. *Apical enlargement:* It has been stated that a larger apical preparation is associated with poor prognosis. Being technique sensitive, extensive apical enlargement is frequently associated with canal transportation, jeopardising canal disinfection. But considering the importance of removing infected root dentin (harbouring intracanal micro-organism), an extensive apical preparation is believed to enhance the disinfection, and favour improved prognosis. Thus, apical enlargement, being technique sensitive, require considerable skill to achieve better results.
c. *Culturing:* A negative culture obtained before root filling may present better prognosis; however, the technique is not followed in routine.
d. *Treatment sessions:* The teeth treated in two sessions or less have a better chance of healing than teeth treated in multiple sessions. It is established that teeth treated at multiple visits are at a greater risk of becoming infected with *E. faecalis* and developing persistent apical periodontitis. Also, single visit root canal treatment presents with a similar healing rate as multiple visit treatment and patients experience less frequency of postobturation pain.
e. *Materials and technique*:
    - Intracanal medicament: Teeth treated with calcium hydroxide heal better than teeth not medicated at all or medicated with other material.
    - Instrumentation technique: Standardized technique gives better results than serial instrumentation technique.
f. *Microbial elimination*: Abundant use of sodium hypochlorite, extensive apical enlargements and dressings with an effective intracanal medicament such as calcium hydroxide provide maximal microbial elimination. As micro-organisms are the primary cause of persistent apical periodontitis; microbial elimination significantly affects prognosis.

Postoperative Factors

Restoration: A well restored tooth that seals coronal cavity effectively and prevents microbial ingress, favours a better prognosis.

FUTURE OF ENDODONTICS

Endodontics is constantly evolving through improvements in our understanding of the nuances of pulp physiology and pathology, coupled with advances in materials and other technological innovations. The future of endodontics lies in exploring the different aspects of the principles of endodontics, facing the challenges and taking the advantage of advancements in research and technology.

The important features are as follows.

Endodontic Imaging

The advent of digital capture systems in the last couple of years have revolutionized the endodontic diagnosis and treatment

The advantages of digital imaging include significant dose reduction, relatively faster image acquisition, ability to enhance images, elimination of wet processing, easier transmission, and archival of images. The digital sensors are slightly smaller than film but sufficient for endodontic purposes.

The future of endodontic imaging relies on wireless sensors, including the newly introduced CMOS-APS sensors (in endodontics, instantaneous images are required, which is best served by CMOS sensors).

The advent of cone beam computed tomography (CBCT) has resulted in widespread adoption of this technology for capturing three-dimensional image. CBCT is useful in diagnosing dental anomalies/ developmental disturbances, anatomic variations, calcified canals, broken instruments, vertical root fractures, resorption (external and internal) etc. and especially useful in implant placement.

Endodontic Visualization

The use of optical magnification instruments enables the endodontist to magnify a specified field, which is usually difficult to perceive by the naked eye. The recently introduced Endodontic Visualization System (EVS) incorporates both endoscopy and orascopy into one unit. The improved EVS II System combines the fiber optic orascope and a rigid endoscope. EVS provides optimal magnification for visualization during endodontic procedures.

A variety of additional upgrades for microscope functions have been introduced. Instead of fixed focal distances that limit the microscope to a certain distance, focal distance adapters are available, allowing for easier adjustments during root canal procedures. Extendable (foldable) binoculars were introduced for better ergonomics. Magnetic arrest functions (clutch) are also available for increased stability with use of microscope. LED lights (emission spectrum, 450–550 nm) offer a significantly longer lifetime; however, brightness is compromised as compared to xenon light.

Root Canal Preparation

The concept of pericervical dentin (PCD) *(defined as the dentin near the alveolar crest; roughly 4.0 mm coronal to the crestal bone and 4.0 mm apical to crestal bone)*, is a critical structure and is crucial during transferring load from the occlusal table to the root. The modification in the traditional straight line access helps to preserve the pericervical dentin. With the modern endodontic molar access, the coronal third of the crown can be flared to gain access to the canal orifices instead of the straight line access. The Endoguide Burs (SS White) revolutionized the traditional access preparation allowing shift from conservation to preservation. Preserving the dentin thickness, right from the access preparation to the root canal instrumentation is considered mandatory for long-term success of treatment.

Various rotary systems like Self-Adjusting File System, V-Taper, Safe Siders, Hyflex Files, NeoNiTi, Protaper Next, Single File Systems (WaveOne, One Shape, Komet F360) have changed the sequence in endodontic instrumentation. Wizard Navigator is a newer file system, which the manufacturer claims to face the endodontic canal challenges. Technologies and file design like the M-wire technology, controlled shape memory, hollow tube designs have great and direct impact on the chemico-mechanical debridement. New devices are being designed in apex locator along with the torque controlled gear reduction handpieces.

Root Canal Disinfection

The delivery of irrigant (irrigation dynamics) within root canal system is crucial to achieve the requisite success in treatment. The mechanism by which fluid dynamics can be improved and also the development of newer-effective antimicrobials are under constant research.

The improved delivery systems are Monoject endodontic needles, ProRinse probes, Micromega 1500, CaviEndo systems, the Max-I-Probe, The Endo-Eze system, etc. New irrigation technology will allow clinicians to conveniently choose, dispense, and more effectively irrigate root canal systems.

The use of ultrasonics along with dental operating microscopes is termed as Microsonics. The use of ultrasonic instruments has revolutionized the art of endodontic retreatment.

A new paradigm shift is the Gentle Wave system which utilizes multisonic ultracleaning technology that can quickly, easily and safely loosen and remove pulp tissue along with debris within few minutes. With introduction of lasers to the field of dentistry, various treatment modalities changed. New laser tips have been designed for endodontic disinfection namely PIPS and X-PULSE. Newer technologies are being studied for better treatment modalities in future.

Apart from biocompatible disinfection, many other frontiers in regenerative endodontic research are being currently investigated. These involve tissue engineering strategies that include the evaluation of suitable scaffolds, growth factors, and harvested stem cells to be used in pulpal regeneration. The use of platelet-rich plasma, platelet fibrin, and a gelatin hydrogel as scaffolds are routinely used in clinics. A recent trial involves harvesting stem cells from a donor site followed by *ex-vivo* expansion, sorting, and auto-transplantation into a recipient tooth to promote the regeneration of the once lost functional pulp-dentin complex. A bright future is in store for the regenerative endodontics.

Nanotechnology

Advancement in the field of nanotechnology in the past has changed the mindset of clinicians opting endodontics as their field of specialization.

Tiny machines, known as nanoassemblers, could be controlled by computer to perform specialized jobs. Nanorobots could also be the part of endodontic kitty. Replacement of the whole tooth, including the cellular and mineral components, is referred to as complete dentition replacement. This therapy is possible through a combination of nanotechnology, genetic engineering, and tissue engineering. Use of nanosponges introduced in blood stream could reduce toxicity; this could be applied in dental pulp revitalization.

A lot has already been achieved in terms of technological advancements in materials, equipment and still a lot has to be achieved in the field of regeneration and improving biocompatibility of materials. Endodontics would always be in demand in future because the preservation of the natural tooth is the best treatment for the patient, which is the principle of endodontic treatment. With so much of research and advancement carried out in this field, one can proudly say that future of endodontics is indeed vivid and exciting.

BIBLIOGRAPHY

1. Blicher B, Baker D and Lin J. Endosseous implants versus non-surgical root canal therapy: a systematic review of the literature. Gen. Dent.: 2008; 56:576–82, 591–592.
2. Friedman S. Prognosis of initial endodontic therapy. Endodontic Topic: 2002; 2, 59–58.
3. Friedman S. Considerations and concepts of case selection in the management of post-treatment endodontic disease (treatment failure). Endodontic Topics: 2002; 1, 54–78.
4. Friedman S and Mor C. The success of endodontic therapy: healing and functionality. J. Calif. Dent. Assoc.: 2004; 32:493–503.
5. Goldman M, Pearson AH, Darzenta N. Endodontic success-Who's reading the radiograph? O. Surg O. Med O. Pathol,: 1972, 33; 432–437.
6. Heffernan M, Martin W and Morton D. Prognosis of endodontically treated teeth? Quint. Int.: 2003; 7:558–561.
7. Hamedy R, Shakiba B, Fayazi S, Pak j G and White SN. Patient-centered endodontic outcomes. A narrative review. Iran Endod J.: 2013; 8, 197–204.
8. Kanaparthy R and Kanaparthy A. The changing face of dentistry: nanotechnology. Int. J. Nanomed.: 2011; 6, 2799–2804.
9. Lenherr P, Allgayer N, Weiger R, Filippi A, Attin T and Krastl G. Tooth discoloration induced by endodontic materials: a laboratory study. Int. Endod. J.: 2012; 45: 942–949.
10. Li X, Kolltveit KM, Tronstad L and Olsen I. Systemic diseases caused by oral infection. Clin. Microbiol. Rev.: 2000; 13:547–558.
11. Miran S, Mitisiadis TA and Pagella P. Innovative dental stem cell-based research approaches: The future of dentistry. Stem Cells Int.:2016; Article. ID7231038: 1–7.
12. Murray CA and Saunders WP. Root canal treatment and general health: a review of the literature. Int. Endod. J.: 2000; 33:1–18.
13. Ng YL, Mann V, Rabbarran S, Lewsey J and Gulabivala K. Outcome of primary root canal treatment: Systematic review of the literature – part 2 – influence of clinical factors. Int. Endod. J.:2008; 41:6–31.
14. Ng YL, Mann V and Gulabivala K. Outcome of secondary root canal treatment: A systematic review of the literature. Int. Endod. J.: 2008; 41:1026–46.
15. Oshima M and Tsuji T. Functional tooth regenerative therapy: tooth tissue regeneration and whole-tooth replacement. Odontology: 2014; 102:123–136.
16. Pallasch TJ and Wahl MJ. Focal infection: new age or ancient history? Endod. Topics: 2003; 4:32–45.
17. Siqueira JF. Aetiology of root canal treatment failure: why well treated teeth can fail. Int Endod J.: 2001, 34, 1–10.
18. Sjogren U, Hagglund B, Sundqvist G, Wing K. Factors affecting the long term results of endodontic treatment. J Endod,:1990, 16; 498–504.
19. Smith DE, Zarb GA. Criteria for success of osseointegrated endosseous implants. J Prosth. Dent.: 1989, 62; 567–572.
20. Smith AJ, Duncan HE, Diogenes A, Simon S and Cooper PR. Exploiting the bioactive properties of the dentin-pulp complex in regenerative endodontics. J. Endod.: 2016; 42:47–56.
21. Trope M. Implant or root canal therapy—an endodontist's view. J. Esthet. Restor. Dent.: 2005; 17:139–140.

Chapter 2

Biology of Dentin–pulp Complex

Dentin is the mineralized connective tissue of the tooth covered by enamel in coronal portion and cementum in roots. The dental pulp is a loose specialized connective tissue in the central portion of the tooth, which is enclosed on its outer surface by dentin. It comprises cells, fibers, ground substance, blood vessels and nerves. The pulp retains the vitality of dentin and dentin provides the necessary support to pulp. The knowledge of biology of these tissues is the basis of 'restorative dentistry' and 'preventive endodontics'. Since both the tissues are inter-related, they are known as dentin–pulp organ or dentin–pulp complex.

The functional grouping of pulp and dentin is explained as follows:

- Pulp and dentin make physiological couple and response collectively to external stimuli.
- Pulp carries nerves; provides sensitivity to dentin.
- Pulpal connective tissues respond to dentinal injuries, may not be directly stimulated.
- Encapsulation in dentin creates a low compliance environment that influences the defense potential of the pulp.

STRUCTURE OF THE DENTIN–PULP COMPLEX

Dentin is composed of closely packed dentinal tubules containing dentinal fluid and the cytoplasmic processes of the cells (the odontoblasts). These most distinctive cells of the dentin–pulp complex lie along the predentin border forming the peripheral boundary of the dental pulp (Fig. 2.1). Under the odontoblasts, there is cell-free zone and beneath that layer present a cell-rich zone. The pulp core with reduced cell density consists of connective tissue, blood vessels and nerves. The interdependence of dentin and pulp is responsible for dentin maturation and protection of tooth.

Despite the differences in structure and composition, pulp and dentin are integrally connected; more so, the physiologic and pathologic reactions in one tissue affect the other. The two tissues have a common embryonic origin and also remain in an intimate relationship throughout the life of the vital tooth. When normal teeth are stimulated thermally, the dentinal fluid expands or contracts causing hydrodynamic activation of intradental nerves. Anything that influences dentin affect the pulp and vice versa.

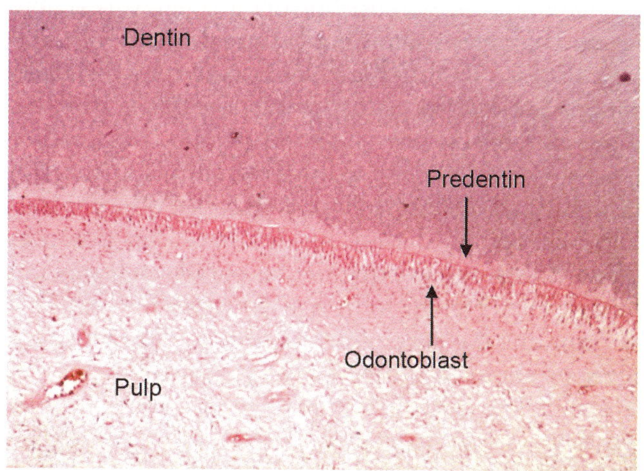

Fig. 2.1 Low-power photomicrograph of the dentin–pulp complex of a tooth illustrating dentin, pulp, odontoblasts (arrow) and prodontin (arrow)

If enamel and cementum are lost for any reason, pulp and dentin become functionally continuous; dentin surface becomes a fluid filled continuum in such conditions. This fluid medium along with microorganisms may diffuse across dentin to produce pulpal reactions. The pulp responds to the short term stimuli by mounting an acute inflammatory response. In response to the long term stimuli, pulpal tissues produce tertiary dentin as a biologic response in an attempt to reduce permeability of the dentin–pulp complex. Thus, these two tissues function as an integrated unit. The concept that dentin–pulp complex functions as an integrated unit is based on embryological and clinical evidences.

DEVELOPMENT OF DENTIN–PULP COMPLEX

Tooth development, initiating at 6th week of intrauterine life, is a process characterized by a series of sequential interactions between oral epithelium and the underlying tissues. Dental epithelium provides instructive signals for initiation of tooth development. Under the influence of cell signals, epithelial cells of the dental lamina at predetermined locations proliferate and project into the underlying neural crest derived ectomesenchyme. This projection gets pronounced in to a cap shape due to proliferation of cells. Further proliferation leads to the enamel organ assuming a bell shape. Simultaneous with the proliferation, there also occurs morpho-differentiation of the cells in the enamel organ. The inner enamel epithelium differentiates into specialized cells called ameloblasts, which lay down enamel. The ectomesenchyme enclosed beneath enamel organ condenses to form dental papilla whose outermost layer subjacent to inner enamel epithelium differentiates into specialized cells called odontoblasts, which lay down dentin. As dentin is laid down by odontoblasts, the existing dental papilla matures into dental pulp. Dental follicle is a mesenchymal tissue surrounding the developing tooth germ. The inner and outer epithelium grows apically to form a two cell layers, called Hertwig's epithelial root sheath, which commences root formation and also determines the shape of the roots. The Hertwig's epithelial root sheath signals adjacent mesenchyme of the dental papilla to differentiate into odontoblasts, which lay down the root dentin. Further, mesenchyme of the dental follicle differentiates into cementoblasts, fibroblasts and osteoblasts.

During developmental processes, the growth factors/morphogens control the events, such as initiation, proliferation, morphogenesis, cytodifferentiation and spatial distribution of cells.

DENTIN

Dentin is the mineralized connective tissue of tooth. It consists of apatite crystals, which act as filler particles in a collagen matrix. This mineralized matrix was formed by odontoblasts, which began secreting collagen at the dentinoenamel junction (Fig. 2.2a and b) and then grew centripetally while trailing odontoblastic processes.

According to the formation, dentin is of three types:

i. Primary dentin
ii. Secondary dentin
iii. Tertiary dentin

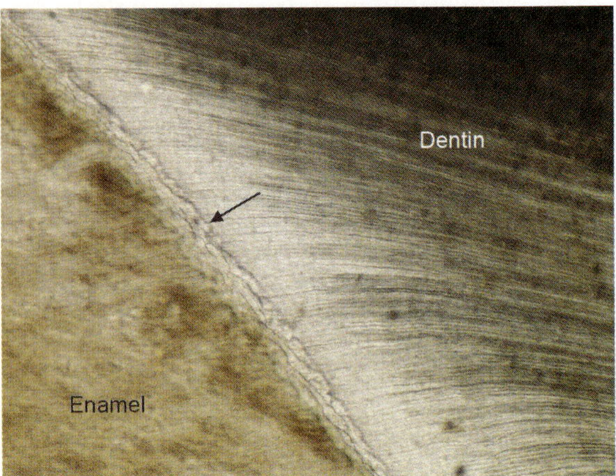

Fig. 2.2a Longitudinal ground section of tooth illustrating enamel, dentin and dentinoenamel junction (arrow)

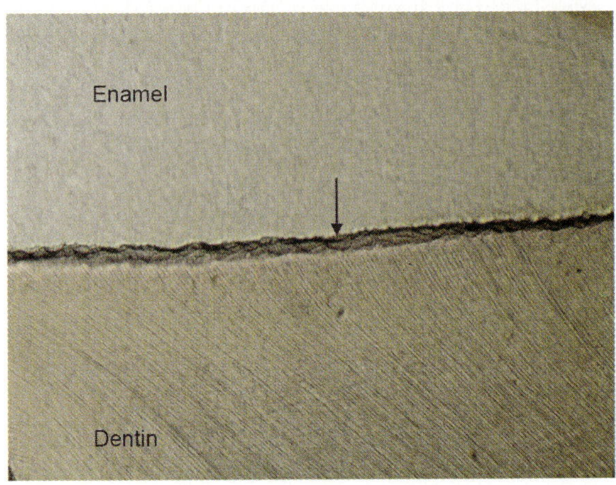

Fig. 2.2b Dentinoenamel junction (arrow) in a ground section. The scalloped nature of the junction when seen in one plane is striking

i. *Primary dentin*: Primary dentin is the original tubular dentin largely formed prior to eruption of tooth. The outer layer of primary dentin, called 'mantle dentin', is slightly less mineralized (about 4%) than regular circumpulpal dentin. Mantle dentin is about 150 µ wide and comprises the first dentin laid down by newly differentiated odontoblasts.

ii. *Secondary dentin*: Secondary dentin is structurally the same as primary dentin; however, secondary dentin is formed after completion of root formation. The difference between secondary and primary dentin is that the secondary dentin is secreted slowly as compared to primary dentin (Fig. 2.3a and b).

iii. *Tertiary dentin*: Tertiary dentin, known as 'irritation dentin', is also known as reactionary, reparative or irregular secondary dentin. It is formed only when dentin has been subjected to trauma or irritation (Fig. 2.4).

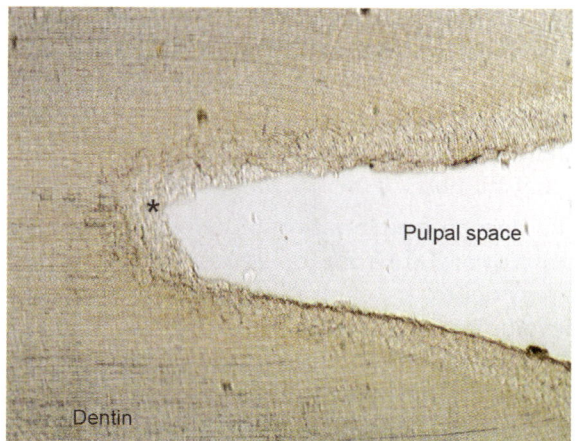

Fig. 2.3a Section of dentin illustrating secondary dentin (*), dentin and pulpal space. The region where dentinal tubules change direction delimits the junction between primary and secondary dentin

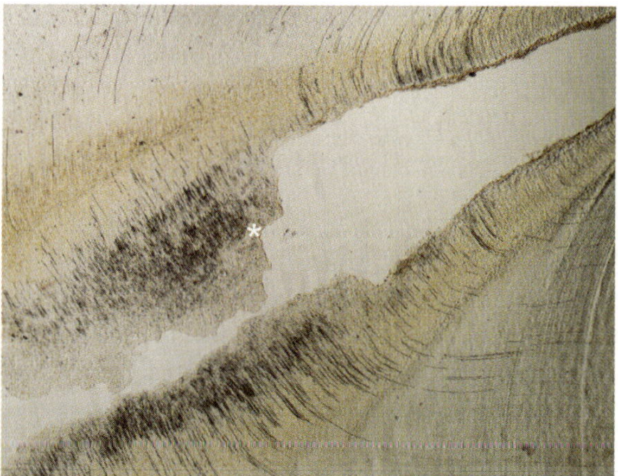

Fig. 2.3b Obliteration of pulpal space (*) by deposition of secondary dentin

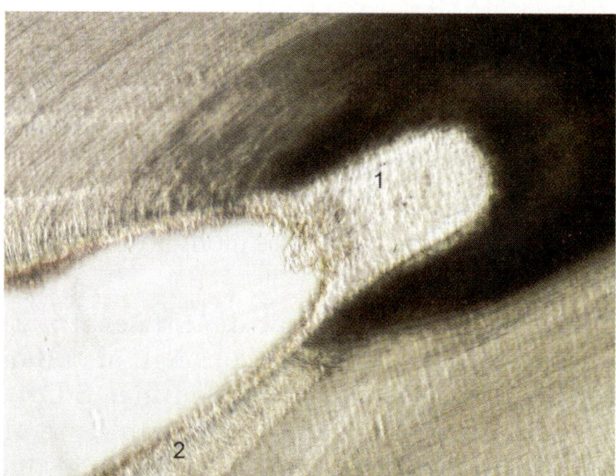

Fig. 2.4 Tertiary (reparative) dentin with a regular tubular pattern and no cellular inclusions. This dentin probably was deposited slowly in response to a mild stimulus. (1) Tertiary (reparative) dentin; (2) Secondary dentin

Chemical Composition

Dentin comprises 70% inorganic, 20% organic and 10% water.

The inorganic phase is carbonate rich apatite crystals of intertubular dentin. The apatite crystals are of small size relative to large apatite crystals in enamel; responsible for the high critical pH of dentin (pH 6.7).

The organic portion of dentin matrix is made up of 90% type I collagen and rest is non-collagenous proteins, growth factors and proteoglycans.

Components of Dentin

i. ***Peritubular dentin:*** Dentin is traversed by 1.0–2.0 μ diameter dentinal tubules. The dentinal tubules in the coronal part of the tooth extend from the enamel to the pulp and are 2.5 to 3.5 mm long. They contain odontoblastic processes and tissue fluid. The tubules have a highly mineralized lining, along most of their length known as the peritubular dentin. The peritubular dentin is formed as a main part of coronal circumpulpal dentin. It is not found in the most pulpal part of dentin in newly erupted teeth. This feature is important in restorative dentistry because the main part of deeply prepared tooth in young individual will comprise cytoplasmic material rather than mineralized dentin matrix.

The continuous growth of the peritubular dentin in the main bulk of dentin leads to obturation of the tubules. Occluded dentinal tubules are referred to as 'dentin sclerosis'. Sclerosed dentin reacts differently to acid etching than normal dentin; causes differences in the collagen mesh when exposed to acid etching. The etching time may have to be modified to provide an adequate hybrid layer of collagen and resin. Dead tracts are also seen in dentin. These are the dentinal tubules in which odontoblasts degenerate either due to caries, trauma or injury during cavity preparation. Under transmitted illumination, the tracts appear dark because air in them refracts the light (Fig. 2.5).

ii. ***Intertubular dentin:*** Intertubular dentin (50 to 60 nm long, 36.4 + 1.5 nm wide and 10.3 + 0.3 nm thick) is the dentin presents in between the dentinal tubules. It is less mineralized than peritubular dentin and can be easily distinguished. Intertubular dentin matrix has a dense collagen matrix; whereas, peritubular dentin matrix contains little collagen. The mineral of peritubular dentin is in the form of carbonate rich hydroxyapatite crystals, having higher crystallinity and are harder than intertubular dentin.

iii. ***Odontoblasts:*** Odontoblasts form a single layer of cells between dentin and pulp; their number may vary

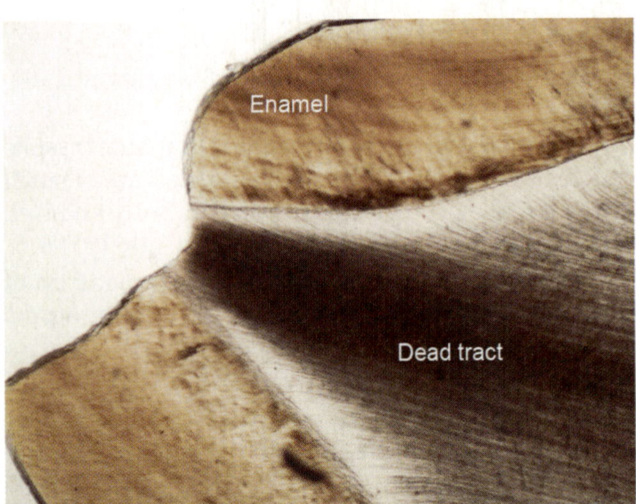

Fig. 2.5 Dead tracts in a ground section of a tooth. Under transmitted illumination the tracts appear dark because air in them refracts the light

from 45000–55000 cells/mm^2. The cell body of odontoblasts is located on the pulp side of dentin and cytoplasmic processes are inserted into tubules of mineralized dentin. A large nucleus is located in the basal portion of the cell, close to the pulp along with Golgi apparatus, mitochondria and endoplasmic reticulum. The cell body is 20–40 μ tall and 3.0–5.0 μ wide, depending upon the dentinogenic activity. They produce the organic matrix of pre-dentin and dentin including Type I collagen and proteoglycans. Odontoblasts intracellularly transport calcium ions to the mineralization front, and have the capacity to degrade organic matrix.

The cytoplasmic feature of the odontoblasts varies according to the functional activity of the cell. Odontoblasts have all the characteristic organelles, which are associated with protein and proteoglycans production. The activity of odontoblasts is reflected in the number and types of organelles present in the cytoplasm.

The adjacent odontoblasts are attached together with extension junctional complexes and with gap junction. The junctional complex consists of tight junction, known as zonula occludens. These tight junctions are thought to contribute in the final polarization of odontoblasts. Unlike other polarized cells, e.g. epithelial cells, the tight junctions in odontoblasts may be related to cell differentiation than to permeability of cell layers. The interodontoblastic collagen fibers (von Korff's fibers) may pass through the odontoblast-predentin layer from pulp into dentin.

2

iv. *Odontoblastic processes*: The odontoblastic processes are the cytoplasmic extension, gradually narrowing, that penetrates into mineralized dentin, falling the lumen of dentinal tubules. The odontoblastic process lacks cell organelle, but contains secretory vacuoles and microtubules. Its diameter is 3–4 μ at the pulp predentin border and gradually narrows as it passes within the dentinal tubules.

The depth of penetration of cytoplasmic processes is controversial. Various studies have observed different depth of penetration. It is hypothesized that in developing young teeth, the processes might be up to dentin-enamel junction, while in other teeth, the processes may only penetrate up to 0.3 mm into coronal dentin (may be slightly more in root dentin).

It is hypothesized that the cytoplasmic process extends about one-third of the distance from predentin to enamel, indicating that vital tissue changes occur only in the inner-third coronal dentin towards pulp. Changes occurring in the outer two-thirds of the dentin may be of physiochemical nature by precipitation of mineral salts within the tubules or growth of the peritubular dentin via components secreted into the periodontoblastic space. These components may diffuse peripherally to form a matrix that will mineralize.

v. *Dentinal fluid*: It has been hypothesized that a transport mechanism exists between blood circulation and dentin. It is suggested that odontoblasts regulate the transport of substances into dentin. Dentin contains several serum proteins, mainly in dentinal tubules. The origin of the fluid in dentinal tubules (either from pulp tissue extracellular space or from blood vessel or both) may not be clear, but the fluid present, containing inorganic and organic constituents, is a significant component of pulp-dentin complex. The space between odontoblast process and the tubule wall is filled with fluid, commonly referred to as '*dentinal fluid*'. The dentinal fluid is under control of odontoblasts, until tissue is damaged because of caries, cavity preparation, etc. It is established that the odontoblastic cell layer forms a functional barrier that restrains the passage of fluid, ions and other molecules along the extracellular pathway.

It has been accepted that dentin sensitivity to extrinsic irritants is mediated through alteration in hydraulic conductance of the dentinal fluid. The accepted hydrodynamic theory implicate fluid movement through dentinal tubules as a transducing mechanism, explaining dentin sensitivity (dentin is more sensitive to outward than inward flow).

Adhesive restorations are also dependent on the dentinal fluid. Increased dentinal wetness and fluid flow make successful bonding more difficult in deep cavities than superficial dentin. Dentinal fluid movement is also affected by other extrinsic factors. A high sucrose diet may depress dentinal fluid flow. Numerous studies have demonstrated that high sucrose diet reduce dentin formation during dentinogenesis. The dentinal fluid flow plays a protective role against bacterial acidogenic challenge.

Caries does affect dentinal fluid. In carious teeth, dentinal fluid act as a protective factor through the occlusion of dentinal tubules and the innate response of the dentin–pulp complex to the deposition of intratubular immunoglobulins [fluid may contain superoxide dismutase 3 (SOD3), considered to be present in lymph and plasma]. The presence of 'SOD3' and the higher concentration of 'Fetuin A' in dentin as compared to serum indicate that the active transport system by the odontoblasts are involved for the serum proteins. The overall permeability of dentin depends upon the integrity of the odontoblastic layer, presence of odontoblastic processes in dentinal tubules and the flow rate/viscosity of dentinal fluid.

Response of Odontoblasts to Injury

Depending on the nature, magnitude and duration of the injury, the odontoblasts may be reversibly or irreversibly damaged. Irreversible injury to odontoblast may occur during cavity preparation or desiccation of exposed dentin surface.

New dentin may eventually laid down on the dentinal wall corresponding to the site of injury by the action of secondary odontoblasts which are differentiated from undifferentiated mesenchymal cells present in the pulp. The new dentin formed in response to an injury is called *'tertiary dentin'*. When tertiary dentin is formed by newly differentiated odontoblasts, it is known as *'reparative dentin'* and when tertiary dentin is formed by the surviving odontoblasts, it is known as *'reactionary dentin'*. Tertiary dentin formation irrespective of type represents an important defense mechanism and a regenerative property of the pulp-dentin organ. The dentin formed locally may vary in structure and composition. The tubules are often more irregular, the dentin is less mineralized and it may have higher content of organic material than primary dentin. Interface dentin, often a tubular dentin forms a barrier between the physiologic secondary dentin and tertiary dentin. This barrier reduces the permeability of the affected dentin and may make it impermeable because the tubules from primary dentin do not cross the interface dentin.

Dentin Permeability

The tubular structure of the dentin provides channels for the passage of solutes and solvents across dentin. The number of dentinal tubules per square millimeter varies from 15,000 at dentinoenamel junction to 65,000 at the pulpal end. The density and the diameter of the tubules increase with dentin depth from the dentinoenamel junction to pulp. The permeability of dentin is lowest at dentinoenamel junction and highest at the pulpal end.

Dentin permeability depends on following factors:

i. Movement of inorganic/organic substances through dentinal tubules
ii. Movements of exogenous substances into the intertubular dentin

Dentin may be regarded both as barrier and as a permeable structure, depending on its thickness, age and amount of inorganic materials. The rate of diffusion of exogenous material across the dentin to the pulp is dependent upon dentin thickness and the hydraulic conductance of dentin. Thin dentin permits more diffusion than thick dentin. It is established that the inward diffusion of materials competes with the outward fluid movement in exposed vital dentin (open tubules). This competition may serve as a protective function mitigating the flow of bacterial products into exposed dentin.

The permeability of the dentin varies widely. Axial dentin is more permeable than occlusal dentin. The gingival floor/gingival extension of the finish lines in tooth preparation are often considered as high dentin permeability regions. The permeability of sclerotic dentin is very low.

The permeability of root dentin and coronal dentin is not uniform. The root dentin has a permeability about 3.0 to 8.0% as that of coronal dentin. It is likely that the relative impermeability of root dentin protects the periodontal tissues from wide variety of potentially cytotoxic compounds that might be used as intracanal medicaments.

The permeability of root dentin itself is not uniform but displays regional differences along its axial length. Cervical and middle root dentin has higher permeability than apical dentin. The permeability of the floor of pulp chamber in the region of furcation is also high because of presence of accessory canals in the furcation area.

Dentin permeability has numerous clinical implications. The dentin disks when soaked in 5.0% sodium hypochlorite solution for one hour produces 105% increase in hydraulic conductance of dentin (important during irrigation). During endodontic instrumentation of root canals, the softest inner dentin is removed. The increase in diameter of the root canal, facilitates thinning of dentin and decreasing the number of the tubules/mm. This may increase the permeability; however, preparation of root canal also creates smear plugs and smear layers on the dentinal surface that decreases its permeability.

The tubule density near the apical dentin is of great importance during apical surgery. During apical surgery, resection of the root at an oblique angle may be favoured to facilitate visibility and placement of a reverse filling. But this angled resection may expose dentinal tubules beneath the retrofilling material, subsequently more chances of leakage. The greater the angle of resection, the greater the potential for microleakage. Thus, minimal angled sections have been advocated to prevent leakage through exposed dentinal tubules.

Smear Layer and Smear Plugs

Smear plugs are composed of ground debris, whose particle size is smaller than the tubule orifice. The presence of ground debris in the tubule orifice lowers the permeability of dentin. It is pertinent to note that sodium hypochlorite does not remove the smear layer because it contains both organic component and inorganic component (sodium hypochlorite removes organic component). Only after removal of inorganic component with ethylenediaminetetraacetic acid (EDTA) or acids, sodium hypochlorite can remove the organic portion. This is why sodium hypochlorite and EDTA in combination are preferred as endodontic irrigants.

Any instrument placed in contact with the root canal will create a smear layer. The presence of the smear layer and smear plugs prevents the entry of sealer or even thermoplasticized gutta-percha into the dentinal tubules.

PULP

Dental pulp is specialized, highly vascularized connective tissue and is in direct communication with periodontium through apical foramen. Pulp is incompressible; volume within pulp cannot be increased (during inflammation, tissue pressure is increased rather the volume). Pulp has the unique ability to form dentin even after the tooth is fully developed. The pulp is relatively rich source of stem cells.

The pulp is divided into four zones (Fig. 2.6a and b).

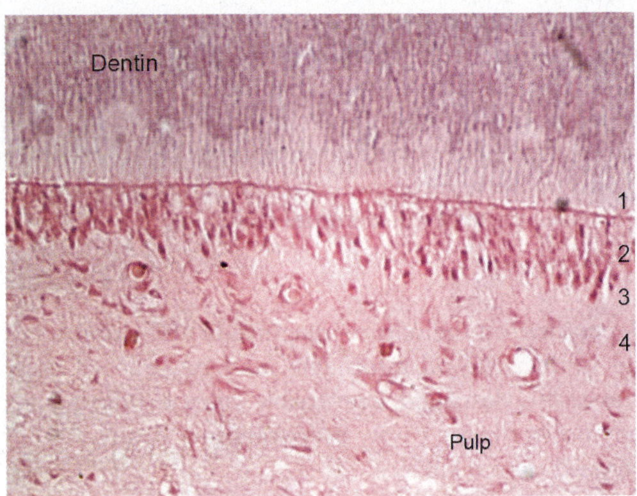

Fig. 2.6a Micropictograph of pulp organ illustrating (1) predentin; (2) odontoblast layer; (3) cell free zone and (4) cell rich zone

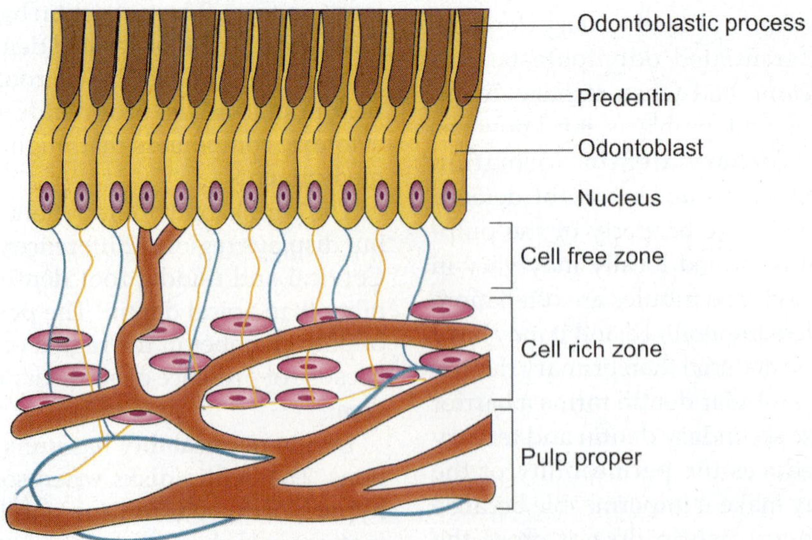

Fig. 2.6b Zones of pulp (diagrammatic)

i. *Zone of odontoblasts*: A layer of odontoblasts, circumscribes the outermost part of the pulp. They form a single layer lining in the most peripheral portion of the pulp. The cytoplasmic extension (odontoblastic process) extends into dentinal tubules. The shape of the cell body of odontoblasts is not uniform, rather these cells are tall and columnar in the coronal pulp, short and columnar in the mid portion of the tooth and cuboidal to flat in root portion. The *primary function* of odontoblasts is to produce and deposit dentin.

ii. *Zone of Weil (cell-free zone)*: Subjacent to odontoblast layer, an area relatively free of cells, known as 'cell-free zone' or 'zone of Weil' is seen. Major constituents of this zone are the rich network of mostly unmyelinated nerve fibers, blood capillaries and few fibroblasts. The function of capillaries is to provide nutrition to the odontoblasts, especially during dentinogenesis; the nerve plexus are involved in the neural sensation of pulp.

iii. *Cell-rich zone*: Next is the cell-rich zone. The constituents of this zone are ground substance, fibroblasts, undifferentiated mesenchymal cells, defense cells (macrophages and lymphocytes), blood capillaries and nerves. The higher density of fibroblasts in this zone is much more prominent in the coronal pulp than in root pulp. The *functions* of cell-rich zone are:

- Fibroblasts form as well as degenerate collagen fibers
- By depositing calcified tissues, they help in reparative dentin formation
- Collagen fibers secreted by odontoblasts form the dentinal matrix; whereas; collagen fibers secreted by fibroblasts support the pulp.
- Ground substance acts as barrier against the spread of bacteria. It acts as transport medium for metabolites and other waste products.
- Collagen fibers collectively protect the neurovascular bundle, especially in the apical third area.
- Undifferentiated mesenchymal cells may differentiate into other cells during repair and regeneration, as per need.

iv. *Pulp proper*: From the cell-rich zone inward is the central connective tissue mass known as pulp proper. This zone contains fibroblasts, larger blood vessels and nerves. Undifferentiated mesenchymal cells and defense cells such as macrophages are frequently located in perivascular area. Collagen fiber bundles are more numerous in root pulp than coronal pulp.

The clinical implication of this higher density of collagen fiber bundles in apical region is the use of barbed broach during removal of pulp. The removal of pulp tissue is facilitated when the broach is passively placed apically engaging these collagen bundles.

The ground substance in pulp, the extracellular matrix, is consisted of polysaccharides, glycoproteins and proteoglycans. The proteins bind to cell surfaces and other matrix molecules. The water content is approximately 90%, which may decrease in aged pulp.

The blood vessels and nerves are embedded in the pulp matrix in the central portion of pulp, emanating branching to the periphery of the pulp. The nerve fibers enter through the apical foramen; whereas, lymphatics and venules exit the pulp mainly through apical foramen.

Components of Pulp

a. Cells

The main cells of pulp are:

i. *Odontoblasts*: Odontoblasts are also part of pulp; the highly differentiated cells of the pulp. The cell body of odontoblasts is located on the pulp side of dentin and cytoplasmic processes are inserted into tubules of mineralized dentin. The cell structure of odontoblasts is described under 'components of dentin'.

ii. *Fibroblasts*: These are the most numerous connective tissue cells with the capacity to synthesize and maintain connective tissue matrix. Synthesis of collagen is a main function of fibroblasts in the pulp. Fibroblasts are also responsible for synthesis and secretion of a wide range of non collagenous extracellular matrix components such as proteoglycans and glycoproteins (fibronectin). In addition to synthetic activity, fibroblasts are also involved in the degradation of extracellular matrix. Fibroblasts are able to phagocytose collagen fibrils and digest them intracellularly by lysosomal enzymes.

iii. *Undifferentiated mesenchymal cells*: These are distributed throughout the cell-rich zone occupying the perivascular area. These cells appear as stellate shaped cells with a relatively high nucleus to cytoplasmic ratio. When stimulated, they may give rise to fibroblasts or odontoblasts as per need (also known as reserve cells). In older pulps, the number of undifferentiated mesenchymal cells may diminish, which reduces the regenerative potential of pulp.

iv. *Immunocompetent cells*: The ability of connective tissue to generate local inflammatory and immune reactions makes it an active participant in host defense. This capacity depends on immune-competent cells, which include lymphocyte, macrophages and dendritic cells. They increase in number during inflammation and may play role in repair process in the pulp.

b. Vascularity of Pulp

The most restrictive anatomic characteristic of the pulp is that it is encased in rigid mineralized tissue. This provides the pulp, a low-compliance environment in which nutrition for the tissue is almost entirely supplied via vessels traversing the narrow apical foramen.

It is clinically important to recognize that many of the capillaries in the pulp are largely non-functional in the normal pulp. The blood flow to specific areas can be increased quickly because of capillaries, i.e. local and general hyperaemia in the pulp can occur almost instantaneously without requiring the ingrowth of the new capillaries.

Arterioles enter and venules and lymphatics leave dental pulp through the apical foramen. Vessels also enter and leave the pulp via accessory lateral canals, which may be located anywhere on the root, but are most commonly found in the apical region. Relatively large arterioles pass through the root pulp to supply the coronal pulp. They branch and terminate as capillaries, which are particularly abundant in the coronal subodontoblastic region.

The structure of blood vessels in the pulp is basically similar to the other blood vessels of body; the blood vessels in pulp are thin walled as compared to the size of lumen. The structural characteristics include discontinuities in the endothelial walls and fenestration of capillaries. They facilitate the exchange of nutrients and waste products between the interstitial tissue fluid and blood plasma. This exchange is particularly important at the time of injury, trauma and carious lesions affecting the pulp and plays an important role in maintaining the fluid balance.

The arterial supply of pulp is from posterior–superior alveolar arteries, infraorbital arteries and inferior alveolar branch of maxillary arteries. Pulp does not have a collateral blood supply. Coronal pulp has nearly twice the capillary blood flow than the root pulp (maximum capillaries are in pulp horns). The arterio-vascular anastomosis connects the arterioles directly to venules, bypassing the capillary bed (small 10 vessels). They play a vital role in regulation of blood flow.

c. Interstitial Fluid Pressure

The interstitial fluid pressure in the pulp is relatively high and it plays a role in sudden pain experience when cavity preparation reaches unaffected dentin. The exposure of dentin causes sudden movement of the contents of the tubules, leading to the activation of nerves adjacent to the odontoblasts and resulting in pain. The fluid flow from the pulp to exposed dentin is dependent on the hydraulic conductance of the dentinal fluid.

d. Nerve Impulses in Pulp

Myelinated and unmyelinated nerves enter the pulp through apical foramen and through accessory canals. They mainly follow the blood vessels as they branch and form a network of terminal endings in the odontoblastic–subodontoblastic region and in the peri-odontoblastic spaces of dentin tubules.

Myelinated A fibers (A-β and A-δ fibers: Ratio is 10:90) and non-myelinated C-fibers constitute the sympathetic nervous system. Both sensory and sympathetic nerve endings may terminate in the walls of the blood vessels in main pulp. They are activated at an early stage in the inflammatory process and initiate vasodilation, which starts the protective response to injury by increasing blood volume and vascular permeability in the affected area. A number of neuroreactive peptides has been demonstrated in the pulpal nerve endings, including neurokinins, substance P and calcitonin generelated peptide. Both sympathetic nerve fibers and sensory nerve fibers have effects on pulpal circulation. The number of nerve fibers and the associated neuropeptides decrease with age, which explains the reduced sensitivity of teeth in adults and older individuals.

It has been suggested that some nerve fibers that terminate in the dentinal tubules may be branches of the same nerves that terminate in the wall of blood vessels. This phenomenon explains the difficulties in localizing pulpal pain.

Nerve activity in the pulp can be modified by anesthetic solutions and epinephrine, which may decrease the releases of neuropeptides. Eugenol, known for its sedative effect on pulpal pain has been shown to have an inhibitory effect on sensory nerve action.

Sensory innervation of pulp through trigeminal ganglion is by means of maxillary nerve and the mandibular nerve. A-fibers transmit fast pain (sharp, piercing) and C-fibers transmit slow pain (dull, aching). A- fibers get stimulated first during electric pup testing, followed by C-fiber, if the intensity of stimulus is increased.

Pulp–Dentin Complex Regeneration: Biological Cues

The pulp–dentin complex plays a key role in the immune defense against the external stimuli and stimulate tissue repair during infection or trauma. The unique anatomic and physiologic nature of pulp–dentin complex makes it a difficult tissue to regenerate. The outcome of regenerative endodontic cases reflect only the ectopic tissue formation in the root canal space. The formation of fibrous connective tissue in the root canal space has been documented. The successful regenerative procedures have resulted in excellent healing of periapical tissues, increased root lengths and to some extent return of vitality.

The clinical regenerative protocol utilizes endogenous stem cells or progenitor cells and the biological molecules released from dentin or by evoking bleeding. Dentin contains variety of biological molecules, viz. growth factors [TGF-β1, bone morphogenetic protein (BMP), growth differentiation factors (GDF), insulin like growth factor (IGF) and platelet derived growth factor (PDGF)], non-collagenous proteins (dentin sialoprotein, dentin matrix protein and osteopontin) and glycosaminoglycans (chondroitin sulphate, and dermatan sulphate). Most of these molecules help in odontoblastic differentiation, cell proliferation and dentinogenesis. A few also helps in cell migration, dentin matrix synthesis and angiogenesis. The induced apical bleeding delivers the biological molecules to the root canal space along with stem cells or progenitor cells, because blood clot contains growth factors like TGF-β, PDGF and IGF, etc. These factors activate the cells and help regeneration of pulp-dentin complex.

The exogenous biological cues are as good as endogenous cues. A few exogenous biological cues with higher concentration, e.g. plasma rich platelet, may augment the regeneration process (PRP has higher concentration of blood-derived factors as compared to apical bleeding).

The biological molecules involved in cell differentiation and tissue formation should have controlled release, so that sustained biological effects can be achieved, especially during later stage of regeneration.

The biological molecules involved in cell migration are not very critical as their role is limited in the initial phase of regeneration (controlled release is referred to as the release of biological factors as a specific rate in a given period of time). It has been established that at the early stage of regeneration, cell mobilization is predominant; whereas, in the later stage cell differentiation and tissue formation are predominant.

The biological factors released from dentin or evoked bleeding usually have high initial burst followed by rapid decrease in delivery. These may not be available at the later stage of regeneration when tissue differentiation and tissue formation are to take place; subsequently, leading to ectopic tissue formation in the root canal spaces. The delivery of biological molecules requires a scaffold or a carrier that allows controlled release of the molecules. The biodegradable scaffold allowing controlled release of growth factors are useful in diverting cellular events towards regenerative rather than repair in regenerative endodontic treatment.

BIBLIOGRAPHY

1. Avery J. Repair potential of the pulp. J. Endod.: 1981; 7: 205–212.
2. Bertassoni LE, Habelitz S, Kinney JH, Marshall SJ and Marshall GW. Mechanical perspective on the remineralization of dentin. Caries Res.: 2009; 43:70–77.
3. Cooper PR, Holder MJ and Smith AJ. Inflammation and regeneration in the dentin–pulp complex: A double-edged sword. J. Endod.: 2014; 40, 546–551.
4. Cooper PR, Takahashi Y, Graham LW, Simon S, Imazato S and Smith JA. Inflammation regeneration interplay in the dentin–pulp complex. J. Dent.: 2010; 38:687–697.
5. Couve E, Osorio R and Schmachtenberg O. The amazing odontoblast: activity, autophagy, and aging. J. Dent. Res.: 2013; 92:765–772.
6. Ferracme JL, Cooper PR and Smith AJ. Can materials interaction with the dentin–pulp complex contribute to dentin regeneration? Odontology: 2010; 98:2–14.
7. Goldberg M and Septier D. Phospholipids in amelogenesis and dentinogenesis. Crit. Rev. Oral Biol. Med.:2002; 13: 276–290.
8. Goldberg M and Smith AJ. Cells and extracellular matrices of dentin and pulp: a biological basis for repair and tissue engineering. Crit. Rev. Oral Biol. Med.: 2004; 15:13–27.
9. Gong T, Heng BC, Lo EC and Zhang C. Current advance and future prospects of tissue engineering approach to dentin/pulp regenerative therapy. Stem Cells Int.: 2016; ID9204574.
10. Goracci G. Mori G. and Baldi M. Terminal end of the odontoblast process: a study using SEM and confocal microscopy. Clin. Oral Investig.: 1999; 3:126–132.
11. Grayson W and Marshall J. Dentin: Microstructure and characterization. Quintessence Int.: 1993; 24:606–617.
12. Hahn CL and Best AM. The pulpal origin of immunoglobulins in dentin beneath caries: an immunohistochemical study. J. Endod.: 2006; 32:178–182.
13. Henry B and Trowbridge O. Pulp Biology: Progress during the past 25 years. Aust. Endod. J.: 2003; 29:5–12.
14. Heyeraas KJ. And Berggreen E. Interstitial fluid pressure in normal and inflamed pulps. Crit. Rev. Oral Biol. Med.: 1999; 10:328–336.
15. Holland GR. The odontoblast process: Form and function. J. Dent. Res.: 1985; 64:499–514.
16. Howard C, Murray PE and Namerow KN. Dental pulp stem call migration. J. Endod.: 2010; 3:1963–1966.
17. Ishizaka R, Lohara K and Murakami M. Regeneration of dental pulp following pulpectomy by fractionated stem/progenitor cells from bone marrow and adipose tissue. Biomaterials: 2012; 33:2109–2118.
18. Jang JH, Lee W, Cho KM, Shin HW, Kang MK Park SH and Kim E. In vitro characterization of human dental pulp stem cells isolated by three different methods. Resto Dent Endod.: 2016, 41:283–295.

19. Jontell M, Okiji T, Dahlgren U and Bergenholtz G. Immune defense mechanism of the dental pulp. Crit. Rev. Oral Biol. Med.: 1998; 9:179–200.

20. Kim G. Biological molecules for the regeneration of the pulp-dentin complex. Dent. Clin. N. Am.: 2017; 61:127–141.

21. Kinney JH, Nalla RK, Peple JA, Breunig TM and Ritchie RO. Age related transparent root dentin: Mineral concentration, crystallite size and mechanical properties. Biomaterials: 2005; 26:3363–3376.

22. Magloire H, Maurin JC, Couble ML, Shibukawa Y, Tsumura M, Thivichon-Prince B and Bleicher F. Topical review. Dental pain and ondotoblasts: facts and hypotheses. J. Orofac. Pain: 2010; 24:335–349.

23. Mjor IA, Sveen OB and Keyeraas KJ. Pulp dentin biology in restorative dentistry. Part I: normal structure and physiology. Quintessence Int.: 2001; 1:26–30.

24. Mjor IA. Dentinal permeability: the basis for understanding pulp reactions and adhesive technology. Braz. Dent. J.: 2009; 20:3–16.

25. Morotomi T, Tabata Y and Kitamura C. Dentin–pulp complex regeneration therapy following pulp amputation. Adv. Tech. Biol. Med.: 2015; 3:1–5.

26. Ninomiya M, Ohishi M, Kido J, Ohsaki Y and Nagata T. Osteopontin in human pulp stones. J. Endod.: 2001; 27:269–272.

27. Pashley DH. Dentin-predentin complex and its permeability: physiologic overview. J. Dent. Res.: 1985; 64:613–620.

28. Pietrzak WS and Eppley BL. Platelet rich plasma: biology and new technology. J. Craniofac. Surg.: 2005; 16:1043–1054.

29. Roberts-Clark DJ and Smith AJ. Angiogenic growth factors in human dentine matrix. Arch. Oral Biol.: 2000; 45:1013–1016.

30. Simon SR, Berdal A, Cooper PR, Lumley PJ, Tomson PL and Smith AJ. Dentin–pulp complex regeneration: from lab to clinic. Adv. Dent. Res.: 2011; 23:340–345.

31. Smith AJ, Duncan HF and Diogenes A. Exploiting the bioactive properties of the dentin–pulp complex in regenerative endodontics. J. Endod.: 2016; 42:47–56.

32. Smith AJ, Murray PE, Sloan AJ, Matthews JB and Zhao S. Trans-dentinal stimulation of tertiary dentinogenesis. Adv. Dent. Res.: 2001; 15:51–54.

33. Smith JA. Vitality of the dentin pulp complex in health and disease: Growth factors as key mediators. J. Dent. Educ.: 2003; 67:678–689.

34. Tjaderhane L and Haapasalo M. The dentin–pulp border: a dynamic interface between hard and soft tissues. Endod. Topics: 2012; 20:52–84.

35. Tjaderhane L, Marcela RC, Breschi L, Tay FR and Pashley DH. Dentin basic structure and composition—an overview. Endod. Topics: 2012; 20:3–29.

36. Tziafas D. Belibasakis G, Veis A and Papadimitriou S. Dentin regeneration in vital pulp therapy: design principles. Adv. Dent. Res.: 2001; 15:96–100.

37. Tziafas D. Dentinogenic potential of the dental pulp: facts and hypotheses. Endod. Topics: 2010; 17:42–64.

38. Tziafas D. The future role of a molecular approach to pulp-dentinal regeneration. Caries Res.: 2004; 38:314–320.

39. Zhu X, Zhang C and Huang GT. Transplantation of dental pulp stem cells and platelet-rich plasma for pulp regeneration. J. Endod.: 2012; 38:1604–1609.

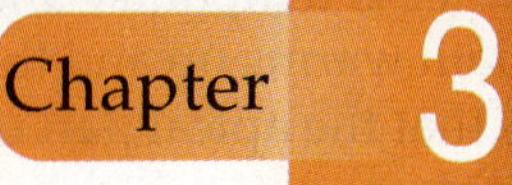

Chapter 3

Pathophysiology of Pain

Pain is unpleasant, sensational, subjective-emotional experience associated with actual or potential tissue damage. It has the function of a warning to tissue damage and also activates the defense mechanism in order to prevent further damage. Pain is not a disease; additional manifestations may be fear, anxiety, pupil dilatation, nausea, vomiting, tachycardia etc. Pain perception is also not constant; varies considerably with environmental conditions. The most common reason for patients to visit dental clinic is pain, which may originate from tooth and associated tissues or may be other non-odontogenic reasons. Thorough anamnesis (recalling the past events) is important to know the history of pain, its frequency and periodicity, etc. Anamnesis should be complimented with clinical examination and relevant tests, as need be, to reach out at proper diagnosis. Pain in orofacial region can be odontogenic or of non-odontogenic reasons.

ODONTOGENIC PAIN

Odontogenic pain has its source from pulp-dentin complex and/or periapical tissues (mainly endodontic). It may be because of preendodontic, interappointment or postendodontic reasons. The causes and effective management of pain encountered at different stages of endodontic treatment are described.

A. Pre-endodontic Pain

The situations arising prior to the removal of the pulp are designated as pre-endodontic pain. Such kind of pain is caused by reparable or irreparable pulpal diseases with or without periapical tissue involvement. 90% patients seeking dental treatment are suffering from pain originating from either pulpal or periapical region (10% may be periodontal or non-odontogenic pain). Based on treatment, pulpal pain can be either from reversible pulpitis or irreversible pulpitis (advanced stages may present as pulp necrosis). Reversible pulpitis require conservative treatment; whereas, irreversible pulpitis and/or pulp necrosis need root canal treatment.

a. Reversible Pulpitis

A pulp with reversible pulpitis, has mild inflammation and is capable of healing once the irritating stimulus is removed. Pain is only felt when a stimulus (usually cold or sweet foods but sometimes heat) is applied to the tooth, and the pain ceases within a few seconds or immediately upon removal of the stimulus. The pain is short and sharp in nature but not spontaneous. There are no significant radiographic changes in the periapical region (radiographic findings may be the cause of the problem, such as caries, a deep restoration, etc.). The pulp's response to cold or heat is exaggerated and brief. Brannstrom described the hydrodynamic theory in which the pathophysiology of dentin sensitivity is related to the sudden rapid movement of fluid into and out of the dentinal tubules as a reaction to certain stimulants. According to this theory, acute pain develops when fluid movement activates A-delta fibers in the vicinity of pulp-dentin junction. These symptoms are resolved by removing the cause. The mild trauma/ stimulus can cause mild inflammation and sufficient mechanical damage to stimulate a nerve reaction; subsequently causing exaggerated response to vitality tests, indicating severe inflammation. This state of pulp is called reversible as inflammation is mild and limited to the area of A-delta nerves; if further infection is prevented, normal state of pulp can be achieved.

Dental caries is the most frequent cause of pulpitis. As caries progresses, the pulp undergoes changes from hyperaemia to pulpitis, and frequently to necrosis. The mechanism by which caries induces pulpitis is probably a combination of direct toxic effects on the pulp and indirect immune reactions (antigen-antibody cellular types). As the lesion progresses, it causes opening of dentinal tubules, subsequently increasing dentin permeability. The increased permeability allows odontoblasts to get affected by toxic bacterial products. The early inflammatory reaction is containment of bacterial growth within the pulp due to phagocytosis by neutrophils but at the expense of pulp tissue. At this stage, since the carious lesion has not penetrated into the pulp, removal and restoration of the lesion will allow the pulp to heal. Certain chemical mediators (bradykinin, serotonin and substance P) sensitize the A-delta fibers and lower their threshold, thereby increasing their response to stimulants.

It is established that the inflammatory mediators, capable of causing pain, are released in the pulp in direct proportion to the insult. Serotonin (5 HT), able to sensitize intra-dental A fibers and Bradykinin have shown to be in significant higher concentration in irreversibly inflamed human pulps. It has also been demonstrated that neuropeptides from the nociceptive nerve fibers present in the pulp [calcitonin gene-related peptide (CGRP), Neurokinin A and substance P] are found in significantly higher concentrations in symptomatic pulp compared with healthy pulps. Sharp pain due to external stimulus like cold which gets relieved after the stimulus is removed, is associated with the pulpodentinal myelinated A-delta neurofibres.

b. Irreversible Pulpitis

The classic symptom of irreversible pulpitis is lingering pain induced by thermal stimuli. Even mild temperature changes (tap water, breathing cold air) may induce pain. The initial reaction is a very sharp pain to hot or cold stimuli, which lingers for a couple of minutes to hours even after the stimulus is removed. The lingering pain is usually a dull ache or a throbbing pain. Spontaneous (unprovoked) pain, which may wake the patient at night and may become worse when lying down, is another hallmark feature of irreversible pulpitis. The more C-fiber-mediated pain (dull, throbbing, poorly localized), the more severe the inflammation and more likely to be irreversible in nature. Patients with irreversible pulpitis may have difficulty locating the precise tooth (source of pain). They may even confuse the maxillary and mandibular arches (but not the left and right sides of the mouth) because of the extensive branching of dental nerve axons and perhaps fewer proprioceptive fibres in the pulp.

Patients may complain of a dull continuous pain, exacerbated by heat but relieved by cold. Exact mechanism is not clear; however, it is speculated that micro-organisms in the infected pulp produce gases, which contract with cold water, relieving pressure on the nerve endings, particularly in the apical portion of the canal. The relief with cold water is temporary and the pain returns as soon as the tooth warms up and the gases expand. It is hypothesized that the apical part of the pulp nerves are the last to necrose.

When the carious lesion penetrates through the dentin and contacts the pulp, the nature of inflammatory response changes from a collection of mostly mononuclear leukocytes to a localized collection of polymorphonuclear leukocytes forming microabscesses within the chronic inflammatory lesion. It is at this stage that reversible pulpitis becomes irreversible. Eventually, initial microabscess leads to numerous other microabscesses. When they are large enough to coalesce, the pulp undergoes liquefaction necrosis.

A few authors suggested that inflammation alone would not cause pulp death. The injured pulp often becomes necrotic even when the injury is minor and intrapulpal pressure rises very high (up to 80 mm Hg). Others opined that the pulp pressure rises initially after injury but declines to its normal level and the pulp may recover.

The increase in pain from inflamed pulps at night or the transformation of the pain from a dull to a throbbing ache has rational physiologic bases. The reduced pressure effect occurs as the head in normal upright posture, is above the heart (gravity keeps the pressure low). When the patient lies down, the gravitational effect disappears, significantly increasing the pulp pressure, over and above that caused by endogenous mediators of inflammation. In the supine position, a higher tissue pressure develops in the pulp, which causes more pain. Another factor contributing to elevated pulp pressure on reclining is the effect of posture on the activity of the sympathetic nervous system. When a person is upright, the baroreceptors (the so-called "carotid" sinus), located in the arch of the aorta and the bifurcation of the carotid arteries, maintain a relatively high degree of sympathetic stimulation to organs richly innervated by the sympathetic nervous system.

Irreversible pulpitis is difficult to diagnose until periradicular tissues are involved. As the periradicular tissues get involved, the tooth becomes sensitive to percussion and the affected tooth can be identified.

c. Pulp Necrosis

The pulp inflammation leads to necrosis followed by infection and eventually loss of tissue because of its ingestion by bacteria. It has been reported that in 50–60% cases, pulps can progress from vitality to necrosis without pain. This phenomenon has been termed as 'painless pulpitis'. It is not known how asymptomatic pulp death can happen; one hypothesis is that the progress of inflammation is so rapid that there is no pain or conversely the inflammation is so slow that the classical inflammatory mediators that participate in the pain process never reach a critical level. It has also been suggested that there may be effective modification by local as well as centrally mediated systems present in pulp (endogenous opioid and adrenergic sympathetic systems do exist in the pulp which may inhibit pulpal pain activation). The effects of the central nervous system (CNS) may be a contributing factor. In pulp necrosis, the pulpal sensory neurons are damaged, that is why it does not respond to thermal and electrical stimuli; however, in case of partial necrosis, pulp can be reactive because C-fibers are more resistant to hypoxia than A-δ fibers (such a phenomenon is common in multirooted teeth).

d. Periradicular Inflammation (Apical Periodontitis)

Periradicular inflammation is the spread of infection from pulp into periradicular tissues.

The presence of bacteria within the root canal system eventually cause a periapical inflammatory response, known as apical periodontitis. This is the response of the body's defense system to the irritation created by the bacteria and their by-products.

Periapical inflammation is the result of interactions between the bacteria in an untreated infected root canal system and the host's defense/immune system. As there is no longer any blood supply to a necrotic pulp, the host's defense cells cannot reach the source of the irritation (i.e. the bacteria in the canal) and, therefore, the body is unable to eliminate the infection. Hence, a chronic inflammatory response develops in the periapical region. Infections of the root canal system usually consist of multiple species of organisms; complex interactions occur where the by-products of some bacteria contribute to the supply of nutrients for other species. Once an infection is established within the root canal system, the number of micro-organisms gradually increase through normal cell reproduction and proliferation mechanisms. The nutritional conditions in each root canal may vary; this explains the different rates at which periapical tissues respond and also why there are varying number of bacterias that can be recovered from root canal system.

Although bacteria are the most common cause of pulp diseases, dental pulps may also get necrosed following trauma when the apical blood vessels are severed. Necrotic debris alone, although stimulating phagocytosis and tissue repair, may not produce enough irritation to the periapical region.

The clinical findings of pulpitis to periradicular inflammation are sensitivity to bite and dull-persisting-pulsating pain. As the inflammatory process progresses to alveolar bone, the patient may report fever, swelling, etc. The inflammation progressing to periosteum is the most painful phase.

Chronic apical periodontitis represents a dynamic balance between exogenous root canal microbiota and their by-products, and the host's defense mechanisms. The chronic lesion, termed as 'periapical granuloma', is made up by mononuclear and polymorphonuclear leukocytes and fibrovascular elements.

The histological appearance of periapical granuloma represent every event of periradicular inflammatory process from the acute response to the end-stage lesion. Neighbouring histological features, i.e. necrotic, exudative, granulomatous and fibrous zones may penetrate into surrounding alveolar bone. According to predominant zones, the lesion can be classified as exudative, granulomatous, granulofibrotic, etc. (Fig. 3.1).

The mountain pass concept: Kronfeld (1955) equated the micro-organisms in the root canal to an army in the 'mountains' which enters the 'plains' through the foramina or 'the mountain pass'. The bacteria in the root canal can be compared to an army waiting behind high, inaccessible mountains, the walls of the canal. Through the mountain pass (the apical foramen), the bacteria (army) try to invade the plain beyond the pass (the periodontium and the bone). The granulation tissue (army of the host) tries to prevent the mountain army from progressing farther. The defending army is represented by the white blood cells and other cells of the granulation tissue. They accumulate near the opening of the apical foramen. For a long time there may be no action. Occasionally, a few soldiers of the mountain army descend through the pass, the apical

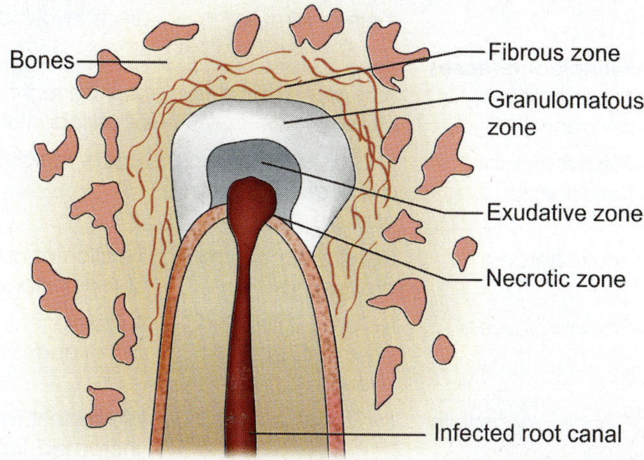

Fig. 3.1 Zones of sequelae of root canal infection

foramen, but they are usually captured and destroyed by the defenders, the white blood cells. Then suddenly the mountain army makes a mass attack and a battle occurs. Such a battle between invading bacteria and body tissues is known as acute inflammation. The outcome of this battle may vary. The bacteria may win and invade the plain; then the clinical manifestation will be an acute periapical abscess. If the defenders (WBCs) are successful, they may overcome the invading bacteria. The bacteria in the canal (mountain army) are eliminated by extraction of the tooth or by sterilization of the root canal (root canal treatment).

The granulations shrink, and the white blood cells (WBCs) leave and return into the general circulation. This explains why the apical granulation tissue disappears after extraction or after successful root canal treatment. So the granuloma is a defense against spread of infection. It is this tissue with its newly formed capillaries (the granulation tissue) which is responsible for repair.

e. Referred Pain

The term *'referred pain'* implies the pain felt in any part of body away from the place of tissue damage. Another term 'odontalgia' refers to the pain caused by pathological changes in other tissues and reflected on teeth.

The mechanism of referred pain is explained by the theory of convergence (the key location is spinal core of trigeminal nerve: Spinal cord is divided into (i) Subnucleus oralis, (ii) Subnucleus interpolaris and (iii) Subnucleus candalis). The nociceptive nerve fibers, conducting the stimuli from head and neck areas converge in the subnucleus candalis (spinal core) of trigeminal nerve. Certain afferent fibers also belong to other cranial nerves.

When the pain (nerve impulses) gets activated and travel the brain centers; these centers may not identify the exact cause of painful stimuli.

The clinical features of odontogenic pain are tabulated in Table 3.1.

B. Inter-appointment Endodontic Pain (Flare-up)

Local anesthesia is an effective means of controlling pain during endodontic treatment, except while treating the *'hot tooth'* (irreversible pulpitis).

Such patients often carry ice water to help control the pain. Such teeth are mostly prevalent in mandibular arch. The inferior alveolar nerve block delivered to attain pulpal anesthesia in such teeth may not be adequate. Even asymptomatic teeth in a mandibular arch are not properly anesthetized by such blocks.

Table 3.1 Clinical features of odontogenic pain

Disease process	*Symptoms*	*Radiographic findings*	*Response to pulp testing*	*Response to percussion/ palpation*
Pulp diseases				
Reversible pulpitis	Slight responsive to thermal stimulus	No change in periapical radiolucency	Respond to pulp tests	Not sensitive to percussion/ palpation
Irreversible pulpitis	Responsive to thermal stimulus: may be pain	No change in periapical radiolucency	Responds (possibly with extreme pain on thermal stimulus)	May or may not have pain on percussion/palpation
Pulp necrosis	Not responsive to thermal stimulus	No change till periapical areas involved	No response	Depends on status of periapical tissues
Periapical diseases				
Acute apical periodontitis	Pain on mastication/ chewing	May be slight widening of periodontal ligament	Usually not responsive	Pain on percussion/ palpation
Chronic apical periodontitis	Mild discomfort on mastication or putting pressure	Apical radiolucency	No response	Mild discomfort on percussion/palpation
Acute abscess	Significant pain: may be swelling	Initiation of appearance of radiolucency	No response	Pain on percussion/ palpation
Chronic abscess	No pain, if draining sinus or pain and swelling	A radiolucent area at the apex	No response	Not sensitive to percussion/ palpation
Condensing osteitis	Symptom less: no pain	Intermittent radiopacity (increased trabecular bone density)	Usually not responsive	Usually not responsive

Central core theory may explain the phenomenon: in the mandible; the outer nerves fibers of the inferior alveolar nerve supply the molars while the nerve fibers for anterior teeth lie deeper. Anesthetic solutions may not be able to diffuse into all the nerve fibers and provide an adequate block. It is observed that local anesthetic failure after a mandibular block was highest in incisors, followed by premolars and molars.

It has also been hypothesized that in symptomatic teeth the inflamed tissue have an altered resting potential and reduced threshold of excitability. It was shown that anesthetic agents were not able to prevent the transmission of nerve impulses because of the lowered excitability thresholds of inflamed nerves. Various strategies like changing the local anesthetic solution or the injection technique were not successful in anesthetizing 'hot teeth'. Accessory nerves have also been implicated as a potential reason for the failure of this nerve block (Fig. 3.2). The mylohyoid nerve is the accessory nerve most often implicated as the cause for mandibular anesthesia failure. However, inferior alveolar nerve block combined with mylohyoid nerve block did not significantly improve the mandibular anesthesia. Combining intraligamentary injection with inferior alveolar nerve block injection was found to be effective.

Causes of Inter-appointment Pain

The frequency of inter-appointment pain is significantly higher in teeth with periradicular lesions as compared to teeth with normal periradicular tissues. Microbial insult is the major cause of inter-appointment pain; however, certain iatrogenic factors do play a key role. Inter-appointment pain is considered a result of imbalance in host-bacteria relationship induced by intracanal procedures.

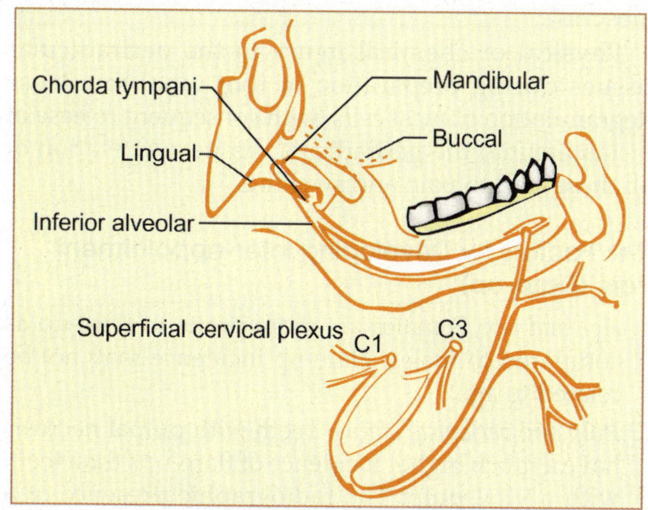

Fig. 3.2 Failure of mandibular nerve block (implications of accessory nerves)

a. Microbial Causes

The factors associated with precipitation of pain by micro-organisms are:

i. *Presence of pathogenic bacteria*: There is no evidence on the qualitative or quantitative shift in the endodontic microbiota that can cause inter-appointment pain. It is hypothesized that the bacterial species associated with such pain are the same as those involved with infected root canals. The change in environment of the bacterial species may be a contributing factor.

ii. *Virulence of the pathogens*: Virulence of endodontic pathogens may not be a predisposing factor for inter-appointment pain; only effective if conditions are created for them to exert pathogenicity. (If the root canal environmental conditions are in some way altered by intracanal procedures and as a result become conducive to the expression of virulence genes, microbial virulence can be enhanced and inter-appointment pain can ensue).

iii. *Microbial synergism:* Most of the endodontic pathogens may show virulence only when in association with other species (synergism), which can certainly influence pain factor.

iv. *Host resistance*: Individuals with poor resistance are more susceptible to postoperative consequences (prone to develop pain after root canal treatment). Poor resistance can be because of varied factors. Herpesvirus infection may be one factor that can diminish host resistance. Herpesviruses have the ability to interfere with the host immune response, which may trigger overgrowth of pathogenic bacteria and/or diminish the host resistance to infection. Herpesviruses may also induce the release of proinflammatory cytokines by host defense cells; subsequently, patients with decreased resistance feel inter-appointment pain.

b. Iatrogenic Causes

Certain iatrogenic causes may lead to inter-appointment pain; the main causes are:

i. *Apical extrusion of debris/chemical agents/over-extended obturating material:* In asymptomatic periradicular lesions associated with infected teeth, there is a balance between infecting endodontic microbiota and the host defense. If during root canal preparation micro-organisms are extruded into the periradicular tissues, the host will have to face a larger number of irritants, disrupting the balance between aggression and defense; consequently, an acute inflammatory response and pain. The risks of inter-appointment pain can be even higher in the event of over-instrumentation; lead to significant extrusion of debris containing micro-organisms along with mechanical injury to the periradicular tissues. The incidence of pain in re-treatment cases with periradicular lesions has been demonstrated to be significantly high. Removal of filling material and also the solvents used during removal of filling may contribute to exacerbation of the periradicular inflammation. Virtually, all instrumentation techniques promote apical extrusion of debris. Crown-down techniques, irrespective by hand or engine-driven instrument, usually extrude less debris; however, qualitative factor is difficult to control (even a small amount of infected debris with virulent micro-organisms may exacerbate periradicular inflammation).

ii. ***Incomplete instrumentation/over-instrumentation***: The microbiota associated with primary endodontic infections is usually established as a mixed consortium, and alteration of part of this consortium will affect both the environment and the remaining species. Incomplete preparation can disrupt the balance within the microbial community by eliminating some inhibitory species and leaving behind other. Such bacteria, if overgrow, may lead to exacerbation of periradicular inflammation. Environmental change (ingress of oxygen in the root canal) may alter the oxidation–reduction potential (Eh) in the root canal; subsequently, lead to acute exacerbation. This theory is based on the fact that the increase in Eh would induce microbial growth pattern to change from anaerobic to aerobic, with consequent overgrowth of facultative bacteria. Overgrowing facultative bacteria might precipitate acute periradicular inflammation.

iii. ***Secondary intra-radicular infections***: Secondary intra-radicular infections are caused by micro-organisms that were not present in the primary infection. They may get entry into the root canal system during treatment, between appointments, or even after the endodontic treatment. If the micro-organisms that gain access to the root canal are successful in surviving and colonizing in a new environment, a secondary infection will establish and may be one of the causes of postoperative pain.

Inflammatory Events Leading to Inter-appointment Pain

Inter-appointment pain is almost exclusively due to the development of acute inflammation at the periradicular tissues in response to the intensity of injury from the root canal system. The inflammatory response to tissue injury may provide potential for repair of the diseased tissues. It may result in undesirable effects such as pain and intensified tissue damage. Chemical mediators released after tissue injury may induce pain due to direct effect on the nerve fibers, or can cause pain indirectly by increasing the vascular permeability; subsequently producing edema and swelling. Bacteria that suddenly gain access to the periradicular tissues may face two lines of defense; complement system and phagocytes (neutrophils and macrophages) present in the chronic inflamed tissue. The encounter of the bacteria with these host defense mechanisms trigger the production and release of chemical mediators of inflammation, which will induce vascular changes in the microcirculation and recruit new phagocytic cells to the site.

Increased vascular permeability along with increased hydrostatic pressure is the hallmark of acute inflammation. The increase in the vascular permeability leads to a marked outflow of fluid, which gets accumulated in the extravascular space. This fluid (inflammatory exudate) may elevate the tissue hydrostatic pressure resulting in swelling and pain.

Exudation induces an increase in tissue hydrostatic pressure, with resultant compression of nerve endings causing pain and swelling.

A sudden egress of a large mass of bacteria into the periradicular tissues represent bacterial cells and their by-products that can cause a massive emigration of neutrophils, which may be unable to phagocytose large bacterial masses and die subsequently. Consequent leakage of lysosomal enzymes and oxygen radicals into the surrounding tissues will lead to pus formation (abscess).

Physical or chemical injury to the periradicular tissues during preparation of root canal can cause degranulation of mast cells, with consequent release of histamine into the periradicular tissues. Activation of all these lead to pain and swelling.

Risk Factors for Developing Inter-appointment Pain (Flare-up)

1. *Age and sex*: Females are more prone to flare-up as compared to males. Flare-up incidence may not be related to age.
2. *Pulp and periapical status*: Teeth with pulpal necrosis have a much higher incidence of flare-ups than teeth with a vital pulp. The radiographic presence of a periapical lesion, particularly larger lesions, also considered as a risk factor for development of

flare-ups. The diagnosis of pulp necrosis and acute apical abscess, is more likely to result in a flare-up than any other pulp and periapical disease.

Interestingly, the presence of a sinus tract virtually ensures that a flare-up will not occur. The tract functions as a relief valve, releases pressure, reduces inflammatory mediators and consequently prevents the sudden onset of pain.

3. *Patient's signs and symptoms*: A patient complaining of pain is considerably more likely to experience an inter-appointment flare-up than a patient without prior symptoms. It is established that patient in pain, which would also increase stress levels; subsequently affect the immune functions.
4. *Treatment factors*: There is no universal agreement as to whether retreatment results in a higher incidence of post-treatment pain/flare-ups than conventional root canal treatment. Incomplete debridement has been traditionally assumed to be a cause of flare-ups; however, not properly documented. Mostly, flare-up/pain occurs before obturation phase.

Antibiotics are commonly administered to patients prior to and after root canal treatment; however, prophylactic antibiotics are contraindicated for prevention of flare-ups.

Treatment of Inter-appointment Pain

The '3D' approach; Diagnosis, Definitive treatment and Drugs has been accepted as treatment protocol for the inter-appointment pain.

a. Diagnosis

The initial phase is diagnosis. Several conditions have been shown to mimic endodontic/odontogenic pain. The current episode of pain may be initiating from another tooth, an unrelated sinus or TMJ-related condition, is to be thoroughly evaluated. The patient's past history of treatment coupled with consultation with the previous dental surgeon help reach out at diagnosis.

b. Definitive Treatment

i. ***Re-treatment***: The involved tooth should be anesthetized prior to re-treatment. The access cavity should then be opened, cleaned and looked for any missed out canal orifice. Enhanced magnification and illumination are beneficial. The obturated material, if any, should be removed. Drainage can be established through the root canal, reducing the localized tissue pressure. It is suggested that the apical constriction be sufficiently enlarged to allow for drainage through the canal.

ii. ***Incision and drainage/trephination***: The rationale for an incision and drainage procedure is to facilitate the evacuation of pus, micro-organisms and toxic products from the periradicular tissues. Moreover, it allows for the decompression of the associated increased periradicular tissue pressure and provides significant pain relief. Detail procedure of incision and drainage/trephination is described in Chapter 23.

iii. ***Intracanal medicaments***: It is established that use of intracanal steroids and a corticosteroid–antibiotic combination has been shown to reduce post-treatment pain.

iv. ***Occlusal reduction:*** The teeth with flare-up condition present with difficulty in biting and chewing, due to increased levels of inflammatory mediators that stimulate periradicular nociceptors. Occlusal reduction may alleviate the mechanical stimulation and relieve pain.

c. Drugs

i. ***Antibiotics***: The advancement in our understanding of the biology of the inflammatory process, along with the known risks associated with antibiotics, it is advised that the clinician should prescribe antibiotics only in case of frank abscess.

ii. ***Analgesics***: The NSAIDs have been shown to be very effective for managing pulpal and periradicular pain. In patients with known sensitivity to NSAIDs or aspirin, acetaminophen is preferred for post-treatment pain. However, NSAIDs are effective in reducing pulpal and periradicular levels of the inflammatory mediator PGE_2. Ibuprofen is also effective for managing pulpal and periradicular pain of inflammatory origin.

C. Post-endodontic Pain

Failure of root canal treatment or sequelae of residual microbial infection leads to pain; soon after root canal treatment or may be after prolonged duration.

Management

- Reducing nociceptive input from the site of injury: pretreating with NSAIDs.
- Attenuating the perception of pain in the central nervous system: pretreat with NSAIDs plus long acting local anesthetic.
- Steroids can be given as an adjunct anti-inflammatory drug.

Pretreatment with either ibuprofen (600 mg) or flurbiprofen (100 mg) is effective for management of post-treatment pain. Some patients do not tolerate

NSAIDs; pretreatment with acetaminophen (1000 mg) is effective for reducing post-treatment pain in such patients.

The long-acting local anesthetics (i.e. bupivacaine, ropivacaine, etc.) can provide an increased duration of post-treatment analgesia beyond the period of anesthesia. The long-acting local anesthetics can provide a duration of analgesia up to 8–10 hours.

NON-ODONTOGENIC PAIN

Odontogenic pain is the most common pain in orofacial region; however, when clinical examination excludes odontogenic cause, other causes of orofacial pain should be considered. Involvement of orofacial organs, such as nose, throat, eye, ear, glands, etc. should be evaluated thoroughly to reach out at diagnosis. Pain in the orofacial region may stimulate as odontogenic pain, posing a diagnostic dilemma for dental practitioner.

Orofacial pains can be acute (trigeminal neuralgia, cluster headache, sinusitis, sialolithiasis, etc.) or chronic (postherpetic neuralgia, TMJ disorder, cheek-muscle pain, etc.).

The nature and duration of acute and chronic non-odontogenic pain is depicted in Table 3.2.

Clinical Characteristics

Clinical characteristics are usually varied and may mimic other pain disorders which may not originate in the orofacial region. The extent of pain may vary from very mild and intermittent pain to severe, sharp and continuous.

Pain may not always originate from dental structures; it is important to distinguish between site and source of pain, which will facilitate correct diagnosis. Pain can be divided into two types:

a. *Primary pain*: The site and source of pain are coincidental and in the same location.

b. *Heterotopic pain*: The site and source of pain are different. It can be divided into three general types:

i. *Central pain*: Pain derived from the central nervous system and perceived peripherally.

ii. *Projected pain*: Pain felt in peripheral distribution of the same nerve that mediated the primary nociceptive input.

iii. *Referred pain*: Spontaneous heterotopic pain, felt at the site of pain with separate innervation to the primary source of pain.

The most important non-odontogenic pains, indirectly related to teeth and surrounding tissues, are described.

1. Pericoronitis

Pain commonly arise from gingiva/mucous membrane around any erupting teeth, which gets infected. Mandibular third molars are usually involved. The pain may be constant or intermittent; biting triggers pain. Acute pericoronitis involves bacterial infection around semierupted mandibular third molar. Trismus may be associated with this tooth because the tooth is close to the mandibular insertion of temporalis muscle.

Analgesics are prescribed to relieve pain and local irrigation of the tissues help in healing. Antibiotics are generally not indicated, unless there are signs of severe infection (fever, malaise, etc.).

Table 3.2 Non-odontogenic pain—nature and duration

Condition	*Nature of pain*	*Trigger zone/stimulation*	*Duration of pain*
Acute			
Trigeminal neuralgia	Lancinating (episodic)	Light touch triggers pain	Few seconds
Cluster headache	Severe ache (episodic)	Rapid eye movement (REM) sleep, alcohol	30–45 minutes
Acute otitis media	Severe ache, throbbing (non-episodic)	Lowering head triggers pain	Few hours; may linger for days
Sinusitis	Moderate ache in maxillary teeth (non-episodic)	Lowering head triggers pain	Continuous for days
Sialolithiasis	Sharp pain (episodic)	Biting induce pain	Pain when triggered
Chronic			
Postherpetic neuralgia	Deep ache, burning	Spontaneous	For long duration
TMJ disorders	Dull ache, sharp	Opening mouth/chewing triggers pain	For long duration
Cheek-muscle pain	Dull ache, severe episodes	Spontaneous	Usually for few weeks
Myalgia	Dull ache	Stress, clenching of teeth	Usually for few weeks

2. Alveolar osteitis

The most common complication of extraction of mandibular teeth is alveolar osteitis (dry socket), which is rarely seen in maxillary teeth. Unhealed socket results in entrapment of food debris, which may aggravate bony nerve endings. Pain is dull and throbbing; usually develops two-three days after extraction.

Irrigating the socket with mild antiseptics along with analgesics are effective in pain control. An obtundent dressing is given to promote healing. Antibiotics are not indicated.

3. Myofascial pain

Myofascial pain is described as non-pulsating and aching pain, which occurs continuously as compared to pulpal pain. Patients are unable to locate the source of pain and often believe pain is originating from the tooth. Tooth sensitivity to temperature, percussion or occlusal pressure may be felt as a result of referred pain from the offending muscle. Pain might be associated with extended muscle use and get exacerbated with emotional stresses. Palpation of the trigger point (a localized hyper-excitable area within the muscle) is able to reproduce the toothache.

Anesthetizing the strained muscle rather than the tooth alleviates pain. Warm or cold compresses, muscle stretching, massage, etc., facilitate relief of pain.

4. Pain of sinusitis

Sinusitis is a common ailment. The roots of the maxillary dentition are usually in intimate contact with and even may be protruding into the sinus cavity. The inflammation and infection in sinus have direct effect on roots of maxillary teeth; and the infectious process in the dentition may effect sinus as an acute or chronic sinusitis. In such cases, patients may present with facial pain and pressure in the maxillary posterior region. Other symptoms such as headache, nasal discharge or congestion and ear pain may also be recognized as sinus disease. Sinus pain can also present as a continuous dull ache or diffuse lingering pain in the maxillary teeth with sensitivity to percussion, mastication and/or temperature. When multiple maxillary teeth feel pain, it indicates pain of sinus origin rather than odontogenic pain.

Pain may be elicited by palpation of the infraorbital regions or when the patient is asked to bow the maneuvering the head to the levels of the knees. The absence of any inflammation around teeth may further lead to the conclusion that there is sinus inflammation.

Treatment should be directed towards the maxillary sinus infection. Mostly acute sinusitis is of viral origin and requires nasal decongestants. In case of bacteria-induced sinusitis, a regimen of antibiotics is additionally prescribed. Antiallergic drugs are also effective.

5. Migraine and trigeminal cephalgia

Headache is the pain localized to cranium. Two primary headache types that may present as toothache are migraine and trigeminal cephalgia. Trigeminal cephalgia is further categorized as cluster headache, paroxysmal hemicranic and neuralgiform headache.

Migraines are typically unilateral, moderate to severe pains of pulsatile and throbbing quality, which may last between few hours and days. Migraine is often accompanied by nausea, vomiting and may present with or without neurological symptoms.

Cluster headache is common in young adults (age 20–40 years). Pain being boring and severe, usually located around orbits. Pain may last for few minutes and may linger for hours.

Collectively, such pains are referred to as neuro-vascular orofacial pain, which is usually treated with symptomatic drugs.

6. Trigeminal neuralgia

The most common branch of trigeminal nerve involved in neuralgia is the mandibular nerve followed by maxillary nerve. The pain in trigeminal neuralgia is often severe and intense. There is often a trigger zone, which when stimulated produces severe pain. Rarely, a tooth can be a trigger zone; if so, can pose a diagnostic challenge. The differences between trigeminal neuralgia and atypical facial pain are explained in Table 3.3.

Table 3.3 Differences between trigeminal neuralgia and atypical facial pain

	Trigeminal neuralgia	*Atypical facial pain*
Age and sex	Older adults; female to male ratio is 2 to 3	Young adults; mostly females
Location of pain	Along distribution of branches of the trigeminal nerve. One sided usually.	One sided; may be on both sides
Duration of pain	Less; in minutes	Constant and more
Quality of pain	Severe (sharp, stabbing, lancinating)	Moderate (diffuse, burning, aching, dull)
Trigger zones	Stimulation of trigger zones	No trigger zone
Treatment of choice	Carbamazepine	Tricyclic antidepressants

Pain originating from abnormalities in the neural structures (neuropathic pain) can be of two types—episodic and continuous.

The clinical presentation of an *episodic neuropathic pain* is severe and shooting, that lasts only a few seconds. Pain may and may not restrict to tooth.

Continuous neuropathic pain is constant and unremitting, which can be of high and low intensity. Such pains when felt in teeth have been referred to as atypical odontalgia or 'phantom toothache'.

The characteristics of continuous neuropathic pain that differentiate it from odontogenic pain are: (a) Diffuse pain, (b) pain not always restricted to a tooth, (c) pain that is continuous dull, aching or throbbing and (d) pain that may not be relieved by local anesthetic block.

7. *Pain due to orofacial malignancies*

Primary squamous cell carcinoma of the oral mucosa (gingiva, vestibule or floor of mouth) may present with pain and sensory disturbances that mimic toothache.

Nasopharyngeal cancers may present with signs and symptoms that can be confused with temporomandibular disorders, parotid gland lesions and other odontogenic infections.

Systemic cancers such as lymphoma and leukemia may have intraoral manifestations that mimic toothache. Orofacial pain has also been associated with metastatic and non-metastatic malignancies. Any soft or hard tissue changes around odontogenic structures must be evaluated and if not related to tooth, other neoplastic (cancer) lesions are suspected.

8. *Cardiac pain*

Cardiac pain is an additional source of referred pain to the teeth and jaw mainly due to cardiac ischemia (pain radiate to the left shoulder and arm). It affects neck, ear, teeth and jaws. Clinical characteristics of pain may vary as episodic lasting from minutes to hours.

If the pain is associated with cardiac or chest pain, it is most often relieved by sublingual nitroglycerin. Patients should be referred to cardiologist for management.

9. *Psychogenic pain*

Psychogenic pain is the pain that is associated with psychologic factors in the absence of any physiologic cause. Pain is diffuse, vague and difficult to localize. Usually, the pain is inconsistent and present without any identifiable pathological causes. In case, the pain is accompanied by any psychological disorder; definite possibility of a psychogenic pain.

Patients should be referred to a psychiatrist for management.

BIBLIOGRAPHY

1. Ajmera K and Mulay S. Non-odontogenic toothache—a clinical dilemma. Int. J. Scientific Study: 2014; 2:90–93.
2. Annino DJ and Goguen LA. Pain from the oral cavity. Otolaryngologic Clinics of North America: 2003; 36:1127–1135.
3. Baad-Hansen L. Atypical odontalgia – pathophysiology and clinical management. J. Oral Rehabil.: 2008; 35:1–11.
4. Balasubramaniam R, Turner LN, Fischer D, Klasser GD and Okeson JP. Non-odontogenic toothache revisited. Open J. Stomato.: 2011; 1:92–102.
5. Bender IB. Pulpal pain diagnosis – a review. J. Endod.:2000; 26:175–179.
6. Benoliel R and Sharav Y. Neurovascular orofacial pain. Cephalalgia: 2008; 28:199–200.
7. Brook I. Sinusitis of odontogenic origin. Otolaryngology – Head and neck surgery: 2006; 1356:349–355.
8. Carius A and Schulze-Bonhage A. Trigeminal pain under vagus nerve stimulation. Pain: 2005; 118:271–273.
9. Christopher JS, John KN, Henry G, Joanna MZ and Richard O. Toothache of trigeminal neuralgia: Treatment dilemmas. J. Pain: 2008; 9:767–770.
10. Clark GT. Persistent orodental pain, atypical odontalgia, and phantom tooth pain: When are they neuropathic disorders? J. Calif. Dent. Assoc.: 2006; 34:599–609.
11. Ehrmann EH. The diagnosis of referred orofacial dental pain. Aust. Endod. J.: 2002; 28:75–81.
12. Hargreaves KM and Keiser K. Local anesthetic failure in endodontics. Mechanisms and management. Endod. Topics: 2002; 1:26–39.
13. Hargreaves KM and Keiser K. Building effective strategies for the management of endodontic pain. Endod. Topics: 2002; 3:93–105.
14. Henry M A and Hargreaves K M. Peripheral mechanism of odontogenic pain. Dental Clinic North Am. 2007, 51, 19–44.
15. Jens CT. Trigeminal neuralgia versus atypical facial pain. Oral Surg., Oral Med., Oral Pathol., Oral Radiol.: 1996; 81:424–432.
16. Jerjes W, Hopper C, Kumar M, Upile T, Madland G and Newman S. Psychological intervention in acute dental pain: Review. Br. Dent. J.:2007; 202:337–343.
17. Koratkar H, Parashar V and Koratkar S. A review of neuropathic pain conditions affecting teeth. Gen. Dent.: 2010; 58:436–441.
18. Kreiner M, Falace D, Michelis V, Okeson JP and Isberg A. Quality difference in craniofacial pain of cardiac vs. dental origin. J. Dent. Res.: 2010; 89:965–969.
19. Kretzschmar DP and Kretzschmar JL. Rhinosinusitis: Review from a dental perspective. Oral Surg., Oral Med., Oral Pathol, Oral Radiol.: 2003; 96:128–135.
20. Kureishi A and Chow AW. The tender tooth. Dentoalveolar, pericoronal, and periodontal infections. Infect. Dis. Clin. North Am.: 1988; 2:163–182.
21. Levin LG, Law AS, Holland GR, Abbott PV and Roda RS. Identify and define all diagnostic terms for pulpal health and disease states. J. Endod.:2009; 35:1645–1657.

22. Linn J, Trantor I, Teo N, Thanigaivel R and Goss AN. The differential diagnosis of toothache from other orofacial pains in clinical practice. Aust. Dent. J.: 2007; 52:100–104.
23. Melis M, Lobo SL, Ceneviz C, Zawawi K, Al-Badawi K, Maloney G and Mehta N. Atypical odontalgia: A review of the literature. Headache: 2003; 43:1060–1074.
24. Namazi MR. Presentation of migraine as odontalgia. Headache: 2001; 41:420–421.
25. Nixdorf R, Moana-Filho EJ, Law AS, McGuire LA, Hodges JS and John MT. Frequency of persistent tooth pain after root canal therapy: A systematic review and meta-analysis. J. Endod.: 2010; 36:224–30.
26. Nixdorf R, Moana-Filho EJ, Law AS, McGuire LA, Hodges JS and John MT. Frequency of non-odontogenic pain after root canal therapy: A systematic review and meta-analysis. J. Endod.: 2010; 36:1494–1498.
27. Oshima K, Ishii T, Ogura Y, Aoyama Y and Katsuumi I. Clinical investigation of patients who develop neuropathic tooth pain after endodontic procedures. J. Endod.:2009; 35:958–961.
28. Perkins FM and Kehlet H. Chronic pain as an outcome of surgery. Anesthesiology.: 2000, 93; 1123–1133.
29. Prpic-Mehicic G and Galic N. Odontogenic pain. Med. Sci.: 2010; 34:43–54.
30. Ram S, Teruel A, Kumar SK and Clark G. Clinical characteristics and diagnosis of atypical odontalgia: Implications for dentists. JADA: 2009; 40:223–228.
31. Renton T. Dental (odontogenic) pain. Reviews in Pain: 2001; 5:2–7.
32. Rosenberg P, Babick P, Schertzer L and Leung A. The effect of occlusal reduction on pain after endodontic instrumentation. J. Endod.: 1998; 24:492–496.
33. Sarlani E, Balciunas BA and Grace EG. Orofacial pain-Part II: Assessment and amanagement of vascular, neurovascular, idiopathic, secondary and psychogenic causes. AACN Clin. Issues: 2005; 16:347–358.
34. Scholz J and Woolf CJ. Can we conquer pain? Nat. Neurosci.:2002; 5:1062–1067.
35. Siqueira JF and Barnett F. Inter-appointment pain: mechanisms, diagnosis, and Treatment. Endod. Topics: 2004; 7:93–109.
36. Slots J, Sabeti M and Simon JH. Herpesviruses in periapical pathosis: an etiopathogenic relationship? Oral Surg., Oral Med., Oral Path.: 2003; 96:327–331.
37. Siqueira JF Jr. Microbial causes of endodontic flare-ups. Int. Endod. J.: 2003; 36:453–463.
38. Trowbridge HO. Review of dental pain histology and physiology. J. Endod.:1986; 12:1–8.
39. Quail G. Atypical facial pain-a diagnostic challenge. Aust Fam Physician.: 2005, 34, 641–645.
40. Weyman BJ. Psychological components of pain perception. Dent. Clin. North Am.: 1978; 22:101–113.

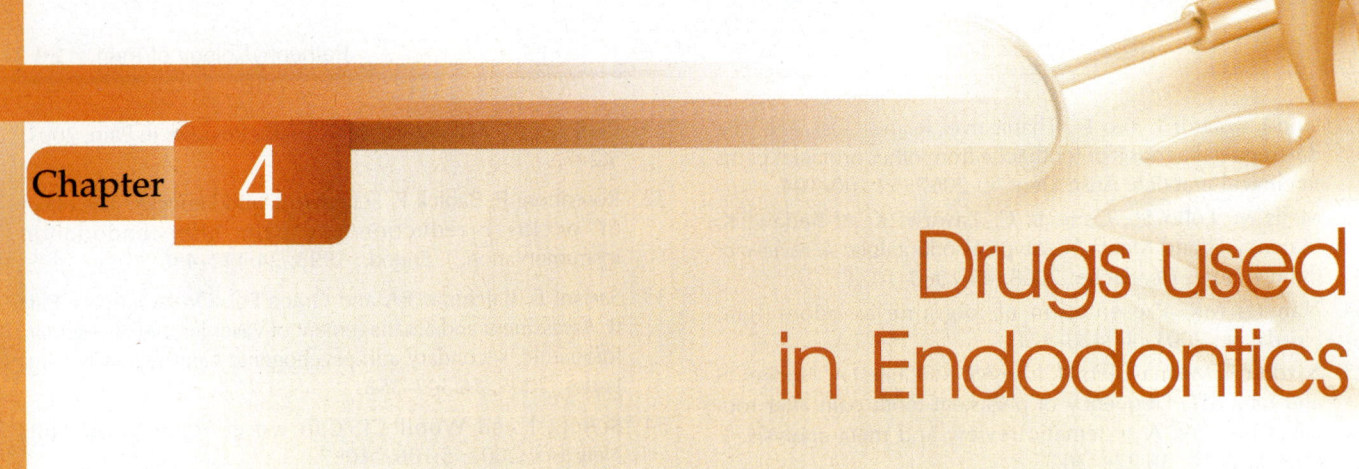

Chapter 4

Drugs used in Endodontics

The primary goal of endodontic treatment is to eradicate micro-organisms along with harbouring sites, so as to achieve requisite healing of the periapical tissues. The treatment may be accompanied by anxiety, pain and/or problem of persistent infection. Certain drugs/medicaments are to be prescribed in such situations. The operator should be aware of the indications, contraindications, actions/reactions and also the side effects of the drugs, which can be prescribed to control pain, anxiety and/or infections. WHO (1966) defined drug as *'any substance or product that is used or intended to be used to modify physiological systems or pathological state for the benefit of the recipient'*. A pharmaceutical medicine or medicinal product is defined as *'any chemical agent intended to be used in the diagnosis, cure, treatment or prevention of disease'*. Various drugs are used before, during and after endodontic procedures.

The drugs used in endodontics are broadly categorized as:

I. Management of fear and anxiety
II. Effective pain control
III. Management of infection
IV. Miscellaneous

I. MANAGEMENT OF FEAR AND ANXIETY

Fear and anxiety can be identified by either behavioural changes or recognizing physical changes, such as dilated pupils, pale skin, excessive sweating, tingling of extremities and increase of blood pressure. The reasons for fear in a dental clinic are fear of pain, belonephobia (fear of needle and injection) and unpleasant past experience of self and peer groups.

The initial management of fear and anxiety is psychosedation (*an act of making calm through psychological motivation*). Psychosedation is mainly through verbal and non-verbal (body language) communication of the doctor, which affects the patient in alleviating fear and anxiety (discussion with patient identifying reasons of fear along with counseling will minimize the fear level). In case psychosedation is not achieved, certain drugs (pharmacosedation) are tried. Anxiolytic sedative-hypnotic drugs can be prescribed in routine; rarely anesthesia is required to manage fear and anxiety.

A. Sedative-hypnotic Drugs

Various drugs are used as sedative-hypnotic to control fear and anxiety in a dental set-up. Apart from relieving anxiety, these drugs are also used for various clinical situations, such as:

- Insomnia
- During treatment of epilepsy
- As a component of balanced anesthesia
- Control of ethanol or other sedative-hypnotic withdrawal state.
- Muscle relaxant in specific neuromuscular disorders.
- Diagnostic aids for treatment in psychiatry.

Side-effects

- Dependence
- Depression of central nervous system functions
- Amnestic effects
- Cause depression when administered with other drugs, including ethanol.

Classification

The sedative-hypnotic drugs are classified as:

a. Barbiturates
   i. Ultrashort acting: Methohexital, thiopental sodium
   ii. Short acting: Secobarbital (Seconal), pentobarbital
   iii. Intermediate acting: Amytal (amobarbital) and Tuinal (secobarbital and amobarbital)
   iv. Long acting: Phenobarbital and barbital.
b. Benzodiazepines
   i. Short acting: Midazolam, triazolam, prazepam

ii. Intermediate acting: Alprazolam, lorazepam, oxazepam
iii. Long acting: Diazepam, nitrazepam, flurazepam.

c. Non-benzodiazepines: Imidazopyridine derivatives; zolpidem, zaleplon, zopiclone.
d. Antihistamines: Diphenhydramine, promethazine, hydroxyzine.
e. Anticholinergic: Glycopyrrolate, atropine/scopolamine.
f. Miscellaneous drugs: Opioids, propofol, chloral derivatives, meprobamate.

a. *Barbiturates*

The varying dose of barbiturates produces different level of CNS depression, such as relaxation (sedation) and drowsiness (hypnosis). Barbiturates enhance the activity of neurotransmitter that inhibits the activity of nerve cells in the brain. At higher doses, barbiturates can produce general anesthesia and even coma.

Barbiturates are mainly used as minor tranquilizers to reduce anxiety levels and mental acuity. Barbiturates were initially used in oral surgery for third-molar extraction; however, their tendency to cause respiratory depression has led to its limited use in the dental clinic. 100–200 mg secobarbital and 15–30 mg pentobarbital thrice daily are effective sedative-hypnotic drugs.

b. *Benzodiazepines*

Benzodiazepines are categorized as non-barbiturate sedatives. These are less potent than barbiturates. The main benefit of using benzodiazepine instead of barbiturate is the decreased occurrence of hangover effect that often accompanies barbiturates. The commonly used benzodiazepines are:

i. *Diazepam (Valium)*: Diazepam effectively reduces anxiety and is a profound amnestic. Diazepam is safe and effective both orally and intravenously. 5.0–10 mg dose is effective orally and 2.5–5.0 mg intravenously. In the case of intravenous sedation, its long duration of action makes it a preferred choice for longer duration surgeries (intravenous and intramuscular injections are generally painful). The elimination time is prolonged, which may lead to some lingering effect (hangover) of sedation.
ii. *Midazolam (Versed)*: Midazolam is about 2.5 times as potent as diazepam and is used both orally and as intravenous injections. The recommended dose is 0.5–1.0 mg/kg orally and 0.05–0.15 mg/kg intravenously. Midazolam has a significantly shorter half-life than diazepam, making it an ideal agent for short procedures. It does not have any 'hangover' effect. Respiratory depression is of concern with the use of midazolam.
iii. *Triazolam (Halcion)*: Triazolam is a potent sedative agent. It is used mainly orally (0.25 to 0.50 mg). One hour prior intake of triazolam is quite effective in producing sedation and amnesia.
iv. *Lorazepam (Ativan)*: Lorazepam has approximately 10–20 hours as half-life. The adult dose for dental sedation range from 0.5 to 4.0 mg depending upon the procedure undertaken. The onset of action occurs within 60 minutes.

The dosage of drugs commonly used for sedation and hypnosis are tabulated in Table 4.1.

c. *Non-benzodiazepines*

Non-benzodiazepines are chemically distinct drugs; however, their effects and clinical profiles are indistinguishable from benzodiazepines. The effects of non-benzodiazepines can be reversed using benzodiazepines antagonist, flumazenil. It is hypothesized that their action is selective (on one subunit out of five BZ receptors), which reduces their potential for cognitive impairment.

The commonly used non-benzodiazepines are:

i. *Zolpidem (Ambien)*: Zolpidem has rapid onset of action (within 30 minutes) and has short half-life. The usual adult dose is 10 mg (5.0 mg is advised for geriatric patients). The 'hangover' effects are minimum.

Table 4.1 Dosages of drugs commonly used for sedation and hypnosis

Sedation		*Hypnosis*	
Drug	*Dosage*	*Drug*	*Dosage*
Alprazolam (Xanax)	0.25–0.5 mg 2–3 times daily	Chloral hydrate (Somnote)	500–1000 mg
Chlordiazepoxide (Equilibrium)	10–20 mg 2–3 times daily	Estazolam (Prosom)	0.5–2.0 mg
Diazepam (Valium)	2.0–10.0 mg daily (5.0 mg twice daily)	Lorazepam (Ativan)	0.25–4.0 mg
Lorazepam (Ativan)	0.25–2.0 mg once or twice daily	Secobarbital (Seconal)	100–200 mg
Oxazepam (Serepax)	15–30 mg 3–4 times daily	Triazolam (Halcion)	0.125–0.5 mg
Phenobarbital (Luminal)	15–30 mg 2–3 times daily	Zaleplon (Sonata)	5.0–20 mg
Propofol (Diprivan)	2.0–2.5 mg/kg daily	Zolpidem (Ambien)	5.0–10 mg

ii. *Zaleplon (Sonata)*: Zaleplon is available in 5.0 mg and 10.0 mg capsules (dose ranges from 5.0 to 20.0 mg). It has faster onset of action and short half-life.

iii. *Zopiclone (Zimovane)*: The average adult dose is 7.5–15.0 mg (available as 5.0 mg and 7.5 mg tablets). It has rapid onset of action and short half-life.

d. *Antihistamines*

Antihistamines cause sedation as a side effect (mainly used to manage allergic reactions). Diphenylhydramine (Benadryl) is commonly used antihistamine for the treatment of allergic cough. It is also effective in the relief of nausea, vomiting and vertigo. The onset of action is within 15–30 minutes and the adult dosage is 20–25 mg for effective sedation. Promethazine (Phenergan) is also used as sedative. The adult dose for sedation is 25–50 mg. Another commonly used antihistamine is hydroxyzine (Atarax), whose onset of action is within 15–30 minutes and the adult dose is 50–100 mg. Hydroxyzine has minimal side effects on cardiovascular and respiratory functions. Mostly antihistamines have anticholinergic properties.

e. *Anticholinergic*

Anticholinergic drugs block acetylcholine from binding to its receptors on certain nerve cells. They inhibit parasympathetic nerve impulses (responsible for involuntary movement in the gastrointestinal tract and other parts of the body). The nerve impulses also control functions such as salivation, digestion, urination, etc. Atropine and scopolamine are effective in blocking short-term memory; depresses CNS, cause amnesia, drowsiness and sleep. These drugs decrease salivary secretions. Glycopyrrolate may be preferred over atropine/scopolamine for its superior anti-sialagogue effects, less pronounced cardiac effects, and poor CNS penetration. The recommended dose of glycopyrrolate is 0.1–0.3 mg intramuscular and 1.0–2.0 mg orally.

Anticholinergic may lead to dry mouth and retention of urine.

f. *Miscellaneous drugs*

i. *Opioids (Morphine)*: Opioids are seldom used alone for sedation. These are effective in producing euphoria, sedation, and analgesia; however, may be accompanied by nausea and respiratory depression. Because of its slow onset and longer duration of activity, it is commonly used in anesthesia for postoperative pain management rather than intravenous sedation.

Meperidine hydrochloride and fentanyl citrate are the most commonly used opioids for intravenous sedation and general anesthesia. The peak effect occurs in 15–30 minutes and the analgesic effect may last for 4 hours.

ii. *Propofol (Diprivan)*: Propofol in low dose is an effective sedative. It is highly lipid-soluble, which accounts for its rapid uptake and short duration of action. It is a potent amnestic and a powerful antiemetic. In an adult, 2.0–2.5 mg/kg (maximum 250 mg) is the recommended dose. Propofol may lead to mild itching/rashes or slight burning.

Premedication with Sedative Drugs

Premedication is advised before any surgical procedure to minimise anxiety and other associated features. The sedatives are preferred as premedication agents prior to anesthesia.

Indications

- Patients undergoing surgical procedures
- Disabilities or special need patients, especially children (Autistic, Asperger's, Down's syndrome)
- Patients having past experience of emergency during anesthesia.

Contraindications

- Anticipated airway difficulty
- Obstructive sleep apnea
- Acute systemic illness, e.g. severe sepsis
- Severe renal or hepatic impairment
- Previous allergy to sedative drugs

Advantages

- Reduces both patient and parental anxiety
- Provide effective anterograde amnesia
- Reduces postoperative behavioural changes

Disadvantages

- Non-compliance by the patient may worsen anxiety
- Some drugs like midazolam may lead to paradoxical reactions
- May potentiate the effect of other sedative drugs, e.g. opioids.

B. Anesthetic Agents

Local anesthetics are the fastest and most effective drugs for the management of fear and anxiety; best suitable for pain control also. A variety of local anesthetic agents is available for specific dental procedures, possessing requisite properties, such as time of onset and duration, hemostatic control and minimum side effects.

The commonly employed anesthetic agents are:

i. *Lidocaine/Lignocaine/Xylocaine*: It is available in three formulations: 2.0% without vasoconstrictor (plain), 2.0% with 1:100,000 epinephrine (vasoconstrictor), and 2.0% with 1:50,000 epinephrine. The onset of action is fairly rapid (3–5 minutes). It is also available as topical solution (20–40 mg/ml) with 2.0% and 5.0% concentrations. Lidocaine without vasoconstrictor has anesthetic effect for 1–2 hours; however, pulpal anesthesia is only for 5 to 10 minutes, so not preferred for most dental procedures. The formulations with the epinephrine (vasoconstrictor) have anesthetic effect for 1–1.5 hours on pulp. The 1:50,000 epinephrine concentrations are advantageous for hemostasis in surgical sites; however, not useful for pulpal anesthesia. The overdose of lignocaine may lead to drowsiness, loss of consciousness and respiratory arrest.

ii. *Mepivacaine*: Mepivacaine is available in two formulations: 3.0% plain solution and 2.0% solution with 1:20,000 levonordefrin (vasoconstrictor). The plain solution has effective anesthetic duration of 20 to 40 minutes for pulpal lesions. The vasoconstrictor containing solution provides the pulpal anesthesia for 1–1.5 hours. The levonordefrin vasoconstrictor is less likely to produce cardiac side effects (palpitations), than epinephrine; however, it has the potential to increase blood pressure.

iii. *Bupivacaine*: Bupivacaine is four times potent than lignocaine, mepivacaine and prilocaine. It is available as 0.5% solution with 1:200,000 epinephrine. Bupivacaine exhibits a remarkable increase in the duration of anesthesia; however, it may display a slightly slower time of onset (5–10 minutes). Bupivacaine is preferred in regional nerve block injection techniques with mandibular blocks. As a block, pulpal anesthesia is effective up to seven hours (preferred in lengthy dental procedures).

iv. *Articaine*: Articaine is one and a half time potent than lignocaine. It is available as a 4.0% solution with 1:100,000 epinephrine. The anesthetic effect remains potent for less than one hour; usually not preferred in dental procedures. It has also shown risk of nerve paresthesia, particularly for inferior alveolar and lingual nerve block injections. The solution is avoided in females who are breast-feeding; may be excreted in milk.

v. *Prilocaine*: Prilocaine is slightly less potent and considerably less toxic than lidocaine. The contra-indications for use of prilocaine, include patients with history of cardiac/respiratory failure due to hypoxia. Prilocaine is available as a 4.0% solution with 1:200,000 epinephrine. The solution is effective for 40 to 60 minutes in case of pulpal involvement. The main advantage is the decrease in side effects due to the lower vasoconstrictor concentration.

These agents alone and in various combinations are being used as topical anesthetic agent. A commercially available EMLA cream (lignocaine and prilocaine: 2.5% each) is a common topical anesthetic agent.

Anesthesia Delivery Systems

The intraoral local anesthesia is associated with certain drawbacks, such as patient's fear of injection and the perception of being painful. New injection delivery techniques, including the computer controlled local anesthetic delivery vehicles, have been introduced that provide reliable anesthesia and do not result in undesirable extraoral soft tissue anesthesia.

The commonly employed delivery systems are:

a. Computer controlled technology
   i. Wand system (Milestone Scientific)
   ii. Comfort Control Syringe (Dentsply).

b. Intraosseous delivery system
   i. Stabident system (Fairfax Dental)
   ii. X-Tip system (X-Tip technology)
   iii. Intraflow system (IntraVantage)

a. *Computer controlled technology*

The systems, which employ computer controlled technology in administration of local anesthesia are:

i. The Wand system utilizes computer microprocessor to control the flow rate and also the fluid pressure. An electronically controlled motor delivers the anesthetic solution at a slow rate. The delivery of anesthetic solution into any injection site is carried out at a rate below the threshold of pain. The small diameter of the syringe/handpiece facilitates stable grip, subsequently less pain to the patient.

ii. The Comfort Control Syringe is an electronic, computer-controlled anesthetic delivery system. The Syringe houses the anesthetic cartridge directly behind the needle, just as in a conventional syringe; facilitating finger tips to control the delivery. It has five pre-programmed speeds for different injection techniques and can be used for all injection techniques.

b. *Intraosseous delivery system*

The technique of delivering local anesthetics directly into alveolar bone (intraosseous) in close proximity to root apices in not new; however, electronic delivery methods have greatly improved the convenience of intraosseous injections. The intraosseous technique is quite reliable for pulpal anesthesia for one or two teeth and is particularly useful to anesthetize the 'hot tooth'. The systems used are:

i. *The Stabident system* is a two-part system with a separate perforated needle. A bur is first used to penetrate the house using a slow speed handpiece after which the anesthetic injection needle is passed through the perforation directly into the cancellous bone.

ii. *The X-Tip system* is also a two-part system; in place of the perforated needle, a cannular guide is used for insertion of the anesthetic injection needle into the cancellous bone.

iii. *The Intraflow system* is a one-step technique utilizes a low-speed handpiece with a foot-pedal control system that permits perforation and injection into the site immediately.

As the intraosseous injections are delivered into the highly vascular cancellous bone tissue; use of vasoconstrictor in anesthetic agents is not advised due to rapid uptake of the agent into the circulatory system, subsequently increasing patient's heart rate.

Techniques of Anesthesia

a. *Conscious sedation*

Sedation is a state of drowsiness or mental relaxation. The operator should evaluate the patient's level of anxiety in a dental clinic. Patients with a history of claustrophobia, low pain tolerance, unpleasant dental experiences in childhood are favourable candidates for sedation.

Conscious sedation is a low level of sedation produced by pharmacologic/nonpharmacologic method. It retains the patient's ability to preserve the airway and the patient reacts to the physical stimulation as in routine. The drugs used in conscious sedation should possess a safety margin, to prevent total loss of consciousness.

b. *General anesthesia*

General anesthesia is a state of controlled unconsciousness, accompanied by loss of protective reflexes. This form of anesthesia is the most dependable anesthesia modality. It is indicated for management of highly anxious and phobic patients undergoing endodontic surgical procedures.

In endodontics, general anesthesia is indicated to drain abscess of painful non-vital tooth. In such instances, a general anesthetic is administered on first sitting; subsequently, after completion of the emergency procedure, the endodontic procedures can be carried out in routine.

The dental procedure, if expected to last longer than an hour, or when considerable water spray is going to be used, the airway can be protected with endotracheal intubation; however, for short duration cases endotracheal intubation is rarely required. A continuous observation and monitoring of the patient must be carried out during general anesthesia to manage the airway.

c. *Oral sedation*

Oral sedation is considered ideal for patients requiring short and moderate duration dental procedures.

For an endodontic procedure, lasting up to one hour, Triazolam, a short-acting benzodiazepine (0.25–0.5 mg), can be given one hour before the procedure. Triazolam provides anxiolytic, hypnotic, and amnesic effects, which are desirable in endodontic patients. It has a relatively short half-life with minor 'hangover' effects. The antihistamines have also been used as sedatives for endodontic procedures. Diphenhydramine (Benadryl 50 mg), hydroxyzine 50–100 mg, promethazine (Phenergan) 25–50 mg may be prescribed one hour prior to the endodontic procedure.

Advantages

- Effective in endodontic procedures
- Favourable patient acceptance
- No fear of implication of intravenous route
- Safe when used in recommended dosages (rarely contraindicated)

Disadvantages

- Inability to modify dose of the drug for individual patients and in specific cases

d. *Intramuscular/intravenous/intranasal sedation*

The intramuscular/intravenous route of drug administration is preferred where oral administration is difficult. Ketamine is an ideal drug to be used via intramuscular route. Midazolam is used for intramuscular and intranasal sedation.

Benzodiazepines followed by an opioid are used to intensify the level of sedation; also provide sufficient analgesia. A benzodiazepine-opioid combination for intravenous sedation is preferred because both are reversible. An adult escort is required along with the patient because recovery from intramuscular/intravenous drugs may be prolonged. Sometimes intravenous administration of flumazenil/naloxone is required to achieve reversal in intramuscular/intravenous drugs.

Advantages

- Maintains control over the patient's level of sedation (dose can be controlled by evaluating sedation).
- Favourable patient's acceptance.

e. *Inhalation*

Nitrous oxide is a colourless and virtually odourless gas with a faint, sweet smell. It is an effective analgesic/

anxiolytic agent causing central nervous system (CNS) depression and euphoria with little effect on the respiratory system. Analgesic effect of nitrous oxide is initiated by neuronal release of endogenous opioid peptides with subsequent activation of opioid receptors. The flow of oxygen is adjusted to 5–6 liters per minute before initiating inhalation process. Nitrous oxide is activated at a flow of one liter per minute; oxygen level is decreased simultaneously. Process is repeated till sedation is achieved.

Inhalation process is practical and effective; however, it is *contraindicated* in certain conditions, such as:

- Chronic obstructive pulmonary diseases.
- First trimester of pregnancy.
- Severe emotional disturbances or drug-related dependency.
- Methylenetetrahydrofolate reductase deficiency.
- Cobalamin deficiency.

f. *Hypnosis*

Hypnosis implies inducing depression in central nervous system, which resembles normal sleep. Agents that produce these effects are referred to as sedative-hypnotics.

Various investigators have confirmed that hypnotherapy prior to dental surgery can significantly help patients to overcome their apprehension and anxiety; also helps them minimize the use of analgesics following the surgery.

II. EFFECTIVE PAIN CONTROL

The International Association for the Study of pain defines pain as *'an unpleasant sensory and emotional experience arising from actual or potential tissue damage or described in terms of such damage'*.

Pain may be categorized as (i) acute pain and (ii) chronic pain.

Features of acute pain

- Generally has a known cause
- May last from seconds to hours
- May be associated with tachycardia and anxiety
- Subsides after removal of the stimulus.

Features of chronic pain

- May last from months to years
- Usually associated with decreased functions

Management of Pain

Acute inflammation is associated with a condition known as hyperalgesia, characterized by spontaneous pain, an exaggerated response to stimulation, and a reduced pain threshold. Blocking the development of hyperalgesia is the first step in management of pain.

Effective management of pain depends upon the following features:

- Diagnosing cause of the pain
- Use of analgesic as premedication along with sedative drugs
- Use of anesthesia, when required
- Acupuncture/laser acupuncture, as per need.

The introduction and subsequent application of analgesic agents to eliminate the physical and psychological effects of pain should be carefully assessed. The specific pathology of pain should be diagnosed before prescribing analgesics.

The types of analgesics used in endodontics are:

1. Non-narcotic/non-opioid analgesics
2. Opioid analgesics
3. Corticosteroids.
4. Alternative analgesics (acupuncture)

1. Non-narcotic/Non-opioid Analgesics

Non-narcotic/non-opioid drugs are the class of drugs which function by inhibiting cyclooxygenase enzymes (COX), which produces prostaglandins. There are two types of COX enzymes, COX-1 and COX-2. Both enzymes produce prostaglandins, responsible for inflammation and pain.

The non-narcotic/non-opioid analgesics are of following types:

a. *Nonselective COX inhibitors [non-steroidal anti-inflammatory drugs (NSAIDs)]*
   - Salicylates: Aspirin, sodium salicylate
   - Propionic acid derivatives: Ibuprofen, naproxen, ketoprofen.
   - Anthranilic acid derivative: Mefenamic acid, flufenamic acid
   - Aryl-acetic acid derivatives: Diclofenac, aceclofenac.
   - Oxicam derivatives: Piroxicam, tenoxicam.
   - Pyrrolo-pyrrole derivative: Ketorolac
   - Indole derivative: Indomethacin.
   - Pyrazolone derivative: Phenylbutazone, oxyphenbutazone
   - Aniline derivative: Acetaminophen (paracetamol) (only analgesic effect)

b. *Preferential COX-2 inhibitors*
   - Nimesulide
   - Meloxicam
   - Nabumetone.

c. *Selective COX-2 inhibitors*
- Celecoxib
- Etoricoxib
- Parecoxib

d. *Analgesic-antipyretics with poor anti-inflammatory action*
- Para-aminophenol derivatives: Paracetamol (acetaminophen)
- Pyrazolone derivative: Metamizol, propyphenazone.
- Benzoxazocine derivative: Nefopam.

a. *Nonsteroidal anti-inflammatory drugs (NSAIDs) (Non-selective COX inhibitors)*

Traditional NSAIDs produce analgesia by their actions on peripherally inflamed tissues as well as on certain regions of the brain and spinal cord. The NSAIDs have been reported to be effective for managing pulpal and periradicular pain. In patients with known sensitivity to NSAIDs or aspirin, and in those who have gastrointestinal ulcerations or hypertension due to renal effects of NSAIDs, acetaminophen should be preferred for such pain. Pretreatment with NSAIDs has been effective in irreversible pulpitis.

The commonly used nonsteroidal anti-inflammatory drugs are:

i. *Salicylates (aspirin)*: Aspirin is considered as the most common remedy for acute pain. It reversibly inhibits cyclooxygenase enzyme, blocking synthesis of prostaglandins. It inhibits migration of polymorphonuclear cells and macrophages into the site of inflammation. It is effective in patients susceptible to stroke and thromboembolic heart attack. Prolonged use of aspirin may lead to gastrointestinal problems and also bleeding from the gut. 300–600 mg, 6–8 hourly dose is effective.

ii. *Acetaminophen*: Analgesic and antipyretic properties of acetaminophen are comparable to those of aspirin. Unlike aspirin, gastrointestinal irritation or prolong bleeding is not the problems with acetaminophen. 300 gm of acetaminophen can effectively produce analgesic effect.

Like opiates, acetaminophen has little anti-inflammatory effect but provide analgesia and antipyretic effects similar to aspirin. 90 to 95% acetaminophens are metabolized in the liver. Four percent may get metabolized into toxic metabolites. Because of this reason high dose and long-term use of acetaminophen may cause liver damage. One main advantage of acetaminophen is that it has no effect on blood platelets.

iii. *Naproxen*: Naproxen is one of the effective analgesic. A 220 mg dose of naproxen sodium (equivalent to 200 mg of ibuprofen) is effective in producing analgesic onset and peak effect, but has a longer duration of action (longer half-life of 13 hours).

iv. *Ibuprofen*: Ibuprofen is one of the most predominantly used analgesic. A 400 mg dose of ibuprofen has longer duration and greater peak analgesic effect than 600 to 1,000 mg of aspirin or acetaminophen. Ibuprofen may cause gastric bleeding and ulceration, especially with high doses and chronic use.

v. *Indomethacin*: Indomethacin is more effective than aspirin and also more toxic. It is usually prescribed in severe pain, like osteoarthritis, etc. Indomethacin is contraindicated in pregnancy.

b. *Preferential COX-2 inhibitors*

Nimesulide is a weak inhibitor of synthesis of prostaglandins. 100 mg dose is effective in relieving mild pain. It is not preferred in children.

c. *Selective COX-2 inhibitors*

Rofecoxib, valdecoxib and celecoxib are commonly available COX-2 inhibitors as pain relieving drugs. The adverse reactions, such as gastrointestinal ulceration and bleeding etc. are minimum with their use.

Rofecoxib is preferred in comparison to celecoxib and valdecoxib because of following advantages:
- It is not contraindicated in patients with a history of sulphonamide allergy.
- The duration of action of rofecoxib is sufficiently long to allow single daily dose.
- 50 mg rofecoxib is comparable to 400 mg of ibuprofen in onset and peak pain relief.

d. Analgesic-antipyretics with poor anti-inflammatory action

Acetaminophen and certain allied derivatives are considered week anti-inflammatory agents, even though they inhibit prostaglandins and reduce fever. Acetaminophens may not adequately block COX in the peripheral nervous system; action mainly on central nervous system.

Commonly prescribed analgesics in endodontic clinic
- Ibuprofen 200 mg, 400 mg, 600 mg
- Paracetamol 650 mg
- Diclofenac 50 mg, 100 mg
- Aceclofenac 250 mg
- Tramadol 50 mg
- Ketorol DT 10 mg
- Nimesulide 100 mg

2. Opioid Analgesics

Opioid analgesics activate receptors that inhibit transmission of the nociceptive signals from the trigeminal nucleus to the higher brain centers and activate peripheral receptors to reduce pain. Their use is limited due to the adverse effects that include nausea, vomiting, drowsiness, dizziness, constipation and respiratory depression; however, by chronic use the patient may develop physical tolerance and dependence.

The opioid analgesics are classified as:

a. *Natural opium alkaloids*: Morphine, codeine
b. *Semisynthetic opiates*: Diacetylmorphine (Heroin), pholcodine.
c. *Synthetic opioids*: Pethidine (Meperidine), propoxyphene (Methadone), tramadol, fentanyl, pentazocine, butorphanol.

Opioid analgesics: Key features

- Opioids are good analgesics, but not good anti-inflammatory agents.
- Codeine is a standard opioid for oral administration. It may produce less analgesia than either aspirin (650 mg) or acetaminophen (600 mg).
- Pentazocine and related opioid have satisfactory analgesic effect. Sedation is a common side effect. Respiratory depression effect may be similar to morphine.
- In addition to relieving pain, opioids may cause nausea, vomiting and constipation.
- Overdoses lead to respiratory depression, and chronic use can culminate into physical dependence.
- Opioid analgesics may decrease or inhibit salivary flow, contributing to the development of caries, periodontal problems, oral candidiasis, etc.

The *commonly used opioid-analgesics* are:

i. *Morphine*: Morphine is a potent analgesic (visceral pain is relieved better than somatic pain). The associated features of pain are also relieved, such as apprehension, fear, etc. The recommended dose is 10–20 mg (2.0–10.0 mg intravenous) depending upon the intensity of pain. The side effects of morphine may be vomiting, respiratory depression, urinary retention, etc. Morphine is not prescribed in renal diseases and hypothyroidism.
ii. *Tramadol*: Tramadol has weak opioid activity, exhibiting less drug dependence, respiratory depression, as well as other side effects commonly associated with opioid use. Effective dose is 50–100 mg every six hours (maximum 400 mg/day).
   Tramadol with acetaminophen is appropriate option, especially for those patients who do not tolerate NSAIDs/opioid analgesics.
iii. *Pentazocine (Fortwin)*: Pentazocine has weak antagonist and marked agonist actions. Sweating, tachycardia and rise in blood pressure are the common side effects. Other adverse effects include dry mouth, alteration in taste, urinary retention and tinnitus, etc. Vomiting is less frequent. Pentazocine is indicated for postoperative and moderate to severe pain in burns, trauma, fracture, cancer, etc. Recommended dose is 25 mg oral or 30 mg/ml intramuscular, as and when required. Pentazocine is a 'ceiling' drug; dose cannot be increased in case of increasing pain.
   Safety and efficacy of pentazocine in children younger than 12 years of age has not been established.
iv. *Butorphanol (Butrum)*: Butorphanol is more potent than pentazocine. It is indicated for postoperative and other short lasting painful conditions. It should be avoided in patients with cardiac ischemia.The duration of action is similar to morphine. The recommended dose is 1.0 mg/ml or 2.0 mg/ml intramuscular or intravenous depending upon pain.

Combination of drugs

A meticulous approach is frequently exercised to enhance the analgesic effects of oral medication by combining two or more drugs having different mechanisms of action. A combination of ibuprofen and opioid is considered effective and safe analgesic.

Even diclofenac plus vitamin B has been more effective to relieve pain than diclofenac alone.

The combination of acetaminophen/NSAID with an opioid allows for increased analgesia because the drugs act through dissimilar mechanisms. Aspirin-opioid combinations are not preferred because of potential NSAID-aspirin interactions.

The clinicians should be conscious about the benefits and risks of the drug combination in the management of pain.

Adverse effects of the combination

- Maximum pain relief is mostly accomplished by single agent. The combination usually leads to adverse effects.
- Combination may lead to added side effects.
- With opioids, the increased analgesia can be obtained by using a larger dose of a single drug; no use of combining with other analgesics.
- Combination of aspirin, phenacetin and caffeine (APC tablet) has been associated with kidney problems.

3. Corticosteroids

Steroids, also refer to as corticosteroids, are usually not used in endodontics because of its immunosuppressive effect (suppress the defence mechanism). It has been established that a single oral dose or local use of steroids (intracanal medicament) might not have any specific harmful effects. Two classes of enzymes, viz. Phospholipase and cyclooxygenase are the basic target site, with intake of analgesics and anti-inflammatory drugs. Phospholipase synthesizes arachidonic acid from phospholipids. Cyclooxygenase synthesizes prostaglandins. Steroids are the group of drugs which function by inhibiting phospholipase A_2, which reduces the production and concentration of prostaglandins and leukotrienes.

Corticosteroids refer to both glucocorticoids and mineralocorticoid (both mimic hormone produced by adrenal cortex). Mineralocorticoid is rarely used; glucocorticoid is used as synonym with corticosteroid.

The differences between glucocorticoids and mineralocorticoids are summarized in Table 4.2.

Glucocorticoids are frequently employed to reduce or to eradicate inflammation. In addition, they can inhibit the progression of inflammation, which ultimately leads to necrosis of pulp tissue.

The compounds of glucocorticoids and mineralocorticoids and their dosage are tabulated in Table 4.3.

Steroids should be used with caution in patients with ulcerative colitis, peptic ulcer, diabetes, pregnancy and pyogenic infections.

Glucocorticoids are contraindicated in patients with systemic fungal infections and those who are known hypersensitive to the drug. Glucocorticoid therapy may lead to psychological disturbances, which can be mild and reversible (insomnia, euphoria/nervousness) or pronounced (schizophrenic psychosis). The severity of adverse effects depends upon the duration and dose of the steroid used.

Intraligamentary/intraosseous, intramuscular and oral administration of steroids have effectively reduced postendodontic pain. Steroids are effective in relieving pain associated with irreversible pulpitis and chronic inflammatory diseases. Intraoral intake of 6.0–8.0 mg of dexamethasone or 40 mg of methylprednisolone is sufficient as anti-inflammatory dose. Dexamethasone is less potent than other corticosteroids, such as triamcinolone.

Steroids have been used systemically to shorten the course of nerve paraesthesia due to endodontic procedures. Intramuscular injections of steroids are also prescribed for the treatment of sodium hypochlorite accidents.

Corticosteroids cause the adrenal glands to slow down or stop the production of cortisol. Hence, they cannot be discontinued abruptly. The adrenal glands take some time to start producing cortisol again. Tapering the dose of corticosteroids gradually allows the body to start producing cortisol.

Local application of steroids

Steroids have been widely used as an intracanal medicament. Hydrocortisone alone and in combination

Table 4.2 Difference between glucocorticoids and mineralocorticoids

Glucocorticoids	*Mineralocorticoids*
• Glucocorticoids compounds are: Cortisol, cortisone, triamcinolone	• Mineralocorticoids compounds are: Aldosterone, deoxycorticosterone
• Control carbohydrates, fat and protein metabolism	• Control electrolyte and water balance of the body
• Secretion is under control of adenohypophyses	• Secretion is under control of renin angiotensin system
• They are anti-inflammatory and anti-allergic	• No such role
• Helpful in repairing injury and stress factor	• Do not help repair and stress factor
• Reduce pain	• Do not manage pain

Table 4.3 Glucocorticoid and mineralocorticoid—dosage and compound

	Compound	*Dose*
Glucocorticoids Short acting	• Hydrocortisone (cortisol)	• 20 mg
Intermediate acting	• Prednisolone • Methylprednisolone • Triamcinolone	• 5.0 mg • 4.0 mg • 4.0 mg
Long acting	• Dexamethasone • Betamethasone	• 0.75 mg • 075 mg
Mineralocorticoids	• Deoxycorticosterone acetate • Fludrocortisone (Florinef) • Aldosterone	• 2.5 mg (sublingual) • 0.2 mg • Not used clinically (necessary for regulation of salt and water in the body)

with antibodies have shown favourable results. It has been established that the combination effectively reduces inflammation in the periapical areas.

The most commonly used steroid-antibiotic combination for local applications are:

i. Ledermix is a combination of a steroid with an antibiotic (1.0% triamcinolone (steroid) and 3.0% demeclocycline (tetracycline in a polyethanol-glycol base). It has been established that the dentinal tubules are the major route of supply of the active components to the periradicular tissues than the apical foramen. The components of ledermix are capable of diffusing through dentinal tubules and cementum to reach periapical tissues. Demeclocycline is quite effective against susceptible bacteria in root canals. The effect of demeclocycline is achieved for all bacteria within the first day of application onto dentinal surface; however, this effect may remain one-tenth after one week. Towards the cementum, the concentration of demeclocycline after one day is not sufficient to eliminate most strains of endodontic bacteria.

ii. Ledermix paste (1.0% triamcinolone and 3.0% demeclocycline-calcium) and Ledermix cement (0.7% triamcinolone, 3.0% demeclocycline with calcium based salts) are effective anti-inflammatory agents when used locally. Both cement and the base do not show any unfavourable side effects.

iii. Ledermix and calcium hydroxide (50:50 mixture) has also been used as intracanal medicaments to eradicate endodontic micro-organisms from root canal walls.

iv. Septomixine forte paste contains steroid and two antibiotics, neomycin and polymixin B sulphate. Both these antibiotics are not suitable against endodontic bacteria because of their inappropriate spectra of activity. Neomycin is effective against gram-negative rods, but ineffective against bacteroids, fungi, viruses, etc. Polymyxin B sulphate is bactericidal against gram-negative bacteria, but not effective against gram-positive bacteria.

The commonly employed anti-inflammatory drugs are tabulated in Table 4.4.

4. Alternative Analgesic (Acupuncture)

Acupuncture and laser acupuncture have been used successfully as an alternative form of analgesia.

Several studies have showed that acupuncture treatment produced equivalent or better results than conventional treatments in the pain management in dentistry.

A study, wherein a laser acupuncture involving a beam from a 2.8–6 mW Helium-Neon laser, was delivered and focused on the selected skin point of the patient. No other sedative or analgesic was administered before or during the operation. Out of total 610 patients studied, no one complained of any side effects.

Factors affecting the prescription of analgesics

i. *Age of the patient*: As the age increases, less dose of analgesics are prescribed, especially in case of opioids (opioid sensitivity is common with advancing age). The regular dose of analgesics should be reduced by 50%.

Table 4.4 Commonly employed anti-inflammatory drugs

Drug	*Presentation*	*Dosage*
Acetylsalicylic acid	Tablets—100 mg and 500 mg	1–2 tablet, 3–4 times/day (maximum dosage 3 gm)
Ibuprofen	Tablets—200 mg, 400 mg, 600 mg	1 to 2 tablets – 3–4 times/day (Maximum – 320 mg/day)
Diclofenac	Capsules/Tablets—50 and 100 mg	1 tablet (3–4 times/day)
Nimesulide	Tablets—100 mg	1 tablet, twice daily
Betamethasone	Tablets—0.5 and 2.0 mg	1 tablet (2–4 times daily)
Dexamethasone	Tablets—0.5, 0.75 and 4.0 mg	0.75 to 15 mg/day (2–4 times daily)
Acetaminophen and Codeine	Tablet 300 mg acetaminophen and 30 mg codeine	1–2 tablets (3–4 times daily) (Maximum 300 mg acetaminophen/ day and 300 mg codeine/day)
Tramadol	Tablet 50 mg	1–2 tablets (3–4 times daily) (Maximum 400 mg/day)
Tramadol and Acetaminophen	37.5 mg tramadol and 325 mg acetaminophen	1–2 tablet (3–4 times daily) (Maximum 3000 mg acetaminophen 400 mg tramadol)

ii. *Paediatric patients*: Ibuprofen oral suspension (100 mg/5.0 ml) every four hours is the effective oral analgesic for children. The dose for 3 to 7 years old children is 5.0 ml (1 teaspoon) every six hours and twice that for children 7 to 12 years old.

iii. *Body size*: The dosage is directly proportional to body size.More the weight and circumference of the patient, more dose of the drug.

iv. *Maintenance of effective drug concentration*: The patient should be directed to take the initial dose as soon as feasible, followed by a fixed dose schedule for 3–5 days depending upon the procedure.

v. Analgesics should be taken before onset of pain, followed by as per instructions of the operator.

III. MANAGEMENT OF INFECTION

It has been established that pulp-periapical infection involves aerobic, facultative anaerobic and anaerobic micro-organisms. The dynamics of dental infections warrants judicious use of antibiotics and that too as an adjunct along with other treatment modalities. Acute lesions accompanied by pain and/or swelling, which can be drained via root canal or soft tissues, do require antibiotic therapy. Chronic infections generally do not require antibiotic therapy. Chronic alveolar infections are associated with pulpless teeth, which do not have blood supply reaching the pulp space. Following systemic intake, the concentration of antibiotics reaching at the site (root canal) is negligible; therefore, systemic antibiotic therapy is not beneficial. Antibiotics are chemical substances produced by either live micro-organisms or synthetic process, aiming at inhibiting the growth and/or destroying the micro-organisms.

Odontogenic infection, including endodontic infections, are polymicrobial involving combination of gram-positive, gram-negative, facultative anaerobes and strict anaerobic bacteria (Table 4.5).

It is hypothesized that microbial resistance to antibiotics is increasing at an alarming rate. The major cause of this problem is the use of antibiotics in an inappropriate manner, leading to dominance of resistant micro-organisms. When bacteria become resistant to antibiotics they may transfer resistance genes from antibiotic–resistance to antibiotic–susceptible micro-organism.

Endodontic sensitivity of endodontic bacteria is gradually decreasing with growing number of resistant strains (*Porphyromonas* spp. and *Prevotella* spp.).

Antibiotics should be employed only for the management of active infectious disease or the prevention of metastatic infection such as infective endocarditis in medically high-risk patients (Table 4.6).

Table 4.5 Commonly reported endodontic microbes

Anaerobic bacteria
I. *Gram-positive rods* • *Eubacterium* spp. • *Propionibacterium propionicus* • *Actinomyces* spp. • *Filifactor alocis* • *Pseudoramibacter alactolyticus*
II. *Gram-negative rods* • Prevotella • Porphyromonas • *Tannerella forsythia* • *Campylobacter rectus* • *Fusobacterium* spp.
III. *Gram-positive cocci* • *Parvimonas micra* • Peptococcus
IV. *Gram-negative cocci* • Veillonella • Dialister spp.
V. *Spirochetes* • *Treponema denticola* • *Treponema socranskii* • *Treponema parvum*
Facultative anaerobic bacteria
I. *Gram-positive rods* • Lactobacillus • Diphtheroids
II. *Gram-positive cocci* • *Streptococcus viridans* • Beta haemolytic streptococcus • Gamma haemolytic streptococcus • *Enterococcus* spp.
III. Gram-negative cocci • *Neisseria dentiae* • *Neisseria oralis*

Indications

The indications of systemic use of antibiotics are:

- Infection is bacterial and not viral (will respond to antibiotics)
- Acute odontogenic and non-odontogenic infections
- As prophylaxis in patients with infective endocarditis and replacement therapy
- As prophylaxis to avoid or minimize systemic spread of infection

Myths of using antibiotics

1. *Antibiotics cure patients*: Antibiotics are not curative; except in immunocompromised patients. They assist in the re-establishment of the balance between the host's defence and the invasive agents.
2. *Antibiotics are substitutes for surgical intervention*: Antibiotics do not provide an appropriate substitute

Table 4.6 Antibiotics as an adjunct in endodontic lesions

• Acute apical periodontitis (pain on percussion/biting)	• No need of antibiotics
• Acute apical abscess (periapical sinus)	• No need of antibiotics
• Pulp necrosis (non-vital tooth)	• No need of antibiotics
• Irreversible pulpitis (pain)	• No need of antibiotics
• Apical abscess with systemic involvement (swelling with fever, lymphadenopathy, etc.)	• Antibiotics required
• Persistent infections (chronic exudate)	• Antibiotics required
• Any lesion with medically compromised patient (systemic diseases causing impaired immunologic functions)	• Antibiotics required

for removal of the source of the infection. When the clinical situation does not allow for immediate curative treatment, an appropriate antibacterial therapy can be implemented.

3. *When and which antibiotic to be used*: The knowledge of invading micro-organisms and their susceptibility establish the choice of antibiotic.
4. *Antibiotics increase the host defence*: A few studies have observed that antibiotics increase the host's defence to infection. Various postulates are:
   - Antibiotics that can penetrate into the mammalian cell (erythromycin, tetracycline, clindamycin and metronidazole) are more likely to affect the host defence
   - Tetracycline may suppress white cell chemotaxis
   - Most antibiotics (except tetracycline) do not depress phagocytosis
   - T- and B-lymphocyte transformation may be depressed by tetracycline.
5. *Multiple antibiotics are superior to a single antibiotic*: It is often assumed that a combination of antibiotics is superior to a single antibacterial agent. The primary indication for combined antimicrobial therapy is a severe infection; major consequences may ensue if antibiotic therapy is not instituted immediately.
6. *Bactericidal agents are always superior to bacteriostatic agents*: Bactericidal agents are required for patients with impaired host defence; however, bacteriostatic agents are equally effective when the host's defence against infections are unimpaired. Post antibiotic effects are more persistent with bacteriostatic agents (erythromycin, clindamycin) than with bactericidal agents (beta-lactamase).
7. *Antibiotic dose and duration of therapy for endodontic infections*: The proper dose and duration of therapy depends upon the microbial pathogen(s) suspected in the infection lesion. In dentistry, the prescription of antibiotics is empirical, as exact nature of pathogens is not known (broad spectrum antibiotics are prescribed on presumptive basis).
8. *All types of infections require a complete course of antibiotic therapy*: A common belief is that prolonged antibiotic therapy is necessary to prevent 'rebound' infections. Orofacial infections usually do not 'rebound' if the source of the infection is eradicated. Patients placed on antibiotic therapy for an orofacial infection should be evaluated periodically.

Classification

Antibiotics are mainly identified as of two types: (i) those that kill bacteria rapidly and (ii) those that kill bacteria slowly by retarding bacterial protein synthesis. The faster-killing antibacterial agents are preferred in endodontic infections.

The antibiotics are classified as:

a. Beta-lactam antibiotics
   i. Benzyl-penicillin (penicillin G)
   ii. Phenoxy-penicillin (penicillin V)
   iii. Penicillinase-resistant penicillin/anti-staphylococcal-penicillin (oxacillin)
   iv. Aminobenzyl-penicillin (ampicillin, amoxicillin)
   v. Ureido-penicillin (broad-spectrum penicillin) (Mezlocillin, Piperacillin)

b. Aminoglycosides (streptomycin, gentamicin, amikacin)

c. Nitroimidazole (metronidazole)

d. Macrolides (erythromycin, clarithromycin, azithromycin)

e. Lincosamide (clindamycin)

f. Quinolones (norfloxacin, ofloxacin, ciprofloxacin, levofloxacin, moxifloxacin)

g. Cephalosporin (first generation—cefazolin, cefadroxil; Second generation—cefuroxime, loracarbef; Third and fourth generation—cefotaxime, ceftriaxone, ceftazidime)

Penicillin, cephalosporin, and metronidazole are the bactericidal antibiotics commonly used against endodontic micro-organisms. The first two kill by integrating and weakening the cell wall; whereas, the latter impedes DNA of the bacterial cell. Both are effective against actively growing organisms. Antibiotics that fight bacteria by slowing their protein synthesis (bacteriostatic antibiotics) are generally not advised.

The commonly prescribed antibiotics in endodontic infections are:

i. *Penicillin*

Penicillin, having a short half-life (about one hour) is a narrow-spectrum antibiotic. The injectable penicillin is Procaine penicillin; whereas, Penicillin V (Phenoxymethyl penicillin) is given by oral route.If penicillin is prescribed by oral route, the patient is instructed to take the required dose one hour before meal. Patients with compromised kidney functions are given reduced dose, since it is excreted through kidney. If the patient is undergoing hemodialysis, the dose is fixed in consultation with the nephrologist. Penicillin is not well absorbed from intestinal tract (70% wastage), with diarrhea as a frequent side effect.

Penicillin is generally non-toxic. If the patient is not allergic, there are no side effects from over-dosage.

Amoxicillin is considered the drug of choice because of its better absorption from the gut. It is preferred for orofacial infection because it is readily absorbed and can be taken with food. One major disadvantage of using penicillin is the possibility of allergic reactions (may be in the form of stomach upset and diarrhea). The recommended dose of penicillin is 1.2–2.4 IV/ 24 hours intramuscularly and amoxicillin is given orally as 500 mg thrice a day.

ii. *Cephalosporins*

Cephalosporins are improved version of penicillin with the ability to kill stubborn infections. Cephalosporins are classified as fuse generation; first-generation cephalosporins are the most effective in endodontic infections, since they kill most of the endodontic pathogens; whereas, second- and third-generation cephalosporins are preferred for respiratory infections.

iii. *Metronidazole*

Metronidazole is a preferred bactericidal drug because of its fast action. It attacks the bacteria's DNA. This drug is more suitable against obligate anaerobe and not against facultative bacteria/aerobes. Metronidazole is often used in combination with another antibiotic, usually amoxicillin, to combat the stomach ulcer-causing bacteria, *Helicobacter pylori*. This combination of two fast-killing drugs help in eradicating endodontic infections. Patients taking metronidazole should be cautioned not to take alcohol during days of drug intake plus one day after to allow the drug to be eliminated properly.

The half-life of metronidazole is 8–10 hours and the recommended dose is 500 mg thrice a day. Side effects include an unpleasant, metallic taste and brown discoloration of the urine. Metronidazole has also been associated with blood dyscrasias and hypersensitivity reactions.

iv. *Macrolides (Erythromycin, Clarithromycin, Azithromycin)*

Erythromycin, clarithromycin and azithromycin are also called macrolides because of their large molecule. Erythromycin kills bacteria by slowing down the synthesis of bacterial protein. Erythromycin is the drug of choice for patients allergic to penicillin. The macrolides kill many gram-positive bacteria but have a limited spectrum for gram-negative bacteria. Use of erythromycin may lead to gastric cramps; however, allergic reactions are rare. The wider-spectrum new macrolides, azithromycin and clarithromycin, are effective for endodontic infections.

It should be noted that clarithromycin is metabolized by both the liver and the kidney. Caution is warranted, in patients with compromised kidney or liver, because the half-life of the drug is prolonged (the half-life of erythromycin is in the range of 1 to 2 hours; whereas, clarithromycin's half-life is 6 hours, and azithromycin has a remarkable 40-hour half-life). The recommended dose of azithromycin is 500 mg daily.

v. *Clindamycin*

Clindamycin is frequently used in endodontic infections, especially for patients allergic to penicillin. It is rapidly and completely absorbed and has a good spectrum of killing endodontic pathogens. Patients being treated with clindamycin who experience diarrhea or any gut problem should immediately be referred to their physician for evaluation.

The average half-life of clindamycin is about three hours. The recommended dose of clindamycin is 300 mg thrice daily or 600 mg intravenous injection. The side effects include gastrointestinal problems, which may become fatal due to development of pseudo-membranous colitis.

vi. *Tetracycline (Doxycycline)*

Tetracycline is least affected by heavy metal ions, such as calcium; so the patient does not have to avoid dairy products. Tetracycline has the ability to kill the broadest spectrum of microbes. Half-life of most tetracycline is about 10–16 hours, allowing dose twice daily.

Tetracycline may cause staining of developing teeth as they bind to calcium during formation of teeth and bones. Their use should be avoided in children and pregnant women. A rare side effect is phototoxicity, where exposure to the sun causes severe sunburn or rash.

vii. *Sulfa drugs*

Sulfa drugs are frequently used for urinary tract infections. Sulfa drugs cannot kill rapidly because they compete with a precursor in the bioformation of folic acid, which many bacteria cannot obtain from other sources. Sulfa drugs are the slowest and poorest of bacteriostatic antibiotics. They are not generally used in endodontic infections.

Use of antibiotics: Key features

- Penicillin is the antibiotic of choice for endodontic infections due to its effectiveness in polymicrobial infections, low toxicity and low cost (only problem of allergic reactions).
- Amoxicillin and amoxicillin plus clavulanic acid demonstrated a higher antibacterial effectiveness than penicillin.
- Clindamycin is the antibiotic of choice for patients allergic to penicillin.
- Metronidazole demonstrated the greatest amount of bacterial resistance and is only effective against anaerobes; should not be used alone (metronidazole in combination with amoxicillin is preferred).
- The host defence may be affected by antibiotics that easily penetrate into the mammalian cell; whereas, bactericidal, non-penetrating agents (penicillin and cephalosporin) affect the least.

The commonly used antibiotics, their dosage and side effects are tabulated in Table 4.7.

Antibiotic Prophylaxis

Systemic diseases compromising the immune system mainly call for consideration of prophylactic antibiotics. The goal of antibiotic prophylaxis is to prevent clinical infection by destroying small numbers of bacteria present before or introduced during treatment. Oral bacteria, especially streptococci can cause heart and artificial joint infections.

The protocol proposed by the American Heart Association states that antibiotics must be administered one hour (oral route) or 30 minutes (intravenous route) before the procedure. The antibiotics of choice are amoxicillin 2.0 grams. Clindamycin 600 mg is preferred for patients allergic to penicillin.

The prophylaxis regime is tabulated in Table 4.8.

The procedures for which antibiotic prophylaxis is recommended are:

- Periodontal procedures (periodontal surgery, deep curettage, scaling and root planing etc.)
- Implant placement
- Difficult extractions
- Replantation of avulsed teeth
- Endodontic surgery
- Intraligamentary/intraosseous injections
- Postoperative suture removal (selected cases)
- Prophylactic cleaning of teeth where bleeding is anticipated

Flowchart 4.1 summarizes protocol of drugs used in endodontics.

Table 4.7 Commonly used antibiotics: Dosage and side effects

Antibiotic	*Route of administration*	*Dose*	*Side effects*
Penicillin	Oral Intramuscular/intravenous	1000 mg initially followed by 500 mg every 6 hourly 1.2–2.4 million IU/24 hours intramuscular	Hypersensitivity reactions, gastric problems
Amoxicillin	Oral	500 mg/8 hours and 1000 mg/12 hours Combination of 250 mg amoxicillin + 125 gm clavulanic acid	Diarrhea, nausea, hypersensitivity reactions
Amoxicillin-clavulanic acid (Augmentin)	Oral/intravenous	500–875 mg/8 hours orally 1000–2000 mg/8 hours intravenous	Diarrhea, nausea, candidiasis, hypersensitivity reactions
Clindamycin	Orally/intravenous	300 mg/8 hours orally 600 mg/intravenous	Pseudomembranous colitis
Gentamicin	Intramuscular/intravenous	240 mg/24 hours	Ototoxicity/Nephrotoxicity
Ciprofloxacin	Oral	500 mg/12 hours	Gastrointestinal disorders
Azithromycin	Oral	500 mg/24 hours	Gastrointestinal disorders
Metronidazole	Oral	500–750 mg/8 hours	Anesthesia/paresthesia of the limbs, incompatible with alcohol intake

Table 4.8 Antibiotic prophylactic regimens for dental procedures

Route of administration	*Antibiotic*	*Dose*	
		Adult	*Children*
Oral	Amoxicillin	2.0 g	50 mg
Oral route not feasible (intramuscular/intravenous route)	Ampicillin	2.0 g intramuscular/intravenous	50 mg intramuscular/ intravenous
	Cefazolin	1.0 g intramuscular/intravenous	50 mg intramuscular/ intravenous
Allergic to penicillin/ ampicillin (oral route)	Cephalexin	2.0 gm	50 mg/kg
	Clindamycin	600 mg	20 mg/kg
	Azithromycin/Clarithromycin	500 mg	15 mg/kg
Allergic to penicillin/ampicillin (oral route not feasible)	Cefazolin	1.0 Gm IV, IM	50 mg
	Clindamycin	600 mg	20 mg

Flowchart 4.1: Protocol of drugs used in endodontics

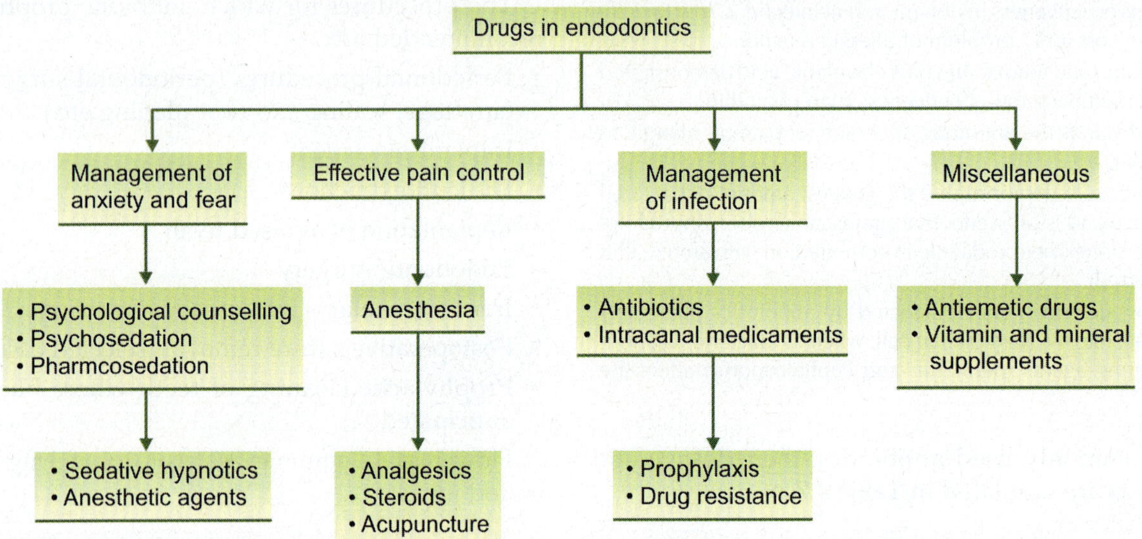

Antibiotic Use: Risk and Precautions

Various clinical conditions warrants use of antibiotics; however, these should be cautiously and judiciously used, especially in certain systemic conditions, such as:

a. *Pregnancy*: Four level of risk during pregnancy has been established:

i. *Category 1*: No evident risk factor (no antibiotic corresponds to this group). A few studies reported no teratogenic effect with the use of penicillin and erythromycin).

ii. *Category 2*: No effect in animals (azithromycin, penicillin V, amoxicillin, erythromycin, metronidazole).

iii. *Category 3*: Effect not established in either animals or human studies (morphine, atropine, corticosteroids, clarithromycin, fluoroquinolones and sulfa drugs).

iv. *Category 4*: Teratogenic effects upon the fetus; however, the potential benefits may be acceptable despite the potential risk (aminoglycosides, tetracycline, carbamazepine, lorazepam). (*Oral contraceptives may be rendered ineffective by penicillin and erythromycin. The patient taking these medicines should be informed that the contraceptive will be ineffective for the duration and also 10 days after its use*).

b. *Kidney failure*: The dose of the antibiotics should be adjusted according to the level of creatinine clearance.

c. *Liver failure*: Antibiotics which metabolized in liver, should be restricted. The dose of erythromycin, clindamycin and metronidazole should be adjusted when administered to patients with liver failure.

The side effects of systemic antibiotics are:

- Hypersensitivity reaction
- Alteration of the bacterial flora
- Toxic to host cells
- Development of resistant strains

4

Drug Resistance

Drug resistance refers to unresponsiveness of a micro-organism to an antimicrobial activity; synonymous with the phenomenon of tolerance.

Resistance can be natural or acquired.

- *Natural resistance*: Some microbes lack the metabolic process or the target site which is affected by the particular drug (*for example*, gram-negative bacilli are normally unaffected by penicillin).
- *Acquired resistance*: The resistance developed by an organism due to the use of an antimicrobial over a period of time (*for example*, gonococci quickly develops resistance to sulphonamides as compared to penicillin. Staphylococci and tubercle bacilli develop rapid resistance to penicillin).

Antibiotic resistance can be microbiological or clinical. Microbiological resistance exists when an organism possesses any resistance mechanism; whereas, clinical resistance is the failure to achieve a concentration of antimicrobial that inhibits the growth of the organism in a particular tissue or fluid.

Multiple drug resistance or multi-resistance is antimicrobial resistance shown by a species of micro-organism to multiple antimicrobial drugs (resistant to multiple antifungal, antiviral, and antiparasitic drugs).

Mechanism of Drug Resistance

Bacterial resistance may be developed by mutation of the DNA molecule or can be acquired from other bacteria by DNA transfer (from one species to another). In addition to enzymatic destruction of antibiotic molecules, as with-lactamase, bacteria may get resistance by not allowing an antibiotic to pass through the cell membrane. Another situation may also lead to resistance when the bacteria can pump out antibiotic molecule faster than it can enter.

Bacteria generally pass on their resistance genes to their offspring. In any clinical situation, it is mandatory to limit antibiotic therapy; the patient should get benefit from the antibiotics and should not facilitate developing 'resistance' amongst the micro-organisms.

Antimicrobial activity can be described in terms of minimum inhibitory concentration. Bacteria can be described as 'sensitive', 'intermediate susceptible' or 'resistant', depending on the intensity of drug required to inhibit growth of the micro-organism. The resistance is related to the serum concentration of a drug that is achieved at the site of infection/tissues. Serum concentration in tissues might not be reproducible between patients or even in the same patient at different sites.

An organism can also acquire resistance to an antibiotic to which it was previously sensitive. This can be due to chance mutation in the genetic material of the cell, or the acquisition of resistance genes from other drug-resistant cells.

The main mechanisms by which micro-organisms exhibit resistance to antimicrobials are:

- Micro-organisms destroying/inactivating/modifying the drug (enzymatic deactivation of penicillin G in some penicillin-resistant bacteria through the production of β-lactamases).
- Micro-organisms making the drugs impermeable/alteration of target site (reduced drug accumulation by decreasing drug permeability and/or increasing active efflux (pumping out) of the drugs across the cell surface).
- Micro-organisms facilitating drug tolerance/alteration of metabolic pathway (some sulfonamide-resistant bacteria do not require para-aminobenzoic acid for the synthesis of folic acid and nucleic acids; instead, they may utilize preformed folic acid).

Prevention of drug resistance

The following features help prevent the drug resistance:

- Inadequate/prolonged use of antimicrobials should be avoided.
- Use the appropriate antimicrobial for an infection (no antibiotics for viral infections).
- Identify the causative organism.
- Select an antimicrobial which targets effectively to the specific organism (do not rely on broad-spectrum antibiotics).
- Organisms notorious for developing resistance must be treated accordingly.
- Complete an appropriate duration of antimicrobial treatment (not too short and not too long).
- Use the correct dose for bacterial eradication (sub-therapeutic dose may lead to resistance).
- Use combination of antimicrobials, if prolonged treatment is required.

Injudicious use of Antibiotics (Antibioma)

Antibiotic resistance has been an established phenomenon; overdose of antibiotics may contribute to development of resistance. Various studies have reported resistance of *Streptococcus viridians* for antibiotics such as clindamycin and macrolides. Broad spectrum antibiotics are generally used in endodontics. Injudicious use of antibiotics for self-limiting infection is a common feature.

'Antibioma' is a common sequelae of injudicious use of antibiotics without concentrating on the underlying pathology. For example, in an abscess, if proper drainage of pus is not established (antibiotics are prescribed for long duration), pus may get covered with thick fibrous tissue. This is known as *'Antibioma'*. The treatment is surgical removal along with curettage of the wound (incision and drainage may not be effective). Antibiotics can be prescribed for fast healing of the socket (for limited period only).

IV. MISCELLANEOUS

a. Antiemetic Drugs

Postoperative nausea and vomiting are one of the most common complaints following surgery. Swallowed blood and secretions stimulate the gag reflex and are potent gastric irritants. Antiemetic medications act by blocking the receptors at the chemoreceptor trigger zones.

Antiemetic drugs are categorized as:

- Anticholinergic (hyoscine, dicyclomine)
- Antihistaminic (chlorpromazine, prochlorperazine)
- Prokinetic drugs (domperidone, metoclopramide)
- Adjuvant antiemetic (dexamethasone, benzodiazepines)
- Newer drugs (ondansetron, bolasterone)

Adverse effects of antiemetic drugs are:

- Sedation
- Extrapyramidal reactions
- Ondansetron may produce headache, mild constipation or diarrhea and abdominal discomfort.

Dexamethasone (8.0 mg) intravenously has been shown to decrease the incidence of nausea/vomiting when given shortly after induction of general anesthesia. Propofol also has antiemetic effects, particularly when administered for maintenance of anesthesia. Avoidance of known nausea triggering agents such as nitrous oxide, ketamine, and longer-acting opioid medications may also reduce postoperative nausea and vomiting.

b. Vitamin and Minerals Supplements

Vitamins (A, B, C, D, E) and mineral (calcium, phosphorous, zinc, iron, magnesium) are prescribed as supplements after endodontic surgeries to combat effects of antibiotics and improving nutrition as well. A plethora of commercial preparation of multivitamins and antioxidants are available in market.

4

BIBLIOGRAPHY

1. Abbott PV, Hume WR and Pearman JW. Antibiotics and endodontics. Aust. Dent. J.: 1990; 35:50–60.
2. Abbott PV. Selective and intelligent use of antibiotics in endodontics. Aust. Endod. J.: 2000; 26:30–39.
3. Ahmad N and Saad N. Effects of antibiotics on dental implants. J. Clin. Med. Res.: 2012; 4:1–6.
4. Aminoshariae A and Kulild J. Evidence-based recommendations for antibiotics usage for endodontic infections and pain: a systematic review. J. Am. Dent. Assoc.: 2016; 147:186–191.
5. Andersson DI and Hughes D. Persistence of antibiotic resistance in bacterial populations. Fems Microbiology Rev.: 2011; 35:901–911.
6. Attar S, Bowles WR, Baisden MK, Hodges JS and McClanahan SB. Evaluation of pretreatment analgesia and endodontic treatment for postoperative endodontic pain. J. Endod.: 2008; 34:652–655.
7. Bangerter C, Mines P and Sweet M. The use of intraosseous anesthesia among endodontists: results of a questionnaire. J. Endod.: 2009; 35:15–18.
8. Baumgartner JC and Xia T. Antibiotic susceptibility of bacteria associated with endodontic abscesses. J. Endod.: 2003; 29:44–7.
9. Cope AL and Chestnutt IG. Inappropriate prescribing of antibiotics in primary dental care: reasons and resolutions. Primary Dent. Care J.: 2014; 3:33–37.
10. Corbett IP, Kanna MD, Whitworth JM and Meechan JG. Articaine infiltration for anesthesia of mandibular first molars. J. Endod.: 2008; 34:514–518.
11. Debelian GJ, Olsen I and Tronstad L. Bacteraemia in conjunction with endodontic therapy. Endod. and Dent. Tramatol.: 1992; 8:248–254.
12. Donaldson M, Gizarelli G and Chanpong B. Oral sedation: A primer on anxiolysis for the adult patient. Anaesth. Prog.: 2007; 54:118–129.
13. Flanagan T, Wahl MJ, Schmitt MM and Wahl JA. Size doesn't matter: needle gauge and injection pain. Gen. Dent.: 2007; 55:216–217.
14. Fouad AF. Are antibiotics effective for endodontic pain—An evidence based review. Endod. Topics: 2002; 2:52–66.
15. Gilbert P, Das J and Foley I. Biofilm susceptibility to antimicrobials. Adv. Dent. Res.: 1997; 11:160–167.
16. Gordon SM, Mischenko AV and Dionne RA. Long-acting local anesthetics and perioperative pain management. Dent. Clinic. North Am.: 2010; 54:611–620.
17. Jayakodi H, Kailasam S, Kumaravadivel K, Thangavelu B and Mathew S. Clinical and pharmacological management of endodontic flare-up. J. Pharm. Bioallied. Sci.: 2012; 4:294–298.
18. Khademi AA, Saatchi M, Minayian M, Rostamizadeh N and Sharafi F. Effect of preoperative alprazolam on the success of inferior alveolar nerve block for teeth with irreversible pulpitis. J. Endod.: 2012; 38:1337–1339.
19. Larsen T. Susceptibility of *Porphyromonas gingivalis* in biofilms to amoxicillin, doxycycline and metronidazole. Oral Microbiol. Immunol.: 2002; 17:267–271.
20. Li C, Yang X, Ma X, Li L and Shi Z. Preoperative and nonsteroidal anti-inflammatory drugs for the success of the inferior alveolar nerve block in irreversible pulpitis treatment: a systematic review and meta-analysis based on randomized controlled trials. Quint. Int.: 2012; 43:209–219.

21. Longman LP, Preston AJ, Martin MV and Wilson NHF. Endodontics in the adult patient: the role of antibiotics. J. Dent.: 2000; 28:539–548.
22. Macy E. Penicillin and beta-lactam allergy: epidemiology and diagnosis. Current Allergy and Asthma Reports: 2014; 14:476.
23. McDonenell G and Russell AD. Antiseptics and disinfectants: activity, action, and resistance. Clin. Microbiol. Rev.: 1999; 12:147–149.
24. Mcmahon RE, Adams W and Spolnic KJ. Diagnostic anesthesia for referred trigeminal pain: Part I. Compend. Contin. Educ. Dent.: 1992; 13:980.
25. Mellor AC, Dorman ML and Girdler NM. The use of an intra-oral injection of ketorolac in the treatment of articaine and lidocaine in the treatment of irreversible pulpitis. Int. Endod. J.: 2005; 38:789–792.
26. Mickel AK, Wright AP, Chogle S, Jones JJ, Kantorovich I and Curd F. An analysis of current analgesic preferences for endodontic pain management. J. Endod.: 2006; 32:1146–1154.
27. Miles M. Anesthetics, analgesics, antibiotics and endodontics. Dent. Clin. North Am.: 1984; 28:865–82.
28. Mohammadi Z. Systemic and local applications of steroids in endodontics: an update review. Int. Dent. J.: 2009; 59:297–304.
29. Nogueira BML, Silva LG, Mesquita CRM, Menezes SAF, Menezes TOA, Faria AGM and Porpino MTM.: Is the use of dexamethasone effective in controlling pain associated with symptomatic irreversible pulpitis? A systematic review. J. Endod.:2018; 1-8.
30. Pak JG and White SN. Pain prevalence and severity before, during and after root canal treatment: a systematic review. J. Endod.: 2011; 37:429–38.
31. Pallasch TJ. Antibiotic prophylaxis. Endod. Topics: 2003; 4:46–59.
32. Parirokh M and Abbott PV. Various strategies for pain-free root canal treatment. Iran. Endod. J.: 2014; 9:1–14.
33. Paxton K and Thome DE. Efficacy of articaine formulations: quantitative reviews. Dent. Clin. North Am.: 2010; 54:643–653.
34. Pochapski MT, Santos FA, Andrade ED and Sidney GB. Effect of pre-treatment dexamethasone on post-endodontic pain. Oral Surg., Oral Med., Oral Path., Oral Radiol. Endod.: 2009; 108:790–795.
35. Ramu C and Padmanabhan TV. Indications of antibiotic prophylaxis in dental practice—review. Asian Pac. J. Trop. Biomed.: 2012; 2:749–754.
36. Remmers T, Glickman G, Spears R and He J. The efficacy of Intraflow intraosseous injection as a primary anesthesia technique. J. Endod.: 2008; 34:280–283.
37. Rocas IN and Siqueira Jr. JF. Detection of antibiotic resistance genes in samples from acute and chronic endodontic infections and after treatment. Ach. Oral Biol.: 2013; 58: 1123–1128.
38. Roda RP, Bagan JV, Bielsa JM and Pastor EC. Antibiotic use in dental practice: a review. Med. Oral Pathol. Oral Cir. Bucal.: 2007; 12:e186–92.
39. Sambandam V and Neelakantan P. Steroids in Dentistry—A review. Int. J. Pharm. Sci. Rev. Res.: 2013, 22:240–245.
40. Sanghavi J and Aditya A. Applications of corticosteroids in dentistry. J. Dent. Allied Sci.: 2015; 4:19–24.
41. Segura-Egea JJ, Gould K, Sen BH, Jonasson P, Cotti E, Mazzoni A, Sunay H, Tjaderhane L and Dummer PMH. Antibiotics in endodontics: a review. Int. Endod. J.: 2016; 1–16.
42. Selden HS. Patient empowerment. A strategy for pain management in endodontics. J. Endod.: 1993; 19:521–523.
43. Silva NM. Systemic medication applied to endodontic treatment: a literature review. RSBO: 2014; 11:293–302.
44. Sivakumar NR. Steroids in root canal treatment. Int. J. Pharm. Pharma. Sci.: 2014; 6:17–19.
45. Stewart PS and Costerton JW. Antibiotic resistance of bacteria in biofilms. Lancet: 2001; 14:135–138.
46. Tong DC and Rothwell BR. Antibiotic prophylaxis in dentistry. A review and practice recommendation. JADA: 2000; 131:366–374.
47. Vera JRM and Gomez-LusCentelles ML. Antimicrobial prophylaxis in oral surgery and dental procedures. Med. Oral Patol. Circ. Buccal.: 2007; 12:44–52.
48. Walton RE and Chiappinelli J. Prophylactic penicillin: effect on post-treatment symptoms following root canal treatment of asymptomatic periapical pathosis. J. Endod.:1993; 19:466–470.
49. Wong JK. Adjuncts to local anesthesia: separating fact from friction. J. Can. Dent. Assoc.: 2001; 67:391–397.
50. Zahed M. Systemic, prophylactic and local applications of antimicrobials in endodontics: an update review. Int. Dent. J.: 2009; 59:175–186.

Chapter 5

Diseases of the Dental Pulp

Dental pulp is the soft connective tissue of mesenchymal origin located in the center of the tooth. It is situated in an enclosure called pulp chamber in the crown and root canal in the root covered with dentin. It contains odontoblasts, fibroblasts and defense cells. The fibroblasts represent the largest cell population, and appear as both inactive and active cells; the latter producing the intercellular substances and collagen precursors. The undifferentiated mesenchymal cells may replace odontoblasts as well as defense cells, and assume their functions; designated as replacement cells.

The *primary function* of the pulp is 'formative'; it gives rise to odontoblasts that not only form dentin but interact with dental epithelium to initiate the formation of enamel. Pulp also provides several *secondary functions* related to tooth sensitivity, hydration, defense, etc.

Certain anatomical features make the pulp a unique tissue which may be responsible for its vulnerability to various physical, chemical, and bacterial insults. Pulp reacts to these irritants as do other connective tissues. Pulpal injury may result in inflammation and subsequent cell death. The degree of inflammation is proportional to the intensity and severity of the irritants. Minor injuries, such as incipient caries or shallow cavity preparations, cause little or no inflammation in the pulp. In contrast, deep caries or extensive operative procedures, usually produce severe inflammatory changes. Depending on the severity and duration of the insult coupled with the host responses, the pulpal response ranges from transient inflammation to necrosis. These changes are usually very slow, without pain and remain unnoticed, till symptoms warrant the patient.

PULPAL INFLAMMATION

The process of inflammation in the pulp is basically the same as in other connective tissues of the body; however, certain features, unique of its kind in pulp, tend to alter the course of this response.

The features are:

- Pulp can produce reparative dentin, which protects pulp from injury and other irritants.
- Pulp is surrounded by hard tissue (the dentin), which does not allow the usual swelling associated with the acute inflammatory process.
- Pulp lacks collateral circulation (few vessels supply the pulp through the apical foramen and another few enter through lateral/accessory canals); compromising healing capacity.

During inflammation, exudates leave the vessels and raise the interstitial pressure. Since the fluid is not compressible and there is little room for edema, this may cause local tissue hypoxia leading to localized necrosis. It is established that increase of pressure in one area does not affect the other areas of pulp. The local inflammation results in increased tissue pressure in inflamed area and not the entire pulp cavity. Limited increase in pressure within affected pulpal area is explained by the following features:

- Increased pressure in inflamed area leads to net absorption of interstitial fluid from adjacent capillaries in uninflamed tissues.
- Increased interstitial pressure lowers the trans-capillary hydrostatic tissue pressure difference, thus limiting the filtration process.
- Increase in interstitial fluid pressure results in increased hydrostatic drainage and keep the pulpal volume almost constant.
- Break in endothelium of capillaries facilitates exchange mechanisms.

Continued spread of local inflammation may lead to total necrosis. Earlier, it was thought that the pulp responded initially by acute inflammation, followed by chronic inflammation, regardless of the etiologic factor. It is established that the initial response might be due to chronic inflammation (most of the irritants progress slowly; however, rapid irritation by operative procedures lead to acute inflammation).

Entry of Irritants to Pulp

Potential antigens include bacteria and their degradation by-products, which directly or via dentinal tubules, can initiate inflammatory reactions. Irritations from any source enter the pulpal tissue through the following portals:

i. Direct extension through the dentinal tubules, as in case of caries or chemicals placed on the dentin.
ii. Extension of periodontal disease into the pulp; in deep periodontal pockets, exposing the lateral canals or apical foramen to the oral environment, may lead to total pulp necrosis.
iii. Extension by process of anachoresis, the localization of blood-borne bacteria within the pulp. This explains why some pulps become necrotic when there is no apparent etiologic factor.
iv. In addition to nonspecific inflammatory reactions, immune responses may also initiate and perpetuate pulpal diseases.

CAUSES OF PULP DISEASES

The causes of pulp diseases are categorized as:

A. *Physical*

a. *Mechanical*

i. Traumatic injuries
ii. Mechanical irritants
iii. Pathologic/physiologic wear
iv. Cracked tooth syndrome
v. Barodontalgia
vi. Lasers
vii. Restorations

b. *Thermal*

i. Cavity preparation
ii. Exothermic setting of cements
iii. Thermal conduction through restorations
iv. Polishing heat

c. *Electrical*

i. Galvanic current from dissimilar fillings

B. *Chemical*

i. Phosphoric acid, acrylic monomer, etc.
ii. Dental erosion (acids)

C. *Bacterial*

i. Toxins associated with caries
ii. Direct pulp invasion from caries/trauma
iii. By blood borne microbes (anachoresis)

A. Physical

a. Mechanical

The mechanical injuries leading to pulp diseases are:

i. *Traumatic injuries*

Traumatic dental injuries may occur at any age; however, mostly young children are affected. The injuries can be because of fights, sports, automobile accidents, house hold accidents, compulsive bruxism, nail biting and opening bobby pin with teeth (Fig. 5.1). Mainly incisors are affected, may be primary or permanent (fractured or displaced incisors).

The severity of trauma and degree of apical closure at the time of trauma are important factors in recovery of the pulp. Mild to moderate trauma or teeth with immature apex have a better chance of pulpal survival. Completed root formation or severe injuries may lead to irreversible changes. The dental procedures, if not carried out properly, may injure the pulp. Such inflammation is usually reversible; however, if not managed on time may lead to irreversible changes.

ii. *Mechanical irritants*

The mechanical irritants are generally carried by occlusal trauma, curettage of deep periodontal pockets and use of dull burs/points during cavity preparation. Continuous cavity preparation using heavy pressure also act as mechanical irritant. Irritation because of mechanical separator and orthodontic movements also affect pulpal tissues.

The damage to the subjacent odontoblast cells in the pulp tissue needs to be avoided. The number of dentinal tubules per unit surface area and their diameter increases as we move closer to the pulp. As a result, dentinal permeability close to the pulp is higher than near the dentinoenamel junction or cementodentinal junction. Therefore, potential for pulpal damage increases as more dentin is removed during the cavity

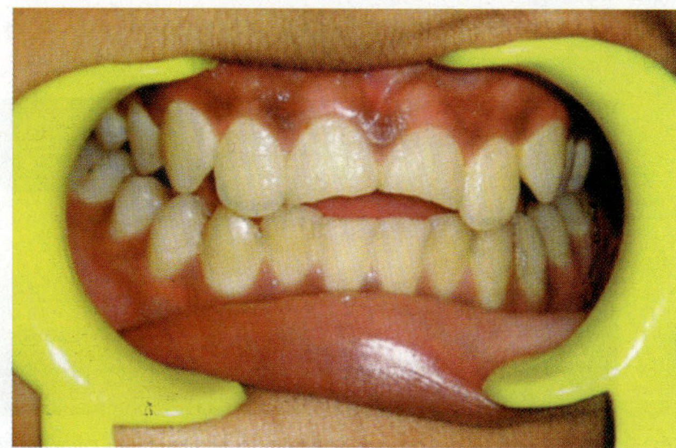

Fig. 5.1 Fracture of maxillary incisors due to trauma

preparation. The most critical factor is the *'remaining dentin thickness'*. Minimal effects are transmitted to the pulp if the remaining dentin thickness is 2.0 mm or more. Pulp damage is considered proportional to the amount of dentin removed and also the depth of removal as well.

iii. *Pathologic/physiologic wear*

Dental pulp has got an excellent reparative power of laying down dentin reacting to clinical situation; however, in some conditions, the reparative capacity of the pulp does not keep pace with the stimulus. In such conditions, the pulp shows irreversible damage; for example, a severely attritioned mandibular incisor may lead to pulpal necrosis.

The abrasion caused by the dentifrices may also be so severe causing pulp exposure. Night clenching or bruxism and occlusal trauma may also show similar involvement of the pulp.

iv. *Cracked tooth syndrome*

Incomplete hair line crack through the body of the tooth (cracked tooth syndrome) may sometime cause severe pain. The patient usually complains of pain, ranging from mild to excruciating at the initiation and release of biting pressure. The most common and reliable diagnostic method is to reproduce the pain. When the patient bites on a cotton applicator, rubber wheels or tooth slooth, the fractured fragments may separate and the pain may be reproduced (Fig. 5.2a and b). Magnified examination of the crown of the tooth may disclose an enamel crack; using operating microscope or transilluminating the tooth by using fiberoptic light. The incomplete fracture of enamel and dentin usually produces mild pain; eventually pain becomes severe when the fracture line touches the pulp.

v. *Barodontalgia (Aerodontalgia)*

The pain experienced by a patient in a recently restored tooth during low atmospheric pressure usually at high altitude is called Barodontalgia (aerodontalgia). This condition can be experienced either during flight or during a test run in a decompression chamber. Barodontalgia can be observed in altitude of over 5000 feet, but attitude of 10,000 feet and above lead to symptoms. A tooth with chronic pulpitis may not produce any symptoms at ground level but it may cause pain at high altitude because of low atmospheric pressure. Giving a layer of cavity varnish or liner under the restoration helps to prevent this problem. Although the process of barodontalgia is not properly understood, it may be related to pulpal hyperaemia or to the gases which are trapped in the teeth following root canal treatment.

vi. *Lasers*

Lasers, especially during cavity preparation may lead to inflammation in pulp. The production of heat and rise in the pulpal temperature can damage the pulp. Electron microscopic studies have shown disruption and degeneration of pulpal peripheral nerve endings, subsequently leading to reduced sensitivity.

vii. *Restorations*

Pulpal pain and subsequent pulp tissue changes may result following the insertion of metallic restoration like gold foil and silver amalgam restoration. Other restorations viz. silicate cements and zinc oxide eugenol cements may produce inflammatory reaction in pulp. Glass-ionomer cements and/or composite resins, especially in deep cavities, have also shown pulpal changes.

b. Thermal

The thermal injuries are usually due to following causes:

i. *Cavity preparation*

The inflammation following cavity preparation may range from reversible to irreversible changes. It is established that deeper the preparation, more extensive is the pulpal inflammation. The main reason is heat produced by cutting/grinding instrument during

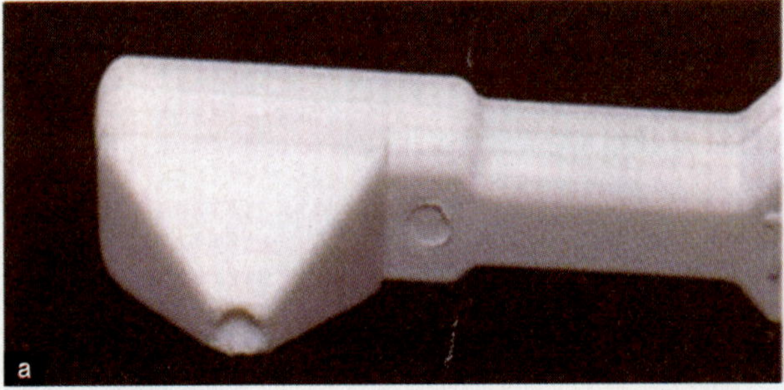

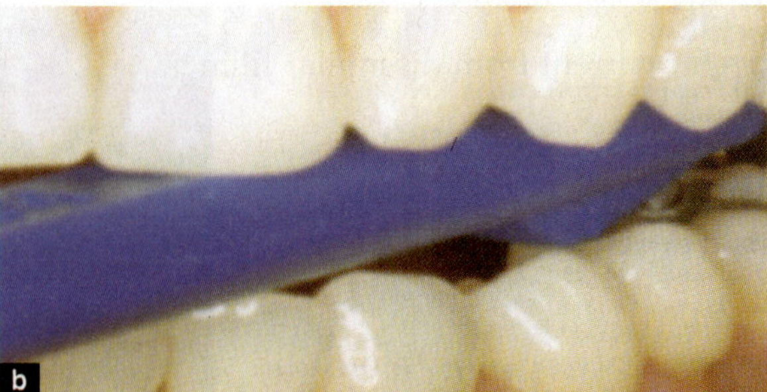

Fig. 5.2 (a) Tooth slooth (a small pyramid shaped plastic bite block with a small concavity at the apex of the pyramid). (b) Patient biting on tooth slooth

cavity preparation, especially if used without coolant. The generated heat may cause the irreparable damage to the pulp. Constant drying with air syringe/chip blowing may also contribute to pulp inflammation and subsequently the necrosis, particularly in a stressed pulp.

The features contributing rise in the pulpal temperature are:

- Amount of force applied by the operator.
- Size, shape and condition of the cutting tool.
- The speed (revolution per minute) of cutting tool.
- Continuous time of usage.

ii. *Exothermic setting of cements*

Certain cements, viz. zinc phosphate cements create exothermic reaction during setting; the heat so produced will lead to changes in pulp tissues.

iii. *Thermal conduction through restorations*

Metallic restorations are positive conductor of heat. Restoration like silver amalgam and gold foil, especially if close to the pulp, may conduct temperature changes to the pulp and cause irreparable damages. Sudden temperature changes because of ice cream/coffee, tea, etc. may contribute to pulpal damage. Remaining dentin thickness under the metallic restoration is the key factor in determining the type of inflammatory changes in the pulp. Dentin is the natural thermal insulator which protects the pulp from thermal insults. The procedures which lead to removal of protective layer of the dentin over the pulp, lead to pulpal inflammation and subsequent changes.

iv. *Polishing heat*

The abrasive instruments, because of their frictional working produce heat, especially when used without coolants. The routine polishing of the restoration produces enough heat, which can be detrimental to pulp. Even interproximal finishing and polishing of the restorations using the abrasive finishing strips without a constant air coolant may also cause similar damage to the pulp.

c. Electrical

Two chemically dissimilar metallic restorations, like silver amalgam and cast gold restoration, when come in contact in presence of saliva, produce electrogalvanism or galvanic shock. As both the restorations are wet with saliva, an electric couple exists, with a difference in potential between the dissimilar restorations. When two restorations come in contact, the potential is suddenly short circuited, resulting in acute changes in pulp and subsequent pain.

B. Chemical

Chemical causes of pulp injury are probably less common. Earlier, arsenic in silicate cement powder and the use of desensitizing paste containing paraformaldehyde accounted for pulp necrosis; however, these materials are no longer in use. It is established that most restorative materials, if properly used, do not cause any damage to the pulp. Some of the materials may contribute to pulpal inflammation; however, the initial inflammatory reaction may subside with time.

A few restorative materials may cause chemical insult to the pulp, such as:

- Phosphoric acid of zinc phosphate cement.
- Acid etching with 37% ortho-phosphoric acid
- Calcium hydroxide, owing to its high alkaline pH, produces low grade irritation.
- Eugenol in zinc oxide eugenol cement
- Dental erosions, if continued, may also lead to pulp involvement.

The remaining dentin thickness plays a crucial role in determining the effect of chemicals on the pulp. The thickness of remaining dentin is inversely proportional to the effect; more the thickness, less detrimental effect. Certain restorative materials are hygroscopic; absorb moisture from the dentin, leading to its desiccation. For example, cavit placed over thin dentin causes desiccation.

C. Bacterial

The role of bacteria in causing pulp inflammation is well established. The ingress of bacteria in the mechanically exposed pulp determines the prognosis of vital pulp therapy.

The bacteria may enter the pulp following different ways as:

- Caries
- Fracture
- Tooth anomalies (dens invaginatus and dens evaginatus)
- Palato-gingival or radicular lingual groove
- Infection caused via periodontal pocket/periodontal abscess
- Haematogenic

The micro-organisms present in the carious lesion are the main sources of irritation of the dental pulp. Bacterial invasion from a carious lesion and/or traumatic exposure frequently cause pulp inflammation. Bacterial invasion is also possible through lateral canals, or periodontal/periapical blood vessels. Once bacteria invade the pulp, the damage is almost irreparable. The species of bacteria recovered from inflamed or infected pulps are many and varied in nature. Although lactobacilli (acidogenic micro-organism) are commonly found in carious dentin, they are seldom recovered from the pulp because of their low degree of invasiveness. Micro-organisms need not be present in the pulp to produce inflammation; the degradation by-products of bacteria are sufficiently irritating to cause inflammatory reaction.

The bacteria most often recovered from infected pulps are streptococci and staphylococci; however, many other micro-organisms (mostly anaerobes) have been isolated from the infected pulp. The molecular analysis of pathogens, have identified several newer species.

Pulpal tissue may remain inflamed for a long period of time; may and may not undergo necrosis. The factors which stimulate pulp necrosis are:

- Virulence of bacteria
- Marked increase in intrapulpal pressure
- Host resistance
- Blood circulation
- Lymph drainage.

Once the pulp is exposed either by caries or trauma, it is considered infected because micro-organisms gain access immediately. The invading bacteria, however, may be confined entirely to the small area of pulp exposure; the body and apical portion of the pulp may remain normal. The initial reaction of the pulp to bacterial invasion is an inflammatory response. Polymorphonuclear cells reach the areas of initial insult, which prevent further dissemination of bacteria deeper into the pulp.

The pulpal reaction to an inflammation differs from other parts of the body as pulp is enclosed in a rigid chamber. The inflammatory exudate facilitates rise in intrapulpal pressure, which strangulates the pulpal blood vessels at the apical foramen. This in turn causes the local tissue hypoxia, eventually leading to pulp necrosis.

Flowchart 5.1 Pulp reactions to various irritants

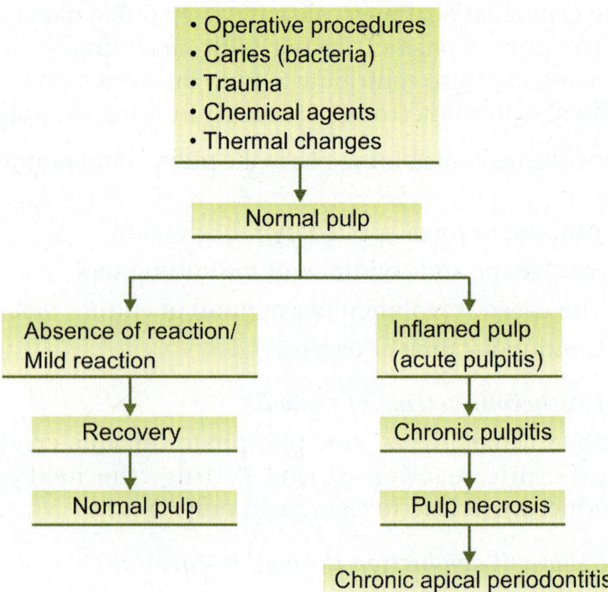

Flowchart 5.1 depicts pulp reactions to various irritants.

The diagnostic criteria for the assessment of pulp and periapical conditions are tabulated in Table 5.1.

CLASSIFICATION OF PULP DISEASES

There is no definite and accepted classification for pulpal diseases. Usual classifications are based on (a) duration and severity of inflammation (acute, subacute, chronic), (b) Presence/absence of symptoms (symptomatic, asymptomatic) and (c) ability to heal (reversible, irreversible).

Table 5.1 Diagnostic criteria for the assessment of pulp and periapical conditions

Stage	*Procedure*	*Outcome*
History	Medical/Dental history Description of present complain Previous treatment, if any	Provisional diagnosis
Clinical examination	Extra-oral/intra-oral signs Individual tooth assessment	Identify and differentiate possible cause(s)
Clinical tests	Pulp sensitivity tests Palpation/percussion, etc.	Provisional diagnosis of the status of the pulp and periapical tissues
Radiographic examination	Periapical radiograph(s)	Analysis of configuration of pulp Provisional diagnosis of the periapical status
Correlation of all above findings	Combine the history, clinical examination, clinical tests and radiographic examination results	Definitive diagnosis

'Acute inflammation' implies inflammatory reactions which are closer to the source of the injury or infection; peripheral chronic activity may and may not be evident. As the intrapulpal or intraperiapical pressure increase beyond the threshold limits of the sensory receptors, varying degree of pain is felt. The absence of pain does not mean that acute inflammatory response is absent. It means that the intrapulpal pressure is below the threshold limits of the pain receptors.

The predominant cells in the acute response are polymorphonuclear leukocytes, neutrophils and tissue macrophages.

'Subacute inflammation' is a stage of hyperactivity between exudative (acute) and proliferative (chronic) inflammatory components as in pulpitis and advanced form of apical periodontitis.

This stage is characterized clinically by period of mild to moderate symptoms.

'Chronic inflammation' is characterized by the formation of granulation tissue in the area peripheral to the exudative zone. This response may arise at the end of acute inflammatory process or may develop from the onset, when a low-grade irritation to the pulp or periapex is neutralized by effective tissue resistance.

The intrapulpal pressure is below the threshold limits of the pain receptors in chronic inflammation (asymptomatic or painless). When the strength of the irritant is reduced, the granulomatous tissue (granulation tissue plus chronic inflammatory cells) becomes hyperactive, leading to repair and healing.

The predominant cells in chronic inflammation are lymphocytes, plasma cells and macrophages.

Pulpal diseases have been classified by various authors; the accepted ones are described:

1. ***Initially Gofung (1928) classified pulpal diseases as***
   A. Acute pulpitis
      a. Partial
      b. General
      c. Purulent
   B. Chronic pulpitis
      a. Fibrous
      b. Hypertrophic
      c. Gangrenous
2. ***Classification by World Health Organization (WHO)***
   A. Pulpitis
      a. Initial (hyperemia)
      b. Acute
         i. Suppurative (pulpal abscess)
      c. Chronic
         i. Ulcerative
         ii. Hyperplastic (pulp polyp)
         iii. Unspecified
   B. Necrosis
   C. Pulp degeneration
      a. Denticles
      b. Pulpal calcification
      c. Pulp stones
   D. Formation of secondary/irregular dentin in pulp
3. ***Grossman's classification***
   A. Hyperaemia
   B. Pulpitis
      a. *Reversible pulpitis*
         i. Symptomatic (acute)
         ii. Asymptomatic (chronic)
      b. *Irreversible pulpitis*
         i. Acute
            - Abnormal response to cold
            - Abnormal response to heat
         ii. Chronic
            - Hyperplastic pulpitis (pulp polyp)
            - Internal resorption
   C. Pulp degeneration
      a. Calcific degeneration
      b. Atrophic degeneration
      c. Fibrous degeneration
   D. Pulp necrosis
      a. Coagulative necrosis
      b. Liquefactive necrosis
      c. Caseation necrosis
4. ***Stock's classification***
   A. Normal pulp
   B. Concussed pulp
   C. Pulpitis
      a. Reversible
      b. Irreversible
   D. Pulp necrosis
   E. Internal resorption
5. ***Walton's and Torabinejad's classification***
   A. Pulpitis
      a. Reversible
      b. Irreversible
      c. Hyperplastic
   B. Pulp necrosis
   C. Pulp calcification
   D. Internal resorption
6. ***Abbot's classification***
   A. Clinically normal pulp (based on clinical examination and test results)
   B. Pulpitis
      a. Reversible pulpitis
         i. Acute
         ii. Chronic

b. Irreversible pulpitis
  i. Acute
  ii. Chronic

C. Pulp necrosis
  a. Necrobiosis (part of pulp is necrotic and inflamed; rest is irreversibly inflamed)
  b. No signs of infection
  c. Infected

D. Pulpless, infected root canal system

E. Degenerative changes
  a. Atrophy
  b. Pulp canal calcification
    i. Partial
    ii. Total
  c. Hyperplasia
  d. Internal resorption
    i. Surface
    ii. Inflammatory
    iii. Replacement

F. Previous root canal treatment
  a. No signs of infection
  b. Infected
  c. Technical standard (based on radiographic appearance)
    i. Adequate
    ii. Inadequate
  d. Other problems, e.g. perforations, fractured instrument, missed canal, etc.

SIGNS AND SYMPTOMS OF PULP CONDITIONS

Each condition of pulp is dynamic in nature; if not treated, progresses to another condition. Therefore, the signs and symptoms overlap between various pulp conditions. During diagnosis, the operator should keep in mind the dynamic nature of pulp and also the limitations of assessing the pulpal status. A 'clinical' normal healthy pulp implies that the pulp has no signs and symptoms suggestive of any disease entity. The term 'clinical' is used, since the pulp may exhibit some histological changes. A clinically normal pulp does not respond to heat stimuli; however it may react to cold stimuli with mild pain, which can last for a minute or so. Dentin sensitivity is also a separate entity, wherein, no pulpal disease is noticed. The pain is consistent with thermal, chemical, tactile or osmotic stimuli when applied on dentin. The discomfort usually lingers till the stimulus is removed.

The pulp conditions following Grossman's classification are described:

1. Hyperemia

Pulpal hyperemia implies excessive accumulation of the blood in the pulp with a predisposition to edema as a result of prolonged vasodilation. An increased blood volume in the confined environment of dental pulp increases the intrapulpal pressure especially in the affected areas. Hyperemia is an initial and potentially reversible pulpal response that sets a stage for inflammatory cycle (Fig. 5.3). Hyperemia is not a disease entity but a symptom. There are two types of hyperemia:

- Active hyperemia
- Passive hyperemia

In active hyperemia, there is an increased arterial flow; whereas, in passive hyperemia, there is a diminished venous flow. Clinically, both active and passive hyperemia are indistinguishable.

Causative Factors

Various factors leading to hyperemia are:

- Trauma induced by dental procedures
- Excessive dehydration of cavity walls
- Irritation of exposed dentin from restorative materials
- Injudicious use of mechanical separators/too rapid orthodontic movements
- Trauma from high fillings

Management

Removal of the causative factor will lead to resolution of hyperemia. The capability for resolution depends upon strength and duration of irritant, extent of pulp tissues affected and prior health status of the pulp itself. The prognosis for the pulp is favorable if the irritant is removed early, otherwise the inflammatory process sets in.

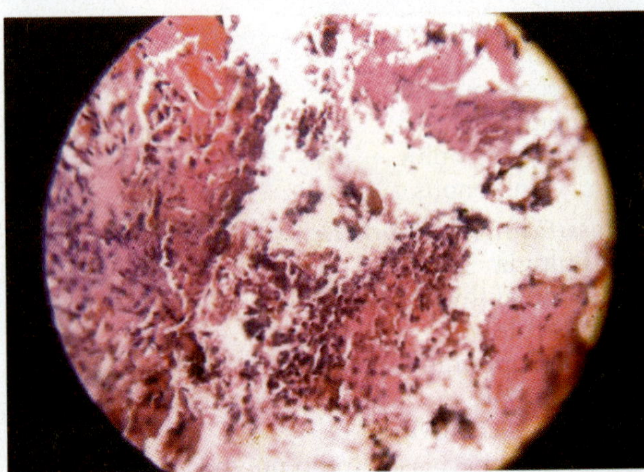

Fig. 5.3 Pulpal hyperaemia

2. Pulpitis

The pulp response in the form of inflammatory process which is a defensive mechanism of the pulp is termed as pulpitis. The inflammatory process in the pulp is more prevalent in younger teeth with larger dentinal tubules as compared to mature teeth with few and occluded dentinal tubules. Pulpitis can be either reversible or irreversible.

a. Reversible Pulpitis

It is a mild to moderate inflammation of the pulp which is capable of returning to the normal state once the stimuli is removed. Pain of brief duration may be produced by stimuli, such as sweet and cold, rarely heat; but the pain subsides as soon as the stimulus is removed.

Etiology

The features causing reversible pulpitis are:

- Accidental trauma/traumatic occlusion
- Quick thermal changes
- Excessive dehydration leading to desiccation of the dentin
- Oral galvanism
- Chemical insults

Clinical symptoms and diagnosis

'Symptomatic reversible pulpitis' is characterized by sharp pain, last for a moment and generally disappears when the stimulus is removed. It is usually brought on by cold, sweet/sour than hot food beverages. It does not occur spontaneously and does not continue when the cause has been removed.

'Asymptomatic reversible pulpitis' may result from incipient caries and is resolved after removal of the caries and restoration of the tooth.

Since the pulp is sensitive to temperature changes, particularly cold; application of cold is an excellent method of localizing and diagnosing the involved tooth. A tooth with reversible pulpitis reacts normally to percussion, palpation, and mobility test and the periradicular tissues appear normal on radiographic examination (Fig. 5.4a). The pulp may recover completely, or the pain may last longer each time, and intervals of relief may become shorter, until the pulp finally succumbs.

The clinical difference between the reversible and irreversible pulpitides is quantitative; the pain of irreversible pulpitis is more severe and last longer. In reversible pulpitis, the cause of the pain is generally traceable to a stimulus, such as cold water; whereas in irreversible pulpitis, the pain sets in without any apparent stimulus.

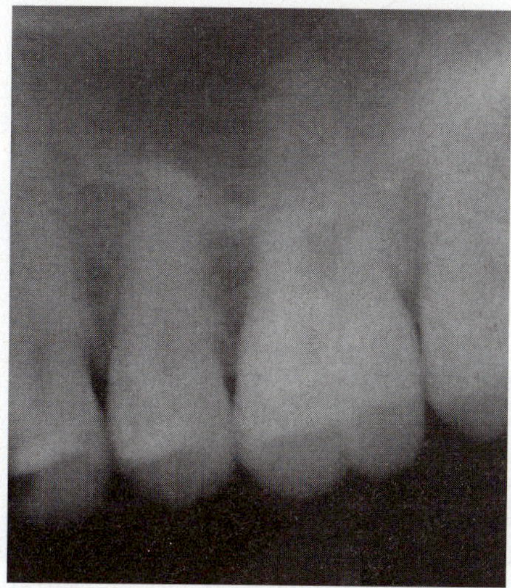

Fig. 5.4a Normal periapical areas

Histopathology

A mild to moderate inflammatory changes, limited to the area of involved dentinal tubules is seen histopathologically. Reparative dentin, disruption of the odontoblast layer, dilated blood vessels, extravasation of edema fluid and presence of immunocompetent chronic inflammatory cells are evident (Fig. 5.4b and c).

Treatment

The removal of irritants is the treatment preferred in reversible pulpitis. Insulating the exposed dentin results in diminished symptoms (if present) leading to reversal of the inflammatory process in the pulpal tissue. However, if irritation of pulp continues or increases in intensity, moderate to severe inflammation develops; subsequently leading to irreversible pulpitis and eventually pulpal necrosis.

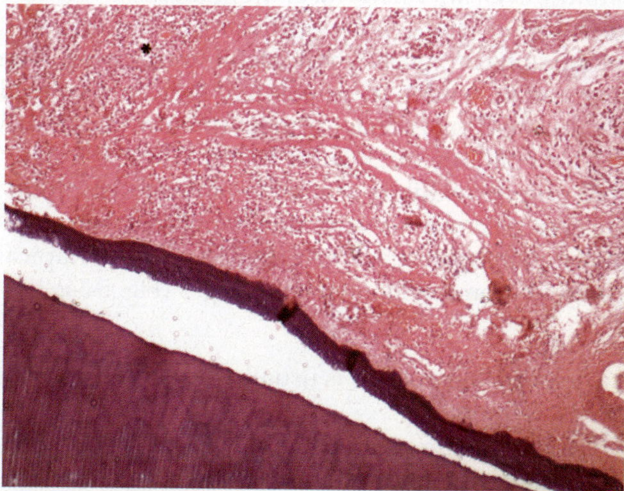

Fig. 5.4b **Acute pulpitis**: Showing diffuse inflammation of pulp

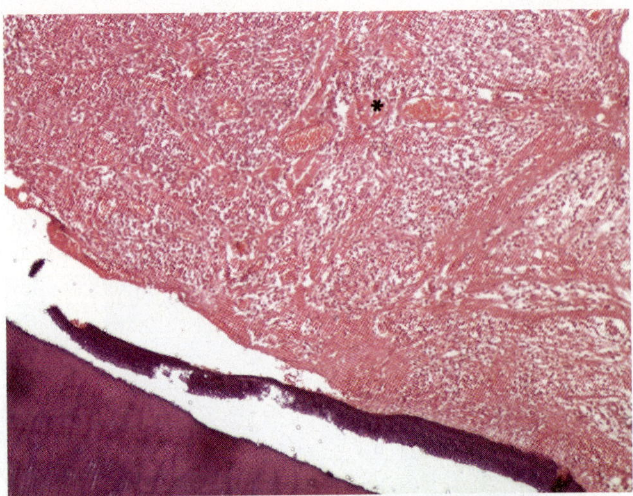

Fig. 5.4c **Acute pulpitis**: Core is composed of purulent exudate consisting of polymorphonuclear leukocytes against a background of fibrin, necrotic tissue debris, vascular dilatations and extravasated red blood cells

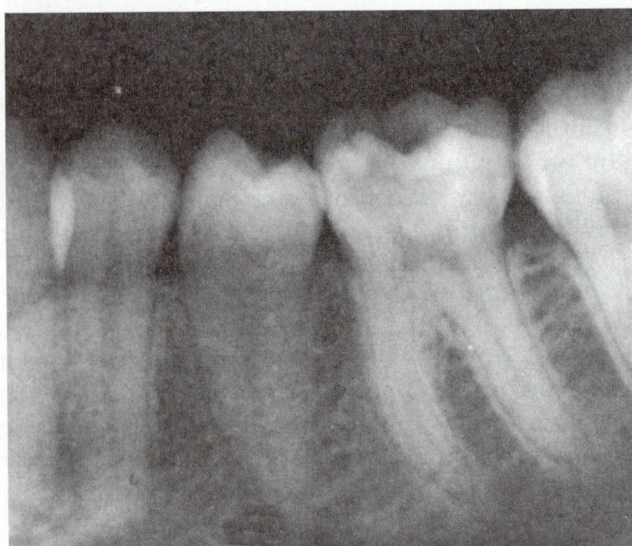

Fig 5.5a Widening of periodontal ligament along with initiation of rarefaction in the periapical area

The prognosis is usually favorable. The status of the pulp is to be reviewed periodically (at least up to 3–6 months) to analyze clinical normal status of pulp. If pulp is free of symptoms and respond normally to pulp tests, it is to be designated as 'normal' (assuming the inflammation has subsided).

b. Irreversible Pulpitis

It is a persistent inflammatory condition of the pulp. Irreversible pulpitis, if untreated, is categorized as symptomatic (acute) or asymptomatic (chronic). The acutely inflamed pulp is symptomatic and the chronically inflamed pulp is asymptomatic. Acute irreversible pulpitis exhibits spontaneous pain induced by hot/cold stimulus. The pain lingers on for several minutes, even after removal of the stimulus. Even mild temperature changes are sufficient to induce pain. Radiographs are usually not useful in diagnosis. The tooth can be tender on percussion, indicating spread of inflammation to periapical areas (pain on percussion may also indicate crack in the tooth). Chronic irreversible pulpitis exhibits the same kind of symptoms; however, pain is less severe and intermittent than continuous as in acute case. Radiographically, periapical changes become evident at later stages (Fig. 5.5a).

Etiology

The irreversible pulpitis is usually a progression from reversible pulpitis.

The most common cause of the irreversible pulpitis is the bacterial contamination; however, chemical, thermal and/or mechanical factor may also cause irreversible pulpitis.

Clinical symptoms and diagnosis

- In the early stages of irreversible pulpitis, pain may be caused by sudden temperature changes (particularly cold), sweet/acidic food. The pressure of packing food into a cavity or even suction exerted by the tongue may also elicit pain.
- The pain is continued and may linger for a longer period even after removal of the cause. Initially the pain is described as sharp, piercing and shooting. It may be intermittent or continuous, depending on the intensity of pulpal involvement. The change of posture (lying down or bending) exacerbates the pain (changes in the intrapulpal pressure may be the cause).
- The pain can be referred to adjacent teeth, to the temporal region when an upper posterior tooth is involved or to the postauricular/preauricular or even to the lower border of the mandible, when a lower posterior tooth is involved.
- The in-built pressure in the pulp, if continued, may lead to gnawing and/or throbbing pain (clinical exposing the pulp provide immediate relief).
- Patients are often awake at night by the pain, which continues to be intolerable. Pain is increased by heat and is sometimes relieved by cold. Apical periodontitis is absent except in the condition where the pulpal inflammation has crossed the apical barrier and involves the periradicular periodontium.

The diagnostic features of pulp diseases are summarized in Table 5.2.

Table 5.2 Diagnostic features of pulpal diseases

Clinical features	*Normal pulp*	*Reversible pulpitis (asymptomatic)*	*Reversible pulpitis (symptomatic)*	*Irreversible pulpitis (asymptomatic)*	*Irreversible pulpitis (symptomatic)*	*Pulp necrosis*
History	No history of pain	No history of pain	No history of spontaneous pain	No history of pain	Spontaneous pain	Pain in advanced stages only
Thermal (cold) test	Mild response to cold; does not linger	Mild response to cold	Quick and sharp response; discomfort may not linger	Quick and sharp response; discomfort may not linger	Exaggerated response to cold; pain lingers	No response
Pain on percussion	Negative	negative	Negative	Negative	May be positive	No response; responsive in late stages
Radiographic findings	Normal	Normal; presence of caries	Normal	Normal periodontal ligament/ thickening of periodontal ligament	Normal periodontal ligament/thickening of periodontal ligament	Normal appearance; may be periapical radiolucency

Histopathology

Irreversible pulpitis may be caused by a long standing noxious stimulus such as caries. As caries penetrates deep into dentin, it causes a chronic inflammatory response in the underlying pulp. If the caries is not removed, the inflammatory changes in the pulp may increase in severity as the caries approaches the pulp. The inflammatory reaction produces micro-abscess. The pulp, trying to protect itself, walls off the areas with fibrous connective tissue. Microscopically, an area of the abscess and a zone of necrotic tissue is evident (Fig. 5.5b). The micro-organisms present in the late carious stage along with lymphocytes, plasma cells and tissue macrophages are also seen. No micro-organisms are present in the center of the abscess because of the phagocytic activity of the polymorphonuclear cells. If the carious process continues to advance and penetrates the pulp, the histological picture changes. It has been established that bacteria needed to be within 1.0 mm of the pulp before inflammatory changes could be observed. Evidence of irreversible pathosis may not be observed until the reparative dentin is invaded. An area of ulceration (chronic ulcerative pulpitis) is evident that drains through the carious exposure into the oral cavity and reduces the intrapulpal pressure, and therefore, the pain. An area of necrotic tissue and zone of proliferating fibroblasts forming the walls of the lesion is also seen.

Differential diagnosis: reversible/ irreversible pulpitis

In reversible pulpitis, the pain is transitory, lasting just for a moment; whereas, in irreversible pulpitis, the pain may last longer. Thermal tests are useful in locating the affected tooth. The electric pulp test requires less current to elicit a response than on a normal tooth.

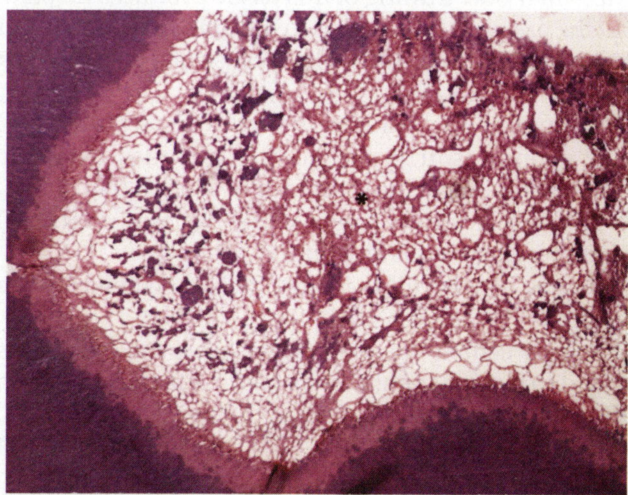

Fig 5.5b Chronic pulpitis: Presence of loose, delicate connective tissue with bundles of dense collagen and diffuse infiltration of chronic inflammatory cells with dystrophic calcification

Reversible pulpitis	Irreversible pulpitis
• Pain traceable to stimulus (cold water/air)	• May not be traceable to stimulus (may be without any apparent stimulus)
• Pain is transitory (last for a moment)	• Pain lasts longer and severe
• Symptoms subside immediately after removal of cause	• Pain usually lingers
• Less current required to elicit pain	• Less current required to elicit pain initially; more current in advanced cases
• Infrequent episodes of pain/discomfort	• Pain is increasing in frequency, to be continuous

Treatment

Root canal treatment is the treatment of choice. The prognosis is favorable.

c. Chronic Hyperplastic Pulpitis (Pulp Polyp)

Chronic hyperplastic pulpitis or proliferative pulpitis is generally recognized as pulp polyp. This is a specific type of inflammatory hyperplasia, which occur in young pulp (with abundant blood supply) due to extensive carious exposure. This disorder is characterized by overgrowth of granulation tissue, resulting from long standing, low grade irritation.

The hyperplastic pulpitis occurs almost exclusively in children and young adults, and both in primary and permanent dentition.

The clinical appearance of the polypoid tissue shows fleshy, reddish pulpal mass, filling most of the pulp chamber or even sometimes extends beyond the confines of the tooth. Polypoid tissue is less sensitive than normal pulp tissue and more sensitive than gingival tissue. Cutting of this tissue produces no pain, but the pressure transmitted to the pulp may cause mild pain. The tissue bleeds easily because of a rich network of blood vessels.

The pulp polyp exhibits the following features:

- A spongy, soft tissue nodule extrudes from the cavitated or fractured surface of a tooth (Fig. 5.6).
- The surface texture (color) varies from smooth (pink) to granular (red and white).
- Polyps usually fill the entire pulpal chamber of the tooth.
- Polyps usually develop in carious primary molars and first permanent molars because, anatomically in young persons, these teeth have large pulp chambers. Less frequently, maxillary central incisors in both dentitions are affected.
- A pulp polyp is a single lesion, but multiple teeth may be affected.
- Teeth with open or incomplete apexification of the root apices are the most susceptible.

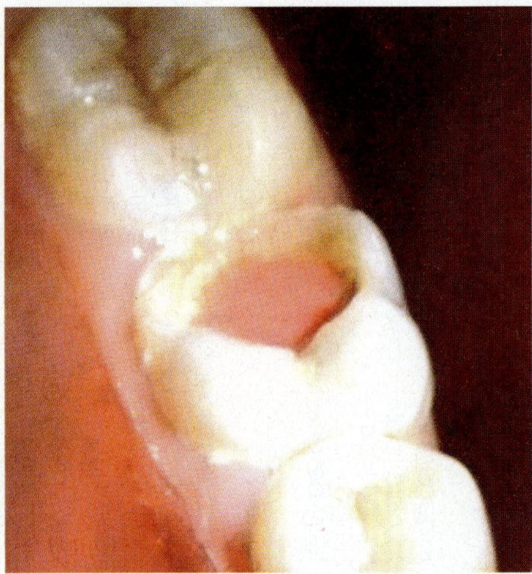

Fig. 5.6 Pulp polyp

Pathophysiology

The pulp polyp is the result of both mechanical irritation and bacterial invasion into the pulp chamber, mainly due to caries or trauma. The large exposure of pulpal tissue to the oral environment followed by bacterial invasion results in a chronic inflammatory response that stimulates an exuberant granulation tissue reaction. The chronically inflamed granulation tissue proliferate from the pulp cavity and is covered by stratified squamous epithelium (Fig. 5.7).

The hyperplastic tissue reaction occurs because the young dental pulp has a rich blood supply and favorable immune response that is more resistant to bacterial infection. Furthermore, because the tooth is open to the oral cavity, transudates and exudates from the inflamed pulpal tissue drain freely and do not accumulate within the restricted and rigid confines of

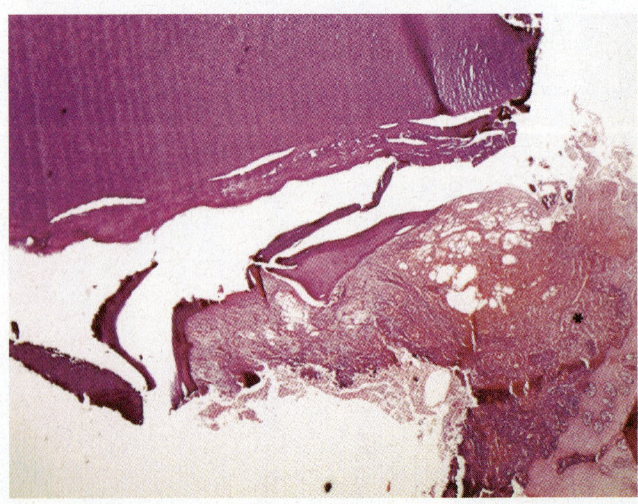

Fig. 5.7 **Chronic hyperplastic pulpitis:** Chronically inflamed granulation tissue proliferating from the pulp cavity and covered by stratified squamous epithelium

the tooth. Tissue necrosis with destruction of the microcirculation that usually accompanies irreversible pulpitis may not occur because of lack of significant intrapulpal pressure. In young teeth with open apices, the risk of pulpal necrosis is minimum. The presence of a rich vascular network in the young pulpal tissue is an important protective mechanism against the inflammatory response that significantly decreases with age.

Etiology

A large open cavity, a young resistant pulp and a chronic low grade stimulus are the causative agents for hyperplastic pulpitis. Mechanical irritation and bacterial invasion often provide the stimulus.

Symptoms

- Pulp polyps reach a maximum size within a couple of months and then remain static.
- Pulp polyps are usually asymptomatic; direct pressure during mastication may cause mild-to-moderate tenderness.
- Localized bleeding may occur, especially when the tissue is traumatized.
- Mobility of the tooth and sensitivity to percussion are usually absent.

Treatment

The root canal treatment is preferred in pulp polyp; however, formocresol pulpotomy has also been tried, especially in primary teeth. The removal of hyperplastic pulpal mass with a sharp spoon excavator, followed by control of bleeding, formocresol dressing and filling can be carried out in young teeth. The prognosis is favorable.

d. Internal/External Resorption

Trauma in the form of an accident or during cavity preparation, are considered as triggering mechanism for internal resorption. Internal resorption, if continued, may lead to pulp necrosis. Internal resorption is categorized in three forms, viz. surface, inflammatory and replacement resorption. Surface resorption usually remains undiagnosed and needs no treatment. Inflammatory resorption is common; occurs because of activation of odontoclasts within the inflamed pulp tissue. Radiographically, an oval-shaped area is seen along the canal walls. Apical periodontitis develops once the canal becomes infected. Replacement resorption is usually uncommon; dentin is resorbed and replaced by bone like tissue. This condition is usually asymptomatic; however, radiographically irregular enlargement of pulp space filled with bone-like tissues is evident.

External root resorption is usually caused by the transmission of bacterial toxins from infected pulp via dentinal tubules to an external root surface that might have been partly denuded of the cementum. Classic cells are stimulated to the region by inflammatory mediators such as prostaglandins and cytokines, which are liberated as part of the inflammatory process. The breakdown of dentin further stimulates pulpal inflammation (details in Chapter 27).

3. Pulp Degeneration

The degeneration of the pulp is seldom recognized clinically, especially at early stages. The degeneration generally affects older people, though teeth of younger people, as a result of persistent and mild irritation, may also get affected.

It may be induced by the attrition of teeth, erosion and bacterial invasion, etc. Once the pulp gets degenerated, the tooth becomes discolored and does not respond to pulp sensitivity tests; however, teeth with partial degeneration respond to external stimuli.

The pulpal degeneration is categorized as:

a. Calcific degeneration
b. Atrophic degeneration
c. Fibrous degeneration

a. Calcific Degeneration

Calcific degeneration (in the form of pulp stones or diffuse calcification) usually occur in response to trauma, caries, periodontal disease, or other irritants (Fig. 5.8a to d). The calcification is generally initiated in the pulp chamber; may involve root canal partially or complete. Complete calcification is referred to as 'canal obliteration'.

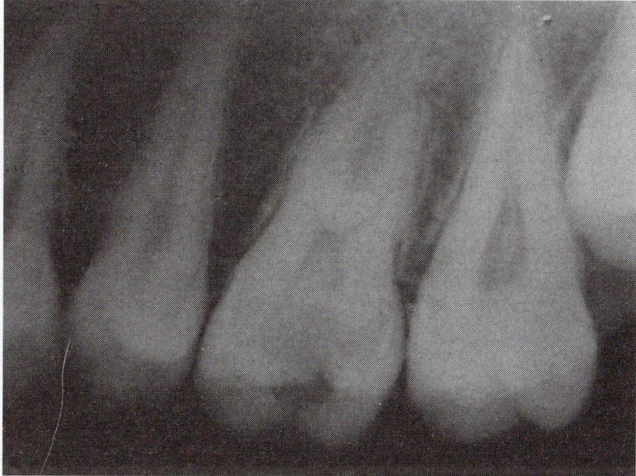

Fig. 5.8a Complete calcification of the pulp chamber and palatal root canal of maxillary first molar (may be due to caries)

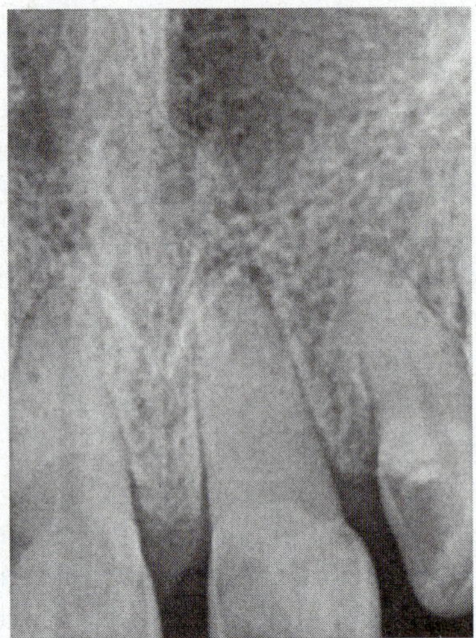

Fig. 5.8b Complete calcification of the pulp chamber and root canal of maxillary incisor (calcific degeneration of pulp: Canal obliteration)

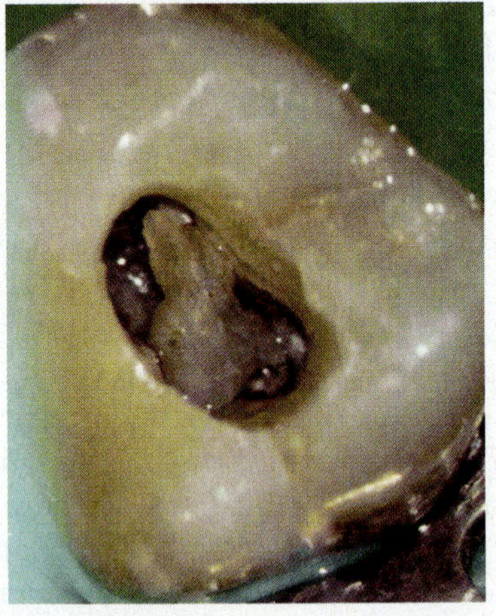

Fig. 5.8c Pulp stone in a coronal chamber under operating microscope

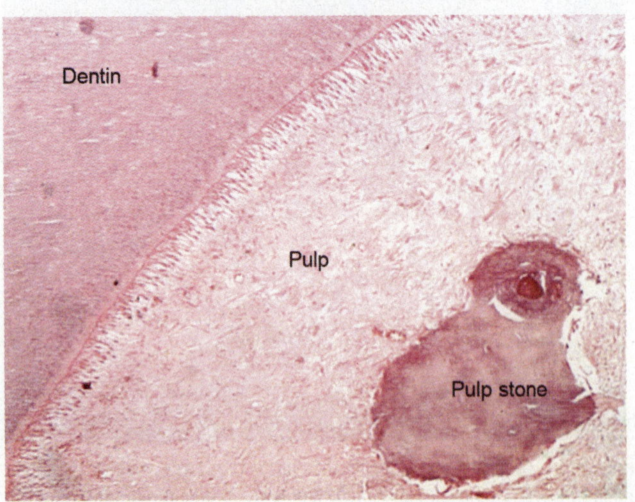

Fig. 5.8d Pulp stones in an aged dental pulp

Calcific degeneration does not represent the pathology of the pulp rather may occur with ageing or low grade irritation. The condition is recognized radiographically. Discrete areas of localized pulp necrosis resulting from small infarctions may be caused by deep scaling that interrupts the blood supply to a lateral canal, often lead to localized calcification as a defense reaction. The teeth are usually asymptomatic but may exhibit less sparkling appearance or looks more opaque and discolored.

Pulp canal obliteration: Key features

- Traumatized anterior teeth usually develop pulp canal obliteration
- Mostly teeth are symptom-free
- Pulp vitality tests are unreliable
- Discoloration is common clinical finding
- Require no treatment in routine; if need of treatment, calcification pose challenge

b. Atrophic Degeneration

Pulpal atrophy normally occurs with the advancing age. With age, the number and size of cells decreases and collagen fiber increases. The aged pulp seems less likely to resist various insults than the young, healthy and normal pulp. No significant clinical/radiographic signs are present. The size of pulp chamber is reduced and pulp may exhibit delayed response to pulp testing. No treatment is indicated.

c. Fibrous Degeneration

In this condition, the cellular content of the pulp is replaced by the fibrous connective tissue, which on removal from pulp gives a leathery fibrous appearance.

4. Pulp Necrosis

Pulp necrosis can be partial or total, depending on whether part or entire pulp is involved. The term 'Necrobiosis' is preferred in case of partial necrosis. It implies presence of bacteria within the necrotic part of the pulp, which may be invading the rest of the pulp tissue. Pulp sensitivity tests are usually inconclusive at this stage. The symptoms are mild/intermittent pain lingering for the last over many weeks. Radiographically signs of apical periodontitis are evident (usual widening of periodontal ligament). Once the pulp is invaded by bacteria, then the bacteria usually spread along the pulp tissue. Micro-organisms grow using pulp tissue as nutrient and slowly render the tooth pulpless. Necrosis is usually a sequel to inflammation (untreated caries, leaking restorations, failed pulp capping); may occur following traumatic injuries in which the pulp is destroyed before an inflammatory reaction takes place. Trauma leads to severing of apical blood supply if the tooth is displaced (luxation/avulsion) or significant damage to apical periodontal ligament (subluxation). The ischemic infarction, which develops may lead to dry gangrenous necrotic pulp (Fig. 5.9a and b). Radiographic changes are not significant unless there is apical involvement. Pain is also not present unless periodontal ligament is affected. Long standing necrosis leads to dull, continuous pain which increases with heat and temporarily subsides by cold. This might be due to the gases generated by bacteria in necrosed teeth, expands by heating causing pain and contract with cold which help to minimize the pain temporarily.

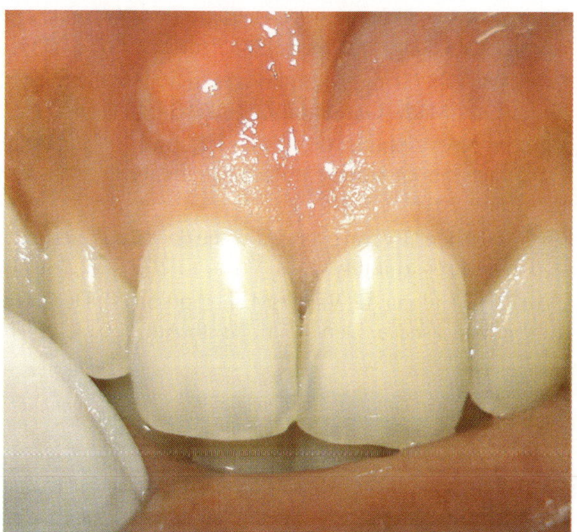

Fig. 5.9a Chronic periapical abscess in relation to maxillary right incisor with sinus formation (clinical)

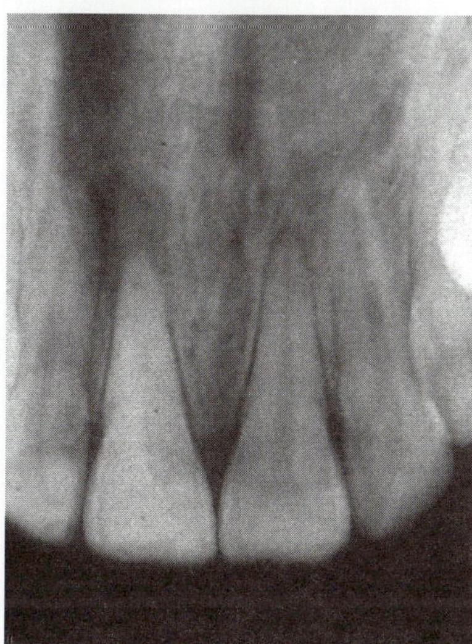

Fig. 5.9b Chronic periapical abscess in relation to maxillary right incisor (radiological)

Types of Pulp Necrosis

a. Coagulative
b. Liquefactive
c. Caseation

a. Coagulative necrosis: It is a type of necrosis caused by irreversible focal injury of pulp, most commonly due to ischemic cessation of blood flow. Soluble portion of pulp tissue is precipitated or converted into a solid mass.

b. Liquefactive necrosis: This type of necrosis of pulp occurs following ischemic injury and bacterial infection. Affected pulp becomes soft and liquefied in the centre containing necrotic debris.

c. Caseation necrosis: It is a form of necrosis wherein combined features of both coagulation and liquefaction necrosis is seen. The pulp tissue is soft, granular and converted into a cheesy mass consisting of coagulated proteins.

The summary of pulp condition and treatment strategies is tabulated in Table 5.3.

Table 5.3 Pulp condition and treatment strategies

Condition of the pulp	*Treatment strategies*
Dentin hypersensitivity	• Occlusion of exposed dentinal tubules with desensitizing agents.
Reversible pulpitis (acute and chronic)	• Removal of the cause • Follow-up to assess healing • If not healed, root canal treatment
Irreversible pulpitis (acute and chronic)	• Routine endodontic treatment
Chronic hyperplastic pulpitis	• Conventional root canal treatment if apices are mature • Formocresol pulpotomy in young teeth
Pulp atrophy	• No treatment required, if physiological • If pathological, remove the cause
Pulp calcification (partial and total)	• No treatment required unless the canal is infected • If infected, conventional endodontic treatment
Root resorption (external/internal)	• Conventional endodontic treatment with regenerative medicaments in the canal
Pulp necrosis	• Conventional endodontic treatment • Surgical intervention, if necessary

The end products of pulp decomposition are those of protein decomposition, namely hydrogen sulfide, ammonia, fatty substances, water and carbon dioxide. The intermediate products such as indole, skatole, putrescine and cadaverine, contribute to the unpleasant odor sometimes emanating from the root canal.

BIBLIOGRAPHY

1. Abott PV and Yu C. A clinical classification of the status of the pulp and the root canal system. Aust. Dent. J. Endod.: 2007; 52:S17–S31.
2. Abott PV. Assessing restored teeth with pulp and periapical diseases for the presence of cracks, caries and marginal breakdown. Aust. Dent. J.: 2004; 49:33–39.
3. Abott PV. Classification, diagnosis and clinical manifestation of apical periodontitis. Endod. Topics: 2004; 8:36–54.
4. Abott PV. The periapical space – dynamic interface. Ann. R Australas Coll. Dent. Surg.: 2000; 15:223–234.
5. Ali SG and Mulay S. Pulpitis: A review. IOSR J. Dent. and Med. Sci.: 2015; 14:92–97.
6. Bender IB. Reversible and irreversible painful pulpitides: diagnosis and treatment. Aust. Endod. J.: 2000; 26:10–14.
7. Dummer PM, Hicks R and Huws D. Clinical signs and symptoms in pulp disease. Int. Endod. J.: 1980; 13:27–35.
8. Dummer PM, Hicks R and Huws D. Clinical signs and symptoms in pulp disease. Int. Endod. J.: 1980; 13:27–35.
9. Goga R, Chandler P and Oginni AO. Pulp stones: a review. Int. Endod. J.: 2008; 41:457–468.
10. Jansson L, Ehnevid H, Lindskog S and Blomlof L. Development of periapical lesions. Swed. Dent. J.: 1993; 17:85–93.
11. Johnson RH, Dachi SF and Haley JV. Pulpal hyperaemia: a correlation of clinical and histologic data from 706 teeth. J. Am. Dent. Assoc.: 1970; 81:108–117.
12. Levin LG, Law AS, Holland GR, Abbott PV and Roda RS. Identify and define all diagnostic terms for pulpal health and disease states. J. Endod.: 2009; 35:1645–1657.
13. Nair PN. Apical periodontitis: a dynamic encounter between root canal infection and host response. Periodontol 2000: 1997; 13:121–148.
14. Oginni AO, Sofowora CAA and Kolawole KA. Evaluation of radiographs, clinical signs and symptoms associated with pulp canal obliteration: an aid to treatment decision. Dent. Traumatology.: 2009; 25:620–625.
15. Paterson RC and Pountney SK. Pulp response to *Streptococcus mutans*. Oral Surg., Oral Med., Oral Pathol.: 1987; 64:339–347.
16. Smith JW. Calcific metamorphosis: a treatment dilemma. Oral Surg., Oral Med., Oral Pathol.: 1982; 54:441–444.
17. Vibhute NA, Vibhute AH, Daule RT, Bsal PP and Aditi M. Hard facts about stones: pulpal calcifications: A review. J. Pat. Care: 2016; 2:1–4.
18. Yu C and Abbott PV. An overview of the dental pulp: its functions and responses to injury. Aust. Dent. J.: 2007; 52:84–116.
19. Zero DT, Zandona AF, Vail, MM and Spolnik KJ. Dental caries and pulpal disease. Dent. Clin. North Am.: 2011; 29–46.

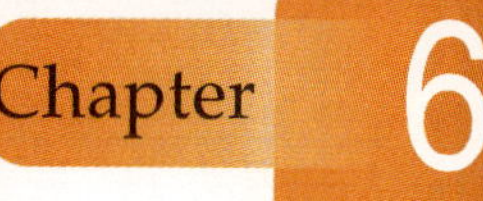

Chapter 6

Diseases of Periradicular Tissues

The periradicular tissues have an unlimited source of undifferentiated cells that participate in inflammation and repair as well. These tissues do have rich collateral blood supply and lymphatic drainage. The rich blood supply usually counter act the destructive activities of the irritants from within and outside the root canal. Depending on severity of irritation, duration and host response, periradicular pathosis may range from mild inflammation to extensive damage of periodontal attachment tissues. The injury leads to cellular damage, releasing specific and non-specific immunologic mediators of the inflammatory process.

Periradicular inflammation gets initiated during pulpal inflammation and even before the pulp is completely necrotic. Micro-organisms, their degradation products, mediators of inflammation and damaging pulpal tissues stimulate the inflammatory reaction in the periradicular tissues. That is why, many a times, the pulp may remain partially vital, along with periradicular pathosis.

The structures surrounding the apex of tooth roots where the apical foramina are located, are known as the *'periradicular tissues'* (peri = around, radicular = root). The tissues around apical foramen/root apex are composed of cementum, periodontal ligament and the alveolar bone. The micro-organisms from infected pulp tissues may invade these periapical tissues via apical foramen and/or lateral/accessory canals trespassing the root cementum. The lesions produced by periapical infection are generally in close proximity to the apices of the teeth. Periapical lesions are mainly recognized during radiographic examination. Clinically, these lesions can be diagnosed by patient's symptoms; however, visual-intraoral examination may not be adequate to identify these lesions.

DEFINITION

Periradicular diseases are defined as *'the diseases occurring around the apex of a tooth, may be of endodontic or non-endodontic origin.'* The periradicular lesions generally are of inflammatory origin; however, a few periradicular lesions may not be due to inflamed/necrotic pulps.

GENERAL FEATURES

The micro-organisms that cause dental caries do not confine to enamel only. The microbes invade dentin and the pulp as they progress and multiply. If caries is not treated during the initial stages, bacteria gain access to the pulp through the dentinal tubules. As they enter the pulp, an inflammatory reaction is produced, which leads to pulpal diseases and subsequently, pulp necrosis. From the pulp, bacteria can enter the surrounding bone through the apical foramen. The ensuing response of the tissues surrounding the apical foramina may result in periradicular diseases.

The periradicular diseases are mainly caused by bacteria prevalent in necrosed pulp. The necrosis of pulp is generally the sequelae of bacterial invasion of pulp or in few cases the cracked teeth. The traumatic injuries, may be in later stages, also lead to pulp necrosis.

Since periradicular inflammation involves the periodontal ligament and the alveolar process (two important components of the periodontium), the term 'periodontitis' is used. More so, if the inflammation is confined to the apical region, the term 'apical periodontitis' is used, which can be acute or chronic.

The periradicular diseases can be of endodontic (pulp) origin or non-endodontic origin. Pulp inflammation may invade the periapical tissues leading to periradicular diseases; periapical tissues may get involved due to periodontal diseases, trauma and/or remnants of odontogenic epithelium causing periradicular cysts, etc. A few iatrogenic causes (chemical irrigants/medicaments, over-instrumentation of root canals) also lead to periradicular diseases.

Periradicular diseases: possible causes

Bacterial
- Infection from pulp
- Infection from periodontium

Traumatic
- Physical trauma (blow)
- Traumatic occlusion
- Aggressive thermal stimulus

Chemical/Iatrogenic
- Irrigants and intracanal medicaments
- Over-instrumentation/overfilling of root canals

CLASSIFICATION

The earlier investigators classified periradicular diseases as:

i. Nonseptic pericementitis
ii. Septic pericementitis
iii. Pericemental abscess (inflammation of periapical tissues without infection)
iv. Alveolar abscess (infection with or without sinus)

The term 'pericementitis' was later changed to 'periodontitis'. Three main categories of periodontitis were recognized, viz. traumatic, chemical/iatrogenic and bacterial. The diseases of periapical tissues have been identified on this categorization.

Over the years the diseases of periapical tissues have been defined and classified by different authors.

The commonly referred classifications are:

Prinz's classification

1. Acute pericementitis
   i. Acute apical pericementitis
   ii. Acute marginal pericementitis
   iii. Acute diffuse suppurative pericementitis
   iv. Acute intraradicular pericementitis
2. Chronic pericementitis
   i. Chronic apical suppurative pericementitis
   ii. Chronic proliferative pericementitis

Coolidge's classification

1. Acute inflammation
   i. Traumatic and chemical periodontitis
   ii. Apical periodontitis from infection
   iii. Acute alveolar abscess
2. Chronic inflammation
   i. Suppurative periodontitis
   ii. Proliferative periodontitis
3. Granuloma
4. Radicular cyst
5. Condensing osteitis

6

Grossman's classification

1. Acute apical periodontitis
2. Acute alveolar abscess
3. Chronic alveolar abscess
4. Subacute alveolar abscess
5. Granuloma
6. Cyst

Later, the classification was modified as follows:

1. Acute periradicular disease
   a. Acute apical periodontitis (vital and non-vital)
   b. Acute alveolar abscess
   c. Phoenix abscess
2. Chronic periradicular diseases
   a. Chronic apical periodontitis
      - Chronic alveolar abscess
      - Cystic apical periodontitis/radicular cysts
   b. Persistent apical periodontitis
3. Condensing osteitis
4. External root resorption
5. Diseases of non-endodontic origin

WHO (World Health Organization) classification

WHO specified periradicular disease by coding; the codes are:

Code 4.4: Acute apical periodontitis (apical periodontitis of pulp origin)

Code 4.5: Chronic apical periodontitis (granuloma)

Code 4.6: Periapical abscess with sinus to maxillary antrum
- Sinus with nasal cavity
- Sinus with oral cavity
- Sinus with skin

Code 4.7: Periapical abscess without sinus (dento-alveolar abscess and periodontal abscess)

Code 4.8: Radicular cyst (apical periodontal cyst, periapical cyst)
- Apical and lateral cyst
- Residual cyst
- Inflammatory paradental cyst

Code 4.9: Unspecified diseases of pulp and periapical tissues

WHO further subdivided the diseases of periapical tissues into four categories:

i. Distribution of inflammatory cells in the lesion
ii. Whether epithelial cells are present or absent
iii. Whether the lesion is transformed to cyst
iv. Relationship of cyst cavity to root canal of the affected tooth

Ingle's classification

Ingle's classified periradicular diseases as painful and non-painful.

1. Painful periradicular diseases
   a. Acute apical periodontitis
   b. Advanced apical periodontitis
      i. Acute apical abscess
      ii. Phoenix abscess
      iii. Chronic apical abscess (suppurative apical periodontitis)
2. Non-painful periradicular diseases
   a. Condensing osteitis
   b. Chronic apical periodontitis
      i. Incipient stage
      ii. Advanced stage
         - Periapical granuloma
         - Suppurative apical periodontitis
         - Apical cyst

The definitions of commonly used terms associated with periradicular diseases are briefed in Table 6.1.

Table 6.1 Periradicular lesions; definitions of commonly used terms

Terms	*Definition*
Normal periapical tissues	The lamina dura surrounding the tooth is intact along with uniform periodontal ligament space (teeth will not be abnormally sensitive to percussion or palpation)
Acute periapical periodontitis	Inflammation of the apical periodontium producing clinical symptoms, viz. painful response to biting and percussion
Sub-acute periapical periodontitis	Inflammation of the apical periodontium producing mild clinical symptoms as compared to acute periapical periodontitis
Cellulitis	Acute and edematous spread of an acute inflammatory process; abscess, which cannot establish drainage, may spread diffusely through fascial planes of soft tissues
Parulis	A mass of subacutely inflamed granulation tissue at the intraoral opening of a sinus tract
Abscess	Localized collection of purulent exudate (pus) in a cavity formed by the disintegration of tissues
Pus	A product of inflammation consisting of leucocyte, degenerated tissue elements, tissue fluids and micro-organisms
Sinus	A hollow space in a bone or other tissues; literally, a hollow cavity in skull connecting with nasal cavity
Sinus tract	A tract leading to a suppurating cavity
Chronic periapical periodontitis	Inflammation and destruction of apical periodontium that is of pulpal origin which does not produce clinical symptoms (a periradicular radiolucent area may be present)
Acute periapical abscess/ Acute apical abscess/ Acute periradicular abscess/ Acute alveolar abscess/ Dentoalveolar abscess	An inflammatory reaction to pulpal infection characterized by rapid onset, spontaneous pain, tenderness, pus formation and eventual swelling of the associated tissues
Chronic periradicular abscess/ Suppurative periradicular periodontitis/ Chronic periapical abscess/ Chronic alveolar abscess/ Chronic dentoalveolar abscess	An inflammatory reaction to pulpal infection and necrosis characterized by gradual onset, little/no discomfort and the intermittent discharge of pus through an associated sinus tract
Periapical scar	The defect created by periapical inflammatory lesion may be filled with dense collagenous tissues rather than normal bony tissue (usually occurs when both facial and lingual cortical plates have been lost)
Condensing osteitis/ Sclerosing osteitis/ Periradicular osteosclerosis/ Focal sclerosing osteomyelitis/ Sclerotic bone	A diffuse radiopaque lesion, representing a localized bony reaction to a low grade inflammatory stimulus, usually seen at the apex of a tooth (or its extraction site, where there might be a long standing pulp pathosis)
Sequestrum	A fragment of necrotic bone that has been separated from the adjacent vital bone

A. PERIRADICULAR DISEASES OF ENDODONTIC ORIGIN

The periradicular lesions of endodontic origin are mainly categorized as:

1. Acute periradicular lesions
2. Chronic periradicular lesions

Periradicular lesions of shorter duration associated with symptoms such as pain are known as acute or symptomatic; whereas, those of longer duration with mild or no symptoms are termed as chronic or asymptomatic.

1. Acute Periradicular Lesions

The initial response of inflammation in periradicular tissues is pain. The polymorphonuclear cells and the edematous fluid fill the space between the tooth and the bone, thereby increasing the pressure, which compresses the nerve endings resulting in severe pain. The pain continues until bone is resorbed creating some space, which accommodates the fluid and releases the pressure.

Acute periradicular lesions are the following types:

a. Acute apical periodontitis
b. Acute apical/alveolar abscess
c. Acute exacerbation of chronic lesion (phoenix abscess)

a. Acute Apical Periodontitis

Acute apical periodontitis is the inflammation of the periodontium as a result of trauma, bacterial infection initiating from within the root canal space, regardless of the pulp being vital or non-vital. The lesions are painful, especially during biting and on percussion.

Causes of acute apical periodontitis in a vital pulp

- Trauma caused by an abnormal or premature occlusal contact (seen in recently placed occlusal restoration).
- Forceful wedging of an object between the teeth; for example, tooth pick, wedge, use of separators during restorative and orthodontic procedures, rubber dam application etc.
- Blow on to the tooth.

Causes of acute apical periodontitis in a non-vital pulp

- As a sequel of pulpal diseases; diffusion of potential irritants from within the pulp spaces.
- Over instrumentation during root canal cleaning and shaping procedure.
- Micro-organism and debris are pushed inadvertently into the periradicular tissues during root canal preparation.
- Forcing of irritating medicaments like formocresol in the periradicular tissues.
- Extension of root canal filling material into the periradicular tissues, which acts as a continuous source of irritation.

Diagnosis

Patient may inform as regard recently placed occlusal restoration. Application of pressure by finger tip or lightly tapping the tooth with the butt end of the mouth mirror results in excruciating pain.

Acute apical periodontitis, as a sequel of pulp necrosis, may not respond to pulp vitality tests; whereas, acute apical periodontitis caused by an abnormal occlusal contact responds normally to the pulp vitality tests.

Differential diagnosis

A differential diagnosis should be made between the acute apical periodontitis and acute apical abscess. The patient's history, signs—symptoms and clinical examination can differentiate between these two periradicular entities.

Signs and symptoms

- Severe pain (throbbing/constant)
- Tender on percussion (pain on biting)
- Tooth may be slightly elevated from its socket because of pressure of fluid collected in the periradicular tissues
- Delayed vitality tests
- No swelling

Radiographic features

The Lamina dura remains intact without any break in continuity, especially in case of vital pulps. The periodontal ligament space may appear normal or slightly enlarged (Fig. 6.1).

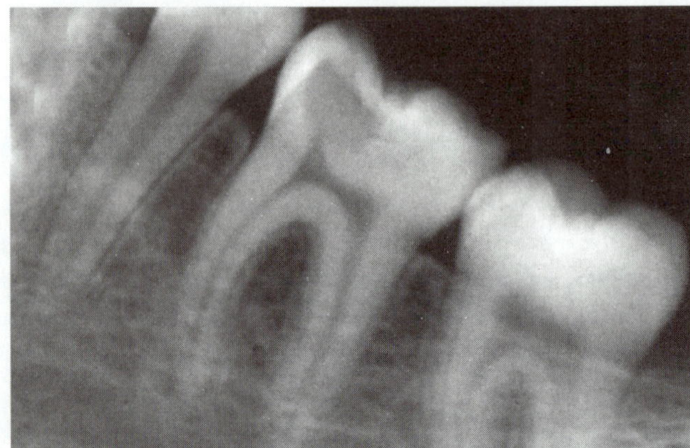

Fig. 6.1 Acute apical periodontitis (slight widening of periodontal ligament in mandibular first molar)

Histological features

Inflammatory reaction leads to dilatation of blood vessels. Polymorphonuclear cells initiate inflammatory response (polymorphonuclear cells and macrophages are visible within a localized area at the apex). Serous exudate accumulates; subsequently leading to distension of periodontal ligament spaces. A small area of liquefaction necrosis may be evident. In case irritation continues, it may lead to bone/root resorption. Initial bone and/or root resorption are not evident radiographically; however, may be identified histologically.

Treatment

It is important to understand whether acute apical periodontitis is associated with a vital or non vital pulp. Determining the cause and relieving the patient's acute symptoms accordingly is the line of treatment. Root canal treatment can be initiated, if pulp is involved. Appropriate anti-inflammatory analgesics can also be prescribed.

Prognosis is usually favorable.

Acute apical periodontitis: Key features
- Tooth may be vital or non-vital
- Throbbing/constant pain
- No swelling
- Pain on percussion (pain on biting)
- Pulp vitality tests can be negative
- Lamina dura remains intact; periodontal ligament can be slightly widened
- Removal of cause should be the priority; root canal treatment in case tooth is non-vital

b. Acute Apical/Alveolar Abscess

Acute apical/alveolar abscess is a localized collection of pus in the alveolar bone around the root apex; the infection following necrosis of pulp extends through the apical foramen into the periapical tissues. The abscess is sequel of the apical periodontitis.

Etiology

- Bacterial invasion from the necrotic pulp
- Traumatic/chemical involvement of pulp
- Mechanical irritation may also lead to acute apical abscess

Signs and symptoms

Depending upon severity of the reaction, patients with acute apical abscess usually have signs/symptoms as:
- Moderate to severe discomfort/swelling
- Systemic manifestations of an infective process such as high temperature, malaise and leukocytosis
- The tooth is often elevated in its socket and interferes in occlusion.
- Spontaneous or throbbing pain
- Tender on percussion

Diagnosis

The affected tooth does not respond to electric and thermal tests. Clinical examination can be effective in diagnosing acute abscess. The tooth may be tender on percussion; apical mucosa is tender on palpation and the tooth may be mobile and extruded.

Radiographic features

The radiographic features range from thickening of periodontal ligament space to a frank resorptive lesion. Initial lesions do not show much changes (only widened periodontal ligament); as hard tissues get involved, definite radiolucency can be seen (Fig. 6.2).

Histological features

Increase in pressure leads to hypoxia of pulp tissues; subsequently formation of pus because of breakdown of polymorphonuclear cells and lysis of pulp remnants.

Histological features show a localized lesion of liquefaction necrosis containing numerous polymorphonuclear cells, debris, cell remnants and an accumulation of purulent exudates.

The abscess is usually surrounded by granulomatous tissues; therefore, the lesion is categorized as an abscess within a granuloma. Significantly, the abscess may not communicate directly with the apical foramen.

Treatment

Usually, acute abscess is an emergency since the patient is in great agony. The main objective of emergency management is to relieve the periradicular pressure by establishing the drainage. Most common approach is

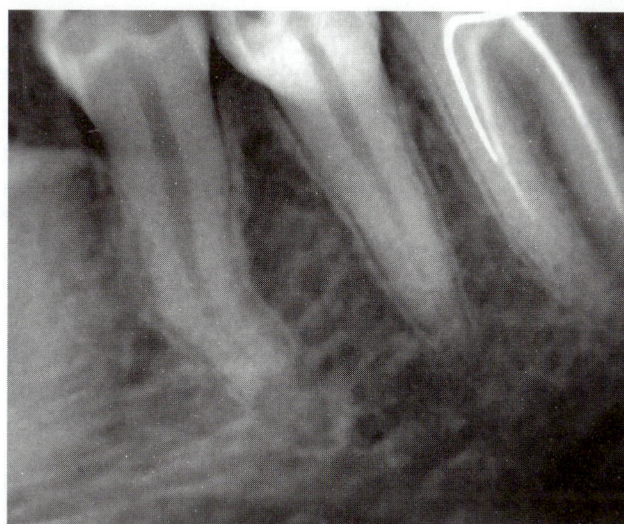

Fig. 6.2 Acute apical abscess (widening of periodontal ligament in mandibular second premolar)

6

to open the tooth and allow purulent exudates to escape through the root canals. After the drainage, the conventional endodontic treatment can be carried out. In case, where the drainage is not established through the root canal, surgical incision and drainage can be carried out through the periapical tissues. Antibiotics and anti-inflammatory analgesics can be prescribed. The tooth should be dis-occluded slightly, if it is extruded from its socket.

Prognosis is usually favourable.

Acute alveolar/apical abscess: Key features

- Non-vital tooth (do not respond to vitality tests)
- Palpable swelling
- Spontaneous/throbbing pain
- Tender on percussion
- Systemic manifestation (fever, malaise, etc.)
- Tooth extruded from socket (not mobile)
- Widening of periodontal ligament to frank radiolucency
- Drainage through root canal or periapical tissues is effective; followed by root canal treatment
- Good prognosis

c. Acute Exacerbation of Chronic Lesion (Phoenix Abscess)

Phoenix Abscess is a condition in which acute suppurative inflammation is superimposed on an existing chronic apical periodontitis (acute exacerbation of a chronic lesion).

The chronic lesions like periradicular granuloma or the cyst, suddenly present acute inflammatory symptoms. The spontaneous metamorphosis from dormant chronicity to a sudden, acute condition gives the analogy of 'Phoenix'. Phoenix, a mythological bird, was destroyed in fire that arose again from the ashes to start another life. Chronic apical periodontitis was equated to the ashes and an acute apical abscess was the Phoenix coming to life.

A phoenix abscess may develop spontaneously and immediately after the initiation of endodontic treatment on an asymptomatic tooth. As the root canals are opened, the equilibrium of environment of chronic periradicular lesion gets altered; inadvertent entry of micro-organism and the debris into the periapical tissues subsequently leads to acute inflammation (the micro-organisms in chronic lesions remain in equilibrium with the surrounding environment).

Signs and symptoms

- Swelling; acute and spontaneous
- Cellulitis of the area (Fig. 6.3)
- Recent history of initiating root canal treatment
- Patient in discomfort; facial asymmetry

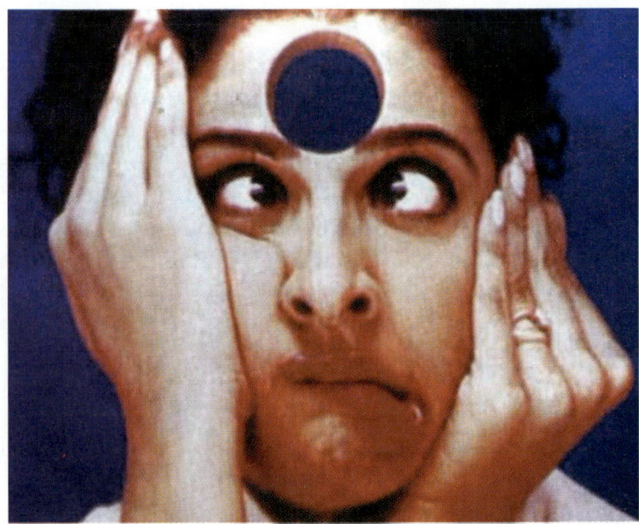

Fig. 6.3 Phoenix abscess (clinical presentation)

Diagnosis

Lack of response to vitality test is indicative of necrotic pulp. In rare cases, a tooth may respond to the electric pulp test because of fluid in the root canal; or in a multi-rooted tooth. Only history and associated symptoms distinguish phoenix abscess from acute alveolar abscess. The tooth is tender on percussion. Cellulitis of the area is evident.

Radiographic features

Radiographs show radiolucent areas as prevalent in chronic periradicular lesions. A well-defined peri-radicular lesion is evident.

Treatment

Only anti-inflammatory drugs including steroids are helpful. Antiallergic drugs (antihistamines) are also effective. Surgical incision etc. is not advised.

Phoenix abscess: Key features

- Acute exacerbation of existing chronic lesion
- Change in equilibrium of microbes; initiation of root canal treatment of long-standing chronic case facilitates ingress of micro-organisms/debris, etc. into periapical tissues
- Cellulitis of the area
- Radiographic picture of chronic lesion
- Pulp vitality tests are negative
- Anti-inflammatory analgesics and antihistamines are effective

2. Chronic Periradicular Lesions

The periradicular lesions mainly develop due to the infected pulp. As the micro-organisms grow and multiply, they start extruding into the periapical area. When bacterial infection or by-products of the micro-organisms enter periapical tissues, the patient's defense usually cope with the irritants. If the micro-organisms are virulent and sufficient in number, acute inflammation (acute apical abscess) sets in; however, in case, micro-organisms are less virulent and/or less in number, the inflammation usually turns into a chronic lesion. If the source of the irritants is not removed, the periapical tissues are continually exposed to these bacterial irritants. The initial acute inflammation, as the time passes, may become chronic. Healing of the periradicular lesion takes place only when the continuous extrusion of the micro-organism is stopped by performing the endodontic treatment procedure. Occasionally, however, an area within a chronic inflammatory reaction may exacerbate (flare up) producing a focus of acute inflammation. If no treatment is initiated, the inflammation progress; the epithelial cell rests of Malassez, which are present in the apical area, start proliferating and the lesion turns gradually into a granuloma. As the granuloma increases in size because of the proliferation of cells within, the central mass starts liquefying and forms an individual small cystic spots. As these cystic spots grow, they coalesce eventually and form a big cystic lesion.

Since, periapical chronic inflammation is long-lasting and is stimulated by continual irritation; different disease entities are possible.

The chronic periradicular lesions are:

a. Chronic apical/alveolar abscess (suppurative apical periodontitis)
b. Periapical granuloma
c. Periapical cyst
d. Apical scar
e. Condensing osteitis

a. Chronic Apical/Alveolar Abscess (Suppurative Apical Periodontitis)

Chronic apical/alveolar abscess is a long standing, low grade infection from within the root canal space that has resulted in an abscess.

Etiology

Chronic apical/alveolar abscess has a pathogenesis similar to the acute apical/alveolar abscess, that is, pulpal necrosis. The abscess may burrow through bone and soft tissues to form a sinus tract on to the oral mucosa (Fig. 6.4a and b) or sometimes, extra-orally (Fig. 6.5). It may also drain through the periodontium into the sulcus.

Signs and symptoms

The condition is usually asymptomatic. Such an abscess is detected only during the routine radiographic examination or because of presence of the sinus tract. The sinus tract may be lined partially or completely by

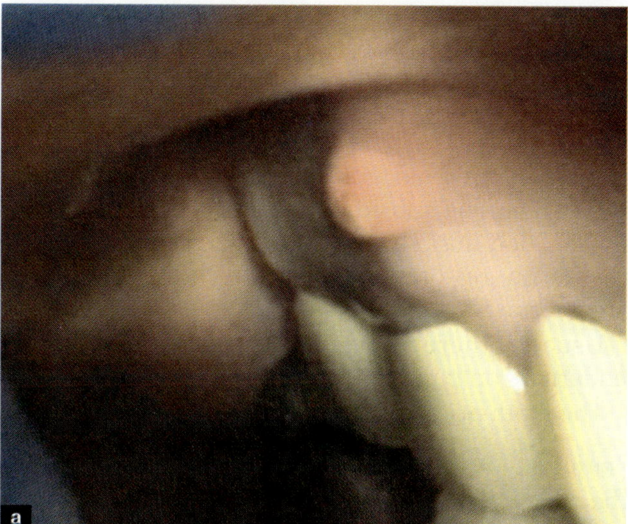

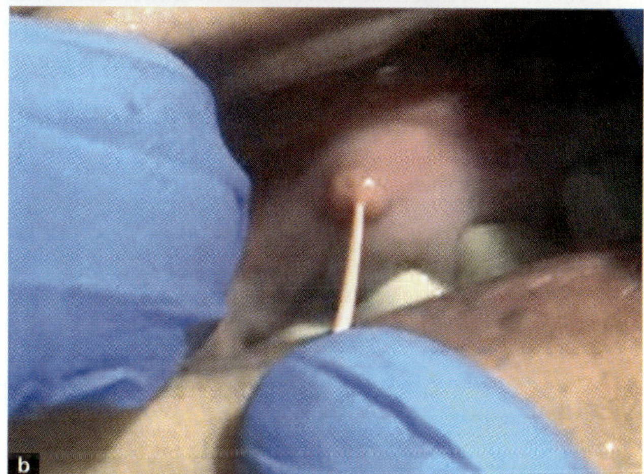

Fig. 6.4 (a) Chronic apical abscess (sinus in oral mucosa); (b) Sinus tract being checked with gutta-percha

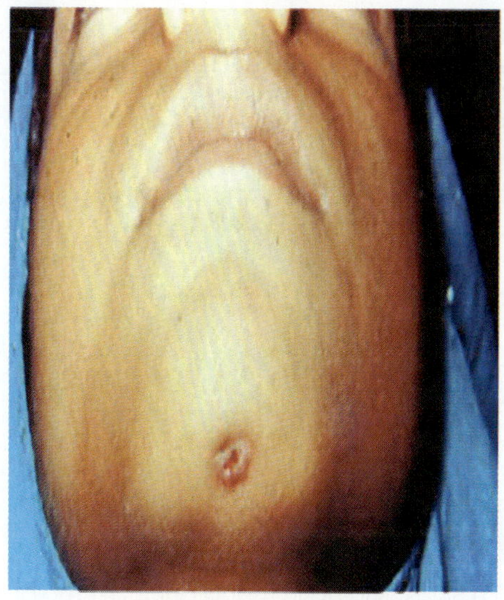

Fig. 6.5 Extra oral sinus

epithelium surrounded by inflamed connective tissues. The sinus tract prevents exacerbation or swelling by providing continual drainage of the purulent exudates.

Diagnosis

The patient presents with past history of sudden sharp pain which has subsided and not recurred. Clinical examination may show a large open carious lesion or large leaky restoration under which the pulp might have necrosed.

Usually, there is no pain on percussion and no tenderness on palpation.

The tooth does not respond to vitality tests.

Radiographic features

The radiograph shows a diffuse area of bone rarefaction; however, it is not a definite diagnosis. Origin of sinus tract can be diagnosed by putting gutta-percha cone in to the sinus and getting a routine periapical radiograph (sinus tracing, Fig. 6.6a and b). Accurate diagnosis can only be confirmed by histopathological examination of the lesion.

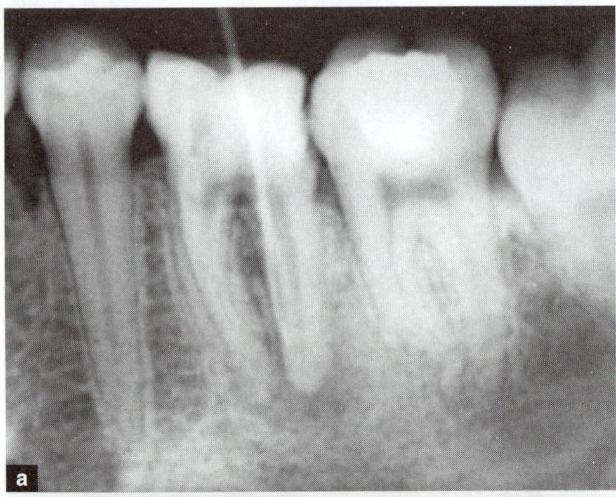

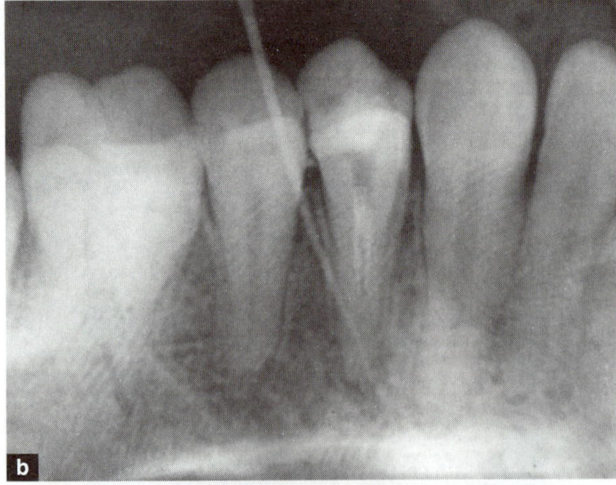

Fig. 6.6 (a) Sinus tracing in mandibular first molar, (b) Sinus tracing in maxillary premolars

Treatment

The routine endodontic treatment eliminates infection from the root canal. The sinus tract also resolves following root canal treatment. The extraoral sinus opening tract may need be surgically excised. Prognosis is usually favourable.

Chronic apical/alveolar abscess: Key features

- Long standing non-vital teeth
- Pulp necrosis elements slowly and continuously irritating; turn to chronic abscess
- Usually asymptomatic
- Mostly associated with sinus tract formation; may be mucosal or extraoral skin
- Vitality tests negative
- Conventional root canal treatment preferred
- Surgical excision of extraoral sinus, if need be
- Source of sinus tract can be diagnosed by putting guttapercha in the tract and getting it radiographed (sinus tracing)

b. Periapical Granuloma

Periapical granuloma is a mass of chronically inflamed granulomatous tissues at the root apex resulting from pulp necrosis and extrusion of the micro-organism and their toxins into the periradicular tissues.

A granuloma contains granulation tissues and chronic inflammatory cells infiltrating its fibrous connective tissue stroma. This is why the term 'granulomatous' rather than 'granulation' is used in referring the granuloma.

A granuloma may be seen as a chronic low grade defensive reaction of the alveolar bone to the irritation from the necrosed pulp. The granulomatous tissues may vary in size from a fraction of millimeter to a centimeter or even larger. It may consist of fibrous capsule which is continuous with the periodontal ligament and a central portion full of loose connective tissues and blood vessels. It is characterized by the presence of lymphocytes, plasma cells, mononuclear and polymorphonuclear cells. The epithelial cells rest of Malassez are also seen within the periodontal ligament, which are derived from the Hertwig's epithelial root sheath.

Etiology

The granuloma is developed from infection/irritation from necrosed pulp; subsequently stimulating cellular reaction at the periapex.

Signs and symptoms

It is usually asymptomatic, except in cases where it breaks down and undergoes suppuration.

Diagnosis

The condition is generally discovered during the routine radiographic examination. The involved tooth is not tender on percussion. The mucosa overlying the apex of the concerned tooth may or may not be tender to palpation.

The tooth does not respond to pulp vitality tests.

Differential diagnosis

A granuloma cannot be differentiated from other periradicular lesion unless the tissue is evaluated histopathologically.

Radiographic features

Initially, periodontal ligament thickening is a common finding. The tooth shows well-defined area of rarefaction at the periapex and there is break in the continuity of the lamina dura (Fig. 6.7a). Root resorption may also be seen at the apical area (Fig. 6.7b).

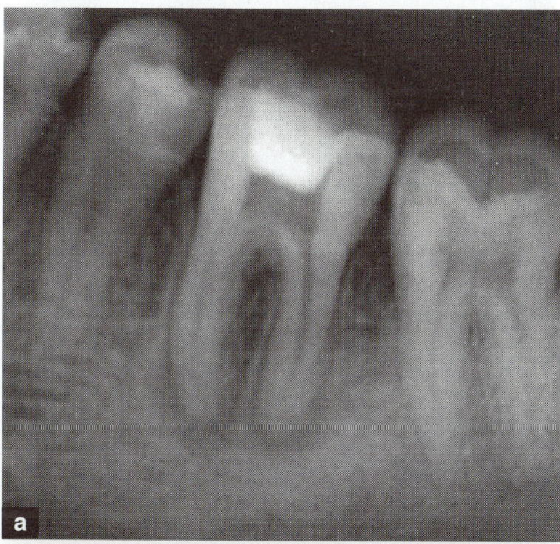

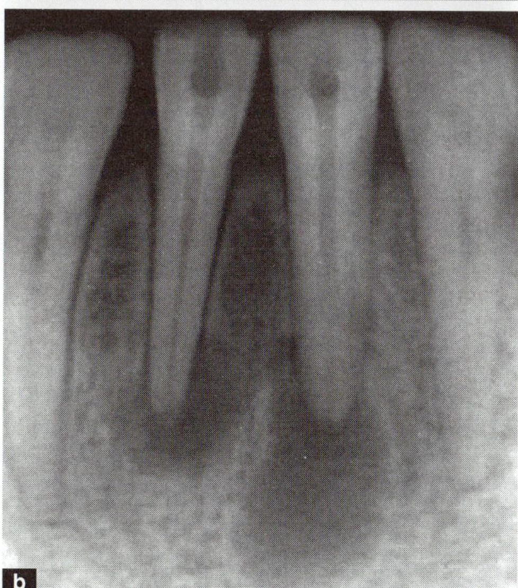

Fig. 6.7 (a) Periapical granuloma in mandibular first molar; (b) Periapical granuloma in mandibular anterior teeth; (Note: Apical resorption)

Histopathological features

The lesion is characterized by predominance of lymphocytes, plasma cells and macrophages surrounded by relatively uninflamed fibrous capsule. The surrounding coverage is made up of collagen, fibroblasts and rich vascular network (Fig. 6.8). As the inflammatory reaction continues, the exudates collect at the expense of the surrounding alveolar bone. At the periphery, fibroblasts actively build fibrous wall. The alveolar bone at the periphery may show resorption due to the presence of osteoclast cells (neutrophils cause localized tissue destruction, stimulating osteoclasts, which cause resorption of bone; periodontal ligament space widens and radiolucency develops). Prolonged inflammation without any treatment stimulates resorption of bone in the affected tooth, resulting in loosening of the tooth.

Treatment

The conventional root canal therapy is the treatment of choice. The patient is evaluated periodically to observe the resolution of periradicular radiolucency. Usually, the healing and establishment of normal periradicular architecture is achieved in 6 months to 1 year. Surgical intervention may be necessary, if not healed.

Prognosis is good.

Periapical granuloma: Key features

- Sequelae to chronic pulpal infection (long standing non-vital tooth)
- Mostly asymptomatic
- No pain on percussion (pain only if it turns to acute stage); no tenderness on palpation
- Chronic inflamed tissue collected at root apex; plenty of cells and fibrous tissue
- Loss of continuity of lamina dura; well-defined area of rarefaction
- Conventional root canal therapy is effective
- Prognosis is good

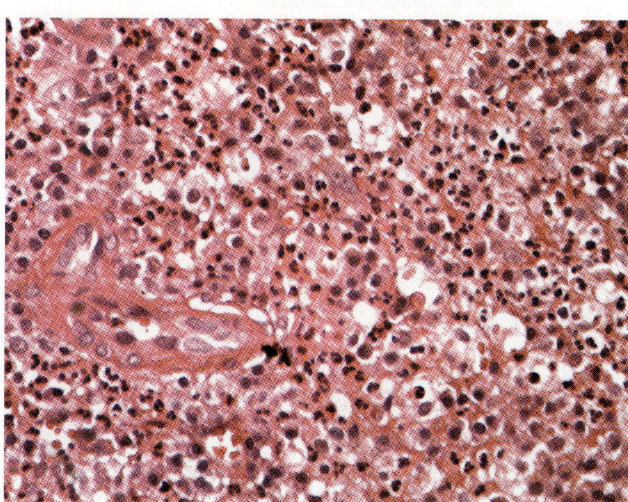

Fig. 6.8 Microphotograph of pyogenic granuloma (H&E x 40)

c. Periapical Cyst

Periapical cyst is a chronic inflammatory response of periapex that develops from a pre-existing granulomatous tissue. It is characterized by a central fluid filled epithelium lined cavity surrounded by granulomatous tissue and peripheral fibrous encapsulation (Fig. 6.9).

Periapical cyst is an acute inflammatory cyst with a distinct pathologic cavity completely enclosed in an epithelial lining (no communication with the root canal); whereas, periapical pocket cyst is an apical inflammatory cyst containing a sac like epithelial lined cavity (communication with the root canal). Cyst may also develop after tooth extraction at the site of extraction (Fig. 6.10).

Signs and symptoms

A periradicular cyst may not present any specific symptom. It may become large enough and present as swelling. The symptoms of necrosed pulp are, however, evident.

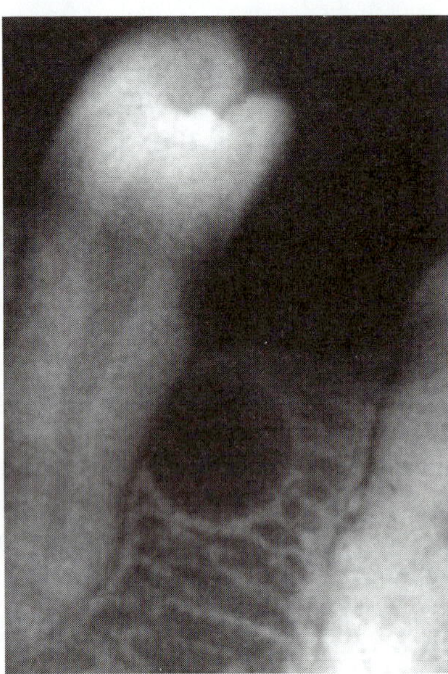

Fig. 6.9 Lateral periodontal cyst

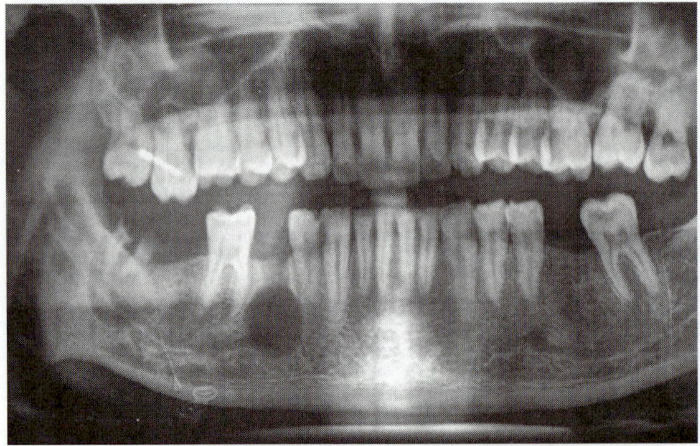

Fig. 6.10 Residual cyst after tooth extraction

Diagnosis

The tooth may not respond to vitality tests; only radiographs are helpful. On radiographic examination, there is loss of continuity of lamina dura with an area of rarefaction.

Differential Diagnosis

The radiograph can be helpful in identifying whether the lesion is granuloma or cyst. If a lesion is radiographically hazy, it is a granuloma; whereas, a well circumscribed lesion with sclerotic border is a cyst (Fig. 6.11a and b).

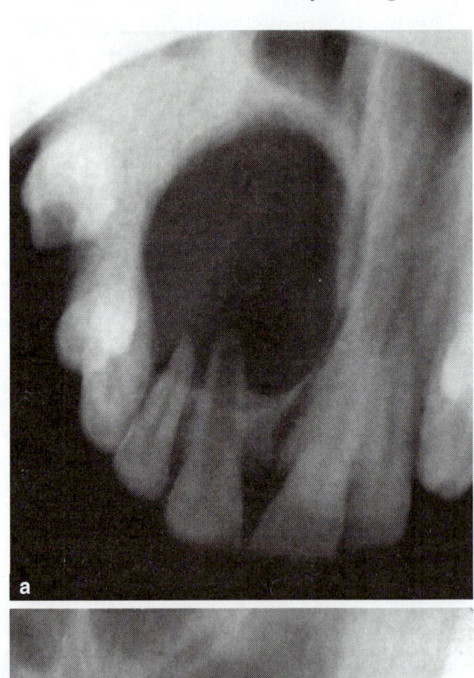

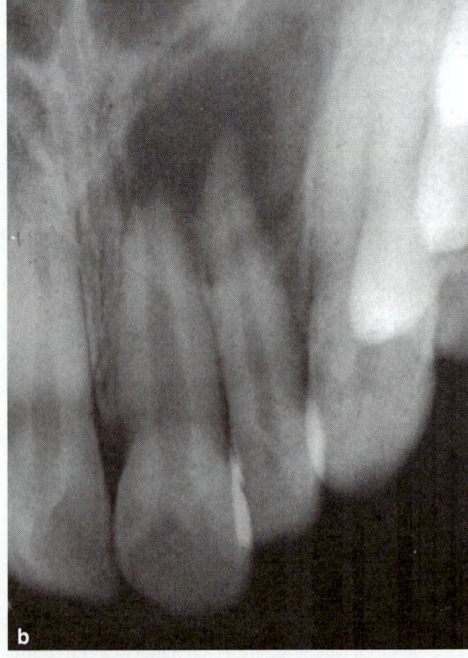

Fig. 6.11a and b Periapical cyst (radiographic appearance)

The radiographic picture of a small cyst may not be differentiated from that of a granuloma. Although positive differentiation between cyst and granuloma cannot be made from radiographs, certain features may suggest presence of cyst:

- Cyst is larger than a granuloma.
- May cause spread of adjacent roots due to continuous pressure from cystic fluid.
- A radiopaque band usually encircles the radiolucent area.

When a periradicular lesion is presented radiographically, it may not be a true cystic or granulomatous lesion; rather, it is a mixed lesion containing the elements of both the cyst and the granuloma. The lesion can therefore be:

- Cyst
- Predominantly cystic with some granulomatous patches
- Granuloma
- Predominantly granulomatous with few cystic patches

Dystrophic calcifications may be seen in long standing cysts. Rarely, cyst may elevate the osseous floor of the sinus and protrude into maxillary sinus.

Histopathological features

A cyst shows inflammation in periradicular tissue along with proliferation of epithelial cell rests of Malassez (Fig. 6.12). In chronically inflamed connective tissue, inadequate nutrition to epithelial cells may lead to their degeneration and death. Intercellular fluid gives the epithelial cells a sponge like characteristic (spaces between cells increase). A definite central cavity develops containing fluid along with number of cells in different stages of degeneration.

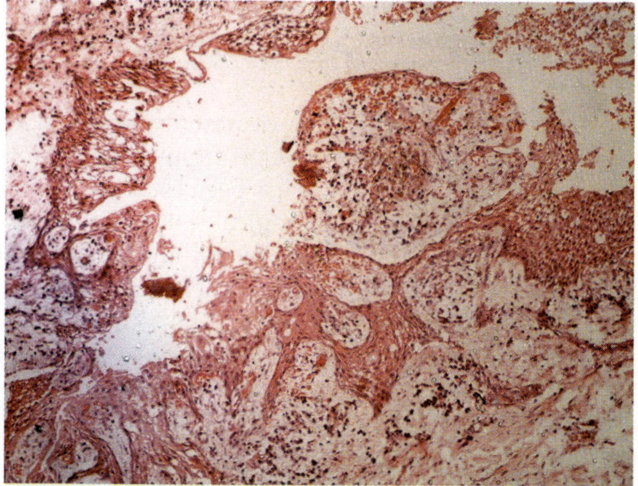

Fig. 6.12 Microphotograph of radicular cyst (H&E x10) illustrating stratified squamous epithelium in arcading pattern and connective tissue

Treatment

The periapical cysts have least potential for healing without surgical intervention as long standing cysts show little evidence of granulomatous tissue. Treatment involves root canal treatment of involved tooth followed by surgical removal of the cystic lesion (marsupialization).

> ***Periapical cyst: Key features***
> - Chronic inflammatory response of granulomatous tissues at the root apex
> - Swelling can be palpable at apex (small cysts are not palpable)
> - Negative response to vitality tests
> - A definite radiographic band encircling the radiolucent area is a diagnostic feature
> - A fluid cavity filled with cells at various stages of the cyst development
> - Surgical intervention (excision of cyst) is the treatment of choice

The recommended guidelines for treatment of periapical lesions are tabulated in Table 6.2.

d. Condensing Osteitis

Condensing osteitis is recognized by a well-defined radiopacity at the apex of a non-vital tooth.

Inflammatory lesions of the periapical region generally result in localized bone destruction and its replacement with inflammatory tissues. In some cases, these inflammatory lesions may result in bone deposition. When this happens, a radiopacity appears on radiographic examination; it is known as *'condensing osteitis'*.

Condensing osteitis is caused by the same irritants (necrotic pulps) that cause other types of periradicular inflammatory disease. It is observed more often in children and teenagers than in adults. Increased

Table 6.2 Recommended treatment for periapical lesions

Periapical lesions: characteristics	*Recommended treatment*
Lesion diameter less than 5.0 mm	Conventional root canal treatment; periodic follow-up
Lesion diameter 5.0–10 mm (endodontic diagnosis)	Conventional root canal therapy; periodic follow-up for long duration
Lesion diameter more than 10 mm	Surgical intervention; if not feasible, resinifying therapy
No healing even 3 months after root canal treatment	Re-treatment; may opt for surgical intervention (retrograde approach)

6

resistance and more abundant blood supply are the usual explanations. Intraoral examination cannot detect condensing osteitis. The patient may have experienced pain and discomfort in the past, which subsided with time.

Radiographic features

The radiographic features are the most characteristic features of condensing osteitis. The lesion is marked by a periapical radiopacity (Fig. 6.13). The radiopacity is usually well-circumscribed; it may be demarcated from the surrounding bone by a narrow radiolucent border.

Histopathological features

Presence of bony tissue intermixed with a fibrous connective tissue stroma along with chronic inflammatory cells are the main histopathological features.

Treatment

The treatment of condensing osteitis is the same; root canal treatment as recommended for other inflammatory periapical lesions. Since the lesion may resolve with conservative means, surgical intervention may not be necessary. Extraction would be the last choice.

Condensing osteitis: Key features

- Long standing non-vital tooth
- Prevalent in young permanent teeth
- Chronic inflammation may occasionally lead to condensation of bony tissues along with fibrous connective tissue (radiopaque on radiograph)
- No pain on percussion
- Patient feel slight discomfort
- Conventional root canal treatment is effective; if not, extraction

e. Apical Scar

Chronic periapical lesions are treated in routine, both surgically and non-surgically. Apical scar is recognized by the persistence of a well-defined radiolucency in the periapical regions following treatment of chronic apical periodontitis. A scar can also form after periapical surgery (Fig. 6.14).

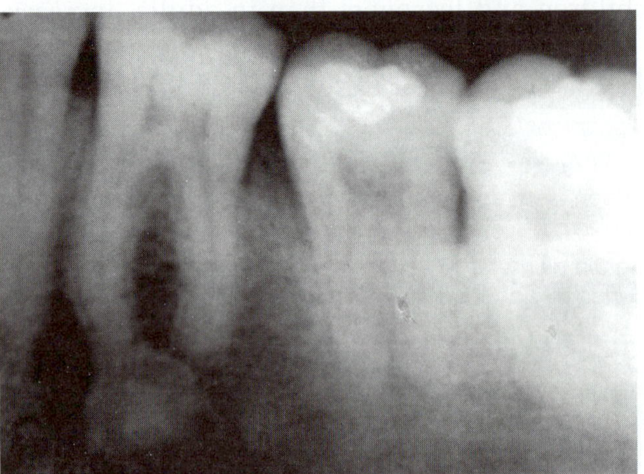

Fig. 6.13 Condensing osteitis in mandibular molar

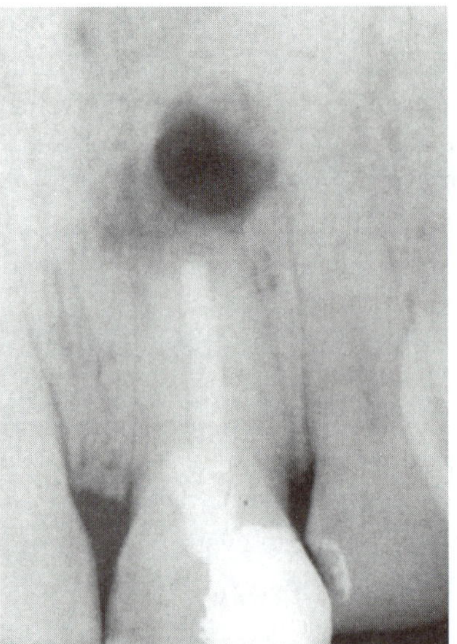

Fig. 6.14 Apical scar

In majority of cases, the void created by lesion-removal is filled with normal bone with time. In few cases, the void may get filled with fibrous connective tissue producing a scar. This occurs most frequently when both facial and lingual cortical plates have been lost. The scar appears as radiolucent area. The periapical radiolucency creates a doubt whether the lesion has healed or the lesion recurred due to failure of the root canal filling. The size of radiolucency should be evaluated periodically along with other signs and symptoms to differentiate between healed and failed cases. Retreatment is usually not required.

B. PERIRADICULAR LESIONS OF NON-ENDODONTIC ORIGIN

Periradicular lesions, though commonly linked with pulp infections, may also develop from the remnants of odontogenic epithelium. It has been established that approximately 10–12% of periapical lesions have non-endodontic origin. In such cases, biopsy and histological evaluations can be helpful. The indications of biopsy are tabulated in Table 6.3.

The characteristic features of periradicular lesions of non-endodontic origin are:

- Vital teeth
- Intact lamina dura
- Distinct radiolucency around periapex
- Organized bone loss/hard tissue loss
- Biopsy confirms the diagnosis

6

Table 6.3 Indications for biopsy of periapical lesions
• Lesion adjacent to the root apex of vital tooth
• Persistent periapical lesion even after one year follow-up of root canal treatment
• Lesion with irregular radiolucency
• Lesions effectively causing mobility without periodontal disease
• Lesion, which separates from root apex by changing radiation angle
• Lesion with unusual symptoms
• Progressively growing lesion with history of malignancy

Most of the non-endodontic periradicular lesions are cystic in nature or of benign jaw lesions. The common ones are:

i. *Traumatic bone cyst*: Traumatic bone cyst is the fluid containing cavity in the jaw bone, which may not have the epithelial cover. The lesion usually mimics chronic periapical inflammatory disease (Fig. 6.15). The involved tooth is vital, without any external resorption. The recommended treatment is the surgical excision.

ii. *Odontogenic keratocyst*: Odontogenic keratocyst arise from the cell rests of dental lamina. The lesion is commonly seen in young individuals between 20 and 40 years of age. The lesion mainly involves the posterior area of the mandible (ramus and body) (Fig. 6.16a and b). The lesion is mostly asymptomatic; however, a few cases may present with pain and/or swelling. The absence of caries and/or pulp involvement can help differentiate this lesion from apical periodontitis. Enucleation is the treatment of choice. Since recurrence is common, long-term follow-up is mandatory.

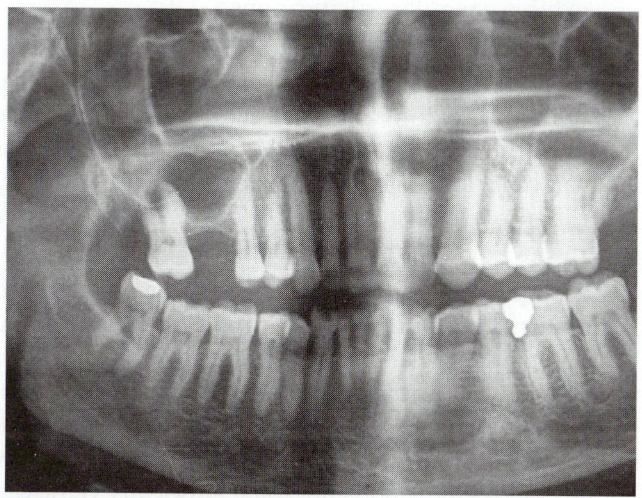

Fig. 6.15: Traumatic cyst

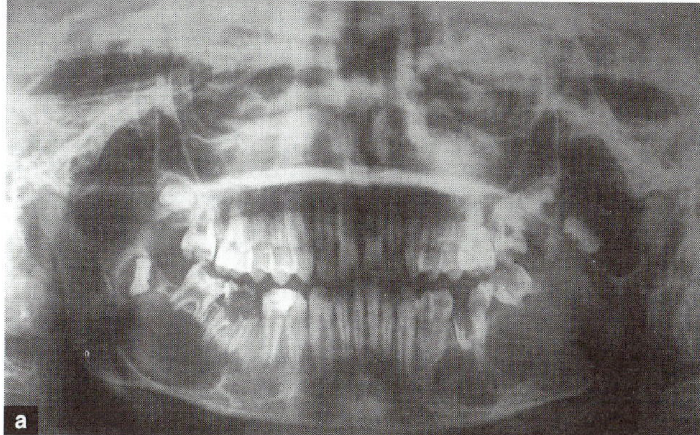

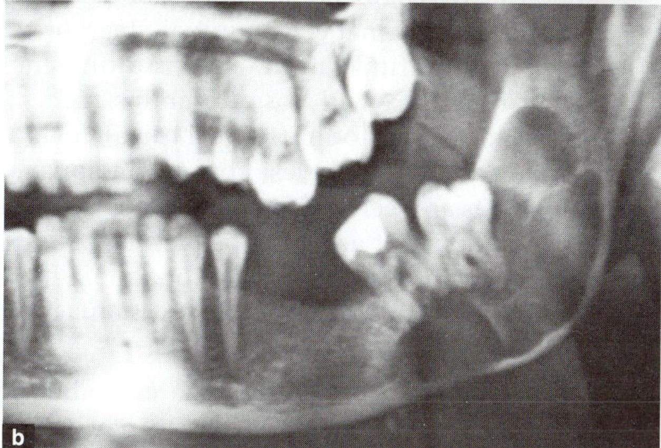

Fig. 6.16 Odontogenic keratocyst: (a) Bilateral; (b) At an angle

iii. *Calcifying odontogenic cyst*: Calcifying odontogenic cyst, is mostly asymptomatic and frequently seen in anterior region of both the jaws (Fig. 6.17). Radiographically, the cyst presents with well-defined radiolucency with occasional diffuse radiopaque areas. Ghost cells have been seen within the epithelial coverage. Enucleation is the treatment of choice.

iv. *Nasopalatine duct/cyst*: Nasopalatine duct/cysts are usually asymptomatic; rarely, may present with

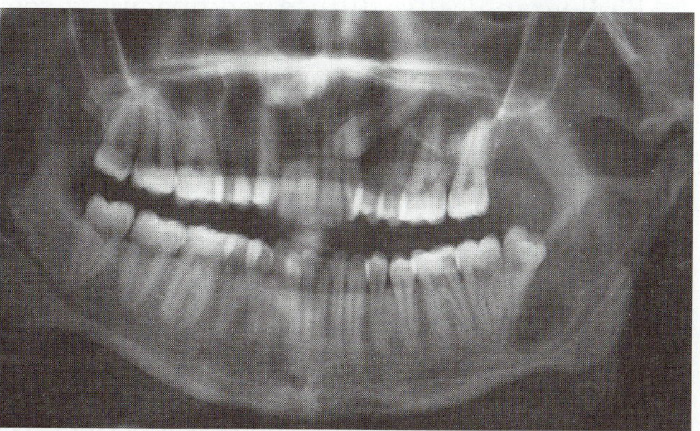

Fig. 6.17 Odontogenic cyst

6

pain and/or swelling. The cystic lesion is often confused with periapical lesion, especially when the lesion is exhibited over the apex of maxillary central incisors. The teeth are vital and the radiolucency may change site with radiographs at different angles. Surgical enucleation is preferred treatment.

v. *Periapical cemental dysplasia (cementoma)*: Periapical cemental dysplasia (cementoma) is due to proliferation of connective tissues within the periodontal membrane. It usually involves the periapical areas of mandibular anterior teeth. The lesion is asymptomatic. The initial stage of the lesion (well-defined unilocular radiolucency around root apex with loss of lamina dura) is similar to the endodontic periapical lesions (granuloma/cyst). As the lesion grows, radiopaque components are seen within the radiolucent areas (mixed radiolucent and radiopaque). Finally, the lesion becomes completely radiopaque. Histopathological evaluation is important to diagnose the lesion.

vi. *Cementoblastoma*: Cementoblastoma is the benign neoplasm of the jaw (neoplasm of cemental origin). The slowly growing, asymptomatic lesions usually affect mandible than maxilla. The expansion of cortical plate of bone is the characteristic feature of cementoblastoma. It presents with well-defined radiopacity with cortical border confined by radiolucent margins. These teeth may and may not respond to pulp vitality testing (later stages of cementoblastoma affects pulp vitality). Hypercementosis is the smaller sized cementoma, wherein, there is no jaw expansion.

vii. *Ossifying fibroma*: Ossifying fibroma is a benign jaw neoplasm affecting mainly the posterior region of the mandible. The lesion is often asymptomatic and rarely swelling of the cortical plates is seen. Radiographically, diffuse radiopacity is seen within a radiolucent area. The lesion is fast growing. Complete excision is the treatment of choice.

viii. *Ameloblastoma*: Originating from odontogenic epithelium, ameloblastoma affects mainly the posterior region of the mandible. These are benign in nature; however, may aggressively erode the adjacent teeth. Mostly, pain and/or swelling may occur. Various types of ameloblastomas have been recognized [multicystic (solid), unicystic, extraosseous (peripheral) and desmoplastic]. The multicystic form is the most common. Radiographs exhibit multilocular radiolucency with soap-bubble, spider-web or honey-comb shape appearance. Variable resorption of bony cortex may be seen (Fig. 6.18). The tumor is resected completely along with additional resection of margins beyond the radiological limits of the tumor.

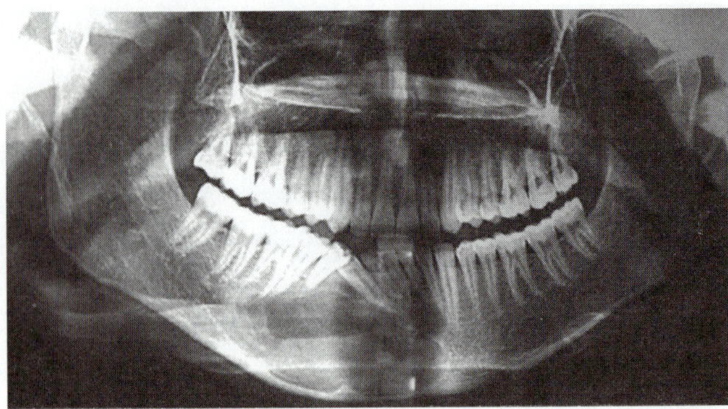

Fig. 6.18 Ameloblastoma

ix. *Giant cell granuloma*: Giant cell granuloma frequently involves anterior segment of jaws. Radiographically, the lesion presents a well-defined unilocular or multilocular radiolucency. Both slow growing and aggressive (fast-growing) lesions are prevalent. The involved teeth are vital. Periapical curettage is an effective treatment for these lesions; however, radicular surgery is required in aggressive type of lesions.

x. *Myxoma*: Myxoma is rare odontogenic tumor that arises from mesenchymal cells. These are benign in nature; however, may aggressively lead to resorption of adjacent roots. Smaller lesions are unilocular, whereas larger lesions are multilocular. Radiologically, the lesion presents with distinct or ill-defined borders. The internal architecture may exhibit irregular calcifications.

xi. *Malignant jaw lesion*: Several malignant lesions in the periapical region mimic endodontic periapical lesions. Lesions such as lymphoma, multiple myeloma, squamous cell carcinoma, chondrosarcoma, and osteosarcoma, etc. are to be properly diagnosed (most of them are misdiagnosed if only radiological findings are analyzed).

Radiographically, these lesions show ill-defined radiolucency without any cortical border. Periodontal ligament widening and loss of lamina dura are common radiological features. It is opined that any unusual symptom of bone destruction adjacent to vital teeth should be considered for biopsy (Table 6.3). Both slow and fast growing lesions are to be surgically removed in consultation with the oncology surgeon.

BIBLIOGRAPHY

1. Abbott PV and Yu C. A clinical classification of the status of the pulp and the root canal system. Aust. Dent J.: 2007; 52:S17–S31.
2. Abbott PV. Diagnosis and management planning for root-filled teeth with persisting or new apical pathosis. Endod. Topics: 2011; 19:1–21.
3. Abbott PV. The periapical space- a dynamic interface. Aust. Endod. J.: 2002; 28:96–107.
4. Al-Hezaimi K. Apical actinomycosis: case report. J. Can. Dent. Assoc.: 2010; 76:a113.
5. Bhaskar SN. Periapical lesions - types, incidence and clinical features. O. Surg., O. Med., O. Path.:1996; 21:657–671.
6. Buonavoglia A, Latronico F and Pirani C. Symptomatic and asymptomatic apical periodontitis associated with red complex bacteria: clinical and microbiological evaluation. Odontology: 2013; 101:84–88.
7. Chala S, Abouqal R and Abdallaoui F. Prevalence of apical periodontitis and factors associated with the periradicular status. Acta. Odontol. Scand.: 2011; 69:355–359.
8. Chang CC, Hung HY, Chang JY, Yu CH, Wang YP and Liu BY. Central ossifying fibroma: a clinicopathologic study of 28 cases. J. Formos. Med. Assoc.: 2008; 107:288–294.
9. Chapman MN, Nadgin RN, Akman AS, Saito N, Sekiya K and Kaneda T. Periapical radiolucency around the tooth: radiologic evaluation and differential diagnosis. Radiographics: 2013; 33:e15–32.
10. Damm DD. Interradicular radiolucency. Lateral periodontal cyst. Gen. Dent.: 2011; 59:395.
11. Eversike R, Su L and El Mofty S. Benign fibro-osseous lesions of the craniofacial complex. A review. Head Neck Pathol.: 2008; 2:177–202.
12. Faitaroni LA, Bueno MR, Carvalhosa AA, Mendonca EF and Estrela C. Differential diagnosis of apical periodontitis and nasopalatine duct cyst. J. Endod.:2011; 37:403–410.
13. Fuji R, Saito Y and Tokura Y. Characterization of bacterial flora in persistent apical periodontitis lesions. Oral Microbiol. Immunol.: 2009; 24:502–505.
14. Garcia CC, Sempere FV, Diago MP and Bowen EM. The post-endodontic periapical lesion: histologic and etiopathogenic aspects. Med. Oral Patol. Oral Cir. Bucal.:2007; 12:585–590.
15. Gutmann JL, Baumgartner C, Gluskin AH, Hartwell GR and Walton RE. Identify and define all diagnostic terms for periapical/periradicular health and disease states. J. Endod.: 2009; 35:1658–1674.
16. Huumonen S and Orstavik D. Radiological aspects of apical periodontitis. Endod. Topics: 2002; 1:3–25.
17. Iqbal M, Kim S and Yoon F. An investigation into differential diagnosis pulp and periapical pain-a PennEndo database study. J. Endod.: 2007; 33:548–551.
18. Jacinto R, Gomes BP and Shah HN. Quantification of endotoxins in necrotic root canals from symptomatic and asymptomatic teeth. J. Med. Micro.: 2005; 54:77–83.
19. Jakovljevic A, Knezevic A and Karalic D. Pro-inflammatory cytokine levels in human apical periodontitis: correlation with clinical and histological findings. Aust. Endod. J.: 2015; 41:72–77.
20. Jansson I, Ehnevid H, Lindskog S and Blomlof I. Development of periapical lesions. Swed. Dent. J.: 1993; 17:85.
21. Kahler B. Traumatic bone cyst suggestive of a chronic periapical abscess: a case report. Aust. Endod. J.: 2011; 37:73–75.
22. Khemaleelakul S, Baumgartner JC and Pruksakom S. Autoaggregation and coaggregation of bacteria associated with acute endodontic infections. J. Endod.: 2006; 32:312–8.
23. Kuc I, Peters E and Pan J. Comparison of clinical and histological diagnosis in periapical lesions. O. Surg., O. Med., O. Path.: 2000; 89:333–337.
24. Mehrazarin S, Alshaikh A and Kang MK. Molecular mechanisms of apical periodontitis: Emerging role of epigenetic regulators. Dent. Clinic. N. Am.: 2017; 61:17–35.
25. Morsani JM, Aminoshariae A and Han YW. Genetic predisposition to persistent apical periodontitis. J. Endod.: 2011; 37:455–459.
26. Nair PN. Apical periodontitis- a dynamic encounter between root canal infection and host response. Periodontol 2000: 1997; 13:121–148.
27. Nair PN. On the causes of persistent apical periodontics: a review. Int. Endod. J.: 2006; 39:249–281.
28. Ortega A, Farina V, Gallardo A, Espinoza I and Acosta S. Non-endodontic periapical lesions: a retrospective study in Chile. Int. Endod. J.: 2007; 40:386–390.
29. Ostavik D, Kerckes K and Erikson HM. The periapical index: a scoring system for radiographic assessment of apical periodontitis. Endod. Dent. Traumatol.: 1986; 2:20–34.
30. Pace R, Cairo F, Giuliani V, Prato LP and Pagavino G. A diagnostic dilemma: endodontic lesion or odontogenic keratocyst? A case presentation. Int. Endod. J.: 2008; 41:800–806.
31. Peters E and Lau M. Histopathologic examination to confirm diagnosis of periapical lesions: a review. J. Can. Dent. Assoc.: 2003; 69:598–600.
32. Radics T, Kiss C and Tar I. Interleukin-6 and granulocyte-macrophage colony-stimulating factor in apical periodontitis: correlation with clinical and histologic findings of the involved teeth. Oral Microbiol. Immunol.: 2003; 18:9–13.
33. Razavi SM, Kiani S and Khalesi S. Periapical lesions: a review of clinical, radiographic and histopathologic features. Avicenna J. Dent. Res.: 2015; 7:e19435.
34. Ricucci D, Mannocci F and Ford TR. A study of periapical lesions correlating the presence of a radiopaque lamina with histological findings. Oral Surg., Oral Med., Oral Pathol., Oral Radiol., Endod.: 2006; 101:389–394.
35. Ricucci D, Siqueira JF and Lopes WS. Extraradicular infection as the cause of persistent symptoms: a case series. J. Endod.: 2015; 41:265–273.
36. Schultz M, von Arx T, Altermatt HJ and Bosshardt D. Histology of periapical lesions obtained during apical surgery. J. Endod.: 2009; 25:634–642.
37. Slots J, Nowzari H and Sabeti M. Cytomegalovirus infection in symptomatic periapical pathosis. Int. Endod. J.: 2004; 37:519–524.
38. Suomalainen A, Apajalahti S, Kuhlefelt M and Hagstrom J. Simple bone cyst: a radiological dilemma. Dentomaxillofac. Radiol.: 2009; 38:174–177.
39. Torabinejad M, Bakland LK and Linda L. Immunopathogenesis of chronic periapical lesions. Oral Surg.: 1978; 46:685–699.
40. West, J D.: Endodontic diagnosis. Mystery or mastery? Dent Today: 2004, 23, 80–87.

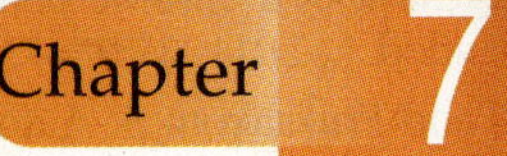

Chapter 7

Rationale of Endodontic Treatment

Physical, chemical or bacterial noxious stimuli can produce reversible or irreversible changes in the dental pulp and periradicular tissues. The changes depend upon duration, intensity and pathogenicity of the stimulus along with the host's ability to resist and subsequently repair the tissue damages. The mild-to-moderate noxious stimuli to the pulp may produce sclerosis of the dentinal tubules, formation of reparative dentin, or reversible inflammation; whereas, irreversible inflammatory changes caused by severe injury can lead to necrosis of the pulp and subsequent pathologic changes in the periradicular tissues. Since the pulp is encased in the rigid hard tissues with virtually no space for expansion coupled with limited portals of entry and exit without any efficient collateral circulation, a clear concept of the fundamentals of inflammation becomes mandatory for understanding diseases of pulp and their extension to the periradicular tissues.

INFLAMMATION

Inflammation is the sequence of basic physiologic and morphologic reactions occurring in the vascular, lymphatic, and connective tissues of the body. The objective of inflammation is to remove/destroy the irritants and to repair the damage caused to the tissues.

Repair of the tissues depends on the severity of injury and host resistance. The injurious agent may cause reversible or irreversible changes to the tissues. Irreversible changes lead to tissue damage; whereas, reversible changes lead to repair. Removal of the irritants, exudates, and cellular debris enhance the reparative process. Fibroblasts from adjacent tissues and capillary buds from adjacent blood vessels proliferate in the area resulting in the production of new collagen fibers matrix and also rich supply of blood vessels to the area of injury to form granulation tissue. The inflammatory process resolves when repair is completed.

Signs and Symptoms

The cardinal signs and symptoms of inflammation are:

1. *Pain (dolor)*

   Pain is due to the action of cytotoxic agents released from humoral, cellular, and microbial elements acting on the nerve endings.

2. *Swelling (tumor)*

   Swelling in affected tissues is due to the ingress of macromolecules and fluid.

3. *Redness (rubor)*

   The redness is due to vasodilatation of vessels (capillaries filled with more blood).

4. *Heat (calor)*

   Heat is produced by vasodilatation of the vessels and rushing of blood to the affected tissues.

5. *Disturbance of functions* (immobility)

   The functions are disturbed (loss of functions) because of the changes in the affected tissue.

In an inflamed pulp, as in any other inflamed organ of the body, all the symptoms are evident; however, 'pain' and 'disturbance of functions' can be recognized clinically.

COMPONENTS OF INFLAMMATION

The characteristic components of inflammation are as follows.

A. Cellular Events

In the pulp and periradicular tissues, inflammation may be either acute or chronic. These two states can be recognized only at the histological level and depend on predominance of cells in the lesion. The main cells of an acute inflammatory lesion are the polymorphonuclear neutrophils. In chronic inflammation, lymphocytes, plasma cells, monocytes, and macrophages are predominant. As a rule, no definite demarcation exists between acute and chronic inflammation. Lesions usually have both types of cells, with either acute or chronic cells predominating.

a. Polymorphonuclear Neutrophils (PMNs)

The polymorphonuclear neutrophils morphologically consist of a nucleus with three or more connected lobules and cytoplasm containing lysosomal and specific granules. They are present during the acute or early stages of inflammation. Their main function is to phagocytize bacteria; may also phagocytize and lyse fibrin and cellular debris. They are attracted to the area of inflammation by chemotactic factors produced by bacteria or by complement, and they are the first cells to migrate from the blood vessels. Serum factors of complement and immunoglobulins called 'opsonins' bind bacteria to the surfaces of the polymorphonuclear neutrophils. During this stage, the bacteria are encapsulated in vacuoles that move into the cytoplasm of the polymorphonuclear neutrophils and come in contact with lysosomal granules, which degranulate and release lysosomal enzymes for lysis of the bacteria. They have a narrow range of life; usually destroyed at the inflammatory site as the tissue fluids fall to a pH of 6.5 due to the increased production of lactic acid during phagocytosis and its release into the tissues during their death. Destruction of the polymorphonuclear neutrophils also causes the release of the proteolytic enzymes, pepsin and cathepsin, with resulting tissue lysis. PMNs with the by-products of cellular lysis and debris, are the principal constituents of pus.

b. Monocytes/Macrophages

Macrophages are derived from circulating monocytes. Immature monocytes in extravascular areas, such as areas of inflammation, differentiate into macrophages. Macrophages are phagocytic cells that ingest cellular debris, micro-organisms, and particulate matter. They secrete certain mediators of inflammation, such as lysosomal enzymes, complement proteins and prostaglandins.

Macrophages enhance the immunologic reaction by ingesting, processing, and degrading antigen before it is presented to the lymphocytes. Their capacity to remove debris from the area facilitates repair. Macrophages are the mononucleated cells; may fuse with other macrophages to produce a multinucleated giant cell at the time of action.

c. Lymphocytes

Lymphocytes appear in the chronic stage of inflammatory reaction, which are related to the immunologic system of the organism. Small lymphocytes have a large, spherical or slightly indented nucleus surrounded by a thin band of cytoplasm containing small granules. Two types of small lymphocytes, i.e. B cells and T cells, are known. Both these cells are derived from the pluripotent haematopoetic stem cells. Stem cells are carried by the blood to the thymus to become immunologically competent T cells. In contrast, B-cells become immunocompetent in the bone marrow.

T cells have a long life span and are the most common cells of the lymphocytic series in the blood. They are responsible for cell mediated immunity and immune surveillance of an organism. They re-circulate through the lymphoid tissues and organs of the body, except through the thymus, and are found in the paracortical areas of the lymph nodes. When T cells are stimulated by an antigen, they develop into sensitized T lymphocytes. These T lymphocytes have various immunologic manifestations, such as:

- *Memory T cells:* They speed up immunologic reaction in subsequent encounters with the same antigen
- *Helper or suppressor T cells:* These stimulate or suppress development of the effector T or B cells
- *Effector T cells:* They may produce cell-meditated immune reactions; for example, the delayed hypersensitivity reaction.
- *Lymphokine:* The sensitized T lymphocytes also release chemical mediators called lymphokines. Lymphokines may activate macrophages, polymorphonuclear leukocytes, and non-sensitized T cells, or they may produce interferon, which inhibits viral replication required by the immune response.

B cells have a shorter life span than T cells. They are found more in the cortical areas of the lymph nodes than in the blood. When activated by an antigen, B cells become larger cells called plasmablasts, which divide to form plasma cells and memory B cells. *The memory B cells* speed the immunologic reaction in subsequent encounters with the same antigen. *The plasma cells* are large, oval and round cells with eccentric nuclei containing chromatic material arranged in a cartwheel form. The plasma cells produce immunoglobulins, called 'antibodies'. B cells are responsible for the humoral immunity of the human beings.

The immunoglobulins (antibodies) have five major classes, i.e. *IgM, IgG, IgA, IgD and IgE.* These are involved in different defense reactions such as:

- Neutralization of bacterial toxins by antitoxins
- Coating of bacteria by antibodies or opsonization to facilitate phagocytosis
- Lysis of bacteria by complement activation
- Agglutination of bacteria
- Combining of the antibody with viruses to prevent their entry into the cells.

d. Eosinophils, Basophils and Mast Cells

Other cells found in pulp and periradicular tissues during the inflammatory response are eosinophilic leukocytes, basophilic leukocytes and the mast cells. The eosinophils are found largely in allergic and parasitic reactions. During the immune response, they are involved in phagocytosis of the antigen-antibody complexes and in the detoxification of histamine. Basophils and mast cells are considered similar cells; basophils are found in the hemopoetic system, and the mast cells are found in tissues. They both contain granules, which de-granulate and release chemical mediators, such as histamine (a vasodilator) and heparin (an anticoagulant) that can initiate an inflammatory or an allergic response.

B. Vascular Changes

The main characteristics of inflammation are the two vascular changes, i.e. vasodilation and increased capillary permeability, which lead to a series of physiologic and morphologic changes in the system. A brief vasoconstriction is followed by vasodilatation of the arteries caused by relaxation of the arteriolar and capillary sphincters. This opens dormant capillary beds and increases the blood supply to the affected area. Proteolytic enzymes released from injured cells, bacterial toxins, coupled with traumatic forces are the injurious agents that may release histamine from mast cells, facilitating vasodilatation of the vessels.

The vasodilatation is accompanied by an increased rate of blood flow and a decrease in flow resistance. These changes increase intravascular pressure, and permeability of capillaries. Histamine enhances the permeability reaction by contracting the endothelial cells of the venules and producing intracellular gaps. This process favors the filtration of plasma and macromolecules from the venules. The blood plasma escaping through the vessel walls is usually less viscous and contains less protein than blood plasma remaining in the blood vessels. In inflammation, the blood plasma that leaks into the tissues and contains plasma proteins such as albumins, fibrinogen, and immunoglobulins is referred to as '*inflammatory exudate*'. This exudate brings the chemical mediators and inflammatory cells to the inflamed site; dilutes bacterial toxins, thereby reducing the potential of tissue damage and helps to form fibrin to complete the inflammatory reaction.

Hageman factor or factor XII of the blood clotting system is released into the tissues in the inflammatory exudates. This factor is activated by collagen, damaged basement membrane of blood vessels, or by an antigen-antibody complex and reacts with prekallikrein of the tissue plasma to produce kinins. These kinins, such as bradykinin, produce vasodilatation and increase the permeability of blood vessels. It also activates the fibrinolytic and blood coagulating systems. Fibrinogen in the inflammatory exudates is acted on by the Hageman factor to produce fibrin, which confines the inflammatory reaction to a limited area. Plasminogen from the plasma found in the inflammatory exudates is activated to plasmin. Plasmin may activate the complement system, digests fibrin and thereby aids in the removal of blood clots or fibrin plugs, or it may activate the kinin system. The inactive serum proteins of complement are also released from the blood in the inflammatory exudates. Immunoglobulins activate the complement cascade to produce anaphylatoxin that acts on mast cells and causes the release of histamine. Complement activation also results in the release of a chemotactic factor, which aids in leukocytosis and lysis of bacteria.

The fluid leaked from the vessels into the tissues accumulates to produce edema. The subsequent increase in tissue pressure causes the venules to collapse and reduces both the venous drainage and the blood flow from that area. The stasis of blood in the venules due to increased viscosity of blood and the increased pressure resistance of the venules cause the leukocytes to migrate from the center of the blood vessels to the periphery. This process is called *margination* of leukocytes. After margination, the leukocytes start adhering to the vessel walls, known as *pavementation*. The next step in the inflammatory reaction is the *emigration* of the leukocytes. The leukocytes are attracted by complement to the site of inflammation and migrate through the vessel walls by amoeboid movement. This migration process is called *chemotaxis*. The polymorphonuclear neutrophils migrate first, followed by the monocytes and lymphocytes. Chemotaxis is also caused by complement, prostaglandins, kallikrein and bacterial products.

Prostaglandins, thromboxanes and leukotrienes are the mediators of inflammation that are derived from membrane phospholipids. Phospholipase, a lysosomal enzyme produced by polymorphonuclear leukocytes, reacts with the cell membrane phospholipids to produce arachidonic acid, which in turn, produces prostaglandins, thromboxanes, and leukotrienes. The polymorphonuclear neutrophils also produce lysosomal enzymes, which give rise to chemotactic substances that attract more leukocytes to the area of inflammation.

The vascular response continues with the aggregation of red blood cells in the vessels. This aggregation increases the resistance of the blood to flow. This resistance, along with the increase in blood viscosity produced by the loss of plasma, causes metabolic changes, such as decrease in the oxygen concentration, an increase in carbon dioxide levels and a lower pH in the inflammatory site. These changes are detrimental to the metabolism of the pulpal tissue, as elsewhere in the body, because they prevent the removal of waste products. The aforementioned changes may spread inflammation to the adjacent tissues; this vicious cycle of inflammation may lead to total necrosis of the pulp.

Syngcuk Kim's Hypothetic Model

The migration of monocytes and lymphocytes renders the inflammatory site capable of an immunologic reaction. As the inflammatory reaction progresses, macrophages necessary to process the antigen, plasma cells derived from B lymphocytes and immunoglobulin/lymphocyte mediators of the immune system can be found at the inflammatory site. Extravascular immunoglobulins found in the inflamed pulp tissues and plasma cells are predominantly IgG type, although IgA, IgE and IgM containing plasma cells are also present. The presence of these immunoglobulins indicates that the pulp possesses the mechanism for immunologic reaction that contributes to pulpal and periradicular disorders.

The recovery of the pulp to insult can be explained by some unique vascular responses. *Arteriovenous anastomoses and 'U-turn loops'* open in the pulpal vasculature, reduce the blood flow to the area of inflammation and thereby decrease the vascular pressure. The increased tissue pressure allows the return of macromolecules and fluids to the venules. These two changes return vascular pressure and stimulate the repair process.

Manifestations of Periradicular Inflammation

An inflammatory response may result in partial or complete necrosis of the pulpal tissue. In such cases, the root canal serves as a pathway for the noxious products and antigens to the periradicular area. The inflammatory and immunologic responses in the periradicular area also occur in a similar way as in the pulp. On reaching the periradicular area, these noxious products produce granulation tissue in place of normal periradicular tissues. The periradicular pathologic tissues contain polymorphonuclear neutrophils, lymphocytes, plasma cells, macrophages and mast cells, along with the immunoglobulins IgG, IgA, IgM, IgE and complement. In the presence of these anaphylactic, cytotoxic, antigen-antibody complex, delayed hypersensitivity reactions may occur in the periradicular area. It is hypothesized that endodontic flare-ups might be mediated by IgE reactions and that bone resorption is mediated by a lymphokine called 'osteoclastic activating factor'. The osteoclastic factor confirmed the role of immunologic reactions in the physiology and pathology of the periradicular tissues.

C. Tissue Changes

Tissue changes following inflammation are either degenerative or proliferative.

a. Degenerative Changes

Degenerative changes in the pulp may be resorptive or calcific. Thrombosis of the blood vessels and release of leukotoxins from the damaged tissue cells lead to degenerative changes; subsequently necrosis of pulp. Another form of degeneration is suppuration. When the polymorphonuclear cells are injured, they release proteolytic enzymes that cause the liquefaction of the dead tissues resulting in suppuration or formation of pus.

Three requisites necessary for suppuration are:

i. Necrosis of tissue cells
ii. Presence of a sufficient number of polymorphonuclear leukocytes
iii. Digestion of the dead material by proteolytic enzymes

If the reaction is not intense, because of weak irritant; the result will be an exudation consisting chiefly of serum, lymph, and fibrin (serous exudates).

All dead cells, particularly polymorphonuclear cells, liberate proteolytic enzymes. Since the enzymes digest not only the leukocytes, but also the adjacent dead tissue, it results in abscess formation. Micro-organisms are not necessary for development of an abscess; a sterile abscess may result from chemical or physical irritation in the absence of micro-organisms.

b. Proliferative Changes

Proliferative changes are produced by mild irritants. Within the same area, a substance acts both as an irritant and a stimulant; for example, calcium hydroxide and its effect on adjacent tissues. In the center of the inflammatory area, the irritant may be strong enough to produce degeneration or destruction; whereas, at the periphery, the irritant may be mild enough to stimulate proliferation. Generally, if the tissue is in apposition, as in the case of an incision for root resection, fibroblastic repair will take place. When a gap is present between two parts of the tissue, granulation tissue repair will predominate. Granulation tissue, itself is resistant to infection. The principal cells of repair are the fibroblasts, which lay down cellular fibrous tissue. If the collagen fibers get substituted, dense acellular tissue is formed. In either case, fibrous repair is the result. Destroyed bone is not always replaced by new bone, but it may be replaced by fibrous tissue.

Endodontic Implications

The reaction of the periradicular tissues to noxious products of tissue necrosis, bacterial products and antigenic agents from the root canal has been described by Fish's phenomenon of foci of infection. He experimented with guinea pigs by drilling in the bone and packing wool fibers saturated with a broth culture of micro-organisms. Four well defined zones of reaction (Fig. 7.1) were found (Zones are considered as the basics of inflammatory reaction in any part of the body; so as in periradicular areas):

1. Zone of infection
2. Zone of contamination
3. Zone of irritation
4. Zone of stimulation

Zone of infection	• Presence of micro-organisms • Presence of polymorphonuclear leucocyte cells • Micro-organisms may invade periradicular areas • Micro-organisms present in the center of the lesion
Zone of contamination	• Cellular destruction around the central zone caused by bacterial toxins • Bacterial toxins may lead to death of bone cells (autolysis) • Infiltration of lymphocytes and round cells
Zone of irritation	• Presence of macrophages and osteoclasts • Bacterial toxins get diluted • Normal bone cells and osteoclasts can survive • Macrophages digest collagen; bone filled with polymorphonuclear cells (sign of repair)
Zone of stimulation	• Abundance of fibroblasts and osteoblasts • Bacterial toxins get diluted and do not act as irritant • Fibroblasts laid down collagen fibres; act as wall of defence around zone of irritation • Epithelial rests of Malassez; if stimulated, can form a cyst, otherwise, granulomatous tissue may be observed showing signs of healing

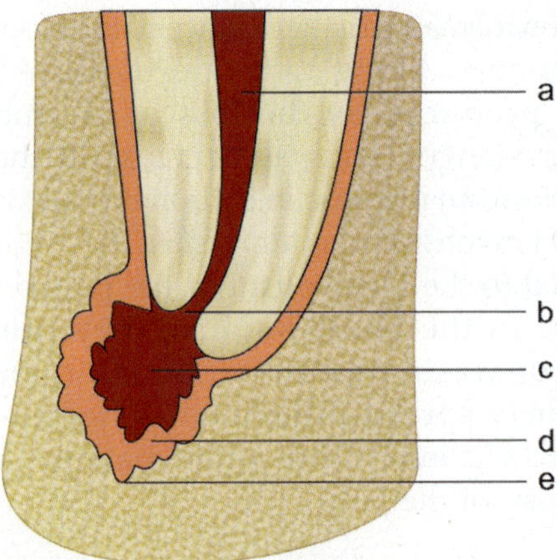

Fig. 7.1 Zones of reaction (diagrammatic): (a) Infected pulp, (b) zone of infection, (c) zone of contamination, (d) zone of irritation, (e) zone of stimulation

1. Zone of infection

This zone is characterized by polymorphonuclear leukocytes. In Fish's study, infection was seen in the center of the lesion; micro-organisms were found only in that area. The micro-organisms not disposed off by polymorphonuclear leukocytes were found in haversian canals or in the fissures made in the bone matrix by the drill.

2. Zone of contamination

This zone is characterized by infiltration of round cells. Around the central zone, cellular destruction, not from bacteria themselves but from the toxins discharged from the bacteria was observed. Whether the toxins were tissue breakdown products or exotoxins was not established. In this area, bone cells had died and had undergone autolysis, so the lacunae appeared empty. Lymphocytes were prevalent everywhere.

3. Zone of irritation

This zone is characterized by macrophages and osteoclasts. Evidence of irritation farther from the central lesion was observed as the toxins became more diluted as the distance increased. In this area, the small round cells, normal bone cells and osteoclasts were found in small numbers. The collagen framework was digested by phagocytic cells, (macrophages), while osteoclasts attacked the bone tissue. The interesting result of their activity is that they open up a gap in the bone all around the center of the lesion; as trees fell to isolate a forest fire. The space, thus obtained gets filled with polymorphonuclear leukocytes and until that has taken place, the danger of widespread necrosis remains. This area presents the histological picture of preparatory activity to repair.

4. Zone of stimulation

This zone is characterized by fibroblasts and osteoblasts. At the periphery, the toxins were mild enough to be a stimulant. In response to this stimulation, collagen fibers were laid down by the fibroblasts, which acted both as a wall of defense around the zone of irritation and as a scaffolding on which the osteoblasts build new bone. This new bone was built in an irregular fashion.

The basis of Fish's experiment can be applied to understand the reaction of the periradicular tissues to a pulpless tooth. The infected root canal is the seat of infection. The micro-organisms in the root canal are rarely motile and do not move from the root canal to the periradicular tissues; however, they can multiply sufficiently to move out of the root canal. As the micro-organisms gain access to the periradicular tissues, a chronic abscess results. The toxic products of micro-organisms and the necrotic pulp in the root canal are irritating and destructive to the periradicular tissues and together with the proteolytic enzymes released by the dead polymorphonuclear leukocytes, help to produce pus.

At the periphery of the destroyed area of osseous tissue, toxic bacterial products may be diluted enough to act as a stimulant. The toxic products from the root canal are diffused from the apical foramen and destroy bone in the immediate vicinity of the root apex. Further away, the toxins are so diluted that they act as a stimulant and form a granuloma. Fibroblasts then build fibrous tissue and osteoblasts around it to delimit the area with a wall of sclerotic bone. If, in addition, the Epithelial rests of Malassez are stimulated, a cyst forms.

Micro-organisms are usually transient in periradicular tissue, even when an area of rarefaction is present radiographically. These transient bacteria can be destroyed by polymorphonuclear leukocytes. Although this phenomenon explains the development of radiolucent areas as a result of infection of the pulp, it may not clarify the development of radiolucent areas following trauma. The pulp may be sterile, even then a radiolucent area may develop because of tissue breakdown products of the pulp that irritate the periradicular tissues.

After the completion of root canal treatment, the reservoir of bacteria or noxious products has been eliminated; repair is initiated and the destroyed periapical bone heals in time.

Implications of Residual Infection before and after Root Canal Treatment

One of the objectives of root canal treatment is to eradicate all types of micro-organisms from the pulp spaces. During cleaning and shaping, this objective is achieved with inherent limitations of cleaning the hidden areas occupied by the micro-organisms. Even after the obturation, some species of micro-organisms survive; especially in apical third of root canals. The possible events in apical area can be:

i. The apical segment may have 'vital' pulp tissue. Such tissue, over a period of time, may get infected and lead to failure of the treatment. It is established that the outcome of treatment would depend upon virulence and the number of bacteria along with host resistance.

ii. The apical segment can be blocked by the dentinal chips during canal preparation. In case, the blockage occurs after canal preparation, or during preparation of vital pulps/non-infected pulp, the dentinal chips can function as a nidus for calcification and closure of the apical foramen. In case of infected pulp, this area of dentinal chips debris can contain micro-organisms, which may affect the outcome of the treatment.

iii. The apical segment of the canal may remain unfilled. It is established that 1.0 mm of unfilled canal may harbor 80,000 micro-organisms; however, in non-infected canal, the free space can be occupied by ingrowth of periodontal ligament tissues. If infection persists, inflammation will set in and hinder with the treatment outcome.

iv. The apical segment can be filled with sealers or pastes. Most endodontic sealers have some antibacterial activity; may help eliminate remaining micro-organisms. The sealer/paste may get solubilized or phagocytized and the space is filled by ingrowth of periodontal tissues. One should also keep in mind that such sealer/paste, if extruded out of apex may cause transient discomfort.

It is accepted that the length of instrumentation of infected canal is critical; should be cleaned up to the terminus. It may involve the possibility of over-instrumentation, which can force infected debris into the periradicular areas.

The apical area of the root canal harbors most of the micro-organisms, which remain in contact with the host tissues through apical foramen and other accessory foramen prevalent in that area. Micro-organisms of the apical area, especially in infected cases, are predominantly anaerobic. It has been established that 90% of bacterial cells remain anaerobic after 8–12 weeks in the apical area; prevalent species being *Prevotella intermedia, Prevotella buccalis, Peptostreptococcus anaerobius* and *Veillonella parvula.*

The apical portion of the root canal system is considered 'critical', with regard to cleaning and obturating the area. The quality and quantity of bacteria remaining in this area, whether can be managed by host defense, is not known to the operator. It is mandatory to prepare the canal to its apical limits so as to achieve 'no-bacteria' environment conducive for healing and repair.

To effectively clean and disinfect the apical portion of canal, it is recommended to use patency files, which can breach the apical area or even pass through the dentinal debris created during instrumentation. A small size file (no. 8 or 10) is placed 1.0 mm beyond the apical terminus area in an attempt to remove dentinal debris from the apical portion of the root canal. It is advised that the smaller files should be passively moved through the apical constriction area without widening the same. It is accepted that patency files keep the apical foramen patent and unblocked; maintaining control over the working length.

Since patency files dislodge debris accumulated in the apical portion, it is speculated that the debris is pushed into the periapical areas. The extruded debris can play a role in inducing postoperative pain and even persistence of periapical lesions. However, the influence of small patency files on the extrusion of debris is questionable; many authors have opined that passive action of patency files do not allow debris extrusion and subsequently pain and discomfort.

In case of retreatment of failed root canal treated teeth, the persistent infection in the apical portion is considered as the major cause of failure. Residual micro-organisms can be located in instrumented areas and even in dentinal tubules. If these micro-organisms could not be counteracted by host's defense; and if in sufficient number and virulence, can develop an inflammatory lesion in the periapical areas.

It has been established that enlarging the root canal, without disturbing the apical terminus, would lead to sufficient removal of micro-organisms and their by-products, thereby improving the chances of better outcome of the treatment.

Implications of extraradicular infections

The most common form of extraradicular infection is the acute periradicular abscess, which is the result of egress of virulent bacteria from the root canal. In normal circumstances (host response), the periradicular inflammation succeed in preventing micro-organisms from gaining access to the periradicular tissues; however, in certain cases, the micro-organisms can overcome the resistance and establish extraradicular infection. Extraradicular infection can also be due to the attached bacteria around root tip surface or independent formation of cohesive colonies within the body of the periapical inflammation. It is established that the extraradicular infection may be dependent on root canal infection (egress of bacteria from the root canal) or independent of the root canal infection (bacterial colonies in the form of biofilm around external root tip surface or persistence of certain bacteria even after resolution of periradicular inflammation).

It has been hypothesized that a few species of endodontic microflora have the ability to challenge the host defense and subsequently survive independently in the inflamed periradicular tissues and cause extra-radicular infection. Many types of putative pathogens have been detected in persistent extraradicular infections, such as *Porphyromonas endodontalis, Porphyromonas propionicum, Fusobacterium nucleatum, Treponema* spp. *and Prevotella* spp. A persistent periradicular infection caused by *Actinomyces* spp. is 'periradicular actinomycosis', which can successfully be treated by surgical intervention.

As the success rate of non-surgical root canal treatment is fairly high, it is presumed that the incidence of extraradicular infections is quite low. It has been seen that much of the persistent infections can be resolved with retreatment of the root canal system. Higher percentage of healing after retreatment proves that the main cause is located within the root canal spaces. Root canal procedures may sometimes favor establishment of extraradicular infection (extrusion of debris: over-instrumentation), which should be prevented by all means, preferably sticking to the accurate working length.

Repair Following Endodontic Treatment

The radiographic picture of periapical tissues of a pulpless tooth; if normal prior to treatment, should remain normal after the root canal treatment. Occasionally, immediately after endodontic treatment, the radiograph may show a slight rarefied area, indicating a response to previous irritation, whether mechanical, chemical or bacterial. This is generally considered a prelude to repair. Repair begins as soon as infection is controlled (Fig. 7.2a and b).

The stages of repair may be described as follows:

a. *Organization of the blood clot*
b. *Formation of granulation tissue*: During this stage, the endothelial loops become canalized by the increased pressure of the blood and open new channels for the circulation. Anastomosis of these loops now occurs,

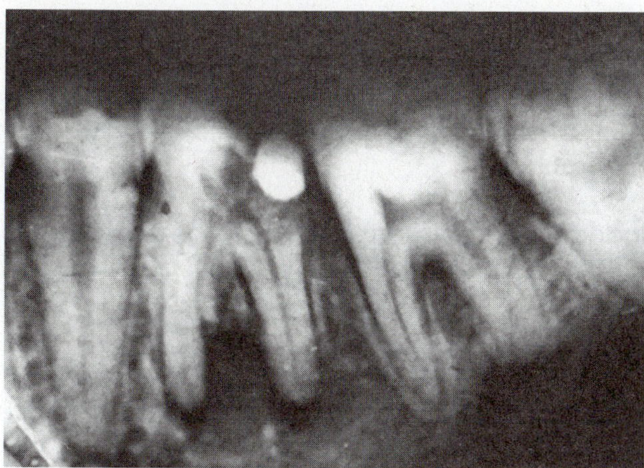

Fig. 7.2a Preoperative

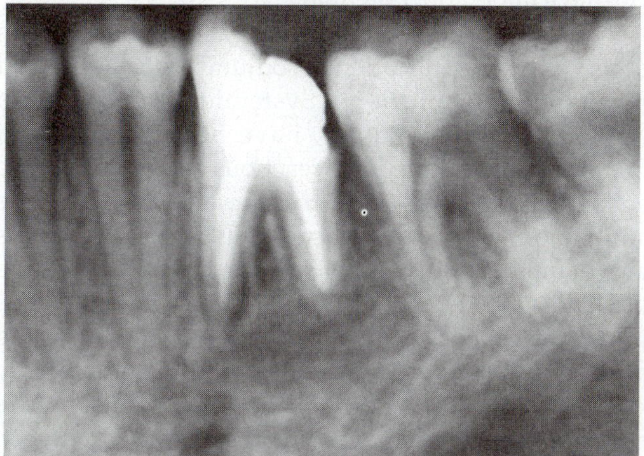

Fig. 7.2b Signs of healing after root canal treatment

forming a rich network of small blood vessels. When an area of rarefaction is present, this stage has already occurred in most cases.

c. *Development of scar tissue*: This stage is present in the soft tissues. Fibroblasts grow along the fibrin strands and help to form the protein matrix by laying down collagen fibers. Both the fibroblasts and the capillaries become fewer in number and vascular fibrous tissue or scar tissue is formed.

In bone, the process is not different; however, it is complicated because soft tissue is to be converted to hard tissue. The protein matrix of bone is formed by osteoblasts, which are specialized fibroblastic cells. The bone matrix fluid is sub-saturated with calcium salts. The osteoblasts produce an enzyme, alkaline phosphatase, which splits off inorganic phosphorous from organically bound phosphorous. The increase in phosphate ions form a saturated solution of calcium phosphate that is precipitated into the matrix. These areas of islands in which the calcium phosphate is precipitated unite to form spongy trabeculae.

Osteoblastic activity is stimulated by stresses and strains, such as exercise of jaw bones during mastication. If a pulpless tooth is already completely out of occlusion, the potential for repair of the periapical tissue is reduced. Moreover, corticosteroids, if given for a prolonged period, inhibit the fibroblastic activity during repair and delay the development of granulation tissue, thus retarding the repair process.

A chronic inflammatory reaction of the periapical tissue is common in the presence of an infected root canal. Shortly after the root canal has been sterilized, the inflammatory reaction subsides, and fibroblasts and osteoblasts become more prominent. Even though some periodontal fibers might have detached, reattachment occurs as the source of infection is removed. Meanwhile, if areas of resorption have developed on the root surface in the region of the destroyed bone, they will be repaired by cementoblasts and these areas will become anchor points for attachment of new periodontal fibers. Resorption and deposition of bone may occur simultaneously. In fact, new bone may even be deposited on old one (new lamellae interwoven with old lamellae can be seen).

It has been observed that when the radiographic examination showed repair, the accuracy of the radiographic interpretation is in concurrence with the histopathologic findings in almost 85% of cases. A reduction in periapical radiolucency and reappearance of bone trabeculae are dependable signs of repair.

The question is often asked whether incompletely developed young teeth will continue to erupt after root canal treatment. It has been observed that endodontic treatment seldom interferes with tooth eruption. Whether to do root canal treatment before or during orthodontic movement is also a question that is occasionally asked. Orthodontic tooth movements do not interfere with the physiology of tooth, even during or after the orthodontic treatment. In most cases, the bands can be left on the teeth because they did not interfere with endodontic treatment. When non-vital teeth are moved with gentle pressure, the tissues remain normal and the repair process is not disturbed. The periodontal ligament is even less likely to be disturbed following endodontic treatment, except when inflammation occurred during treatment. In such cases, it is preferred to elapse at least one week before continuing the orthodontic treatment.

Following endodontic treatment, repair generally occurs in 6 months to one year, depending on the intensity of damage prior to treatment. In some cases, repair may take longer; the area of rarefaction did not disappear completely even after 8 years of endodontic treatment as reported in few studies (areas refer to as 'apical scar').

A persistent area of rarefaction following endodontic treatment is not necessarily indicative of infection as repair might have been completed by connective tissues rather than by bone regeneration. In some cases, the connective tissue matures into dense fibrous tissue instead of bone. Once this occurs, trabeculated bone will not be formed. Clinical cases have been described, in which an area of rarefaction was present, but histological examination depicted dense avascular fibrous connective tissue. Such areas are designated as 'Apical scar'.

Endodontic Infections and Systemic Reactions

The theory of focal infection, as regard causal relationship between oral infections and systemic conditions, remained controversial due to lack of substantial evidence. There is no definite evidence that bacteria from infected root canals can cause bacteremia; however, some specific patients may be at risk.

It has been established that bacteremia can occur as a result of routine activities like chewing, brushing, etc. Since bacteremia can occur from daily activities, it is not possible to exactly determine whether the bacteremia emanated from root canal infection or from other activities. Whatever the origin, bacteremia is usually transient; however, it is prudent to avoid certain situations that could predispose to bacteremia, such as over-instrumentation in endodontics.

Infected root canals and also oral micro-organisms have been considered as potential foci of infection. It is documented that these foci are co-related with systemic diseases, such as coronary heart diseases, bacterial endocarditis, brain abscess, etc. during endodontic procedures; studies have confirmed that bacteremia occur only in case of over-instrumentation and if instruments remain in confines of root canals, bacteremia do not occur. A few authors, however, opined that bacteremia can occur even if instrumentation is maintained within the canal system; hypothesizing that apical debris extrusion is induced by all instrumentation techniques (quantity may vary). Such debris, if infected, can get into periradicular tissues and subsequently into the blood circulation.

It is established that root canal infection may lead to bacteremia, but whether that bacteremia is sufficient to cause diseases or subside with time, has not been confirmed (very few bacterial species of root canal origin survive for longer time in other parts of body).

Further research is warranted to confirm whether bacteria from oral cavity can be involved in focal infections (other body locations); however, antibiotic prophylaxis is advised in patients at risk to develop infective endocarditis. Antibiotic prophylaxis should also be considered for immunosuppressed patients or patients who have undergone surgical procedures in the recent past.

Endodontic Treatment and Allergic Reactions

Endodontic treatment involves series of biomaterials with varying degree of contact with soft tissues and blood circulation. Endodontics may have limited risk of provoking allergic reactions associated with materials; however, ingredients of various materials have been classified as allergens. Materials like iodine, chlorhexidine, sodium hypochlorite, formaldehyde, chloramine, zinc oxide preparation, resin preparations, etc. have allergenic potential.

The most frequent allergic reactions have been observed after application of sodium hypochlorite and formaldehyde solutions. Systemic reactions, both immediate and delayed, have been reported in literature. The immediate reactions are based on the encounter between the intruding allergens and the antibodies released by plasma cells. Type 1 reactions are usually involved; based on release of active mediators by interaction between IgE immunoglobulins in mast cells, eosinophils, platelets and the intruding allergens. Delayed responses may be elicited by haptenic substances, such as metal ions in the endodontic materials (cell mediated delayed reactions). Metal ions (excluding instruments) are limited to silver alloy used in core material and as retrograde filling materials. In addition, metal salts may be present in endodontic sealers (added to enhance radiopacity).

It is hypothesized that minute quantities of chemical substances associated with endodontic therapy may establish contact with immunocompetent host tissue via apical foramen. The direct soft tissue contact is limited to the apical end or accessory canals; overfilled sealers and retrograde fillings, increase the contact considerably.

It is established that sensitization of non-allergic patient by the endodontic materials is least likely; however, allergic reactions in a previously sensitized individual is possible. The apparently low prevalence of such reactions are explained by three factors; small apical exposure, limited possibility of passage through dentinal tubules and the availability of minute quantity of allergens.

Healing of Sinus Tract

Sinus is a tract leading from an enclosed area of inflammation to an epithelial surface, and is one of the sequelae of inflammatory disease. A sinus tract is a drainage duct for the suppuration produced by abscesses (Fig. 7.3a and b). The suppuration from the periapical inflammatory process may be resorbed by the host organism. Otherwise, it will flow through the less resistant tissue area, creating winding trajectories. Then it will spread through the bone marrow, periosteum, loose connective tissue among the muscle fascias, and finally drain onto the epithelial tissue through either a mucosal or, occasionally, a cutaneous sinus tract. Cutaneous sinus tracts cause discomfort to the patient due to frequent drainage on the face and an unpleasant aesthetic appearance. Cutaneous sinus tracts are seen more often in adults than in children. They are usually present on the chin and cheek and 80% of the reported cases are associated with the mandibular teeth. Cutaneous sinus tracts of dental origin are encountered more frequently than sinus tracts of other pathological conditions; therefore, dental infection must be the primary suspect in the differential diagnosis of sinus tracts of the face and neck.

Sinus tract adjacent to teeth or near the apex of the tooth is usually considered to be of endodontic origin and root canal therapy is the primary treatment to achieve its healing. However, stoma of a sinus tract may not always exit opposite the lesion; at times, it may have associated periodontal lesion and require combined endodontic periodontal treatment. Rarely, the etiologic factor may be involving or aggravated by orthodontic reasons. Slutzky-Goldberg et al. found chronic periapical abscess as the most prevalent cause for the origin and existence of the sinus (71.0%) followed by broken restoration (53.0%). The most frequent site of orifices was buccal (82.4%), followed by lingual or palatal (12.0%). According to them, lesions mainly originated from maxillary teeth (63.1%) while mandibular teeth were found responsible for only 38.9% cases. The presence of a sinus tract in the oral cavity is usually considered of pulpal origin, but it can also be caused by periodontal disease, however, the prevalence and incidence of periodontal abscess is lesser than periapical abscess.

The sinus tract itself has been treated with several different therapies, ranging from phenol cauterisation to apicoectomy combined with fistulous trajectory curettage.

Currently, cutaneous sinus tracts of endodontic origin, as well as sinus tracts with either mucosal or nasal drainage, require no special therapy because they heal after appropriate endodontic therapy. A fibrosis of the sinus tract trajectory is not uncommon, mainly in the older sinus tract. In these cases, fibrosis develops peripherally, spreading along the whole trajectory, and its surgical removal is necessary.

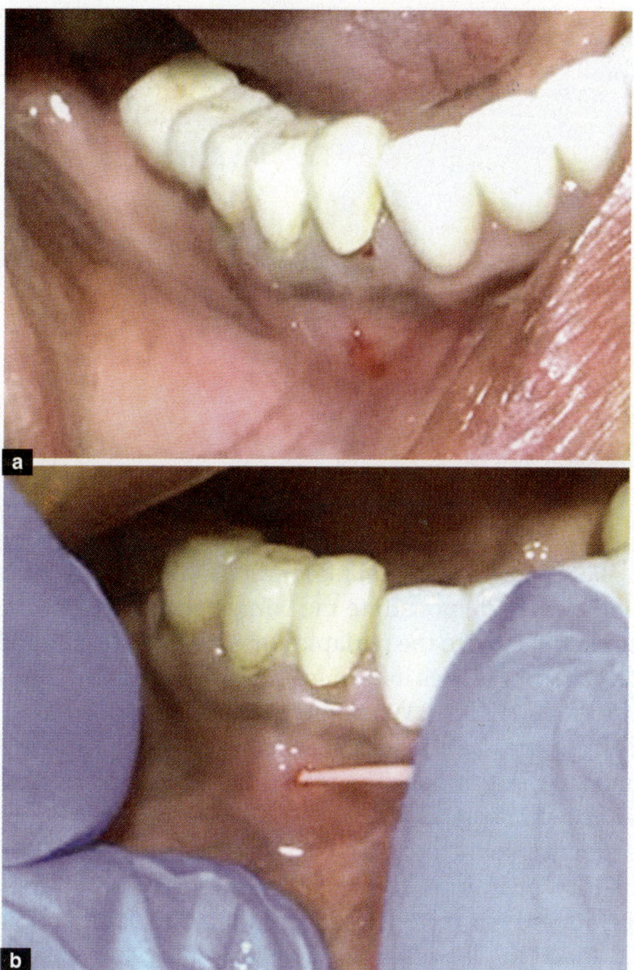

Fig. 7.3 (a) Draining sinus; (b) Sinus tract being checked with gutta-percha

Clinical Assessment

Clinically the sinus opening resembles a small ulcer, but its appearance varies according to the phase of the periapical abscess. During the active phase, the sinus tract is patent and discharges pus. Water soluble radiopaque media can be injected into the patent sinus tract or occasionally, the tract may allow the insertion of a gutta-percha cone or a diagnostic probe (Fig. 7.4).

Table 7.1 Draining sinus v/s healed sinus

Draining sinus	*Healed sinus*
• Sinus is active with pus discharge	• Sinus has healed with pus discharge absent
• Surrounding mucosa is reddish pink in color	• Surrounding mucosa presents normal tissue coloration
• Gutta-percha point can be inserted	• Gutta-percha point cannot be inserted

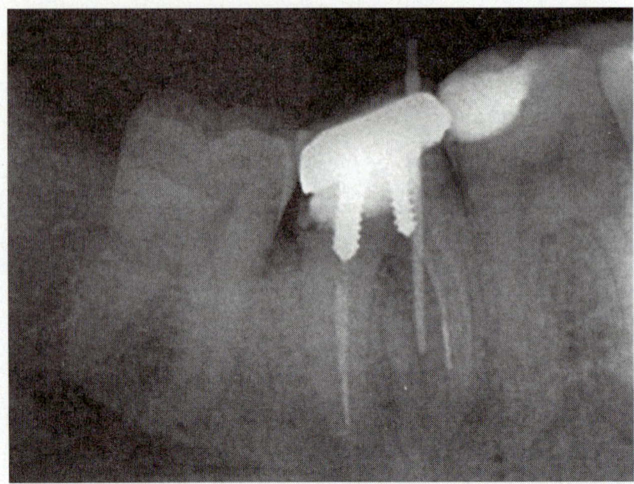

Fig. 7.4 Sinus tracing with gutta-percha

Periapical and lateral radiographs taken at this time will clearly demonstrate the course and extent of the sinus tract. Once the periapical abscess has discharged its contents, it goes into an inactive phase and the sinus tract tends to heal. When there is another exacerbation of the abscess, the sinus tract once again becomes patent and discharges pus. The offending tooth will be non-vital and may be tender. It may have a fracture or caries extending to the pulp, or, the patient will at least give a history of trauma to the tooth or surrounding area. Treatment is directed towards elimination of the source of infection. The offending tooth is removed if it is too badly/grossly decayed, or if there is extensive loss of the surrounding alveolar bone. In most cases, the sinus tract heals spontaneously if the infected pulp is removed, and the root canal debrided and filled (Table 7.1). Some chronic sinus tracts heal leaving behind a small residual scar. Excision of the residual scar may not be required unless its appearance is of concern to the patient.

BIBLIOGRAPHY

1. Baumgartner JC and Fakler WA. Bacteria in the apical 5 mm of infected root canals. J. Endod.: 1991; 17:380–383.
2. Bystrom A, Happonen RP, Sjogren U and Sundqvist G. Healing of periapical lesions of pulpless teeth after endodontic treatment with controlled asepsis. Endod. Dent. Traumatol.: 1987; 3:58–63.
3. Card SJ, Sigurdsson A, Orstavik D and Trope M. The effectiveness of increased apical enlargement in reducing intracanal bacteria. J. Endod.: 2002; 28:779–783.
4. Chugal NM, Clive JM and Spangberg LSW. Endodontic infection: some biologic and treatment factors associated with outcome. Oral Surg., Oral Med., Oral Pathol., Oral Radiol. Endod.: 2003; 96:81–90.
5. Dandakis C, Lamrianidis T and Boura P. Immunologic evaluation of dental patient with history of hypersensitivity to sodium hypochlorite. Endod. Dent. Traumatol.: 2000; 16:184–187.
6. Flanders DH. Endodontic patency. How to get it. How to keep it. Why it is so important. NY. State Dent. J.:2002; 68:30–32.
7. Goldman M, Rankin C, Mehlman R and Santa CA. Immunological implications and clinical management of prophylactic endodontic treatment. Compendium: 1989; 10:462–464.
8. Hamann C, Rodgers PA, Alenius H, Halsey JF and Sullivan K. Cross-reactivity between guttapercha and natural rubber latex. Assumption vs. reality. J. Am. Dent. Assoc.: 2002; 133:1357–1367.
9. Hensten A and Jacobsen N. Allergic reactions in endodontic practice. Endod. Topics: 2005; 12:44–51.
10. Hensten-Pettersen A, Orstavik D and Wennberg A. Allergic potential of root canal sealers. Endod. Dent. Traumatol.: 1986; 1:61–65.
11. Kunisada M, Adachi A, Asano H and Horikawa T. Anaphylaxis due to formaldehyde released from root canal disinfectant. Contact Dermatitis: 2002; 47:215–218.
12. Orstavik D, Qvist V and Stoltze K. A multivariate analysis of the outcome of endodontic treatment. Eur. J. Oral Sci.:2004; 112:224–230.
13. Penick EC. Periapical repair by dense fibrous connective tissue following conservative endodontic therapy. Oral Surg., Oral Med., Oral Pathol.: 1966; 14:239.
14. Seltzer S, Soltanoff W, Sinai I, Goldenberg A and Bender IB. Biologic aspects of endodontics. Part III. Periapical tissue reactions to root canal instrumentation. Oral Surg., Oral Med., Oral Pathol.: 1968; 26:694–705.
15. Sinai I, Seltzer S, Soltanoff W, Goldenberg A and Bender IB. Biologic aspects of endodontics. Part II. Periapical tissue reactions to pulp extirpation. Oral Surg., Oral Med., Oral Pathol.: 1967; 23:664–679.
16. Siqueira JF. Strategies to treat infected root canals. J. Calif. Dent. Assoc.:2001; 29:825–837.
17. Siqueira JF. Reaction of periradicular tissues to root canal treatment: benefits and drawbacks. Endod. Topics: 2005; 10:123–147.
18. Siqueira JF and Lopes HP. Bacteria on the apical root surfaces of untreated teeth with periradicular lesions: a scanning electrone microscopy study. Int. Endod. J.:2001; 34:216–220.
19. Siqueira JF and Rocas IN. Polymerase chain reaction-based analysis of microorganisms associated with failed endodontic treatment. Oral Surg., Oral Med., Oral Pathol., Oral Radiol.: 2004; 97:85–94.

20. Siqueira JF, Rocas IN. Aves FRF and Santos KRN. Selected endodontic pathogens in the apical third of infected root canals. A molecular investigation. J. Endod.: 2004; 30:638–643.

21. Siqueira JF, Rocas IN, Favieri A, Machado AG, Gahyva SM, Oliveira JCM and Abad EC. Incidence of postoperative pain following intracanal procedures based on an antimicrobial strategy. J. Endod.: 2002; 28:457–460.

22. Stock C. Endodontics-position of the apical seal. Br. Dent. J.: 1994; 176:329.

23. Spangberg LSW and Haapasalo M. Rationale and efficacy of root canal medicaments and root filling materials with emphasis on treatment outcomes. Endod. Topics: 2002; 2:35–58.

24. Sundqvist G and Figdor D. Life is an endodontic pathogen. Ecological differences between the untreated and root-filled root canals. Endod. Topics: 2003; 6:3–28.

25. Tronstad L, Barnett F, Riso K and Slots J. Extraradicular endodontic infections. Endod. Dent. Traumatol.: 1987; 3:86.

26. Wu MK, Wesselink PR and Walton RE. Apical terminus locations of root canal treatment procedures. Oral Surg., Oral Med., Oral Pathol., Oral Radiol. Endod.: 2000; 89: 99–103.

27. Yusuf H. The significance of the presence of foreign material periapically as a cause of failure of root treatment. Oral Surg., Oral Med., Oral Pathol.:1984; 54:566.

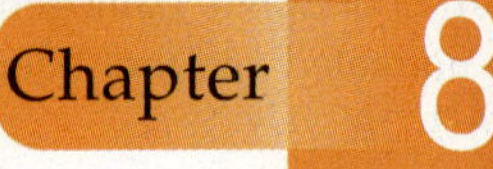

Endodontic Microbiology

The root cause of virtually all diseases of pulp and periapical tissues is micro-organisms. Knowledge of the quality of micro-organisms coupled with their pathological potential is necessary to understand endodontic disease process and to effectively manage such infections.

Molecular biology analysis has established the involvement of both gram-positive and gram-negative bacteria in intraradicular and periradicular infections. In addition to bacteria, fungi, archaea, and viruses have also been observed in intracanal infections. Viruses usually do not survive in necrotic pulp environment (replication depends upon viable host cells); however, human cytomegalovirus and Epstein-Barr virus have been observed in intracanal infections.

The microbes in the normal oral flora are opportunistic pathogens, that is, if they gain access to a normal sterile area of the body such as dental pulp, they may produce disease. The steps in the development of an endodontic infection include microbial invasion, multiplication and pathogenic activity. The intensity of the pathogenic activity is dependent upon host response. It has been reported that endodontic bacteria might be involved in extraoral complications, such as maxillary sinusitis, orbital cellulitis, infective endocarditis, etc.

'Pathogenicity' is a term used to describe the capacity of a microbe to produce disease; whereas, *'virulence'* describes the degree of pathogenicity. Bacteria have a number of virulence factors that may be associated with the disease process. Failure in endodontic therapy may be due to the persistence of infections. The problem is not of the presence of the bacteria, but the specificity of microbial species. Another important concern is that microbes in root canal, despite of growing in aggregate, may form biofilms consisting of a network of different micro-organisms. Biofilms are thin layered condensation of microbes, composed of different bacterial colonies distributed in a matrix. The matrix, constituting about 85% of the total volume, consists of exopolysaccharides, proteins, salts and cell material. The morphology of root canal favors this type of growth.

MICROBES IN ENDODONTIC DISEASE

WD Miller, the father of oral microbiology, was the first researcher to associate presence of bacteria with pulpal disease. Leeuwenhoek, the inventor of a single-lens microscope, was the first to observe oral microbiota from dental plaque and from an exposed pulp cavity.

Invasion of the pulp cavity by bacteria is most often associated with dental caries. Bacteria invade and multiply within the dentinal tubules. Dentinal tubules range in size from 1.0–4.0 μ in diameter, whereas the majority of bacteria are less than 1.0 μ in diameter.

A tooth with a vital pulp is resistant to microbial invasion. Movement of bacteria in dentinal tubules is restricted by viable odontoblastic processes, mineralized crystals, and various macromolecules within the tubules. Caries remains the most common portal of entry for bacteria and bacterial by-products into the pulpal space.

Many studies demonstrated inflammatory reactions adjacent to the exposed dentinal tubules. Although the inflammatory reactions could result in pulpal necrosis, the majority of pulps were able to undergo healing and repair. Following trauma and direct exposure of the pulp, inflammation and bacterial penetration may not be more than 2.0 mm into the pulp. In contrast, a necrotic pulp is rapidly invaded and colonized. Peritubular and reparative dentin may impede the progress of the micro-organisms. However, the empty dentinal tubules, following dissolution of the odontoblastic processes, may allow easy passage of the microbes into the pulp cavity.

Microbes may reach the pulp via direct exposure of the pulp from restorative procedures or trauma or from pathways associated with anomalous tooth development. It is established that changes in the pulp may have correlation with periodontal disease, but pulpal necrosis occurs only if the apical foramen is involved. A few authors are of the opinion that bacteria concurrent in both root canal and periodontal pocket suggests that the periodontal pocket is the source of bacteria in root canal infections.

Anachoresis is the phenomenon by which blood-borne bacteria, dyes, pigments and other materials are attracted and fixed to specific areas of inflammation (process by which microbes may be transported in the blood/lymph to an area of inflammation). It may be the mechanism through which traumatized teeth with intact crowns become infected. The process of anachoresis has been associated with bacteremia and infective endocarditis.

Although more than 150 species of bacteria have been identified in infected root canals, a considerable variation is observed in different individuals with distinct clinical conditions (Fig. 8.1a to d).

Most of the bacteria in an endodontic infection are strict anaerobes. These bacteria grew only in the absence of oxygen but vary in their sensitivity to oxygen. They function at low oxidation-reduction potentials and generally lack the enzymes superoxide dismutase and catalase. Microaerophilic bacteria can grow in an environment with oxygen but predominantly derive their energy from anaerobic energy pathways. Facultative anaerobes grow in the presence or absence of oxygen; possess the enzymes superoxide dismutase and catalase. Obligate aerobes require oxygen for growth; possess the enzyme superoxide dismutase and catalase.

The root canal system is a selective habitat that allows growth of certain bacterial species in preference to others. Tissue fluid and the breakdown products of necrotic pulp provide the requisite nutrients. The nutrients (polypeptides and amino acids), low oxygen tension, and bacterial by-products determine the preferential presence of the bacteria.

A difference exists between the flora of infected root canals, which are open to environment and the one which are closed or freshly opened. The flora is usually polymicrobial, dominated by obligate anaerobic bacteria. Among aerobic micro-organisms, α-hemolytic streptococci are the most commonly recovered organisms. Streptococci mitis and *Streptococcus salivarius* are commonly present in infected root canals.

Although absolute correlation could not be made between any species of bacteria and severity of endodontic infections, several species have been implicated with different clinical signs and symptoms. These species

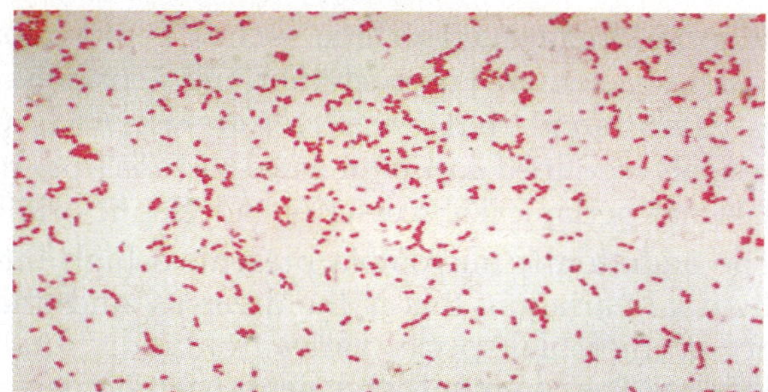

Fig. 8.1a Smear showing Acinetobacter (gram-negative cocci)

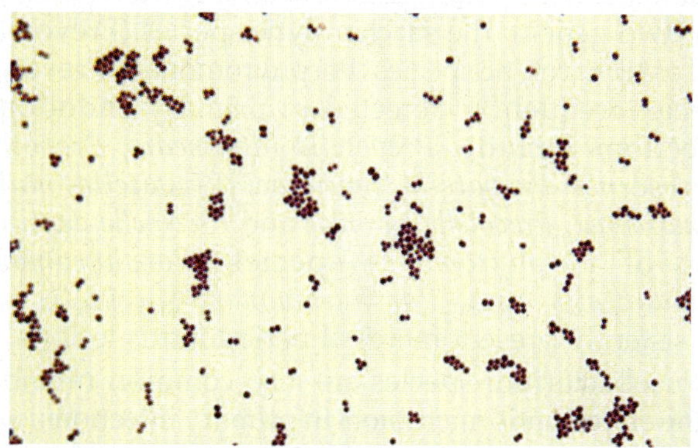

Fig. 8.1b Smear showing *Staphylococcus aureus* (gram-positive cocci)

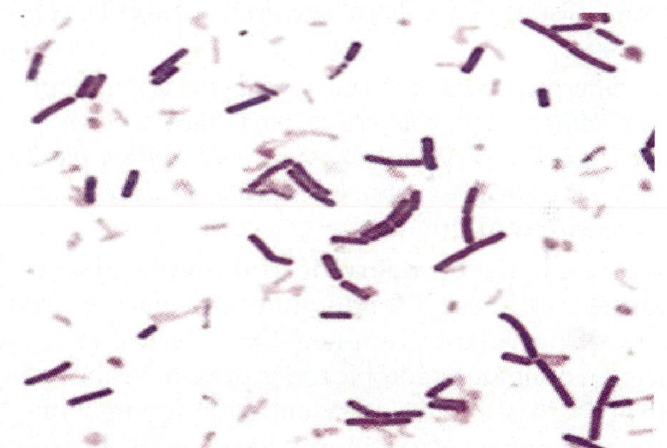

Fig. 8.1c Smear showing Clostridium (gram-positive bacilli)

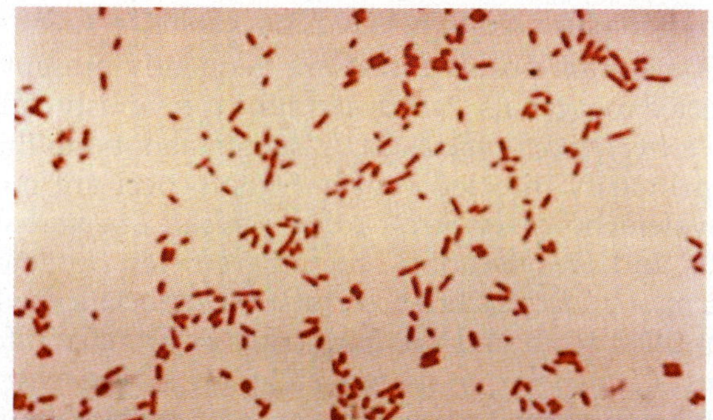

Fig. 8.1d Smear showing *Escherichia coli* (gram-negative bacilli)

include dark-pigmented bacteria, such as, Peptostreptococcus, Eubacterium, Fusobacterium and Actinomyces. It is established that *Prevotella nigrescens* is the commonly identified dark pigmented bacteria from root canals and periapical abscesses of endodontic origin.

The endodontic microbiota presents a high interindividual variation; that is the diversity and abundance of microbial species varies from individual to individual. The commonly prevalent anaerobic bacteria are: Black-pigmented gram-negative anaerobic rods, which include species formerly known as *Bacteroides melaninogenicus*. Later, these bacteria were reclassified into two genera: the saccharolytic species (Prevotella) and asaccharolytic species (Porphyromonas). Prevotella species frequently detected in primary endodontic infections include, *Prevotella intermedia, Prevotella nigrescens, Prevotella tannerae, Prevotella multisacharivorax, Prevotella baroniae* and *Prevotella denticola*. Out of *Porphyromonas* species, *Porphyromonas endodontalis* and *Porphyromonas gingivalis* are consistently present in apical periodontitis lesions.

Fusobacterium species are also common members of the endodontic microbiota in primary infections, with *Fusobacterium nucleatum* being the most prevalent.

Spirochetes are highly mobile spiral-shaped bacteria, falling under genera, Treponema. The most prevalent *Treponema* species are *Treponema denticola* and *Treponema socranskii*.

To differentiate the abscess of periodontal origin from that of endodontic origin, the key factor is the enumeration of spirochetes. The periodontal abscess may contain plenty of spirochetes (30–58%); whereas, endodontic abscess contain less spirochetes (0–10%).

Gram-positive anaerobic rods have also been identified. Of these, Pseudoramibacter alactolyticus is the most prevalent gram-negative species. Filifactor alocis, an obligate anaerobic rod is present in about one-half of the cases of primary endodontic infections. A high prevalence of Actinomyces species, Propionibacterium propionicum, *Olsenella* species, *Slackia exigua, Mogibacterium timidum*, and *Eubacterium* species have also been observed in infected root canals.

Some gram-positive cocci are frequently present in infected root canals. *Parvimonas micra* (previously called *Peptostreptococcus micros*) is present in about one-third of primarily infected canals. Streptococci are most prevalent; however, *Streptococcus gordonii, Streptococcus mitis* and *Streptococcus sanguis* are often detected. *Enterococcus faecalis* has been found in association with root-filled teeth and not frequently in primary infections. *Campylobacter* species including *Campylobacter rectus* and *Campylobacter gracilis*, and gram-negative anaerobic rods have been detected in primary endodontic infections; however, their prevalence is low.

Catonella morbid, a saccharolytic obligate anaerobic gram-negative rod associated with marginal periodontitis, has been found in about 1/4th of the cases of primary endodontic infections. Other bacteria detected sporadically in primary infections include *Veillonella parvular, Eikenella corrodens, Granulicatella adiacens, Neisseria mucosa, Centipede periodontii, Gemella morbillorum, Capnocytophaga gingivalis, Corynebacterium matruchotii, Bifidobacterium dentium* and *anaerobic lactobacilli*.

Gemella morbillorum and *Gemella haemolysans* have been isolated from primary endodontic infections although they do present in persistent infections also.

Studies using broad range PCR associated with clone library analysis or P-RFLP have indicated that many yet-to-be cultivated bacteria can participate in endodontic infection. More than 40–50% of the endodontic microbiota is composed of bacterial phylotypes that are yet to be cultivated belonging to genera synergist, TM7 Dialister, Megapharea, Solobacterium, Olsenella, Eubacterium, cytophaga as well as phytotypes related to family lachnospiraceae.

Yet-to-be cultivated species:

- Synergistes oral clone Ba121
- Synergistes oral clone BH017
- Synergistes oral clone Wo90
- TM7
- Dailister invisus
- Dialister pneumosintes
- Solobacterium
- *Olsenella* spp.
- *Megaspharea* spp. Oral clone CS025
- Eubacterium oral clone BP1-89
- *Eubacterium infirmum*
- *Eubacterium saphenum*
- Cytophaga
- Lachnospiraceas oral clone 55A34
- Lachnospiraceas oral clone MCE760

Endodontic bacteria, broadly belong to 8 of the 12 phyla that have oral representatives, namely firmicutes, bacteroides, spirochetes, fusobacteria, actinobacteria, proteobacteria, synergistes and TM7. Member of the two latter phyla and several representatives of the other phyla still remain to be cultivated.

Rare Endodontic Infections

The micro-organisms rarely seen in endodontic infections are:

Fungi: *Candida* species have been occasionally found in primary root canal infections; mainly identified from persistent root canal infections.

Archaea: It is a highly diverse group of prokaryotes. Archaea, usually not described as a human pathogen, has been detected in 25% root canals of teeth with chronic apical periodontitis.

Virus: Viruses rarely infect root canals. Of the 8 human herpes viruses currently identified, the human cytomegalovirus (HCMV) and Epstein-Barr virus (EBV) have been linked to pathogenesis of periodontal diseases.

MICROFLORA OF ROOT FILLED TEETH

It has also been established that the outcome of the endodontic treatment is significantly influenced by the presence of bacteria in the root canals, especially at the root canal filling stage. This suggests that persistent bacteria can survive in treated root canals and sustain periapical tissue inflammation.

It is important to understand some aspects related to the significance of bacteria found in post-treatment samples. Studies investigating bacteria remaining in the canals after chemomechanical procedures or intra-canal medication provide a prospective view; that is, bacteria found in these samples have the potential to influence the treatment outcome. The percentage of most prevalent bacteria after use of different irrigants and intracanal medicaments is depicted in Table 8.1.

Table 8.1 Studies showing percentage of bacteria after use of various irrigants and intracanal medicaments

Study (author and year)	*Irrigant used*	*Intracanal medicament used*	*Sample taken after*	*Most prevalent species*	*Presence of bacteria (percent)*
Brystrom and Sundquist (1981)	Saline	No	Chemomechanical preparation	*Peptostreptococcus anaerobius* *Lactobacillus* species	70
Bystrom and Sundquist (1985)	0.5% Sodium hypochlorite	No	Chemomechanical preparation	*Fusobacterium* species *Streptococcus* species *Eubacterium* species *Porphyromonas gingivalis* Prevotella species	45
Bystrom and Sundquist (1985)	5% Sodium hypochlorite	No	Chemomechanical preparation	*Streptococcus* species *Fusobacterium nucleatum*	50
Bystrom and Sundquist (1985)	5% Sodium hypochlorite and EDTA	No	Chemomechanical preparation	Streptococci species	75
Gomes et al (1996)	2.5% Sodium hypochlorite	No	Chemomechanical preparation	Streptococci species *Peptostreptococcus micros* *Lactobacillus* species	80
Sjögren et al (1997)	0.5% Sodium hypochlorite	No	Chemomechanical preparation	*Pseudoramibacter alactolyticus* *Fusobacterium nucleatum* *Campylobacter rectus* *Peptostreptococcus micros*	62
Peters et al (2002)	2.0% Sodium hypochlorite	No	Chemomechanical preparation	Actinomyces species *Prevotella intermedia* *Peptostreptococcus micros* *Eggerthella center* *Prevotella oralis*	58
Peters et al (2002)	2.0% Sodium hypochlorite	Calcium hydroxide	Intracanal medication	*Propionibacterium* species *Peptostreptococcus micros* *Veillonella* species *Bifidobacterium* species *Capnocytophaga* species	61
Chavez de Paz et al (2003)	0.5% Sodium hypochlorite	Calcium hydroxide	Intracanal medication	*Lactobacillus* species *Enterococcus* species *Propionibacterium* species	88
Chu et al (2006)	0.5% Sodium hypochlorite	Calcium hydroxide	Intracanal medication	*Neisseria* species *Staphylococcus* species *Capnocytophaga* species *Actinomyces* species	60

It is established that the major factor influencing the outcome of the endodontic treatment is the presence of micro-organisms in the canal at the time of filling. When no bacteria are recovered from the canal at the filling stage, healing of apical periodontitis occurs uneventfully. Therefore, the discussion on the topic "One visit versus multiple visits" should focus on how many visits are required for the canal to be predictably disinfected. Total eradication of bacteria can practically be achieved after chemomechanical procedures; however, certain micro-organisms may be able to survive the chemomechanical effects.

EXTRARADICULAR INFECTIONS

Apical periodontitis lesions are formed in response to intraradicular infections. In most situations, apical periodontitis inflammatory lesions succeed in preventing micro-organisms from gaining access to the periapical tissues. The most common form of extraradicular infection is the apical abscess, characterized by purulent inflammation in the periapical tissues in response to a massive egress of virulent bacteria from the root canal. Most oral micro-organisms are opportunistic pathogens and only a few species have the ability to challenge and overcome host defense mechanism and establish an extraradicular infection.

For instance, it is recognized that some *Actinomyces* species and *Propionibacterium propionicum* have the ability to participate in extraradicular infections and cause a pathological entity called *'apical actinomycosis'*. Some other putative oral pathogens, such as *Treponema* species, *Porphyromonas endodontalis, Porphyromonas gingivalis, Prevotella* species and *Fusobacterium nucleatum*, have also been detected in persistent apical periodontitis lesions.

The major cause of failure after root canal treatment is the persistence of micro-organisms in the apical part of the root filled teeth. Certain species present in normal endodontic infections are capable to survive under nutrient-deficient conditions of the root filled teeth. The microflora of teeth with persistent disease can be enterococci, streptococci followed by lactobacilli, Actinomyces, Propionibacterium, Dialister and Filifactor. The endodontically treated teeth requiring re-treatment have shown a higher prevalence of facultative bacteria, especially *Enterococcus faecalis*, instead of strict anaerobes. In untreated root canal, Enterococci constitute about 5.0% of micro-organisms. Due to change in root canal environment, this micro-organism grow in higher and recoverable proportion. Studies have reported that *Enterococcus faecalis* has some special characteristics which allow them to survive under unfavorable conditions. *Enterococcus faecalis* and allied species enter the canal during treatment, especially when the canal is left open. It is also reported that capacity to withstand wide pH range (up to 11.5) of intracanal medicaments such as calcium hydroxide, make enterococci more viable in root filled teeth. Another characteristic of enterococci is an ability to survive even in the environment of low nutritional supply.

Another micro-organism which has been identified in persistent periapical lesions is *Candida albicans*. Such infections are same in untreated root canals, unless these canals are open to oral environment. *Candida* species can also grow in low-nutrient environment and can resist calcium hydroxide medicaments.

Actinomyces are also prevalent in resistant retreatment cases. *Actinomyces israelii* and *Actinomyces meyeri* are more frequently found in resistant cases and may involve in periapical actinomyces. Recently, Actinomyces radicidentis has been identified. *Propionibacterium propionicus (Arachnia propionica)*, a facultative anaerobe, has been associated with persistent infections that do not respond to conventional root canal treatment (Table 8.2).

Table 8.2 Bacterial species commonly found in infected root canals

Gram-positive cocci	*Gram-positive rods*	*Gram-negative cocci*	*Gram-negative rods*
• *Streptococcus anginosus* • *Streptococcus sanguis* • *Streptococcus mitis* • *Streptococcus mutans*	• *Actinomyces israeli* • *Actinomyces naeslundii*	• *Veillonella parvula* • *Acidaminococcus* spp.	• *Prevotella intermedia* • *Prevotella melaninogenica* • *Prevotella denticola* • *Prevotella buccalis* • *Prevotella oralis*
	• *Eubacterium alactolyticum* • *Eubacterium nodatum* • *Eubacterium limosum*	• *Neisseria mucosa*	• *Porphyromonas endodontalis* • *Porphyromonas gingivalis*
• *Enterococcus faecalis* • *Enterococcus faecium*	• *Propionibacterium propionicus* • *Propionibacterium granulosum*		• *Fusobacterium nucleatum*
• *Parvimonas micra*	• *Lactobacillus* spp. • *Corynebacterium matruchotii*		• *Bacteroides gracilis* • *Campylactobacter rectus* • *Campylobacter curvus* • *Capnocytophaga ochracea*

MICROBIAL DIAGNOSTIC TECHNIQUES

Endodontic infections, being polymicrobial in nature, present problems in identification. Previous studies utilized only aerobic cultivation method, ignoring anaerobic bacteria. Recent techniques revealed broader spectrum of bacteria, including viruses, archaea and fungi etc.

Several methodologies have been used for identification of endodontic infections. Sample collection is important feature for analyzing any endodontic infection.

Sample Collection

The patient is asked to rinse thoroughly. Isolate the tooth with rubber dam. Disinfect both tooth and the rubber dam using 5–10% tincture iodine. The nearby environment is also kept sterile (a live flame is kept in the nearest vicinity of the tooth). To sample a dry canal, a syringe is used to place culture medium into the canal. A file is then used to scrape the canal walls to suspend micro-organisms with the medium. In case of draining canals, a paper point can be kept in the root canal for 30 seconds and shifted to the medium. A syringe after air aspiration can also be used.

A small gauge needle is used to aspirate and collect sample in case of abscess. If aspiration is not possible, the exudates can be collected on a swab. The sample is quickly transferred to the requisite medium.

I. Culture

The type of culture medium influences the results of root canal cultures. Various media have been used in endodontics. These include, brain heart infusion broth (with and without 0.1% agar), thioglycollate broth, glucose ascites, cooked meat and Moller's medium. Glucose ascites medium is preferred since agar allows for growth of aerobes and anaerobes and the ascitic fluid stimulates the growth of fastidious organisms; and glucose help growth of acidogenic species.

Advantages

- Broad range; unexpected species can be identified.
- Allow quantification of major viable micro-organisms.
- Physiological and pathogenicity studies are possible.
- Widely accepted.

Limitations

- Large number of bacterial species cannot be cultured.
- All viable bacteria may not be recovered.
- Once isolated, bacteria require further identification using a number of techniques.
- Low sensitivity.
- Strict dependence on the mode of sample transport.
- Samples require immediate processing.
- Identification of anaerobic bacteria may take several days.
- Costly, time-consuming and laborious.
- Cultivation of strict anaerobe is difficult.

Reasons for bacterial unculturability

- Lack of essential nutrients/growth factors in the artificial culture medium.
- Toxicity of the culture medium may inhibit bacterial growth.
- Other species present in a mixed consortium may produce substances inhibitory to the target micro-organisms.
- Metabolic dependence on other species for growth.
- Disruption of bacterial intercommunication systems induced on culture media.
- Bacterial dormancy (a state of low metabolic activity that some bacteria develop under stressful conditions/starvation) in bacterial cells do not allow them to divide or to form colonies on culture medium.

II. Microscopic Examination

Microscopic examination observes the presence/absence of micro-organisms (infection). Gram stains reveal morphology of microbes; whereas, gram reaction reveals the gram-positive or negative of microbes. Phase contrast microscopy and dark field microscopy are better tools for identifying various species of micro-organisms, including spirochetes.

Advantages

- Supplements culture method.
- Provides rapid information about the flora.

Limitations

- Has limited sensitivity (relatively large number of cells are required before they are seen under microscope).
- Has limited specificity (inability to specify micro-organisms based on pleomorphic morphology).

III. Immunological Methods

The enzyme linked immunosorbent assay (ELISA) and the direct or indirect immunofluorescence tests are commonly used immunological methods for microbial identification.

Advantages

- Takes few hours to identify the microbial species.
- Low cost.
- Can detect dead micro-organisms.

Limitations
- Detect only the target species.
- Low sensitivity.
- Specificity is variable.

IV. Molecular Methods

The commonly encountered micro-organisms are categorized as:

a. Prokaryocytes (prokaryotes)
   - Examples are bacteria, archaea
   - Does not have membrane binding nuclei
   - No mitochondria and Golgi apparatus present
   - Cells have 70s ribosomes (30s–50s subunits containing 16S rRNA and 23S rRNA molecules)

b. Eukaryocytes (eukaryotes)
   - Example is fungi
   - Membrane bound nucleus
   - Cells have 80s ribosomes (40s–60s subunits containing 185 rRNA and 25s rRNA molecules).

The limitations of culture method have led to the introduction of molecular method for identifying uncultivable species. A number of bacteria, such as Bacteroids and Treponemas could be identified from root canals following molecular methods.

It has been established that more than 50% bacterial species are uncultivable. Molecular methods could identify many previously unknown pathogens. Molecular approaches rely on the fact that certain genes contain the microbial identity (ribosomes are intracellular particles composed of rRNA and proteins; sizes are represented by Svedberg (s) units; bacterial cells may have 40s ribosomes with small and large subunits genes. These genes are used in molecular analysis).

There are a plethora of molecular methods for the study of micro-organisms; main being Polymerase chain reaction (PCR) and DNA-DNA hybridization.

Polymerase Chain Reaction (PCR)/ Molecular Amplification

Polymerase chain reaction/molecular amplification is able to amplify one gene to millions of copies of that gene. The strategies are, target nucleic acid amplification, nucleic acid probe amplification and amplification of the probe signal. PCR has the ability to locate and amplify small quantity of specific nucleotide sequence, which might have lost in large ground of nucleic acid (Fig. 8.2).

The PCR method, based on DNA replication, involves three steps, viz. denaturation of target nucleic acid, primer annealing and extension of primer-targets.

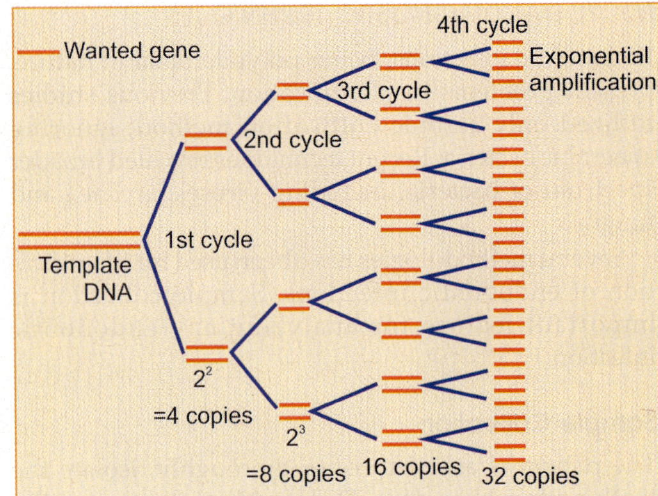

Fig. 8.2 Exponential amplification

- Denaturation of target nucleic acid occurs at 90–95°C, whereby DNA strands get separated.
- Primer annealing occurs at lower temperature (55–60°C) whereby short sequence nucleotide is annealed to a particular nucleic acid target, resulting in duplex formation.
- Extension of primer-target occurs at 70–75°C, whereby two duplex strands are formed with the help of enzyme polymerase.

Reverse transcription polymerase chain reaction (RT-PCR), a variant of polymerase chain reaction (PCR), is a technique commonly used in molecular biology to detect RNA expression (Fig. 8.3). Reverse transcriptase PCR (RT-PCR), involves exploiting the ability of reverse transcriptase enzyme to synthesize complementary DNA (cDNA) from mRNA transcripts, and then using PCR to amplify regions of interest. RT-PCR is used to clone expressed genes by reverse transcribing the RNA of interest into its DNA complement through the use of reverse transcriptase. Subsequently, the newly synthesized cDNA is amplified using traditional PCR.

Various derivatives of PCR technology have been developed; the commonly used PCR-derived assays are:

i. *Multiplex PCR*: Multiplex PCR assay permits the simultaneous detection of different microbial species. Two or more sets of primers specific for different targets are introduced. Primers having similar annealing temperatures are selected for multiplication.

ii. *Nested PCR*: This approach provides increased sensitivity. The first PCR product is subjected to second round of amplification with a separate primer set and anneals accordingly. However, Nested PCR has one drawback; high probability of contamination during transfer of first round product to the second one.

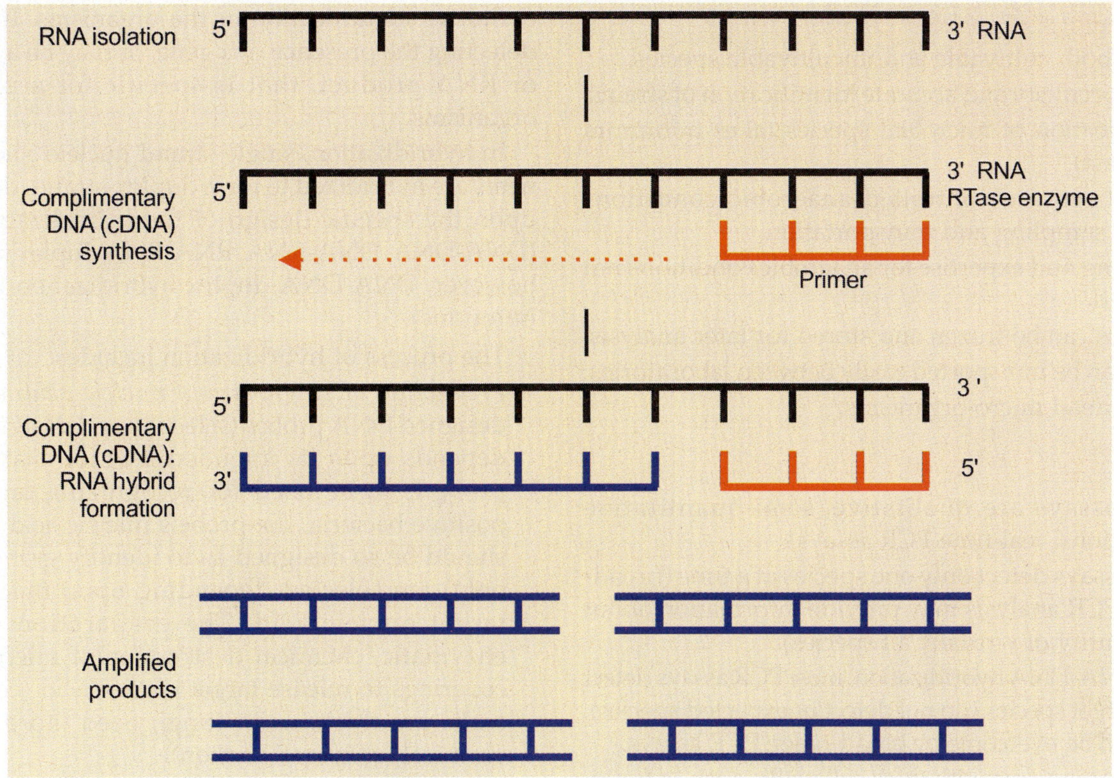

Fig. 8.3 Reverse transcriptase-PCR (RT-PCR)

iii. *Real time PCR*: Real time PCR assay allows for quantification of individual target species and also the total number of bacteria in a clinical sample. The process is fast and contamination of nucleic acid is limited as no manipulation is carried out after initial amplification (overcome disadvantage of Nested PCR).

iv. *Arbitrarily primed-PCR (AP-PCR)*: AP-PCR is relatively fast PCR based fingerprinting (genomic) technique used to determine whether two isolates of the same species are epidemiologically related. The technique is also known as random amplified polymorphic DNA (RAPD). The advantage of AP-PCR includes its ability to furnish specific DNA profiles without knowing the DNA sequences. Clonal analysis of micro-organisms may help to know whether certain strains of a given species are associated with a disease process and also help tracking the origin of micro-organism infecting a particular site.

v. *Broad-range PCR*: Broad-range PCR can identify several novel, unexpected and uncultivable bacterial pathogens directly from the diverse human sites. The technology is used to investigate the whole microbial diversity in a given environment. In PCR broad-range technique, primers are so designed that are complementary to conserved regions of a particular gene that are shared by a group of micro-organisms.

Denatured Gradient Gel Electrophoresis (DGGE)

The genetic fingerprinting of complex microbial communities implies extracting and amplification of rDNA using broad range primers and then analyzing the amplified PCR products by denaturing gradient gel electrophoresis (DGGE). The DGGE technique is based on electrophoresis of PCR amplified rDNA fragments in polysaccharide gel containing increasing gradients of DNA denaturants.

In DGGE technique, multiple samples can be analyzed concurrently and possible to compare the structures of microbial community of different areas. Temperature gradient get electrophoresis (TGGE) uses the same principle as of DGGE, but temperature gradient is used in TGGE as compared to chemical denaturants in DGGE.

Terminal Restriction Fragment Length Polymorphism (T-RFLP)

Terminal restriction fragment length polymorphism, a modified version of conventional RFLP, wherein rDNA from different species in a community is PCR amplified using primers labelled with fluorescent dye. (The fluorescent dyed primer limits the analysis to only the terminal fragment of the enzymatic process.) T-RFLP has greater resolution than gel based techniques (DGGE/TGGE). The technique effectively assesses genetic differences between microbial strains and also provide insight into the structure and function of microbial communities.

Advantages of PCR Derived Techniques

- Detect both cultivable and uncultivable species.
- High specificity and accurate identification of strains.
- Identification of microbial species takes minimum time (fast).
- Do not require controlled anaerobic conditions during sampling and transportation.
- Handling and expertise for anaerobic conditions not required.
- Samples can be frozen and stored for later analysis.
- DNA can be transported easily between laboratories.
- Detect dead micro-organisms.

Limitations of PCR Derived Techniques

- Most assays are qualitative/semi-quantitative (exceptions: real-time PCR assays).
- Most assays detect only one species at a time (broad-range PCR analysis may provide information about the identity of virtually all species).
- Like DNA-DNA hybridization, most PCR assays detect only target species (do not detect unexpected species). This can be overcome by broad-range PCR assays.
- Micro-organisms with thick cell walls, such as fungi, may be difficult to break open and may require additional steps for lysis and consequent release of DNA.
- Some assays can be laborious and costly.
- Hybridization assays using whole genome probes detect only cultivable species.
- Possibility of false positive and false negative results.

DNA-DNA Hybridization

The basic principle is the presence of a specific gene/particular nucleic acid sequence, interpreted as a definitive identification of the organisms. It involves detecting the presence of a gene, or may be a part of it, or RNA product, that is specific for a particular organisms.

In hybridization, single-strand nucleic acid components are hybridized to form duplex-strand, depending upon the specific design of the hybridization assay (DNA-DNA, DNA-RNA, RNA-RNA duplex may form; however, DNA-DNA duplex hybridization is formed in routine).

The process of hybridization includes:

- *Production of single-strand nucleic acid*: Specially designed DNA probes (selection and design of probe depends upon its intended use; for example, if a probe is to be used for recognizing only gram-positive bacteria, the probe's nucleic acid sequence should be so designed as to identify gram-positive only) are selected depending upon the intended target nucleic acid. The preparation involves enzymatic/chemical destruction of microbial cell coverings to release target nucleic acid (certain cell walls are thick, as in fungi; need more time for chemical/enzymatic action).
- Hybridization of target and probe nucleic acid: Hybridization involves radiography (mixing in radiographic film) or non-radioactive means, such as, colorimetry and fluorescence.

In DNA-DNA hybridization technology, the microbial species are not cultivated, nor their DNA amplified. The method permits simultaneous determination of the presence of multitude of bacterial species in single/multiple samples (check-board method).

The main features of microbial identification methods are tabulated in Table 8.3.

Table 8.3 Microbial identification methods: Main features

Culture method	*Microscopic examination*	*Immunological method*	*Molecular analysis*
• Easily identifies bacterial number	• Identify location and density of micro-organisms	• Enzyme linked assays detect even dead cells	• Accurately analyze microbial virulence, and gene expressions
• Effective in study of microbial virulence and antibiotic resistance	• Especially useful for some fastidious organisms (spirochetes are observed under dark-field microscope)	• Low sensitivity, allow detection of specific micro-organisms	• Protein expression can estimate the total bacterial load
• Shows microbial viability	• Allows determination of live and dead cells		• Better sensitivity of microbial detection, taxonomy of micro-organisms and identification of pathogenic strains
• Facilitate *in vitro* testing and experiments	• Allows differentiating microbial forms, shapes and other features		

MICROBIAL INTERACTIONS IN INFECTED ROOT CANALS

a. Host-Microbe Interactions

As the carious activities progress, inflammatory reaction develops in the pulp. The dentin permeability help carry bacterial products to the pulp.

Several physiochemical factors in the root canal have the potential to influence the pathogenicity of bacteria and may modulate the host defense mechanism.

The immune competent cells of pulp provide the necessary signals to activate T-lymphocytes, responsible for local immune defense. Human dental pulps have immune competent cells, such as, helper/inducer T cells, cytotoxic/suppressor T cells, macrophages and class II antigen-expressing cells essential for the initiation of immune responses.

When the host immune system is compromised, or the invading micro-organisms are pathogenic, disease can develop (*Pathogenicity implies ability of an organism to cause disease in another organism*). The pathogens in any form (bacteria, fungi, virus, etc.) can cause tissue destruction directly or indirectly.

Endotoxins, enzymes and associated metabolites affect directly; whereas, indirect damage is caused by disturbing host defense mechanism, induced by bacterial components, which include lipopolysaccharide (LPS), peptidoglycans (PG), lipoteichoic acid (LTA), fimbriae, exotoxins and certain cell membrane proteins. The degree of depth of pathogenicity (disease producing ability) is known as 'virulence'. The characteristics of certain virulence factors playing effective role in endodontic infections are:

- Lipopolysaccharide (LPS), also known as endotoxin, is a part of cell wall of gram-negative micro-organisms.
- Peptidoglycans (PG), a part of cell wall of gram-positive micro-organisms, react with innate immune system inducing inflammatory cytokines in T cells.
- Lipoteichoic acid (LTA), a part of cell wall of gram-positive micro-organisms, composed of lipids and echoic acid; binds with target cells and interact with circulating antibodies.
- Exotoxins, released by living cell, can trigger aberrant activation of T cells (can be bactericidal to other bacteria).
- Fimbriae, thin hair like projections made up of proteins found on cell surface of many gram-negative bacteria; involved in interactions with other bacteria.
- Extracellular proteins, released during bacterial cell lysis; neutralize immunoglobulins and complement components.

A couple of virulent factors, such as polyamines, fatty acids, capsule and extracellular vesicles also participate in host-microbe interactions.

b. Interaction among Micro-organisms

Another mechanism by which the micro-organisms modulate the infection process include ability of some bacteria to inactivate killing mechanism of phagocytic cells. A few bacteria may even genetically vary their surface antigens, causing difficulty for immune system to target these bacteria.

i. Gene Transfer Systems

Chromosomal DNA usually carries genes necessary for cell survival. Bacteria also carry accessory genetic elements, collectively describes as *'horizontal gene pool'*, which include plasmids, bacteriophages, transposons and insertion sequences. These provide movement of genetic information between different bacteria. Plasmids can carry genes that code for antibiotic resistance and also genes capable of transfer from one bacterial cell to another. Transposons, a segment of DNA, can move from one location to another (jump from one DNA molecule to another, refer to as 'jumping genes'). The basic methods by which bacteria can transfer DNA are transformation, transduction and conjugation (cells providing DNA are 'donor' cells and cells receiving DNA are 'recipient').

The genetic transformation of bacteria involve active uptake of DNA and incorporation into the recipient (the recipient cell gets transformed). Natural transformation has been observed in gram-positive bacteria, viz. *Streptococcus mutans*, *Streptococcus gordonii*, and *Streptococcus pneumoniae*.

Transduction involves bacteriophages, which have been isolated from *Actinomyces actinomycetemcomitans* and other *Actinomyces* species in dental plaque and from *E. faecalis* in saliva. Conjugation is considered as the most efficient principle in gene transfer; DNA is transferred between cells that are in cell-to-cell (physical) contact. Conjugative plasmids and conjugative transposons (jumping genes) are transferred between cells that are in physical contact. They are ubiquitous in gram-negative bacteria as well as in gram-positive enterococci, streptococci, staphylococci, Listeria, Bacillus, Clostridium, and Rhodococcus. Conjugation can occur between bacteria and eukaryotic cells. Two groups of conjugative plasmids (pAM 1 and pIP501) have been recognized in gram-positive bacteria (earlier, studies observed conjugative plasmids only in gram-negative bacteria). The conjugate plasmids can transfer from prokaryote *E. coli* to eukaryote yeast,

Saccharomyces cerevisiae, as well as to high eukaryotes such as Chinese hamster ovary cells (CHOC).

The pheromones are secreted by a potential 'recipient' cell which 'activates' the transfer system of a potential 'donor' cell. Pheromone-responding plasmids in *E. faecalis* can carry genes related to antibiotic resistance as well as virulent traits.

ii. Antibiotic Resistance and Virulence associated with Plasmids

In addition to antibiotic resistance, a diverse range of products that may potentially contribute towards 'Virulence' such as cytotoxins, adhesions, and certain metabolic enzymes are also often encoded by plasmids. Genes on plasmids that encode cytolysins have been observed in *E. faecalis*, in most of clinical samples.

iii. Plasmids in the Oral/Endodontic Microbiota

In the oral microbiota, studies have focused on the identification and epidemiology of plasmids in streptococci, black-pigmented anaerobic bacteria, *P. nigrescens*, *F. nucleatum*, oral spirochetes and *E. faecalis*. Plasmids were found in 26.7% *F. nucleatum* strains. Plasmids were isolated from 7 to 11 oral *E. faecalis* strains recovered from endodontic patients. It is also shown that gene transfer can occur from *T. denticola* to *S. gordonii* in experimental biofilms.

Several studies have reported the positive and negative association of bacteria and pairs of bacteria with various clinical signs and symptoms. For example, positive associations were found between *F. nucleatum* and *P. micra*, *P. endodontalis*, *Selenomonas sputigena*, and *Campylobacter rectus* in teeth with apical periodontitis. In contradiction, species of Streptococci, *P. propionicum*, *Capnocytophaga ochracea* and *Vibrio* spp. could not show any association with other bacteria.

BIOFILMS IN ENDODONTIC INFECTIONS

Biofilm is defined as '*a sessile, multicellular microbial community, characterized by cells that are attached to a surface and collectively enmeshed in a matrix of polymeric substances (usually polysaccharides), their own secretions*'. Literally, biofilm implies a thin layer of condensed microbes, which may occur in any surface structure in nature. The primary source for organization of this biofilm is the free-floating bacteria (called planktonic bacteria), which exist in any aqueous environment. The excreted products of these bacteria, especially the adhesive substances like polysaccharides and proteins are the pre-requisite for initial attachment of organisms and also binding different bacteria in the film. The matrix constitutes approximately 85% of biofilm, rest are the cells. It is established that biofilms assume a stronger pathogenic potential as compared to organisms in planktonic stage. Formation of biofilms challenge the host-defense system and also therapeutic anti-microbial treatment measures.

The scanning microscopic evaluation observed micro-colonies of micro-organisms in the biofilms that contain open water channels, within which flow of water and nutrients occurs. Bacteria living in community life style has several advantages, as bacteria functioning together in biofilm are able to degrade large complex nutrient molecule that would not be degraded by an individual bacteria. Glycoproteins and other proteins supplied by oral fluids act as source of nutrition for the microbial communities.

The sessile micro-organisms in biofilm are 1000 times resistant to anti-microbial agents as compared to same organisms in planktonic form. It is established that the physiological properties of bacteria in biofilms are different from those of same bacteria in other environment (Phenotype of biofilms bacteria is distinct from that of planktonic bacteria). Oral micro-organisms have the capacity to adapt to changing environment. With respect to environmental heterogenicity within biofilm, it is likely that different biofilm harbor different phenotypes of micro-organisms. The diverse physical-chemical nature depends upon concentration of nutrients, available of end-products, oxygen and associated growth factors.

Another important feature of biofilm is 'Quorum sensing', a bacterial cell-to-cell communication mechanism for controlling cellular function in a dense aggregates of bacteria. Quorum sensing is useful in controlling environmental stresses and is involved in the regulation of several microbial properties. Micro-organisms like Streptococci, Porphyromonas, Fuso-bacterium, etc. possess the ability of quorum sensing and subsequently effectively optimize phenotype properties of biofilm bacteria in root canals.

The biofilm matrix also contain extracellular DNA (eDNA). It is reported that eDNA originates from the intracellular DNA under conditions where lysis is not observed. eDNA is mostly due to native secretion and not due to cell death; however, high concentration of eDNA is attributed to cell lysis leading to release of DNA into extracellular medium.

Development of Biofilm

The stages involved in biofilm formation are:

Stage I: The first stage involves absorption of organic and inorganic molecules in the planktonic stage to the surface, known as 'conditioning layer'. This conditioning layer is composed of proteins and glycoproteins from saliva and gingival crevicular fluid. It promotes adhesion of newer micro-organisms on selective bases, influencing the microbial composition of biofilm.

Stage II: Second stage involves the adhesion and co-adhesion of micro-organisms to the conditioning layer. The early colonizers are important and crucial for additional adhesion of micro-organisms.

Stage III: Third stage involves multiplication and metabolism of attached micro-organisms. The characteristics of micro-organisms and the environment influence the growth and multiplication of micro-organisms in the biofilm (Fig. 8.4).

Stage IV: Fourth stage involves detachment of micro-organisms from the biofilm; concurrently with attachment process. The localized detachment of micro-organisms starts with initial adhesion and increases as the number of micro-organisms increase with time. The detachment of micro-colonies can be because of 'erosion' of small portion of biofilm and because of 'sloughing', whereby invasive area of biofilm is lost. The detachment of micro-organisms leads to spreading and colonizing other sites.

Types of Biofilm

Biofilms in endodontics are divided into (i) intracanal biofilm, (ii) external root (cementum) surface biofilms, (iii) periapical biofilm and (iv) biomaterial surface biofilms.

i. Intracanal Biofilm

The characteristics of intracanal biofilm (attached to root dentin) are:

- Multilayer biofilm attachment on dentinal wall of root (attachment thickness vary at different sites)
- Major bulk of organisms existed as loose collection of cocci, rods, filaments, etc.
- Dense aggregates of micro-organisms also observed
- Extracellular matrix of bacterial origin can fill the spaces between bacterial species and colonies

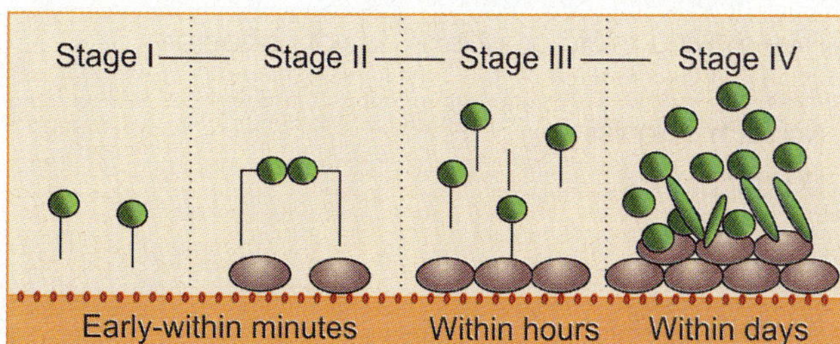

Fig. 8.4 Stages of biofilm formation

- *Enterococcus faecalis* can develop biofilm under any condition of root canal (Fig. 8.5a and b); i.e. aerobic, anaerobic. Nutrient rich (aerobic/anaerobic) environment facilitates *E. faecalis* to produce typical biofilms with aggregate of bacterial cells and water channels; whereas, nutrient deficient (aerobic/anaerobic) environment facilitate formation of biofilm, which is irregular, unorganized and may contain dead cells along with viable cells. Mineralization/calcification of *E. faecalis* biofilms has been observed because of interaction of root dentin structure with *E. faecalis* (pressure of calcium and phosphate ions help precipitation of bacterial-induced apatite ion mature biofilm). The ability of *E. faecalis* to form calcified biofilm on root canal

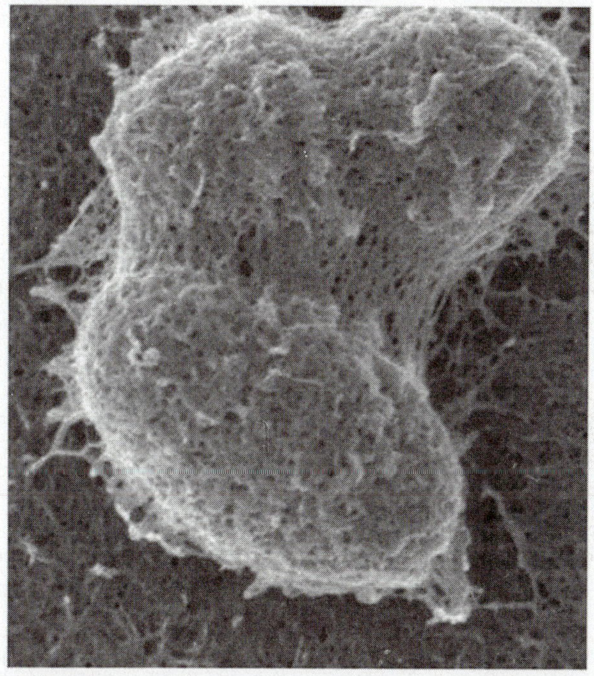

Fig. 8.5a *Enterococcus faecalis* biofilm (initial stage)

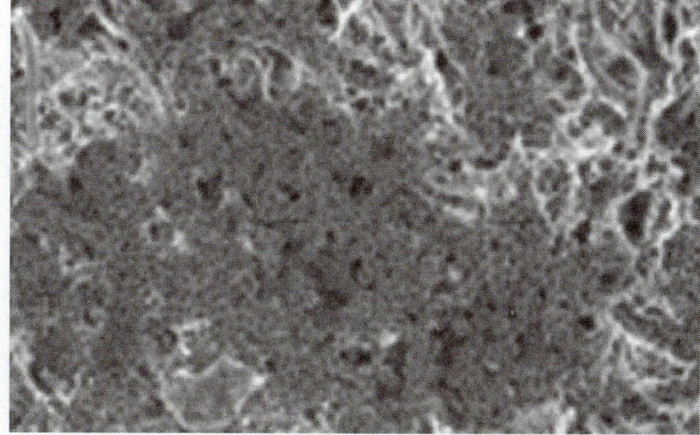

Fig. 8.5b *Enterococcus faecalis* biofilm (late stage)

dentin may be a contributing factor for its persistence. Co-aggregation interactions of other micro-organisms, especially *Fusobacterium nucleatum*, also contribute to persistent endodontic infections.

ii. External Root (cementum) Surface Biofilms

The characteristics of external root (cementum) surface biofilms are:

- Formed on external surface (cementum) of root apex.
- Apex of root adjacent of apical foramen is coated with continuous, smooth layer of variety of micro-organisms held together by extracellular matrix material.
- Calcified biofilms on the apical root surfaces have also been reported in case of persistent apical infective and delayed healing of periapical lesions.
- A few authors opined that external root surface aggregation of bacteria might not be a common occurrence in teeth with infected pulps (biofilm composed of cocci, bacilli, and filaments present only on teeth with apical periodontitis).

iii. Periapical Biofilms

The characteristic features of periapical biofilm are:

- Periapical biofilms may and may not be dependent on the root canal infections (usually root canal microbiota are opportunistic pathogens and do not survive host's defense in the periapical area).
- Rarely, a few microbial species or their strains may survive and infect periapical tissues (*Actinomyces* spp. and *Propionibacterium* spp. have been observed in periapical tissues after endodontic treatment).
- The microbial adherence can be as in external root surface biofilm or within the body of the inflammatory lesion.
- *Actinomyces* spp. usually have fimbrial structure that help in bacterial congregation, which survive in periapical environment by clinging to host cells and other bacteria, if present (Actinomyces usually live in equilibrium with host tissues and do not induce persistent infection; mostly lead to chronic periapical inflammation).

iv. Biomaterial Surface Biofilms

Biomaterial surface biofilms implies formation of bacterial adhesive layers onto a biomaterial surface, which may be inside or outside the root canal. Such biofilms are known as foreign body centered biofilm or biomaterial centered infections.

The *characteristic features* are:

- Biomaterial surface biofilm is mainly associated with root canal obturating materials, posts, implants and implant supported prosthesis.
- Bacterial adhesion on biomaterial surface involves conventional stage, viz. transport of bacteria to biomaterial surface, non-specific adhesion process followed by specific adhesion phase.
- Biofilm on root canal obturating materials, may be intraradicular or extraradicular, involves mainly *E. faecalis*, *Streptococcus* spp. and *Staphylococcus* spp. on gutta-percha points; whereas, *Propionibacterium* spp. and *Fusobacterium* spp. do not form biofilm on gutta-percha (mainly gram-positive facultative anaerobes colonies on gutta-percha points).

Characteristics of Biofilm as a Community

Considering biofilm as a community of micro-organisms, it should possess the following features:

- Ability to self-organize (autopoiesis)
- Ability to resist environmental disturbances (homeostasis)
- Should be effective in association than singly (synergy)
- Face environmental challenges collectively and not in isolation (communality)

The differences between biofilm and planktonic cells are tabulated in Table 8.4.

Table 8.4 Differences between biofilms and planktonic (free-cells)

Biofilm (community structure)	*Planktonic (free-cells)*
• Community of various micro-organisms co-operating each other	• Free-moving micro-organisms do not cooperate
• Arranged in microcolonies	• No such colonies
• Micro-organisms adhered in matrix of lipopolysaccharide/glycoproteins, etc.	• No adherence
• Intraspecies and interspecies communicate with each other	• No such communication
• Gradient of pH, nutrient and oxygen tension	• No such gradient
• Effective resistance to antibiotics	• Less resistance to antibiotics

ENTEROCOCCUS FAECALIS: SIGNIFICANCE IN ENDODONTICS

Enterococcus faecalis (E. faecalis) is the most commonly implicated micro-organisms in persistent endodontic infections. It is established that major cause of failure of root canal treatment is the survival of micro-organisms in the apical end of root filled teeth. *E. faecalis* has been found in high percentage of root canal failures and is able to survive in the post-filled challenges.

Characteristics and Strains

Enterococci are gram-positive cocci that can occur singly or in pairs. They are facultative anaerobes (ability to grow in absence and presence of oxygen) seen in human intestinal lumen and faeces (Fig. 8.6a and b). They are also prevalent in female genital tracts and are normal inhabitant of oral cavity. *E. faecalis* is associated with both primary endodontic infections and persistent infections (prevalence in persistent infections are much more; nine times more than primary infections). Enterococci can survive harsh environment, viz. salt concentration and alkaline pH. They can survive at temperature of 60°C (usually 10–45°C is the comfort zone temperature for *E. faecalis*). Molecular studies have confirmed 23 Enterococci spp. A few subtypes of *E. faecalis* have also been identified by molecular analysis techniques.

E. faecalis can survive prolonged periods of nutritional deprivation. It exhibits widespread genetic polymorphism (possesses protease, gelatinase and collagen binding proteins, which help them binding to dentin and invading even the dentinal tubules). It utilizes serum as the nutritional source (originates from periodontal ligaments and alveolar bone). It has the ability to suppress the action of lymphocytes, subsequently altering the host-immune system. *E. faecalis* biofilms are much resistant to phagocytosis and antimicrobial.

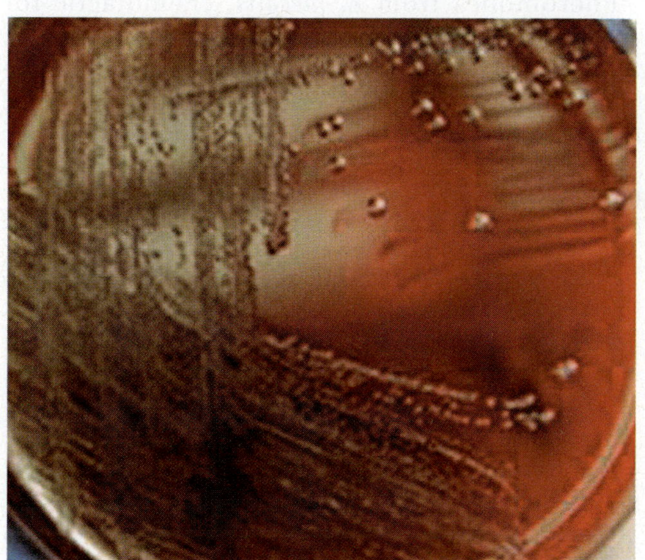

Fig. 8.6a Colonies of *Enterococcus faecalis*

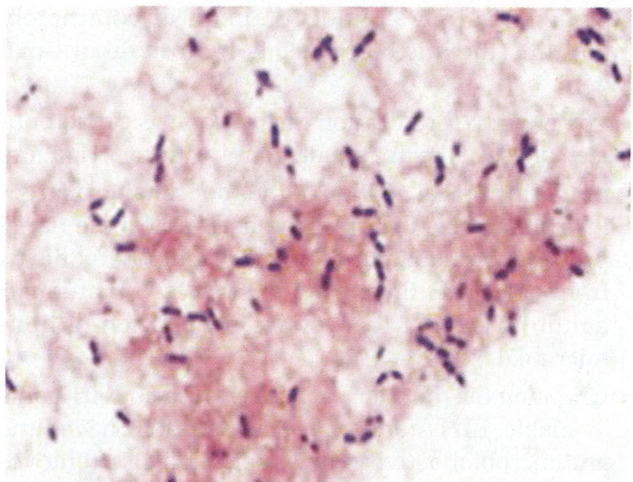

Fig. 8.6b *Enterococcus faecalis*

Virulent factors are summarized as:
- Survive prolonged periods of nutritional deprivation
- Binds to dentinal surface and invade dentinal tubules from 1000 to 1500 μ depending upon availability of nutrition
- Suppresses action of lymphocytes, subsequently alters host-defense response
- Utilize serum from alveolar bone and periodontal ligament as nutritional source
- Possesses lytic enzymes like cytolysin and lipoteichoic acid
- Compete with other cells
- Helps in biofilm formation and get associated
- Resist intracanal medicament by maintaining hemostasis

E. faecalis biofilms include formation of microcolonies and adherence of micro-organisms followed by dissolution of mineral (calcium and phosphate) fraction from dentin, resulting in initial calcification. Later, *E. faecalis* biofilms show carbonated-apatite structure, which are resistant to eradicate. These micro-organisms can effectively inactivate antimicrobial agents. *E. faecalis* co-aggregates with *Fusobacterium nucleatum* resulting in further aggravation of endodontic infections. *E. faecalis* biofilms have been observed to be thicker than biofilms produced by other organisms.

Methods of Eradication

Enterococcus faecalis may enter root canal system during treatment, in-between appointments and even after the completion of the treatment. It is important to prevent entry of *E. faecalis* at any phase of the treatment and the treatment regime should be aimed at completely eradicating the micro-organisms from the root canal system.

The effective eradication of *E. faecalis* is carried out at each phase of the treatment, mainly during irrigation.

- Preparing apical portion of the root canal to a larger instrument size than initial master apical file (large preparation facilitate removal of micro-organisms from apical dentin substrate; removes intratubular dentin, which further allows penetration of antimicrobials).
- Irrigating the root canal spaces with various irrigants available. EDTA and citric acid solutions have little antimicrobial activity; however, their use removes the smear layer, which facilitates irrigation solution access to dentinal tubules.
  - 2.0% chlorhexidine is effective in eliminating or at least minimizing *E. faecalis* from the root canal spaces and dentinal tubules.
  - 3.0 to 5.35% sodium hypochlorite, when used in adequate amount, has the ability to destroy *E. faecalis*.
  - MTAD (tetracycline isomer, an acid and a detergent) effectively destroys *E. faecalis* because of its anticollagenase activity, low pH and ability to be released gradually with time.
  - Combination of two irrigants has been tried successfully. Combining 2.0% chlorhexidine with calcium hydroxide can achieve pH of 12.8, which can eradicate *E. faecalis* (calcium hydroxide alone is not effective to that extent).
  - Other irrigants as ozonated and superoxide water and lasers are also effective in eradicating *E. faecalis*. Stannous fluoride has also shown great efficacy.
  - Intracanal medicaments, such as Metapex (silicone oil based calcium hydroxide paste containing 38% iodoform effectively disinfect dentinal tubules. Iodine potassium iodide is more effective intracanal agent than calcium hydroxide.
- Chlorhexidine and iodoform impregnated gutta-percha have shown little effects against *E. faecalis*. A few authors have claimed 5.0% chlorhexidine in gutta-percha can be effective in eradicating *E. faecalis*.
- Various sealers, such as AH plus, Grossman sealer, Roth 811 sealer (zinc oxide eugenol based) and silicone based sealers have shown positive results in eradicating *E. faecalis*.
- Plasma dental probe, photodynamic therapy/light activated therapy are also effectively used to eradicate *E. faecalis* biofilms.

8

E. faecalis should be prevented from re-entering root canal system during or after treatment. Oral rinsing with 2.0% chlorhexidine, disinfecting gutta-percha with sodium hypochlorite before obturating root canals along with completely sealing the coronal aspects of the tooth are the effective measures.

Potential role of Enterococci in unsuccessful root canal treatment

It has been hypothesized that in periapical infections that involve *E. faecalis*, tissue damage may be predominantly caused by the host response to the bacteria rather than direct damage from bacterial products. Viable but not culturable *E. faecalis* produces stress proteins in adverse environmental factors, such as sodium hypochlorite, salt, bile salts, acid and heat, alkaline stress, glucose starvation, elevated temperatures, and in tap water.

Enterococci have low sensitivity to antimicrobial agents. It is established that the proficiency with which *E. faecalis* can invade dentinal tubules facilitates protection from chemomechanical root canal preparation and intracanal dressing technique. In the presence of human serum, *E. faecalis* bound better to collagen.

Co-aggregation (formed by *E. faecalis*) interactions occurring in biofilms may provide an effective means by which *E. faecalis* remain in root canals; as these biofilm mature, they exhibit the ability to calcify which may facilitate their stability.

Virulence factors identified in Enterococci recovered from infected root canals are: Enterococcus surface protein and collagen-binding protein, which contribute to ability to bind the dentin.

Pheromones from *E. faecalis*, chemotactic for neutrophils may trigger superoxide formation. Overall, possession of the above 'virulence traits' might provide advantage over other species enabling survival in the infected root canals.

BIBLIOGRAPHY

1. Aamdal SA and Petersen FC. The biofilm concept: consequences for future prophylaxis of oral disease. Crit. Rev. Oral Biol. Med.: 2004; 15:4–12.
2. Alabdulmohsen ZA and Saad AY. Antibacterial effect of silver nanoparticles against *Enterococcus faecalis*. Saudi Endod. J.: 2017; 7:29–35.
3. Al-Mahdi A and Balto HA. The synergistic effect of ultrasonic activation and irrigation on *Enterococcus faecalis* biofilm. Saudi Endod. J.: 2016; 6:1–8.
4. Araki AT, Ibraki Y, Kawakami T and Marques JL. Er:YAG laser irradiation of the microbiological apical biofilm. Braz. Dent. J.: 2006; 17:296–299.

5. Auschill TM, Arweiler NB, Neutuschil L, Brecx M, Reich E and Sculean A. Spatial distribution of vital and dead microorganisms in dental biofilms. Arch. Oral Biol.:2001; 46:471–476.
6. Baumgartner JC, Khemaleelakne SU and Xia T. Identification of spirochetes (Treponema) in endodontic infections. J. Endod.: 2003; 29:794–797.
7. Baumgartner JC, Watkins BJ, Bal KS and Xia T. Association of black pigmented bacteria with endodontic infections. J. Endod.:1999; 25:413–415.
8. Baumgartner JC, Watts CM and Xia T. Occurrence of candida albicans in infection of endodontic origin. J. Endod.: 2000; 26:695–698.
9. Baumgartner JC. Microbiologic aspect of endodontic infections. J. Calif. Dent. Assoc.: 2004; 32:459–468.
10. Chavez de Pax LE. Redefining the persistent infection in root canals: Possible role of biofilm communities. J. Endod.: 2007; 33:652–662.
11. Chavez de Paz LE, Dahlen G, Molander A, Moller AJR and Bergenholtz G. Bacteria recovered from teeth with apical periodontitis after antimicrobial endodontic treatment. Int. Endod. J.: 2003; 36:500–508.
12. Chavez de Paz LE, Molander A and Dahlen G. Gram positive rods prevailing in teeth with apical periodontitis undergoing root canal treatment. Int. Endod. J.: 2004; 37:579–587.
13. Chen V, Chen Y and Li H. Herpesviruses in abscesses and cellulitis of endodontic origin. J. Endod.: 2009; 35:182–188.
14. Chiniforush N, Pourhajibagher M, Shahabi S and Bahador A. Clinical approach of high technology techniques for control and elimination of endodontic microbiota. J. Lasers Med. Sci.: 2015; 6:139–150.
15. Chugal N, Wang JK, Wang R, He X, Kang M and Li J. Molecular characterization of the microbial flora residing at the apical portion of infected root canals of human teeth. J. Endod.: 2011; 37:1359–1364.
16. Costerton JW, Lewandowski Z, DeBeer D, Caldwell D, Korber D and James G. Biofilms, the customized microniche. J. Bacteriol.: 1994; 176:2137–2142.
17. Cvitkovitch DG, Li YH and Eller R. Quorum sensing and biofilm formation in Streptococci infections. J. Clin. Invest.: 2003; 112:1626–1632.
18. Dahle UR, Sunde PT and Tronstad L. Treponemas and endodontic infections. Endod. Topics: 2003; 6:160–170.
19. De Paz LC. Gram-positive organisms in endodontic infections. Endod. Topics: 2004; 9:79–96.
20. Distel JW, Hatton JF and Gillespie MJ. Biofilm formations in medicated root canals. J. Endod.: 2002; 28:689–693.
21. Evans M, Davies JK, Sundqvist G and Figdor D. Mechanisms involved in the resistance of *Enterococcus faecalis* to calcium hydroxide. Int. Endod. J.: 2002; 35:221–228.
22. Fenno JC and McBride BC. Virulence factors of oral treponemas. Anaerobe: 1998; 4:1–17.
23. Fouad AF and Barry J. The effect of antibiotics and endodontic antimicrobials to the polymerase chain reaction. J. Endod.: 2005; 31:510–513.
24. Fouad AF. Endodontic microbiology and pathobiology: Current state of knowledge. Dent. Clinic N. Am.: 2017; 61:1–15.
25. Ghigo JM. Natural conjugative plasmids induce bacterial biofilm development. Nature: 2001; 412:442–445.
26. Giardino LO, Ambu E, Savoldi E, Rimondini R, Cassanelli C and Debbia EA. Comparative evaluation of antimicrobial efficacy of sodium hypochlorite, MTAD, and Tetraclean against *Enterococcus faecalis* biofilm. J. Endod.: 2007; 33:852–855.
27. Gomes BPA, Jacinto RC and Pinheiro ET. Molecular analysis of Filifactor alocis, *Tannerella forsythia* and *Treponema denticola* associated with primary endodontic infections and failed endodontic treatments. J. Endod.: 2006; 32:937–940.
28. Gomes BPA, Montagner F, Jacinto RC, Pinheiro ET, Zaia AA, Ferraz CCR and Souza-Filho FJ. Gemella morbillorn in primary and secondary/persistent endodontic infections. O. Surg., O. Med., O. Path.: 2008; 105:519–525.
29. Gomes BPA., Pinheiro ET, Gade-Neto CR, Sousa EL, Souza-Filho FJ, Ferraz CC and Zaia AA. Microbiological examination of infected root canals. Oral Microbiol. Immunol: 2004; 19:71–76.
30. Grohmann E, Muth G and Espinosa M. Conjugative plasmid transfer in gram-positive bacteria. Microbiol. Mol. Biol. Rev.: 2003; 67:277–301.
31. Guven K and Orstavik D. Virulence factors of *Enterococcus faecalis*: Relationship to endodontic disease. Crit. Rev. Oral Biol. Med.: 2004; 15:308–320.
32. Haisao WW, Li KJ and Liu Z. Microbial transformation from normal oral microbiota to acute endodontic infections. BMC Genomics: 2012; 13:345.
33. Hamada S, Amano A, Kimura S, Nakagawa I, Kawabata S and Morisaki I. The importance of fimbriae in the virulence and ecology of some oral bacterial. Oral Microbiol. Immunol.: 2004; 13:129–138.
34. Hashioka K, Yamasaki M, Nakane A, Horiba N and Nakamura H. The relationship between clinical symptoms and anaerobic bacteria from infected root canals. J. Endod.: 1992; 18:555–561.
35. Jakovljevic A and Andric M. Human cytomegalovirus and Epstein-Barr virus in etiopathogenesis of apical periodontitis: a systematic review. J. Endod.: 2014; 40:6–15.
36. Jhajharia K, Parolia A, Shetty KV and Mehta LK. Biofilm in endodontics: a review. J. Int. Soc. Prev. Comm. Dent.: 2015; 5:1–12.
37. Jung IY, Choi BK, Kum KY, Yoo YJ, Yoon TC, Lee CY and Park DS. Molecular epidemiology and association of putative pathogens in root canal infections. J. Endod.: 2000; 26: 599–604.
38. Jung IY, Choi BK, Kum KY, Yoo YJ, Yoon TC, Lee SJ and Lee CY. Identification of oral spirochete at the species level and their association with other bacterial in endodontic infections. O. Surg., O. Med., O. Path.: 2001; 92:329–334.
39. Kalfas S, Figdor D and Sundqvist G. A new bacterial species associated with failed endodontic treatment: identification and description of actinomyces radicidentis. Oral Surg., Oral Med., Oral Pathol., Oral Radiol. Endod.: 2001; 92:208–214.

40. Kaufman B, Spanberg L, Berry J and Fouad AF. *Enterococcus* species in endodontically treated teeth with and without periradicular lesions. J. Endod.: 2005; 31:851–856.
41. Khemaleelakul S, Baumgartner JC and Pruksakorn S. Identification of bacteria in acute endodontic infections and their antimicrobial susceptibility. Oral Surg., Oral Med., Oral Pathol., Oral Radiol. Endod.: 2002; 94:746–755.
42. Kolenbrander PE, Andersen RN, Blehert DS, Egland PG, Fosters JS and Palmer RJ. Communication among oral bacterial. Microbiol. Mol. Biol. Rev.: 2002; 66:486–505.
43. Leonardo MR, Rossi MA, Silva LAB, Ito IY and Bonifacio C. EM evaluation of bacterial biofilm and microorganisms on the apical external root surface of human teeth. J. Endod.:2002; 28:815–818.
44. Loo CY, Corliss DA and Ganeshkumar N. *Streptococcus gordonii* biofilm formation: Identification of genes that code for biofilm phenotypes. J. Bacteriol.: 2000; 182:1374–1382.
45. Love RM. *Enteroroccus faecalis*—a mechanism for its role in endodontic failure. Int. Endod. J.: 2001; 34:399–405.
46. Love RM. Invasion of dentinal tubule by root canal bacteria. Endod. Topics: 2004; 9:52–65.
47. Martinez JL and Baquero F. Interactions among strategies associated with bacterial infection: pathogenicity, epidemicity, and antibiotic resistance. Clin. Microbiol. Rev.: 2002; 15:647–679.
48. McHugh CP, Zhang P, Michalek S and Eleazer PD. pH required to kill *Enterococcus faecalis* in vitro. J. Endod.: 2004; 30:218–219.
49. Mohammadi Z, Palazzi F, Giardino L and Shalavi S. Microbial biofilms in endodontic infections: An update review. Biomed.: 2013; 36:59–70.
50. Munson MA., Pitt-Ford T, Chong B, Weightman A and Wade WG. Molecular and cultural analysis of the microflora associated with endodontic infections. JDR: 2002; 81:761–766.
51. Nair RPN and Schroder HE. Periapical actinomycosis. J. Endod.: 1984; 10:567–570.
52. Nakata K, Yamasaki M, Iwata T, Suzuki A, Nakane A and Nakamura H. Anaerobic bacterial extracts influence production of matrix metalloproteinases and their inhibitors by human dental pulp cells. J. Endod.: 2000; 26:410–413.
53. Narayanan LL and Vaishnavi C. Endodontic microbiology. J. Conserv. Dent.: 2010; 13:233–239.
54. Neves MA, Provenzano JC and Rocas IN. Clinical antibacterial effectiveness of root canal preparation with reciprocating single-instrument or continuously rotating multi-instrument systems. J. Endod.: 2016; 42:25–29.
55. Neves MA, Rocas IN and Siqueira JF. Clinical antibacterial effectiveness of the self-adjusting file system. Int. Endod. J.: 2014; 47:356–365.
56. Noiri Y, Katsumoto T, Azamai H and Ebius S. Effect of Er:YAG laser irradiation on biofilm-forming bacteria associated with endodontic pathogens in vitro. J. Endod.: 2008; 34:826–829.
57. Olsen I and Dahlen G. Salient virulence factors in anaerobic bacteria, with emphasis on their importance in endodontic infections. Endod. Topics: 2004; 9:15–26.
58. Peciuliene V, Maneliene R, Baleikonyte-Drukteinis S and Rutkunas V. Micro-organisms in root canal infections: a review. Stomatologic-Baltic Dental and Maxillofacial J.: 2008; 10:4–9.
59. Portenier I, Waltimo TMT and Haapasalo M: *Enterococcus faecalis*—the root canal survivor and 'star' in post treatment disease. Endod. Topics: 2003; 6:135–159.
60. Priester JH, Horst AM, Van de Werfhorst LC, Saleta JL, Mertes LA and Holden PA. Enhanced visualization of microbial biofilms by staining and environmental scanning electron microscopy. J. Microbiol. Methods: 2007; 68:577–87.
61. Provenzano JC, Antunes HS, Alves FRE, Rocas IN, Alvs WS, Silva MRS and Siqueira JF. Host-bacterial interactions in post-treatment apical periodontitis: A metaproteome analysis. J. Endod.: 2016; 42:880–885.
62. Rocas IN, Siquiera JF Jr, Santos KR and Coelho AM. 'Red Complex' (*Bacteroide forsythus, Porphyromonas gingivalis* and *Treponema denticola*) in endodontic infections: a molecular approach. O. Surg., O. Med., O. Path.: 2001; 91:468–471.
63. Rocas IN, Siquiera, JF Jr and Santos KR. Association of *Enterococcus faecalis* with different forms of periradicular diseases. J. Endod.: 2004; 30:315–320.
64. Rolph HJ, Lennon A, Riggio MP, Saunders WP, MacKenzie D, Coldero L and Bagg J. Molecular identification of micro-organisms from endodontic infections. J. Clin. Microbiol.: 2001; 39:3282–3289.
65. Sakamoto M, Siqueira JF Jr, Rocas IN and Benno Y. Molecular analysis of the root canal microbiota associated with endodontic treatment failures. Oral Microbiol. Immunol.: 2008; 23:275–81.
66. Santos AL, Siqueira JF and Rocas IN. Comparing the bacterial diversity of acute and chronic dental root canal infections. PLoS One: 2011; 6:e28088.
67. Sedgley C and Clewell DB. Bacterial plasmids in the oral and endodontic microflora. Endod. Topics: 2004; 9:37–51.
68. Sedgley C, Lennan SL and Clewell DB. Prevalence, phenotype and genotype of oral Enterococci. Oral Microbiol. Immunol.: 2004; 19:95–101.
69. Shelburne CE, Gleason RM, Germaine GR, Wolff LF, Mullally BH, Coulter WA and Lpatin DE. Quantitative reverse transcription polymerase chain reaction analysis of Porphyromonas gingivalis gene expression in vivo. J. Microbiol. Methods: 2002; 49:147–156.
70. Shibata Y, Hiratsuka K, Hayakwa M, Shiroza T, Takguchi H, Nagatsuka Y and Abiko Y. A 35-kDA coaggregation factor is a hemin binding protein in porphyromonas gingivalis. Biochem. Biophys. Res. Commun.: 2003; 300:351–356.
71. Shreshtha A, Shi Z, Neoh KG and Kishen A. Nanoparticulates for antibiofilm treatment and effect of aging on its antibacterial activity. J. Endod.: 2010; 36:1030–5.
72. Silver S. Bacterial silver resistance: Molecular biology and uses and misuses of silver compounds. FEMS Microbiol. Rev.: 2003; 27:341–353.
73. Siqueira J and Rocas CI. Molecular detection of black pigmented bacteria in infection of endodontic origin. J. Endod.: 2001; 27:563–566.

74. Siqueira J and Rocas I. Cultivable bacteria in infected root canals as identified by 16S rRNA gene sequencing. Oral microbiology and Immunology: 2007; 22:266–271.

75. Siqueira J and Rocas I. Oral Treponemas in primary root canal infections as detected by nested PCR. Int. Endod. J.: 2003; 36:20–26.

76. Siqueira J and Rocas I. *Peptostreptococcus micros* in primary endodontic infections as detected by 16sr DNA based PCR. J. Endod.: 2003; 29:111–113.

77. Siqueira J and Rocas IN. Polymerase chain reaction-bases analysis of micro-organisms associated with failed endodontic treatment. Oral Surg., Oral Med., Oral Pathol., Oral Radiol. Endod.: 2004; 97:85–94.

78. Siqueira J and Rocas IN. The oral microbiota: general overview, taxonomy, and nucleic acid techniques. Methods Mol. Biol.: 2010; 666:55–69,

79. Siqueira J, Alves KRF and Rocas IN. Pyrosequencing analysis of the apical root canal microbiota. J. Endod.: 2011; 37:1499–1503.

80. Siqueira J, Rocas IN, Cunha CD and Rosado AS. Novel bacterial phylotypes in endodontic infections. J. Dent. Res.: 2005; 84:565–569.

81. Siqueira JF and Rocas IN. Bacteroides Forsythus in primary endodontic infections as detected by nested PCR. J. Endod.: 2003; 29:390–393.

82. Siqueira JF and Rocas IN. PCR-based identification of *Treponema maltophilum T. amylovorum, T. medium* and *T. lecithimolyticum* in primary root canal infections. Arch. Oral Biol.: 2003; 48:495–502.

83. Siqueira JF and Rocas IN. Uncultivated phylotypes and newly named species associated with primary and persistent endodontic infections. J. Clin. Microbiol.: 2005; 43:3314–3319.

84. Siqueira JF and Sen BH. Fungi in endodontic infections. O. Surg., O. Med., O. Path.: 2004; 97:632–641.

85. Siqueira JF, Rocas IN, Moraes SR and Santos KR. Direct amplification of rRNA gene sequences for detection of putative oral pathogens in root canal infetions. Int. Endod. J.: 2002; 35:345–351.

86. Siqueira JF. Endodontic infections: concepts, paradigms and perspectives. O. Surg., O. Med., O. Pathol.: 2002; 94:281–293.

87. Siqueira JF. Periapical actinomycosis and infection with Propionibacterium propionicum. Endod. Topics: 2003; 6: 78–95.

88. Spratt DA. Significance of bacterial identification by molecular biology methods. Endod. Topics: 2004; 9:5–14.

89. Steinberger RE and Holden PA. Extracellular DNA in single- and multiple-species unsaturated biofilms. Appl. Environment. Microbiol.: 2005; 71: 5404–5410.

90. Stuart CH, Schwartz SA, Beeson TJ and Owatz CB. *Enterococcus faecalis*: its role in root canal treatment failure and current concepts in retreatment. J. Endod.: 2006; 32:93–98.

91. Sunde PT, Tronstad L, Eribe ER, Lind PO and Olsen I. Assessment of periradicular microbiota by DNA-DNA hybridization. Endod. Dent. Traumatol.: 2000; 16:191–196.

92. Svensater G. and Bergerholtz G. Biofilms in endodontic infections. Endod. Topics: 2004; 9:27–36.

93. Thoma VC, Hiromasa Y, Harms N, Thurlow L, Tomich J and Hancock LE. A fratricidal mechanism is responsible for eDNA release and contributes to biofilm development of *Enterococcus faecalis*. Mol. Microbiol.: 2009; 72:1022–1036.

94. Tronstad L and Sunde PT. The evolving new understanding of endodontic infections. Endodontic topics: 2003; 6:57–77.

95. Usha HL, Kaiwar A and Mehta D. Biofilm in endodontics: New understanding to an old problem. Int. J. Contemp. Dent.: 2010; 1:44–51.

96. Vineet RV, Nayak M and Kotigadde S. Association of endodontic signs and symptoms with root canal pathogens: A clinical comparative study. Saudi Endod. J.: 2016; 6:82–86.

97. Waltimo T, Haapsalo M, Zehnder M and Meyer J. Clinical aspects related to endodontic yeast infections. Endod. Topics: 2005; 9:66–78.

98. Wang BY, Chi B and Kuramitsu HK. Genetic exchange between *Treponema denticola* and *Streptococcus gordonii* in biofilms. Oral Micorbiol. Immunol.: 2002; 17:108–112.

99. Williamson A, Cardon JW and Drake DR. Antimicrobial susceptibility of monoculture biofilms of a clinical isolate of Enterococcus faecalis. J. Endod.: 2009; 35:95–97.

100. Zehnder M and Belibasakis GN. On the dynamics of root canal infections—what we understand and what we don't. Virulence: 2015; 6:216–222.

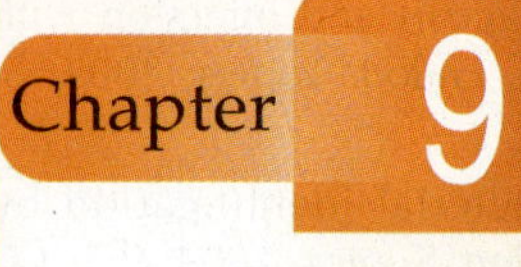

Chapter 9

Diagnosis and Diagnostic Aids

The success in endodontic treatment depends upon correct diagnosis, meticulous preparation and three-dimensional obturation of root canal system. The Hippocratic Oath, *'do no harm'* should be strictly followed by the operator. Dental treatment in any form, should never be embarked upon until the diagnosis is established. Diagnosis is the most critical aspect of patient care since adequate treatment planning depends on accurate diagnosis. The process of diagnosis involves collection of information, observing signs and symptoms, thorough clinical examination and accurate interpretation of objective testing. Various scientific devices can be used to gather information and the thoughtful interpretation of the collected information help arriving at diagnosis. An accurate diagnosis is a result of the synthesis of scientific knowledge, clinical experience, intuition and also common sense.

Diagnosis and Prognosis

Diagnosis is considered as the cornerstone in the practice of healing art. It is the correct determination and logical appraisal of conditions observed during the examination, as evidenced by distinct signs and characteristics of health/disease. This is accomplished through sensory and mental processes used in evaluation of the findings observed during examination. Diagnosis is defined as *'the utilization of scientific knowledge for identifying a diseased process and to differentiate it from other diseased processes'*. Literally, the art of identifying a disease from its signs and symptoms is *'diagnosis'*; whereas, *prognosis* is pre-determination of the probable course and outcome of the disease.

Diagnostician

Diagnostician is a qualified person, who has the scientific knowledge of normal and abnormal conditions of the body; who is authorized to identify the disease process by taking relevant history, performing thorough clinical examination and is able to analyze the data obtained from various diagnostic aids.

The diagnostician should have sympathetic ears to hear, eyes to see, hands to feel, nose to smell, brain to analyze and clinical experience to derive proper diagnosis. He/she should have:

- Knowledge of disease process
- Interest in the subject
- Concern for patient care
- Curiosity to find the details
- Intuition to suspect unusual
- Patience to finalize the diagnosis.

PATIENT ASSESSMENT

The moment patient enter the dental clinic, the process of patient's assessment starts. The doctor should observe and analyze the patient as regard his/her gait, posture and attitude. The patient's dress sense and also the way of communication at the front office should also be evaluated. All these features are carefully observed and managed in a friendly manner; affects treatment outcome.

Personal record

Patient record is usually maintained for identification, legal and medical record purposes.

This record should have all personal details, medical history, past dental experience and the patient's expectation. The informed consent should be secured in one note.

With digitalization, the patient data, fingerprints and signature can be kept on a computer; alternatively a scanned sheet can be attached to the patient's file.

Social and psychological review

- Attitude of the patient
- Financial status
- Patient's expectations
- Patient's motivation.

Personal history

- Diet (vegetarian or non-vegetarian): Non-vegetarian diet requires more chewing that may affect teeth and muscles of mastication
- Brushing habits (faulty tooth brushing may lead to damage to teeth and gums)
- Alcohol and smoking habits.

Past dental history

- Previous visit to a general practitioner and/or endodontist
- What procedure was carried out?
- Frequency of visiting dental surgeon
- Past dental experience (difficulty in tolerating certain procedure)
- Attitude of the patient towards dental treatment

Occupational history

- Occupation may lead to some dental problems, such as:
  - Abrasion cavities in tailors and cobblers due to pin holding habit in between front teeth
  - Erosion in acid factory workers.

Family history

- Assess family attitude towards oral health
- Assess inherited problems, as:
  - Malocclusion
  - Dentinogenesis imperfecta/amelogenesis imperfecta, etc.

Chief complaint

Chief complaint(s) of the patient should be recorded in patient's own words which helps the clinician to concentrate on the problem for which patient seeks dental treatment.

The patient must be encouraged to discuss his/her problems for developing good rapport; subsequently adequately diagnosing the disease process.

"Listen to your patient; presenting you the diagnosis"

History of present illness

History taking is a very important phase of the diagnostic procedure. The operator should analyze the following aspects:

i. *Nature of the problem*: Generally the problem is pain, swelling, and loss of function or esthetics. Pain and swellings related to pulp necrosis and/or traumatized teeth imply endodontic involvement of the tooth; but, non-odontogenic pain should also be considered.

ii. *Onset*: Chronicity of the problem may indicate underlying histopathologic changes in the pulp or periradicular tissues. Onset being spontaneous or provoked, sudden or gradual should also be analyzed. *(Reversible pulpitis is characterized by pain which is caused by a specific irritant and the pain subsides when the irritant is removed. In case of irreversible pulpitis, the pain lingers on.)*

iii. *Intensity*: Dull, aching, pulsating, throbbing, radiating, stabbing, etc. are descriptions of pain usually associated with irreversible pulpal changes.

After pulp necrosis, the intensity of pain may be mild or none; still indicating endodontic intervention. (Diagnosis is a combination of all subjective and objective tests.)

iv. *Duration*: Episodes of pain of long duration are usually associated with irreversible pulpitis or partial pulpal necrosis. Reversible pulpitis is usually characterized by pain of short duration.

v. *Frequency*: More frequent the occurrence of painful episodes; more severe the pathologic condition of the pulp.

vi. *Aggravating factors*: Factors like cold, hot, sweet, sour, chewing, etc. may aggravate pain; viz. dentin exposure (sensitivity type of pain), reversible pulpitis (pain to cold stimulus or sweets).

vii. *Relieving factors*: Factors such as cold, hot water bath, analgesics, etc. may relieve pain, viz. reversible pulpitis (pain relieved by removal of stimulus), irreversible pulpitis (pain lingering even after removal of stimulus).

History of present illness: Key features

- Nature of the problem: Pain, swelling, etc. (endodontic or non-odontogenic)
- Onset: When did the problem start?(acute or chronic)
- Intensity: How painful is it? (mild, moderate or severe)
- Duration: How long it hurts? (pain of short or long duration)
- Frequency: How often does it hurt?
- Aggravating factors: Cold, hot, sweet, sour, etc.
- Relieving factors: Cold, hot water bath, analgesics, etc.

Medical history

Thorough medical history is mandatory as it affects dental diagnosis and also the treatment outcome. Details given in Chapter 10.

Clinical Examination

Clinical examination implies careful inspection and accurate investigation of the condition prevailing in a patient. It is 'hands on' process of observing both normal and abnormal conditions in the patient's oral cavity.

Vital signs such as blood pressure, pulse rate, respiratory rate and temperature should be recorded prior to clinical examination.

The intraoral and extraoral tissues are thoroughly examined and properly recorded. The recorded data provides following features:

a. Provides information for accurate/comprehensive treatment plan
b. Help in third party communication
c. Assessing quality of infrastructure/instrumentation in clinic
d. May be required in legal proceedings
e. Useful for forensic matters, if need be

The recorded data should be:

- *Uncomplicated*: Should be effective and accurate means of recording oral conditions (easily understood by others)
- *Comprehensive*: All oral conditions, both normal and abnormal along with associated tissues to be noted
- *Accessible*: The patient record should be easily accessible for reference, during and on recall appointments
- *Current*: Continually updating the patient's features as the treatment is progressed.

SOAP format of recording

- **S:** Subjective (patient symptoms)
- **O:** Objective (signs)
- **A:** Assessment
- **P:** Planning of treatment

Extraoral Examination

The operator should examine:

- Eyes—for fear, apprehension and systemic disease like anemia, etc.
- Facial asymmetry or distentions—for swellings or other abnormality.
- Lip (competency, ulcerations, presence of mucocele, lip line, mobility, etc.)—provides information for esthetics.
- Temporomandibular joint—any deviation, clicking sound, pain in the morning (especially in patients with occlusal disturbances and bruxers).
- Salivary glands (swelling, blockage, etc.).
- Lymph nodes (size, mobility, tenderness).
- Muscles of mastication (palpation of these muscles may reveal muscle fatigue, common in patients with bruxism).

Intraoral Examination

Examination of soft tissues (Fig. 9.1a to d)

- Buccal mucosa: Any ulceration (lichenoid reaction, white patch etc.)
- Buccal vestibule (swelling or sinus opening)
- The intraoral sinus tract should be traced to its origin
- Hard palate/soft palate: Swelling, ulceration, smoker's palate
- Frenum: Size and configuration (important during diastema closure)

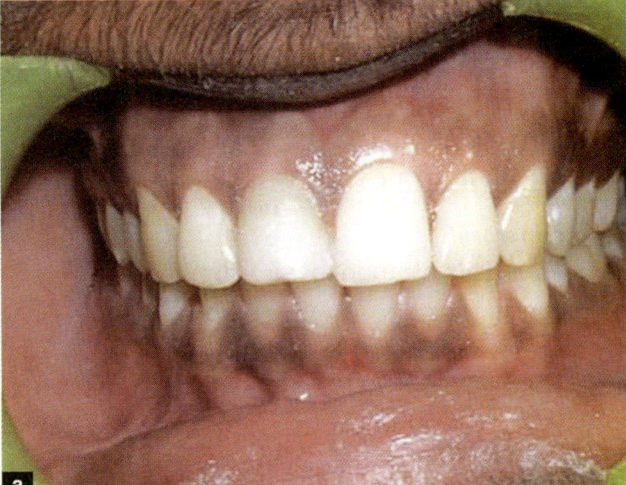

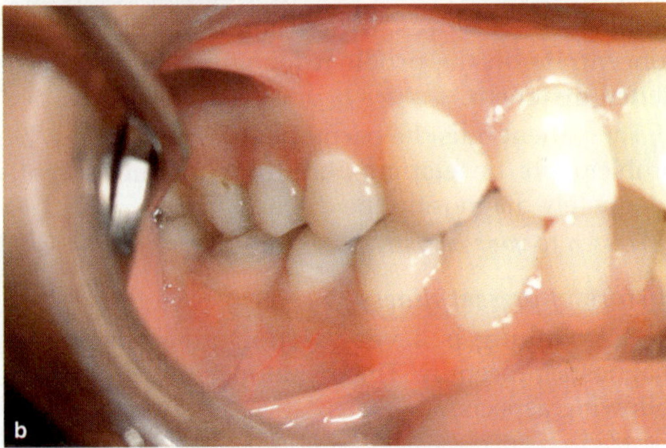

Fig. 9.1a and b Gingival examination

- Floor of mouth and tongue (dorsal, ventral and lateral aspects)
- Gingiva (color, contour, consistency, surface texture, size and shape)
- Oropharynx.

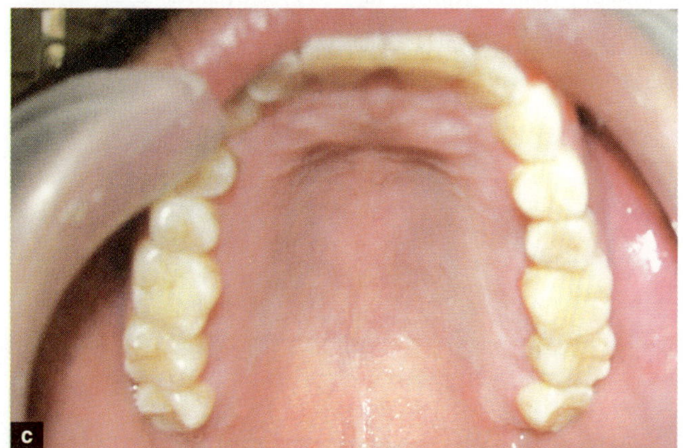
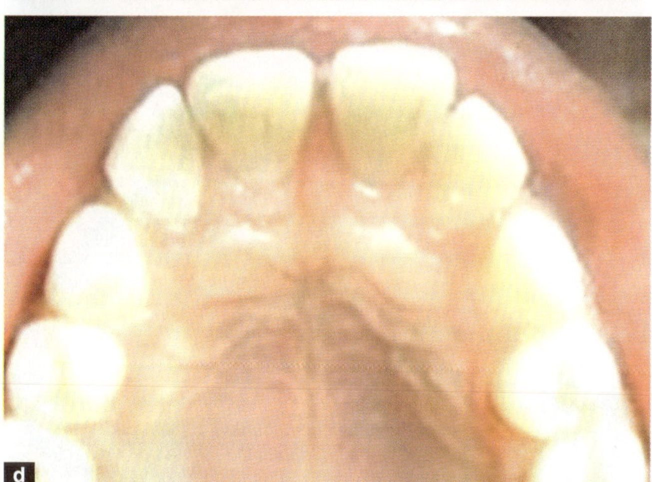

Fig. 9.1c and d Examining the palatal surface

Examination of hard tissue (teeth) (Fig. 9.2a and b)

Teeth are recorded using any denotation system.

Number of missing restored, retained and deciduous teeth are noted. Teeth are carefully examined for caries, enamel fracture, discoloration, etc.

The various methods which can be used in endodontic diagnosis are tabulated in Table 9.1.

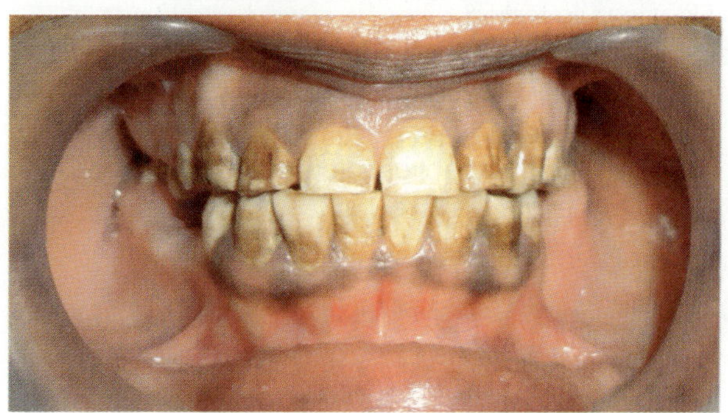

Fig. 9.2a Generalized discoloration

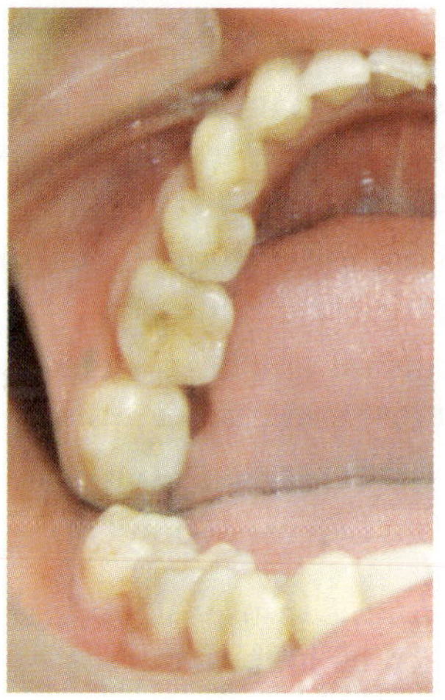

Fig. 9.2b Microcracks in mesiobuccal cusp

Table 9.1 Methods used in endodontic diagnosis

Clinical inspection methods	*Radiographic techniques*
• Visual inspection	• Conventional radiography
• Magnification	• Radiovisiography (RVG)
• Dyes	• Xeroradiography
• Palpation	• Digital subtraction radiography
• Percussion	• Computerized tomography (CT)
• Mobility and depressibility	• Magnetic resonance imaging (MRI)
• Periodontal Probing	• Cone beam computerized tomography (CBCT)
• Bite test (occlusal pressure test)	• C-arm imaging
• Test cavity	
• Anesthesia test	
• Videography/Intraoral camera	
• Fiberoptic transillumination	

(Contd...)

Table 9.1 Methods used in endodontic diagnosis (*Contd.*)

Clinical inspection methods	*Radiographic techniques*
Pulp vitality tests	*Tests measuring tooth temperature*
Tests assessing the neural status of pulp • Thermal test – Cold test – Heat test • Electric pulp testing *Tests assessing the blood supply of pulp* • LASER Doppler flowmetry • Pulse oximetry • Dual wavelength spectrophotometry • Optical reflection vitalometer • Photoplethysmography	• Cholesteric liquid crystal • Electronic thermography • Infrared thermography (Hughes probeye camera)
Newer methods • Ultrasound imaging • Computer expert system (COMENDEX) • LASER optical disc storage	

CLINICAL INSPECTION METHODS

1. ***Visual inspection***: It involves visual examination of teeth and associated structures, evaluating the following features:

- *Color*: Discoloration of the teeth, uniform or localized caries, fractures/craze lines
- *Contour*: Unusual anatomy, defective restorations, cervical lesions/non-carious lesions
- *Consistency*: Caries, resorption, etc.
- *Supra-eruption*: Extrusion of teeth.

2. ***Magnification***: The use of optical magnification instruments such as loupes, microscopes, endoscopes and orascopes enables the operator to magnify a specified treatment field beyond that perceived by the naked eye.

3. ***Dyes***: Use of dyes helps in the detection of caries and fractures. Methylene blue dye, India ink, crystal violet and erythrosine red are used to diagnose the presence of crown or root fractures.

(A very small amount of the dye is placed on a small cotton pellet and the crown/root is coated with it. The dye on the surface is washed away; in case of fracture, the dye remains within the crack and can be observed through loupes or a dental operating microscope.)

4. ***Palpation***: Palpation implies moving index finger tip around the soft tissues to identify tissue consistency and any discomfort, etc. (Fig. 9.3). The features of palpation are:

- Should be carried out bilaterally at the same time

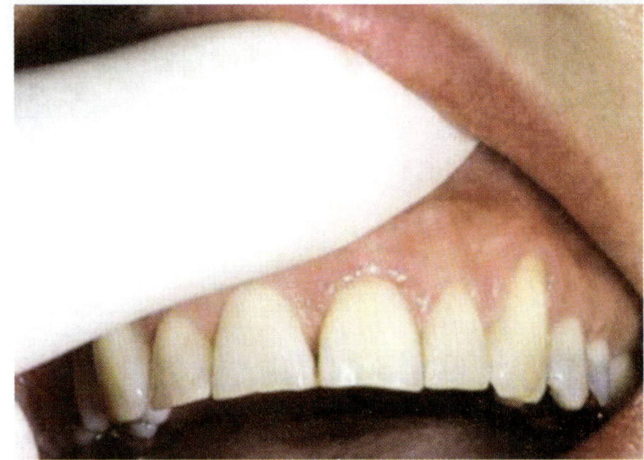

Fig. 9.3 Palpation

- Aids in locating a swelling, intensity and location of pain
- Evaluate presence of lymphadenopathy
- Evaluate presence of bony crepitus.

5. ***Percussion***: Percussion implies striking the tooth with a quick, moderate blow of low intensity with finger, followed by mirror handle to determine tenderness (Fig. 9.4). The contralateral tooth is percussed prior to the questionable tooth. Percussion evaluates following features:

- Periodontal status (periodontal ligament)
- Pain on percussion can be due to periradicular pathosis, fractures, periodontal disease, traumatic occlusion, sinusitis (pain in two or more teeth in the upper jaw), or any other condition that affects the periodontal ligament.

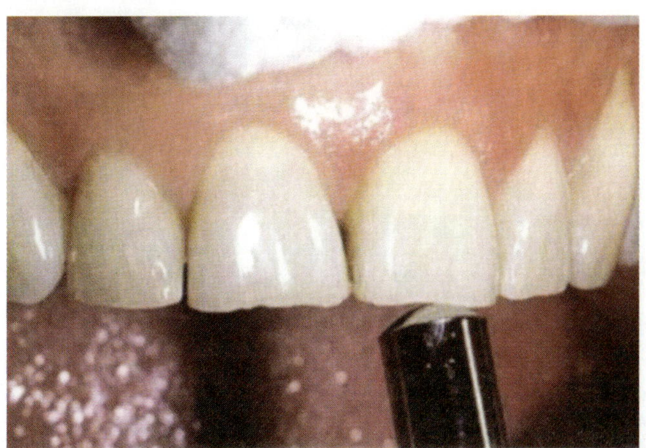

Fig. 9.4 Percussion

Key features of percussion test are summarized in Flowchart 9.1.

> ***Percussion test: Key features***
>
> *Positive response*
> - Rapid orthodontic movement
> - High points on restorations
> - Occlusal trauma
> - Lateral periodontal abscess
> - Apical periodontitis, periapical abscess
>
> *Negative response*
> - Healthy tooth
>
> *Sounds during percussion*
> - Dull note (abscess formation)
> - Sharp note (inflammation)
> - Metallic note (ankylosis)

6. ***Mobility and depressibility***: The tooth is moved buccally/lingually using handles of two instruments (Fig. 9.5).

Two index fingers can be used, but effective only in grade III mobility. To evaluate depressibility, apply pressure apically on the occlusal or incisal aspects.

Mobility and depressibility evaluate the integrity of the attachment apparatus.

Grades of mobility

Grade I: Noticeable movement within the socket

Grade II: Lateral movement within 1.0 mm range

Grade III: More than 1.0 mm lateral movement and/or depressibility

The mobility may be due to apical abscess, periodontal disease, horizontal fracture in the middle/coronal third of the root, vertical fracture, chronic bruxism or clenching.

> *Palpation, percussion, mobility and depressibility check the integrity of the attachment apparatus; not the condition of pulp*

7. ***Periodontal probing***: Periodontal probing evaluates:

- Health of periodontium (Fig. 9.6a and b)
- Furcation involvement, palatogingival groove, etc.
- Differentiate disease of periodontal origin from pulp origin.

8. ***Bite test (occlusal pressure test)***: Bite test is useful in identifying teeth with symptoms of apical periodontitis, abscess or cracks.

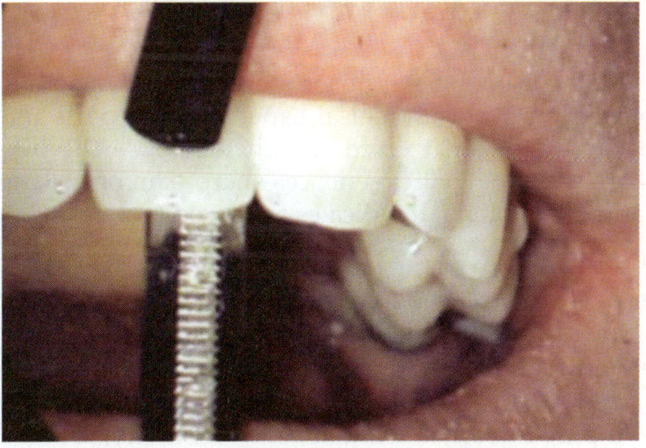

Fig. 9.5 Mobility and depressibility

Flowchart 9.1: Key features of percussion test

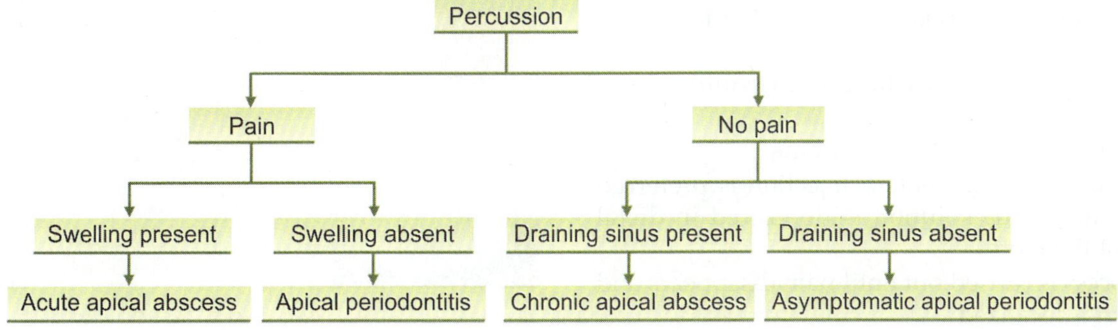

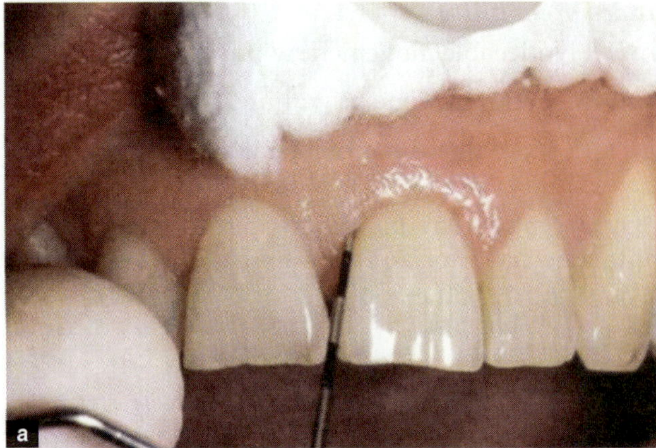

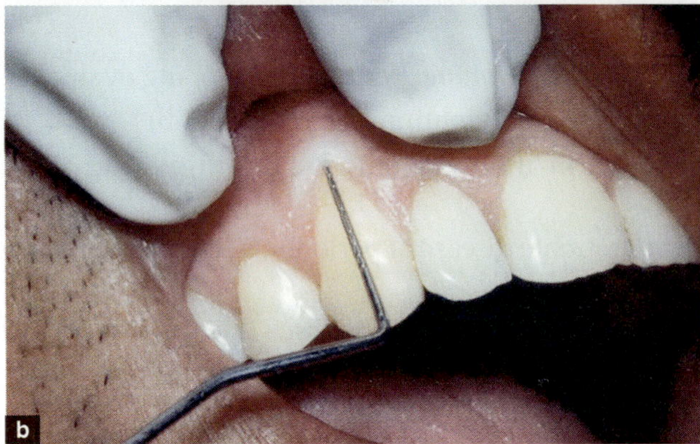

Fig. 9.6a and b Periodontal probing

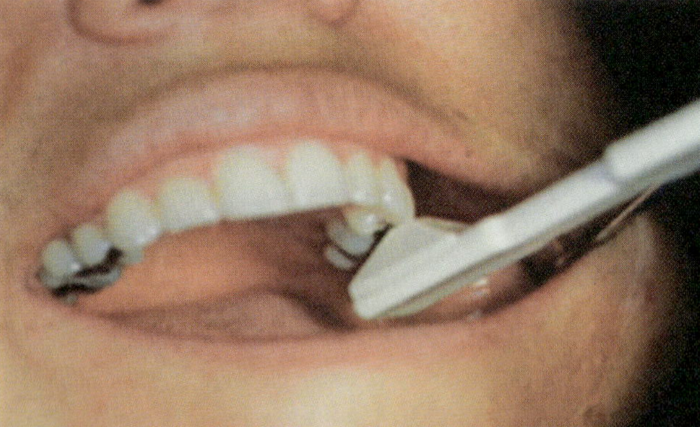

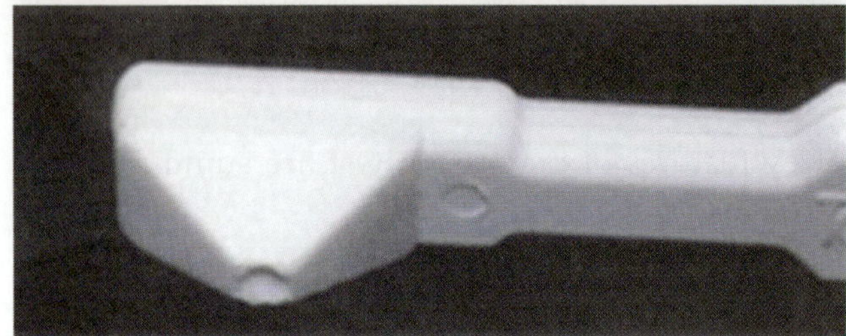

Fig. 9.7 Tooth slooth placed in posterior region

Orangewood stick, rubber wheel or tooth slooth is placed on occlusal/incisal aspect of the tooth and patient is asked to bite and then release the bite (Fig. 9.7). If patient experiences sharp pain on release rather than biting, it indicates a cracked tooth.

9. Test cavity

- A cavity is prepared deep into dentin without anesthesia and without coolant (Fig. 9.8a and b)
- Pain/sensitivity during cavity preparation indicates vital pulp
- If pulp is reached without pain/sensitivity, proceed with root canal treatment
- The cavity test is used as the last resort, being subjective.

10. Anesthesia test

- Anesthesia test is carried out when other tests have failed
- Restricted to patients where pain could not be localized
- Single tooth is anesthetized at a time
- Infiltration/intraligamentary injection is preferred (0.2 ml anesthetic solution is deposited in distal sulcus of the tooth)
- The process is carried out until pain disappears and the tooth is localized.

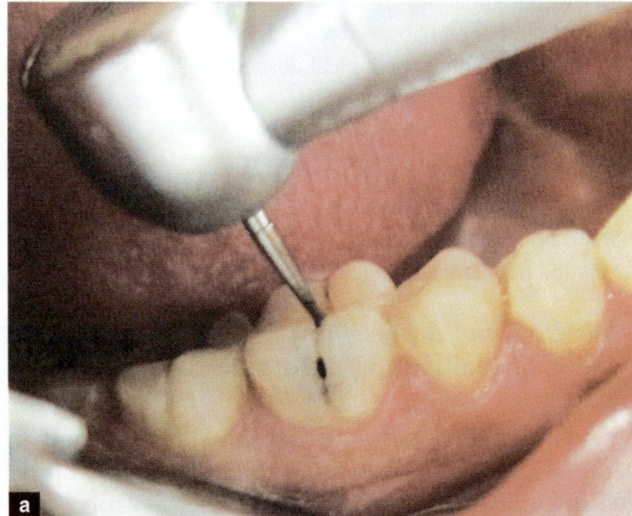

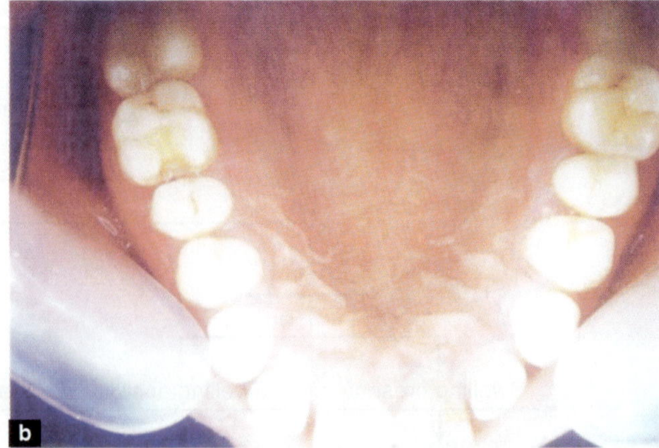

Fig. 9.8a and b Test cavity

11. Videography/*intraoral camera*: Miniature color charged coupled devices (CCD) with fiberoptic probes (video camera) are used to examine teeth and the surrounding soft tissues in the oral cavity. The smaller probes can be inserted into root canals to view root canal intricacies. Images are captured and then displayed on TV screen.

12. *Fiberoptic transillumination*: Fiberoptics (optical fibers) refers to flexible, thin cylindrical fibers of high quality glass/plastic (0.1 mm). Individual fibers are grouped together to form fiberoptic bundles. Fiberoptic transillumination works on the principle that caries, calculus, restorative materials, sound tooth structure, inflammatory exudates and healthy periodontium have different indices of light transmission.

Since caries has a lower index of light transmission than sound tooth structure, an area of decay and its spread along the path of dentinal tubules will be displayed as a dark shadow.

Periapical tissue may be similarly transilluminated; teeth with a periapical pathology reveal a shadow around the apex.

Fiberoptic transillumination is primarily used to:

- Detect cracks, discolorations, calcification in crown (a calcified crown will appear more dull/opaque than a tooth with a healthy pulp chamber).
- Aid in the determination of pulp vitality. In teeth with necrotic pulps, the shadow of the pulp chamber will appear darker.
- Detect caries, calculus and soft tissue lesions.

The fiberoptic probe should be held on the linguo-cervical area and an observation should be made by direct vision (Fig. 9.9a and b). If the probe is held on the labio-cervical area, then lingual surface should be viewed with a mirror. During transillumination, the main lights of the clinic and the dental unit should be switched off.

PULP VITALITY TESTS

Pulp vitality testing is an important aid in the diagnosis of pulp and periapical diseases (apical periodontitis). The ideal test should be accurate, reproducible and non-injurious. The commonly used tests are thermal and electrical tests, indicative of the neural status of the pulp; also called 'Pulp Sensibility Tests'.

The pulp vitality tests, indicative of the blood supply of pulp, are laser Doppler flowmetry, pulse oximetry, etc.

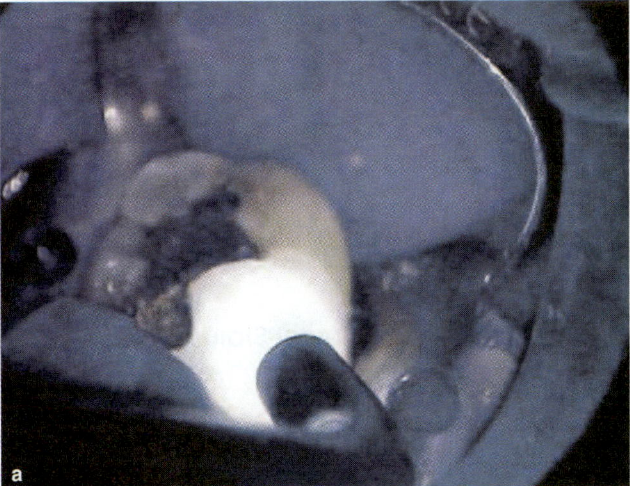

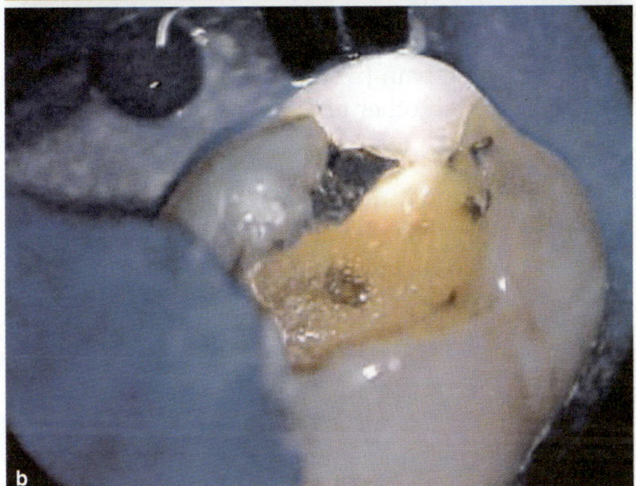

Fig. 9.9a and b Transillumination

In clinical practice, the key areas of pulp testing are:

i. *Localization of pain*: The origin of pain in tooth is mainly because of involvement of pulp. The pain is to be identified (testing pulp status), differentiating from other non-odontogenic pains (normal response to pulp testing eliminates the diagnosis of pulp pathology).

ii. *Identifying radiolucent areas*: Radiolucent areas at the periapical region are generally indicative of pulp pathology. If pulp response is normal, other reasons, such as periodontal abscess, cysts, etc. can be considered. Normal anatomical structures, such as mental foramen may also present as periapical radiolucency.

iii. *Preoperative assessment*: Vitality tests are important to assess the pulp status prior to planning any treatment for pulp/periapical pathology.

iv. *Postoperative assessment*: The teeth treated with pulp capping/pulpotomy procedures are periodically tested for pulp vitality. In case of no response, the treatment is considered as 'failed', and other treatment modality can be planned.

v. Vitality testing is important in finalizing the treatment plan in traumatized teeth (traumatic teeth need to be assessed periodically).

The commonly employed tests are categorized as follows.

A. Tests Assessing the Neural Status of Pulp

a. Thermal Test

Thermal tests are carried out to assess the status of the pulp. The patient's response help to decide whether the pulp is healthy or inflamed; identifying the offending tooth when the patient is unable to locate the source of the pain (results of thermal tests should be correlated with other tests to ensure vitality).

Advantages

- Easily performed
- More reliable than electric pulp testing.

Guidelines

Before commencing the thermal tests, follow the guidelines as:

- Explain the implications of test to the patient. Demonstrate on a normal tooth. Explain the type of sensation, which patient may feel.
- The site of performing the test is cervical-third of the buccal surface of the posterior tooth and in anterior teeth, center of middle and cervical-third of labial surface (*thermal tests are not effective in posterior teeth; amount of dentin may act as insulator*).
- The pain may be replicated by the tests; so be prepared to relieve the pain, if sets in.
- There may be delayed response from few teeth. Wait for a minute before testing the next tooth.
- The response from crowned teeth will vary.
- Instruct patient on how to respond (e.g. raise your finger when pain is felt).
- The concerned teeth should be isolated, dried with a gauze or cotton (should not be dried with a blast of air); salivary ejector is placed.
- The results should be recorded.

The response of thermal tests (heat and cold) is attributed to different phenomena in pulp. The response to cold stimulus is attributed to the hydrodynamic theory (contraction of fluid in the dentinal tubules and the subjacent pulpal tissues). Such a movement deforms intratubular and peripheral (A-δ) nerves fibers, which activates an action potential.

In cases of advanced acute pulpitis, indicating varying degrees of necrosis, cold may not exacerbate the painful symptoms. If the peripheral coronal A-δ fibers are not viable, they cannot be activated by fluid movement.

The cold may relieve symptoms of acute pain; the vasoconstriction will reduce the blood volume thereby reducing the high intrapulpal pressure.

Hot stimulation causes vasodilation and subsequent increase in intrapulpal pressure. Intrapulpal pressure rises when heat is applied to the tooth. In an intact pulp, a specific pulpal temperature should be reached before pain is felt.

In normal teeth, there is a delayed response to heat; whereas, in inflamed pulp, an increased intrapulpal pressure already exists. Therefore, the immediate painful response to sudden/gradual heat is expected.

Thermal tests can be conducted as:

i. Cold test

The cold test (Fig. 9.10) helps:

- To differentiate between reversible and irreversible pulpitis
- To identify the necrosed teeth
- If the pain subsides immediately after removing the stimulus; suggestive of hypersensitivity or reversible pulpitis
- Lingering pain (even after the stimulus is removed), suggests irreversible pulpitis.

Agents used in cold test

- Air blast
- Ice water bath
- Ice stick
- Ethyl chloride spray (4°C), dichlorodifluoromethane (–21°C), tetrafluoroethane (refrigerant spray) (–15°C to –26°C)
- Carbon dioxide snow (dry ice) (–78°C)

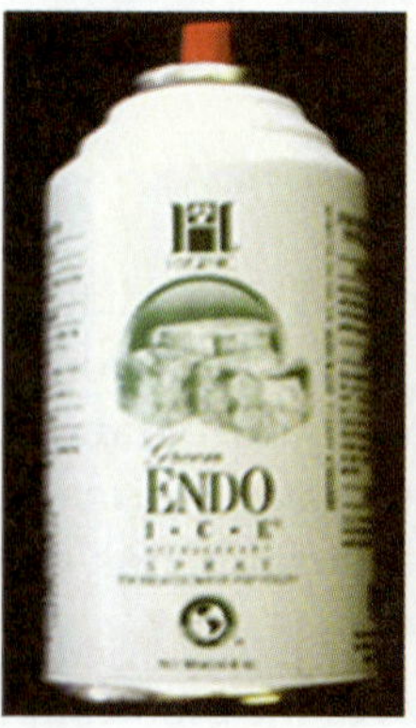

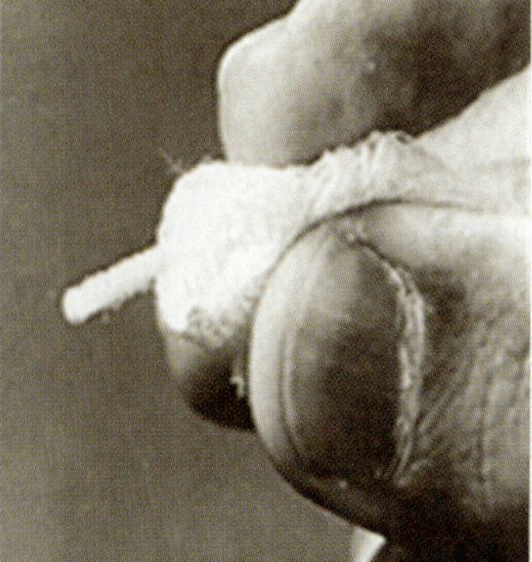

Fig. 9.10 Cold test—endo-ice (refrigerant spray: Tetrafluoroethane)

The *routinely used agents in cold test* are:

- *Ice stick*: It should be applied at the junction of cervical and middle third of labial surface of tooth. Pencils of ice can be made by filling discarded anesthetic carpules with water and kept in refrigerator.

  Disadvantages
  - Cold water may drip onto the gingiva (false positive)
  - Not as cold as other agents, viz.

  Ethyl chloride spray (4°C) dichlorodifluoromethane (–21°C) and tetrafluoroethane (refrigerant spray) (–15°C to –26°C)

  The agent is sprayed on cotton pellet held in cotton pliers and applied on tooth surface at the stipulated site. Spraying these agents directly on tooth surface is not recommended.
- *Carbon dioxide snow (dry ice)*: Solid stick of carbon dioxide is prepared by delivering carbon dioxide gas into a specially designed plastic cylinder. The carbon dioxide stick (–78°C) is applied to the stipulated site on the natural tooth or over the crown for five seconds.

  Disadvantages
  - May cause infarction lines on enamel, causing pitting even in five seconds.
  - May damage the surface of ceramic restorations.

ii. Heat test

Agents used in heat test (preferred temperature: 65°C)
- Hot water bath
- Hot air
- Hot burnisher
- Hot gutta-percha
- Hot impression compound
- Rubber wheel mounted on a mandrel
- Heating devices (system B – 150°F)
- LASER

Response to thermal test
- No response: Non-vital pulp or false negative
- Mild to moderate response, subsides within one to two seconds after removal of stimulus: **Healthy pulp**
- Strong momentary painful response, subsides within one to two seconds after removal of stimulus: **Reversible pulpitis**
- Moderate to painful response that lingers for several seconds after removal of stimulus: **Irreversible pulpitis**

The *routinely used agents in heat tests* are:

- *Hot burnisher/gutta-percha*: The tooth is lubricated with thin layer of cocoa butter/petroleum jelly. The tip of gutta-percha stick is heated for two seconds till it becomes shiny and placed at the junction of cervical and middle third of labial surface (Fig. 9.11). The test is convenient and easily manipulated.
- *Hot water technique*: Isolate the tooth with rubber dam, pour hot water from a conventional syringe for five seconds or until patient begins to feel pain.

Advantages
- Simulates the existing conditions experienced by the patient on taking hot food
- Effective in penetrating porcelain fused to metal crowns
- *Heating devices and LASER*: Heating devices, viz. Gutta-percha cutters, system B and pulsed Nd:YAG Laser are accepted alternative to hot gutta-percha method.

  The pain produced is mild and tolerable.

b. Electric Pulp Testing

The parts of electric pulp tester are: main device, electrode probe tip and lip clip attachment (Fig. 9.12). It is available either as battery operated or with

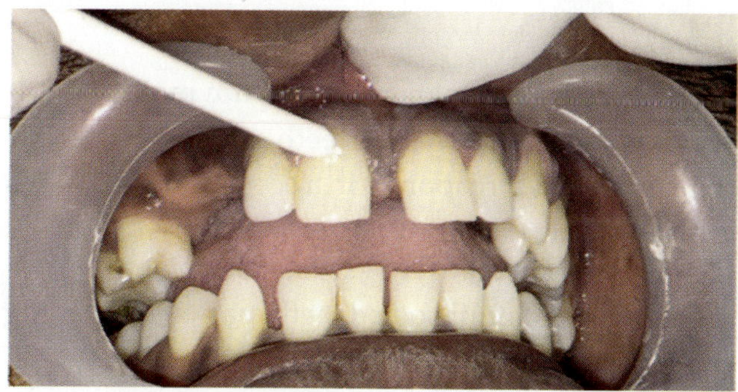

Fig. 9.11 Heat test with gutta-percha stick

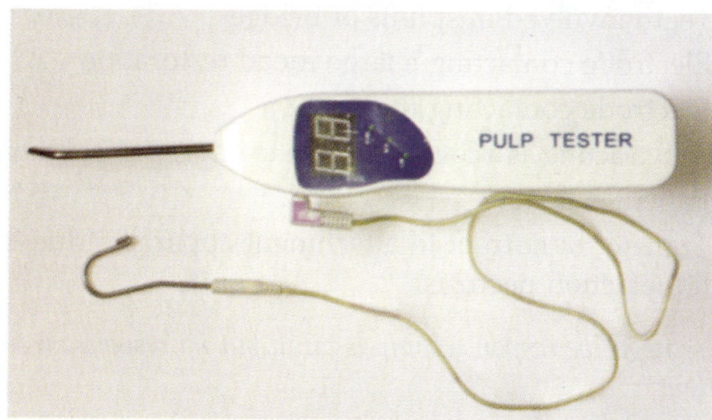

Fig. 9.12 Electric pulp tester

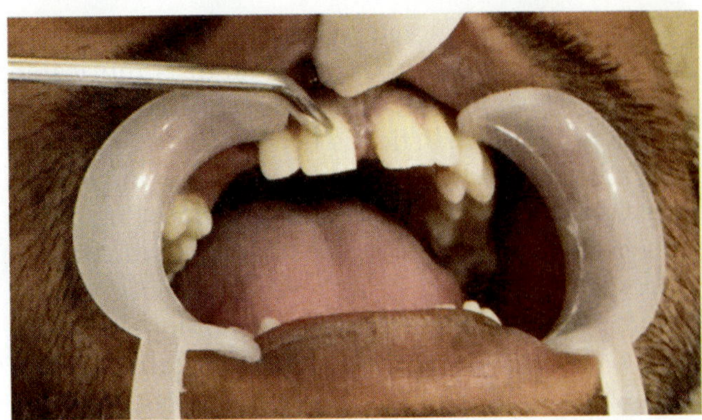

Fig. 9.13 Electric pulp testing

cords that plug into electric outlets; it stimulates response by electrical excitation of the neural elements (Aδ fibers) within pulp. It does not provide any clue on the vascular supply of the tooth which is a real indicator of pulp vitality. Electric pulp testers are difficult in teeth restored with full crowns and are contraindicated in patients with cardiac pacemakers (Fig. 9.13).

Advantages

- Electric stimulus is comfortable
- Digital display on electric pulp testers is instant, easy and reliable
- Provides a quantitative reading

Disadvantages

- Cannot be used in patients with pace makers
- False reading in immature teeth
- False negative response in recently traumatized teeth
- No indication regarding vascular supply
- Reading from multi-rooted teeth may be misleading (partial necrosis).

False positive response (pulp is necrotic, but patient gives a response)

- Teeth involved in splints or bridges
- Electrode contacting a large metal restoration
- Electrode contacting the gingiva
- Saliva acting as a conductor due to improper isolation
- Patient's anxiety
- Transfer of current to attachment apparatus due to liquefaction necrosis.

False negative response (pulp is vital, but no response from patient)

- Heavily pre-medicated patient (tranquilizers, narcotics, etc.)
- Inadequate contact with tooth surface (inadequate conductor, composite restoration, large restoration with bases)
- Recently traumatized teeth
- Young teeth with immature apices
- Older teeth with sclerotic dentin
- Excessive calcification in the canals
- No current (dead batteries).

Electric Pulp Testing Technique

Check the gadget prior to use

↓

Coat electrode with good conductor gel

↓

Adjust lip clip attachment

↓

Adjust the rheostat to minimum current (gradually increase the current during use)

↓

Ask the patient to indicate tingling sensation (raising hand or any other sign)

↓

Start the procedure on control tooth (antagonist or adjacent tooth)

↓

Place the electrode tip at the junction of cervical and middle third of labial/buccal surface (less effective in posterior teeth)

↓

(Junction of middle and cervical third of anterior teeth and the mesiobuccal cuspal tip on molar teeth is the optimal site to determine the lowest response threshold)

↓

Gradually increase the current (up to 4.0 mA)

↓

Note the patient's response

↓

Take at least two readings and record the average

↓

Do not repeat the stimulus for more than twice; nerve tissue may react at a lower threshold

Limitations of Pulp Sensibility (Thermal and Electrical) Tests

- Tests remain inconclusive in children. Children do not respond to a stimulus and the subjective symptoms. Children avoid painful stimulus and their ability to properly respond to pulp testing is limited.
- Thermal and electrical tests measure only nerve responses and not the blood flow.
- Not effective in aged patients (reduced neural component, reduced volume and deposition of secondary dentin making dentinal tubules narrow). The response is weaker as compared to more innervated and less calcified dentinal tubules in younger individuals.
- Less reliable in immature teeth; also in teeth following traumatic injuries.
- The response is different on different days, even at different hours of the same day (tests lack reproducibility).
- Extensive restorations, pulp calcification, pulp recession may create difficulty in interpreting pulp status.
- The results of the tests may not correspond to the histopathological studies.

B. Tests Assessing the Blood Supply of Pulp

The thermal and electric tests assess the response of Aδ nerve fibers in pulp dentin complex. If Aδ nerve fibers get stimulated, the patient responds as feeling pain/tingling from the tooth. A positive response indicates functioning of Aδ fibers; however, no indication of blood flow in pulp tissues. In case of no blood flow, Aδ fibers cease to function; however, there are instances, such as trauma, where there is blood flow in pulp, but A fibers are not functioning.

Consequently, tests which measure blood flow are considered ideal. Tests assessing the pulpal vascularity are:

a. Laser Doppler Flowmetry

The laser Doppler flowmetry is a noninvasive technique that detects red blood cell movement in a small volume of tissue (about 10 mm^3). It can measure blood flow in very small blood vessels of pulp; measuring micro-circulation of pulp (Fig. 9.14a and b).

Principle

It utilizes light beam from a He-Ne laser (632.8 nm), which is carried to the tissues by a fiberoptic probe that carries light by one fiber and receives back the scattered (reflected) light by another fiber to the instrument.

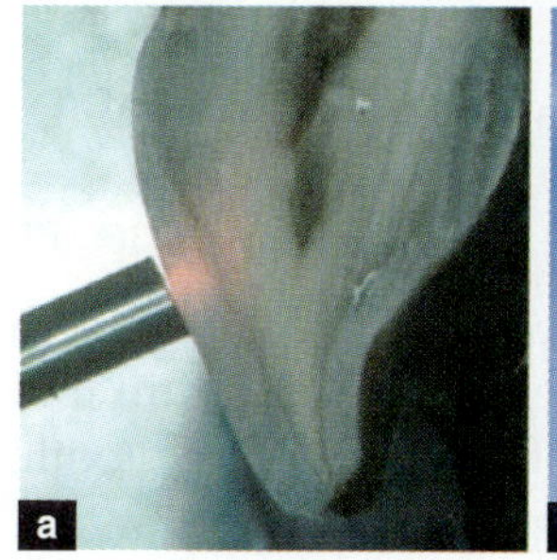

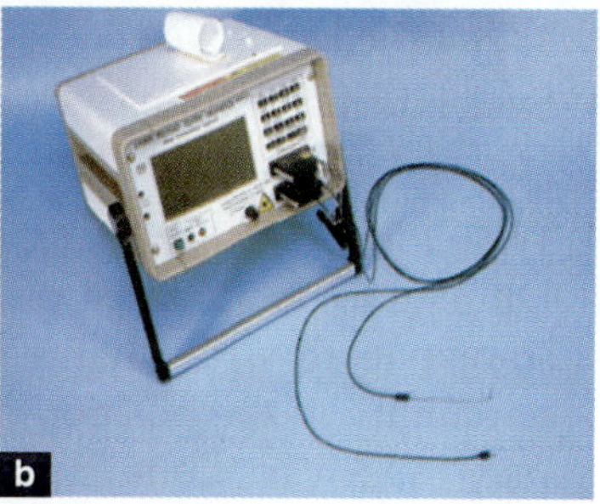

Fig. 9.14 Laser Doppler flowmetry: (a) Laser Doppler flowmetry (clinical); (b) Laser Doppler flowmeter

Fraction of light which is scattered back (Doppler shift) is detected; output is proportional to the number and velocity of blood cells and produce a signal that is a function of the red cell flux (volume of cells illuminated × mean cell velocity).

Color power Doppler flowmetry, a modified version, detects and elicits direction of blood flow within the tissues (contrast media is injected to improve observation). Power Doppler enhances the sensitivity of the technique measuring blood flow.

Laser Doppler Flowmetry Technique

Place rubber dam to avoid interference of gingival tissues

↓

Place fiberoptic probe on the tooth surface

↓

Project monochromatic laser beam on to the crown to the pulp

↓

The reflected light in accordance with movement of blood cells is received by the meter

↓

Scattered light is processed producing output signal

↓

Output signal can be displayed on digital board and/or printed

Advantages

- Reflects vascularity of pulp
- No problems with apprehensive patients
- Noninvasive procedure
- Provides accurate reading in case of recently erupted teeth or traumatized teeth (effective in pulp testing of children)
- Effectively monitor revascularization of replanted teeth.

Disadvantages

- Systemic medications may alter blood flow in pulp; subsequently, the readings
- Sensitivity to motion
- Difficult to obtain laser reflection from certain teeth (molar teeth with thicker enamel and dentin and variability in the position of pulp within the tooth, may cause variations in pulpal blood flow)
- Differences in sensor output and inadequate calibration by the manufacturer may dictate use of multiple probes for accurate assessment
- Gingival blood vessels can give false readings
- Need custom fabricated jig to hold sensor
- Equipment is expensive.

b. Pulse Oximetry

Pulse oximetry determines the oxygen saturation of circulating arterial blood. It analyzes changes in light transmission through any pulsating vascular area; the changes calculate pulse rate and the oxygen saturation. As the hemoglobin is oxygenated, it increases transmission of light. Well-oxygenated blood appears bright red.

The device consists of a probe containing two light emitting diodes that emit light in two wavelengths; (i) Red light (660 nm) and (ii) Infrared light (800 nm) to measure the absorption of oxygenated and deoxygenated blood respectively.

The device may be 'reflectance' type or 'transmission' type depending upon the type of light incident on the detector (Fig. 9.15).

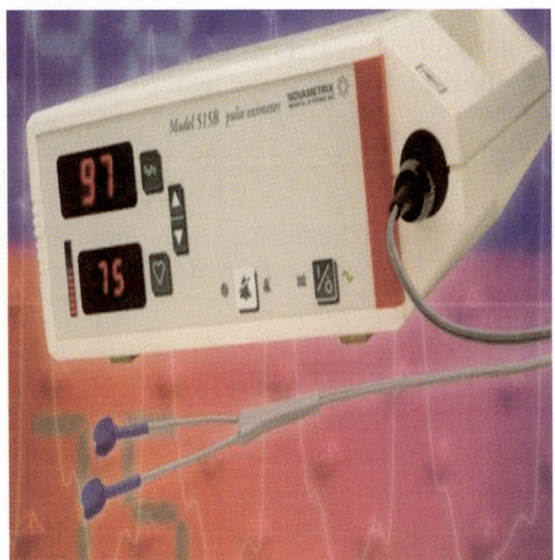

Fig. 9.15 Pulse oximetry

Tooth is sandwiched between a photoelectric detector and an LED of red/infrared lights. It measures oxygen pressure of erythrocytes (providing pulp vitality), following two principles:

i. Light absorbance of oxygenated hemoglobin is different from that of reduced hemoglobin, at the oximeter's two wavelengths, red and infrared light.
ii. The absorbance of both wavelengths has a pulsatile component, which is due to the fluctuations in the volume of arterial blood between source and the detector.

The relationship between the pulsatile change in the absorption of red light and infrared light is assessed by the oximeter to show the saturation of arterial blood.

Advantages

- Effectively detects pulpal blood flow
- Pulp circulation can be detected independent of gingival circulation
- Useful in traumatic injuries
- Easy to reproduce pulp pulse reading.

Disadvantages

- Reliability—mixed results
- Pulpal blood flow is not pulsed, as arterioles are present
- Pulp is insulated by enamel and dentin, difficult to detect pulsations by the probe
- In addition to the absorption; refraction and reflection also occur; some light reaches photo detector diode without passing through the tissue bed
- Only detect bound hemoglobin (hemoglobin bound to other gases may give false results).

c. Dual Wavelength Spectrophotometry

Dual wavelength spectrophotometry measures oxygenation changes in the capillary bed rather than in the supply vessels. It does not depend on a pulsatile blood flow. The presence of arterioles in pulp, coupled with its covering by dentin, make it difficult to detect a pulse in the pulp. However, various studies have approved the efficacy of dual wavelength spectrophotometry in pulp testing (Fig. 9.16).

Advantages

- Yield objective test results
- Instrument is small, portable and inexpensive

9

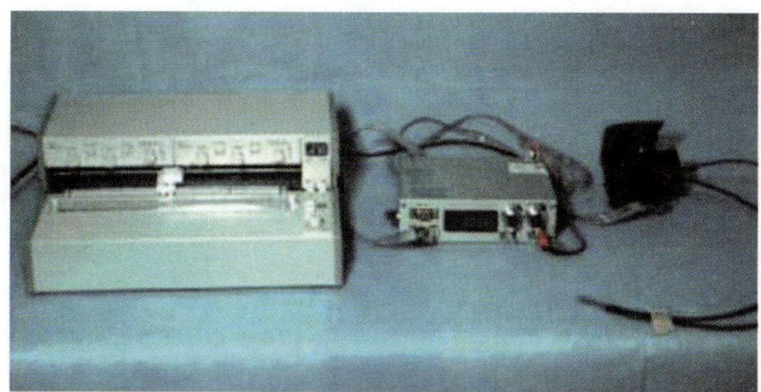

Fig. 9.16 Dual wavelength spectrophotometry

- Uses visible light that is filtered and guided to tooth by fiberoptics (eye protection not required as in laser light).

d. Optical Reflection Vitalometer

Optical reflection vitalometer (ORV) is based on the same principle of pulse oximetry; uses reflected light instead of transmitted light.

It measures oxygen in tissues by means of light, which is based on the fact that photons passing through the human tissue are attenuated by absorption. Absorption is spectrally sensitive especially infrared range where organometallic molecules such as hemoglobin have characteristic absorption spectra that shifts with oxygenation.

Difference between Optical Reflection Vitalometer (ORV) and pulse oximetry; ORV uses reflected light instead of transmitted light as in Pulse oximetry

e. Photoplethysmography

Photoplethysmograhy is a non-invasive method to detect vascularity (Fig. 9.17). It uses a light source and a photoconductive cell with peak intensity for red and infrared light to detect optical density changes. The technique is used to detect circulating anomalies in the human dental pulp. The components required are: a light source to illuminate the tissue (tooth) and a photodetector to measure the changes, if any. A selected band of light is passed through tooth, while continuously monitoring the intensity of transmitted light. The specific wavelength of light is absorbed by hemoglobin, while the remaining light is passed through the tooth and is detected by the receptor.

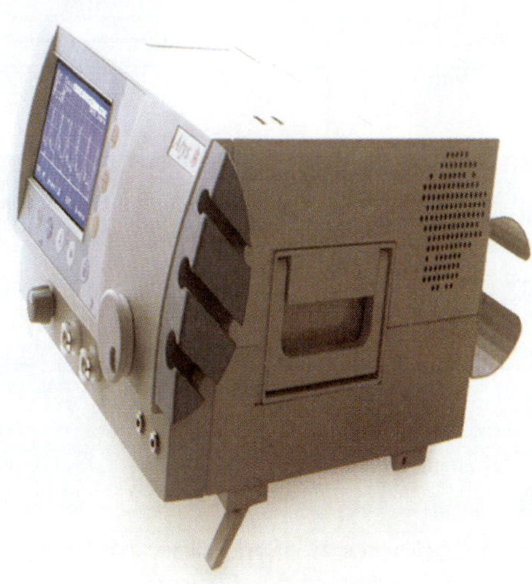

Fig. 9.17 Photoplethysmography

RADIOGRAPHIC TECHNIQUES

Various radiographic techniques are employed to diagnose pathological changes in teeth and the surrounding tissues (*refer* to Fundamentals of Dental Radiology; 4th ed: Vimal K Sikri, for details of radiographic techniques).

1. Conventional Radiography

Use of conventional radiography is vital for diagnosis and follow-up in endodontics. It is a reliable source for gaining information regarding the pulp canal space and the periapical tissues.

Ideal Requirements of a Radiograph

- Image of tooth to be evaluated should be in centre of radiograph.
- Image should show 4.0–5.0 mm beyond the apex of the tooth and the surrounding bone or the pathologic condition.
- Should present an accurate image of the tooth; no elongation or fore-shortening.
- Should exhibit good contrast, so that all pertinent structures are readily identifiable?
- In multi-rooted teeth with curved canals, at least two radiographs should be taken; one at a normal vertical and horizontal angulations and other with a 20° horizontal angulations, either in mesial or distal direction.

How to 'Read' a Radiograph

Proper illumination and magnification gadgets (X-ray viewer with magnification lens) are essential for reading a radiograph. A radiograph should be thoroughly evaluated from one corner to the other.

The radiographs provide information as:

i. Integrity of the crown and the roots

- Proximal caries, secondary caries, root caries
- Number of roots/extra roots

- External resorption
- Crown/root fracture.

ii. Internal anatomy of the tooth

- Size of the pulp chamber and its proximity to the restoration/caries
- Depth of the restoration: pulp capping, pulpotomy (remaining dentin over pulp)
- Pulp stones
- Dystrophic calcifications
- Internal resorption
- Blunderbuss canals
- Root canal system
  - Length of the root
  - Mesiodistal width of the pulp canal space
  - Position of canal (s)
  - Mesial/distal curvature of the root
  - Hint towards position of the apical foramen
  - Apical radiolucency
  - Lateral radiolucency (indicating lateral canals)
  - Physiological radiolucency (mental foramen, etc.)
- Periodontal defects.

***iii. Integrity of the lamina dura*:** The lamina dura is a thin white line seen around the root with the radiolucent periodontal ligament in between. It is the thin cortical bone into which the periodontal fibers are embedded.

The strain on the teeth or expansion of pulpal disease can be observed as a thickening of the lamina dura.

There may be break in continuity of lamina dura, which indicates spread of the disease with visible breach in the cortical bone plate.

iv. *Trabecular pattern of bone and the surrounding structures*: It is important to be familiar with normal bone trabecular pattern; to be able to identify the changes which may occur due to diseases.

The height and pattern of alveolar crest, the appearance of normal radiographic features and other regular findings will help in identifying the abnormal findings.

Buccal Object/SLOB/Clark's Rule

This rule is based on the principle that, the root or canal farthest from the film (buccal) moves the greatest distance on a radiograph taken with the cone angled in the horizontal plane. If the cone is pointed from the mesial aspect toward the distal when a bi-canaled bicuspid is radiographed, the buccal root image will move more than lingual and appear distal to the lingual root image on the film.

9

Mesial/distal angulations further reveal:

- Number of roots
- Number of root canals
- Presence of buccal/lingual canal curvature
- Differentiate the true dental lesions from the false ones.

The ***techniques used in conventional radiography*** are:

a. *Paralleling cone technique/long cone technique*: X-ray film is supported parallel to long axis of the teeth and central ray of the X-ray beam is directed at right angles to the teeth and film. Placing X-ray film parallel to long-axis in maxillary posterior teeth is difficult; a cotton pellet is placed in between film and the tooth to make the technique semi-parallel. This modified paralleling technique is preferred in maxillary molars (Fig. 9.18a and b).

Advantages

i. *Dimensional accuracy*

- Minimal distortion
- No superimposition of shadow of zygomatic arch on maxillary molars
- Teeth apices and maxillary sinus better visualized
- Length of teeth can be easily measured.

ii. *Simplicity*: Beam alignment device eliminates the need for dental radiographer to determine horizontal and vertical angulation.

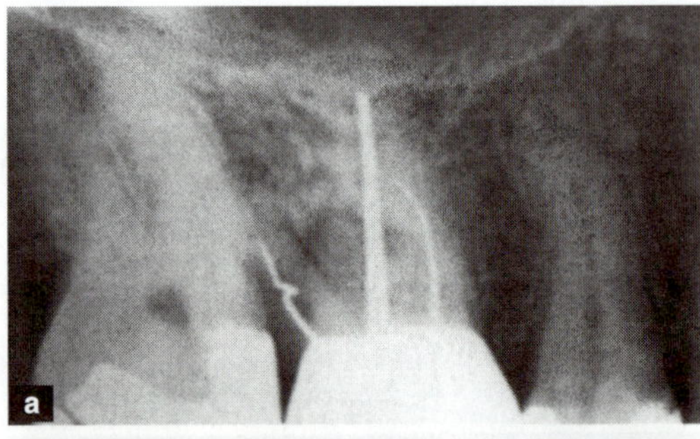

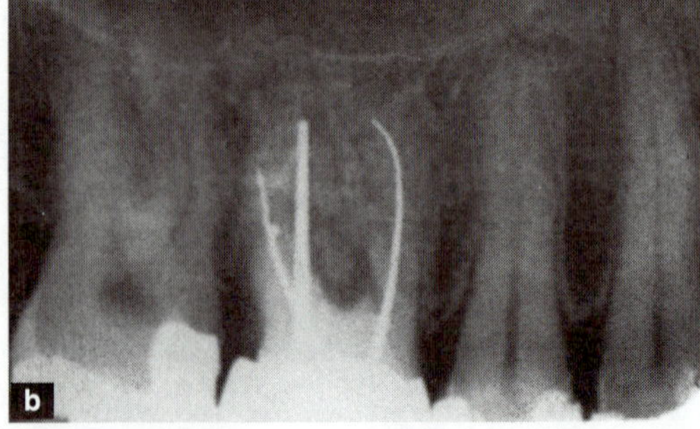

Fig. 9.18 (a) Radiograph of maxillary molar by bisecting technique; (b) Radiograph of same tooth by modified paralleling technique

iii. *Duplication*: Easy to standardise; can be accurately duplicated when serial radiographs are indicated.

Disadvantages

- Difficulty in film placement in child patient and also in adult patient with a small mouth opening or shallow palate.
- Discomfort (film holding device may impinge on oral tissues)
- Expensive.

b. ***Bisecting technique/short cone technique***: The central ray is directed perpendicular to the bisector of the angle between film and the tooth (Fig. 9.19a to d).

Advantage

- Can be used in patients with shallow palate, bony growths.

Disadvantages

- Image distortion
- Difficulty in determining the angulation: any error in vertical angulations lead to image distortion.
- Unnecessary exposure of the patient's hand to X-rays.

c. ***Bitewing technique***: Bitewing radiographs are used to evaluate mainly the changes in the coronal tooth structure. The cone, kept parallel to the film, provides image of the crown and the alveolar crest. The technique is useful for diagnosing proximal caries and morphology of coronal pulp (Fig. 9.20).

Limitations of conventional radiography

- Two-dimensional image of three-dimensional object
- State of pulpal health cannot be ascertained
- Periapical pathology can be evident only after 33% of bone destruction
- Vertical root fractures cannot be diagnosed
- Anatomic structures can mimic radiolucency
- Extent of caries or periapical pathology is much larger than what is seen on the radiographs
- Bony trabeculae can be misinterpreted for horizontal root fractures.

Sinus tracing: The presence of long-standing chronic periradicular diseases may lead to sinus formation with opening in the vestibule. It is essential to locate the origin of the sinus tract (the offending tooth) so that proper treatment can be carried out. In this technique, gutta-percha point is inserted through the sinus tract opening till it moves towards the lesion, followed by intraoral radiograph to determine the exact point of origin of the lesion (Fig. 9.21). Sinus tracing helps:

- To localize endodontic lesion to a specific tooth
- To differentiate endodontic from periodontal lesions.

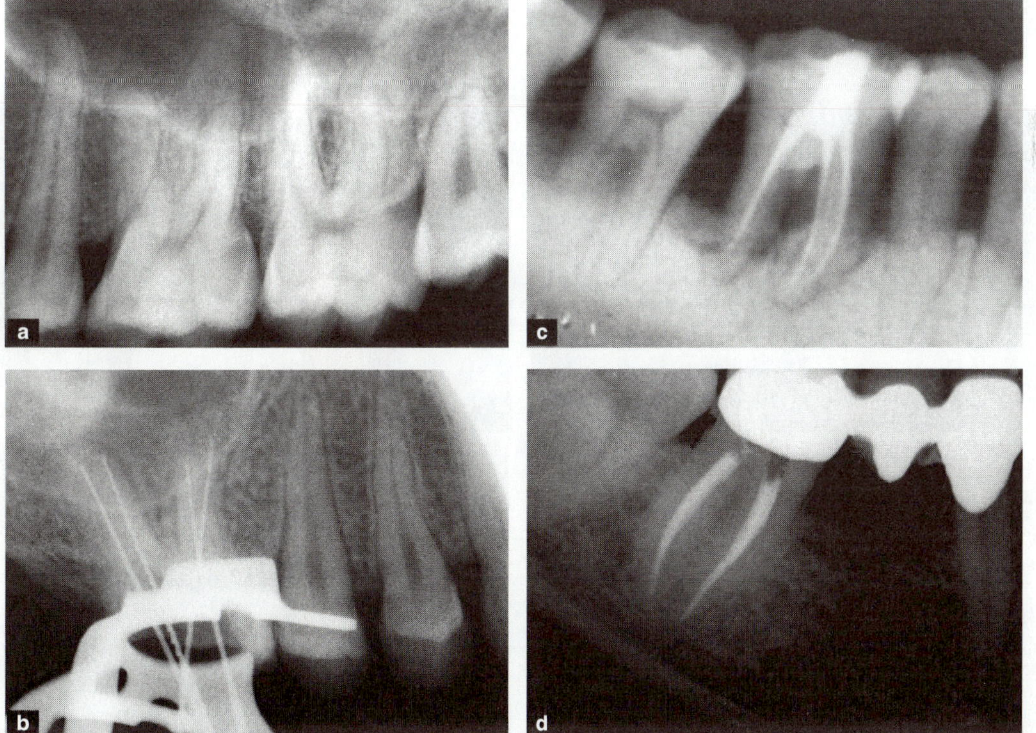

Fig. 9.19 Bisecting technique: (a) Radiograph of maxillary molars; (b) Diagnostic radiograph of maxillary first molar; (c) Radiograph of mandibular molar; (d) Obturated mandibular molar

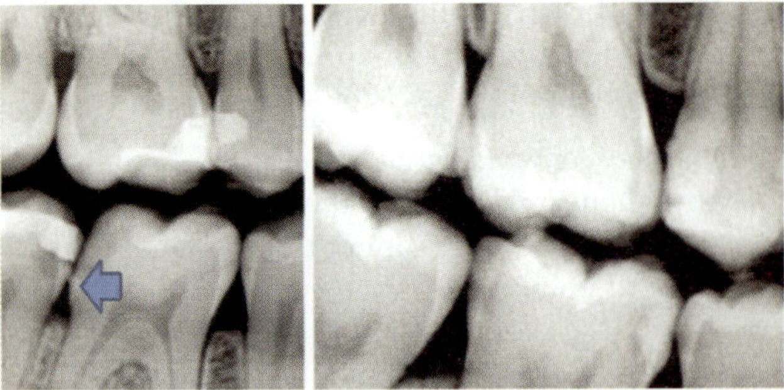

Fig. 9.20 Bite wing radiograph (arrow showing caries)

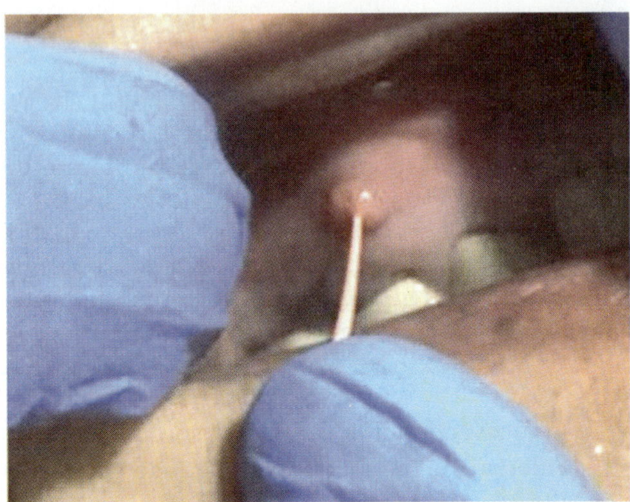

Fig. 9.21 Sinus tracing in maxillary first molar

2. Radiovisiography (RVG)

Radiovisiography digitizes ionizing radiation that provides instant image on a video monitor. The technique reduces radiation exposure by 80%.

It has *three* components:

- *Radio*: Consists of a hypersensitive *intraoral sensor* and an X-ray unit
- *Visio*: Video monitor and display processing unit
- *Graphy*: High resolution video printer.

Two kinds of detectors are used in radiovisiography:

- Charged coupled device (CCD)
- Photo-stimulable phosphor (PSP).

Image is captured directly on charged couple device (CCD) placed in a patient's oral cavity.

Signal from the CCD computer is digitized into 256 gray levels, displaying the image on monitor; enhanced by varying contrast (Fig. 9.22).

Advantages

- Elimination of X-ray film and processing errors
- Decreased radiation exposure (up to 80% less)
- Manipulation of image as varying contrast is possible
- Image can be duplicated and stored in a computer
- Lesser time for images.

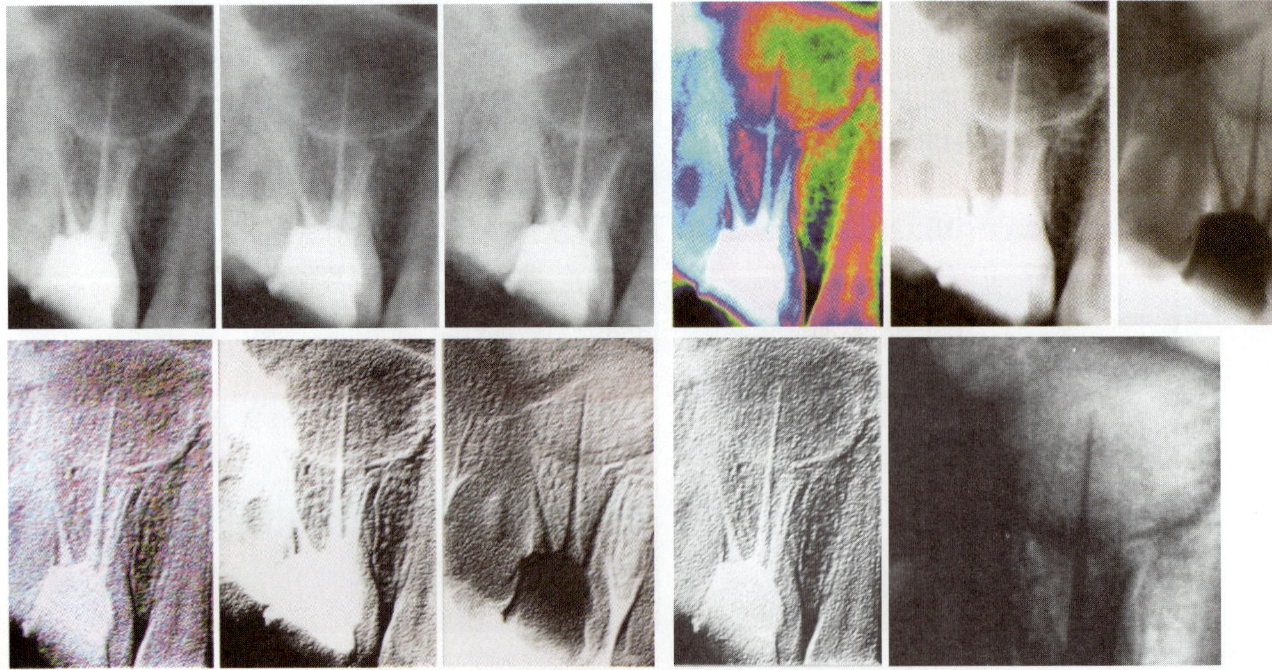

Fig. 9.22 Radiovisiography image and their modified forms

Disadvantages

- High cost
- Size of the sensor
- Low doses can impair image quality
- Inability to sterilize the sensor
- Manipulation of data possible
- Incompatibility with some existing X-ray machines.

3. Xeroradiography

Xeroradiography involves the production of a visible image utilizing a charged surface of a photoconductor as the detecting medium (selenium applied to sheet of aluminium known as xerographic plate); partially dissipating the charge by exposure to X-rays (25 seconds) to form a latent image and making the latent image visible by xerographic processing.

It is a complex electrostatic process and needs a photoconductor.

Advantages

- High contrast
- Edge enhancement
- Greater ability to resolve fine structure
- Choice of positive and negative display
- Display fine details of bone and teeth.

Disadvantage

- High chances of artefacts.

4. Digital Subtraction Radiography

Digital subtraction radiography depicts diagnostic information without background noise (those structures with no diagnostic importance). It is performed by subtracting the gray level values of one radiograph from the corresponding gray levels of another radiograph; what remains after subtraction is an image of the differences between the two images (Fig. 9.23 a to c).

The technique is mainly used for reviewing the progress of caries and periapical lesions.

Advantages

- Ability to remove structured noise
- Detection of changes
- Reduces sources of error
- Can detect loss of cancellous bone
- Helps in monitoring bone healing
- Evaluation of internal and external resorption
- Evaluation of periapical scars.

Disadvantages

- No geographic reproducibility of X-ray source-to-object relationship (intraoral stent to X-ray source)
- Expensive.

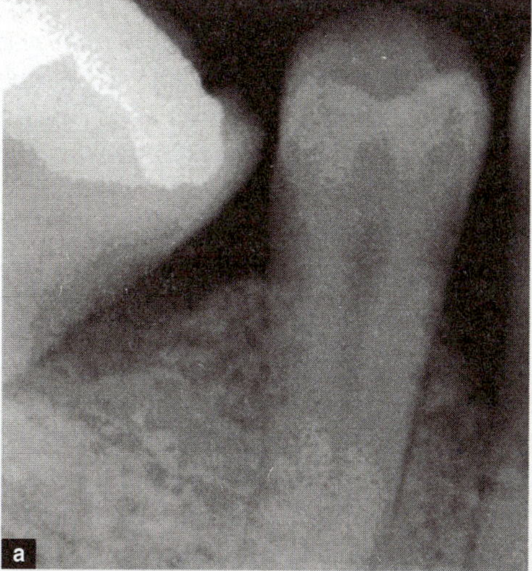

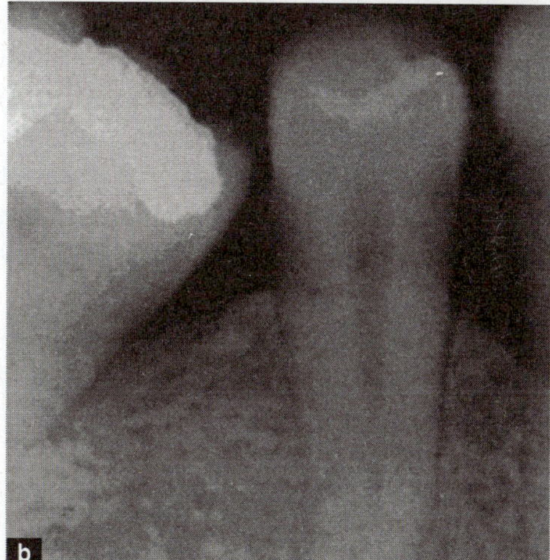

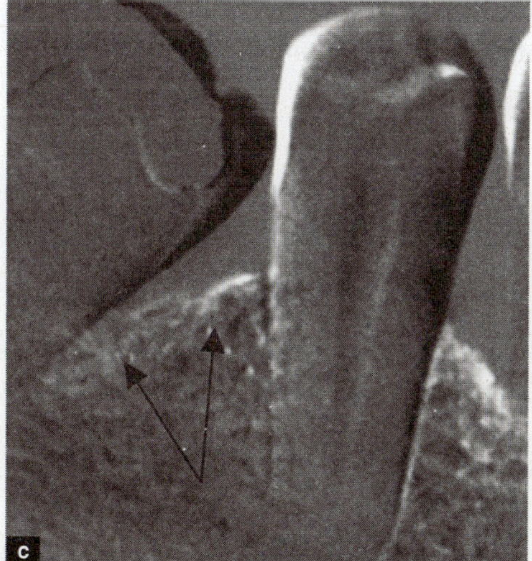

Fig. 9.23a to c Digital subtraction radiography: (a) Preoperative radiograph before periodontal surgery showing bone loss mesial to first molar; (b) Postoperative radiograph after periodontal surgery (four months) showing bone mineralization mesial to first molar; (c) Digitally subtracted radiograph showing detailed areas of bone mineralization (white areas—arrows)

(In digital subtraction radiography, it is difficult to improve sensitivity or speed of detecting periapical changes. The densitometry assessment of separate radiograph, where the gray value measurements are used to provide numerical data on the progress/healing of apical lesions).

5. Computed Tomography (CT)

Computed tomography (CT) provides three-dimensional image of an object. CT images have the ability to evaluate the target tissue in thin slices (1.0–2.0 mm thick). The location of the slides can be predetermined by the operator. Earlier CT scanners utilized single detector to capture X-ray beams. Later, more than one detector were popularized with arc-shaped and circular detectors. Current CT scanners use multiple (64) detectors, which simultaneously detect images. Computed tomography detects mesiodistal as well as labiolingual extent of the pathology. In endodontics, it is useful in diagnosing number of canals, morphological abnormalities, calcification of root canal, three-dimensional image of root canal, such as root curvature and diameter of root canal (Fig. 9.24a and b).

Advantages

- Detects three-dimensional image of root canals
- Reveals thickness of the cortical bone
- Eliminates anatomical noise.

Disadvantages

- Radiation dose is high
- Geometric resolution is inadequate
- Expensive.

Micro Computed Tomography

In micro computed tomography (Micro CT), X-radiations are converged over the sample and captured by a sensor. The projected rays are converted to digital images. The volumetric pixel (voxel) provided by micro CT ranges between 5 and 50 µm. Micro CT allows the use of same sample for different tests without destruction of sample; however, it permits the examination of specimens of limited size, limited to *in vitro* specimens.

The technique is useful for *in vitro* analysis of internal anatomy of teeth, root canal instrumentation, retreatment of failed root canals, etc. (preferred in preclinical training of students for learning endodontic procedures).

Spiral Computed Tomography

Spiral computed tomography acquires projection data with a spiral sampling three dimensional reconstruction. This technique is useful to reconstruct overlapping structure at arbitrary intervals, increasing the ability to resolve small objects.

The technique is used in endodontic applications, such as evaluation of root fracture, analysis of root resorption, location of extra/aberrant root canals and other pulp space anomalies.

Tuned-aperture Computed Tomography (TACT)

Tuned-aperture computed tomography (TACT) is advantageous because the images produced have less anatomical noise and absence of artefacts. The technique has been utilized to detect vertical fractures and also aberrations in root canal anatomy; however, TACT is rarely used for endodontic applications.

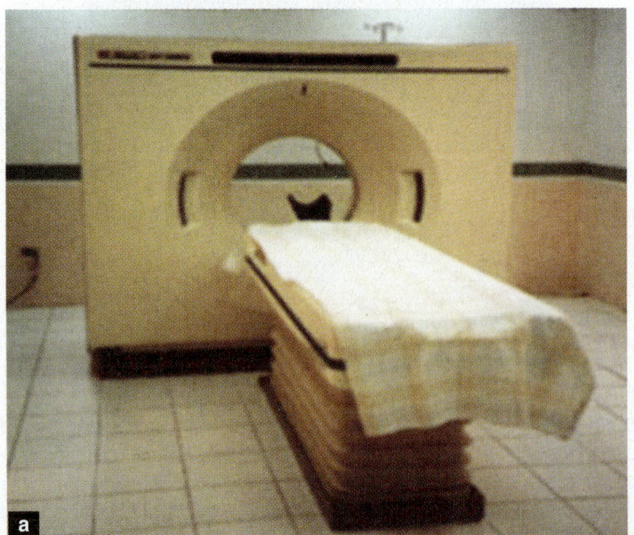

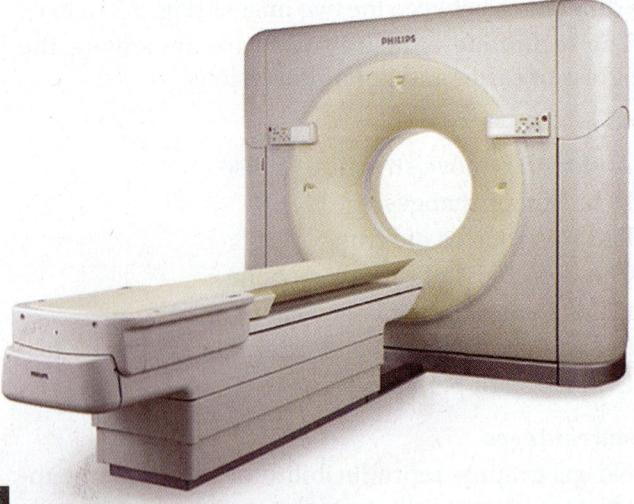

Fig. 9.24a and b Computed tomography (CT) scanners

6. Magnetic Resonance Imaging (MRI)

Magnetic resonance imaging (MRI) is a noninvasive imaging technique, which uses radio waves in spite of ionizing radiations. MRI is best suited in evaluating soft tissues; whereas, it does not provide good details of bony structures.

In endodontics, MRI is effective in differentiating small branches of neurovascular bundle entering apical foramen. It also evaluates periapical lesions as well as thickening of cortical bone. MRI scans are not affected by artefacts caused by metallic restorations, contrary to the CT technology.

Advantages

- No ionizing radiation involved
- Direct multiplane image is possible without re-orienting the patient
- Resolution of soft tissues is good
- Safe in pregnant ladies and infants
- Image can be manipulated.

Disadvantages

- Imaging time is long
- Metal present in the vicinity of the imaging magnet can be hazardous
- Contraindicated in patients with pace makers
- Expensive.

A recently developed MRI method, SWIFT (sweep imaging with Fourier transformation), overcomes many difficulties of detecting fast relaxing signals. The technique offers three-dimensional analysis of hard and soft tissues without subjecting the patients to ionizing radiations.

7. Cone Beam Computed Tomography (CBCT)

Cone Beam Computed Tomography (CBCT) serves as a bridge from 2D to 3D with lower irradiation than computed tomography (Fig. 9.25). CBCT produces 3D images at a low cost and least radiation exposure. It utilizes a cone beam instead of a fan-shaped beam of conventional CT, acquiring images of the volume as desired. Limited volume CBCT scanners can capture 40 mm × 40 mm volume of the data (data acquired is captured in term of 'volume', which is made up of voxels (3D pixels)). The technique elicits a high spatial resolution of bone and teeth along with adjacent tissues.

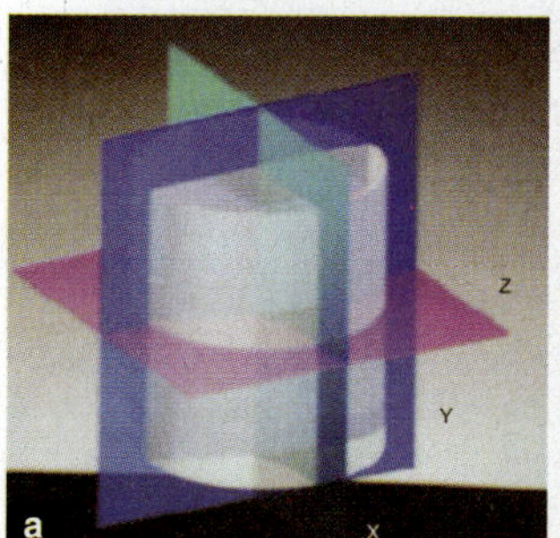

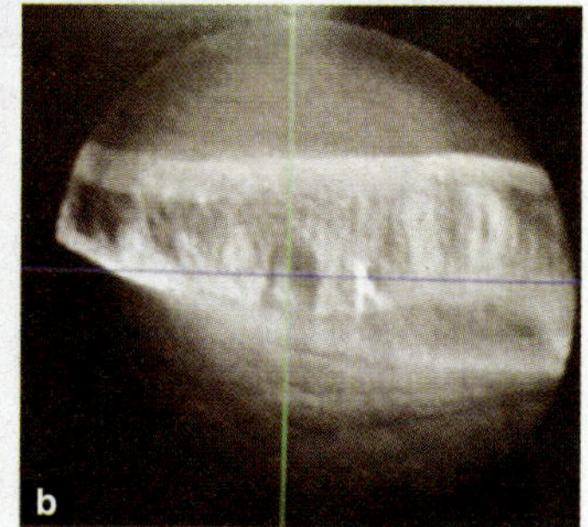

Fig. 9.25a and b Cone beam computed tomography (CBCT)

The limited volume CBCT machines are most appropriate for examining individual teeth for fracture/periapical disease/endodontic applications and are preferred over large volume CBCT for the following reasons:

- Provides objective and accurate representation of osseous changes overtime.
- Increased spatial resolution to improve the accuracy of endodontic-specific tasks like visualization of accessory canals and root fractures.
- Least radiation exposure to the patient.
- Time saving.

Limitations of CBCT

- CBCT images lack resolution of conventional radiographs
- Metal crowns and posts affect the image quality and diagnostic efficacy
- Presence of artefacts
- Radiation dose is higher than conventional radiographic level.

Utility of CBCT in Endodontics

a. ***Hidden periapical lesion***: The clinical and radiographic assessment, many a times remain inconclusive to differentiate the offending tooth (Fig. 9. 26). Limited

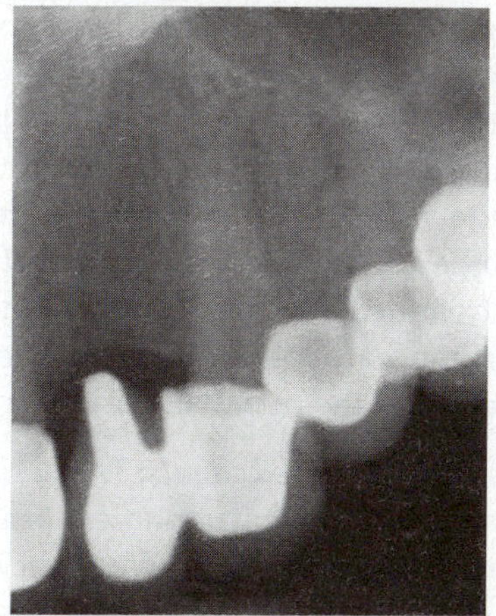

Fig. 9.26 Periapical radiograph not showing any periapical pathosis

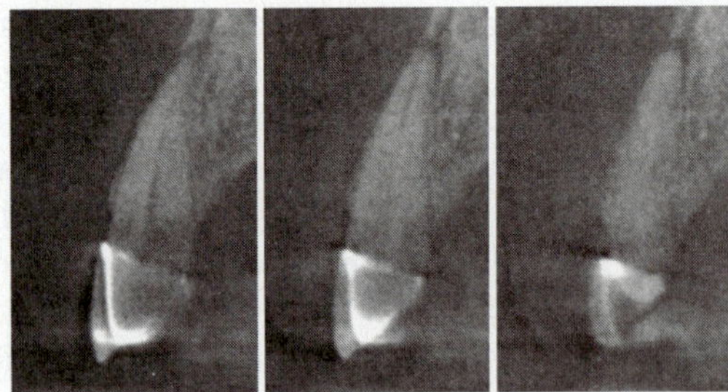

Fig. 9.27 CBCT showing periapical radiolucency (maxillary canine)

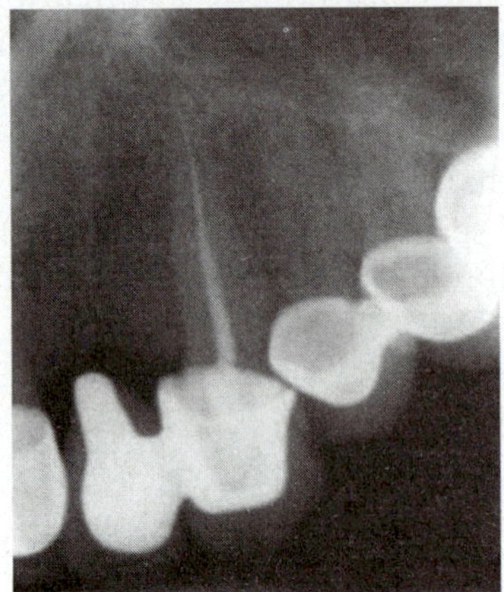

Fig. 9.28 Root canal treated maxillary canine

volume CBCT clearly showed a lesion at the apex of upper left canine (Fig. 9. 27). The length of the tooth was accurately measured using the CBCT, thus allowing precise placement of the root canal filling material (Fig. 9.28).

b. *Sinus infection secondary to periapical infection*: The conventional CT scan could not reveal definite pathological lesion (Fig. 9.29). The periapical radiograph of the region also did not clearly show any pathosis (Fig. 9.30). Cone beam CT scan of the region (Fig. 9.31) showed a periapical lesion at the apex of upper first molar. The lesion had perforated the floor of the maxillary sinus suggesting that the maxillary sinus infection was secondary to an infected pulp and periapical abscess associated with upper left first molar. Endodontic treatment was carried out on the tooth. This illustrates an intimate relationship between maxillary posterior teeth and the maxillary sinus.

c. *Hidden lesion and missed canals*: The periapical radiograph shows a radiolucent periapical lesion in endodontically treated upper first molar (Fig. 9.32a and b). Limited volume CBCT revealed a missed fourth canal in the mesial buccal root of upper first molar (Fig. 9.33) and also radiolucent lesion and four canals

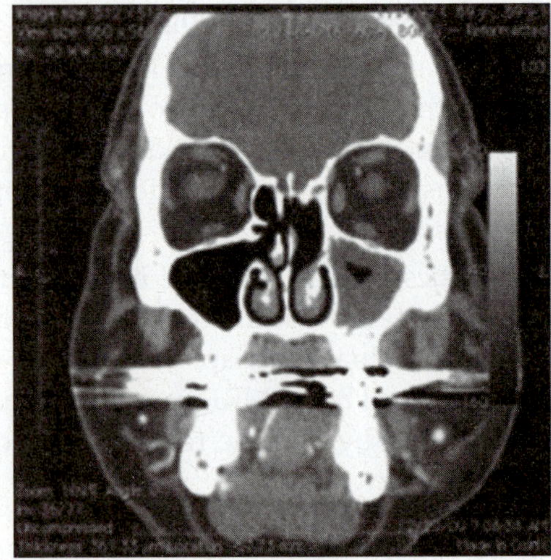

Fig. 9.29: No pathology in conventional CT

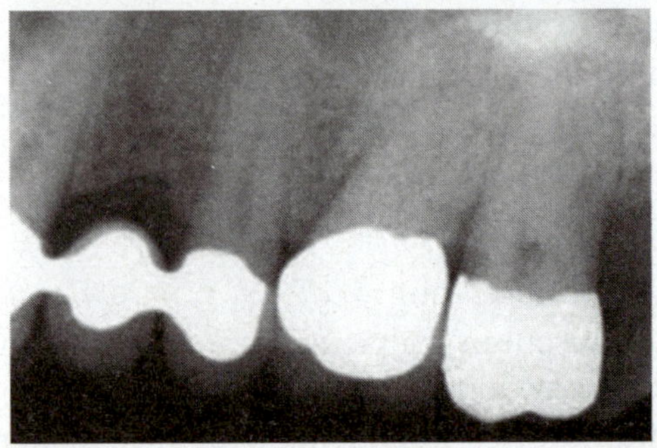

Fig. 9.30 No pathology in periapical radiograph

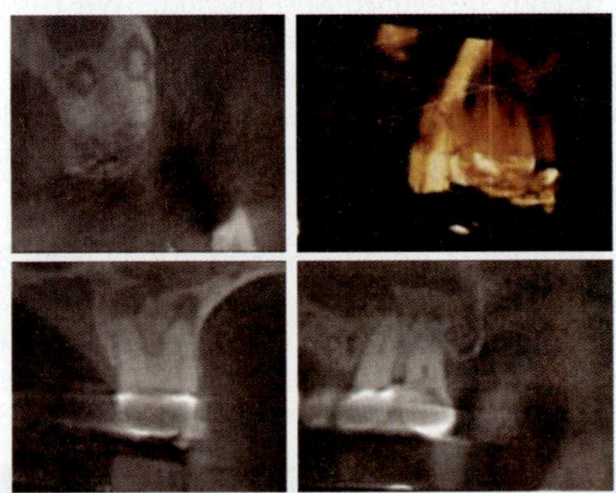

Fig. 9.31 CBCT showing perforation in maxillary sinus

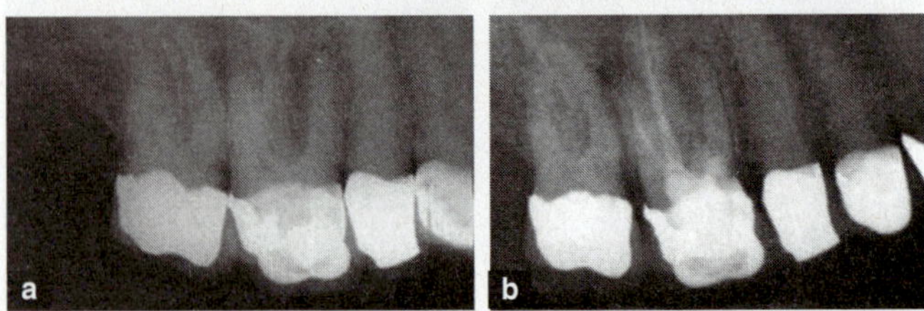

Fig. 9.32 (a) Preoperative (maxillary first molar); (b) Root canal treated (maxillary first molar)

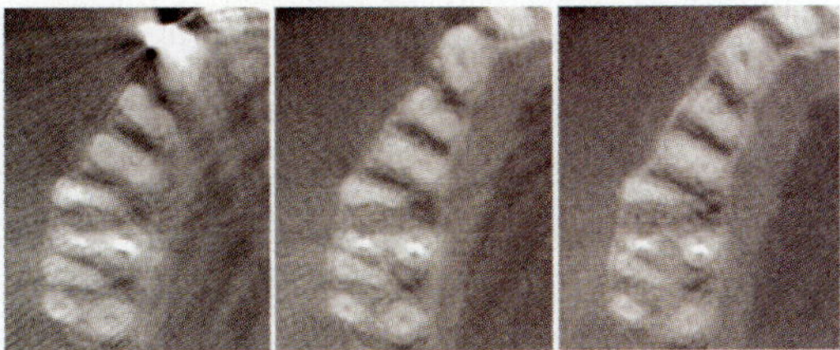

Fig. 9. 33 CBCT showing missed fourth canal

associated with roots of upper right second molar. CBCT is useful to locate hidden periapical lesions and also to determine the number of roots and root canals.

The periapical radiograph did not reveal extra root canal in mandibular first molar (Fig. 9.34). Limited field view CBCT revealed that mandibular first molar had five canals and an additional canal (distolingual) was missed (Fig. 9.35). The tooth was accordingly retreated (Fig. 9.36a and b).

d. ***Additional roots***: The periapical radiograph of maxillary left lateral incisor shows a diffuse radiolucency in the cervical region of upper left lateral incisor, which was endodontically treated (Fig. 9.37a and b). CBCT axial, reformatted panoramic and cross-sectional images showed a second untreated missed root, mesial and buccal to the treated root (Fig. 9.38a and b). When the second root was treated and filled, the tooth healed uneventfully (Fig. 9.39).

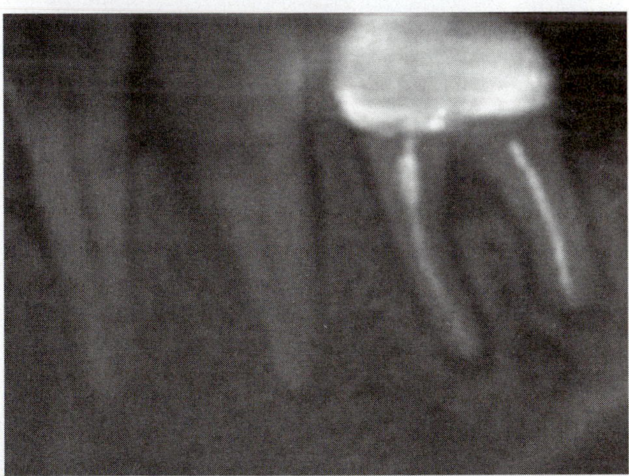

Fig. 9.34 Preoperative

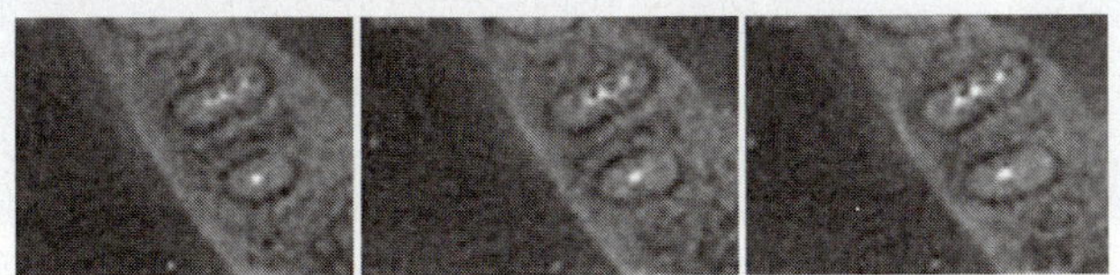

Fig. 9.35 CBCT showing extra canal

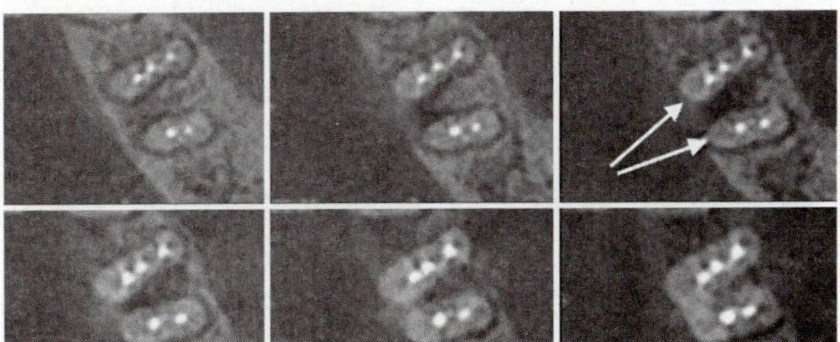

Fig. 9.36a Extra canal treated

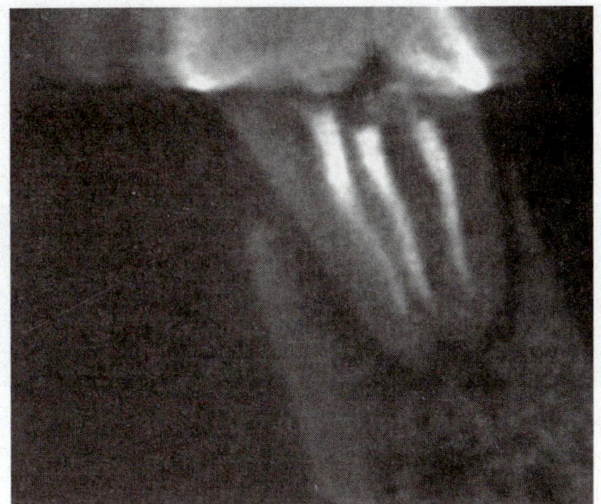

Fig. 9.36b Tooth retreated

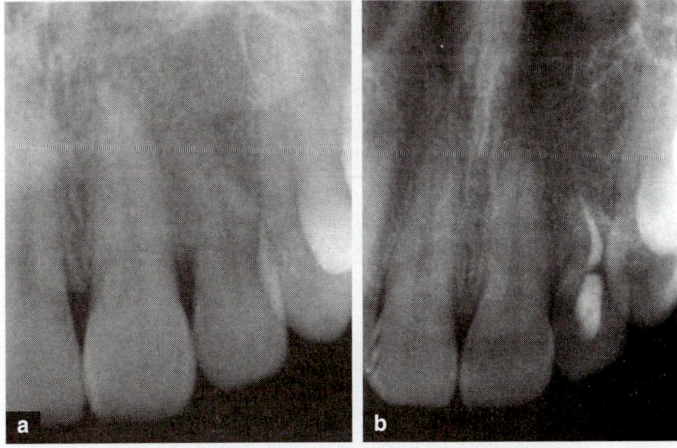

Fig. 9.37 Maxillary lateral incisor: (a) Preoperative; (b) Root canal treated

e. ***Dehiscence***: The periapical radiograph of maxillary molar does not show any definite finding (Fig. 9.40); whereas, CBCT coronal slices (Fig. 9.41) revealed that the apices of the buccal roots were outside the buccal cortical plate of bone. Apicoectomy was performed on both the roots (Fig. 9.42) and the patient was relieved of symptoms.

f. ***Planning endodontic surgery***: The periapical radiograph shows proximity of the apices of first and second molars to the mandibular canal (Fig. 9.43). CBCT

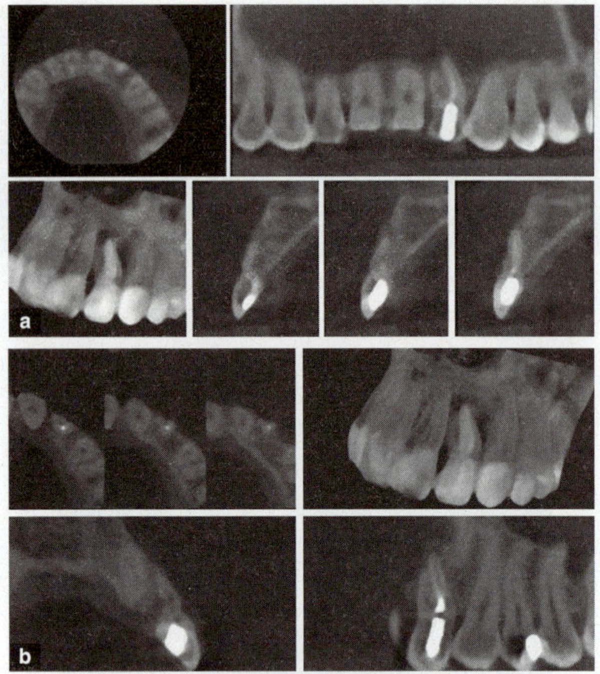

Fig. 9.38a and b CBCT showing extra canal in lateral incisor

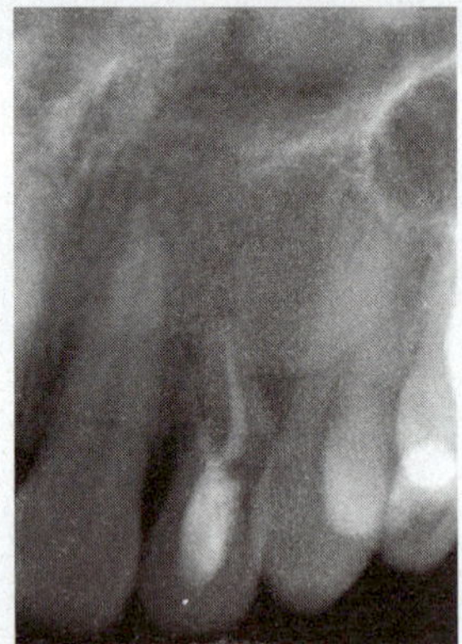

Fig. 9.39 Treated tooth

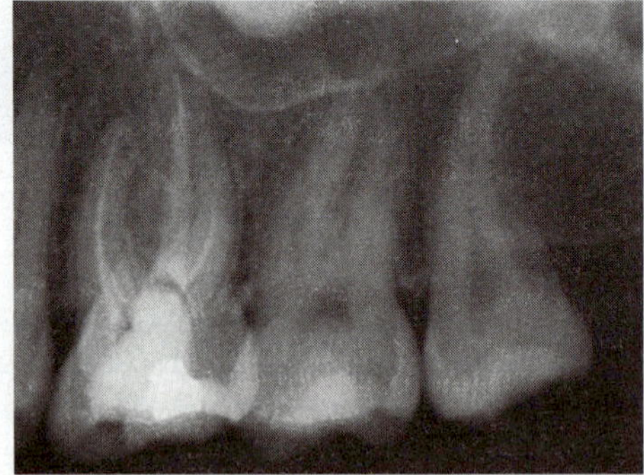

Fig. 9.40 No definite finding in maxillary molar

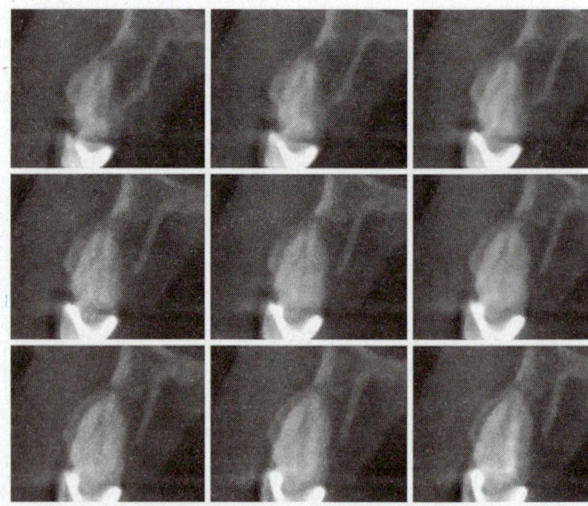

Fig. 9.41 CBCT showing roots outside buccal cortical plate

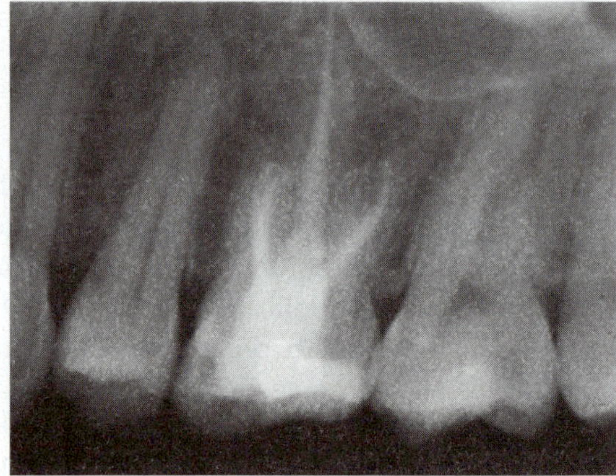

Fig. 9.42 Tooth after apicoectomy

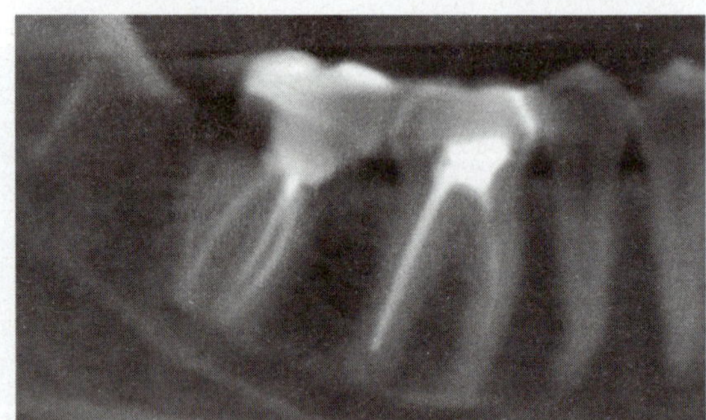

Fig. 9.43 Proximity to mandibular canal

imaging (cross-sectional view) shows widening of periodontal ligament at the apex of distal root of second molar and its close proximity to the mandibular canal (Fig. 9.44). Apical surgery could be risky, so extraction was planned.

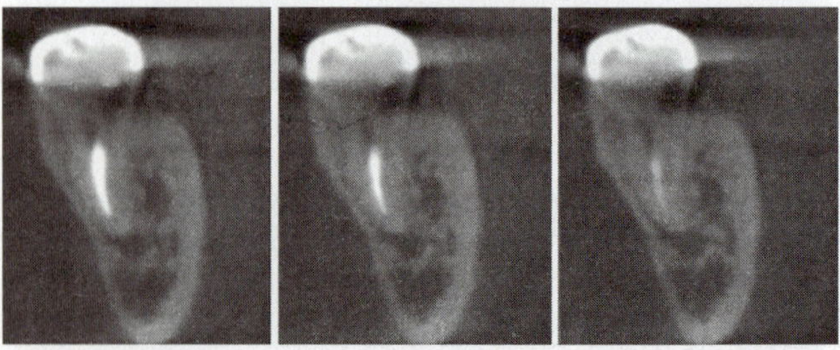

Fig. 9.44 CBCT confirming close proximity to mandibular canal

g. ***Evaluating vertical fracture***: The periapical radiograph of lower left first molar (Fig. 9.45) failed to show any pathosis; whereas, CBCT (cross-section view) of the region showed the loss of bone all along the distal surface of the mesial root of mandibular left first molar consistent with vertical root fracture (Fig. 9.46). This case clearly illustrates the value of CBCT when compared to 2D intraoral periapical radiography for detecting bone loss secondary to vertical root fracture.

h. ***Cervical root resorption***: The periapical radiographs of the tooth shows a diffuse area of radiolucency in the cervical region of the tooth (Fig. 9.47). CBCT images (cross-section view) shows areas of resorption both on the facial and the lingual surfaces (Fig. 9.48). The lesion on the lingual aspect of the tooth was not detected clinically and its location could not be predicted from the periapical radiograph.

i. ***Internal root resorption***: The periapical radiograph of lower first molar revealed an area of decreased density in the coronal region (Fig. 9.49). CBCT images (cross-section view) revealed a large resorptive defect which had perforated the lingual aspect of the tooth below the crest of bone (Fig. 9.50). The different

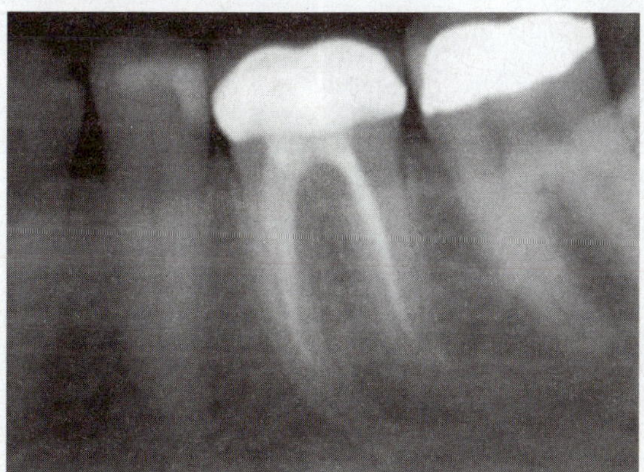

Fig. 9.45 Mandibular first molar (no pathological finding)

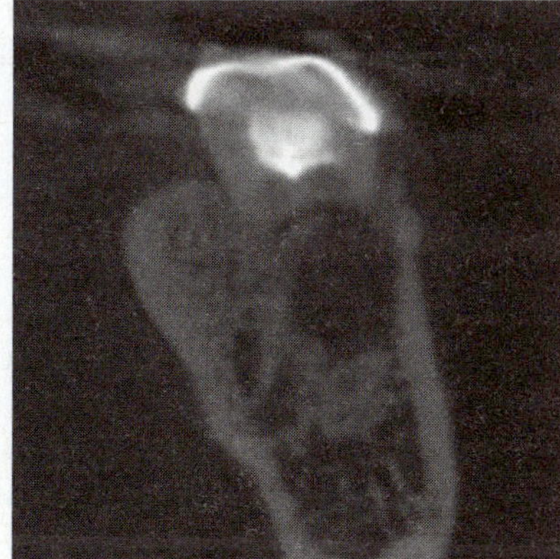

Fig. 9.46: CBCT (cross-section view) showing vertical root fracture

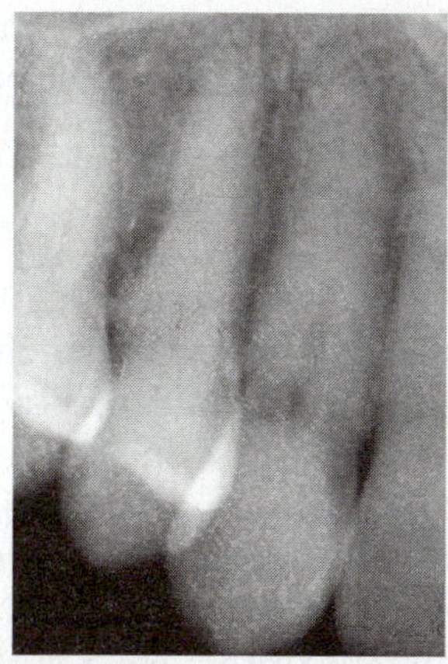

Fig. 9.47 Diffuse radiolucency in cervical areas of maxillary canine and first premolar

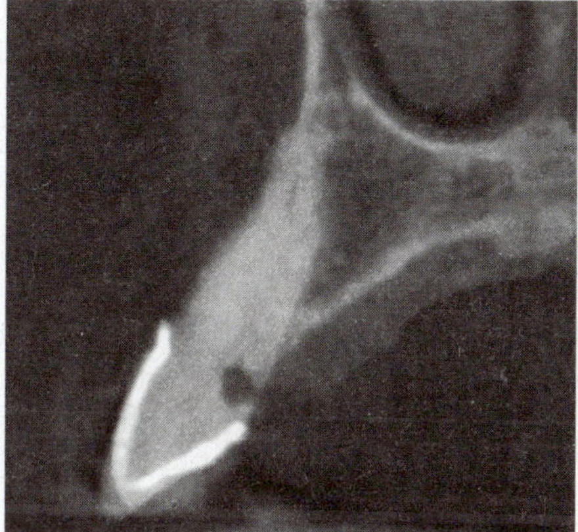

Fig. 9.48 CBCT (cross-section view) showing resorption

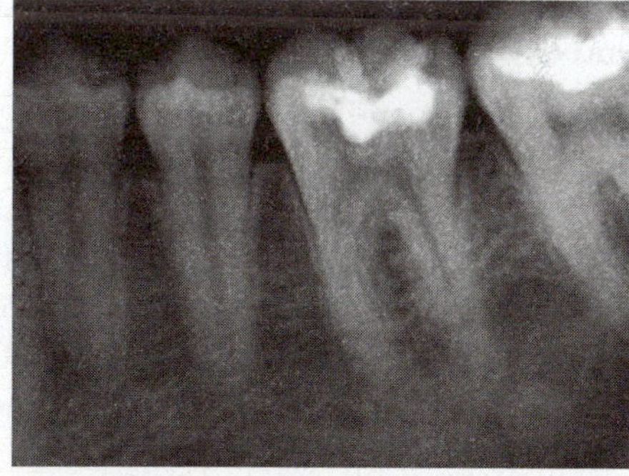

Fig. 9.49 Decreased density in coronal region of mandibular first molar

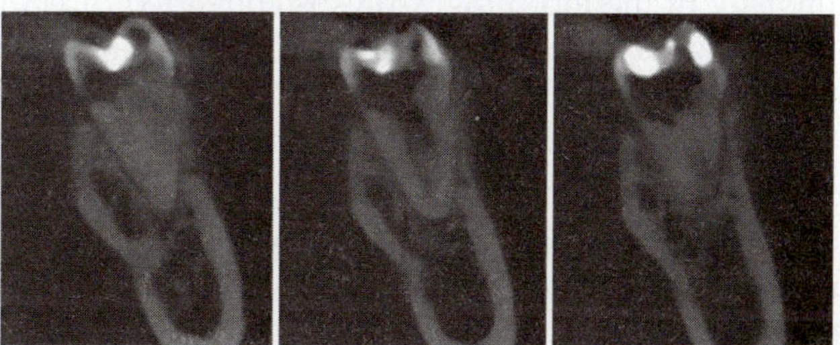

Fig. 9.50 CBCT (cross-section view) revealing resorption

slices reveal the extent and location of the defect which could not be determined by the periapical radiograph.

8. C-Arm Imaging

C-arm imaging is a new, dynamic, innovative and moving real time imaging technique, that differs from conventional dental radiography which is static. Clinicians can observe live imaging event, while in previous imaging techniques, the operator could monitor treatment progress by making radiographs before and after the procedure. C-arm imaging system in endodontic practice provides a cutting edge over existing methods because of its advantage of real time imaging.

C-arm cone beam computed tomography (CT) is an advanced imaging technique that uses C-arm flat-panel fluoroscopy systems to acquire and display three-dimensional (3D) images. It provides high and low contrast soft tissues (CT-like) images in multiple viewing planes.

Images intensifying principles have considerably reduced harmful effects of radiations. An image intensifier, also provides real-time imaging, facilitating position of the patient and to visualize pathology of interest. To keep the radiation dose from becoming a health hazard, the exposure rate in C-arm CT image intensification is much less than in conventional radiography. As per the manufacturers, the maximum radiation dose for the present system used is 0.25 mSv for 5 second exposure time.

In case of analog image intensifiers, the X-ray strikes a fluorescent surface after being attenuated to different degrees through the patient body. Depending upon the strength of radiation, the surface can glow more or less bright. A vacuum tube captures the glow and displays this on the monitor. Due to curved surface of the tube, the accuracy of image diminishes towards the edges, leading to distortions.

The modern flat-panel technology is the digital development of image intensifier technology. The intensity of the incoming X-rays is converted directly into a digital value. Dispensing with electron optics allows distortion free images, hence improving the overall image quality.

C-arm imaging (capturing 3D images) comprises a stand and a C-arm to which the detector, X-ray tube and collimator are attached. The C-arm keeps the X-ray tube, collimator, and a flat-panel detector exactly aligned under varying view angles. C-arm systems provide high positioning flexibility and excellent patient access.

C-arm imaging systems with automated exposure control adjust X-ray exposure parameters, such as detector entrance dose (*detector entrance dose is the X-ray dose measured behind the antiscatter grid; whereas, system dose is the detector entrance dose evaluated at a reference detector zoom format*). The detector entrance dose for C-arm imaging is about half the system dose.

C-arm 3D real time imaging is helpful in routine treatments, especially in aberrant canal anatomy. The technique is also useful in by-passing the separated instruments and instrument (post) retrieval during retreatment procedures. Procedural errors are also effectively managed by this system (Fig. 9.51a to d).

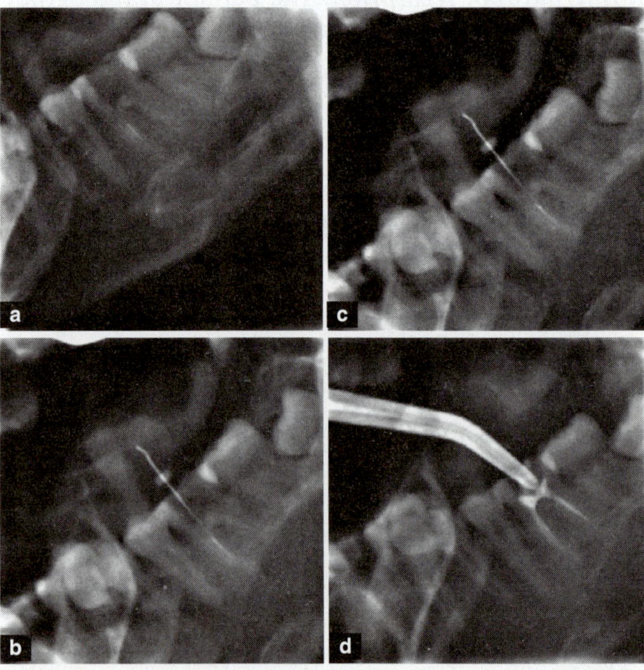

Fig. 9.51 C-arm imaging: (a) Preoperative (mandibular first molar); (b) Negotiating separated instrument; (c) Endosonic file widening the dentin around separated instrument; (d) Postobturation

TESTS MEASURING TOOTH TEMPERATURE

The temperature measurement of teeth provides valuable information of the integrity of the underlying pulp. The underlying principle is that the teeth with vital pulps (effective blood flow) are warmer as compared to nonvital teeth (no blood flow). A few authors (Fenibunda, 1986) reported that there was no difference in the surface temperature of vital and non-vital teeth. He opined that the effect of blood supply in a tooth is masked by the environmental factors. He further stressed that the time taken to reach equilibrium (rate of return of surface temperature to normal after the application of thermal change) depended upon the pulp blood supply. The gadgets used in measuring surface temperature are thermocouple, thermistor, infrared thermometer and cholesteric liquid crystals.

1. Cholesteric Liquid Crystals

Howell et al (1970) employed color change of cholesteric liquid crystals applied to surfaces of the teeth as diagnostic modality (Table 9. 2). Crystalline cholesteric crystals (cholesteric compounds in 10% solution in chlorinated hydrocarbon solvent) heated to its melting point become cloudy liquid, exhibiting crystal like properties under polarized light. Changes in temperature alter the pitch and period of helical structure; subsequently new colors are produced.

The major advantages of cholesteric liquid crystal technique include simplicity of use. It is hypothesized that vital pulp even in apical third area can maintain the surface temperature of tooth. This technique is no longer advocated now.

2. Electronic Thermography

The components of electronic thermography are infrared sensor, control unit, thermal image computer, software, color monitor and printer (Fig. 9. 52). It is used to check pulp vitality by electronically measuring the change in temperature onto the tooth surface.

3. Infrared thermography (Hughes Probeye Camera)

Infrared thermography can detect temperature changes as small as 0.1°C, measuring the pulp vitality. It consists of thermal video system and the silicon close-up lens.

The *disadvantages* of surface temperature measurement technique are that the patient should be at rest and get acclimatized prior to testing. Proper isolation is also necessary.

Table 9.2 Color changes and pulp vitality status using cholesteric liquid crystals

Color change	*Vitality status*
Blue-green Green-blue	Vital
Red-green Green	Vital
Red Yellow-red Yellow	Nonvital

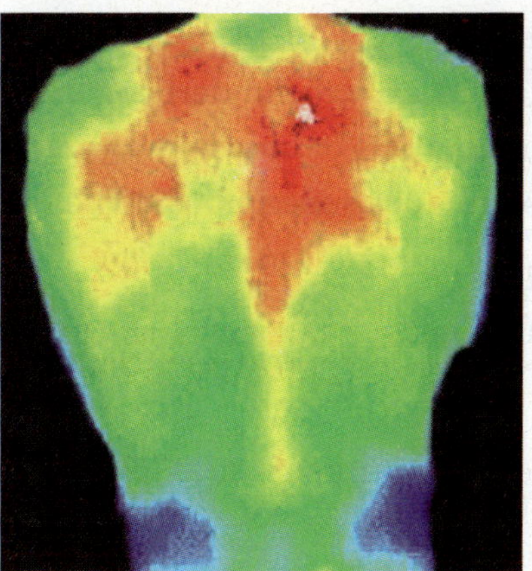

Fig. 9.52 Electronic thermography

NEWER METHODS

1. Ultrasonic Imaging

Ultrasound imaging or ultrasonography is being tried in endodontics to overcome the limitations of computed tomography (high cost and greater dose of radiations). It is based on the reflection of sound waves (the interface of tissues have different acoustic properties); the frequency is above the range of human hearing (1–20 kHz). The echoes are converted into electrical signal by the transducer, producing white and gray shades on the screen. Hard tissues (bone and teeth) produce high echo intensity (hyperechoic) and are white; whereas, soft tissues, which do not reflect ultrasound energy (anechoic) are dark in reflection.

- Low echo signal: Dark spots
- High echo signal: Bright/white spots.

- Hypoechoic/transonic: Low echo intensity
- Anechoic: No reflection of echoes (occurs in any area filled with fluid)
- Hyperechoic: High echo intensity (bone)

Ultrasound imaging is considered as a safe method, but the ultrasound energy which produces heat in the tissue should be controlled. This limitation is quite less as compared to techniques using ionizing radiations.

In endodontics, the technique can be useful in evaluating periapical lesions and also the vascular supply of these lesions; however, lesions covered by cortical plates are difficult to evaluate.

Ultrasound imaging differentiates between cyst and granulomas; reveals nature of bony lesion content:

- *Cystic lesion: Hypoechoic, well contoured cavity surrounded by bony walls, filled with fluids (do not exhibit vascular supply in color Doppler examination)*
- *Granulomas: Poorly defined lesion, can be hypo or hyperechoic (exhibit vascular supply in color Doppler examination)*

Advantages

- Accurately identify the underlying disease process
- No harmful effects of ultrasound waves
- Does not produce superimposition of structures.

Disadvantages

- Ultrasound image cannot evaluate periapical lesion unless there is discontinuity in the buccal cortical bone
- Provides two-dimensional picture; however, certain software may convert the image to three-dimensions.
- Not feasible in posterior region because of thick cortical plate (thick cortical plate prevents ultrasound waves from traversing in those areas).

2. Computer Expert System (COMENDEX)

In computer expert system, diagnostic case facts are entered into the computer and then computer analyzes and report the diagnosis.

It helps in diagnosis of selected pulp pathology (reversible pulpitis, irreversible pulpitis, and necrotic pulp).

3. LASER Optical Disc Storage

Laser optical disc storage has superior diagnostic advantage. It can store 10,000 images on 8 inches optical disc with 0.5 seconds retrieval and display time. Image is recorded by a focused LASER beam, heating a thin film of tellurium suboxide at specific points on the optical disc.

The clinical usage and limitations of various diagnostic tools used in endodontics are summarized in Table 9.3.

Table 9.3 Clinical usage and limitations of diagnostic tools in Endodontics

Diagnostic technique	*Clinical usage*	*Limitations*
Thermal tests	• Assess vitality of pulp (neural based) • Help in identifying the offending tooth when patient is unable to locate the source of pain	• Assess only neural aspects and not blood supply • Difficult in posterior teeth • Difficult in crowned teeth
Electrical tests	• Assess vitality of pulp (neural based) • Electric stimulus is considered comfortable as compared to thermal	• No clue of vascular supply • Difficult in teeth restored with full crowns and even in normal posterior teeth
Pulse oximetry	• Determines oxygen saturation of pulp blood • Effectively detects pulp blood flow even in traumatized teeth	• Blood in arteries is not pulsed; may not be effective • Some refracted light may give false response
Laser Doppler flowmetry	• Detects red blood cell movement even in smaller tissues • Effectively measures microcirculation of pulp	• Systemic medication affect blood flow in pulp; may give false response • Different sensors may need multiple probes for accurate assessment
Computed tomography (CT)	• The clinical usage include excellent visualization of maxillary sinus and adjacent teeth • Evaluate periodontal ligament vis-à-vis periodontitis • Detects vertical root fractures or split teeth (periapical radiographs can rarely detect such lesion) • Can be used to localize foreign bodies in the jaws	• High radiation dose • Expensive software • Low resolution of image • Metallic crowns/posts affect quality of image
Cone beam computed tomography (CBCT)	• Diagnosis of endodontic lesions • Assessment of the non-endodontic lesions and hidden lesions, evaluation of root fractures and trauma • Analysis of external, internal root resorption • Analysis of cracks, dehiscence, etc.	• Artifact formation • Less resolution • Metal crowns/post affect image quality
Magnetic resonance imaging (MRI)	• Smaller branches of the neurovascular bundle can be identified entering apical foramina • Assess the nature of endodontic lesions before and after periapical surgery	• Poor resolutions as compared to conventional radiographs • Long scanning times
Ultrasound imaging	• Detects soft tissue lesions (assess lesion before and after surgery) • Differentiates between cyst and granuloma (reveals nature of bony lesion contents)	Difficult to use in the posterior region because of thick cortical plate (thick plate prevents ultrasound waves from traversing on that area)

BIBLIOGRAPHY

1. Abd-Elmeguid A and Yu DC. Dental pulp neurophysiology: Part 2: Current diagnostic tests to assess pulp vitality. J. Can. Dent. Assoc.: 2009; 75:139–143.
2. Allen J. Phyotoplethysmography and its application in clinical physiological measurement. Physiol. Meas.: 2007; 28:R1–39.
3. Aoyagi T. Pulse oximetry: Its invention, theory, and future. J. Anesth.: 2003; 17:259–266.
4. Arnheiter CSW and Farman AG. Trends in maxillofacial cone-beam computed tomography usage. Oral Radiol.: 2006; 22:80–85.
5. Arun A, Mythri H and Chachapan D. Pulp vitality tests - an overview on comparison of sensitivity and vitality. Int. J. Oral Sci.: 2015; 6:41–46.
6. Bender IB, Landau MA, Fonsecca S and Trowbridge HO. The optimum placement-site of the electrode in electric pulp testing of the 12 anterior teeth. J. Am. Dent. Assoc.:1989; 118:305–310.
7. Bender IB. Reversible and irreversible painful pulpitis: Diagnosis and treatment. Aust. Endod. J.: 2000; 26:10–14.
8. Bhosale S and Rameshkumar M. Endodontic imaging-recent advances: a review. Int. Dent. J. Stud. Resch.: 2016; 4:1–14.
9. Braz AK, Kyotoku BB and Gomes AS. In vitro tomographic image of human pulp-dentin complex: optical coherence tomography and histology. J. Endod.: 2009; 35:1218–1221.
10. Chambers IG. The role and methods of pulp testing in oral diagnosis: a review. Int. Endod. J.: 1982; 15:1–5.
11. Chan M, Dadul T, Langlais R, Russel D and Ahmad M. Accuracy of extraoral bite-wing radiography in detecting proximal caries and crestal bone. JADA: 2017; pp 1–7.
12. Chen E and Abbott PV. Dental pulp testing: A review. Int. J. Dent.: 2009; Article ID 365785.
13. Cotti E. Advanced techniques for detecting lesions in bone. Dent. Clin. North Am.: 2010; 54:215–235.
14. Cotton TP, Geisler TM, Holden DT, Schwartz SA and Schindler WG. Endodontic applications of cone-beam volumetric tomography. J. Endod.: 2007; 33:1121–1132.
15. Ehrmann EH. Pulp testers and pulp testing with particular reference to the use of dry ice. Aust. Dent. J.:1977; 22: 272–279.
16. Emshoff R, Mosehen I and Strobl II. Use of laser Doppler flowmetry to predict vitality of luxated or avulsed permanent teeth. Oral Surg., Oral Med., Oral Pathol., Oral Radiol. Endod.: 2004; 98:750–755.
17. Fanibunda KB. The feasibility of temperature measurement as a diagnostic procedure in human teeth. J. Dent.: 1986; 14:126–129.
18. Farman AG. ALARA still applies. Oral Surg., Oral Med., Oral Pathol., Oral Radiol. Endod.: 2005; 100:395–397.
19. Fleury A and Regan JD. Endodontic diagnosis: clinical aspects. J. Ir. Dent. Assoc.: 2006; 52:28–38.
20. Fuss Z, Trowbridge H, Bender IB, Rickoff B and Sorin S. Assessment of reliability of electrical and thermal pulp testing agents. J. Endod.: 1986; 12:301–305.
21. Gopikrishna V, Pradeep G and Venkateshbabu N. Assessment of pulp vitality: a review. Int. J. Pediatr. Dent.: 2009; 19:3–15.
22. Gumru B and Tarcin B. Imaging in endodontics: an overview of conventional and alternative advanced imaging techniques. J. Marmara Uni. Inst. Health Sci.: 2013; 3:55–64.
23. Howell, RM, Duell RC and Mullaney TP. The determination of pulp vitality by thermographic means using cholesteric liquid crystals. A preliminary study. Oral Surg., Oral Med., Oral Pathol.: 1970; 29:763–768.
24. Ingolfsson AE, Tronstad L and Riva CE. Reliability of laser Doppler flowmetry in testing vitality of human teeth. Endod. Dent. Traumatol.: 1994; 10:185–187.
25. Jafaradeh H and Abbott PV. Review of the pulp sensitivity tests. Part I: General information and thermal tests. Int. Endod. J.: 2010; 43:738–762.
26. Jafaradeh H and Abott PV. Review of the pulp sensitivity tests. Part 2: Electric pulp tests and pulp cavities. Int. Endod. J.: 2010; 43:945–958.
27. Jafaradeh H and Rosenberg PA. Pulse oximetry: review of a potential aid in endodontic diagnosis. J. Endod.: 2009; 35:329–333.
28. Jafaradeh H, Udoye CI and Kinoshita J. The application of tooth temperature measurement in endodontic diagnosis: A review. J. Endod.: 2008; 34.1435–1440.
29. Jafaradeh H. Laser Doppler flowmetry in endodontics: a review. Int. Endod. J.: 2009; 42:476–490.
30. Kamburoglu K, Ilker Cebeci AR and Grondahl HG. Effectiveness of limited cone-beam computed tomography in the detection of horizontal root fracture. Dent. Traumatol.: 2009; 25:256–261.
31. Katkar RA, Tadinada SA, Amechi BT and Fried D. Optical Coherence Tomography. Dent Clin N Am.: 2018; 62: 421–434.
32. Kells BE, Kennedy JG, Biagioni PA and Lamey PJ. Computerized infrared thermographic imaging and pulpal blood flow: Part 1. A protocol for thermal imaging of human teeth. Int. Endod. J.: 2000; 33:442–447.
33. Kocasarac HD and Angelopoulos C. Ultrasound in Dentistry: Towards a future of Radiation-free imaging. Dent Clin N Am.: 2018; 62: 481–489.
34. Lee JY, Yanpiset K, Sigurdsson A and Vann WF. Laser Doppler flowmetry for monitoring traumatized teeth. Dent. Traumatol.: 2001; 17:231–235.
35. Lin J and Chandler NP. Electric pulp testing: A review. Int. Endod. J.: 2008; 41:365.

36. Lin J, Chandler NP, Purton D and Monteith B. Appropriate electrode placement site for electric pulp testing first molar teeth. J. Endod.: 2007; 33:1296–1298.

37. Lindberg LG, Tamura T and Oberg PA. Photoplethysmography. Part 1. Comparison with laser Doppler flowmetry. Med. Biol. Eng. Comput.: 1991; 29:40–47.

38. Lino Y, Ebihara A and Yoshioka T. Detection of a secondary mesiobuccal canal in maxillary molars by Swept-source optical coherence tomography. J Endod.: 2014; 40: 1865–1868.

39. Ludlow JB, Laster WS, See M, Bailey LJ and Hershey HG. Accuracy of measurements of mandibular anatomy in cone beam computed tomography images. Oral Surg., Oral Med., Oral Pathol., Oral Radiol. Endod.: 2007; 103:534–542.

40. Mainkar A and Kim SG.: Diagnostic accuracy of 5 dental pulp tests: a systematic review and meta-analysis. J. Endod.:2018; 44:694–702.

41. Mickel AK, Lindquist KAD, Chogel S, Jones JJ and Curd F. Electric pulp tester conductance through various interface media. J. Endod.: 2006; 32:1178–1180.

42. Miwa Z, Ikawa M, Iijima H, Saito M and Takagi Y. Pulpal blood flow in vital and non-vital young permanent teeth measured by transmitted-light photoplethysmography: a pilot study. Pediatr. Dent.: 2002; 24:594–598.

43. Mohammedi Z. Laser applications in endodontics: An update review. Int. Dent. J.: 2009; 59:35–46.

44. Morea C, Dominguez GC and Coutinho A. Quantitative analysis of bone density in direct digital radiographs evaluated by means of computerized analysis of digital images. Dentomaxillofac Radiol.: 2010; 39: 356–361.

45. Myers JW. Demonstration of a possible source of error with an electric pulp tester. J. Endod.: 1998; 24:199–200.

46. Nair MK and Nair UP. Digital and advanced imaging in endodontics: a review. J. Endod.: 2007; 33:1–6.

47. Nair MK, Nair UDP, Grondahl HG, Webber RL and Wallace JA. Detection of artificially induced vertical radicular fractures using tuned aperture computed tomography. Eur. J. Oral Sci.: 2001; 109:375–379.

48. Nair MK, Seyedain A, Agarwal S, Webber RL, Nair UP, Piesco NP, Mooney MP and Grondahl HG. Tuned aperture computed tomography to evaluate osseous healing. J. Dent. Res.: 2001; 80:1621–1624.

49. Nardo D, Gambarini G, Capuani S and Testarelli L.: Nuclear magnetic resonance imaging in endodontics: a review. J. Endod.: 2018; 1–7.

50. Newton CW, Hoen MM, Goodis HE, Johnson BR and MacClanahan SB. Identify and determine the metrics, hierarchy and predictive value of all the parameters and/or methods used during endodontic diagnosis. J. Endod.: 2009; 35:1635–1644.

51. Nivesh KR and Pradeep S. Recent diagnostic aids in endodontics – a review. Int. J. Pharma. Clin. Resch.: 2016; 8:1159–1162.

52. Pantrea EA, Anderson RW and Pantera CT%. Reliability of electric pulp testing after pulpal testing with dichloro difluoromethane. J. Endod.: 1993; 19:312–314.

53. Patel S, Dawood A, Whaites E and Pittford T. New dimensions in endodontic imaging: part I. Conventional and alternative radiographic systems. Int. Endod. J.: 2009; 42:447–462.

54. Petersson A, Axelsson S, Davidson T, Frisk F, Hakeberg M, Kvist T, Norlund A, Mejare I, Portenier I, Sandberg H, Tranaeus S and Bergenholtz G. Radiological diagnosis of periapical bone tissue lesions in endodontics: a systematic review. Int. Endod. J.: 2012; 45:783–801.

55. Pittford T and Patel S. Technical equipment for assessment of dental pulp status. Endod. Topics: 2004; 7:2–13.

56. Radhakrishnan S, Munshi AK and Hegde AM. Pulse oximetry: a diagnostic instrument in pulpal vitality testing. J. Clin. Pediatr. Dent.: 2002; 26:141–145.

57. Roberts JA, Drage NA, Davies J and Thomas DW. Effective dose from cone beam CT examinations in dentistry. Br. J. Radiol.: 2009; 82:35–40.

58. Rowe AHR and Pittford TR. The assessment of pulpal vitality. Int. Endod. J.:1990; 23:77–83.

59. Sainsbury AL, Bird PS and Walsh LJ. Diagnodent laser fluorescence assessment of endodontic infection. J. Endod.: 2009; 35:1404–1407.

60. Scarfe WC, Farman AG and Sukovic P. Clinical applications of cone-beam computed tomography in dental practice. J. Can. Dent. Assoc.: 2006; 72:75–80.

61. Schnettler JM and Wallace JA. Pulse oximeter as a diagnostic tool of pulp vitality. J. Endod.: 1991; 17:488–490.

62. Severinghaus JW and Aoyagi T. Discovery of pulse oximetry. Anesth. Analg.: 2007; 105:S1–S4.

63. Shemash H, van Soest G and Wu M. Basic research technology: Diagnosis of vertical root fractures with optical coherence tomography. J Endod.: 2008; 34: 739–742.

64. Shemesh H, van Soest G, Wu MK, van der Sluis LW and Wesselink PR. The ability of optical coherence tomography to characterize the root canal walls. J. Endod.: 2007; 3369–3373.

65. Shulze R, Heil U and Gross D. Artefacts in CBCT: a review. Dentomaxillofac Radiol.: 2011; 40: 265–273.

66. Smith E, Dickson M, Evans AL, Smith D and Murray CA. An evaluation of the use of tooth temperature to assess human pulp vitality. Int. Endod. J.: 2004; 37:374–380.

67. Swain MV and Xue J. State of the art of Micro-CT applications in dental research. Int. J. Oral Sci.: 2009; 1:177–188.

68. Tutton LM. MRI of the teeth. Br. J. Radiol.: 2002; 75: 552–562.

69. Tyagi SP, Sinha DS, Verma R and Singh UP. New vistas in endodontic diagnosis. Saudi Endod. J.: 2012; 2:85–90.

70. Tyndall DA and Kohltfarber H. Application of cone beam volumetric tomography in endodontics. Aust. Dent. J.: 2012; 57:72–81.

71. Weisleder R, Yamauchi S, Caplan DJ, Trope M and Teixeira FB. The validity of pulp testing: A clinical study. J. Am. Dent. Assoc.: 2009; 140:1013–1017.

72. West JD. Endodontic diagnosis: Mystery or mastery? Dent. Today: 2004; 23:80.

73. Wilder-Smith PE. A new method for the non-invasive measurement of pulpal blood flow. Int. Endod. J.:1988; 21:307–312.

74. Yanpiset K, Vongsavan N, Sigurdsson A and Trope M. The efficacy of laser Doppler flowmetry for the diagnosis of revascularization of reimplanted immature dog teeth. Dent. Traumatol.: 2001; 17:63–70.

75. Yoon DC, Mol A, Benn DK and Benavides E. Digital Radiographic image processing and analysis. Dent Clin N Am.: 2018; 62: 341–359.

76. Yoon MJ, Kim E, Lee SJ, Bae YM, Kim S and Park SH. Pulpal blood flow measurement with ultrasound Doppler imaging. J. Endod.: 2010; 36:419–422.

Chapter 10

Endodontic Case Selection: Treatment Planning

Case selection and treatment plan are important aspects of endodontic treatment. The treatment plan is based upon the knowledge and skill of the operator coupled with patient's preference. Each case is to be treated as 'individual', since there is no definite principle, which can be applicable to every patient.

Once appropriate diagnostic tests have confirmed the pulpal and/or periradicular lesion, immediate treatment should be directed towards relieving the pain. After the emergency treatment, the operator should decide as regard the prognosis of the concerned tooth. Two important questions the operator must ask himself/herself are (i) whether root canal treatment is the best suited approach as compared to implant placement and (ii) whether the operator is competent enough to manage the case or some 'specialist' is to be called or the patient be referred to the skilled operator. The increasing number of dental surgeons are now opting for extraction and implant placement rather than root canal treatment and postendodontic restorations. High commercial gains might be one of the reasons for the same; or root canal treatment being technique sensitive and time consuming, might not be as viable as implants.

Efficiency, profitability and also patient's satisfaction are the results of well-planned procedures. Endodontic treatment results are a by-product of the clinicians' knowledge, planning and execution of the procedures. It is essential to consider patient's needs, attitude and willingness to undergo the specific treatment regime. The patient's general health and the medical conditions should also be taken into account during planning a case for endodontic procedure.

ENDODONTIC TREATMENT *VS* OSSEOINTEGRATED IMPLANTS

It is always challenging to decide whether to pursue endodontics (especially for a complicated tooth) or extraction and implant as replacement. Till date, there is no definite documentation comparing endodontic therapy with single-tooth implant. Both are predictable procedures when treatment is appropriately planned and executed.

It is emphasized that every effort is to be made to retain the natural tooth and the implant is planned only if the root canal is contraindicated or the prognosis is questionable.

The teeth with reasonable coronal structure and adequate root with sufficient surrounding alveolar bone are considered appropriate candidate for root canal treatment. The outcome of primary root canal therapy depends upon the conditions, such as, absence of periapical radiolucency, root obturated three-dimensionally within the working length and also satisfactory coronal restoration. Various studies have confirmed that primary endodontic treatment was more successful in teeth without apical periodontitis than in teeth with apical periodontitis. Even teeth that have failed initial endodontic treatment can be successfully retreated using non-surgical/surgical procedures. Re-treatment has also been successful as long-term treatment outcomes. The major technological and biological advances have resulted in the development of new treatment modalities in both surgical and non-surgical endodontics. Over the year, the success rate in endodontic treatment has improved.

In osseointegrated implants, sufficient quantity and quality of bone, free from any disease, should be available for implant placement. It is important to evaluate the location of vital anatomical structures that can interfere with implant placement (inferior alveolar canal, mental foramen, maxillary sinus, etc.). Immediate placement of implants offers advantages over delayed placement techniques. The advantages include preservation of existing bone and maintenance of the gingival form and contours.

In certain situations, implants are considered better therapeutic alternative than compromised restorations. A large number of factors, which facilitate the clinician to take right decision are mandatory to be considered in the beginning.

The factors are:

- Patient's need and expectations, finances, esthetics and also the patient's compliance
- Severity of periodontal conditions; pocket depth, tooth mobility and bone loss, etc.
- Furcation involvement; severity of furcation defects, anomalies of root and root canals, etc.
- Treatment factors; unfavorable crown-root ratio, faulty restorations, fractures, lack of remaining tooth structure, etc.
- Systemic diseases affecting the healing process; radiation therapy, Parkinson's disease, multiple myeloma, etc.

It is also emphasized that implants resist dental caries, periodontal diseases and are able to restore structural deficiencies. Endodontic therapy with adequate restoration present better way to preserve function as compared to implants, which can be placed only where prognosis of endodontic treatment is poor. Another advantage of endodontic therapy is early restoration of the patient's function and esthetics (in implants, restoration may be delayed while waiting for bone integration).

Before deciding for extraction, possibility of 'dental implant' should also be considered, which can be a predictable alternative procedure depending upon the condition of the concerned tooth and the patient's systemic health. All options should be considered on the basis of sound biologic principles and finalized on case to case basis.

The decision-making as regard endodontic treatment or osseointegrated implants is depicted in Flowchart 10.1.

Flowchart 10.1: Endodontic treatment *vs* osseointegrated implant: Decision-making

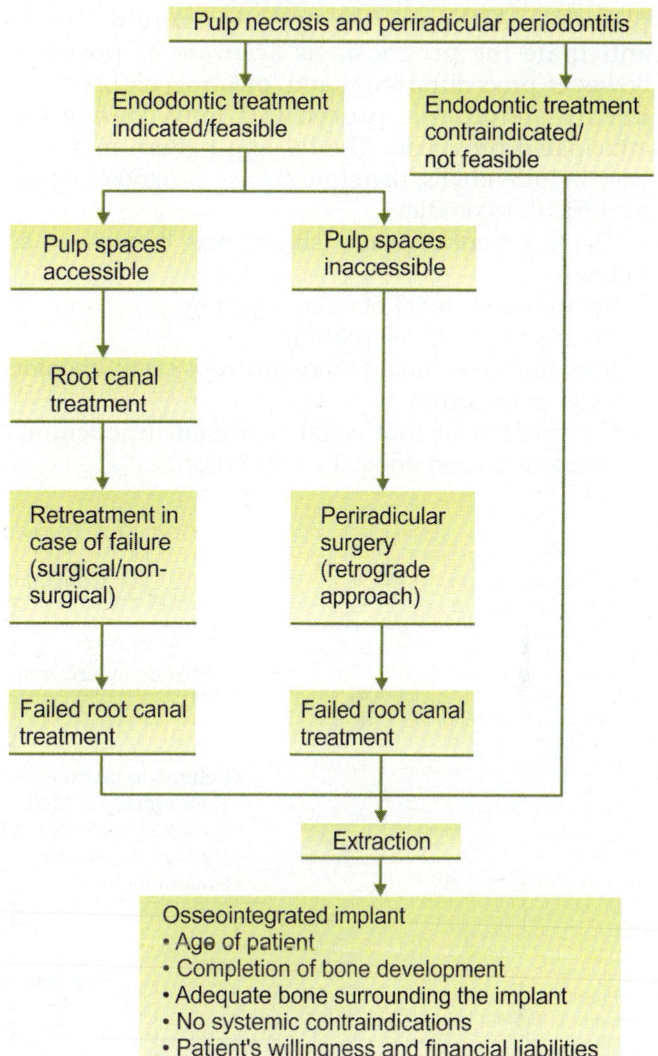

CASE SELECTION (TREATMENT PLANNING) IN ENDODONTICS

Many root canals are treated today than before because of a greater interest of operators to save endodontically involved teeth, which can be restored as a single unit and/or can be used as abutments for fixed prosthesis. The treatment plan remains simple if only one tooth is involved and the status of rest of the dentition is acceptable. It is mandatory to provide symptomatic relief of the pain and swelling prior to root canal treatment.

The remaining tooth structure should be analyzed thoroughly after removing the existing restoration/ filling, if any. The presence of residual caries, cracks/ fracture lines should also be examined before planning the root canal treatment.

The choice of postendodontic restoration may also influence the outcome of endodontic treatment. The restoration should provide adequate coverage to reinforce and protect the endodontically treated tooth. Improper restoration may allow microorganisms to invade the filled root canal spaces. It has been established that both root canal filling and the coronal restoration serve as a barrier against fluid and bacterial penetration into the periapical area. A number of studies have shown that inadequate root canal filing and coronal restorations were associated with an increased incidence of apical periodontitis; however, the technical quality of the root canal preparation and obturation has definite impact on the outcome of treatment as compared to technical quality of the coronal restoration.

The prognosis of the tooth/teeth after endodontic treatment must be taken into account in the treatment planning. Although the operator would like to anticipate the prognosis as accurate as possible; however, procedural errors and/or iatrogenic problems during endodontic procedures may change the anticipated prognosis. The healing pattern may also vary in individuals; therefore correct prognosis might be difficult to predict.

The treatment sequence (stages) may be planned as follows:

- Symptomatic relief of pain/swelling
- Emergency pulp extirpation
- Initiating root canal treatment (root canal opening relieves pressure)
- Completion of root canal treatment (meticulous preparation and adequate obturation)
- Restoration of the treated tooth (leakage-resistant restoration preferred)
- Measures to prevent the recurrence.

Flowchart 10.2 displays the sequence of treatment planning.

Indications and Contraindications

Endodontic treatment may be carried out in any tooth, except when it is not contraindicated by the patient's health; also the anatomy of that tooth permits the requisite instrumentation. The root canal treatment is indicated where pulp and periapical tissues are involved. It may be due to infection or traumatic injuries. In rare cases, intentional endodontic treatment is carried out to facilitate placement of restoration. It is easy to enumerate the contraindications to root canal treatment than to list the indications.

Flowchart 10.2: Sequence of treatment planning

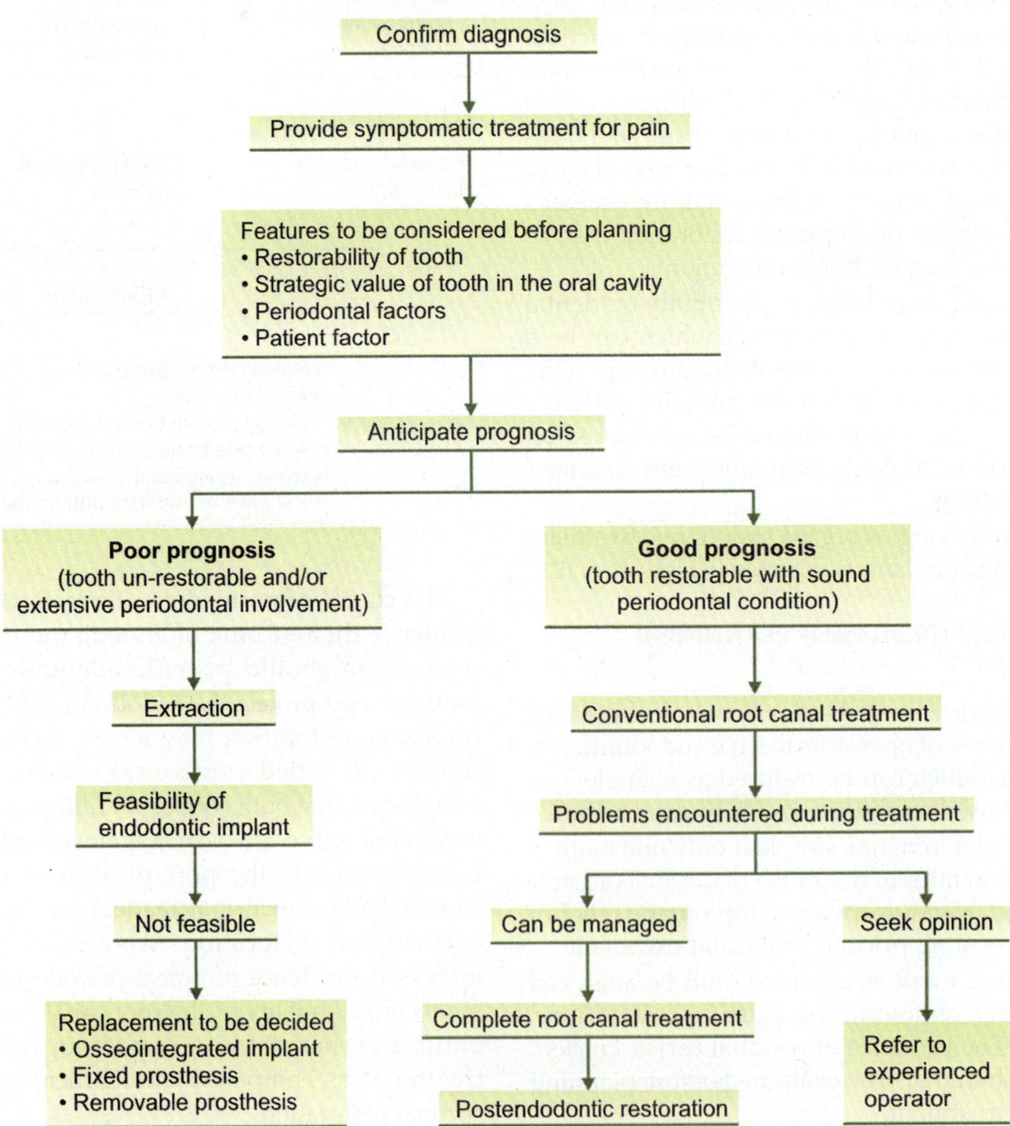

The main *contraindications* are:

- Non-restorable tooth: If the tooth cannot be restored to function following root canal treatment (extensive root caries, massive resorption, unfavorable crown-root ratio), extraction is inevitable followed by replacement options.
- Grade III mobility and/or insufficient periodontal support.
- Vertical root fracture; such teeth have poor endodontic prognosis.
- Tooth with no strategic importance even in future should not be root canal treated.

The major contraindication in endodontics is '*where the tooth cannot be restored*'; however, certain cases warrant the operator to take extra care to carry out the endodontic procedures. Additional treatment modalities should be considered to achieve successful outcome of the treatment. The cases which warrant additional care are:

1. *Extensive destruction of the periapical tissues*: The statement 'excessive destruction' is arbitrary; since, an area of rarefaction of any extent can undergo repair. It has been observed that the greater the amount of bone destroyed, the less will be the likelihood of repair. It is established that the periapical lesions less than 10 mm in diameter are more likely to show evidence of repair than those over 10 mm. The involved tooth should be treated non-surgically and monitored until repair occurs; if no signs of healing, surgical intervention becomes necessary. In young individuals, repair of any rarefied area occurs more readily than in older ones.
2. *Root canal obstructions (secondary dentin, a pulp stone that cannot be removed/bypassed, a calcified/partially calcified canal, a malformed tooth, or a broken instrument)*: In such cases, it is difficult to clean, disinfect and fill the root canal properly; subsequently, the prognosis remains doubtful. The apical third of the root canal is critical and therefore must be prepared and disinfected properly so that the microorganisms harbouring in apical areas cannot reach the periapical tissues. If the apical portion of the canal is blocked, repair of the damaged bone is unlikely to occur because microorganisms can egress into the periapical tissues and hinder with the repair process. In such cases, endodontic treatment of the patent portion of the root canal is completed and a retrograde apical filling is placed to seal the remainder of the inaccessible root canal; alternatively the blocked part of the root is removed surgically.
3. *Incomplete development of the root apex (immature apex).* In such cases, achievement of hermetic apical seal is difficult due to persistent seepage from the periapical areas. Apexification should be attempted and as the apical stop is created, the root canal can be obturated. The tooth has to be kept under observation. Regenerative treatment procedures are also being tried to achieve vascularization in such teeth.
4. *Root perforation*: Perforation of the root surface can be accidental/iatrogenic or as sequel to internal/external resorption. In case of perforation, an effort should be made to induce repair by means of mineral trioxide aggregate (MTA) and other bioceramic materials. A surgical approach may be necessary to wall off the perforation in some cases.
5. *Uncontrolled/persistent periapical exudates*: The uncontrolled/persistent periapical exudate hinders with the success of root canal treatment. This is generally managed by repeated dressings of calcium hydroxide/iodoform, creating alkaline environment in the root canal. If seepage cannot be controlled with an iodoform/calcium hydroxide dressings, then surgical intervention is warranted.
6. *Root canal treated tooth exhibiting an acute infection*: If the infection persists, the root canal is to be retreated. The old filling is removed, the canals are enlarged, prepared and obturated again. Surgical intervention may be necessary in some failed cases.
7. *Foreign body in the periapical tissues*: The presence of a foreign body increases the difficulty of eliminating infection by intracanal treatment alone. Periapical curettage should be carried out along with the root canal treatment.
8. *Root fractures*: Root fracture may not be a good reason for endodontic treatment. The extraction of fractured segment is contraindicated if the pulp is vital and the tooth can be stabilized. When the fracture is in the apical third, with nonvital pulp, endodontic treatment should be carried out. When the apical fragment cannot be placed in line with the main root canal, the endodontic treatment is completed till the fractured segment, and apical root tip is removed surgically. If an area of rarefaction develops, the root fragment should be removed. The fractured segments can be stabilized by using endodontic stabilizers.
9. *Existing restorations*: Full veneer crowns may not exhibit same anatomy as of the underlying crown, creating difficulty in orifice location during retreatment of failed endodontic case. In case of long span bridges, it is always difficult to gain

access from the overlying restoration. All kinds of existing restorations should be removed before initiating endodontic procedures.

10. *Malpositioning of tooth*: Third molars, mostly maxillary third molars, are difficult to treat, especially in patients with limited mouth opening. Such teeth are usually tipped or rotated and pose difficulties in executing endodontic treatment. In extreme cases, extraction is the only option for the clinicians.
11. *Patient motivation*: Patients should be self-motivated and understand the importance of retaining a tooth in the arch. He/she should also be aware of the implications involved during and after endodontic treatment, including financial liabilities. Patients must be convinced and fully trust the operator as regard outcome of the endodontic procedure.

SYSTEMIC DISEASES INFLUENCING TREATMENT PLANNING

It has always been an area of concern for the dental surgeons, precisely the endodontists, to decide whether the tooth with necrosed pulp should be extracted or treated. The focal infection theory is no longer accepted as 'explanatory' for associating oral infection with systemic diseases. Certain systemic diseases do affect pulp and periapical tissues, may be directly or indirectly.

In deciding whether to retain or to extract a pulpless tooth, following features should be considered:

- Pulpless teeth generally do not contribute to systemic disease.
- Systemic diseases, such as active diabetes, tuberculosis, etc. may affect healing pattern; potential for repair is reduced in such patients, compromising with the treatment outcomes.
- Extraction may be contraindicated because of an existing systemic condition of the patient, such as leukemia or radiation necrosis.

A thorough medical history should be recorded, analyzing the probability of any systemic disease. Communicable diseases are also to be identified.

Communicable diseases
- Herpes
- Hepatitis-B
- HIV
- Tuberculosis
- Mumps
- Oral candidiasis

(Transmissible through body fluids, such as blood and saliva, pose great risk to the doctor and the staff.)

Systemic conditions affecting Endodontic treatment
- Asthma
- Bleeding disorders
- Cardiovascular diseases
- Diabetes
- Hypertension
- Medication
- Liver and kidney problem
- Immunosuppressive drugs
- Pregnancy

Physiological changes with age
- Behavior changes
- Diet intake may be less
- Oral and systemic health may deteriorate
- Skin and blood vessels lose elasticity
- Delayed healing
- Bones become brittle
- Alteration in taste/smell
- Change in tooth anatomy
- Variations in pulpal physiology
- Color changes
- Continuous thickening of cementum
- Gingiva becomes edematous and friable; loss of stippling
- Salivary flow decreases

The patient's physician should be consulted before initiating endodontic treatment, especially elderly patients and others suspected of any systemic involvement.

The systemic conditions which warrant extra attention before endodontic treatment are:

a. ***Cardiovascular diseases*:** When a patient has a history of rheumatic fever with valvular heart damage, endodontic treatment should be preferred rather than the extraction. Hypertensive and patient taking anticoagulants are generally treated with utmost care. Special consideration should be given to all such patients. In any case where the patient is at risk, endodontic treatment should be carried out under antibiotic premedication. The recommended antibiotic regime (Table 10.1) is as follows:

- 2.0 gm penicillin V, one hour before the procedure followed by 1.0 gm every 6 hours postoperatively; or

Table 10.1 Antibiotics regimen for cardiac patients

Patient	*Drug (Dose)*
Conventional	Erythromycin (500 gm every 6 hourly) Ampicillin (1.0 gm every 6 hourly)
Allergic to conventional medication	Clindamycin (600 mg every 12 hourly) Azithromycin (500 mg every 12 hourly)

10

- 1.0 gm erythromycin, one hour before the procedure and 500 mg every 6 hours postoperatively.

Mouthwash with 5.0% betadine/chlorhexidine is advised before rubber dam placement to avoid any possibility of bacteremia due to injury to gums.

Vasoconstrictors should not be administered to patients with unstable angina, recent myocardial infarction, recent stroke, recent arrhythmias and hypertensive patients. Local anesthetic agents without vasoconstrictor or minimal vasoconstrictors are preferred for nonsurgical endodontic procedures.

Vasoconstrictors should also be minimized in patient's undergone coronary bypass surgery, especially in first three months. These patients may not require antibiotic prophylaxis unless there are other complications.

Patients with artificial heart valves are considered highly susceptible to bacterial endocarditis. Such patients should be given prophylactic antibiotics before initiating endodontic treatment.

It is a common belief that endodontic treatment should be delayed in patients taking anticoagulant therapy to prevent hematologic complications. Various investigators do not support the routine withdrawal of anticoagulant therapy before endodontic treatment. The endodontist must be familiar with local methods of controlling hemostasis both during surgery and post-operatively. The patient's physicians should be consulted to alter the anticoagulant regime if need be. The patient should also be informed of the possible complications associated with anticoagulants and/or bleeding.

- Check whether hypertension is under control or not
- Carefully administer local anesthesia.

  [Even though adrenaline is contraindicated in hypertensives, amount available in 1:100000 solutions is safe. As anesthetics without vasoconstrictors have a less profound effect and shorter duration of action, slow injection (one minute for 1.8 ml) using 26 or 27 gauge needle is preferred.]

b. *Pregnancy*: Unless emergency treatment is warranted, it is advisable to defer elective endodontic treatment, especially during the first trimester because of the potential vulnerability of the fetus. The second trimester is the safest period during which any procedure can be carried out. Treatment planning should be directed at eliminating pain symptoms during pregnancy.

The postpartum period, wherein the mother breast-feed the child should also be considered. The clinician should avoid any drug harmful to the infant.

Patient's gynecologist should be consulted as regard treatment needs of the patient and also the drug regime.

- Proper chair position for the comfort of the patient.
- Organogenesis is taking place in first trimester; any medication has to be cleared by the gynecologist. Second trimester is relatively safe. Third trimester is also safe but care has to taken with chair position as the fetus is growing and postural hypotension may develop.
- To prevent supine hypotensive syndrome in the dental chair, the pregnant woman should have the right hip elevated 10 to 12 cm or placing the patient in a 5.0 to 15% tilt on her left side can relieve pressure on the inferior vena cava. If hypotension is still not relieved, a full left lateral position may be needed.

c. *Malignant lesions*: The presence of a well-defined apical radiolucency is assumed to be because of non-vital pulp. Many a times, the radiolucency can be due to malignant lesions of the jaws mimicking periapical radiolucency. For example, a definitive diagnosis of a periradicular osteitis can be made only after biopsy. Whenever, there is a discrepancy between initial diagnosis and the clinical findings, the patient should be referred for second opinion. Patient undergoing chemotherapy and/or radiation to the head and neck may have impaired healing responses (endodontic treatment can be performed if the platelet count is more than 50,000/mm). The endodontic treatment should be initiated in consultation with patient's physician/oncologist.

d. *Human immunodeficiency virus (HIV)*: It has been established that the potential of developing hepatitis B/hepatitis C from a needle-stick injury is much higher than developing HIV. A major consideration for the management of patients with HIV/acquired immunodeficiency syndrome (AIDS) is the CD4 lymphocyte count. Patients with CD4 count above 400 mm^3 are considered asymptomatic HIV candidates and can be treated in routine. The endodontic procedures for HIV infected patients can be initiated in consultation with the medical specialist. The intake of medicine should also be noted and can be modified during endodontic procedures.

e. *Renal diseases (dialysis)*: Patient with renal failure and other kidney dysfunction may not be able to metabolize certain drugs. Hemodialysis tends to aggravate bleeding tendencies through physical destruction of platelets. It is important to review the patient's undergoing dialysis before initiating endodontic procedures. The patients, who have had hemodialysis session generally have bleeding tendencies and are fatigued. The elective endodontic treatment should be postponed till a day after hemodialysis. The operator should also be aware of the fact that hemodialysis removes certain drugs from the circulating blood and can shorten the effect of prescribed medications. The drugs used during endodontic procedures may have to be avoided or their doses are to be adjusted. Penicillin V and cephalexin requires increase in dosage; however, erythromycin requires no adjustment. The patient's physician should be consulted as regard specific drug requirements during endodontic treatment.

f. ***Epilepsy***: Epileptic patients should take proper medication before endodontic procedures. The possibility of attack is to be minimized. Inadvertent injection of local anesthetic into vein may trigger an attack of epilepsy.

g. ***Diseases of adrenal cortex and thyroid***: In case of low level of corticosteroids (Addison's disease) and in high level of corticosteroids (Cushing's disease), the patient is unable to handle stress; also the healing is impaired making the patient susceptible to infections. In hypothyroidism, patients have diminished resistance to infection and in hyperthyroidism, epinephrine in local anesthetic may contribute to thyroid crisis. Prophylactic antibiotics are effective during endodontic procedures.

h. ***Diabetes***: The controlled diabetic patients, free from complications like renal failure, hypertension and/or coronary atherosclerotic disease, can be endodontically treated in routine. The standard protocol is followed, wherein prophylactic antibiotics are prescribed. In case the patient does not respond to the prescribed antibiotics, culture sensitivity tests can be performed; subsequently, modifying the antibiotic prescription.

The appointments in endodontic clinic should be scheduled considering the patient's normal meal and insulin schedule protocol. A treatment plan that includes periradicular surgery requires consultation with the patient's physician to review the systemic implications and also the schedule of drugs.

- Check whether diabetes is under control or not (stage of diabetes)
- Patients with diabetes are prone to infection and delayed healing; hence, necessary precautions should be taken
- Schedule early morning appointments where the patient has had medication and meals, so that the risk of hypoglycemia is minimized.

10

i. ***Blood dyscrasia***: It is opined that endodontic procedures are preferred in case of blood dyscrasias (hemophilia, hyperthyroidism, Paget's disease, etc.) as compared to extraction. Also, in patients with acute/ chronic leukemia and rheumatic heart diseases, the endodontic treatment is preferred. The systemic disorders are not definite contraindications for executing endodontic procedures; however, the operator should be conscious of the implications of these diseases.

- Check bleeding and clotting time
- Less traumatic procedure should be carried out.
  (Most challenging is to treat a patient with hemophilia as there is always the risk of puncturing blood vessel and inducing internal bleeding particularly with inferior alveolar nerve blocks. If vital pulp extirpation has to be carried out, gradual fixation of pulp tissue followed by removal in multiple visits is the preferred choice. Care should be exercised in placing rubber dam clamps so that they do not impinge on gingival tissue. Notches may be placed on the labial and lingual surfaces into which the clamps prongs will fit).

j. ***Asthma***

- Asthma, hay fever, skin rashes etc. indicate hypersensitivity problems and the patients should be managed accordingly.
- The patient's medication and nebulizer should be kept ready. The rubber dam application should be modified and removed after short interval of time.
- Clinic set up should be aerosol free.
- Patients with very high blood pressure need physician clearance and medication before anesthesia and even in routine procedures.

k. ***Medications***

- Whether patient is on medication: if yes, for which problem?
- Whether the medication was prescribed by any qualified doctor? This helps in identifying patient attitude towards his/her ailments.
  (Some medication may be interfering with the antibiotics and analgesics, need to be analyzed.)
- Allergic to any drug.

PERIODONTAL DISEASES INFLUENCING TREATMENT PLANNING

Certain cases, such as a combined periodontic-endodontic lesion (an infected pulpless tooth communicates with the periodontal tissues or periodontal infections communicate to the pulp tissues) should be planned keeping in mind the timings of treating one tissue and its effect on the other tissue. It is established that if destruction of the periodontal attachment is considerable, the periodontal fibres may not get repaired even after endodontic treatment.

In case of severe periodontal involvement, extensive alveolar resorption and/or unfavorable crown-root ratio, the planning should be aimed at improving the periodontal status of the tooth. In case of class III mobility, extraction of the tooth should be preferred because the prognosis of the periodontal repair may remain poor even after the endodontic treatment. However, if the tooth is firm despite of the radiographic evidence of bone resorption, endodontic treatment is not contraindicated.

An effort should be made to determine whether the concerned tooth is strategically important or not. This is important in case the patient is already wearing a partial denture, or a partial denture is being planned for the patient. Extraction of the tooth in such cases may allow for a better design of denture, save time and be more economical in the long run.

When more than one focus of infection is present in the oral cavity, each one should be treated in coordination. Such a situation arises when two adjacent untreated pulpless teeth are present, or when pulpal and periodontal disease of the same tooth are coexistent, or when sinus is also involved along with rarefaction, especially in molars.

The existing ailments should be treated in coordination to achieve better treatment outcome.

The treatment planning is summarized in Flowchart 10.3.

FINAL PHASE OF TREATMENT PLANNING

The final phase of case selection and treatment planning involves considering the following factors:

i. Restorability of the tooth
ii. Strategic value of tooth in the oral cavity
iii. Periodontal factors
iv. Patient preference

Flowchart 10.3 Treatment planning

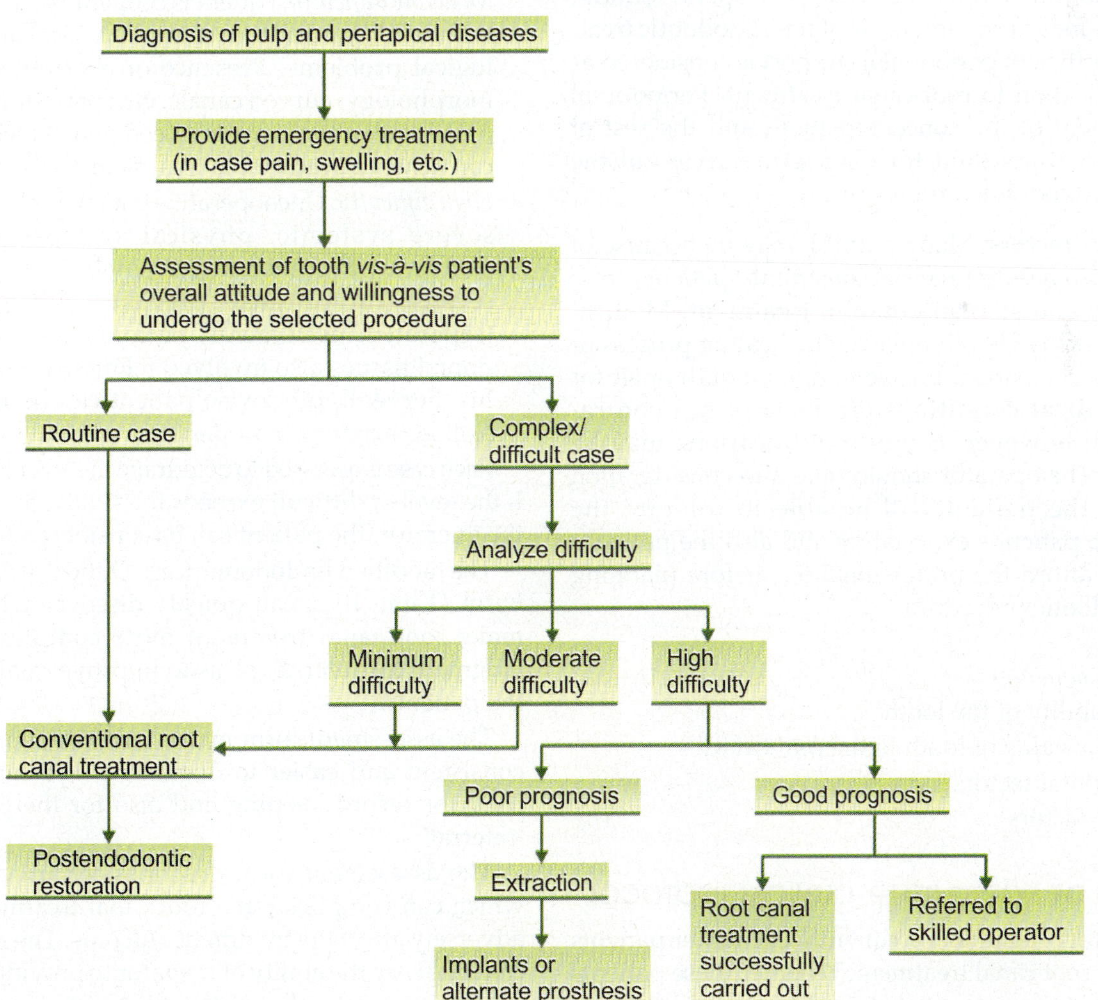

i. *Restorability of the tooth*: The purpose of endodontic therapy is to provide biologically acceptable restoration that will support the stomatognathic system.

The tooth must be assessed for any restorative challenges that may create difficulty in restoration or make the tooth unrestorable following root canal treatment. If the tooth cannot be restored to its functions (reasons may be extensive root caries, massive resorption or unfavorable crown-root ratio), the endodontic treatment should not be planned.

ii. *Strategic value of tooth in the oral cavity*: The strategic considerations include structural integrity, morphology and dimensions of the root, level of surrounding bone/periodontal support and the remaining tooth structure. The tooth having no function in the oral cavity or even in future should not be planned for endodontic treatment. The strategic value of tooth vis-à-vis overall functioning of the stomatognathic system should be given priority in treatment planning.

iii. *Periodontal factors*: The health of the periodontium affects the long-term prognosis of the endodontic treatment. Insufficient periodontal support is considered as contraindication to root canal treatment. Periodontal management of the concerned tooth and the rest of dentition is important for long-term success of the planned endodontic procedure.

iv. *Patient factors*: Many a times, may be because of lack of awareness or financial constraints, patient prefer extraction rather than curative treatment. Medical conditions may also complicate the healing process or may make the patient unable to open mouth or sit for long. Medical conditions are usually not contraindicated; however, certain modifications may be required. The operator should take into consideration whether the patient will be able to tolerate the treatment, patient's expectation and also the patient's ability to afford the professional fee, before planning for endodontic procedure.

Issues to consider
- Restorability of the tooth
- Strategic value of tooth in the oral cavity
- Periodontal factors
- Patient factors

TO REFER OR NOT TO REFER: CLINICAL PROTOCOL

10

The general practitioner frequently encounter patients requiring root canal treatment. Whether these patients be referred to an endodontist or be treated locally is an important decision that impacts the quality of the patient care. Similarly, the beginners in the field of endodontics should also assess the patient accordingly. The decision depends on case to case by taking into account the local and systemic conditions of the patient as well as the prognosis of the planned treatment.

To provide guidance on how to evaluate an endodontic case, the American Association of Endodontists (AAE) has created an Endodontic Case Difficulty Assessment Form (the assessment form is modified for convenience) that helps the operator to evaluate the difficulty of each case and weight it against their endodontic experience.

The level of difficulties are categorized as minimum, moderate and high difficulty.

- *Minimum difficulty*: Patient is cooperative; no systemic, physical or psychological problems. Patient exhibiting normal morphological features; conventional diagnosis along with normal associated tissues. (Budding clinician with limited experience can achieve predictable treatment results.)
- *Moderate difficulty*: Patient is cooperative, but anxious, with mild/moderate systemic, physical and psychological problems. Presence of aberrant root canal morphology, curved canals, etc.; periodontal tissues may involve (only experienced and skilled clinician can achieve predictable treatment results).
- *High difficulty*: Uncooperative patient with moderate/severe systemic, physical and psychological problems. Presence of extremely inclined teeth/severely curved canals; previously failed treatment (separated instruments, perforations, etc.); periodontal tissues also involved (clinician should assess his/her skill, otherwise patient can be referred to skilled/experienced operator).

Each case is assessed to determine the level of difficulty. If the level of difficult exceeds the skill and expertise of the operator, the patient can be considered for referral.

The modified Endodontic Case Difficulty Assessment Form (Table 10.2) can quickly discover what factors make root canal treatment more complex; provide judgment for referral, so as to improve quality care to the patients.

The assessment form makes case selection efficient, consistent and easier to document. The same can be used for record keeping and also for the purpose of 'referral'.

The assessment form describes certain conditions, which can complicate the root canal treatment or can adversely affect the treatment outcome. The risk factors can influence the ability of operator to provide adequate care at a consistently predictable level.

Table 10.2 Endodontic Case Difficulty Assessment Form (*Adapted from* American Association of Endodontists)

Criteria	*Minimum difficulty*	*Moderate difficulty*	*High difficulty*
		A. Patient considerations	
Medical history	No medical problem	One/few medical problems	Complex medical problem/serious illness/disability
History of allergies	• No history of reactions to anesthetic agents • No history of allergy	• Intolerance to vasoconstrictors • Allergic to certain drugs	• Anesthetic medicaments not suitable • Allergic to plenty of objects/drugs
Patient cooperation	• Cooperative and compliant • No problem of mouth opening • No problem of gag reflex	• Anxious but cooperative • Slight limitation in mouth opening • Gags occasionally	• Uncooperative • Significant limitation in mouth opening • Extreme gag reflex
Emergency conditions	Minimum discomfort (pain/ swelling)	Moderate pain/swelling	Severe pain/swelling
		B. Treatment considerations	
Diagnosis	Signs and symptoms consistent with diagnosis (diagnosis easily arrived at)	Extensive differential features (diagnosis not easily achieved at)	Complex signs and symptoms (difficult to diagnose)
Radiographic assessment	Obtaining/interpreting radio-graphs easy	Difficulty in obtaining/interpreting radiographs (problem of mouth opening)	Superimposed anatomical structure; pose difficulty in interpreting radio-graphs
Position of tooth	Anterior teeth (may be slight inclination/ rotation (less than 10°)	Premolars/first molar [may be moderate inclination/rotation (10–30°)]	2nd or 3rd molar [may be extreme inclination/rotation (more than 30°)]
Ease of Isolation	Rubber dam placement in routine	Modification required for rubber dam placement	Extensive modification required or rubber dam placement not feasible
Accessibility	Normal crown morphology	• Full coverage restoration • Extensive coronal destruction	Significant deviation from normal tooth (dens-in-dente, fusion, etc.)
Root canals morphology	• Straight or curvature less than 10° • Canals visible in radiographs	• Moderate curvature (10–30°) • Canals partially visible	• Extreme curvature (more than 30°) or S-shaped curve • Canal divides in the middle or apical third • Deviated canal morphology • Canals not visible
Resorption	No resorption	Minimal apical/ Internal/External resorption	Extensive apical/internal/external resorption
		C. Miscellaneous considerations	
Traumatic injuries	• No fracture • Uncomplicated crown fracture	• Complicated crown fracture • Subluxation/Intrusion	• Complicated crown fracture • Horizontal root fracture • Luxation • Avulsion
Endodontic treatment	No previous treatment	Previous treatment without complications	• Previous treatment with complica-tions (e.g. Perforation, non-negotiated canal, ledge, separa-ted instrument) • Surgical intervention required
Periodontal-endodontic condition	None or mild periodontal involvement	Moderate endodontic/ periodontal involvement (may be concurrent)	• Concurrent endodontic/perio-dontal involvement • Root amputation/hemisection prior to endodontic treatment

A few clinicians prefer to concentrate on restorative dentistry and avoid endodontics; whereas, others opt to treat endodontic cases of minimal to moderate difficulty. Even budding endodontists do not prefer 'enthusiastic endodontic intervention'.

Over the years, with the advent of operating microscope and other gadgets, the clinicians are now attempting to manage complicated endodontic cases. However, certain features should be thoroughly analyzed before initiating endodontic procedures.

The features that can make root canal treatment difficult and warrant the clinician to opt for referral are:

- Extreme inclination/rotation of the tooth
- Significant curvature of the root and root canal
- Radiographic obliteration of pulp chamber and root canals
- Multiple furcated root canals. Aberrant root canal anatomy
- Retreatment of a case restored with post-core restoration.

In case surgical intervention is necessary and that too under general anesthesia, the anesthetist should be consulted in every case; surgery should be carried out under the supervision and instructions of the anesthetist.

American Society of Anesthesiologists (ASA) has classified patients undergoing surgical interventions with general anesthesia.

Class 1: No systemic illness. Patient healthy: No modification required in dental treatment.

Class 2: Patient with mild degree of systemic illness; but without functional restrictions (well-controlled hypertension, diabetic, asthma, etc.): Usually no modification required in dental management.

Class 3: Patient with severe degree of systemic illness which limits activities; but does not immobilize the patient (cardiovascular diseases, unstable angina, hemophilia, etc.): Require modifications in dental management and in drug intake.

Class 4: Patient with severe systemic illness that immobilizes the patient; may sometimes be life threatening (kidney failure, liver failure, etc.): Require definite modifications in dental management.

Class 5: Patient may not survive for more than 24 hours; whether or no surgery.

10

The ASA classification is widely used to assess pre-anesthetic condition of the patient. The clinician should also consider associated factors such as age, obesity, etc. before initiating endodontic procedures under general anesthesia.

BIBLIOGRAPHY

1. Al Shareef AA and Saad AY. Endodontic therapy and restorative rehabilitation versus extraction and implant replacement. Saudi Endod. J.: 2013; 3:107–113.
2. Carrotte P. Endodontics: Part 2 – Diagnosis and treatment planning. Br. Dent. J.: 2004; 197:231–238.
3. Curtis DA, Lacy A and Chu R. Treatment planning in the 21st century: what's new? J. Calif. Dent. Assoc.: 2002; 30:503–510.
4. Dawson AS and Cardaci SC. Endodontics versus implantology: To extirpate or integrate? Aust. Endod. J.: 2006; 32:57–63.
5. Friedman S and Mor C. The success of endodontic therapy – healing and functionality. J. Calif. Dent. Assoc.: 2004; 32:493–503.
6. Friedman S. Considerations and concepts of case selection in the management of post-treatment endodontic disease (treatment failure). Endod. Topics: 2002; 1:54–78.
7. Friedman S. Prognosis of initial endodontic therapy. Endod. Topics: 2002; 2:59–88.
8. Heling I, Gorfil C, Slutzky H, Kopolovic K, Zalkind M, Slutzky-Golberg I. Endodontic failure caused by inadequate restorative procedures: review and treatment recommendations. J. Prosth. Dent.: 2002; 87:674–678.
9. Iqbal MK and Kim S. A review of factors influencing treatment planning decisions of single-tooth implants versus preserving natural teeth with non-surgical endodontic therapy. J. Endod.: 2008; 34:519–529.
10. John V, Chen S and Parashos P. Implant or the natural tooth – A contemporary treatment planning dilemma? Aust. Dent. J.; 2007; 52:S138–50.
11. Kirkevang LL and Horsted BP. Technical aspects of treatment in relation to treatment outcome. Endod. Topics: 2002; 89–102.
12. Marshall FJ. Planning endodontic treatment. Dent. Clinic. North Am.: 1979; 23:495–518.
13. Messer HH. Clinical judgement and decision making in endodontics. Aust. Endod. J.: 1992; 25:124–132.
14. Ng Y, Mann V, Rahbaran S, Lewsey J and Gulabivala K. Outcome of primary root canal treatment: Systematic review of the literature-Part I. Effects of study characteristics on probability of success. Int. Endod. J.: 2007; 40:921–939.
15. Ng Y, Mann V, Rahbaran S, Lewsey J and Gulabivala K. Outcome of primary root canal treatment: Systematic review of the literature-Part 2. Influence of clinical factors. Int. Endod. J.: 2008; 41:6–31.

16. Ng YL, Mann V and Gulabivala K. Outcome of secondary root canal treatment: a systematic review of the literature. Int. Endod. J.: 2008; 41:1026–1046.

17. Ng YL, Mann V and Gulabivala K. Tooth survival following non-surgical root canal treatment: a systematic review of the literature. Int. Endod. J.: 2010; 43:171–189.

18. Parirokh M, Zarifian A and Ghoddusi J. Choice of treatment plant based on root canal therapy versus extraction and implant placement: a mini-review. Iran. Endod. J.: 2015; 10:152–155.

19. Pothukuchi K. Case assessment and treatment planning: what governs your decision to treat, refer or replace a tooth that potentially requires endodontic treatment? Aust. Endod. J.:2006; 32:79–84.

20. Ree MH, Timmerman MF and Wesselink PR. An evaluation of the usefulness of two endodontic case assessment forms by general dentists. Int. Endod. J.: 2003; 36:545–555.

21. Ricucci D, Grondahl K and Bergenholtz G. Periapical status of root-filled teeth exposed to the oral environment by loss of restoration of caries. Oral Surg., Oral Med., Oral Pathol., Oral Radiol. Endod.: 2000; 90:354–359.

22. Saunders WP. Treatment planning the endodontic-implant interface. Br. Dent. J.: 2014; 216:325–330.

23. Tang CS and Naylor AE. Single-unit implants versus conventional treatments for compromised teeth: a brief review of the evidence. J. Dent. Educ.: 2005; 69:414–418.

24. Yeng T, Messer HH and Parashos P. Treatment planning the endodontic case. Aust. Dent. J. Endod. Suppl.: 2007; 52:S32–S37.

Chapter 11

Endodontic Instruments

The successful endodontic procedures are being achieved by use of various instruments, strictly following the biological principles. Over the years, the hand instruments with one make or the other, have been successful in achieving the biological healing of periapical tissues. In the recent past, automated and mechanized instruments are being tried to improve upon the speed and efficiency of the treatment. The design of basic hand instrument was patented by Kerr company in 1915, comprising 2% taper and 16 mm long cutting surfaces.

Later, flexible nickel-titanium (Ni-Ti) instruments were introduced. They are both engine driven and hand instruments. The advent of rotary instruments with respective advantages and disadvantages, have revolutionized the endodontic treatment procedures. The knowledge of anatomy and basic biological principles coupled with use of modern instruments has led to predictably better quality of root canal treatment.

The International Organization for Standardization (ISO) and American National Standard Institute (ANSI) pertain to standardization of endodontic instruments. ISO deals with instruments for preparation (No. 3630-1) and obturation (No. 3630-3) of root canal; whereas, ANSI denotes different numbers for different instruments. ANSI designated instruments as: K-type files and reamers (no. 28). Hedstrom files (no. 58). Barbed broaches and Rasps (no. 63) and condensers, pluggers and spreaders (no. 71).

STANDARDIZATION OF ENDODONTIC INSTRUMENTS

Earlier the root canal instruments were manufactured without adhering to any pre-established criteria. No definite specification regarding diameter, taper or length of cutting blades were followed. Significant differences in configuration of instrument of same sizes were observed when they were measured with a µm-measuring scope.

Ingle proposed standardization of instruments after getting consent from other manufacturing units. The proposal was:

- Instruments shall be numbered from 10 to 100, the numbers to advance by 5 units to size 60 then by 10 units to size 100 (later number up to 140 were accepted).
- Each number shall be representative of diameter of instrument in 100th of mm at the tip (No. 10 is 10/100 or 0.1 mm at tip).
- The flutes shall begin at the tip [designated as $D_1(D_0)$] and shall exactly extend 16 mm up the shaft, [designated as $D_2(D_{16})$] [D_0 and D_{16} denote length while D_1, D_2 denote diameter]. The diameter of D_2 shall be 0.32 mm greater than D_1. This sizing ensures a constant increase in taper of 0.02 mm per mm (Fig. 11.1).
- The tip angle of an instrument should be 75° ± 15°.
- Instrument size should increase by 0.05 mm at D1 between no. 10 and 60. The increase is 0.1 mm from no. 60 to 100.
- Instrument handles be color coded (Fig. 11.2).

Later, the greater taper instruments having taper more than 2% were introduced. They were available in 4, 6, 8 and 10% taper. This means that for every mm gain in length of cutting blade, width of instrument increases by 0.04, 0.06 and 0.08 mm/mm rather than earlier standard of 0.02 mm/mm. These new instrument allow for greater coronal flaring than 0.02 instrument. Instrument having half sizes, i.e. 12.5, 17.5, 22.5, 27.5, 32.5 and 37.5 have also been introduced.

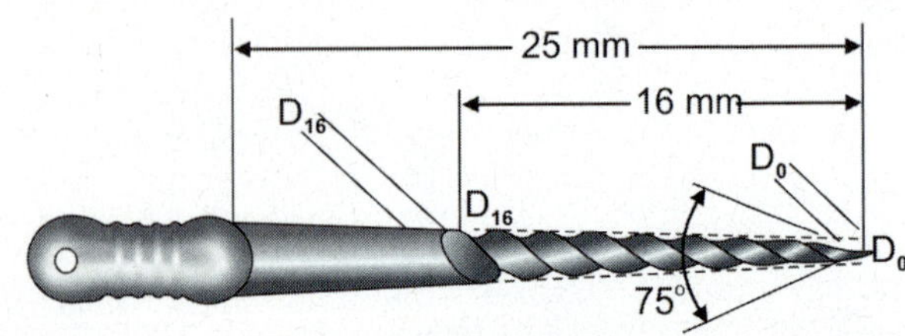

Fig. 11.1 ISO standardization

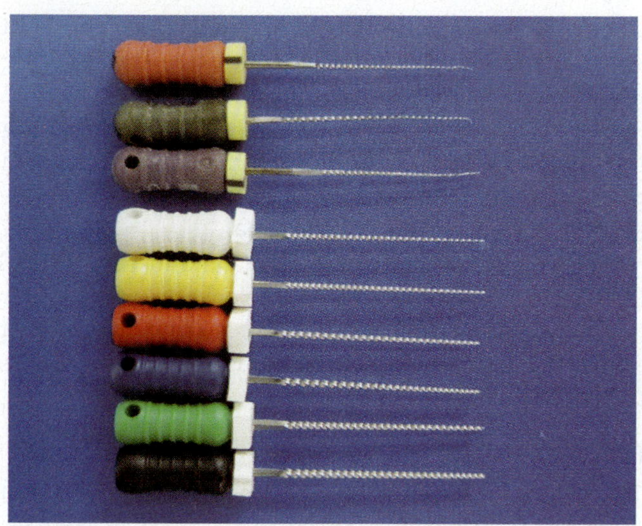

Fig. 11.2 Color coding of K-files

The full extent of shaft (up to handle) comes in 3 lengths, i.e. short (21 mm), standard (25 mm) and long (31 mm). The size of the instrument, their corresponding color and diameter at D_1 and D_2 is depicted in Table 11.1.

Table 11.1 Instrument sizes, diameter at D_1 and D_2 and color coding

Instrument size	*D_1 (mm)*	*D_2 (mm)*	*Color of handle*
06	0.06	0.38	Pink
08	0.08	0.40	Gray
10	0.10	0.42	Purple
15	0.15	0.47	White
20	0.20	0.52	Yellow
25	0.25	0.57	Red
30	0.30	0.62	Blue
35	0.35	0.67	Green
40	0.40	0.72	Black
45	0.45	0.77	White
50	0.50	0.82	Yellow
55	0.55	0.87	Red
60	0.60	0.92	Blue
70	0.70	1.02	Green
80	0.80	1.12	Black
90	0.90	1.22	White
100	1.00	1.32	Yellow
110	1.10	1.42	Red
120	1.20	1.52	Blue
130	1.30	1.62	Green
140	1.40	1.72	Black
150	1.50	1.82	White

MAKE OF ENDODONTIC INSTRUMENT

Earlier instruments were made of carbon steel and stainless steel. These instruments were having good cutting efficiency; however, they lack flexibility. Nickel-titanium alloy was introduced in dentistry by Naval Ordinance Laboratory, earlier known as nitinol. Earlier nickel and titanium were added in the ratio of 50 : 50. Later nickel (54–56%) and titanium (44–46%) were found to be more effective and useful for endodontic use. Traces of cobalt and boron have been added to improve surface hardness. 5.0% aluminium was added at the expense of nickel to improve upon the cutting efficiency; however, these instruments did not show much improvement in cutting efficiency, more so, they lack super-elasticity.

There are two basic categories of Ni-Ti rotary instruments: Active and passive. *'Active instruments'* have active cutting blades; whereas, *'passive instruments'* have a radial land between cutting edge and flute.

Active instruments cut more effectively and aggressively and have a tendency to straighten the canal curvature. Passive instruments perform a scrapping or burnishing rather than a real cutting action; remove dentin slower and have less tendency of canal straightening. Profile, light speed, etc. are 'passive instruments' and Flexmaster, RaCe, Protaper, Hero 642, K_3 etc. are 'Active instruments'.

The comparison of stainless steel and Ni-Ti instruments is tabulated in Table 11.2.

Table 11.2 Comparison of Ni-Ti and stainless steel instruments

Ni-Ti	*Stainless steel*
Softer than stainless steel	Harder than Ni-Ti
Not heat treatable	Heat treatable
Have low modulus of elasticity	Have high modulus of elasticity
Show super-elasticity and shape memory	Do not show elasticity and sharp memory
More flexible (two to three times than stainless steel)	Not flexible
Resist fracture	Fracture easily
Good corrosion resistance	Corrosion resistance fair
Better biocompatibility	Biocompatibility fair
Cutting efficiency less	Cutting efficiency more (60% more than Ni-Ti)
Gives no indication of fracture	Gives indication of fracture

EVOLUTION OF NICKEL-TITANIUM INSTRUMENTS

Over the years the researchers have been trying to improve upon the make and shape of Ni-Ti instruments so as to achieve the requisite root canal preparation without any procedural error; and also without affecting the surrounding periodontium. The evolution is categorized as:

First Generation

The first generation Ni-Ti files have passive cutting radial lands and tapers of 4 and 6%. The passive radial land facilitates a file to stay centered in canal curvatures during root canal preparation. Earlier instruments required numerous files to achieve the preparation objectives; later greater taper (GT) files became available, (taper of 6, 8, 10 and 12%). The *'passive radial land'* is the important characteristics in first generation instruments.

Second Generation

The second generation of Ni-Ti rotary files require fewer instruments to prepare a canal. To minimize screw effect, EndoSequence and RaCe instrument system provide files with alternating contact points. These files have fixed taper along the active blades. The advent of ProTaper (multiple increasing/decreasing percentage tapers) revolutionized the file design. The system provides shorter sequence of files to adequately shape the canal walls.

To increase resistance to fracture, the files are electropolished to remove surface irregularities; however, electropolishing may lead to dullness of the sharp cutting edges. Different cross-sectional designs were tried to improve upon the cutting efficiency of these instruments.

Third Generation

The third generation instruments focused on utilizing heating and cooling methods to reduce cyclic fatigue and improve safety. The desired phase transition between martensite and austenite can be utilized to produce a more optimal metal. Examples of files that offer heat treatment technology are twisted file (Axis/ SybronEndo), HyFlex (Coltene), Vortex, and WaveOne (Dentsply Tulsa Dental).

Fourth Generation

The next generation Ni-Ti instruments utilizes reciprocation (repetitive up and down/back-and-forth motion). M4 (Axis/SybronEndo), and Endo-Eze (ultradent products) are examples of systems that use reciprocation. A reciprocating file that utilizes an equal clockwise and counter clockwise movement may not cut as efficiently as a same-size rotary file. The augering of debris with these files is also limited.

Self-adjusting files (SAF) were introduced, having compressible open tube design that exerts uniform pressure on the dentinal walls, regardless of the cross-sectional configuration of the canal.

The single-file concept, WaveOne and RECIPROC (VDW), drives the file in unequal clockwise and counter clockwise direction. This reciprocating movement allows a file to efficiently cut along with augering the debris effectively.

Fifth Generation

The fifth generation design is such that the center of mass and/or the center of rotation are offset. In rotation, offset design produce a mechanical wave of motion that travels along the active length of the file. Such instruments enhance augering debris out of the canal and improves flexibility.

The examples of such designs are Revo-S (Medidenta), One Shape, and ProTaper next.

TERMS USED WITH ENDODONTIC INSTRUMENTS

The reader should have clear concept of the 'terms' used with endodontic instruments for better understanding of the working of these instruments.

The terms are:

Elastic limit: Elastic limit is the maximum stress that can be applied to a metal without producing permanent deformation. When external forces act on a metal, they tend to form internal stresses, which cause deformation. If the stresses are not much, the metal will return to its original dimensions on removal of the stresses.

Stress: The force acting across a unit area in a solid material (stress is quotient of force divided by an area).

Strain: The amount of deformation a metal undergoes is termed strain.

Elastic deformation: The reversible deformation that does not exceed the elastic limit.

Shape memory: Shape memory is the property whereby the alloys when heated returns to their original shape after having been deformed.

Taper: Taper is the amount of instrument diameter increase each millimeter along its working surface from tip to the handle.

Core: Core is the cylindrical center part of the instrument. The circumference is bordered by the depth of flutes. The diameter of the core is important in determining the flexibility and resistance to torsion.

***Helix angle*:** The angle that the cutting edge makes with the long-axis of the instrument is called helix angle.

***Flute*:** Flute is the groove in the working surface between the cutting blades. The soft tissues and dentin tips are collected here from the canal walls.

***Land*:** The land is the surface that projects axially from the central axis as far as cutting edge between the flutes (plane surface immediately following the cutting edge). It is also known as marginal width.

***Relief*:** The surface area of the land that rotates against the canal wall may be reduced to form relief. The relief reduces the frictional resistance and also aid in protecting the instrument from over engagement and separation.

***Pitch*:** It is the space or distance between one cutting edge and the corresponding adjacent cutting edge along the working area. The smaller the pitch, the more spirals the file will have and also the greater helix angle.

***Rake angle*:** If is the instrument is sectioned perpendicular to the long-axis, the angle formed by cutting edge and the radius of the instrument is the rake angle. The cutting edge has two surfaces: the rake face (surface of the cutting blade on the leading edge) and the clearance face (surface of the blade on the trailing side). If the angle formed by the cutting edge (rake face) and the surface to be cut is obtuse, it is '*positive rake angle*'. If the so angle is acute it is '*negative rake angle*'. If the angle is 90°, this is radial rake angle (neutral rake angle). The positive rake angle is for 'cutting' and the negative rake angle is for 'scrapping'.

Sometimes the term 'cutting angle' is used, which is the angle formed by the cutting edge and the radius when the instrument is sectioned perpendicular to the cutting edge.

FRACTURE OF Ni-Ti INSTRUMENTS

The prevalence of mean clinical fracture frequency of rotary Ni-Ti instruments is approximately 1.0% with a range of 0.4 to 3.7%.

Considerable research has been carried out to understand mechanism of alloy failure and also to minimize operator related issues of fracture of instruments. The main causes of fracture of endodontic instruments (Ni-Ti) are:

a. Metallurgy of Alloy

Nickel-titanium alloys are popular because of their biocompatibility and corrosion resistance. One of the disadvantage of Ni-Ti alloy is its low tensile and yield strength compared with stainless steel, making it more susceptible to fracture. The stress concentration in alloy metallurgy lead to flexure fatigue and subsequent fracture.

b. Factors predisposing to fracture

The rotary Ni-Ti instrument can fracture because of incorrect or excessive use. Many other factors also predispose to fracture of these instruments. The factors affecting susceptibility for fracture of rotary Ni-Ti instruments are:

i. ***Manufacturing process*:** During manufacturing of Ni-Ti alloy, a variety of inclusions (oxide particles), may get incorporated into the metal resulting in their weakness. Manufacturing process even results in many irregularities, which act as areas of stress concentrations and crack initiation during use. Ion implantation and electropolishing methods are used to improve the strength of rotary Ni-Ti instruments.

ii. ***Instrument design*:** The design of instrument may affect its resistance to fracture, especially when subjected to flexural/torsional load. An increase in cross-sectional area may contribute to increased resistance to torsional failure. It has been reported that instrument with a U-flute design and smaller cross-section area are more flexible than the triangular helix design.

   The design features that affect instrument fracture include instrument taper, size of cutting blade, number and depth of flutes, etc.

iii. ***Frequency and speed of instrument use*:** The speed at which instruments operate may not have any effect on the number of cycles to fracture; however, higher speed reduces the period of time required to reach the maximum number of cycles before fracture.

   Light apical pressure and brief use in the canal may contribute to prevention of fracture of rotary Ni-Ti instruments.

iv. ***Preparation technique*:** The clinician need to develop modified instrumentation sequences to avoid binding and threading of instruments in the root canal; sequential use of instruments is preferred in routine. Preflaring of the root canal with hand instruments before use of rotary Ni-Ti instrument creates a glide path for instrument tip and is a major factor in reducing the fracture rate of rotary Ni-Ti instruments.

v. ***Root canal curvatures*:** As the radius of curvature decreases or the angle of curvature increases, the chances of file fracture, even with fever rotation is increased.

The prolonged clinical use of rotary Ni-Ti instruments significantly reduces their cyclic flexural fatigue resistance. Partially fatigued instruments when flexed, reveal fractures associated with surface flaws. No correlation has been found between number of uses and frequency of fracture of instruments.

vi. ***Sterilization procedures***: The influence of sterilization of instruments on their resistance to fracture is still uncertain; may not be an important factor as regards fracture of Ni-Ti instruments.

CLASSIFICATION OF ENDODONTIC INSTRUMENTS

Different classifications for endodontic instruments have been proposed by various authors; however, none is universally accepted. The earlier classifications are:

a. *Harty's classification*

i. Instruments used for access cavity preparation
- Basic instruments
- Rubber dam
- Burs

ii. Instruments used for root canal preparation
- Hand instruments
- Power assisted instruments
- Electronic measuring devices
- Instruments for retrieving broken instruments/posts

iii. Instruments used for filling root canals

iv. Equipment used for storing instruments

v. Equipment for sterilization of endodontic instruments

vi. Equipment for improving visibility.

b. *Grossman's classification*

i. Exploring instruments
- Smooth barbed broach
- DG-16 explorer

ii. Debriding instruments
- Barbed broaches

iii. Shaping instruments
- Reamers
- Files

iv. Obturating instruments
- Plugger
- Spreader
- Lentulo spirals.

The easy way to classify endodontic instruments is according to their sequence of usage. The instruments are classified as:

A. Diagnostic instruments
B. Exploring instruments
C. Extirpating instruments
D. Shaping instruments
E. Obturating instruments
F. Miscellaneous.

A. DIAGNOSTIC INSTRUMENTS

Traditional instruments used in conventional operatory are modified for endodontic use. A typical set of endodontic instruments include a mouth mirror, endodontic explorer, cotton pliers, spoon excavators, spreaders/pluggers, plastic instrument, hemostat, periodontal probe and a ruler.

A number of specialized devices are necessary to evaluate the status of pulp and the surrounding tissues. Magnifying loops and microscopes are used to enhance the visibility and improve upon the diagnostic skills. Pulp vitality testers and the radiographic equipment is described in Chapter 9.

B. EXPLORING INSTRUMENTS

i. *Smooth broach*: The smooth broaches are used to explore the patency of root canals (Fig. 11.3). These are tapered instruments made of soft steel. The conventional taper is 0.007–0.01 mm/mm with variable lengths.

ii. *DG16 and JW17 microexplorer*: Conventionally DG-16 explorer (named after the scientist, David green) was used to explore the root canals; however, its diameter at the tip was large enough to penetrate narrow canals (Fig. 11.4). JW 17 microexplorer is narrower than DG16 and easily penetrates the canals (Fig. 11.5). It slides through the mud or collagen collected at the opening of the canal; whereas, DG16 may push the mud/collagen more apically. Modified forms of DG16 explorer are also being used. (DG 16/17 and DG 16/23). Another

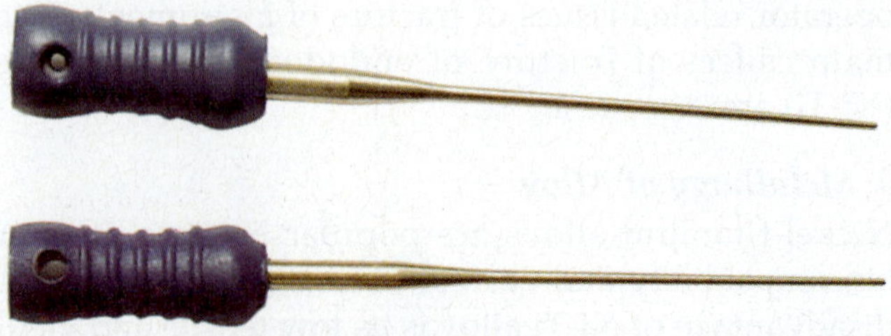

Fig. 11.3 Smooth broach

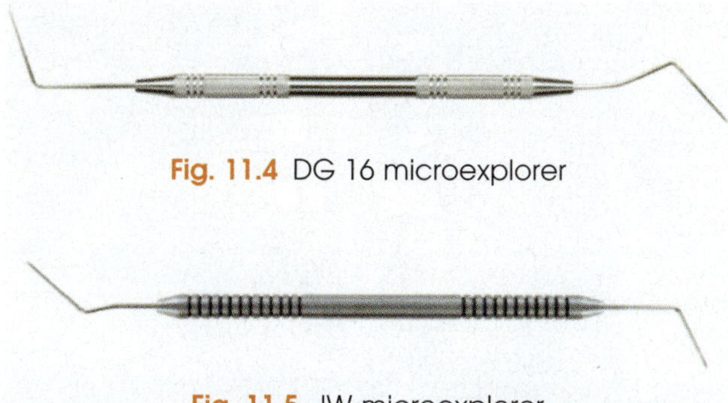

Fig. 11.4 DG 16 microexplorer

Fig. 11.5 JW microexplorer

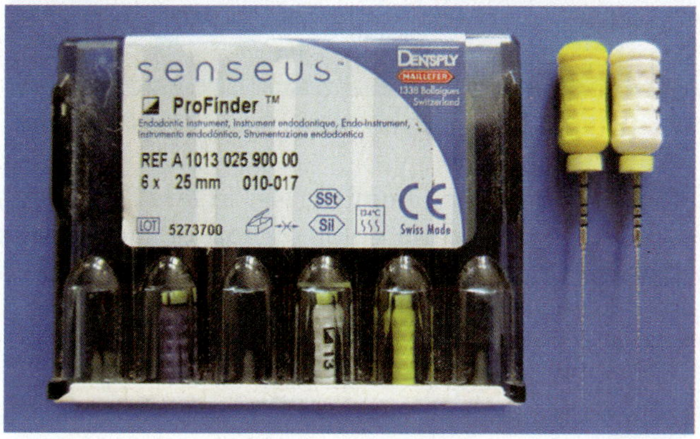

Fig. 11.6 Pathfinder

explorer KC-33, much heavier and sturdier, is also available for canal exploring.

iii. *Pathfinder files*: The smaller number files (No. 6 and 8) are used to negotiate the patency of root canals, known as pathfinders (Fig. 11.6).

iv. *Micro-opener*: Micro-opener is K-file having greater taper characterized by a shank that is bent at an angle of about 200° along with a long plastic handle. It is ideal for the posterior teeth. The Micro-opener series comprises three instruments with tip diameter 0.10, 0.15 and 0.20 mm and a taper of 0.02, 0.04 and 0.06 respectively (Fig. 11.7a).

v. *Micro-debrider*: Micro-débrider is Hedstrom file characterized by a shank that is bent at an angle of 200° along with a long plastic handle. They are available in ISO sizes, 20 and 30 and taper 0.02 (Fig. 11.7b).

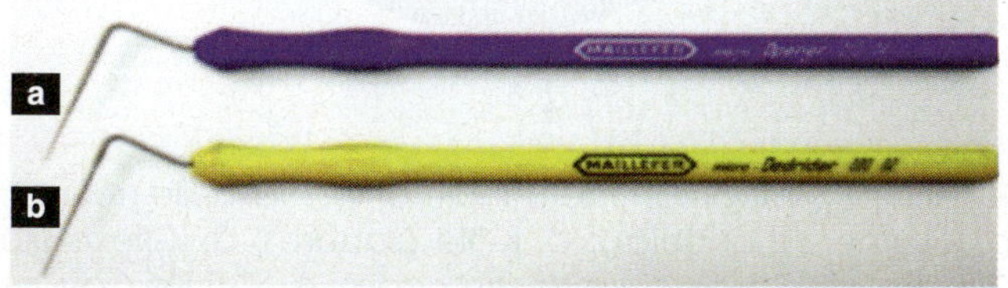

Fig. 11.7 (a) Micro-opener; (b) Micro-debrider

C. EXTIRPATING INSTRUMENTS

i. *Barbed broaches and rasps*

Broach is a tapered instrument made of soft steel. In case of barbed broach, the shaft is notched by a shredder to produce sharp barbs extending outward from the shaft.

The barbed broaches are used to remove soft tissues, cotton and paper points, etc. (Fig. 11.8). The barbed broaches are available in three sizes depending upon the configuration of barbs. These are 'X' (coarse), 'XX' (medium) and 'XXX' (fine). Recently, seven types of color coded broaches have been introduced. Black (coarse), green (medium), blue (fine), red (extra fine – XF), yellow (double extra fine – XXF), white (triple extra fine – XXXF) and purple (quadri extra fine XXXXF).

The instrument is carefully inserted through the access cavity, till approximate canal length is reached. The broach is slightly withdrawn, then rotated a few revolutions and removed. The soft tissue and debris get engaged on barbs and is removed. The canal is débrided of bulk contents before further preparation. The instrument should never be inserted with force. Once the dentin wall is felt, the broach should not be pushed further. The broach should be used in canals which are at least 20–25 number file size. Vital pulps, being low in collagen, are difficult to remove in toto with broaches. Formaldehyde treated pulps become fibrous and can be removed easily using barbed broaches.

Size of the broach is important. Too wide a broach may push the pulpal tissue apically and may bind in the canal and subsequently break. Too narrow a broach may not be able to engage the pulpal tissue properly. Many a times, two small broaches are inserted and twisted in the root canal, thereby engaging and removing the pulp tissue.

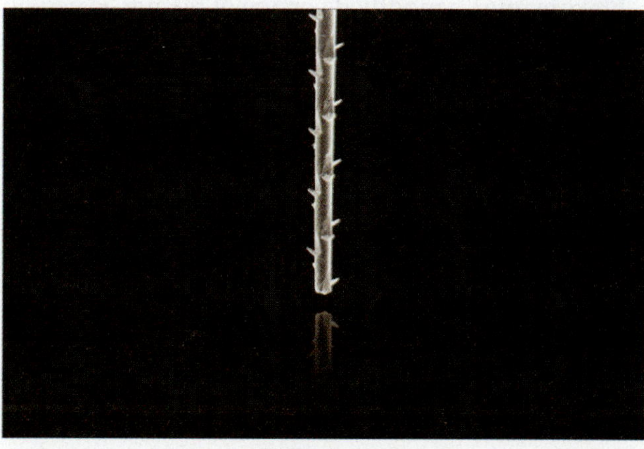

Fig. 11.8 Barbed broach

Barbed broaches and rasps, although similar in design, have significant differences in taper and barb size. The barbed broach has a taper of 0.007–0.010 mm/mm and rasp has a taper of 0.015–0.020 mm/mm. The barb height is much larger in broach than in rasp. The barb of broach comes out of instrument core, so barb is a much weaker instrument than rasp (Table 11.3).

Disadvantages

- Barbs are the weak links; may break within the canal
- Do not help in preparation of root canal.

D. SHAPING INSTRUMENTS

The basic instruments used for cleaning and shaping, as designed by Kerr Company are reamers, files and Hedstrom files.

i. Reamers

Reamers are identified by a *'triangle'* symbol on the handle. These are manufactured by twisting stainless steel wire into triangular blanks to produce cutting edges. Because each angle of blank is approximately 60°, a sharp knife edge is available to shave the canal walls. The cross-sectional area of blank allows a fair degree of flexibility in the reamer. The reamer has lesser flutes per unit length than file (Fig. 11.9). Being less twisted, it is more flexible than file. The instrument has cutting tip which makes the reamer suitable for straight canals only. In curved canals, ledge can occur if the instrument is not precurved.

How to Use

The reamer is used with pushing and rotating motion. Reaming involves placement of instrument towards apex until some binding is felt and then revolving the handle clockwise. Clockwise turning will remove dentin chips and debris from the canal wall; however, counter-clockwise turning may force the same apically.

Flexoreamer, a modified version of reamer, is usually used in curved canals. Flexoreamer has non-cutting tip. It is distinguished from the normal reamer by having different color of the number, e.g. in size 30 reamer, 30 is written in white color on top of the handle; whereas, in flexoreamer, 30 is written in blue color on top of the handle.

Table 11.3 Differences between broach and rasp

Broach	*Rasp*
Taper is 0.007–0.01 mm/mm	Taper is 0.015–0.02 mm/mm
Usual barb height is half the core diameter (other sizes available)	Usual barb height is one-third the core diameter
Barbs are deep and sharp	Barbs are shallow and round
Weaker as compared to rasp	Stronger as compared to broach

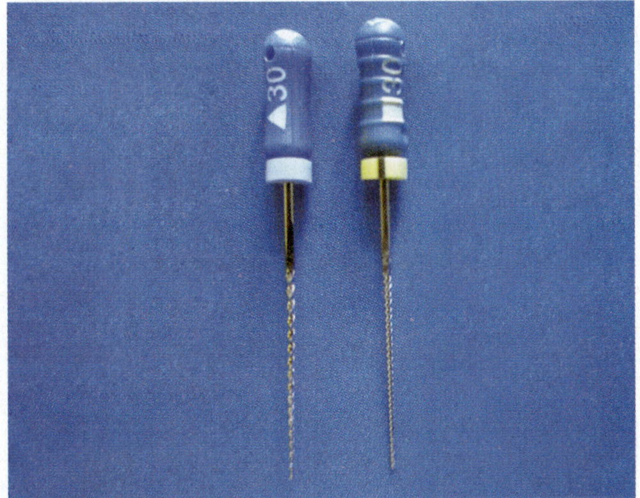

Fig. 11.9 Reamer (left) has lesser flutes than file (right)

ii. Files

Files are identified by a *'square'* symbol on the handle. The triangular blank of reamer is replaced with square blank in files and was twisted more to give greater number of cutting edges (Fig. 11.10).

The square blank has an angle of 90°; the cutting efficiency is less than reamer. A reamer has one to one and a half flute per mm; whereas, files have one and

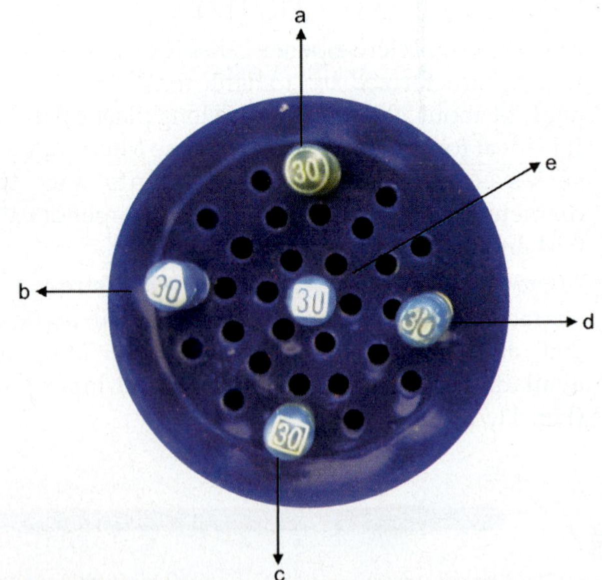

Fig. 11.10 Symbols on the handle of files: a. H-file (round); b. Reamer (triangular); c. K-file (square); d. K-flexo file (square with same color of size code); e. Ni-Ti file (square with half colored)

half to two and a half flutes per mm and thus having many more cutting edges. The cross-sectional area of file (from one angle to opposite angle in the blank) is greater than that of reamer, making it less susceptible to breakage. The greater cross-sectional diameter of file decreases its flexibility.

The progressive taper may enhance the cutting action while decreasing rotational friction between blade of the file and the dentin.

The non-cutting tip design allows each instrument to safely follow the secured portion in the canal, while small flat area on the tip enhances its ability to find its way through soft tissue and debris.

The differences between reamers and files are summarized in Table 11.4.

How to Use

The file is used with pulling motion. Filing involves placement of instrument in the root canal until some binding is felt. The instrument is removed by scrapping against the side wall with little or no revolution. The dragging against one side of the wall is also referred to as rasping action. The withdrawal of instrument by dragging the flutes on dentin walls effectively prepares the canal.

'Pistoning' the file (moving up and down) forcefully in the canal should be avoided. This motion tends to pack dentinal filings at the apex and may create ledges, etc.

The instrument should preferably be moved first towards the buccal side of canal, then reinserted and moved slightly mesially; then, towards the lingual aspect and finally to the distal. This is known as *'circumferential filing'*.

Table 11.4 Differences between reamers and files

Reamers	*Files*
• Made from triangular blank of wire	• Made from square blank of wire
• Number of flutes are 1–1½ per mm	• Number of flutes are 1–2½ per mm
• Cutting angle is 60° (sharp cutting)	• Cutting angle is 90° (less sharp cutting)
• Used with reaming motion	• Can be used with reaming and rasping motion
• Chip space is 60% (more clearing space)	• Chip space is 36% (does not allow much removal of loosened material: less clearing space)
• Produce canal round in shape	• Produce canal irregular in shape
• Less efficient	• More efficient
• More flexible	• Less flexible

It is established that the instrument, rather than its use, determines the general shape of canal preparation. Therefore, reaming action produces a canal that is relatively round in shape; whereas, filing action may produce irregular and eccentric canal shape. Smaller size files (up to number 20) have sufficient flexibility to retain canal shape. However, larger files, being not flexible, may alter the canal shape.

Flexofiles, a modified version of files, is usually used for curved canals. Flexofile has non-cutting tip. It is distinguished from the normal file by having different color of the number on top of the handle (Fig. 11.11); for example, in size 30 file, '30' is written in white color on top of the handle; whereas, in flexofile, '30' is written in blue color on top of the handle.

iii. Hedstrom Files

Hedstrom files are identified by the 'circle' symbol on the handle. These files were manufactured with the idea of having superior cutting efficiency. These files have flutes that resemble successively smaller triangles set on one another (Fig. 11.12). They are manufactured by using sharp rotating cutter that gouges triangular segments out of a round shaft. This produces sharp cutting edges at the base of each cone, which cut tooth

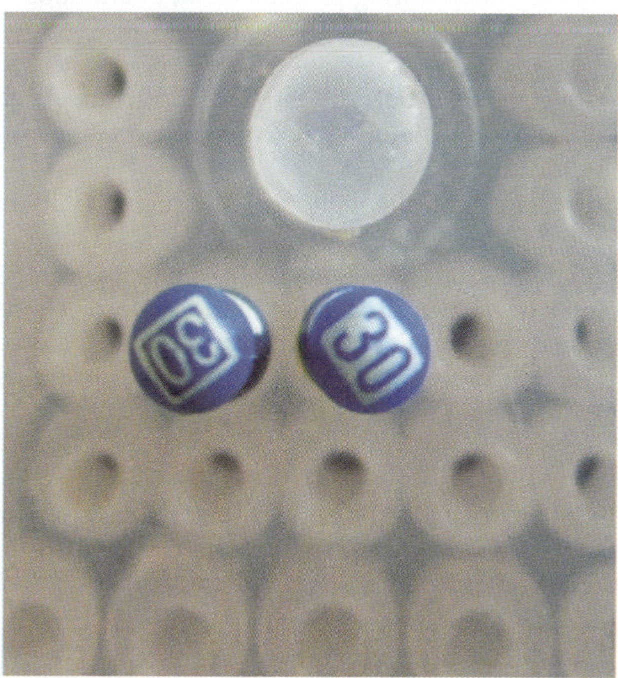

Fig. 11.11 K-flexo file (right): Blue color code on top of handle; K-file (left): White color code on top of handle

11

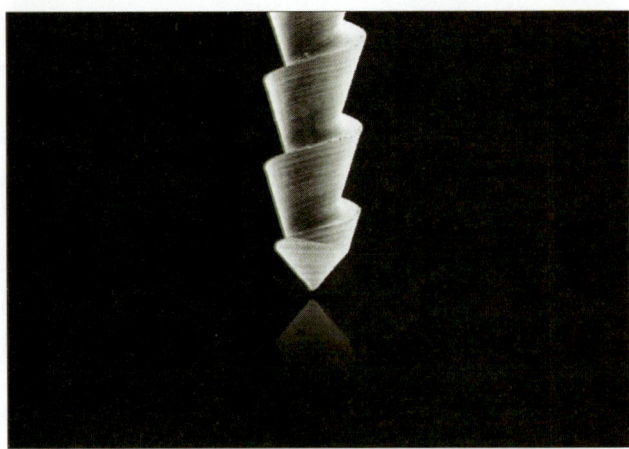

Fig. 11.12 Apical end of H-file

structure on pulling only. The cross-section of H-file shows coma-shaped (tear drop) appearance with one cutting edge. As the cutting efficiency is increased, the flexibility is compromised (flexibility is minimum).

Indications

- Instrumentation of immature teeth with wide canals, which may harbor considerable debris.
- To remove silver points or loose broken instruments from canals. The file is placed alongside the instrument, rotated and pulled occlusally.
- To widen coronal portion of curved canals.
- For widening the orifices of any canals for easy manipulation during preparation and obturation.

Drawbacks

- Gouging in the root canal may lead to fracture if bind in dentin (only 'pull' stroke is allowed; rotation lead to fracture).
- If screwed apically with force, the susceptibility of root fracture increases.

R-file (Rat-tail file), though not commonly used, is similar to barbed broach having metal projections perpendicular to the instrument shaft with pointed polyhedron cross-section. The file fracture easily during working, so not used in routine.

Modification in Files

The initial designs could not clean and shape the entire canal space while retaining the preoperative shape of the canal. The modifications in file system are:

i. Modification in instrument design
ii. Modification in numbering system
iii. Modification in method of manufacturing
iv. Modification in instrument material

i. Modification in Instrument Design

- *Flex-R file*: The square cross-section of file was modified to triangular cross-section. The modified form provides advantages such as, increase in cutting efficiency, increase in flexibility and holding more debris. The tip is flattened, i.e. non-cutting tip. The non-cutting tip decreases the chances of canal transportation and ledging during enlarging curved canals.
- *K-flex file*: The square cross-section of the K-file is changed to rhomboid cross-section. The cutting edge is formed of two acute angles and two obtuse angles. The acute angle increases sharpness, whereas obtuse angle provides more space for debris removal. The overall flexibility is also increased.
- *S-file/Uni-file*: A second blade is added to the single blade of the H-file. A third blade addition (*Helifile*) is also tried. These files are more aggressive in cutting efficiency; however, flexibility is poor. The decreased depth of S-file/Uni-file significantly decreases the tendency of these files to break inside the canal.
- *U-file*: The U-file has two 90° cutting edges at each of the three points of the blade. The flat cutting surface, referred to as 'radial', allow instrument to be used in 360° motion.
- *Canal master file*: The cutting segment of the instrument is reduced from 16 to 1.0–3.0 mm. Such reduction in cutting segment reduce the chance of canal transportation and ledging during enlargement of the curved canals.
- *C-files*: These files are ideally suited for sharply curved or calcified canals. These are available in ISO sizes 8, 10 and 15 with lengths of 18, 21 and 25 mm. The files are of stainless steel, having a square cross-section and a blunt, non-aggressive tip, which allow the instrument to safely follow the canal to the apex (Fig. 11.13).

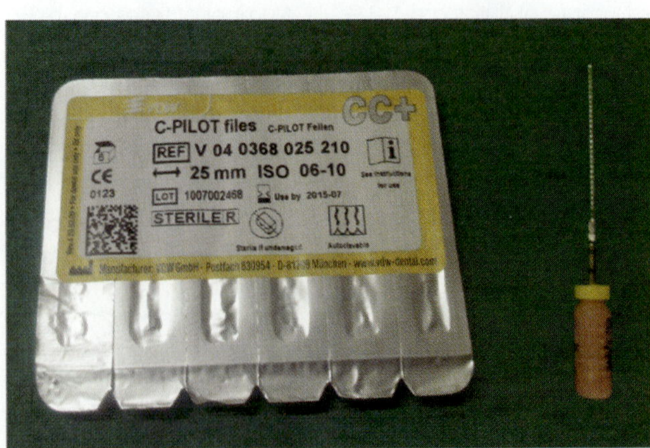

Fig. 11.13 C-file

- *Path finder files*: The smaller number K files (K6 and K8) are used to negotiate the patency of root canals, known as *'path finders'*. Profinder system provides files numbering 10, 13 and 17.
- *Triple-flex files*: The Triple-flex file is obtained by twisting a steel wire with triangular cross-section. Triangular design offers exceptional flexibility and efficient cutting ability. The Triple-flex file is available in ISO sizes from 08 to 80 and lengths 21, 25 and 31 mm.

ii. Modification in Numbering System

- *Intermediate size files*: Many a times, the standard size of the file is to be modified as per requirement of the operator. 1.0 mm apical cutting of the file number 10 makes it number 12 file and size 15 becomes size 17 (Fig. 11.14). Such files are made available in sizes of 12, 17, 22, 27 and so on. Later, these odd number files were manufactured so that, the operator did not have to clip the file. The drawback in this file system is that every file may not be, exactly of the standard size, since a deviation of 0.02 mm is acceptable. Therefore, a size no. 10 instrument may be as small as 0.08 or as large as 0.12 mm. This explains why the operator may have difficulty moving from one size to next size, especially in narrow/curved canals.
- *Golden mediums*: The files are identical to the K-Flexofiles, except that they have intermediate sizes as compared to ISO standard sizes. The files are pre-sterilized with color-coded, plastic handle. They are only available in sizes 12, 17, 22, 27, 32 and 37; the lengths remain 21, 25 and 31 mm. Their use is recommended in those canals, which need intermediary file sizes.
- *Series 29*: Another file system is 'Series 29', whereby instead of increasing each small file by 0.05 mm between sizes, it should be increased by 29% (Schilder named it as Profile 29 series). Let us keep file number 10 as a key size. The file smaller than it would be 0.071 mm at D_0 and file larger would be 0.129 mm at D_0. This system works well in small sizes; however, in larger sizes this much increase was not possible. The system provides *two advantages*: first constant increase in instrument diameter and second, it provides fewer number of instruments as compared to ISO system.

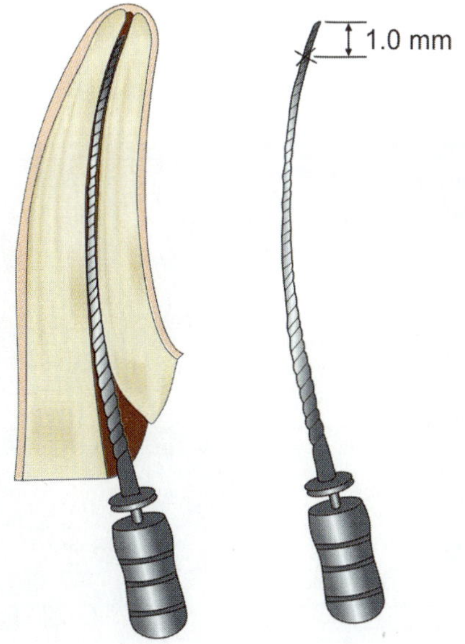

Fig. 11.14 Modification of instrument

iii. Modification in Method of Manufacturing

Instead of instrument twisting, the flutes are created by grinding or milling to decrease the internal stresses induced in the instrument during twisting process.

Later computer assisted milling technique provided files with sharper flutes and also deeper spaces between the flutes.

- *Flex-R file*: These files are manufactured following computer assisted milling technique. The flutes are sharper and the tip is rounded.
- *Ultra-flex file*: These files are also manufactured following computer assisted milling technique using Ni-Ti alloy. The flutes are less sharp than Flex-R file.
- *Sure-flex file*: Similar to ultra flex with sharper flutes.

iv. Modification in Instrument Material

Initial instruments were fabricated from carbon steel; however, due to decreased flexibility and low corrosion resistance of carbon steel, instruments were fabricated in stainless steel. Path finder is the only instrument that is still manufactured from carbon steel. The poor flexibility of stainless steel led to the advent of Ni-Ti instruments. Ni-Ti instruments offer better flexibility; however, its cutting ability is compromised.

E. OBTURATING INSTRUMENTS

i. Spreaders and Pluggers

Spreaders and pluggers are used for root canal obturation. Spreaders are designed for lateral condensation, while pluggers are for vertical condensation.

They are made of stainless steel or chromium plated brass and generally have long handle. These instruments can either be of a uniangular or bayonet style. Root canal spreaders are usually of the bayonet style.

The instrument with long handles are potentially dangerous, because the tips of the working ends are offset from the long-axes of the handles. This may result in strong lateral wedging forces on the working end if the instrument is not operated carefully.

Finger Pluggers and Finger Spreaders were introduced having small handle (Fig. 11.15). These are manufactured both in Ni-Ti and stainless steel. These are available in ISO sizes 15 to 80. The length is 21 mm and 25 mm and the taper is 2%. Pluggers have flat tip, whereas spreaders have sharp tip (Fig. 11.16).

Modifications

- *Heat carriers and pluggers*: The heat carrier and pluggers are designed exclusively for the warm vertical gutta-percha technique. These are machined from a special stainless steel and are angled inward for easy insertion. They are available in anterior and posterior configurations to allow for easier access.

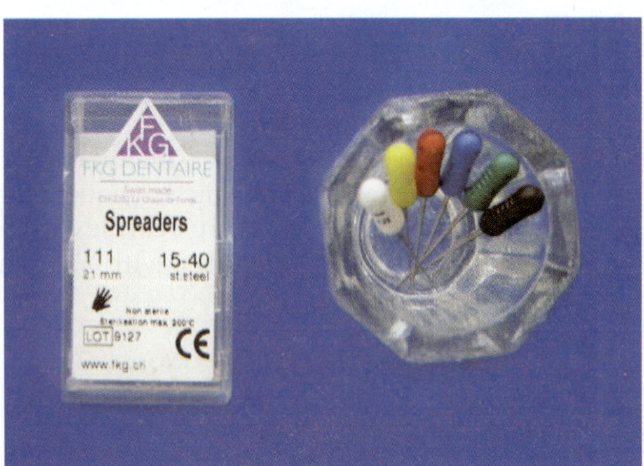

Fig. 11.15 Spreaders

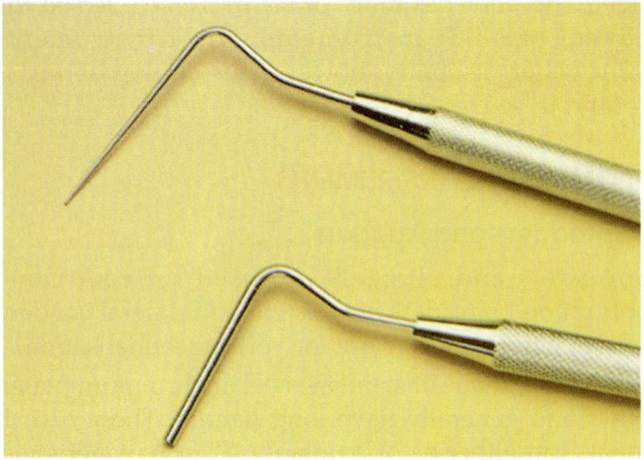

Fig. 11.16 Spreader (top) and plugger (bottom)

- *Spreader dryer*: The spreader dryer has a metal heat retention bulb for longer working time. It is made of stainless steel and available in sizes #2(30), #3(40) and #5(50). The vertical and lateral condensation in warm gutta-percha technique is better performed using these spreaders.
- *Roeko spreader and plugger*: Roeko spreaders are available in stainless steel (size 20 to 50) and Ni-Ti (size 15–35) having rings on the handle, which signifies their size. The flexible tips of Ni-Ti spreaders facilitate lateral condensation of gutta-percha even in curved canals. The spreaders have mm length graduation on the tip.
- *M-series pluggers and spreaders*: The M-series is the first calibrated plugger and spreader system sized to match standard ISO files and gutta-percha points. The ISO-sizing and tapering virtually eliminate binding and allow deeper penetration for better apical seal. The ISO color-coded instruments are available in either a single-ended or double-ended spreader/plugger combination.

ii. Paste Fillers (Lentulo Spiral)

The routinely used paste filler is Lentulo spiral, which is available in three lengths, 17, 21 and 25 mm with size 15–40. The metal handle is color coded. Both hand and rotary versions are available (Fig. 11.17).

The modified version of paste filler has also been introduced, viz. DYNA (length 21, 25 mm; size 25–40), Medidenta (length 21, 25 mm; size 25–70), Sensipast (length 21 mm; size 25–40) and Roydent (length 21 mm and 25 mm; size 25–40). Short length (18 mm) paste fillers are also available.

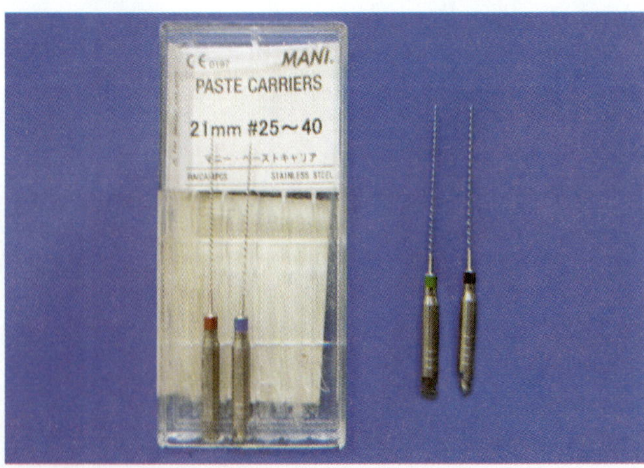

Fig. 11.17 Lentulo spiral

Automated Devices

Automated devices are the instruments which revolve fully/partially or reciprocate around an axis and work under higher speeds.

Advantages

- Significantly quicker
- Canal shape is smooth, well-centered
- Better removal of smear layer
- Less debris extruded apically
- Less operators' fatigue.

Disadvantages

- Lack of tactile sensation
- Susceptible of perforation/ledges, etc.
- Susceptible of file breakage.

The automated devices are categorized into three variants:

1. *Reciprocating*: Imparts partial rotation and/or back and forth movement to cutting instruments (Giromatic, Canal finder system/Endo pulse, etc.)
2. *Vibratory*: The instrument vibrates in the canal [Ultrasonic (Cavi Endo) and Sonic (MM 1500)]
3. *Rotary*: Provides continuous rotation of cutting instruments at a fixed speed (Profile, Light speed, RaCe, etc.)

The rotation/reciprocation is carried out with the help of another gadget known as 'Handpiece'. The handpiece gets rotational energy from engine driven motors. Three types of contra-angle handpiece are usually used, viz. (i) a full rotary handpiece either latch or friction grip; (ii) a reciprocating/quarter-turn handpiece and (iii) special handpiece that imparts a vertical stroke along with reciprocating quarter-turn.

i. A full rotary handpiece allows straight line drilling and/or side cutting. The burs or diamond points used with full rotary contra-angle handpieces can be used to achieve coronal access.

ii. A reciprocating handpiece provides quarter-turn to the instrument. It accepts only latch type instruments. Recently, M4 Safety handpiece having 300 reciprocating motions has been introduced. It has unique chuck that locks regular hand files in place by their handle. Safety Hedstrom instruments are recommended to be used with M4 handpiece. The Endo-grapper is a similar handpiece, with a 10:1 gear ratio and a 450 turning motion.

iii. A vertical stroke handpiece (canal finder) delivers a vertical stroke ranging from 0.3–1.0 mm. The depth of vertical stroke depends upon the free movement of the instrument in the canal. The handpiece also has a *quarter-turn* reciprocating motion along with a vertical stroke.

1. Reciprocating Instruments

a. Giromatic

Girofiles and Girobroaches are used along with Giromatic handpiece (Fig. 11.18a and b). The handpiece is designed to rotate the instrument a *quarter-turn* in an alternate direction. The root canal instruments are activated in the root canal at a speed of up to 3000 cycles/minute. Manufacturers claim that the working is fast with Giromatic; however, studies could not observe much difference between Giromatic and the hand files. The loss of tactile sensation, as with other power driven handpieces, may lead to zipping, over instrumentation and even breakage of the instrument. M4 safety handpiece and Endo-grapper are modified versions of Giromatic handpiece.

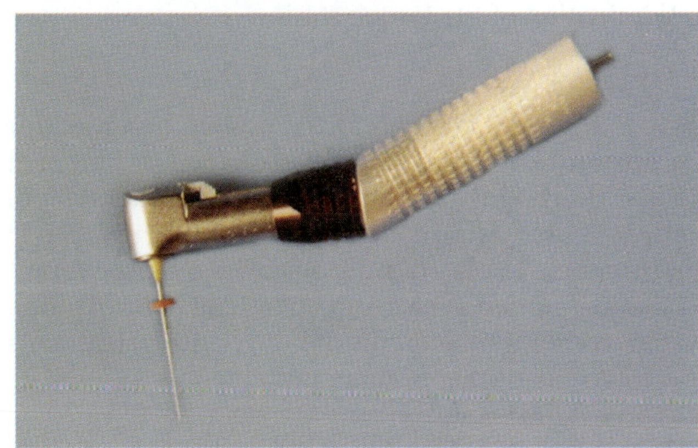

Fig. 11.18a Giromatic handpiece

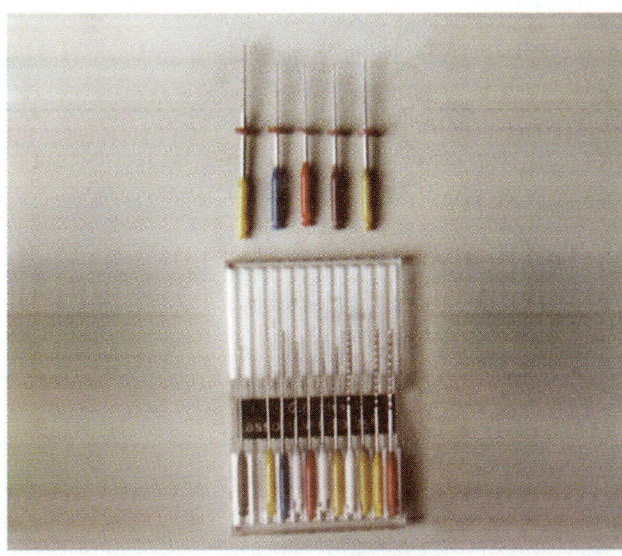

Fig. 11.18b Girofiles

b. Canal Finder System/Endo Pulse

The canal finder system utilizes handpiece, which runs the instrument in a 0.4 mm up and down motion with an additional full turn movement when pressure is applied. The handpiece offers continued irrigation to flush out dentinal chips and can be operated in a wide range of reciprocal speeds.

The file used with canal finder system is A-file. The file has 40° helical angle; which provides efficient cutting. It has non-cutting tip; allows the file to follow the canal lumen without encroaching the outer walls. The tip is longer and more rounded than traditional files. The canal finder system is used for other purposes also, such as, root canal obturation, removal of broken instruments, etc.

The vertical reciprocation has the following *advantages*:

- Reduction of file separation
- Ni-Ti files are not required (stainless steel files are used)
- Elimination of file torque strain.

c. Endo-Eze System

Endo-Eze system is a hybridized system designed for the preparation of curved, ribbon-shaped or flattened canals along with the straight canals. The system combines the benefit of stainless steel and Ni-Ti instruments. These files are used in reciprocating/oscillating motion in each direction. The hybridization system combines the merits of both hand instruments and rotary instruments along with the merits of Ni-Ti files and stainless steel files.

The system consists of the following:

- Three stainless steel shaping files, viz. Purple (10/02), white (13/03) and yellow (13/04) with respective size and taper.
- Three Ni-Ti transitional files (25 mm and tapers 0.08, 0.04 and 0.02) and two hand K-type stainless steel files (size 15 and 20) are also provided.
- Endo-Eze contra-angle handpiece, reciprocating at 30° with 4:1 reduction motor at the speed of 5000 rpm.

Technique

- The glide path is achieved with stainless steel file, followed by Ni-Ti files, especially in curved apical areas.
- Working length is determined using small number hand files.
- The first instrument (apical instrument) that feels resistance at the working length is determined. Once the canal is negotiated, mechanical reciprocating instrumentation is begun using Endo-Eze handpiece. The reciprocating shaping files are used in a circular motion or upward brushing stroke against the canal walls. The preparation is completed following Endo-Eze files in sequence. Continuous irrigation and recapitulation is mandatory.
- The apical one-third is prepared using Ni-Ti transitional files. The apical preparation is completed with hand Ni-Ti files, usually three to four sizes larger than the initial apical instrument.

Advantages

- Simple and reliable.
- Anatomical variations and pathological conditions seldom affect its results.
- Hybridization concept uses technology and rapidity of the systems; maximizing the traditional nature of hand instrumentation.
- Non-circular instrumentation and ability to adapt/follow the natural anatomy of coronal and middle-third of the canal length virtually eliminates the complications like ledging, zipping, canal transportation, unnecessary tooth structure removal and file separation, etc.
- Because of small tip diameter of the active portion, the files are very much flexible and permit instrumentation without deviations, especially in curved canals.

d. EZ-Fill Safesider

These are series of non-circular instruments having a flat side, which extends the entire length of cutting edge. These are available as a file or reamer (length 21 and 25 mm), both for manual and reciprocating (Endoexpress handpiece) use. Both stainless steel (size 08 to 40) and Ni-Ti (30/04: Orange, 25/08: Brown and 25/06: Pink) variants are available. The size, taper, make and color are tabulated in Table 11.5.

Table 11.5 Size, make, color and taper of EZ-Fill Safesiders

Size	Make	Color	Taper
08	SS	Grey	02
10	SS	Purple	02
15	SS	White	02
20	SS	Yellow	02
25	SS	Red	02
30	SS	Blue	02
35	SS	Green	02
40	SS	Black	02
30	Ni-Ti	Orange	04
25	Ni-Ti	Pink	06
25	Ni-Ti	Brown	08

The flat surface makes the instrument easy to use, prevents accumulation of debris, reduces stress and increases the flexibility of the instrument.

With this system, coronal one-third of canal is shaped with peeso reamers leaving the apical one-third for Safesiders and hand files. A peeso reamer called 'Pleezer' (size 2 of peeso reamer) is provided, which straighten the coronal curves of the canal more easily and with less resistance.

Significance of flat surface

- Flat surface reduces the amount of cutting surface in contact with the canal wall. It may decrease the efficiency for time being, but the manipulation is much easier and with less fatigue.
- Dentin debris created can be removed easily.
- Because less instrument is cutting at any time, less stress is given to the instrument; subsequently, less chances of breakage.
- Increases the flexibility of the instrument.

2. Vibratory Instruments

a. Ultrasonic

The endodontic treatment by ultrasonic, sonic or subsonic systems is termed 'Endosonic'. The equipment creates a synergistic system, whereby canal preparation cleaning, irrigation, disinfection, and filling are all accomplished with the same device. An ultrasonic device converts electrical energy into ultrasonic waves of certain frequency by magnetostriction and by Piezoelectricity.

Ultrasonic endodontics is based on a system in which sound as an energy source at 20–25 kHz activates an endodontic file, resulting in three-dimensional activation of the file in the surrounding medium.

The ultrasonic devices derive energy from instruments vibrating and using either electromagnetic or piezoelectric power sources. Magnetostriction is generated by deformation of ferromagnetic material subjected to a magnetic field; whereas, piezoelectricity is the generation of stress in dielectric crystals subjected to an applied voltage. Magnetostrictive transducers produce an elliptical motion at the working tip, while piezoelectric transducer produces longitudinal or transverse linear motions.

***Method of action*:** Ultrasonic cleaning was described initially as implosion or cavitation. Cavitation occurs when ultrasonic file vibrates in a liquid to produce alternate compressions and rarefactions of pressure. A negative pressure develops within the exposed cells of intracanal materials (pulp tissue, bacteria, debris, etc.). This causes breaking of cells leading to their destruction. The broken cell parts are washed out and removed from the canal system.

Removal of dentin for canal preparation and elimination of unwanted intracanal materials is accomplished in less time and with better efficiency with ultrasonic files (Fig. 11.19) as compared to hand files. Ultrasonic endodontics is particularly effective for larger canals and canals that are interconnected.

Ultrasonic tips have been broadly classified as follows:

a. *Non-surgical*
   - Access refinement tips (used for access preparation and refinement)
   - Vibratory tips (used to remove post and core)
   - Bulk removal tips (remove dentin and core material quickly)
   - Troughing tips (used for instrument retrieval)

b. *Surgical*
   - Surgical retro-tips (used for root end preparation).

The most frequently used ultrasonic electromagnetic unit is 'Cavi-endo'. For dental use, piezoelectric units are much more powerful than electromagnetic units. They are effective in removing silver points and posts from root canal space. The most frequently used piezoelectric unit is 'Enac'.

Removal of smear layer may be accomplished more readily with ultrasonics, but site where the tip actually touches the canal wall produces a new smear layer. It is suggested that ultrasonic device should be used after canal preparation by hand and the file should remain in the center of canal away from walls. File must be small and loose in canal, particularly in curved canals, to achieve optimum cleaning.

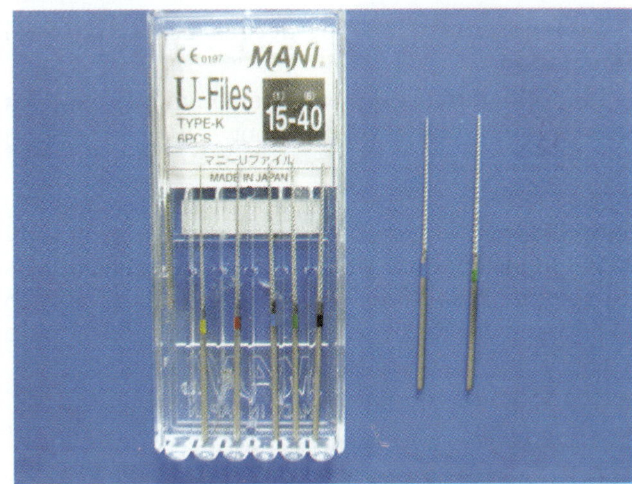

Fig. 11.19 Ultrasonic files

***Sonic handpieces*:** The sonic endodontic handpiece available is Micromega 1500 (or 1400). Like air rotor handpiece, it attaches to regular airline at a specified air pressure. The air pressure may be raised with an adjustable ring on the handpiece to give an oscillatory range of 1500–3000 cycles per second. The irrigant/coolant is delivered into preparation site from the handpiece. The three types of files that are used with Micromega 1500 are *Heliosonic, Shaper* and *Rispisonic*. The Shaper and Rispisonic are barbed while Heliosonic has a fluted cutting edge. The Heliosonic and Shaper files are numbered 15–40; whereas, Rispisonic files are numbered 1–6. All these instruments have safe ended non-cutting tips.

Sonic instruments produce an elliptical pattern of transverse oscillation when operated in air, a pattern similar to those powered ultrasonically (magnetostrictive). However, this large transverse motion is eliminated entirely and replaced by a true longitudinal vibration of the file, when the file is activated and loaded in the canal.

Ultrasonic and sonic instruments are similar in design in that they consist of a driver onto which endosonic file is clamped. The oscillatory pattern of the driver determines the nature of movement of the attached file. Although, the main driver oscillates longitudinally, the file vibrates transversely. This sets up a characteristic pattern of nodes and antinodes. Ultrasonic files of varying lengths are available to be used with the ultrasonic unit.

3. Rotary Instruments

Rotary instruments are constantly rotated at a fixed speed. They require another gadget known as handpiece for carrying the rotation. The rotary instrument can mainly be divided into two categories.

I. Instruments used for access cavity/coronal preparation

The following instruments are commonly used for access cavity/coronal preparation:

a. Burs

Conventional burs are used initially for access cavity preparation. Long shank burs and extra long shank burs are used in endodontics during preparation of deep pulp chamber and even preparation of coronal pulp spaces. These burs can also be used to remove the gutta-percha from the coronal aspect of the root canal.

The modified burs used in endodontics are:

***Endo Access bur*:** A specially designed bur *'Endo Access Bur'*, is a combination of round and cone-shaped coarse diamond, which allows access into the pulp chamber and also prepares the chamber walls (Fig. 11.20).

***Endo-Z bur*:** It is a long, tapered bur for easy access in pulp chamber after initial preparation. It has a non-cutting safe tip, which prevents its penetration in the pulp chamber. The cutting surface length is 9.0 mm and total length is 21 mm (Fig. 11.21).

***Munce Discovery bur*:** It has long, narrow, stiffer shaft design (Fig. 11.22) for better visibility, reduced impingement on deep walls and positive troughing control (34 mm for deep troughing and 31 mm for shallow troughing). It is available in 6 head sizes (#¼, #½, #1, #2, #3, #4).

***LN bur*:** It is a unique ½ round bur on a long neck (length 28 mm). Its design allows for deep drilling along side post or broken instruments (Fig. 11.23).

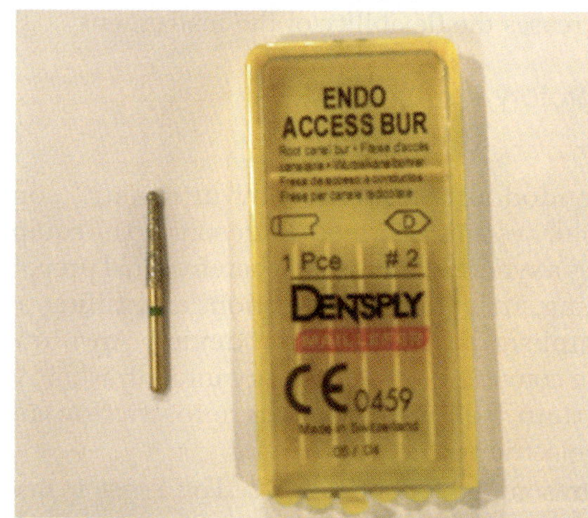

Fig. 11.20 Endo Access bur

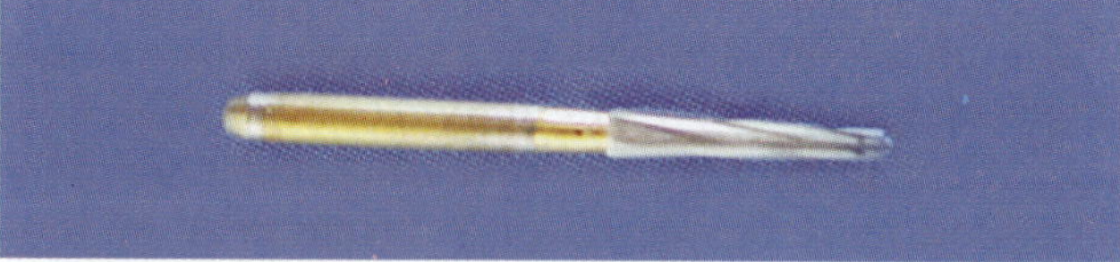

Fig. 11.21 Endo-Z bur

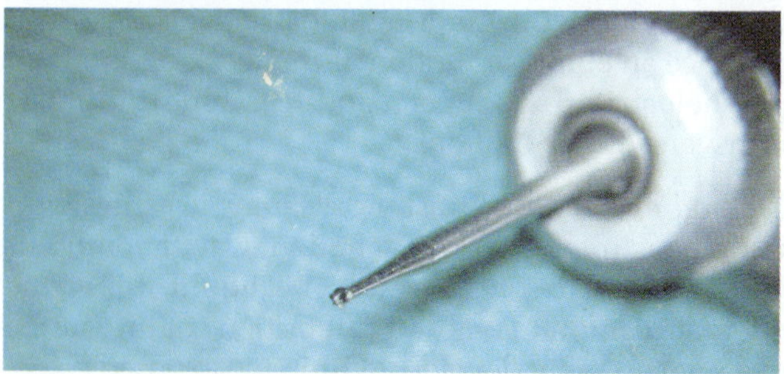

Fig. 11.22 Munce Discovery bur

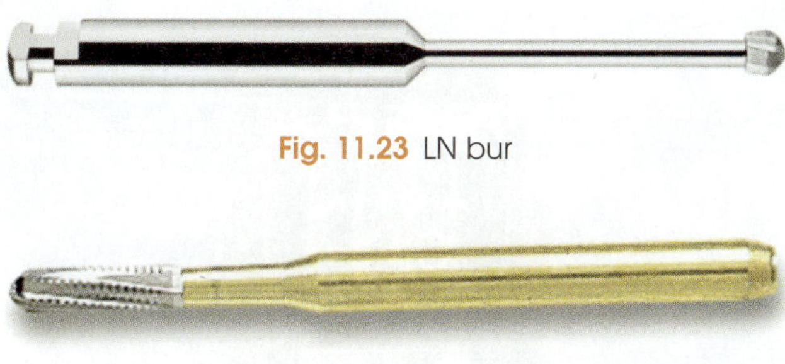

Fig. 11.23 LN bur

Fig. 11.24 Transmetal bur

Transmetal Bur: It is an extra fine cross-cut shape bur, which is designed to remove an old amalgam filling or to cut through metal/metal fused to porcelain crowns without shattering the porcelain or breaking the bur. The cutting surface is 5.0 mm and total length is 19 mm (Fig. 11.24).

b. Gates Glidden (GG) Drills

Gates Glidden drills are made of stainless steel and are available in two sizes, viz. short (28 mm) and regular (32 mm). They are number 1–6 (Fig. 11.25). The number on both the Gates and Peeso are denoted by the number of circumferential grooves located on the shaft just below the cut-out for the latch. The Gates Glidden drill is used to expand the canal orifice for easier instrumentation and obturation. It may be used to expand the coronal portion of root canals. Judicious use of the instrument is mandatory, since, it is liable to fracture.

c. Peeso Reamers

The make and number of the Peeso Reamers are same as that of Gates Glidden drill (flute length 8.5–9.0 mm). Peeso reamer is stiff instrument and does not follow root canal even if there is slight curvature. Its main use is to prepare the root canal for post and core preparation because of its effective lateral cutting. The recommended speed is 400–800 rpm. Gates Glidden drill and Peeso reamers are not end-cutting instruments (by definition they should be reamers and not drills). There is a nipple at the end of these instruments, which prevents cutting at the tip. When the nipple engages the wall of a curved canal, the drill just spins and does not cut apically (Fig. 11.26).

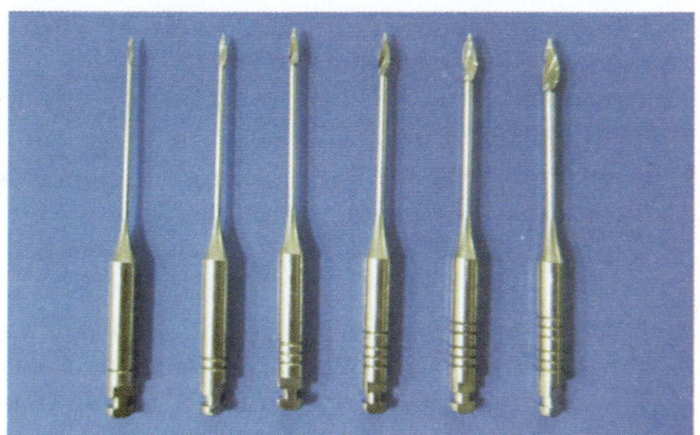

Fig. 11.25 Gates Glidden drills

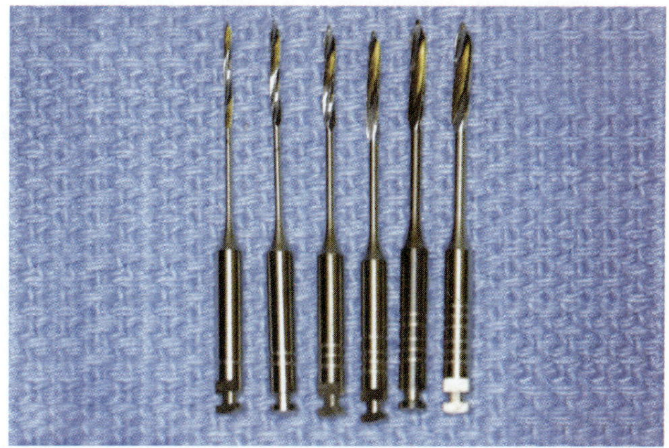

Fig. 11.26 Peeso Reamer

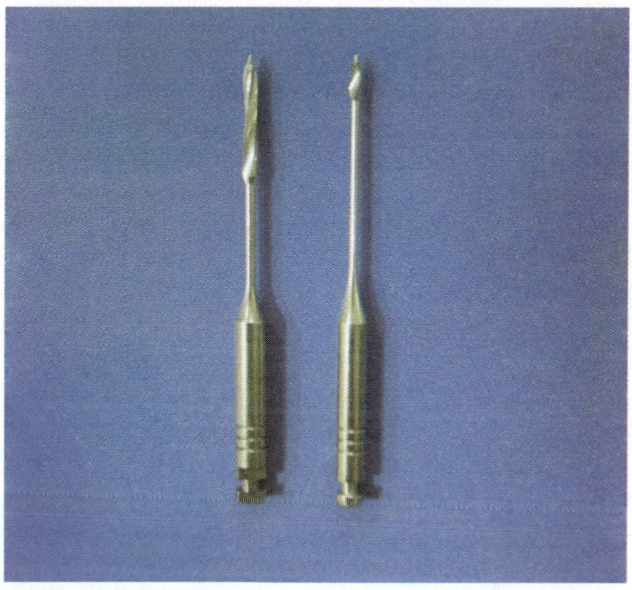

Fig. 11.27 Gates Glidden drill (right) has smaller head than peeso reamer (left)

The differences between Gates Glidden drills and Peeso reamers are:

i. Cutting head is much smaller on Gates Glidden drill as compared to Peeso reamers (Fig. 11.27)
ii. The shaft is thinner on Gates Glidden drill
iii. The diameter of heads are different for the same number instrument (Table 11.6) (Peeso reamer number 2 and Gates glidden drill number 3 are equivalent to size 90 files)

Table 11.6	Difference of sizes of Gates glidden drill and Peeso Reamer	
Size No.	*Gates glidden drill (mm)*	*Peeso Reamer (mm)*
1	0.5	0.7
2	0.7	0.9
3	0.9	1.1
4	1.1	1.3
5	1.3	1.5
6	1.5	1.7

II. Instruments used for root canal preparation

There are numerous rotary systems currently being used for preparation of root canals. Some systems also provide irrigation and obturation facility. The main are:

a. Profile System

Profile instruments, available both in stainless steel and Ni-Ti are the first product of Series 29 (Table 11.7). Initially hand instruments with 0.02 taper were marketed. Later, rotary instruments with 0.02 taper and also with 0.04 and 0.06 taper were developed (Fig. 11. 28). The size varies from 2 (0.129) to 10 (1.0 mm). The greater taper instruments were designated as *'orifice shaper'*.

Later, a series of greater taper files having 0.06, 0.08, 0.10 and 0.12 taper were designed, which provide continuous shape and requisite flare in the coronal one-third area.

The characteristic features are:

- The cross-sectional geometry is created by machining three equally spaced U-shaped grooves around the shaft of a tapered Ni-Ti wire.
- It has symmetric radial lands, which allow file to remain self-centered in the canal.
- There is a central parallel core that may account for enhanced flexibility compared with 'Quantec' and 'Protaper', which possesses a tapered central core.

Table 11.7	Series 29 instruments	
Number	*Size (mm)*	*Color code*
2	0.129	Silver
3	0.167	Gold
4	0.216	Red
5	0.279	Blue
6	0.360	Green
7	0.465	Brown
8	0.600	Silver
9	0.775	Orange
10	1.000	Red

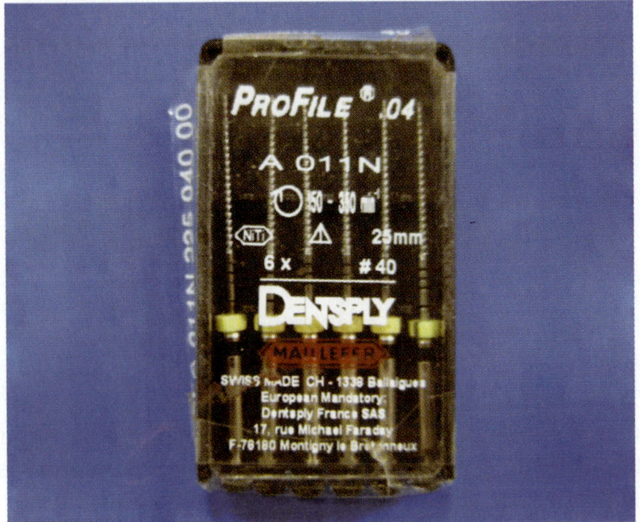

Fig. 11.28 Profile system

- It has 20° negative rake angle at cutting edge. The non-cutting tip guides the instrument into canal.

Clinical Performance

The clinical performance of the instrument is based on following features, viz. cutting efficiency, shaping ability, cleaning efficacy and effect of sodium hypochlorite.

i. *Cutting efficiency*: Cutting efficiency has been defined as *'the procedure of removal of simulated canal/ tooth structure with fluted instrument'*.

   The profile system has passive cutting blades. The slight negative rake angle and radial lands make file cut less aggressively than those having active cutting blades (Protaper, Hero 642, RaCe and POW-R) and those having semi-active cutting blades (Quantec).

ii. *Shaping ability*: It is established that the Ni-Ti rotary files stay centered and maintain canal curvature better than stainless steel hand files.

   Canal shaping with profile usually result in a round preparation and smear layer formation. It is shown that about 35–40% of canal surface remains untouched after complete instrumentation.

iii. *Cleaning efficiency*: The cleaning efficiency is comparable to hand files. The profile 'Series 29' files can be effective up to 70%, if used along with irrigant.

iv. *Effect of sodium hypochlorite*: Sodium hypochlorite irrigation may corrode the Ni-Ti instrument. The micropitting on instrument surface may lead to areas of stress concentration and crack formation.

Technique

The recommended sequence of use of profile instruments is as follows:

- Estimate working length of the canal.
- Create a glide path with a size 10–15 stainless steel K-files.
- Use appropriate sized *'Orifice Shapers'* in coronal one-third.
- Prepare root canal following crown-down technique [use profile instrument (taper/size) of 0.06/30, 0.06/25, 0.04/30 and 0.04/25 up to the resistance].
- Perform apical preparation with taper/size of 0.04/25 and 0.04/30.
- Finish with taper/size (0.06/25) short of working length, blending middle and apical portion.

b. Protaper System

The Protaper system provided less number of files. The number of files with a progressive taper (Protaper) was decreased to a set of six instruments: three shaping files for crown-down procedure and three finishing files for apical shaping. They are available as both hand (Fig. 11.29) and rotary files (Fig. 11.30).

The three shaping files are characterized by increasing taper over the whole length of their cutting blades. The finishing files are available in different diameters and a fixed taper over 3.0 mm to finish apical preparation.

The file design provides ideal and efficient shaping of coronal aspects of root canal.

The first file of Protaper system is called shaper X or SX. It lacks identification ring and is given gold colored handle. SX is available with cutting blade of 14 mm and a tip diameter of 0.19 mm.

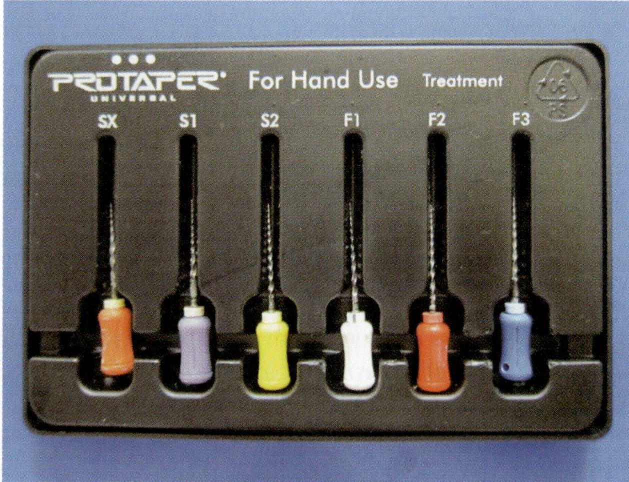

Fig. 11.29 Hand protaper

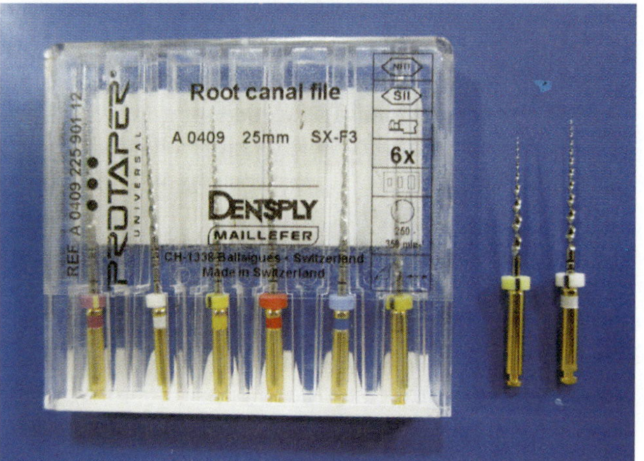

Fig. 11.30 Rotary protaper

Shaping file S1 has a purple identification ring and S2 has a white ring. The diameter at tip of S1 is 0.19 mm and of S2 is 0.20 mm. Both instruments have an increasing taper over whole working range, although the increase is not as aggressive as that of SX. S1 is designed to shape mainly in coronal section of root canal and S2 for middle section.

The finishing files F1, F2 and F3 are marked with a yellow, red and blue ring respectively. Their dimensions at D_0 are 0.20, 0.25 and 0.30 mm respectively.

The characteristic features are:

- The convex triangular cross-section reduces the contact area between blade of file and dentin, and serves to enhance the cutting action and improve safety by decreasing the torsional load.
- These files have a continuously changing helical angle and pitch over 14 mm of cutting blades. This effectively allows its blades to auger debris out of canal and prevents the instruments from inadvertently screwing into the canals.
- The shaping files have progressively tapered design which clinically improves flexibility and cutting efficiency.
- Increasing D_0 diameter and percentage taper correspondingly increases the stiffness of the instrument.
- All protaper shaping files have a progressively increasing taper; SX has the highest increase. At D_6, D_7, D_8 and D_9 the cross-sectional diameter increases from 0.50, 0.70, 0.90 and 1.10 mm respectively. The total increase of taper in SX from D_0 to D_9 is nine different tapers from 3.5 to 19%. S1 has an increasing taper from 2% on D_1 to 11% on D_{14}. S2 has an increasing taper from 4% on D_1 to 11.5% on D_{14}.

- The three finishing files have a fixed taper in first 3.0 mm from D_0 to D_3. (F1 7%, taper F2 8% taper and F3 of 9% taper. The remaining length of cutting blade has the reverse taper. The decreasing taper ensures a continuing flexibility within a file. The instruments provide better apical preparation in addition to shaping middle section also.
- The modified tip allows the instrument to follow the canal and find its way through loose tissues without damaging root canal walls.
- Protaper files have short (1.25 mm) handles as compared to other standard files (1.5 mm). Short handle serves to improve access into posterior regions.

Technique

- Initially 10 or 15 size hand file is used to negotiate the patency of the canal. The working length is established following routine procedures.
- Coronal shaping is carried out with SX file. If a light resistance is felt, the file is withdrawn and worked in a brushing motion against the root canal walls.
- S2 file is inserted preparing the middle half of the root canal. It can be used for apical preparation also. Apical preparation is carried out with finishing files.
- A uniform taper of 7% is produced in apical portion of canal using finishing files. The apical diameter of root canal is gauged with size 20 K-file. The instrument is inserted passively into the canal to working length. If the file binds in apical region, preparation is completed. If file is loose, F2 is used up to working length.

Protaper can be helpful in retreatment cases; finishing files are useful in complete removal of gutta-percha.

c. Light Speed (LSX) System

The light speed instruments are available in different sizes (size varies from 20 to 140). In between sizes such as 22.5, 27.5 and 32.5 respectively between 20 and 25, 25 and 30 and between 30 and 35 and so on are also available. The half sizes are color coded exactly as previous size along with white or black markings or engraved rings on instrument handles (Fig. 11.31). The instruments are available in three lengths, viz. 21, 25 and 31 mm.

The characteristic features are:

- Light speed cutting heads are short and have three radial lands and three U-shaped special grooves between radial lands.

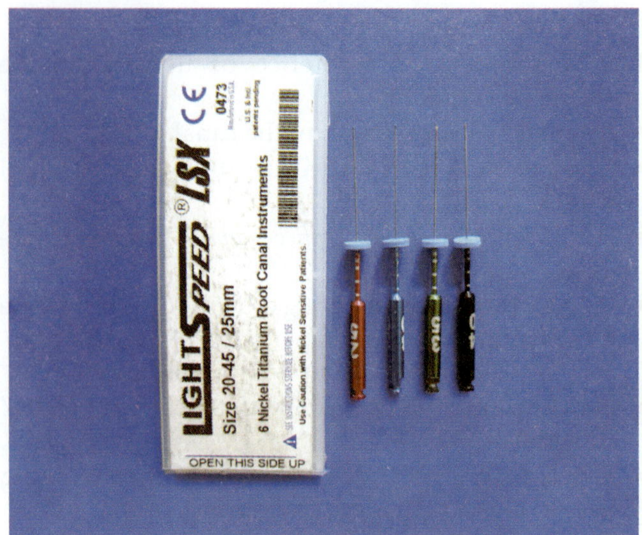

Fig. 11.31 Light speed instruments

- The cutting heads are 0.25 mm (size 20) and 2.25 mm (size 40) long. Light speed is only rotary system whose cutting heads have three different geometric shapes. The first five light speed instruments have short, non-cutting pilot tip and 75° cutting angle. The size 32.5 instrument has a slightly longer non-cutting pilot tip and 33° cutting angle. All other instruments have longer non-cutting pilot tips and a 21° cutting angle.
- The instruments have thin, taperless, non-cutting shafts (this design maximizes flexibility and enables the instrument to negotiate curves.)
- The shank is marked with rings that indicate distances from the instrument's tip. For 21 and 25 mm instruments, junction of shaft and shank is 18 mm from tip and for 31 mm instrument, distance is 22 mm.
- 21 mm instruments have only one ring in shank (20 mm from tip) and 25 mm instruments have three rings indicating distance of 20, 22 and 24 mm from tip. In contrast, 31 mm instruments have four rings indicating distance of 24, 26 and 28 and 30 from tip junctions.

The differences in light speed and conventional hand files are tabulated in Table 11.8.

Technique

Light speed instruments require a straight line access to mid-root areas. The root canal walls are shaped using H-files, which facilitate rotating instruments unhindered to mid-root area. The working length should be recorded using small sized K-files.

Once a light speed instrument has reached its desired length, do not linger at that point and immediately

Table 11.8 Differences in light speed and conventional hand files

	Light speed instrument	*Conventional hand files*
Metal/alloy	Ni-Ti	Stainless steel
Length of cutting head	0.25 to 2.25 mm	16 mm
Tip angles	Varies 21, 33 and 75°	Similar for all files
Non-cutting pilot tip	Present	Absent
Intermediate sizes	Available	Not available
Minimum size	20	08
Maximum size	140	140

withdraw the rotating instrument from the canal. Sequence of instrument is important as for other techniques.

There are three methods of using light speed instruments:

i. Conventional technique
ii. Zurich technique
iii. Hybrid technique

i. *Conventional technique*

The conventional technique involves four steps:

Step 1. Determining initial light speed size: A light sped instrument can reach working length if its cutting head is smaller than canal's diameter at the constriction. For example, size 25 light speed instrument if reaches working length indicates that canal's diameter is larger than size 25. Gauging continues with sequentially larger sizes until a light speed instrument does not reach working length. If size 25 reaches working length but size 27.5 does not, then size 27.5 is termed 'first light speed instrument'.

Step 2. Determine master apical size: After determining the first light speed instrument size, appropriate size of instrument required for apical preparation is determined. The instrument that takes at least 12 pecks to reach working length is 'master apical instrument'. This is known as *"12 Pecks Rule"*.

Step 3. Complete apical instrumentation: After determining master apical instrument size, complete the apical preparation by using next light speed size that is 4.0 mm shorter than working length. If obturating with standard gutta-percha cones, step-back 4.0 mm with sequentially larger light speed instrument so that each length is 1.0 mm shorter than previous instrument. This prepares the apical 5.0 mm of canal with a taper matching that of a standardized cone. Half size instrumentation is also carried out in routine.

If master apical size is 40, step back in 1.0 mm increment to at least size 65 (25 plus initial master apical size).

Step 4. Recapitulation: The canal is recapitulated using respective master apical instrument to working length.

ii. *Zurich technique*

The steps followed in this technique are:

Step 1. Coronal pre-flaring: After canal orifices are located, their coronal openings are enlarged using Gates glidden drills. Initially, 4.0–6.0 mm coronal flaring is achieved.

Step 2. Determining initial apical instrument: Working length is determined using size 15 stainless steel K-files. Then light speed instruments are used. The first few light speed instruments may not bind within the canal. The instrument which first feels resistance in the canal is termed *'Initial apical instrument'*.

Step 3. Determining master apical instrument: All light speed instruments used after initial apical instruments are called *'binding instruments'*. They are used with controlled forward (1.0–2.0 mm) and backward (2.0–4.0 mm) *'pecking movement'*. The forward motion reams the canal; whereas, backward motion tends to clean as it retreats into fresh irrigant. These instruments are used sequentially from smaller to large size. The last instrument used to prepare apical area (may be 6–12 light speed instruments larger than the initial instrument) termed *'Master apical instrument'*.

Step 4. Step back and recapitulation: After master apical instrument is finalized, the step back preparation is initiated. The last step-back instrument is termed *'Final instrument'*.

Finally, the canal is recapitulated using respective master apical instrument to working length.

iii. *Hybrid technique*

As the name indicates, initial preparation is carried out with hand instruments and final preparation with light speed ones.

d. Quantec System

The Quantec system provides graduated taper technique, whereby a series of varying tapers are used to prepare a single canal. The instruments are used in high torque, gear reduction and slow speed handpiece. Quantec files consist of series of 10 graduated Ni-Ti taper files; taper ranges from 0.02 to 0.12. The files are used in conventional crown-down fashion. Taper design 0.08, 0.10 and 0.12 are used for coronal flaring and others for middle and apical areas accordingly. These are available in two types of tip design, viz. non-cutting (LX) and safe-cutting (SC). The LX (non-cutting) tip is ideal for routine cases and in delicate apical areas, whereas SC (safe-cutting) tip is utilized for calcified and constricted canals.

The characteristic features are:

- Slightly positive rake or blade angle (designed to shave rather than scrap dentin).
- Flute design includes a 30° helical angle.
- Wide radial lands prevent crack formation and reduce the rotational friction.

e. Hero 642

As the name implies, the files are available in 0.06, 0.04 and 0.02 taper (642). 0.06 taper is available in 21 and 25 mm length; whereas, 0.04 and 0.02 taper are available in 21, 25 and 29 mm length. The routinely used speed is 300–600 rpm. The progressively increasing diameter and distance between the flutes facilitate smooth guiding without binding in the canal wall. Hero 642 can be combined with sonic MM 1500 handpiece.

The characteristic features are:

- Triangular cutting edges with no radial land
- Positive rake angle (effective cutting)
- Bigger inner core (better resistance to fracture)
- Variable pitch
- Safe tip (stays in centre of the canal).

Hero apical: Hero apical instruments are used for the enlargement of apical one-third of root canals, especially where greater diameters and tapers is required then offered by Hero 642 and Hero shapers. The Hero apical series comprises two instruments both with size of 0.30 mm with a taper of 0.06 and 0.08 respectively.

Endoflare: Endoflare is Ni-Ti instrument used for coronal flaring. The Endoflare is limited to the coronal-third of the canal. The instrument has tip diameter of 0.25 mm and 0.12 taper. The endoflare has same characteristics as that of Hero shaper. It has a safe non-active tip.

Technique

- Crown-down technique is followed in routine.
- Half of the working length is prepared using 0.06 taper.
- 0.04 taper is used 3.0–4.0 mm short of apex and 0.02 taper is used at the apical end.

In difficult canals, smaller size of instrument is preferred.

f. K3 System

The K3 system (Ni-Ti instrument, triple fluted and asymmetrical) includes K3 files and K3 body shapers (Fig. 11.32). The files are available in taper 0.02, 0.04 and 0.06; whereas, body shapers have taper 0.08, 0.10 and 0.12. The body shapers have a shorter taper length (apical 8.0 mm). The fluting on straight (non-tapered) shank do not cut effectively. The remaining flutes are parallel, which increase file flexibility. A modified version, K3 XF, provides better flexibility and resistance to cyclic fatigue (R-phase technology). The differences of U-file and K3 file are tabulated in Table 11.9.

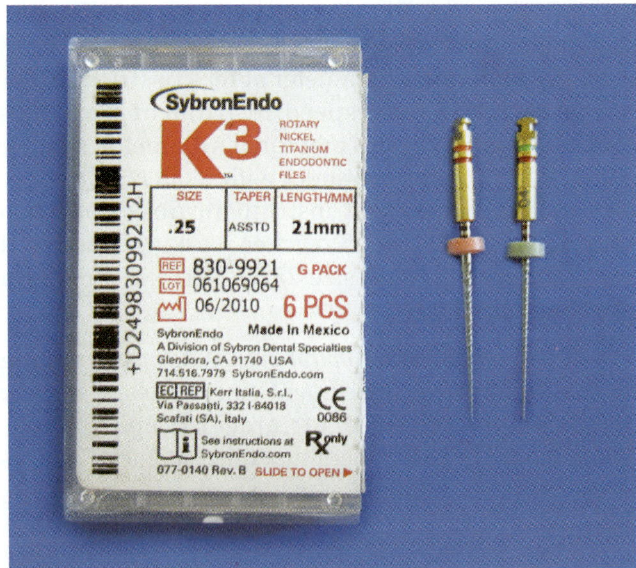

Fig. 11.32 K3 system

Table 11.9 Differences in U-file and K3 file

U-file (profile, GT, light speed)	*K3 file*
• Symmetrically placed lands	• Asymmetrically placed lands
• Equal land widths, flute widths and depths	• Unequal land widths; flute widths and depth
• Negative rake angle	• Positive rake angle
• Symmetrical cross-section	• Asymmetrical cross-section

The characteristic features are:

- Color coding to distinguish between different tip sizes and tapers [0.04 (green) 0.06 (orange)].
- A slight positive rake angle provides more effective cutting.
- A variable core diameter enhances flexibility over the entire cutting length.
- A series of three radial lands with a relief behind two of three lands reduces friction on canal walls.
- Asymmetrical flutes provide superior canal tracking; virtually eliminating transportation and aid in preventing the file from screwing into canal.
- A safe-ended cutting tip.
- Short file handle (access handle—5.0 mm short) without affecting working length of file.

Technique

- K3 body shapers are used to enlarge coronal one-thirds of the root canal. Different taper can be utilized in varying diameter of canals.
- Initial exploration should be carried out in the presence of EDTA gel along with repeated irrigation. The initial chosen body shaper is followed by successively smaller body shaper. Used in succession, K3 files may take the operator to junction of middle and apical third. The subsequent K3 files (0.02, 0.04 and 0.06 taper) allow greater penetration into apical area.
- The apical area is explored first with hand instrument to determine the apical canal diameter, curvatures, calcification, patency and ease of negotiation. Beginning with size 6 to 10 K files, operator should slowly and gently attempt to reach estimated working length as determined by tactile sense and radiographic interpretation.
- After true working length is established, a glide path for subsequent K3 files is established to approximate size 15 to 20 K files. Irrigation and recapitulation should be frequent during apical preparation. K3 files are introduced with larger to smaller tip sizes till working length is reached.

g. Endo Sequence System

The Endo Sequence system is available in both 0.04 (size 15–60) and 0.06 (size 15–50) taper files, with lengths of 21, 25 and 31 mm. It is also available in both single instrument packs and procedural packs (small, medium and large). An initial rotary instrument called an 'Expeditor' is included with the system, which determines the initial canal diameter. The expeditor is a size-27 file (length 21.0 mm and taper 0.011). These files are best suited at a speed of 500–600 rpm.

The characteristic features are:

- The file design provides for alternating contact points, along the instrument's cutting length. The alternate contact points limit its contact with the dentinal walls (thereby reducing torque) and simultaneously promote disengagement.
- The file has precision non-cutting tip that becomes fully engaged 1.0 mm from the tip (D_1).
- The file utilizes variable pitch and variable helical angles. The files with a constant pitch have a tendency to create 'suck-down' (tendency of the file to be pulled apically as it engages the canal walls). Constant helical angles may lead to debris accumulation, subsequently leading to file separation. Variable helical angles aid in removing debris coronally out of the canal.

Technique

- The patency of root canal is confirmed with a small sized file.
- The expeditor is introduced into the canal and taken to initial engagement. If engagement is met within the apical half of the Expeditor's cutting shank, the 'small' Endo Sequence package is opened. If Expeditor advance to midway point before engagement is met, then a 'medium' package is selected. If the Expeditor does not meet any engagement, or is loose at full insertion, then a 'large' package is utilized.
- Begin the crown-down process with the largest file from the selected package. After the second largest rotary file has been used, determine the working length with a size 10 hand file (working length is generally determined after the second rotary file).
- Once the working length has been determined, complete the preparation in a straight crown-down fashion, taking each rotary file to engagement. The first Endo Sequence file to reach working length with resistance completes the preparation.

h. RaCe

'RaCe', is acronym for reamer (R) with alternating (a) cutting (C) edges (e). The instrument is available in 0.02, 0.04, 0.06, 0.08 and 0.10 taper design (Fig. 11.33a and b).

The cross-section of the instrument is triangular with large flutes. These instruments are flexible. The electro-chemical surface polishing decreases distortion and fatigue.

The flutes of RaCe instruments with regular helical angles will only touch the inner surface of elbow of a canal curvature for a short distance. The straight part (straight flutes, no helical angles) of a RaCe instrument might touch the inner surface of an elbow, which causes file strengthening.

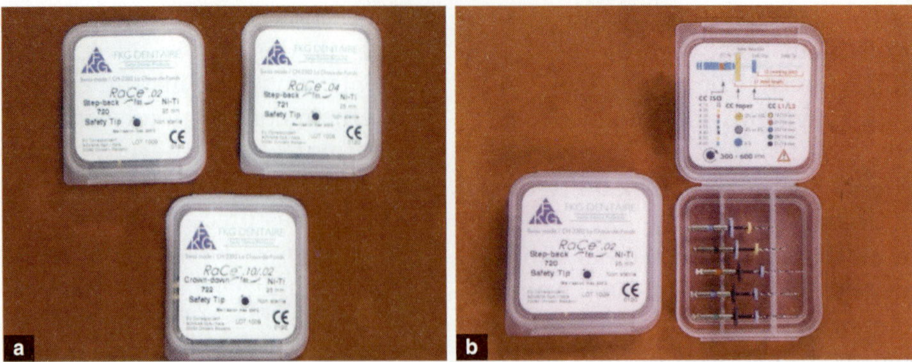

Fig. 11.33a and b RaCe file

The characteristic features are:

- Special torque controlled motor not required.
- Alternate cutting edges provide anti-screwing design.
- The safety tip ensures guidance/centering in the canal.
- Safety memory disc help discarding the instrument at right time (Fig 11.34).

Technique

- The manufacturer has provided the gadget (Fig. 11.35), which measures the curvature of the root canal. Only three types of curvatures are recognized, viz. simple (S), medium (M) and difficult (D). The gadget is placed over the preoperative radiograph and the coinciding curvature is noted (Fig. 11.36).

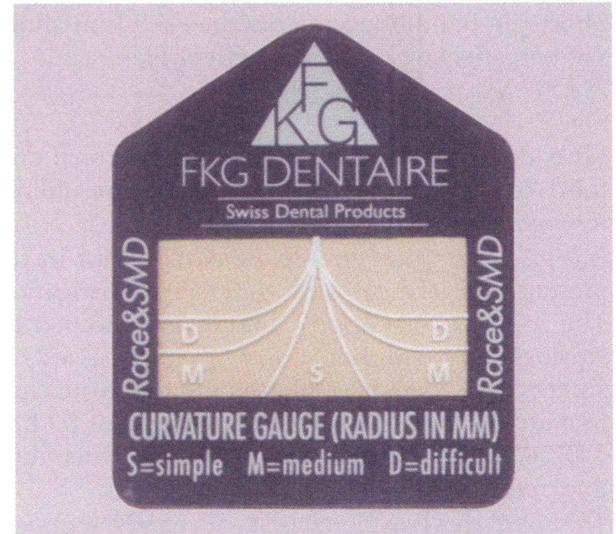

Fig. 11.35 Gadget to measure curvature

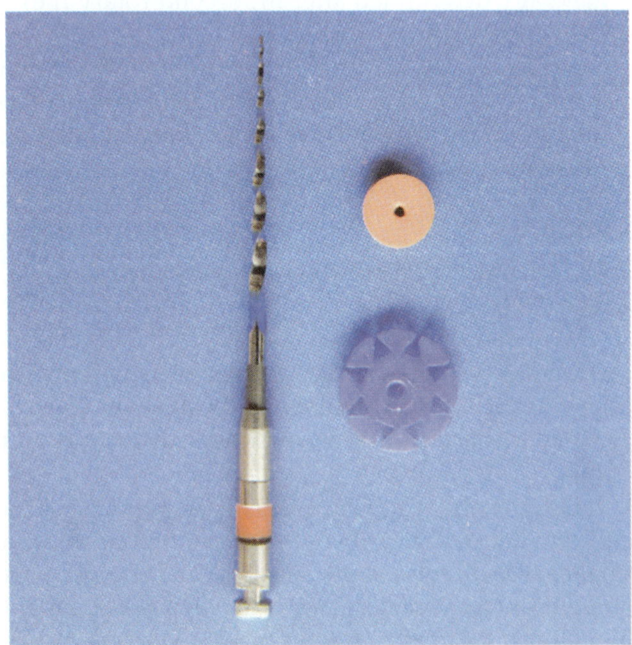

Fig. 11.34 Components of RaCe file (blue-safety memory disc)

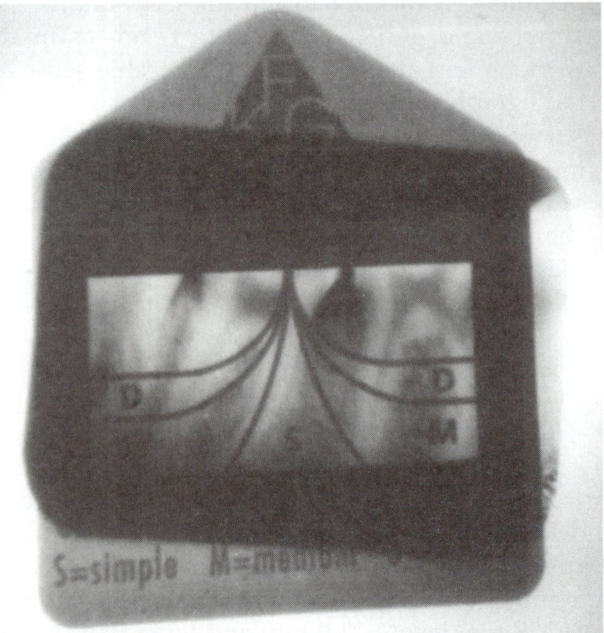

Fig. 11.36 Measuring curvature

- The manufacturer has also provided the charts, which signifies the timings as to when the instrument is to be discarded (Fig. 11.37a and b). For example, using 0.02 taper RaCe instrument (no. 15), in simple curvature canals, two petals of safety memory disc are to be torn. (This means such an instrument in these similar conditions can be used only for four times, since safety memory disc has only eight petals.) Similarly, 0.04 taper RaCe instrument (no. 25) in difficult curvature can be used for only once, since all eight petals need to be torn after use.
- The coronal flaring is carried out with 0.10 taper instrument, followed by 0.08 taper. Subsequently, mid preparation is carried out with 0.06, 0.04 taper and apical preparation with 0.04 and 0.02 taper [the initial instrument can be modified depending upon the canal dimensions; however, sequence must be followed (Fig. 11.38a to f)].

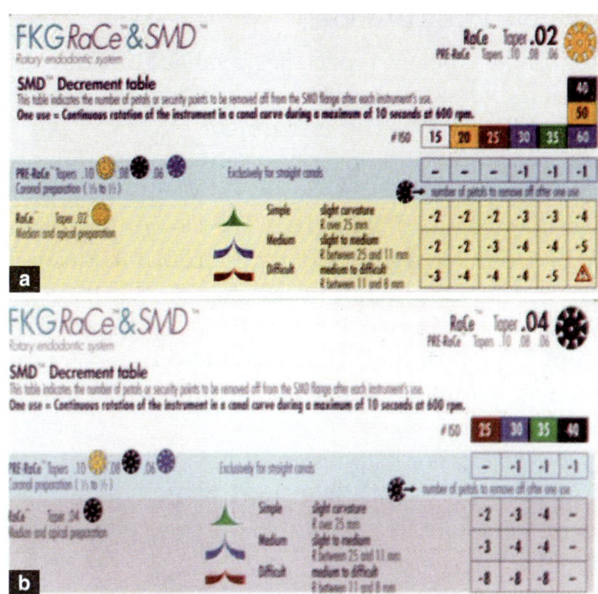

Fig. 11.37a and b Charts guiding the operator as to when discard the instrument

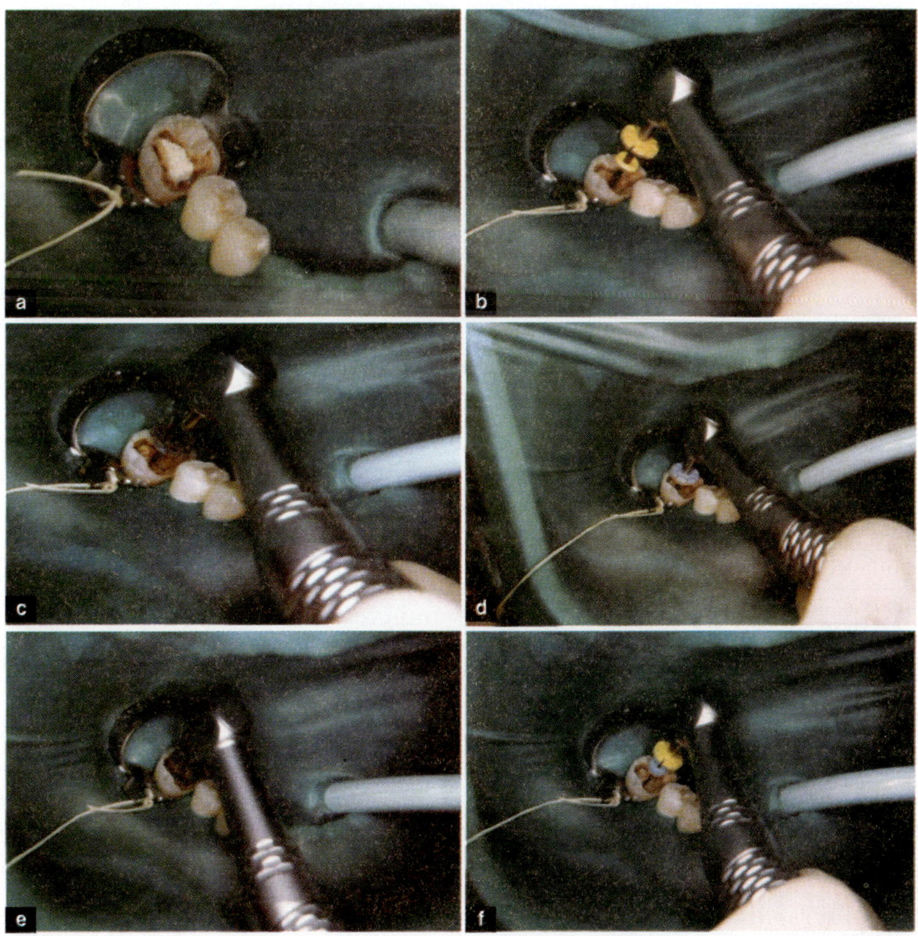

Fig. 11.38 Clinical use of RaCe: (a) Preoperative; (b) Canal preparation with 0.10 taper RaCe file; (c) Canal preparation with 0.08 taper RaCe file; (d) Canal preparation with 0.06 taper RaCe file; (e) Canal preparation with 0.04 taper RaCe file; (f) Canal preparation with 0.02 taper RaCe file

11

i. Variable Taper (V-taper)

The variable taper (V-taper) files, available in both hand and rotary versions, are having short handle and color coding (Fig. 11.39). The instrument facilitates deeper apical shapes with more conservative access. Files are available in three sizes (length 21, 25 and 29 mm) and apical diameter 0.2, 0.25 and 0.3. The files are designated as V10 (from 0 to 4 mm 10% taper; from 4 to 8 mm 5% taper and from 8 to 12 mm 2% taper), V8 (from 0 to 4 mm 8% taper; from 4 to 8 mm 4% taper and from 8 to 12 mm 2% taper) and V6 (from 0 to 4 mm 6% taper; from 4 to 8 mm 3% taper and from 8 to 12 mm 2% taper).

The characteristic features are:

- Parabolic cross-section makes the instrument extremely safe, resistance to fracture, efficient and flexible.
- Tip is non-cutting (prevent ledging and transportation)
- Neutral rake angle
- Variable pitch eliminates screw-in effect and breakage
- No radial land (land causes dragging, friction and heat build-up).

Technique

The preparation is completed with less number of files [30/10, 25/08, 20/06], for large, medium and small canal respectively.

j. Liberators

Liberator is a straight fluted file (all rotary files are helical fluted). The chances of self-threading into canal and separation decrease with the use of liberator (Fig. 11.40). Helical flutes are responsible for self-threading of the instrument into the canal, subsequently separation. Usually used for retreatment, since gutta-percha removal is easy.

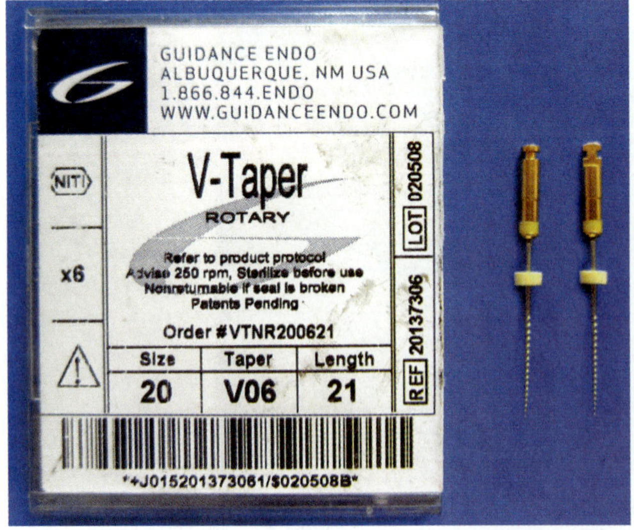

Fig. 11.39 V-taper rotary files

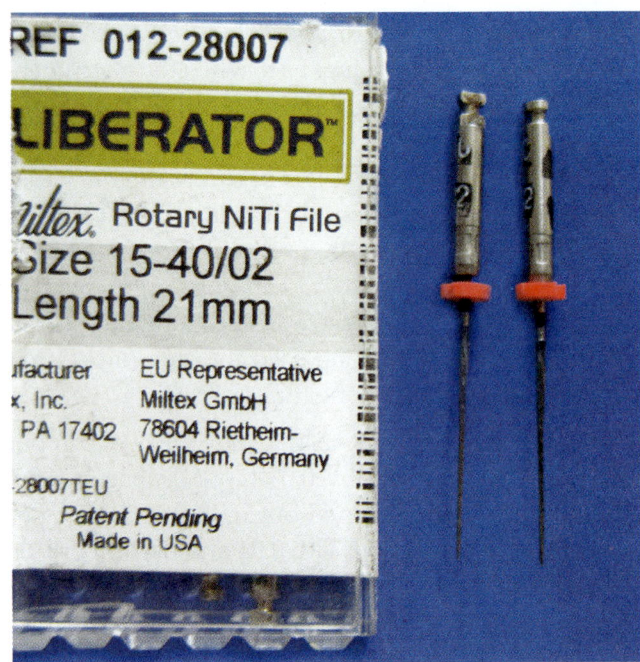

Fig. 11.40 Liberator rotary files

The characteristic features are:

- Cross-section is triangular and lacks radial land, which provides sharp cutting edges.
- File operates at higher speeds (1000–2000 rpm).
- Tip is non-cutting, which minimizes ledging, transportation and helps centering the file in the canal.
- Debris removal is easy.

Technique

The liberator can be used both for step-back technique and crown-down technique.

- Initial exploration/glide path is achieved by smaller number hand files.
- Gates glidden drills are used for coronal preparation, starting from larger number to smaller number.
- The middle and apical-third is prepared following the sequence as followed in routine crown-down technique.
- For step-back technique, the sequence apical to coronal is followed, with smaller number files to larger number files.
- Continuous irrigation is preferred.

11

k. MTwo

These are Ni-Ti files; the initial set includes four instruments with variable tip sizes ranging from size 10 to size 25 and taper ranging from 0.04 to 0.06 (Fig. 11.41a and b). The instrument is available in three sizes; i.e. 21, 25 and 31 mm with 16 mm cutting blade. Extended cutting blades up to 21 mm are also available for simultaneous cutting of coronal and middle parts. MTwo retreatment files are also available, viz. MTwo R 15/0.05 and MTwo R 25/0.05 with active tip, which penetrates better in obturating material.

The characteristic features are:

- Colored ring on handle identifies the size.
- Number of groove rings on handle identifies instrument taper [one ring (04 taper), two rings (05 taper), three rings (06 taper) and four rings (07 taper)].
- Tip is non-cutting, minimizing ledging, transportation, etc.
- Helical angle is variable and spiral pitch is constant for smaller instruments.

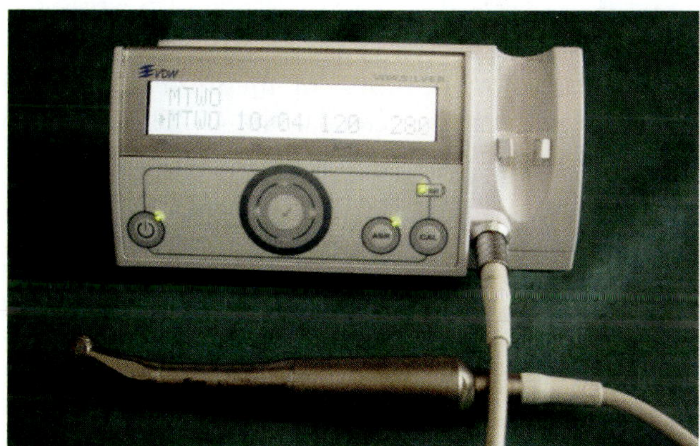

Fig. 11.41a MTwo motor and handpiece

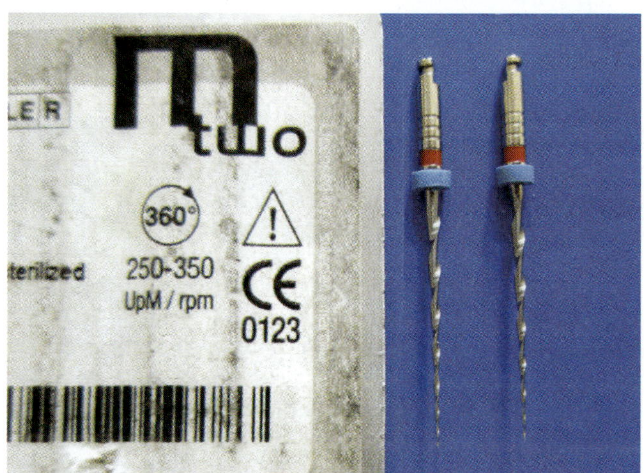

Fig. 11.41b MTwo files

Technique

- Instrument is used at the speed of 300 rpm.
- Glide path is established using small stainless steel K-files.
- The basic sequence of MTwo files is followed, which provides 25/06 shape to the canal. If need be, larger instruments with 0.07 taper can also be used. The technique employed with MTwo is designated as *'simultaneous technique'*, wherein crown to apex preparation protocol is followed (using smaller instruments before using larger instrument as is carried out in step-back technique).

l. EndoWave System

The EndoWave system provides improved quality and increased efficiency. The files can adapt to different shapes of canal, reducing the risk of canal aberrations even in curved canals.

The files are available in sizes 15 to 35 for normal canals and 15 to 25 for curved canals. Corresponding taper 0.02 to 0.08 is available for normal canal and taper 0.02 to 0.06 for curved canal. The usual length of the file is 19, 21 and 25 mm. The ISO color coding identifies the size.

The characteristic features are:

- Triangular design provides sharp cutting edges.
- Negative rake angle.
- Rounded (non-cutting) tip ensures maximum safety.
- Files are conditioned electrochemically, making them smooth and harder (can be used at higher speed).

Technique

Crown-down technique is followed with EndoWave files. Coronal preparation is carried out with size 35 | 08 taper followed by middle and apical preparation with 30 | 06 and 25 | 06 files. Curved canals can be prepared with 0.04 taper or 0.02 taper depending upon the need.

m. FlexMaster

Flexmaster is a rotary Ni-Ti instrument having a convex triangular cross-section with sharp cutting edges. The instrument is available in three tapers, viz. 0.02, 0.04 and 0.06. A FlexMaster initial instrument (Introfile) has a taper of 11. The tip is rounded and self-centric. Taper 0.02 instruments are available in size 20 to 70, while taper 0.04 and 0.06 are in sizes 20 to 40. The different tapers are identified by the number of grooves/rings in the shaft. The sizes are ISO color coded.

Technique

- A torque control motor is required (the recommended speed is 150–300 rpm).
- The usual sequence followed is size 30 | 06 followed by 25/06, 20/06 and 30/04. The same can be modified depending upon the canal size.
- The apical shaping is carried out with 20/02, 25/02, 30/02 and 35/02 size taper of files.

n. Miscellaneous Rotary Systems

i. Rigid Body Shapers (RBS)

Rigid body shapers consist of a series of four Ni-Ti rotary reamer, viz. No.1 (0.61 mm at tip), No. 2 (0.66 mm at tip), No. 3 (0.76 mm at tip) and No. 4 (0.86 mm at tip). These instruments develop a parallel canal shape.

ii. Pow-R Files

Pow-R files are available in both 0.02 and 0.04 taper. These instruments are available in standard ISO sizes as well as in half sizes 17.5, 22.5, 27.5, 32.5 and 37.5. They follow standard ISO color codes as well.

iii. Titanium Rotary Files

The files are having a gradual taper to accommodate the cross-cut design in middle and coronal one-third of file which optimizes canal flare and increases flexural strength. This design makes the instrument highly efficient. All the instruments and stoppers are color coded with groove marked shanks and depth markers. The files are available in a box containing six instruments. The box has a measurement gauge incorporated on one side.

The usual taper of the file is:

- For shaping coronal one-third
  - Orifice widener (14% taper)
  - Coronal shaper (9% taper)
- For shaping middle one-third
  - M file (4–7% taper)
- For shaping apical-third
  - (Blue) A-file (apical finisher for straight canals) (3–6%)
  - (Red) AF file (apical finisher for curved canals) (3–6%)
  - (Yellow) AXF file (apical finisher for severely curved canals) (3–6%).

The characteristic features are:

- Non-cutting tip which minimizes risk of apical and lateral perforations as well as ledge formation.
- Variable helical angle which prevents wedging during canal preparation.
- Cross-cut design incorporated into middle and coronal one-third of instrument, results in rapid débridement with no pressure. It makes the instrument highly efficient and fast.
- Triangular cross-section ensures efficient cutting.

iv. Hyflex X-file

Hyflex X-file provides unique double-fluting, which enhances cutting efficiency for quick and easy instrumentation. The file is available in sizes 8 to 80 in 21 or 25 mm length with ISO color coded handles. The tip is non-cutting and the rake angle is negative (Fig. 11.42).

v. Xtreme Reamer with Rapid Safe Shaping

The instrument is meant for aggressive use even at higher revolutions because of hybrid cutting flute design and annular groove safety feature. The annular ring is present near shaft where fracture normally occurs.

The routine crown-down technique is followed. Orifice opener (30/0.09 taper) can be used to create a funnel shape coronal aspect. Appropriate sized reamer is used to shape the canal; For example, no. 25 (red) for small canals, no. 30 (blue) for medium canals and no. 35 (green) for large canals. No. 40 (black) is also available for very large canals.

vi. Plastic Endo

Plastic Endo is polymer endodontic instruments covered with diamond coatings. The available instruments are F-file, P-file, P-Tip Surgical and Vibe Ultrasonic Piezo unit. The files are for single use only.

The files have unique design and diamond coating; enable the file to agitate sodium hypochlorite and remove remaining dentinal debris without further enlarging the canal.

The design features of current rotary systems are summarized in Table 11.10.

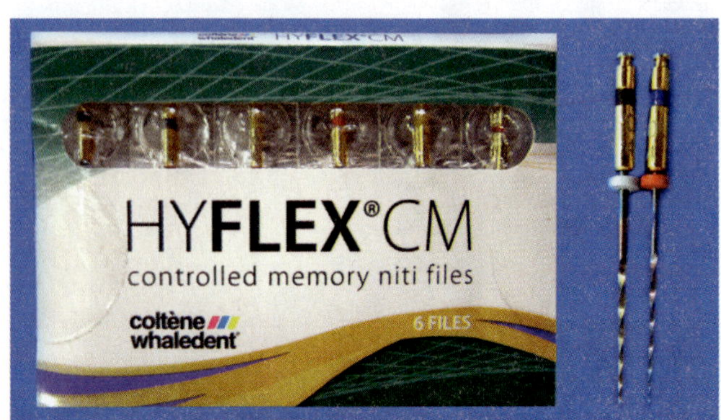

Fig. 11.42 Hyflex file

Table 11.10 Current rotary systems: cross-section design, taper and other characteristic features

Rotary system	*Manufacturer*	*Cross-sectional design*	*Diagrammatic representation*	*Tip design*	*Taper*	*Characteristic features*
ProFile	Dentsply	• Triple-U shape • Neutral rake angle		Non-cutting	Fixed taper (2, 4 and 6%)	• 20-degree helix angle • Constant pitch
ProTaper	Dentsply	• Triangular cutting edges • No radial lands • F3, F4, F5 files (finishing files) have U-flutes		Non-cutting	Variable taper	• Balanced pitch and helix angle • Better flexibility • No problem of screw-in effect in the root canal
ProTaper Next	Dentsply	• Variable cross-section (increasing and decreasing taper design) • Rectangular cross-section except in Protaper next 1, which has square cross-section		Non-cutting	PT Next 1 Tip 0.17 mm/04 taper PT Next 2 Tip 0.25 mm/06 taper PT Next 3 Tip 0.3 mm/07 taper PT Next 4 Tip 0.4 mm/06 taper PT Next 5 Tip 0.5 mm/06 taper	• M-wire technology reduces fatigue and resist fracture • Improved flexibility
Light speed instruments	San AntonioTX	• Triple-U shape • Radial lands		Non-cutting	Uniform taper Produces a tapered shape	• Thin, flexible non-cutting shaft • Short cutting head
Quantec Series	Sybron Endo	• S-shape design • Double helical flute • Positive rake angle • Two wide radial lands		Cutting (SC) Non-cutting (LX)	Fixed taper (2, 4, 6, 8, 10 and 12%)	• Progressively larger flute space as moved towards distal to the cutting blade
Hero 642	MicroMega	• Triangular shape • No radial land • Positive rake angle		Non-cutting	Fixed taper (2, 4 and 6%)	• Variable pitch • 12–16 mm cutting portion • Improved cutting efficiency
K3	Sybron Endo	• Positive rake angle • Three radial lands		Non-cutting	Fixed taper (2, 4 and 6%)	• Variable pitch • Variable core diameter • Improved cutting efficiency and minimum friction
FlexMaster	VDW	• Triangular shape • No radial lands		Non-cutting	Fixed taper (2, 4 and 6%) 11% taper in initial file	• Individual helical angles prevents screw-in effect
RaCe	FKG	• Triangular shape (except RaCe 15/02 and 20/02 which have a square shape) • Two alternating cutting edges • No radial lands		Non-cutting	Fixed taper (2, 4, 6, 8 and 10%)	• Alternating cutting edges improves cutting efficiency • Flexibility is not effective, especially in large files

(Contd...)

Table 11.10 Current rotary systems: cross-section design, taper and other characteristic features (*Contd.*)

Rotary system	*Manufacturer*	*Cross-sectional design*	*Diagrammatic representation*	*Tip design*	*Taper*	*Characteristic features*
EndoWave	J. Morita	• Triangular shape • Negative rake angle		Non-cutting	Fixed taper (2, 4, 6 and 8%)	• Continuous wave design (reduce screw-in effect)
Mtwo	Padova	• S-shape design • No radial lands • Minimum core width		Non-cutting	Fixed taper (4, 5, 6 and 7%)	• Variable pitch • Steep helical angle
Endosequence	Brasseler	• Triangular shape		Non-cutting	Fixed taper (4 and 6%)	• Alternating contact points • Variable pitch • Variable helical angle • Precision tip
V-taper	Guidance endo	• Safe core parabolic		Non-cutting	• Variable taper	• Variable pitch • No radial land
Liberator	Miltex	• Triangular shape		Non-cutting	Fixed taper (2, 4, 6, 8 and 10%)	• Straight fluted file • Variable pitch, no radial land
WaveOne/Wave One Gold	Dentsply	• Convex triangular cross-section • Tips modified to follow canal curvatures • Reciprocation movements		Non-cutting	• Sizes 21, 25, 31 mm • Taper (6 and 8%)	• Wave One Gold has improved flexibility • Reciprocation prevents instrument advancing to its plastic limits
Reciproc system	VDW	• S-shaped cross-section • Two cutting edges		Non-cutting	• Three sizes R25, R40, R50 • Taper 08, 06, 05	• Instrument provide greater flexibility • Increases resistance to cyclic fatigue and improved cutting efficiency
Twisted Files	Kerr	• Triangular cross-section • Positive rake angle		Non-cutting	• Available in five tapers 04, 06, 08, 010 and 012 • Length 23 and 27 mm	• Improved flexibility with less resistance in the canal • R-phase technology resist fracture
OneShape file	Micromega	• Variable cross-section along the blade • 3-cutting edge (apical) 2-cutting edge (coronal)		Non-cutting	• One shape Endoflare 25 mm/012 • One shape glide path 14 mm/03 • One shape shaping 25 mm/06, 30/06, 37/06	• Minimum risk of separation • Flexible, preferred in curved canals

Clinical Recommendations

The operator should follow certain principles in order to avoid or minimize fracture and other associated problems with the use of instruments:

- New instruments should be checked for any metal residues or surface debris prior to use. Such residue may act as areas of stress concentration and lead to fracture.
- The angle and canal curvature should be assessed properly. The operator should proceed cautiously during preparation of curved canals.
- A straight line access should be achieved prior to instrumentation.
- The patency of the canal is to be established using glide path. This will reduce the torsional stresses acting on the tip of the file. In case of delicate apical anatomy or acute curvatures, prefer hand instruments (avoid rotary instruments).
- Torque control electric motors should be used. The torque settings and manufacturer's instructions are to be followed strictly for better results.
- A crown-down sequence should be followed. This will result in less vertical force and torque; also minimizes stress on tip of the instrument.
- The rotary instrumentation should be limited to about 5 to 10 seconds.
- The files should not be apically forced and clinician should pull back at the first sign of resistance in the canal. The files should be used in approximately 1.0 to 2.0 mm deeper increments relative to the last instrument.
- Adequate irrigation and lubrication should be used during preparation to avoid clogging and frictional resistance.
- The flutes of the file should be wiped after every use. Dipping in 6% hydrogen peroxide and wiping with sterilized cloth will be beneficial.
- Examine files regularly before, during and after use under magnification. If the file is stretched or has a shiny spot, it should be discarded.
- It is advisable to use new instruments/system on extracted teeth before routine clinical use.

The Do's and Don'ts for the clinicians are summarized in Table 11.11.

o. Newer Rotary Designs

i. One Shape Single Rotary File

One shape single rotary file system is Ni-Ti with innovative design features. It is preferred in curved canal negotiation with an easy dynamic. Its non-working (safety) tip ensures an effective apical progression avoiding obstructions which may lead to instrument separation. The single file system works in continuous rotation. The preparation is rapid (four times faster than conventional rotary system). The conventional rotary motor is used in a simplified manner.

One shape files are available in different sizes and taper.

One shape Endoflare (25 mm/012)

One shape Glide path (14 mm/03)

One shape shaping (25 mm/06, 30 mm/06 and 37 mm/06).

Design features

The instrument presents a variable cross-section along the blade. The three different cross-section zones are:

- First zone presents 3 cutting-edge design.
- Second (middle) zone has a cross-section that progressively changes from 3 to 2 cutting edges.
- Last (coronal) zone has 2 cutting edges.

Advantages

- Minimum fatigue along the length of the file eliminating the risk of separation.
- No prior sterilization before use (economical).
- One file is used for the treatment of one tooth.
- Controls risk of infections: Safety for patients and staff.
- Easy handling.

Table 11.11 Do's and Don'ts for clinicians

Do's	*Don'ts*
• Assess canal anatomy thoroughly	• Forceful instrumentation
• Achieve straight line access prior to instrumentation	• Dry instrumentation
• Use glide path for patency of canal	• Rotation for long
• Follow crown-down sequence	• Staying in the canal for long
• Use files for 5–10 seconds	• Use of same files repeatedly
• Adequate irrigation and lubrication	• Use of unclean files
• Wipe flutes after each use (dip in hydrogen peroxide)	
• Examine files before, during and after use	

ii. ProTaper Next

The ProTaper Next system comprises five instruments. The file design depicts an increasing and decreasing percentage tapered design. The multiple progressive taper helps to reduce contact between the cutting flutes of the instrument and the dentin wall, subsequently reducing the possibility of screw-in effect. It also increases flexibility and cutting efficiency.

The first instrument in the system is the ProTaper Next X1 with a tip size of 0.17 mm and a 4% taper. This instrument is used after achieving glide path preferably by means of hand instruments. The ProTaper Next X2 (0.25 mm tip with 6% taper) is used to prepare root canal with adequate shape and taper for optimal irrigation and root canal obturation. Both X1 and X2 have an increasing and decreasing percentage tapered design over the cutting areas.

The last three finishing instruments are the ProTaper Next X3 (0.3 mm tip with 7 % taper); ProTaper Next X4 (0.4 mm tip with 6% taper); and ProTaper Next X5 (0.5 mm tip with 6% taper). All three have a decreasing percentage taper from the tip to the shank. These files are used to either create more taper in a root canal or to prepare wider root canals (Fig. 11.43).

The ProTaper Next files have a bilateral symmetrical rectangular cross-section offset from the central axis of rotation (except in the last 3.0 mm of the instrument). The exception is the Pro-Taper Next X1, which has a square cross-section in the last 3.0 mm segment providing core strength in the apical half.

The files are manufactured from M-Wire (not from a traditional Ni-Ti alloy), reducing the cyclic fatigue by 400%. These files are more flexible and resist fracture during preparation.

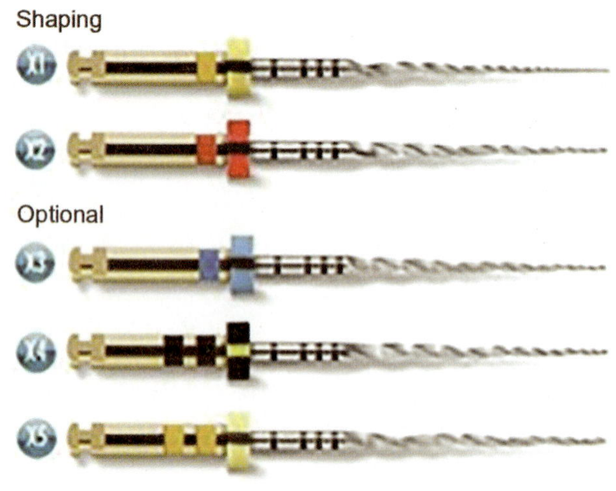

Fig. 11.43 ProTaper Next

iii. Self-Adjusting File (SAF)

The Self-Adjusting File (ReDentNova) is a hollow file, designed as a compressible, thin-walled pointed cylinder (hollow tube—1.5 or 2.0 mm in diameter), with a rough outer surface (Fig. 11.44). SAF does not have a solid metal shaft. The internal part of the hollow tube is composed of Ni-Ti lattice. The file has an asymmetrically positioned tip (conventional Ni-Ti rotary files tip is symmetrically centered). The continuous flow of irrigant is provided through the hollow tube. SAF files have been approved for clinical use. Initial clinical studies have observed better canal preparation with minimum chances of the separation. The radiographic picture of root canal obturations using SAF were comparable to other rotary systems.

Procedure

- The 1.5 mm file may easily be compressed and inserted into any canal previously prepared/ negotiated with a # 20 K-file. The 2.0 mm file will easily compress into a canal that was prepared with a #30 K-file.
- The file attempts to regain its original dimensions, thus applying a constant delicate pressure on the canal walls.
- When inserted into a root canal, it adapts itself to the canal's shape, both longitudinally (as will any Ni-Ti file) and along the cross-section. In a round canal, it will attain a round cross-section; whereas, in an oval or flat canal it will attain a flat or oval cross-section, providing a three-dimensional adaptation.
- The surface of the lattice threads is lightly abrasive, which allows it to remove dentin with a back-and-forth grinding motion.
- The SAF is operated with transline (in and out) vibrating handpieces with 3,000 to 5,000 vibrations per minute and an amplitude of 0.4 mm. Such a handpiece may be the GENTLEpower (360° free

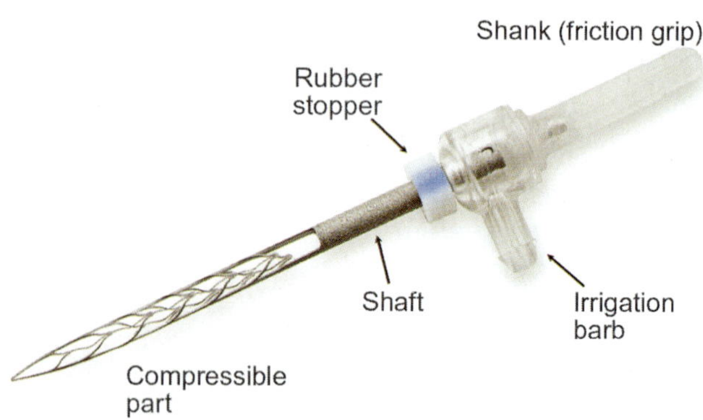

Fig. 11.44 Self-adjusting file (SAF)

rotation; Kavo, Germany), MK-Dent head (360° free rotation; MK-Dent, Germany) or RDT3 head (80 rpm when free and stops rotating when engaging the canal walls, ReDentNova).

- The irrigation tube is connected to a continuous-flow source and has an on-off switch.
- The vibrating movement combined with intimate contact along the entire circumference and length of the canal removes a layer of dentin with a grinding motion.
- The hollow design allows for continuous irrigation throughout the procedure. A special irrigation device (VATEA, ReDent-Nova) is connected by a silicon tube and provides continuous flow of the irrigant (irrigant is the choice of the operator) at a low pressure and at flow rates of 1.0 to 10 ml/minute.
- Alternatively, any physiodispenser type of irrigation device that is primarily designed for implantology, may also be used.
- The SAF is inserted into the canal while vibrating and is delicately pushed in until it reaches the predetermined working length.
- It is then operated with in-and-out manual motion and with continuous irrigation using two cycles of 2 minutes each for a total of 4 minutes per canal.
- This procedure will remove a uniform dentin layer (60–75 mm thick) from the canal circumference.
- The SAF file is designed for single use.

Advantages and characteristics

- ***Adapts itself to the three-dimensional anatomy of root canals:*** Most rotary file systems follow the widest part of the canal and gradually machine it; whereas, the SAF is used as a single file (1.5–2.0 mm diameter) that is narrow and compressed shaped, gradually expands in the canal while removing a uniform layer of dentin from its walls. Because the file adapts itself to the cross-section of a given canal, a canal with a round cross-section is enlarged as a round canal; whereas, an oval canal is enlarged as an oval canal.
- ***Uniform removal of the remaining dentin wall thickness:*** Ni-Ti rotary files may result in uneven thickness of the remaining dentin wall especially in flat canals. In places where round bore has been created, the remaining dentin will be thinner in the mesial and distal aspects than in the untreated areas, which is a predisposing factor for vertical root fractures. On the other hand, SAF removes a uniform layer of dentin from the canal walls, thus resulting in a relatively uniform remaining dentin thickness.
- ***Prevention of canal transportation:*** The SAF file being extremely flexible and pliable, does not impose its shape on the canal, rather complies with its original shape. The rotary Ni-Ti files have a tendency to transport the canal to the outer side of the curvature, especially in curved canals. SAF maintains the apical part of curved canals closer to its original shape and configuration.
- ***High durability:*** The SAF file does not have a core as do other Ni-Ti instruments. Any strain applied to it is distributed along the delicate lattice structure. Fatigue tests have confirmed that SAF can be rotated for more than 150 hours at 900 rpm with a 5.0 mm deflection with no mechanical failure; whereas, some of the Ni-Ti rotary instruments separated within the first hour. It is also important that the structural failure was not of the separation type that is encountered with other nickel-titanium files. Detachment of one of the arches at one of its ends was the typical mechanical failure. The damaged file can be retrieved from the canal without any difficulty.
- ***Continuous irrigation:*** The SAF operates with a continuous flow of the irrigant during preparation. The vibration of the file's metal lattice within the irrigant facilitates its cleaning and débridement effects. Any irrigant solution can be used along with SAF. Vibrating action of the metal lattice facilitates irrigant supply at the critical apical areas.
- ***Removal of the smear layer:*** Smear layer should be removed in order to allow intimate, unobstructed contact of irrigants with bacteria at the orifices of dentinal tubules and also to facilitate sealer's adaptation to the canal walls. When 3.0% sodium hypochlorite and 17% EDTA were used as alternating irrigants with the SAF file, the root canal surface (including its apical third) was rendered clean of debris and the smear layer (SAF allows uniform distribution of irrigant solution).

iv. WaveOne/WaveOne Gold

The WaveOneNi-Ti file system utilizes single file to prepare the root canal.WaveOne Gold replaces original WaveOne series, by improving upon its flexibility (Fig. 11.45).

The specially designed WaveOneNi-Ti files work on reverse *'balanced force'* action using a preprogrammed motor to move the files in a back and forth *'reciprocal motion'*. The files are manufactured using M-Wire technology, improving strength and resistance to cyclic fatigue.

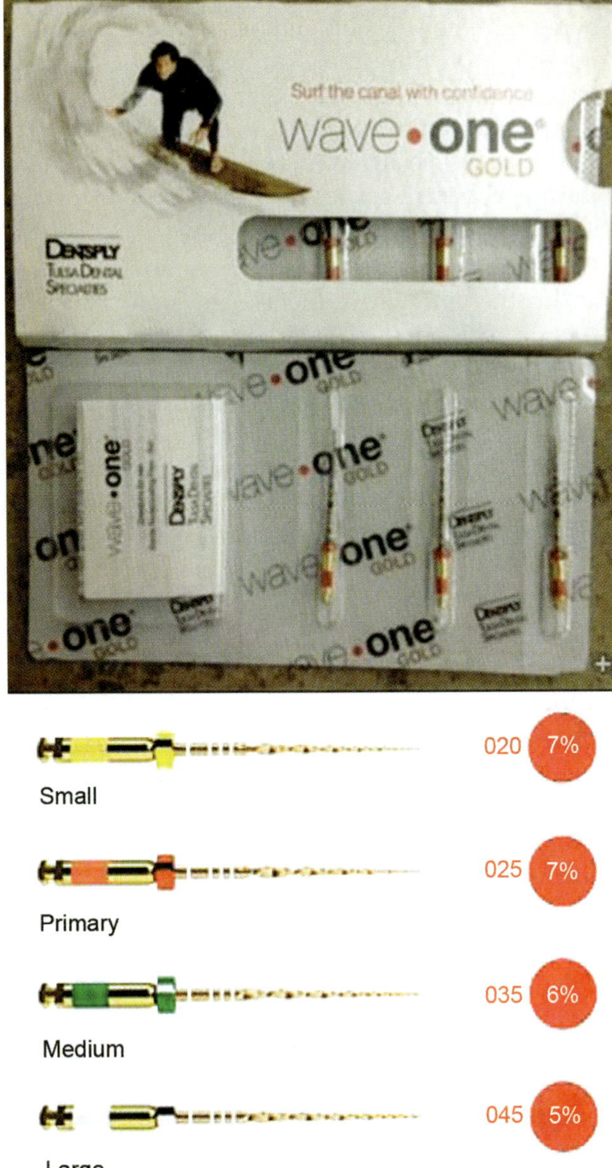

Fig. 11.45 WaveOne Gold files

There are three files available in lengths of 21, 25 and 31 mm in the WaveOne single-file reciprocating system:

- *WaveOne Small file* is used in fine canals. The file size is 21 mm with a continuous taper of 6%.
- *WaveOne Primary file* is used in the majority of canals. The file size is 25 mm with an apical taper of 8% that reduces towards the coronal end.
- *WaveOne Large file* is used in large canals. The file size is 31 mm with an apical taper of 8% that reduces towards the coronal end.

The WaveOne files are designed to work with a reverse cutting action. All instruments have a *modified convex triangular* cross-section at the tip and a *triangular* cross-section at the coronal end. This design improves instrument flexibility; the variable pitch improves safety. The tips are modified to follow canal curvature accurately.

It is hypothesized that root canal instruments cannot be sterilized property; therefore, the concept of root canal files in single use became popular. The plastic colour coding in the handle become deformed once sterilized, preventing the file from being placed back into the handpiece.

The single use file has the advantage of reducing instrument fatigue (one file can carry out preparation, which in routine performed by three or more rotary Ni-Ti files).

The *WaveOne motor*, as supplied by manufacturer is rechargeable; battery operated with a 6 : 1 reduction handpiece. The motor work on the principles of reciprocation, which can be preprogrammed. The counter-clockwise movement (advances the instrument/ cutting the dentin) is greater than the clockwise (disengages the instrument). Three reciprocating cycles complete one reverse rotation; the instrument advances into the canal with minimum apical pressure.

Selection of WaveOne files

The resistance of first hand file into the root canal aids in selection of the WaveOne file as:

- If a 10 K-file feels resistant, use WaveOne small file.
- If a 10 K-file moves to working length easily (loose at constriction), use WaveOne primary file.
- If a 20 K-file or larger touches working length, use WaveOne large file.

Irrigation is continually carried out during root canal preparation. The hand file is inserted to working length and confirm with an apex locator and radiograph. Take WaveOne file to working length.Confirm apical area preparation with hand file and the same size as WaveOne file; if snugly fit, the preparation is complete. If foramen diameter is larger than WaveOne primary file, consider the next larger WaveOne file.

Guidelines

- WaveOne files should be used with a progressive up and down movement with little pressure (not more than three to four times).
- The field should be cleaned continuously.
- Smaller WaveOne file should be used first, followed by the next in size.
- Glide path can be used, if required.
- In curved canals, apical area is prepared by hand files.
- Constant irrigation is mandatory throughout the preparation.

Advantages

- One Ni-Ti file is required per root canal/per tooth.
- Single use file overcomes the problem of sterilization and cross-contamination.
- Less instrument separation (reciprocating movement prevents the instrument advancing to its plastic limit).
- The canals can be shaped as per requirements.
- Eliminates procedural errors by using a single file rather than using multiple files.
- Easy to manipulate.
- Cost-effective.

v. RECIPROC® System

The RECIPROC system utilizes reciprocation movement wherein the root canal is prepared by using only one file. RECIPROC Endomotor is also available for reciprocating movements. The use of glide path is also not advised. The file is available in three sizes R25, R40 and R50.

R25 (Taper 08) color–red

R40 (Taper 06) color–black

R50 (Taper 05) color–yellow; non-cutting lips

The RECIPROC file is moved in a cutting direction and then reverses to release the file. The 360° rotation is completed in several reciprocating movements. The centering ability of the reciprocation technique allows the instrument to follow the path of least resistance, especially in curvatures (Fig. 11.46).

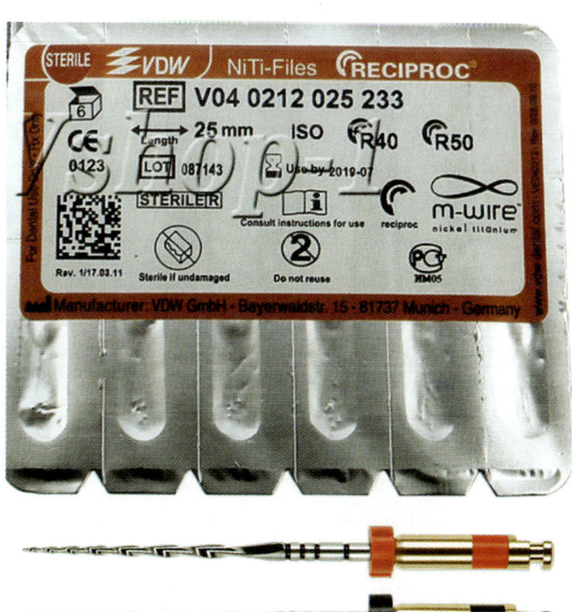

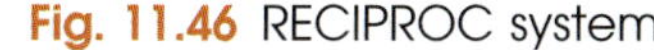

Fig. 11.46 RECIPROC system

RECIPROC® instruments are designed (S-shaped cross-section) using M-wire technology with Ni-Ti. The instrument provides increased resistance to cyclic fatigue and greater flexibility. The deeper flutes facilitate excellent removing of debris from the root canal. The S-shaped cross-section with two cutting edges provides high cutting ability.

vi. Twisted Files

The twisted files are created by taking a raw Ni-Ti wire in the austenitic crystalline form and transforming the same into the rhombohedral (R-) phase by a heat treatment process. The transformation of the wire from austenite to R-phase takes place on cooling to the R-phase transition temperature. R-phase technology provides good superelasticity and shape memory effect; Young's modulus is also lower than that of austenite, making it more flexible. It also provides adequate strength to the file.

Twisted files track the root canal with excellent tactile control and the canal can be shaped in limited insertions.

Twisted files are available in five tapers (0.12, 0.10, 0.08, 0.06, 0.04); and two lengths, 23 and 27 mm.

Large pack includes 0.10, 0.08, 0.06 tapers and small pack 0.04, 0.06, 0.08 taper. Generally, the large pack is used in straight and easily negotiable canals; whereas, small pack is used in small and curved canals.

Tip: Non-cutting pilot tip

Rake angle: Positive rake angle

Speed: 500 rpm

Cross-section: Triangular

Advantages of twisted files

- Triangular cross-section enhance flexibility and generates less friction inside the canal.
- Variable pitch minimizes 'screw-in' effect and appropriate flute width and flute depth effectively collect debris from the canal.
- One piece design (file is manufactured from one piece Ni-Ti) minimize 'wobble' during rotation. One piece file provides more structural integrity.
- Surface conditioning maintains the surface hardness and the sharpness of edges.

Advantages of R phase technology

- Overcomes limitations of grinding file technology.
- Improves properties of Ni-Ti alloy.
- Crystalline structural modification provide maximum flexibility and resistance to breakage.

vii. TRUShape 3D Conforming Files

TRUShape 3D is a new file system that preserves more tooth structure (removes 36% less dentin as compared to conventional files).The file prevents apical transportation, producing predictable apical shape.

It has 'S'-shaped design facilitating flexibility and creating an envelope of motion that better disrupts polymicrobial biofilms.

It is used in conjunction with TRUShape orifice modifiers. The file design provide active cutting cross-section, a fluted length of 7.0 mm, fluted diameter of 0.75 mm and Ni-Ti for strength and flexibility. The files are available in four tip sizes of 20, 25, 30, 40 and lengths 21, 25 and 31 mm.

viii. Vortex Blue

Vortex blue is a new file system, which provides greater resistance to cyclic fatigue, greater strength and reduced shape memory; also conforms to canal curvatures.

The 'Blue Color' of the file is due to an optical effect, created by light rays interacting with a Titanium oxide layer on the surface of the file.

It is triangular in cross-section with safe ended tip and variable helical angle. The lower helical angle (less flutes) in the coronal portion of the file facilitates efficient debris removal and higher helical angle (more flutes) in the apical portion of file provides increased strength.

The files are available in lengths 21, 25 and 30 mm and 4 and 6% taper (packs of six files: color varies with file number, Table 11.12).

In conventional canals, 30/04 file is used up to working length; 40/04 file is used in wider canals and 15–20/04 file is preferred in narrow canals. If resistance is encountered before working length, the next smaller file is chosen following same protocol until working length is achieved. Between each rotary files, recapitulate with no. 10 or 15 hand file to maintain glide path.

Advantages

- Vortex blue files remain centered in the canal, due to reduced shape memory effect.
- Greater resistance to fracture due to cyclic fatigue.
- Increased torque strength.

Table 11.12 File number and color (Vortex blue)

4% and 6% taper	
White	15
Yellow	20
Red	25
Blue	30
Green	35
Black	40

ix. F360 file system

F360 file system is designed with a unique double-S shape cross-section, sharp cutting edges and larger flute spaces. The design ensure better cutting efficiency and removal of infected debris. The system utilizes two files for preparation of most of the root canals (size 25/04 – red and size 35/04 – green). Additional file sizes (size 45/04 – white and size 55/04 – red) are used for wider canals. The length available are: 21, 25 and 31 mm. Corresponding sized paper points and gutta-percha are also available.

The presterilized, single-use files are designed to prevent cross-contamination, easy to maintain sterility and less chances of fracture due to cyclic fatigue.

Advantages

- Improved flexibility
- No canal transportation or other procedural errors
- Resist fracture
- Single-use (saves time and cross-contamination)
- No need to sterilize the file.

x. NeoNi-Ti

NeoNi-Ti is a new file system having rectangular section along the blade, which provides progressive flexibility to better negotiate the root canal curves. The file also provides better cutting efficiency and less smear layer formation.

Appropriate heat treatment of the files can increase the flexibility and resistance to fatigue. The single file technique is easy to use. Recommended speed is 300–500 rpm.

Two variants are available:

NeoNi-Ti C1: It is an orifice-opener. Diameter at tip: 0.25 mm with taper of 12%. Length of file: 15 mm.

NeoNi-Ti A1: Single file used for shaping of root canal in continuous rotation. Diameter at tip can be 0.20, 0.25, and 0.40 mm with taper 8%. Length of file: 21 and 25 mm.

xi. ProTaper Gold Rotary Files

ProTaper Gold files have same features and predictable performance as ProTaper Universal (Fig. 11.47).

The files provide greater flexibility and have greater resistance to cyclic fatigue and enhanced durability.

The 11 mm short handle provides better accessibility.

The system includes series of 'shaping' and 'finishing' files that create the predictable ProTaper Shape (Table 11.13).

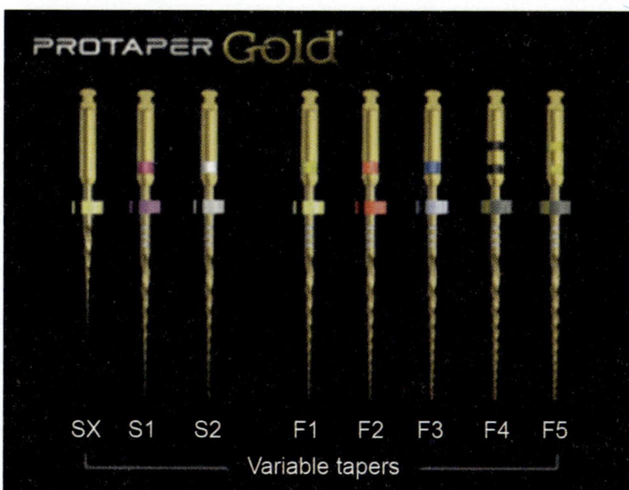

Fig. 11.47 ProTaper gold files

Table 11.13 ProTaper gold finishing files	
Shaper X : 0.19/4%	Finisher 1 : 0.20/7%
Shaper 1 : 0.18/2%	Finisher 2 : 0.25/8%
Shaper 2 : 0.20/2%	Finisher 3 : 0.30/9%
	Finisher 4 : 0.40/6%
	Finisher 5 : 0.50/5%

Due to their metallurgy, ProTaper gold files may appear slightly curved when removed from the package. This is not a defect but rather, an advantage.

F. MISCELLANEOUS INSTRUMENTS

i. *Endobox*: A small box, an organizer for placement of endodontic files, reamers, pluggers, spreaders, etc. and are sorted by sizes.
ii. *Endometer*: These are metal or plastic autoclavable rulers for measurement of root canal preparation and obturation.
iii. *Rubber dam kit*: Rubber dam kit and rubber dam accessories are explained in Chapter 14.
iv. *Stieglitz forcep*: Steiglitz forceps, available with tips bending at 45, 60 and 90°, are used to remove fragmented/separated instruments from the coronal half of the root canal.
v. *Perf paddles*: Perf paddles are mainly available in two sizes, viz. 1 and 2; used to repair perforations inside root canal.
vi. *LC-condenser*: LC-condenser, available in two sizes, is used to condense material in root-end cavities (surgically prepared cavities).
vii. Flap retractors, needle holder, burnishers, currettes, etc. of various shapes and sizes are available for respective usage.

BIBLIOGRAPHY

1. Adiguzel O. A literature review of self adjusting file. Int. Dent. Res.: 2011; 1:18–25.
2. Alapati SB, Brantley WA, Svec TA, Powers JM, Nusstein JM and Daehn GS. Proposed role of embedded dentin chips for the clinical failure of nickel-titanium rotary files. J. Endod.: 2004; 30:339–341.
3. Baugh D and Wallace J. The role of apical instrumentation in root canal treatment: A review of literature. J. Endod.: 2005; 31:333–340.
4. Baumann MA. Nickel-titanium: options and challenges. Dent. Clin. North Am.:2004; 48:55–67.
5. Cheung GSP. Instrument fracture: mechanisms, removal of fragments, and clinical outcome. Endod. Topics: 2009; 16:1–26.
6. Diemer F and Calas P. Effect of pitch length on the behavior of rotary triple helix root canal instruments. J. Endod.: 2004; 30:716–718.
7. DiFiore PM. A dozen ways to prevent Nickel-titanium rotary instrument fracture. JADA: 2007; 138:196.
8. Fayyad DM and Elhakim AA. Cutting efficiency of twisted versus machined nickel-titanium endodontic files. J. Endod.: 2011; 37:1143–1146.
9. Gambarini G, Plotino G and Grande NM. Mechanical properties of nickel-titanium rotary instruments produced with a new manufacturing technique. Int. Endod. J.: 2011; 44:337–341.
10. Guttman JL and Gao Y. Alteration in the inherent metallic and surface properties of nickel-titanium root canal instruments to enhance performance, durability and safety: a focused review. Int. Endod. J.: 2012; 45:113–128.
11. Haapasalo M and Shen Y. Evolution of nickel-titanium instruments: from past to future. Endod. Topics: 2013; 29:3–17.
12. Hof R, Perevalov V, Eltanani M, Zary R and Metzger Z. The self-adjusting file (SAF) Part 2: Mechanical analysis. J. Endod.: 2010; 36:691–696.
13. Hubscher W, Barbakow F and Peters OA. Root canal preparation with Flexmaster: canal shapes analyzed by microcomputed tomography. Int. Endod. J.: 2003; 36:740.
14. Linsuwanont P, Parashos P and Messer HH. Cleaning of rotary nickel-titanium endodontic instruments. Int. Endod. J.: 2004; 37:19–28.
15. Metzger Z, Teperovich E, Zary R, Cohen R and Hof R. The self-adjusting file (SAF) Part 1: Respecting the root canal anatomy—a new concept of endodontic files and its implementation. J. Endod.: 2010; 36:679–690.
16. Metzger Z, Teperovich E, Zary R, Cohen R, Paque F, Hulsmann M and Hof R. The self-adjusting file (SAF) Part 3: Removal of debris and smear layer—a scanning electron microscope study. J. Endod.: 2010; 36:697–702.
17. Montalvao D, Alcada FS, Fernandes FM and Vilaverde-Correia S. Structural characterization and mechanical FE analysis of conventional and M-wire Ni-Ti alloys used in endodontic rotary instruments. The Sci. World J.: 2014; Article ID976459:1–8.

18. Paque F, Barbakow F and Peters A. Root canal preparation with Endo Eze AET: Changes in root canal shape assessed by micro-computed tomography. Int. Endod. J.: 2005; 38:456.

19. Parasbos P. Rotary Ni-Ti instrument fracture and its consequences. J. Endod.: 2006; 32:1031–1043.

20. Peters OA and Paque F. Current developments in rotary root canal instrument technology and clinical use: A review. Quint. Int.: 2010; 41:479–488.

21. Plotino G, Grande NM and Porciani PF. Deformation and fracture incidence of Reciproc instruments: a clinical evaluation. Int. Endod. J.: 2015; 48:199–205.

22. Plotino G, Pameijer CH, Grende NM and Somma F. Ultrsonics in endodontics. A review of literature. J. Endod.: 2007; 33:81.

23. Saber SEM. Factors influencing the fracture of rotary nickel-titanium instruments. Endod. Practice: 2008; 2:273.

24. Sattapan B, Nervo GJ, Palamara JEA and Messer HH. Defects in rotary nickel-titanium files after clinical use. J. Endod.: 2000; 26:161–165.

25. Shen Y, Jeffrey MC, John A, Wang Z, Hieawy A, Yang Y and Haapasalo M. WaveOne rotary instruments after clinical use. J. Endod.: 2016; 42:186–189.

26. Shen Y, Zhou H and Zheng YF. Metallurgical characterization of controlled memory wire nickel-titanium rotary instruments. J. Endod.: 2011; 37:1566–71.

27. Shen Y, Zhou H and Zheng YF. Current challenges and concepts of the thermomechanical treatment of nickel-titanium instruments. J. Endod.: 2013; 39:163–172.

28. Shen Y, Zhou H, Coil JM, Aljazaeri B, Buttar R, Wang Z, Zheng Y and Haapasalo M. ProFile Vortex and Vortex Blue Nickel-Titanium rotary instruments after clinical use. J. Endod.: 2015; 41:937–942.

29. Thompson SA. An overview of Nickel-Titanium alloy used in dentistry. Int. Endod. J.: 2000; 33:297–310.

30. Vallabhaneni S, More GR and Gogineni R. Single File Endodontics. Ind. J. Dent. Adv.:2012; 4:822–826.

31. Varela-Patino P. Alternating versus continuous rotation: a comparative study of the effect on instrument life. J. Endod.: 2010; 36:157–159.

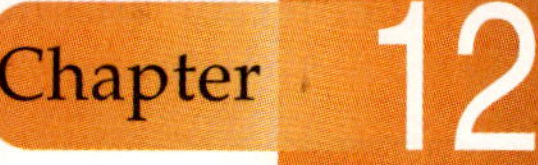

Chapter 12 Sterilization of Endodontic Instruments

The word 'sterile' means absence of any living organisms. A disinfectant is a chemical substance that kills microorganisms on any object, may be instruments, tables, lights, etc. An antiseptic is a chemical that is applied to inhibit the growth of microorganisms (asepsis is absence of micro-organisms in living tissues). Sterilization of operating field and the instruments is mandatory for any successful procedure. It is mandatory to sterilize endodontic instruments so as to achieve successful results. The wide range of endodontic instruments are sterilized following different modalities and kept in a sterile field prior to use on patients. The effectiveness of sterilization is the beginning of successful endodontic procedures. Aseptic techniques were performed in early nineteenth century; later, the use of surgical gloves, masks and gowns became a routine procedure.

STERILIZATION OF OPERATING ROOM

The operating area/chamber is to be sterilized for better clinical outcome. The complete eradication of bacteria may not be possible in operating room. The source of bacteria can be from air, patients attending the area, articles in the room, working equipment, etc.

The methods used to keep the operating area bacteriologically safe are:

i. Air flow is filtered; circulating purified air and continuously removing the contaminated air. The patients are allowed in the area 'off shoes' and preferably in sterilized gowns.
ii. Standard cleaning and disinfection procedures should be followed, which minimizes the bacterial growth.
iii. Fumigation of the area with formalin fumes. Since formalin is pungent, the procedure is carried out overnight in a closed environment. The room is kept closed for 12–14 hours and is ready for use once all the fumes are out. Formalin is usually neutralized with ammonia (2-hour contact) prior to use of the room.

    Formalin use (fumigation) is obsolete in many countries because of its potentially carcinogenic nature. Frequent use of inhalation is hazardous. Newer agents are being used to sterilize the room.
iv. Newer agents for sterilization of operating area are:
    - *Bacillocid rasant* (composition: Glutaraldehyde, Benzalkonium chloride and dimethyl ammonia). It is formalin-free disinfectant with excellent cleaning properties and is cost-effective. It provides complete asepsis within one hour; closing the room for 12 hours is not required.
    - *Virkon*: It is non-aldehyde compound (composition potassium monosulphate, sulfamic acid and sodium dodecyl-sulfonate), considered safe virucidal and fungicidal. It is effective within 30–40 minutes.

STERILIZATION OF INSTRUMENTS

The sterilization of instruments involves the following features:

Processing of Instruments Prior to Sterilization

This includes pre-soaking and cleaning, rinsing, drying and packaging before the instruments are being sterilized.

Presoaking and Cleaning

Presoaking of contaminated instruments keeps them wet until a thorough cleaning can be carried out. This prevents drying of blood, saliva and debris on instruments, which facilitates cleaning. In endodontics, all debris must be removed from instruments prior to sterilization, since it may interfere with the effectiveness of the procedure. The files possess complex design, which facilitates the debris accumulation along the flutes.

The methods used for cleaning are:

i. Manual Scrubbing

Manual scrubbing involves:

- Use of stiff nylon cleaning brushes
- Use of neutral pH detergents
- Brush delicate instruments carefully and slowly; the general instruments are cleaned separately
- Wipe the endodontic instruments with suitable sized gauze moistened with hydrogen peroxide/alcohol
- Heavy utility gloves should be worn while processing contaminated instruments
- The instrument surfaces should be visibly clean and free from stains and tissues.

ii. Ultrasonic Cleaners

The ultrasonic cleaners use vibratory energy, carried as sound waves in the fluid, creating suction, which in turn removes biological matter from the instruments.

An ultrasonic cleaning device should have a lid, a well-designed basket and an audible timer. The device should prevent electronic interferences with other electronic equipment and office communication systems (Fig. 12.1).

Advantages

- *Faster*: Easier in cleaning
- Removes dried blood and saliva
- Minimizes the direct handling of contaminated instruments, subsequently the accidental injuries to hands.

iii. Washer Disinfector

Washer disinfector helps in effective physical cleaning due to high flow of water, (both volume and pressure), which is sprayed all over the instruments. Temperature is maintained below 45°C to avoid any protein coagulation during the flushing stage.

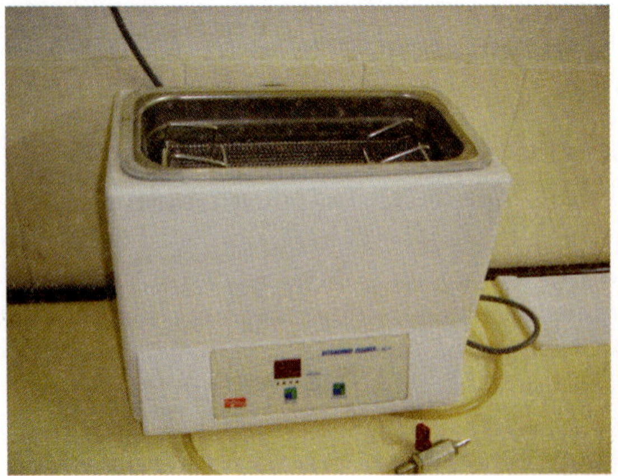

Fig. 12.1 Ultrasonic cleaner

The detergent used in washer disinfector should have:

- Anti-lipid action at high temperatures
- Anti-protein action at low temperatures
- Enzymatic action.

For disinfection process, the temperature of water is elevated gradually to almost its boiling point. The phases of disinfection are:

- *Initial microbial activation phase (45 to 52°C)*: Endospores enter vegetative phase.
- *Microbial inactivation phase (85 to 95°C)*: Pathogenic microorganisms are inactivated or killed. Vegetative endospores are also killed. The contact time is reduced as the temperature increases.

Disadvantage

- Maintenance of disinfected instruments is difficult since, they are obtained in a wet and unwrapped state.

iv. Enzyme Cleaners

Enzymes are powerful tools for cleaning endodontic instruments. A properly selected enzyme cleaner can effectively improve cleaning of instruments. Enzymes accelerate the biological process of the chemicals, and are specific in their catalytic behavior. Some enzymes are effective on specific proteins while others may act on a broad-spectrum of proteins, e.g. KLENZYME cleaners.

Since, the enzymes normally used for instruments cleaning do not attack metals; they are well-suited for cleaning the reusable instruments.

Disadvantages

- Enzymes may lead to corrosion, rust, discoloration and loss of elasticity of the instruments.
- Improper use of cleaning solutions can also lead to stained surfaces.
- Another important attribute of enzyme cleaners is their rinsability. In case enzymes cling to instrument surface, rather than rinse off easily under running water, they can interfere with sterilization process by hiding bacterial contamination. The residual enzymes may also interfere with sterilization.

Packaging

After cleaned instruments have been rinsed and dried, they are to be packed in functional sets before sterilization. This packaging protects the instruments from contamination after sterilization and before use at chairside. A variety of packaging materials are available, with self-sealing paper-plastic and peel pouches being the most convenient.

Studies have shown that it is difficult to remove organic debris from endodontic files despite using automated cleaning devices. It is important to ensure that instrument holders, such as cassettes or file holders have perforations and allow adequate space between instruments to allow access to all instrument surfaces during the cleaning process.

Because of the challenges of cleaning files, deterioration of the cutting surfaces during cleaning and sterilization, and wear during normal use, the Centre for Disease Control and Prevention (CDC) suggest considering endodontic files as single-use devices.

Sterilization

The techniques used for sterilization of instruments are:

1. Flaming
2. Boiling
3. Cold sterilization
4. Autoclave
5. Dry heat sterilization
6. Glass bead sterilizer
7. Hot salt sterilizer
8. Ethylene oxide sterilization
9. Plasma sterilization

1. Flaming

The instruments are sterilized by dipping in alcohol (3 parts of ethyl alcohol and 1 part formalin) and passing over the flame 2–3 times. The process destroys even spores. The tips of tweezers, scissors, etc. can be sterilized using this method; however, root canal files reamers, etc. should not be sterilized by this method.

2. Boiling

Boiling in water for fifteen minutes will kill most vegetative bacteria and inactivate viruses; however, boiling is ineffective against many bacterial and fungal spores. It is considered unsuitable for complete sterilization.

3. Cold Sterilization

Cold sterilization (Fig. 12.2) uses chemical solutions such as:

i. *Quaternary ammonia compounds*: Useful for vegetative microorganisms.

ii. *Ethyl alcohol and isopropyl alcohol*: Useful for vegetative bacteria and tubercle bacilli.

iii. *Alcohol-formalin solution*: Useful for vegetative bacteria, tubercle bacilli and spores.

iv. *Orthophenylphenol and benzyl-para chlorophenol*: Useful for vegetative bacteria, tubercle bacilli, certain fungi and viruses, but not on spores.

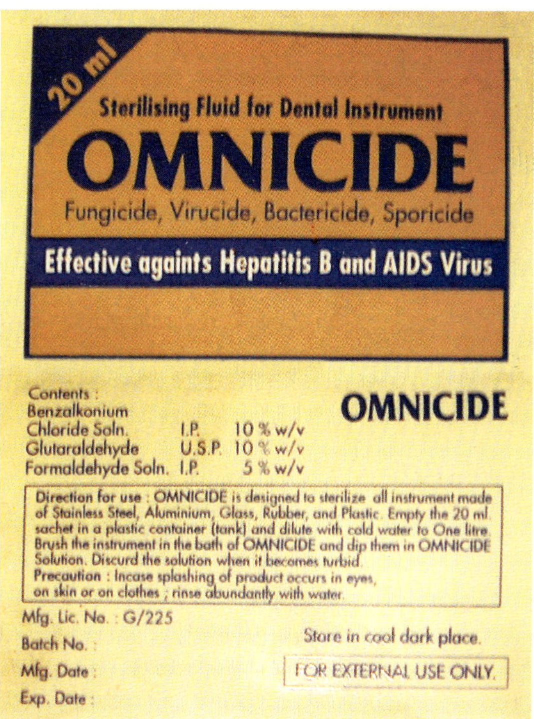

Fig. 12.2 Cold sterilizer

v. *Sporicidin (phenol 7.05%, sodium tetraborate 2.35%, Glutaraldehyde 2% and sodium phenate 1.2%)*: Disinfects instruments in 10 minutes at room temperature and sterilizes in 6.75 hours.

Disadvantages

- Not effective against all varieties of microbial life
- Time taken is long (minimum 20 minutes for proper sterilization).

4. Autoclave

Autoclaving is one of the most rapid and effective method for sterilization.

Sterilization in an autoclave (Fig. 12.3) is carried out with steam (250°F or 121°C) under pressure (15 lb). For a light load of instruments, the time required is fifteen minutes. The burs can be protected by keeping them submerged in a small amount of 2.0% sodium nitrite solution. Carbon steel instruments tend to rust with autoclaving. Handles of endodontic hand instruments are made up of high quality plastic which can bear high temperature exposures. A few manufacturers claim that the plastic of their instruments are high heat resistant which can be used even in dry heat sterilizers.

Advantages

- Most rapid and effective method
- Good penetration of heat.

12

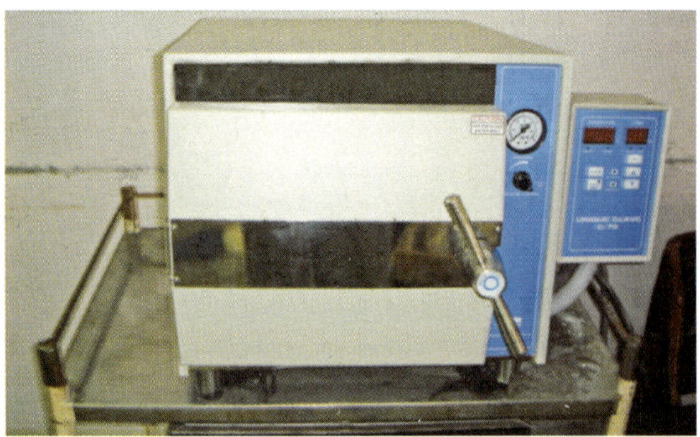

Fig. 12.3 Autoclave

Disadvantages

- Plastic and rubber cannot be sterilized
- Tend to rust carbon steel instruments.

5. Dry Heat Sterilization

Dry heat sterilization effectively kills bacteria without changing the sharpness of the instruments. It works without pressure, steam or chemicals, which increases safety (Fig. 12.4). Utility trays can be sterilized with lids on and stored without contamination. It is economical to use and requires no routine cleaning.

Advantages

- Maintenance of sharp edges of cutting instruments
- No corrosion of instruments
- Packs are dry after sterilization
- Rapid cycles at higher temperature possible
- Less expensive.

Disadvantages

- Poor heat conduction by air (prolonged time)
- High heat damages plastic and rubber items
- Sterilization prolonged at lower temperature.

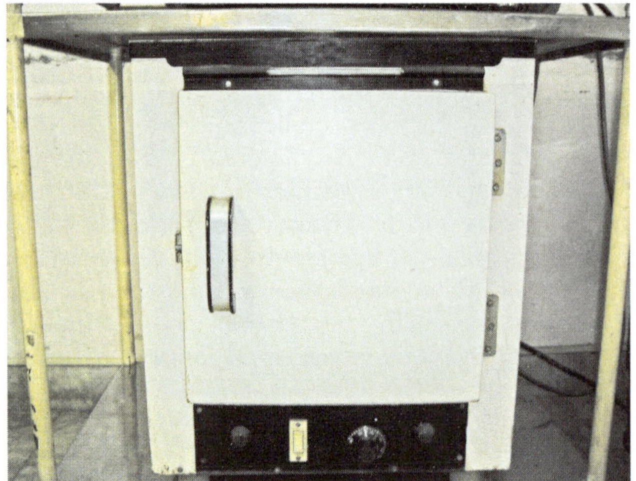

Fig. 12.4 Dry heat sterilizer

6. Glass Bead Sterilizer

Glass bead sterilizer (Fig. 12.5) contains glass beads, less than 1.0 mm in size because larger beads are not effective in transferring heat due to large air spaces between the beads. The instruments to be sterilized are immersed into the heat-up glass beads (temperature 218–280°C) and left for a specific period of time. The time specified for each instrument is:

- Root canal instruments: 5 seconds
- Absorbent points and cotton pellets: 10 seconds
- Long-handled instruments, tips of cotton pliers, blades of scissors and tips of other surgical instruments: 5 seconds.

Disadvantages

- The glass beads (less than 1.0 mm in diameter), sometimes get stuck in the instruments like broaches or cotton pellets, which may get introduced into the root canal and hamper root canal preparation.
- Costlier than the salt sterilizer.
- Considered effective only as auxiliary method of sterilization.

7. Hot Salt Sterilizer

Hot salt sterilizer is used to sterilize absorbent points, broaches, files, reamers and other root canal instruments. The method is preferred to sterilize root canal instruments immediately before start of the treatment.

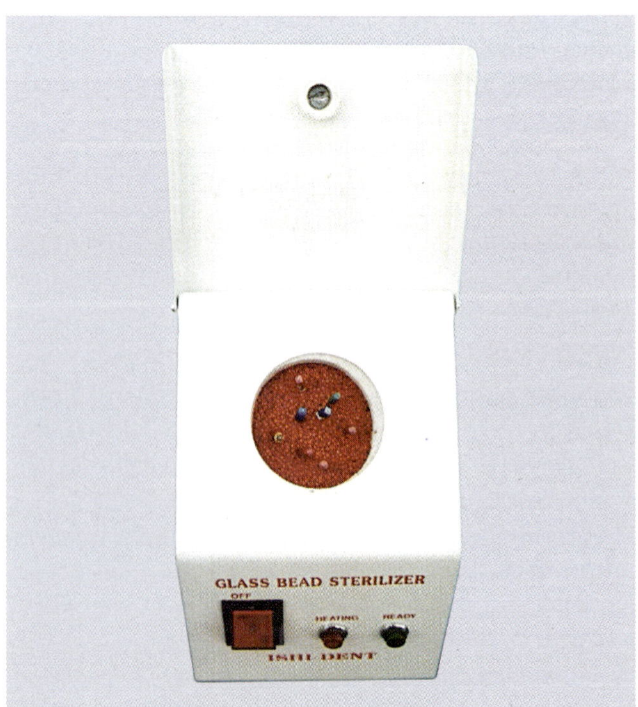

Fig. 12.5 Glass bead sterilizer

Technique

The instruments desired to be sterilized are put into the sterilizer and left for a stipulated period of time (different instruments have different time limits); Broaches, files and reamers are sterilized in 5 seconds; whereas absorbent points and cotton pellets in 10 seconds. The hottest part of the salt bath is along the outer rim, starting at the bottom. Immerse instrument at least a quarter inch below salt's surface and in the peripheral area. It consists of a metal cup in which table salt is kept at a temperature of 425°F [218°C] to 475°F [246°C]. Use of thermometer to monitor temperature of the salt is necessary. It is considered superior to molten metal sterilizer and glass bead sterilizer because the metal or the glass beads occasionally cling to the wet instrument and tend to clog the root canals.

Advantages

- Use of table salt (readily available).
- Contains small amounts of sodium silicoaluminate, magnesium carbonate or sodium carbonate, so it pours readily and does not become fused under heat.
- Any salt carried into root canal can be irrigated easily.
- Salt should be changed every week; or more often depending on the degree of humidity.
- Cost-effective (salt is cheap and easily available).

8. Ethylene Oxide (ETO) Sterilization

Ethylene oxide sterilization is a lengthy process. It is generally carried out at temperatures (30 and 60°C) with relative humidity above 30%. The gas concentration is maintained between 200–800 mg/l for at least 3 hours (Fig. 12.6). The process also involves a period of poststerilization to remove any toxic residues. The gas is extremely dangerous at ambient oxygen levels and its mixtures with air are explosive. When heated, it may rapidly expand causing fire and explosion. Hence, its use has been discarded.

9. Plasma Sterilization

Plasma is basically ionized gas. Plasma sterilization is fast evolving into a promising alternative to standard sterilization techniques. It uses a technique, which involves UV irradiation, photodesorption and chemical etching. The spores are made up of atoms like carbon, oxygen, hydrogen, nitrogen and the like. The radicals react with these atoms to form compounds like carbon dioxide, which can be subsequently flushed out. When the organism loses such atoms that are intrinsic to its survival, it dies (Fig. 12.7).

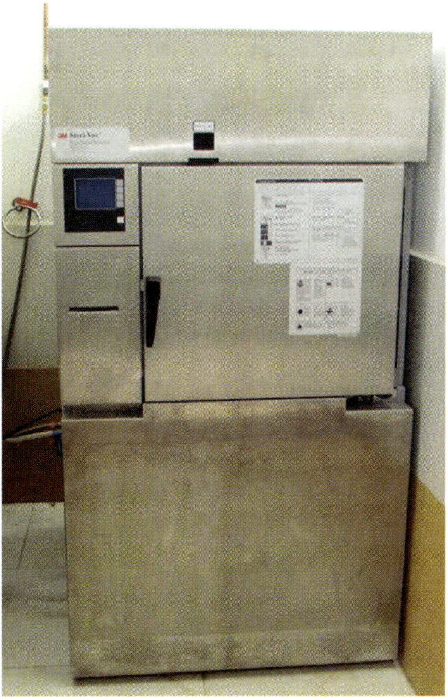

Fig. 12.6 Ethylene oxide sterilizer

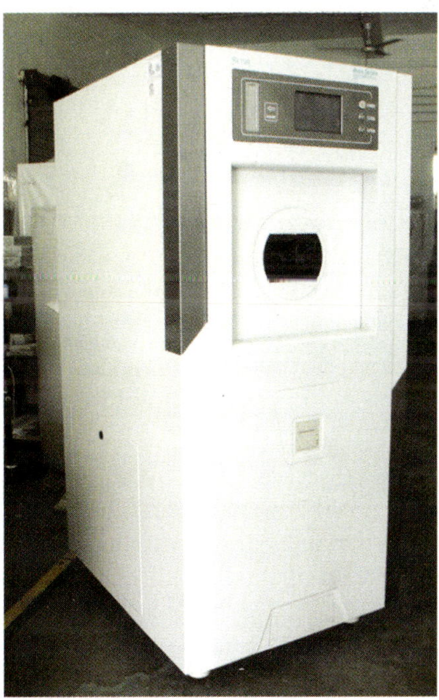

Fig. 12.7 Plasma sterilizer

Advantages

- The process is carried out usually at room temperature and hence poses no dangers associated with high temperatures.
- It does not involve any chemicals and hence is non-toxic (unlike ethylene oxide).
- Time of treatment is fast (one minute or less).
- It is versatile and can sterilize almost any instrument.

10. Laser Sterilization

Carbon dioxide laser has been widely used as one mode of sterilization. It is considered effective in complete eradication of the bacteria from the instrument surfaces. Argon layer and ND:YAG have also been used to sterilize endodontic instruments. Argon Laser is considered better than the other two lasers.

STERILIZATION OF HANDPIECE AND TURBINES

The dental handpiece and turbines (waterlines) due to constant contact with oral fluids are contaminated on both external and internal surfaces.

a. Sterilization of Handpiece

Sterilization of handpiece is carried out as:

- Wipe the handpiece clean with an alcohol soaked soft tissue.
- Never clean the handpiece with boiling water, chemical solution, ultrasonic cleaner or with wire brushes.
- The manufacturer's instructions for cleaning and lubrication must be followed to reduce the risk of turbine degradation. Various cleaning solutions and foam are available to lubricate inner surfaces. Automate devices are also available for cleaning and lubricating. Failure to lubricate handpiece (except tube-free handpiece) contribute significantly to early bearing failure.
- It is best sterilized by autoclaving for no longer than 20 minutes at 121°C (250° F) or 15 minutes at 132°C (270°F).
- Keep the handpiece away from water vapour or mist that may settle and cause premature damage to the bearings.
- Ethylene trioxide has been used as an alternative method for sterilization of dental handpiece as it is less corrosive than steam. However, its effectiveness has not been established.
- Most handpieces require lubrication before sterilization (except tube-free handpiece).
- It is advised to wrap the handpiece in a piece of cloth before placing it in the autoclave. An unwrapped handpiece should be used immediately or sterilize again before use.
- Chemical vapour pressure sterilization (chemiclave) is recommended for ceramic bearing handpieces.
- Dry heat sterilization of handpieces is generally not recommended.
- Ultraviolet radiations are used for maintenance of previously sterilized handpieces (Fig. 12.8).

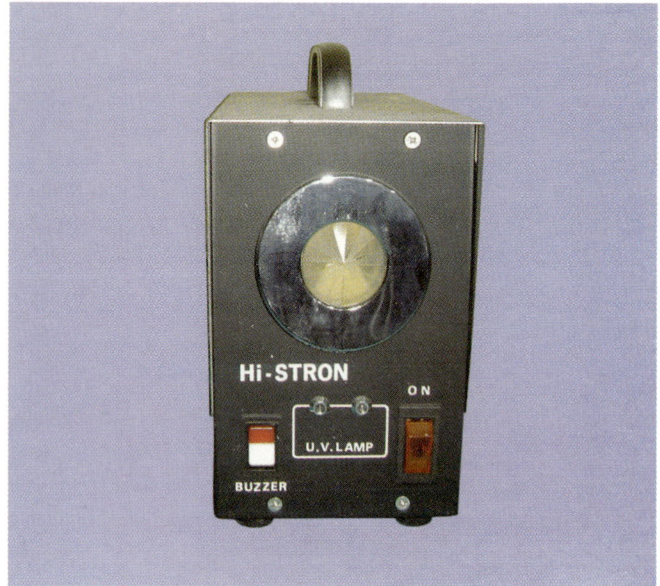

Fig. 12.8 Ultraviolet lamp

b. Sterilization of Dental Unit Waterlines

It is established that dental personnel are constantly exposed to water borne microorganisms. There are various ways by which waterborne microorganisms can cause infection in a patient undergoing dental treatment, viz. homogenous spread during surgical procedures, local mucosal contact, ingestion and inhalation. A range of microbiological flora has been identified in dental unit waterline samples which holds potential to infect healthy dental patients.

A number of products are being used to help control the problem:

- *Filters*: Filters provide physical barrier to the passage of microorganisms. Filters do purify water before it enters the dental unit. Certain fillers are impregnated with iodine, which is gradually released into the water during use of the handpiece; minimizing bacterial counts.
- *Supply of autoclaved water*: The sterile water is supplied in each component of the delivery system. Practically this method is difficult and not cost-effective; moreover, sterile water in pipes becomes contaminated soon, because of inherent biofilm inside the pipes.
- *Chemical disinfectant*: The disinfectants are allowed to remain in waterlines overnight and then powder, if used, should be kept in the pipes for shorter time and then rinsed with fresh water. Rinsing out water lines of the unit with Tween 80 and Ponceau 4R dye lead to a marked reduction in microorganisms.

Canadian Dental Association guidelines for maintenance of dental unit waterlines

- Avoid heating water for the dental unit
- At the beginning and after each patient, purge all lines by removing handpiece, air/water syringe, ultrasonic tips etc. Flushed thoroughly with water (decrease in bacterial count with purging is established).
- Run high speed handpiece for 20–30 seconds after each patient to purge all air and water.
- Use sterile water/saline when flushing open vascular sites and/ or cutting bone during invasive surgical procedures.
- Follow manufacturer's instructions for daily/weekly maintenance, if using bottled water or other special delivery system.

STERILIZATION OF MISCELLANEOUS INSTRUMENTS

- *Burs* must be clean before sterilization. The burs should be presoaked in a container of soapy water to loosen debris. The enzymatic solution is used to clean the diamond points. Ultrasonic system can also be used. After rinsing, the burs must be thoroughly dried by placing them on absorbent towel. Burs, especially the surgical burs, are sterilized by heat. Cold sterilization is not recommended for burs, since the oxidizing agents may weaken carbide burs. Steam autoclaves effectively sterilize burs.
- *Glass slab* can be sterilized by swabbing with tincture of thimerosal, followed by a double swabbing with alcohol.
- *Gutta-percha cones* may be kept in sterile screw capped vials containing alcohol. (To sterilize gutta-percha cone freshly removed from the box-immerse in 5.2% sodium hypochlorite for one minute, then rinse with hydrogen peroxide and dry between two layers of sterile gauze.)
- *Silver cones* are sterilized by passing them through a flame 3–4 times or by immersion in hot salt sterilizer for 5 seconds.
- *Dappen dishes* can be sterilized before use by swabbing with tincture of thimerosal under pressure.
- *Infected endodontic instruments* exposed to three seconds to a laser beam destroys microorganisms including spores.

How does an effective sterilization take place?

Each process of sterilization has certain parameters such as temperature, time, humidity and saturation/ concentration of chemical agent, if used. If an effective sterilization is to be achieved, running a full cycle is not enough; it must also be established that the cycle was run under conditions following all the parameters.

Indicators for Sterilization

1. ***Biological indicators***: The spores of *Geobacillus stearothermophilus* ATCC 7953 and *Bacillus atrophaeus* ATCC 9372 are exposed to sterilization and thereafter incubated. There should be no trace of living spores in case of effective sterilization.
2. ***Chemical indicators (integrators)***: These are chemical compounds which indicate process completion by a color change. As compared to biological indicators these give instant results. These are available in the form of chemical indicator tapes although the change in color does not signify effective sterilization; it merely signifies process completion.
3. ***Process challenge device***: The hollow devices, such as catheters, needles, aspiration syringes, drills, etc. need both outer surface and inside to be sterilized. Hence, this device was created to simulate hollow instruments. It has a long tube connected to a capsule. A chemical integrator is placed inside the capsule and then closed. It thus takes the shape of one end open device. A successful change in color of the chemical integrator inside the process challenge device on completion of the process of sterilization, guarantees sterilization of inside of all hollow devices. The presence of all parameters of sterilization inside the sterilizer, further guarantees sterilization of both the surfaces.

Biological indicator needs to be used after certain interval of time or after major maintenance and repair of the sterilizer as part of process of Validation. Routine monitoring on day to day basis is best carried out by chemical integrators through process challenge device.

BIBLIOGRAPHY

1. Dallolio L,Scuderi A, Rini MS, Valente S, Farruggia P, Sabattini MA, Pasquinelli G, Acacci A, Roncarati G and Leoni E. Effect of different disinfection protocol on microbial and biofilm contamination of dental unit waterlines in community dental practices. Int. J Environ. Res. Public Health: 2014; 11:2064–2076.
2. Gasparini R, Pozzi T, Mangeli R and Fatighenti D. Evaluation of *in vitro* efficacy of the disinfectant Virkon. Eur. J Epidemiol.: 1995; 11:193–197.
3. Ghinzelli GC, Souza MA, Cecchin D, Farina AP and de Figueiredo JA. Influences of ultrasonic activation on photodynamic therapy over root canal system infected with Enterococcus faecalis—an *in vitro* study. Photodiagnosis Photodyn. Ther.: 2014; 11:472–478.
4. Harsoor SS and Bhaskar SB. Designing an ideal operating room complex. Indian J Anaesth.: 2007; 51:193–197.
5. Herd S, Chin J, Palenik CJ and Ofner S. The *in vivo* contamination of air-driven low-speed handpieces with prophylaxis angles. J Am. Dent. Assoc.: 2007; 138:1360–1365.

6. Hooks TW, Adrian JC, Gross A and Bernier WE. Use of carbon dioxide laser in sterilization of endodontic reamers. Oral Surg.: 1980; 49:263–265.
7. Hurt CA and Rossman LE. The sterilization of endodontic hand files. J Endod.: 1996; 22:321–322.
8. Johnson MA, Primack PD, Lushine RJ and Craft DW. Cleaning of endodontic instruments. Part 1. The effect of bioburden on the sterilization of endodontic instruments. J Endod.: 1997; 23:32–34.
9. Kabbin JS, Shwetha JV, Sathyanarayan MS and Nargarathnamma T. Disinfection and sterilization techniques of operation theatre: a review. Int. J Curr. Res.: 2014; 6:6622–6626.
10. Linsuwanont P, Parashos P and Messer HH. Cleaning of rotary nickel-titanium endodontic instruments. Int. Endod. J.: 2004; 37:19–28.
11. Mayur L, Adish S, Ashish M, Deepak J, Sudha M and Rushikesh M. Endodontic instrument sterilization procedures followed by dental practitioner. Uniq. J Med. and Dent. Sci.: 2014; 2:106–111.
12. Miller C. Tips on preparing instruments for sterilization. Am. J Dent.: 2002; 16:66.
13. Miller CH and Sheldrake MA. Sterilization beneath rings on dental instruments. Am. J Dent.: 1991; 4:291–294.
14. Miller CH. Presence of micro-organisms in used ultrasonic cleaning solution. Am. J Dent.: 1993; 6:27–31.
15. Morrison A. Dental burs and endodontic files: Are routine sterilization procedures effective? J Can. Dent. Assoc.: 2009; 75:39a–39d.
16. Nagi M and Takakuda K. Influence of number of dental autoclave treatment cycles on rotational performance of commercially available air-turbine handpieces. J Med. Dent. Sci.: 2006; 53:93–101.
17. Neelakantan P, Cheng CQ, Mohanraj R, Sriraman P, Subbarao C and Sharma S. Antibiofilm activity of three irrigation protocols activated by ultrasonic, diode laser or Er: YAG laser in vitro. Int. Endod. J:2015; 48:602–610.
18. Parker HH and Johnson RB. Effectiveness of ethylene oxide for sterilization of dental handpiece. J Dent.: 1995; 23:113–115.
19. Perakaki K, Mellor AC and Qualtrough AJ. Comparison of an ultrasonic cleaner and a washer disinfector in the cleaning of endodontic files. J Hospital Infect.: 2007; 67:355–359.
20. Rutala WA and Weber DJ. Health care infection control practices advisory committee. Guidelines for disinfection and sterilization in health care facilities. cdc.gov/ncidod/guidelines/Disinfection.
21. TanomaruFilho MT, Leonardo MR, Bunifacio KC, Dametto FR and Silva IA. The use of ultrasound for cleaning the surface of stainless steel and nickel-titanium endodontic instruments. Int. Endod. J: 2001; 34:581–585.
22. Todd RP, Scuott WI and Stephen WG. Microbial contamination of endodontic files received from the manufacturer. J Endod.: 2006; 32:649–651.
23. Whitworth CL, Martin MV, Gallagher M and Worthington HV. A comparison of decontamination methods used for dental burs. Br. Dent. J: 2004; 197:635–640.
24. Zmener O and Spielberg C. Cleaning of endodontic instruments before use. Endod. Dent. Traumat. :1995; 11:10–14.

Chapter 13

Anatomy of Pulp Spaces

The pulp cavity is the cavity within a tooth, which is entirely enclosed by dentin, except at apical foramen. The pulp tissue in the coronal portion is known as pulp chamber and in radicular portion as the root canal. In anterior teeth, the pulp chamber gradually merges into root canal making no distinction. In multirooted teeth, the pulp cavity consists of a single pulp chamber and varying number of root canals.

Much of knowledge of anatomy of pulp spaces is based on the exhaustive work by Hess. The vulcanite preparation of almost 3000 permanent teeth showed minute detail of extensions, ramifications and branching as well as shape, size and number of root canals in different teeth.

For convenience, pulp space is divided into two:

a. *Coronal pulp* (lies within the crown of the tooth)

b. *Radicular pulp* (lies in the anatomic root).

a. Coronal Pulp

The coronal pulp chamber is a box like space surrounded by dentin and located in the anatomical crown. The outer (towards cusps) surface is known as *'roof'* and the inner (towards root) is known as *'floor'*. Influx of the pulp chamber directly under a cusp or a developmental lobe is known as *'pulp horn'*. These pulp horns can extend just under cusp tips or incisal edges in young individuals but as the age advances these become less prominent. The floor of the pulp chamber lies perpendicular to the long-axis of the tooth and is formed as a result of fusion of the diaphragm during the development of the tooth. The canal orifices originate in this pulpal floor. The canal orifices are not separate structures but are continuous with both pulp chamber and root canals (Fig. 13.1). The walls of pulp chamber derive their names from corresponding walls of tooth surfaces, such as the buccal wall of a pulp chamber.

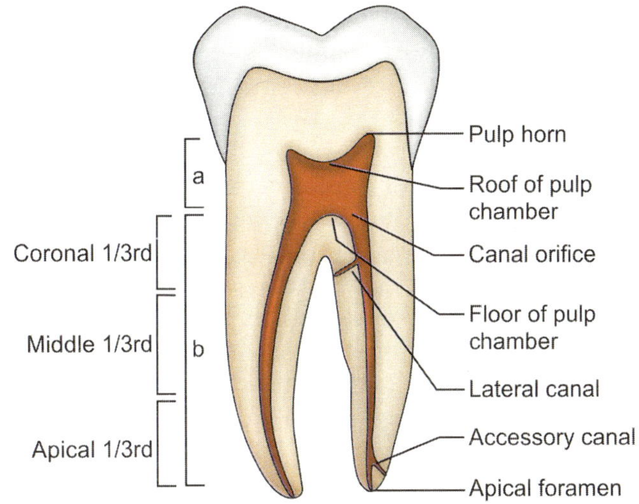

Fig. 13.1 Components of root canal system a. coronal pulp; b. radicular pulp

b. Radicular Pulp

The portion of pulp tissue from the canal orifice to apical foramen is the root canal (radicular pulp). It may be sectioned as coronal, middle and apical third. Accessory/lateral canals are branching of main root canal. The distinction between an accessory canal and a lateral canal is that lateral canal is a canal that branches to lateral surfaces of the root (usually visible on a radiograph); whereas, accessory canal is branch of main canal at apical third/furcation area (usually not visible on radiograph) (Fig. 13.1).

The root canal begins as a funnel shaped orifice, generally at the level or slightly apical to the cervical line and ends at the apical foramen. Most canals tend to curve in the faciolingual direction. These curvatures can be viewed in a radiograph taken at different angles.

A straight root canal extending the entire length of root is not a common feature. Usually, the canals are curved; the curvature may be a uniform curvature of entire canal or a sharp curvature of canal near apex.

Double curvature in form of letter 'S' may also occur. Curvature in narrow root canals may be difficult to negotiate; whereas, curvature of even 30° can be negotiated in wider root canals.

In most cases, number of root canals corresponds with number of roots, but a root may have more than one canal.

Relationships of Pulp Chamber to Clinical Crown

Krasner and Rankow (2004) proposed certain anatomic laws, which correlate the relationships of pulp chamber to the clinical crown:

- *Law of centrality*: The floor of the pulp chamber is always located in the centre of the tooth at the level of cementoenamel junction (Fig. 13.2).
- *Law of concentricity*: The walls of the pulp chamber are always concentric to the external surface of the tooth at the level of the cementoenamel junction (Fig. 13.3a and b).
- *Law of cementoenamel junction*: The cementoenamel junction is the most consistent, repeatable landmark for locating the position of the pulp chamber (Fig. 13.4).
- *Law of symmetry*:
  - *First law*: Except for maxillary molars, the orifices of the canals are equidistant from a line drawn across the floor of the pulp chamber in a direction from mesial to distal (Fig. 13.5a).
  - *Second law*: Except for the maxillary molars, the orifices of the mesial canals can be found on a line perpendicular to a line drawn in a mesiodistal direction in the middle of floor of the pulp chamber (Fig. 13.5b).
- *Law of color change*: The color of floor of pulp chamber is always darker than the walls (Fig. 13.6).
- *Law of orifice location*
  - The orifices of root canals are always found at the junction of walls and the floor (Fig. 13.7).

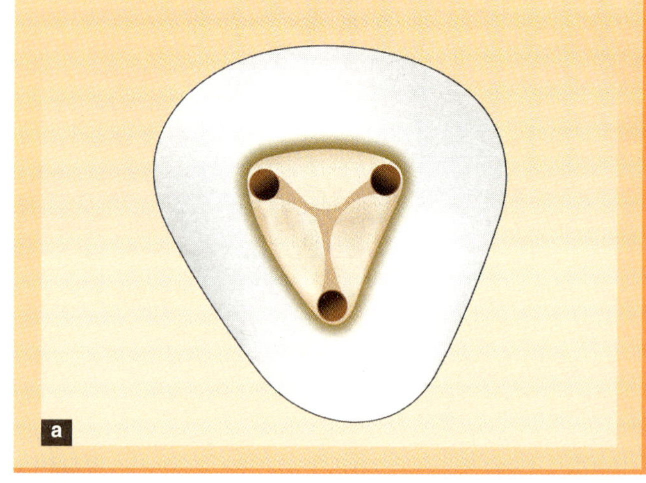

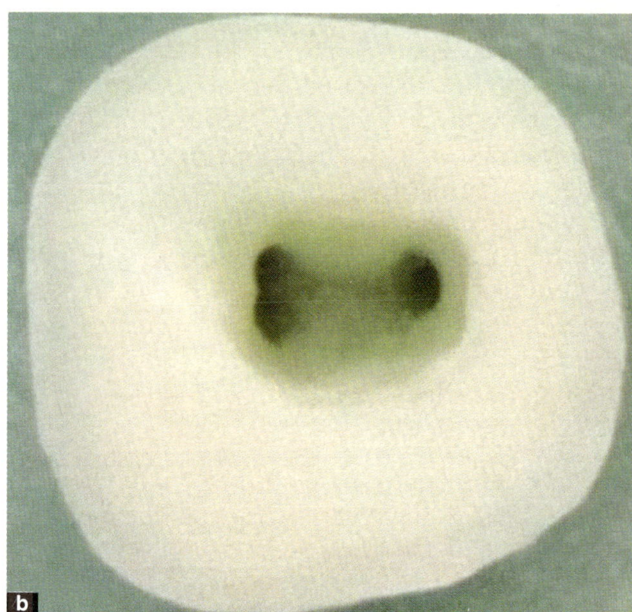

Fig. 13.3 Law of concentricity: (a) Diagrammatic; (b) Clinical

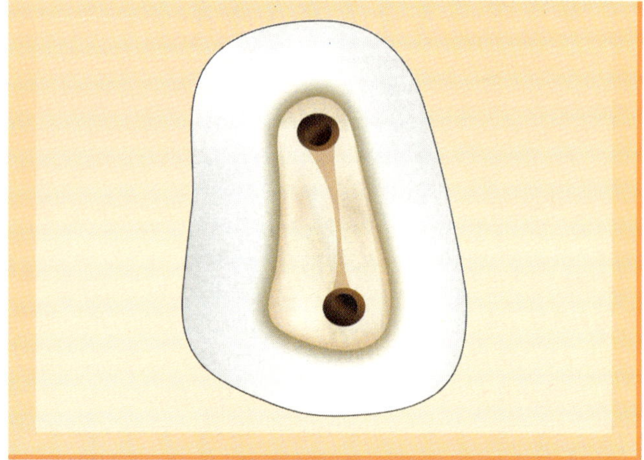

Fig. 13.2 Law of centrality (diagrammatic)

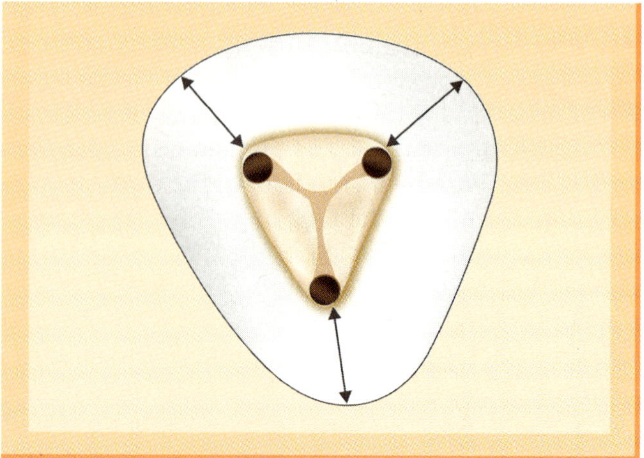

Fig. 13.4 Law of cementoenamel junction (diagrammatic)

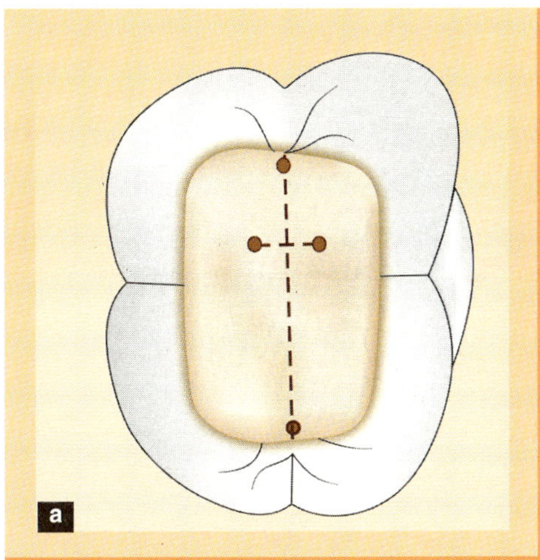

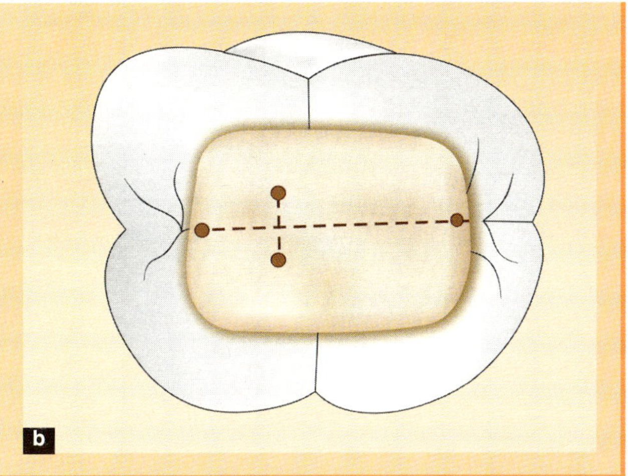

Fig. 13.5 Law of symmetry (diagrammatic): (a) Orifices are equidistant from the mesiodistal line; (b) Orifices are perpendicular to the mesiodistal line

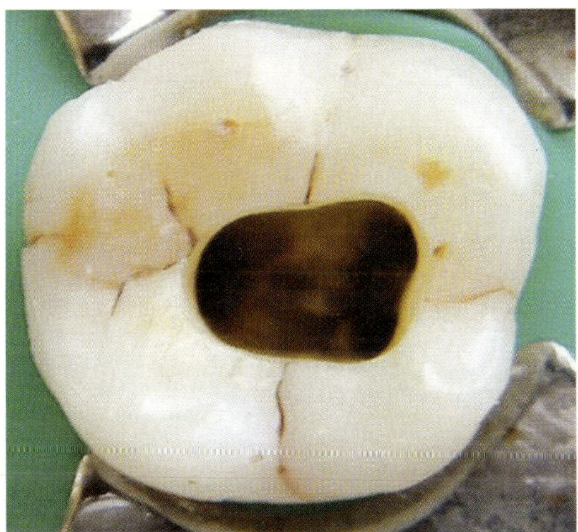

Fig. 13.6 Law of color change (dark at floor of pulp chamber)

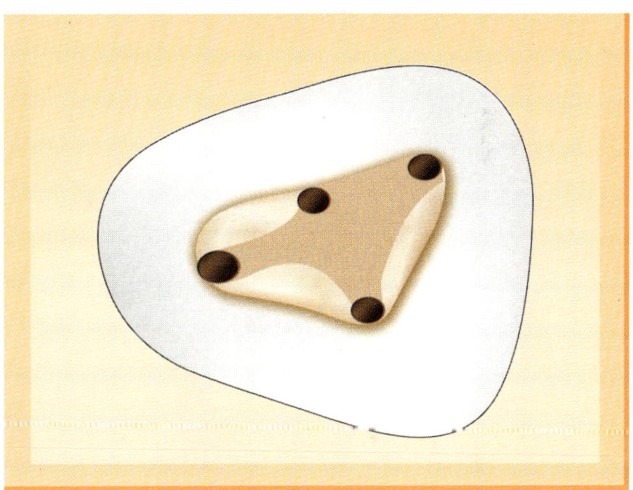

Fig. 13.7 Law of orifice location (orifices at the junction of wall and the floor)

– The orifices are located at the angles of two walls and the floor, coinciding with the developmental fusion lines of the root.

Anatomy of Apical-third of Root Canal

The knowledge of anatomy of apical-third of root canal (Fig. 13.8) is mandatory to carry out successful endodontic procedures. The apical root canal anatomy can be differentiated into three landmarks (Fig. 13.9):

a. *Apical constriction*

The apical constriction is the apical portion of the root canal system having the narrowest diameter, usually referred to as the '*Minor apical diameter*' or '*apical stop*'. It generally lies 0.5 to 1.5 mm short of the apical foramen. Violation of this area by root canal instruments lead to postoperative discomfort and also delay healing. The root canal instrumentation and obturation should be up to this constriction as it would serve as 'apical dentin matrix'.

Dummer et al described the configuration of apical constriction as of following shapes (Fig. 13.10):

- *Type A*. Typical single constriction.
- *Type B*. Tapering constriction with the narrowest portion near the actual apex.
- *Type C*. Constriction followed by another constriction (multiconstrictions).
- *Type D*. Long parallel constriction.

A fifth type has also been reported, wherein the canal is completely blocked with secondary denting and/or cementum.

b. *Cementodentinal junction*

The cementodentinal junction is the meeting point of dentin and cementum, where the pulp tissue ends and periodontal tissue begins. Due to deposition of cementum, the location and diameter of the cementodentinal junction differ considerably (Fig. 13.11). The

13

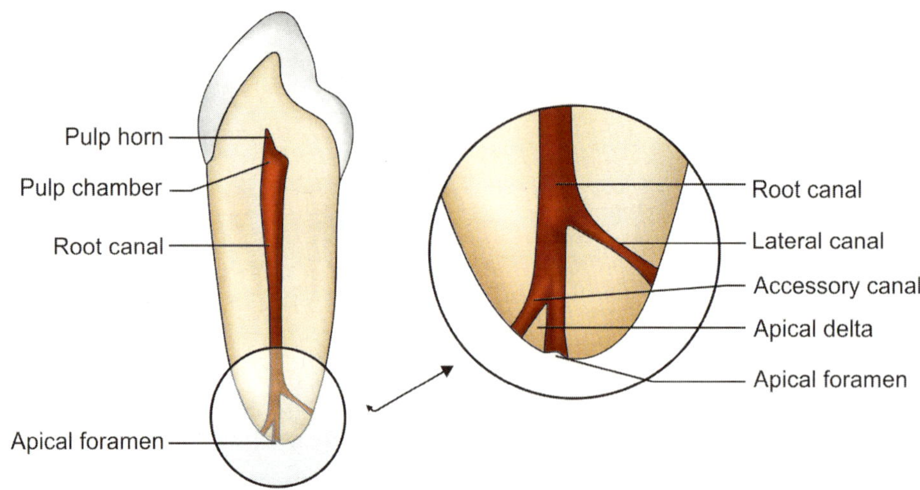

Fig. 13.8 Apical-third of root canal: Diagrammatic representation

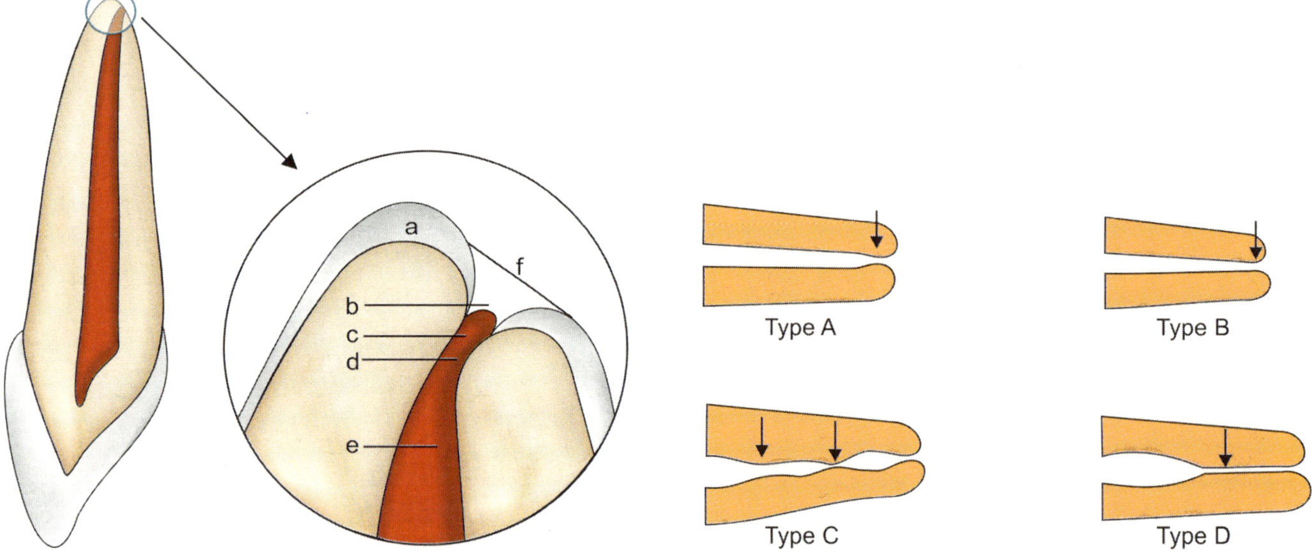

Fig. 13.9 Root end anaomy diagrammatic: (a) Cementum, (b) apical formation, (c) cementodentinal junction, (d) minor constriction, (e) root canal, (f) major opening

Fig. 13.10 Shapes of apical constriction: Type A: Single constriction, Type B: Tapering constriction, Type C: Multiple constrictions, Type D: Parallel constriction

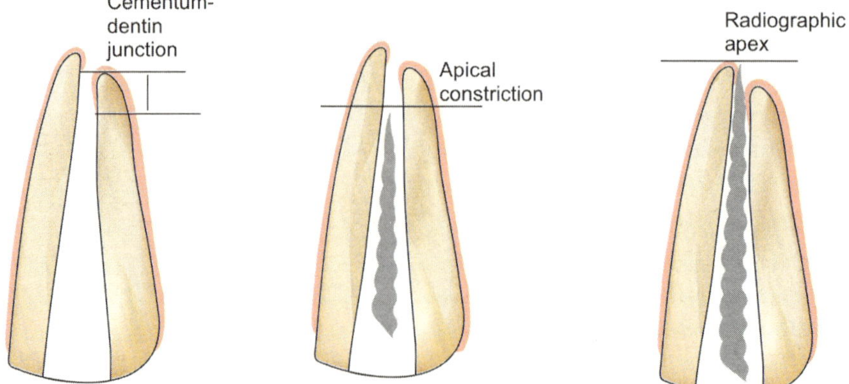

Fig. 13.11 Location of cementum-dentin junction (CDJ). Level may vary on opposite side of the root canal wall, not coinciding with the apical constriction

exact position of the cementodentinal junction can only be determined histologically, but for clinical purpose, it is accepted that it almost coincides with the apical constriction (minor apical diameter). The location may not be the same as apical constriction area; on an average 1.0 mm short of apical foramen. The diameter of canal at cementodentinal junction vary considerably in different teeth.

c. *Apical foramen*

The apical foramen is defined as *'an edge or end that differentiates the termination of canal to the exterior surface of root'*.

Apical foramen, also known as *'major apical diameter'*, is an opening at or near the apex of the root, through which blood vessels and nerves of the pulp enter and exit the canal (Fig. 13.12). Generally, the apical foramen do not exit at apex (mostly 0.5–1.0 mm offset from centre), may be mesial, distal, lingual or labial. In young incompletely developed tooth, the apical foramen is funnel shaped, with the wider portion extending outward known as 'Blunder buss apex'. At that stage, the mouth of the funnel is filled with periodontal tissue that is later replaced by dentin and cementum. As the root develops the apical foramen become narrower and farther from the apex. The space between the apical constriction and apical foramen takes a hyperbolic shape that resembles a 'morning glory' flower. The mean distance between major and minor apical diameter (apical foramen and apical constriction) has been found to be 0.5 mm in young teeth and 0.65 mm in older teeth.

Apical foramen is usually asymmetrical. This occurs due to functional influences on the tooth, viz. occlusal stress, tongue pressure, mesial/distal drift, etc. This leads to exertion of pressure on the surrounding walls, subsequently causing resorption and laying down of cementum, which changes the shape and location of the foramen. The size of apical foramen vary considerably (average size in maxillary permanent teeth is 0.4 mm and in mandibular permanent teeth is 0.3 mm).

ANATOMIC COMPLEXITIES IN ROOT CANAL SYSTEM

1. Radix Entomolaris and Radix Paramolaris

An extra root present distolingual to mesial root of mandibular molar is termed *'Radix entomolaris'* (Fig. 13.13a and b); whereas, additional root at the mesiobuccal side of the distal root of mandibular molar is called *'Radix paramolaris'*. In case of radix entomolaris, the extra root is usually smaller, lingually placed and more curved. It often has a sharp apical hook toward the buccal. It has 100% (1-1) canal configuration. The canal exits the pulp chamber with a marked lingual orientation. Radix paramolaris occurs less frequently than radix entomolaris.

Maxillary first molar may have four roots; two palatal, mesiobuccal and distobuccal.

The two palatal roots (one is normal and the other is supernumerary) are referred to as mesiopalatal or distopalatal. They have also been referred to as *'radix mesiolingualis'* and *'radix distolingualis'*.

Classification

Carlsen and Alexandersen (1990) classified radix entomolaris into following four types according to the location of the cervical part of radix entomolaris:

Type A: Distally located cervical part of radix entomolaris with two distal root components.

Type B: Distally located cervical part of radix entomolaris with one distal root component.

Type C: Mesially located cervical part.

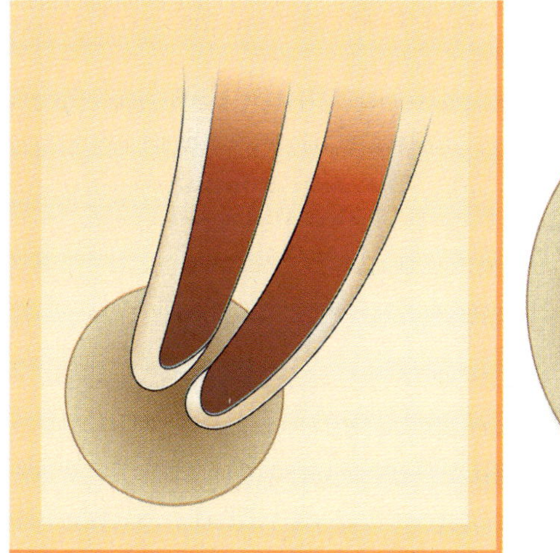

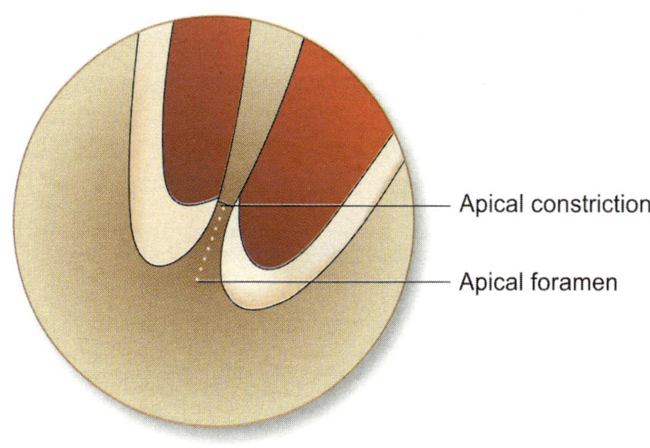

Fig. 13.12 Anatomy of the apical root

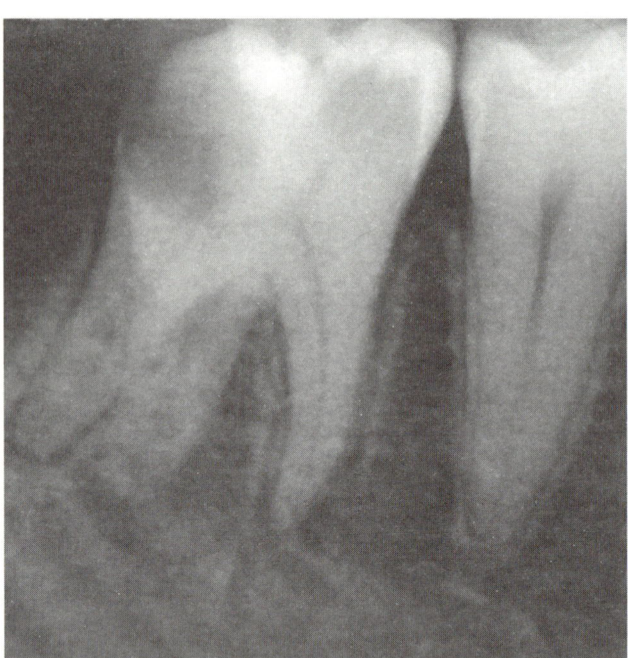

Fig. 13.13a Radix entomolaris (preoperative)

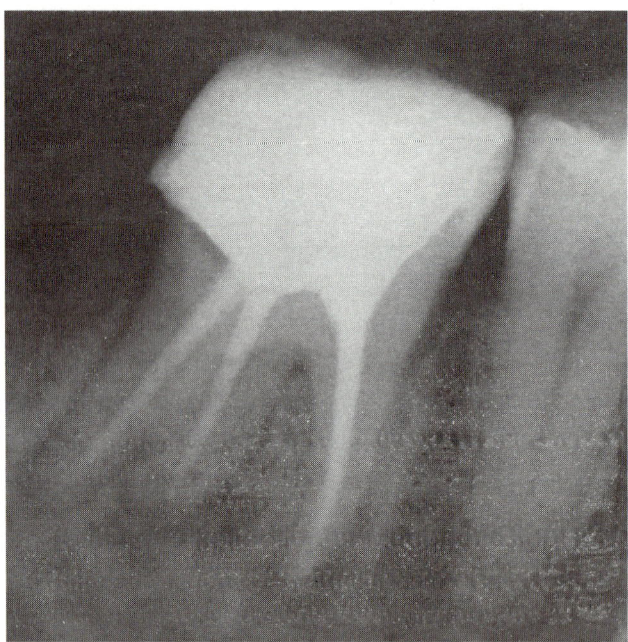

Fig. 13.13b Radix entomolaris (postoperative)

Type AC: Central location (between distal and the mesial root components).

De Moor et al (2004) also classified radix entomolaris into following three types based on the curvature of the separate radix entomolaris variants in buccolingual orientation.

Type I: Straight root/straight root canal.

Type II: Initially curved entrance, which continues as a straight root canal.

Type III: Initial curve in the coronal third of the root canal; second curve beginning in the middle and continuing to the apical third.

Carlsen and Alexandersen (1991) classified radix paramolaris into following two types:

Type A: Mesial part of root complex consists of three cone-shaped macrostructures: Facial, medial and lingual. It can be separate or non-separate.

Type B: Facial part of the root complex consist of three cone-shaped structures: central, mesial and distal. It can be separate or non-separate.

Versiani et al (2012) classified maxillary molars with two palatal roots into following three types:

Type 1: Palatal roots widely divergent, longer and tortuous (buccal roots may be 'cow-horn' shaped).

Type 2: Palatal roots run parallel to each other and comparatively shorter.

Type 3: Palatal roots are less divergent and often shorter than buccal roots.

2. C-shaped Canals

C-shaped canal is one of the important anatomic variation of root canal system. First documented by Cooks and Cox (1979), C-shaped canals are so named because of the cross-sectional morphology of the root canals.

- These are mostly seen in mandibular second molar followed by other mandibular molars and maxillary molars respectively (Fig. 13.14a and b).
- Formed due to failure of Hertwig's epithelial root sheath to fuse on buccal or lingual root surface, leading to fusion of mesial and distal root on buccal and lingual aspect. The C-shaped root may also be formed by coalescence because of deposition of cementum in-between.
- Roots with C-shaped canals usually have conical or square configuration.
- With interrupted/irregular fusion, the two roots stay connected by an interradicular ribbon.
- The shape 'C' can be continuous throughout the root length or two/three distinct canals may be seen in C-shaped groove.

Classification of C-shaped Canals

C-shaped canals have been classified by various authors. The accepted classifications are:

a. Melton classification

Melton et al (1991) classified C-shaped canals, based on cross-sectional canal configuration, into three types (Fig. 13.15).

13

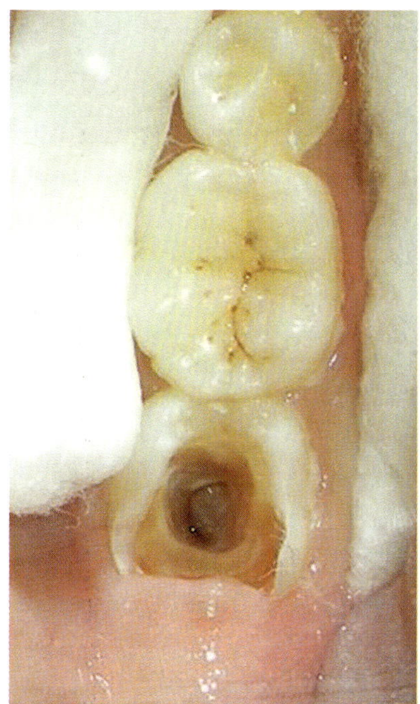

Fig. 13.14a C-shaped canal (clinical)

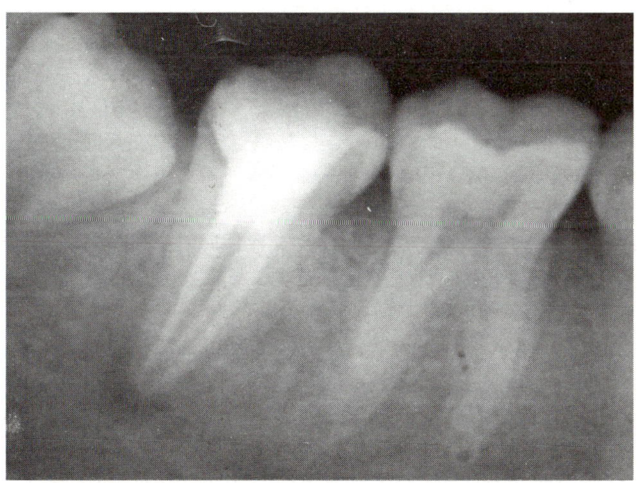

Fig. 13.14b C-shaped canal (obturated)

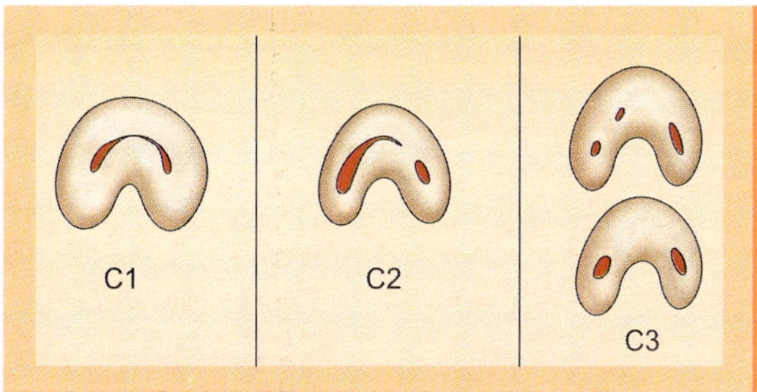

Fig. 13.15 Melton's classification

Type I (C1): The continuous C-shaped canal from pulp chamber to the apex without any separation.

Type II (C2): The semicolon shaped canal, where dentin separates one main distinct canal from a mesial/buccal/lingual canal.

Type III (C3): Two or more (usually two) discrete and separate canals.

- *Subdivision 1*: C-shaped orifice in coronal third, which divides into two or more canals, joining apically.
- *Subdivision 2*: C-shaped orifice in coronal third, which divides into two or more canals from mid-root to the apex.
- *Subdivision 3*: C-shaped orifice in coronal third, which divides into two or more canals from coronal to the apex.

b. Fan classification

Fan et al (2004) modified Melton's classification and categorized C-shaped canals based on anatomic and radiological appearances.

i. Anatomical consideration (Fig. 13.16)

Category I (C1): Uninterrupted C-shape with no separation/division.

Category II (C2): Discontinuation of shape 'C' (semicolon shape); angle β should not be less than 60° (Fig. 13.17a).

Category III (C3): Two/three separate canals; both angles α and β less than 60° (Fig. 13.17b).

Category IV (C4): Only one round/oval canal in the cross-section.

Category V (C5): Canal lumen not visible (mostly in apical area only).

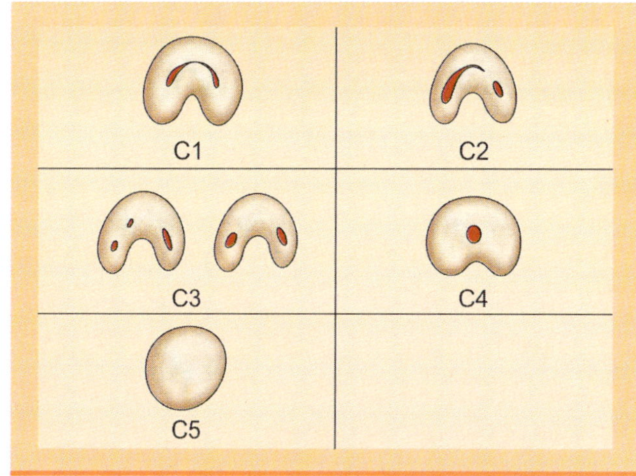

Fig. 13.16 Fan's classification (anatomic)

13

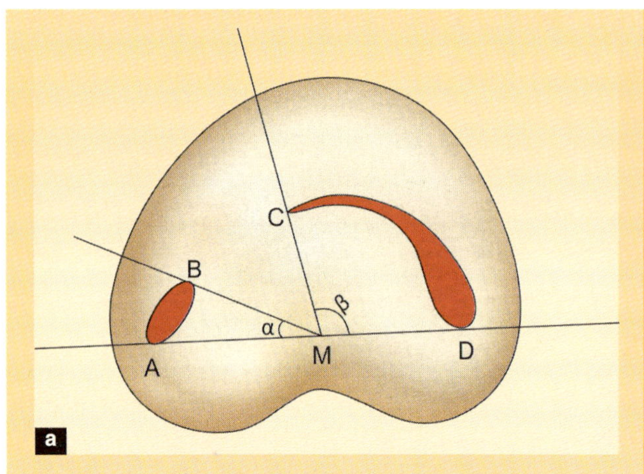

Fig. 13.17a Measurement of angles for C2 canal. Angle β is more than 60°. (A and B) End of one canal cross-section: M, middle point of line AD: α, angle between line AM and line BM; β, angle between CM and DM

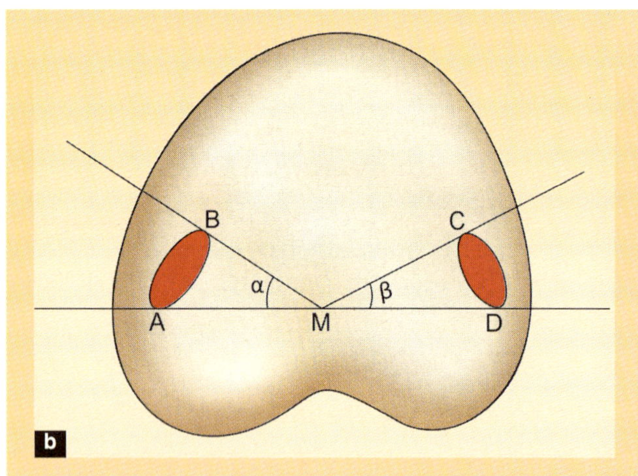

Fig. 13.17b Measurement of the angles for C3 canal. Both angle α and β are less than 60°. (A and B) End of one canal cross-section, (C and D) ends of the other canal cross-section: M, middle point of line AD: α, angle between line AM and line BM; β, angle between CM and DM

ii. Radiographic consideration (Fig. 13.18)

Type I: Conical or square root with a vague, radiolucent longitudinal line separating the root into mesial and distal parts. There are mesial and distal canals that merge into a single canal before exiting at the apical foramen.

Type II: The two canals are separate all along the root and exit separately.

Type III: One canal superimposes on the separation line and the other canal appears to continue to the apex.

13

3. Accessory/Lateral Canals

These are minute canals that extend haphazardly from the radicular pulp to the periodontium. Though found anywhere along the root surface, they are most prominent at the apical third. They contain shreds of connective tissue and blood vessels but do not supply the pulp with collateral circulation.

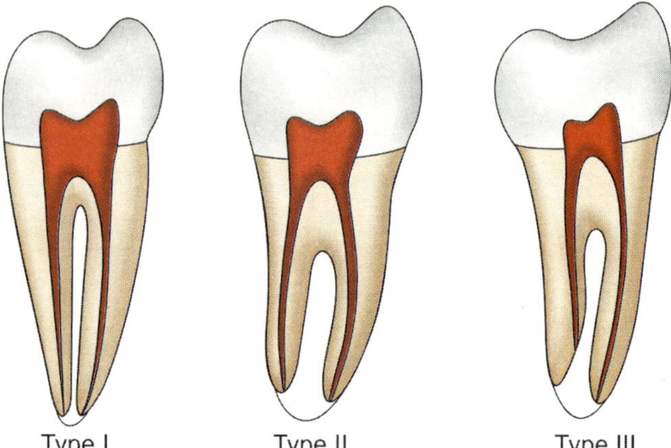

Fig. 13.18 Fan's classification (radiological)

Accessory foramina are the openings of accessory and lateral canal on root surface. These openings are very small; average mean diameter is 6.0–60 µ. The periodontal vessels curve around the root apex of a developing tooth and often become entrapped in Hertwig's epithelial root sheath with resulting formation of lateral canals and accessory foramina during calcification. Lateral canals may also occur in area of bifurcation or trifurcation of multi-rooted teeth as a result of entrapment of periodontal vessels during fusion of parts of the diaphragm that become floor of the chamber. Incidence of lateral canals ranges from 27 to 35% (the apical one-third 70–75%, middle one-third 12–14% and the cervical one-third 15–18%).

Minute canals may also be present in the bifurcation or trifurcation area of a multi-rooted tooth as a result of entrapment of periodontal vessels during fusion of the diaphragm, known as furcation canals.

The following radiological findings indicate the presence of accessory/lateral canals:

- Widening of periodontal ligament space in the middle of root (usually an ovoid radiolucent area is evident at the exit point of accessory canal).
- Bulbous root tip (pulp forming extradentin) is clear indication of extracanal.
- In oral-shaped root and root canal; if file is not in center, there is possibility of accessory canals.
- Sudden disappearance of radiolucency also indicates furcated canals.
- Inner curvature of root, mainly at the apical area; mostly presence of accessory and tortuous canals.

4. Apical Delta

Apical delta refers to a condition where the root canal exits through more than one tiny canals, instead of a single canal. If root canal break-up into many tiny canals at the exit point, the complexity is known as *'Apical delta'*. Usually, these canals cannot be observed on radiographs.

5. Isthmus

An isthmus is a narrow, ribbon-shaped communication between the root canals that contains pulp or pulpally derived tissues. A few authors have named it as 'transverse anastomosis', 'corridor' and simply as 'lateral connection'. Since, the isthmus houses pulpal tissue, it might serve as a potential site for bacterial growth. Usually isthmuses merge into main canal within 3.0 mm from the apex. Whenever two canals are present in one tooth, an isthmus should be suspected and attempt should be made to débride the same.

Classification

Hsu and Kim (1997) classified isthmus into following five types (Fig. 13.19):

Type 1: An incomplete isthmus with a faint communication between two canals (barely traceable).

Type 2: A complete/definite connection between two canals (may be straight or C-shaped).

Type 3: A complete, but short connection between two canals.

Type 4: An incomplete or complete connection between three or more canals.

Type 5: Two or more canal openings without any visible connection.

Studies have reported higher incidence of isthmus in mesial root of mandibular molars (80% at 4.0 mm from apex). Incidence varies in other teeth; 16% in maxillary premolars (1.0 mm from apex), 52% in maxillary premolars at 6.0 mm from apex, 30–40% mandibular premolars at varying levels from apex.

Mehrvarzfar et al (2014) evaluated isthmus prevalence, location and types in mesial roots of mandibular molars in an Iranian population and observed as: 83% mandibular molars had isthmus in mesial root; 90% at 6.0 mm from the apex and 70% at 2.0 mm from the apex. They emphasized upon using newer technologies to clean and fill these areas.

Isthmus is of great importance during apicoectomies of molars as well as other teeth. The retrograde cleaning of these areas is usually difficult; however, with the advent of microultrasonics coupled with better viewing, these areas are cleaned and obturated for better treatment results.

6. Root Canal Curvatures

Root canal curvature is quite common in radicular pulp space. The curvature can be uniform (gradual) in the entire canal; abrupt curve (sharp curvature) near the apical half or even S-shaped (double curvature) in the middle of root canal (Fig. 13.20).

Root canal curvatures should be determined prior to start of root canal procedures so as to avoid procedural errors and subsequent failure of root canal treatment.

Various authors have classified root canal curvatures based on their devices to measure the curvature. The accepted methods of measuring root canal curvatures are:

a. Schneider's Method

Preoperative radiograph of the concerned tooth is scanned. A midpoint is market at the center of canal

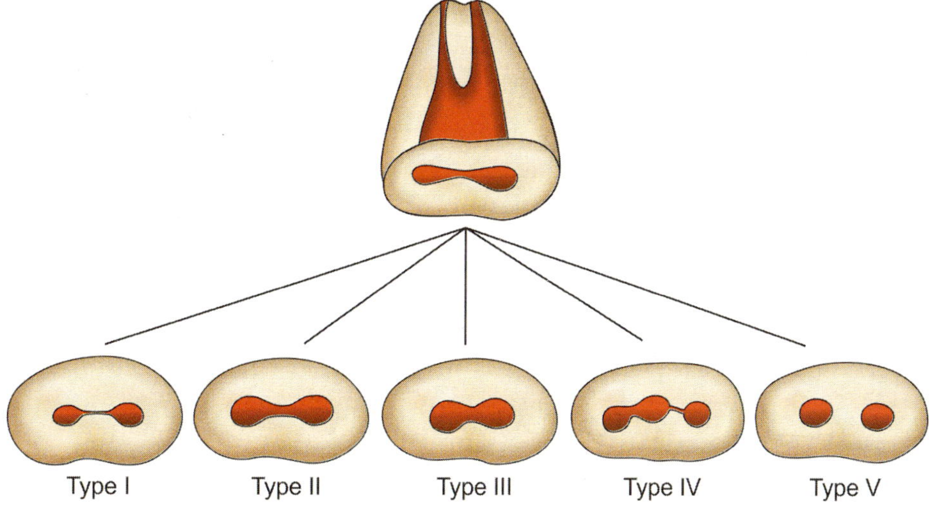

Fig. 13.19 Hsu and Kim's classification of isthmus

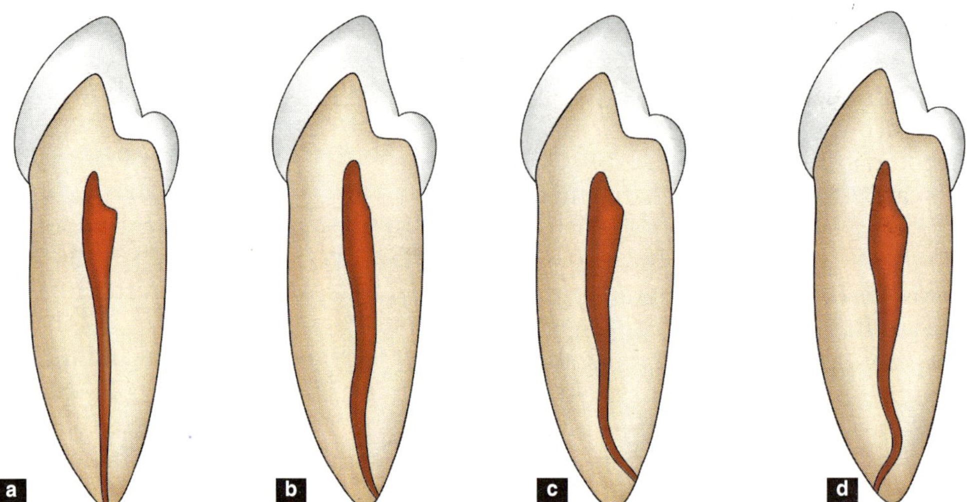

Fig. 13.20 Root canal curvatures: (a) Straight; (b) Minor curvature at apex; (c) Acute curvature in apical area; (d) Double curvature

orifice as 'A'. Another point 'B' is marked at the deviation of the canal. A third point 'C' is marked at the apical foramen. Line AB and BC are joined intersecting each other. Angle formed by this angulation (α) is the angle of curvature (Fig. 13.21a).

Based on angle (α), the curvature is classified as:

- *Straight*: Angle is less than 50°.
- *Moderately curved*: Angle is 5–20°.
- *Severely curved*: Angle is more than 20°.

The double curvatures have also been determined following Schneider's method; whereby, angle 'X' is for first curvature and angle 'Y' is for second curvature (Cunningham and Sonia).

b. Weine's Method

Weine simplified the method by taking long-axis of coronal canal as line AB and long-axis of canal from apex to deviation as CD. The intersection of the two is the angle of root canal curvature (Fig. 13.21b).

c. Lutein Method

Lutein modified Schneider method by identifying four geometrical points. Point A is marked at the center of canal orifice and point B is marked 2.0 mm below the orifice along the long-axis of canal. Point A and B are joined and extended. Point C is marked 1.0 mm coronal

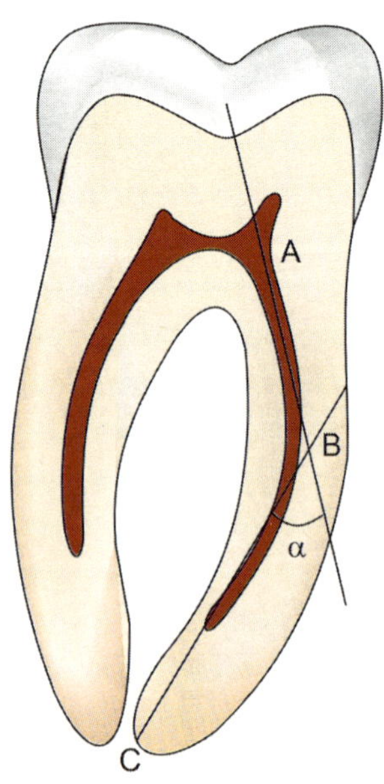

Fig. 13.21a Schneider's method

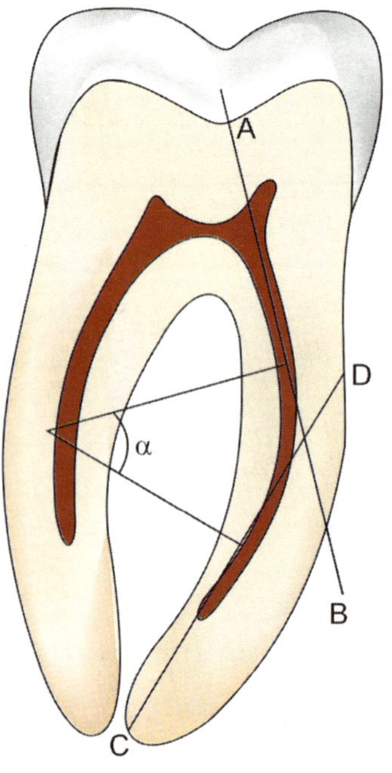

Fig. 13.21b Weine's method

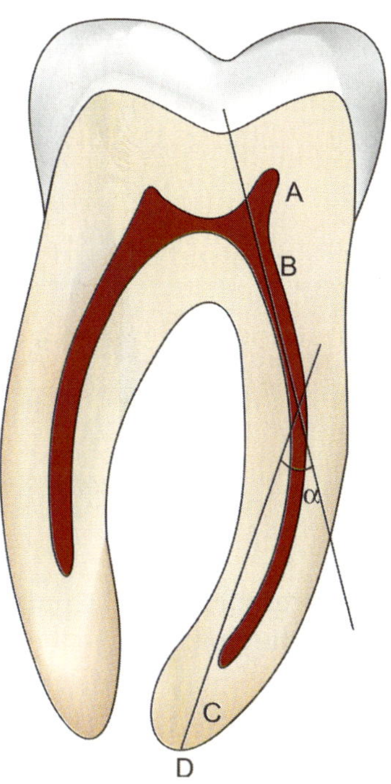

Fig. 13.21c Lutein method

to the apical foramen. Point D is marked at the apical foramen and the line CD is joined and extended. The angle formed by intersection of these two lines is the angle (α) of curvature. He used the same classification as of Schneider (Fig. 13.21c).

d. CBCT Imaging

CBCT provides better view of canal morphology as compared to periapical radiographs (3D imaging of canal curvature; buccolingual curvatures are better seen in CBCT imaging).

A software, provided with CBCT, can measure the radius of root canal curvatures. The smaller the radius, the greater the curvature; more complexities in pulp space anatomy. Based on curvature, the canal curvature is classified as:

Large radius (more than 8.0 mm): Mild curvature

Intermediary radius (between 4.0 and 8.0 mm): Moderate curve

Small radius (less than 4.0 mm): Severe curvature

A few authors prefer simple terms for curvatures as apical curve, sickle-shaped curve, bayonet curve and dilacerated curve; and also I (straight), J (apical curve), C (entirely curved) and S (multicurve).

7. Horizontal Dimensions of Root Canals

Very few studies have documented horizontal status of root canals at varying levels of root. Horizontal dimensions are important parameters, for effective cleaning and shaping of the canal spaces so as to achieve successful results (Figs 13.22 and 13.23).

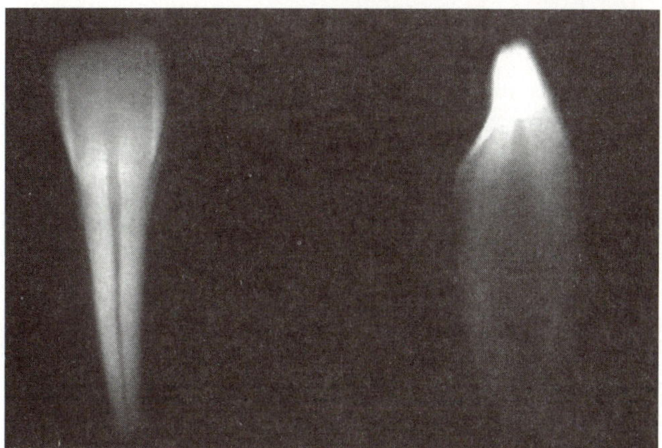

Fig. 13.22 Horizontal dimensions of root canal

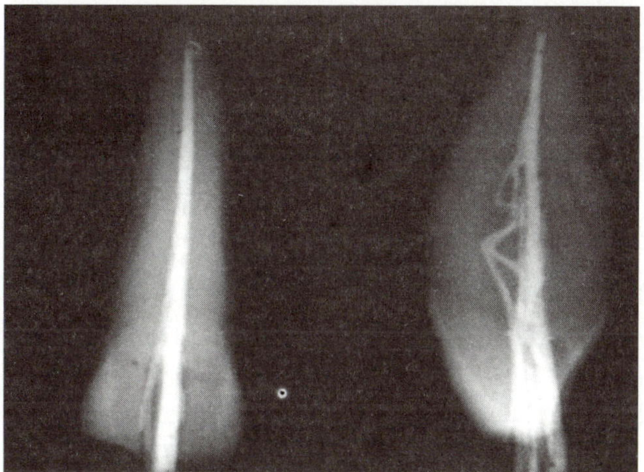

Fig. 13.23 Horizontal dimension of root canal (after obturation)

The horizontal dimensions are classified as:

- Round (maximum initial working width is equal to minimum initial working width).
- Oval (maximum initial working width is up to two times greater than minimum initial width).
- Long oval (maximum initial working width is up to four times more than the minimum initial working width).
- Flattened (maximum initial working width is more than four times greater than the minimum initial working width).
- Irregular (unspecified maximum and minimum working widths).

Circumferential filing is preferred to clean and shape the horizontal dimensions of canal spaces.

Classifications of Root Canal Anatomy

The root canal anatomy has been classified by various authors. The accepted classifications are:

a. Weine's classification (Fig. 13.24)

Type I: A single root canal extends from the pulp chamber to the apex (1-1)

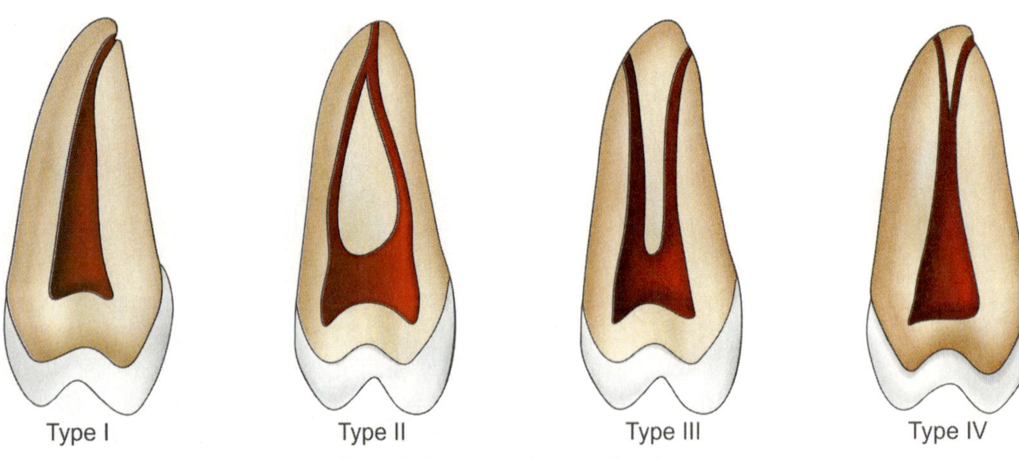

Fig. 13.24 Weine's classification

Type II: Two separate root canals leave the pulp chamber and join short of the apex to form one canal (2-1)

Type III: Two separate canals leaving the chamber and exiting the root in separate apical foramina (2-2)

Type IV: One canal leaving the pulp chamber but dividing short of the apex into two separate and distinct canals with separate apical foramina (1-2).

b. Vertucci classification (Fig. 13.25)

Type I (1-1): A single canal extends from the pulp chamber to the apex.

Type II (2-1): Two separate canals leave the pulp chamber and join short of the apex to form one canal.

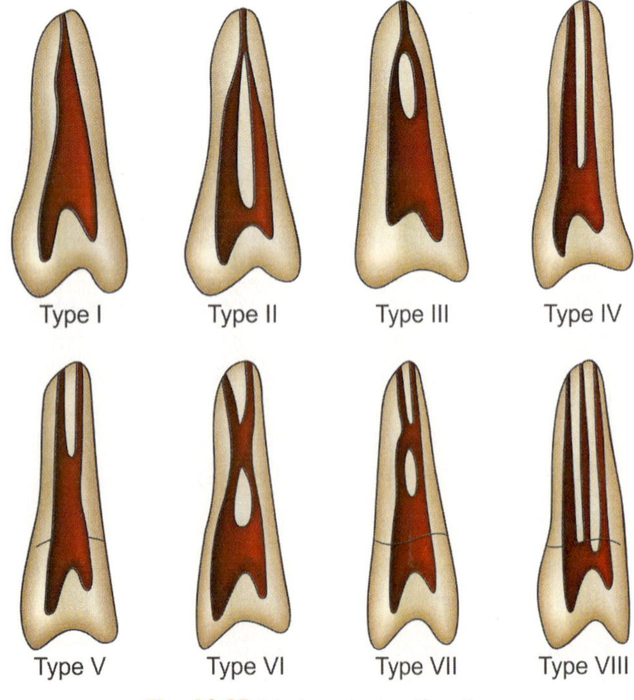

Fig. 13.25 Vertucci classification

Type III (1-2-1): One canal leaves the pulp chamber and divides into two in the root; the two then merge to exit as one canal.

Type IV (2-2): Two separate, distinct canals extend from the pulp chamber to the apex.

Type V (1-2): One canal leaves the pulp chamber and divides short of the apex into two separate, distinct canals with separate apical foramina.

Type VI (2-1-2): Two separate canals leave the pulp chamber, merge in the body of the root, and re-divide short of the apex to exit as two distinct canals.

Type VII (1-2-1-2): One canal leaves the pulp chamber, divides and then rejoins in the body of the root, and finally redivides into two distinct canals short of the apex.

Type VIII (3-3): Three separate, distinct canals extend from the pulp chamber to the apex.

Gulabivala et al extended the types as follows:

Type IX (3-1): Three separate canals merging into one at apex.

Type X (2-1-2-1): Two canals join to form one canal, again bifurcate into two and join at apex (exit as one).

Type XI (4-2): Four separate root canals, merging into two and existing as two at apex.

Type XII (3-2): Three separate canals, exiting two at apex.

Type XIII (2-3): Two separate canals, bifurcate and exit on three at apex.

Type XIV (4-4): Four separate canals, exiting separately at apex.

Type XV (5-4): Five separate canals exiting as four at apex.

Sert et al added two more types:

Type XVI (1-3): One root canal, bifurcating into three at apex (exiting as three).

Type XVII (1-2-3-2): One canal separating to two, than three and exiting as two at apex.

Peiris et al added another two types:

Type XVIII (1-2-3): One canal bifurcating to two and exiting as three at apex.

Type XIX (3-1-2): Three canals merge as one in middle and exiting as two at apex.

Al-Qudah and Awandeh further added four types:

Type XX (2-3-1): Two canals bifurcating into three and exiting as one at apex.

Type XXI (2-3-2): Two canals bifurcating into three and exiting as two at apex.

Type XXII (3-2-1): Three canals bifurcating into two and exiting as one at apex.

Type XXIII (3-2-3): Three canals bifurcating into two and exiting as three at apex.

Rather than following the classification system, the variations in root canals should simply be designated as 1-1, 1-2, 2-1, 2-2 and so on; i.e. the number of canals extending from pulp chamber (if one: write '1'; if two: write '2' and so on) to the number of canals exiting from the roots (if one: write '1'; if two: write '2' and so on). This becomes 1-1, 1-2, etc. In case it divides further in between, the expression can be 1-2-1, 2-1-2, etc.

c. Ahmed and Dummer classification: Citing limitations of present classification system (Weine and Vertucci), Ahmed and Dummer (2017) proposed a new classification, describing details of number of roots, root canals, their deviation and even presence of accessory canals.

In Vertucci's classification, buccal and palatal posts of maxillary premolars are not specified; for example, one rooted maxillary premolar with two separate canal and double rooted premolar with one canal each are designed as Type V (2-2).

The proposed classification describes as number of tooth (11, 12, 13 etc.), number of roots ($^{1}13$, $^{2}13$, etc.) and number of canals ($^{1}14^{2}$, $^{2}14\,B^{1}P^{1}$, etc.). For example, symbol $^{2}15B^{1}P^{2}$ describes as, maxillary second premolar (15), with two roots ($^{2}15$), one canal in buccal root and two canals in palatal root ($B^{1}P^{2}$). These canal configuration can further be referred as 1-1, 2-2, 1-2, 2-1, etc. Accessory canals are shown as A^{1}, A^{2} etc.

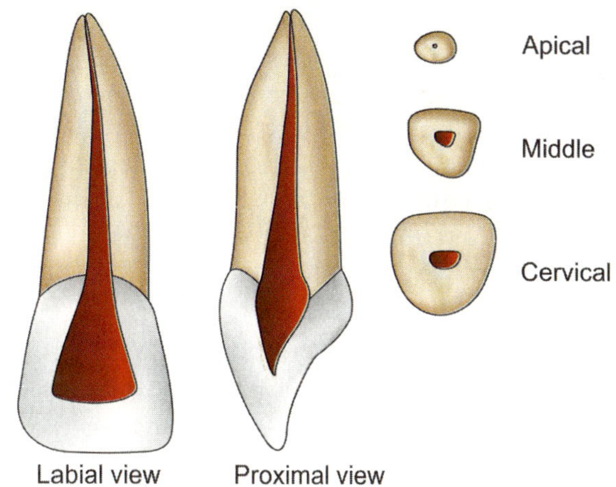

Fig. 13.26 Maxillary central incisor

CONFIGURATION OF PULP SPACES IN INDIVIDUAL TEETH

A. MAXILLARY TEETH

a. Maxillary Central Incisor

- In *labiolingual section*, the pulp cavity is pointed near the incisal edge; wider at the centre and then tapers from cervical area up to apex.
- In *mesiodistal section*, the pulp cavity is wider in the centre, with pulp horns (usually three) extending towards the incisal area. The canal tapers from cervical area up to apex (Fig. 13.26).
- Pulp floor is oval; root canal is continuous with pulp chamber without any distinction.
- Cross-section of root canals is ovoid at cervical end; whereas, round in middle and apical area.
- Variation includes fusion/germination and dens invagination.
- Rarely two or more canals present.
- The configuration of roots, root canals, their deviations and ramifications, curvatures and inclination, etc. are depicted below.

Maxillary Central Incisor							
Length of tooth	*Number of roots*	*Number of root canals*	*Lateral/ accessory canals*	*Apical ramifi-cations*	*Cross-section of root*	*Root curvature*	*Inclination*
23.3 mm (average) 25.6 mm (maximum) 21.0 mm (minimum)	1	1 +1 (rare)	20–45%	13–15%	Coronal (ovoid) Middle (round) Apical (round)	Straight: 75% Distal: 8% Mesial: 4% Labial: 9% Lingual: 4%	Mesial-axial: 2% Palatal-axial: 10%

13

Kasahara et al (1990) evaluated root canal anatomy of 510 extracted maxillary central incisors after making them transparent. They observed accessory canals in 60% specimens (branches were usually very small; only (3%) thicker than the size 40 file). 45% teeth showed apical foramen away from apex (within 1.0 mm from the apex). Vast majority of canal were straight (curvature less than 10°); few were curved towards the labial surface.

Almeida-Gomes et al (2012) reported a rare case of one-rooted maxillary central incisor with four root canals.

b. Maxillary Lateral Incisor

- Pulp chamber is similar to maxillary central incisors but smaller. It has two pulp horns corresponding to developmental mamelons (pulp horns may be absent).
- Cross-section of root canal at the cervical area is ovoid (sometimes round); whereas round at middle and apical area (Fig. 13.27).
- Variation includes fusion/germination, dens invagination (dens in dente).
- One root and more than one canal or two roots and two canals may be present.
- Deviation of root canal system is depicted in Fig. 13.28a to c.

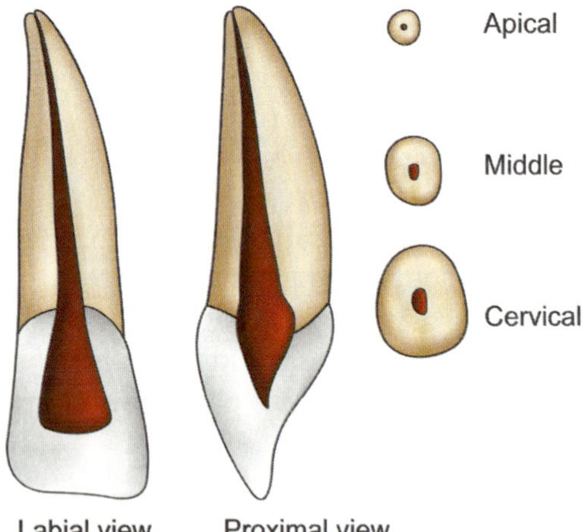

Fig. 13.27 Maxillary lateral incisor

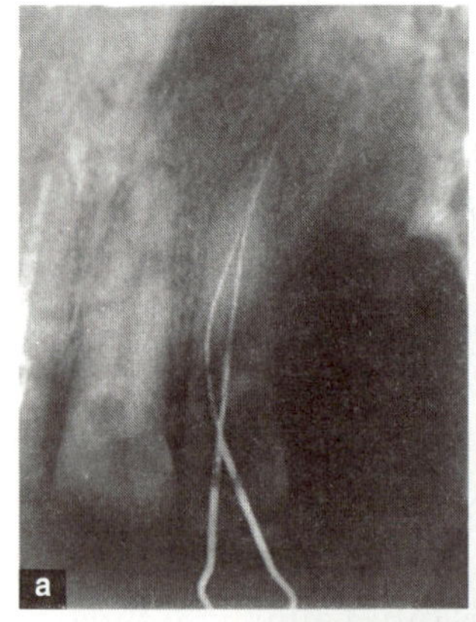

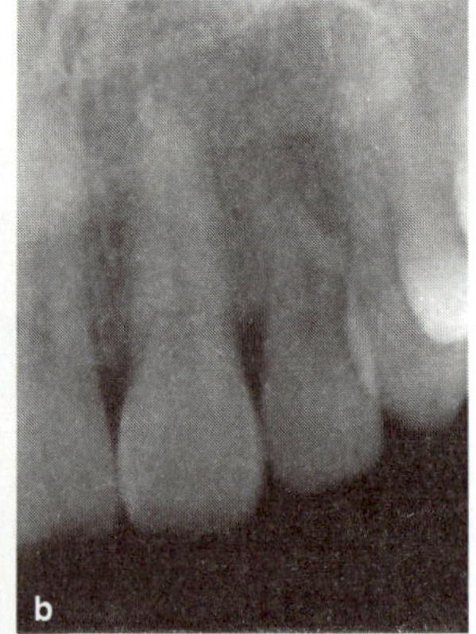

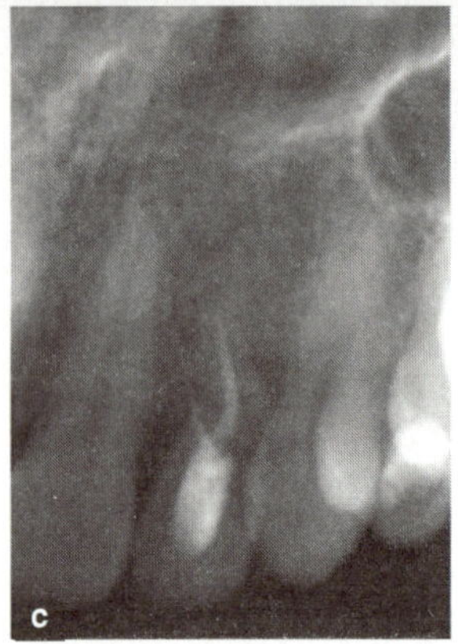

Fig. 13.28a to c Two root canals in maxillary lateral incisor

- The configuration of roots, root canals, their deviations and ramifications, curvatures and inclination, etc. are depicted below.

Peix-Sachez and Minana-Latiga (1999) reported maxillary lateral incisor with three canals.

Mupparapu and Singer (2004) reported a rare case of bilateral dens invagination (dens in dente) in maxillary lateral incisors (same patient exhibited dens invagination in mandibular lateral incisor also).

Mohan et al (2012) reported a case of maxillary lateral incisor with two curved roots and two separate canals. Lee et al (2013) reported three cases of maxillary lateral incisors evaluated by CBCT imaging (i) one root and two canals (ii) two roots and two canals (iii) one root and three canals.

Maxillary Lateral Incisor							
Length of tooth	*Number of roots*	*Number of root canals*	*Lateral/ accessory canals*	*Apical ramifi-cations*	*Cross-section of root*	*Root curvature*	*Inclination*
22.3 mm (average) 25.1 mm (maximum) 20.5 mm (minimum)	1	1 +1 (rare)	10–12%	12–15%	Coronal (ovoid) Middle (ovoid) Apical (round)	Straight: 30% Distal: 53% Mesial: 3% Labial: 4% Bayonet curve: 6%	Mesial-axial: 16% Palatal-axial: 29%

13

Maxillary Canine							
Length of tooth	*Number of roots*	*Number of root canals*	*Lateral/ accessory canals*	*Apical ramifi-cations*	*Cross-section of root*	*Root curvature*	*Inclination*
26.0 mm (average) 28.9 mm (maximum) 23.1 mm (minimum)	1	1 +1 (Rare)	20–25%	8–10%	Coronal (ovoid) Middle (ovoid) Apical (round)	Straight: 39% Distal: 32% Mesial: 0% Labial: 13% Lingual: 7% Bayonet curve: 7%	Mesial-axial: 6% Palatal-axial: 21%

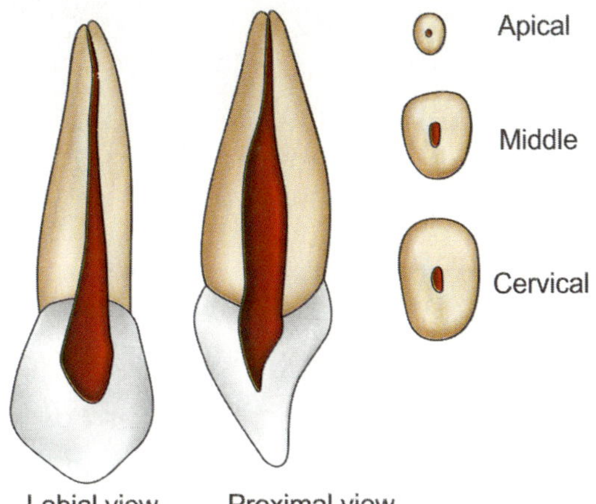

Fig. 13.29 Maxillary canine

c. Maxillary Canine

- Pulp chamber wider labiolingual than mesiodistal, without any pulp horns.
- Cross-section at cervical area is oval labiolingually. It is also oval-shaped in middle and round at the apical area (Fig. 13.29).
- Variation includes two roots and two root canals; roots may be dilacerated and presence of dens invagination (dens in dente).
- The configuration of roots, root canals, their deviations and ramifications, curvatures and inclination, etc. are depicted below.

A number of studies have reported two canals in maxillary canines.

Shin et al (2011) reported a case of maxillary canine evaluated with CT scans, showing two separated root canals (root canals also showed communication at the mid-point).

Nagesh and Sharat (2011) reported single root canal morphology of 250 permanent maxillary canines using CBCT imaging. They observed 81.6% samples exhibited 1-1 canal configuration; 11.6% (1-2-1), 2.8% (2-1), 2% (1-2) and 1.6% (2-1-2-1).

Nikhita et al (2014) studied root canal morphology of 250 permanent maxillary canines using CBCT imaging. They observed 81.6%, 1-1 canal configuration, 11.6% (1-2-1), 2.8% (2-1), 2% (1-2), 1.2% (2-1-2-1) and 0.08% (2-2).

Mupalla et al (2015) reported unusually lengthy canine (31 mm) with two separated root canals (labial-palatal canal orifice) which joined at the apical third (2-1 configuration).

d. Maxillary First Premolar

- In the labiolingual section, pulp horn usually extend farther incisally under the buccal cusp as latter is usually better developed than the lingual cusp.
- In mesiodistal section, pulp horns appear blunt and pulp chamber is in continuation with the root canals. (Fig. 13.30).
- Root canals are generally curved in apical third area.
- Cross-section in cervical area is ovoid or kidney-shaped; whereas, slight ovoid in mid-root and round in apical area.
- Apical end of roots may be nearing maxillary sinus (thin bony separation); judicious instrumentation is advised.
- The incidence of one canal is 10–15%.
- Mostly two canals are present (80%) and the possibility of third canal is 0.5–1.0%.
- Deviations of root canal system of maxillary first premolar are depicted in Fig. 13.31a and b.

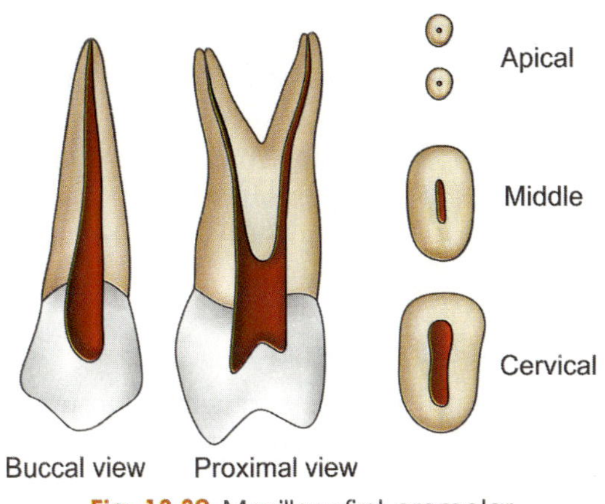

Fig. 13.30 Maxillary first premolar

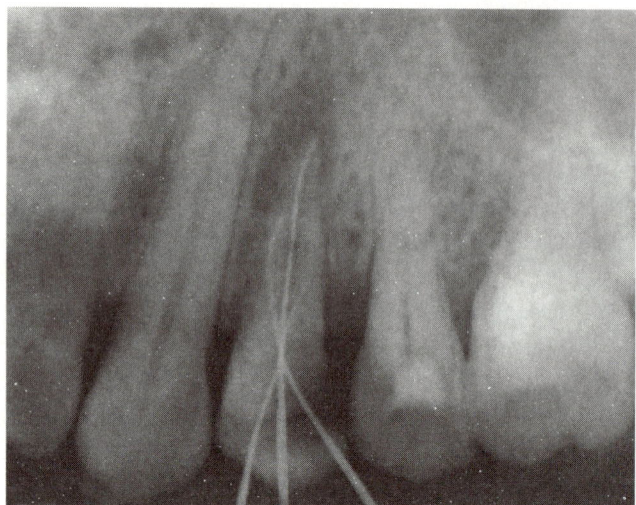

Fig. 13.31a Three canals in maxillary first premolar (diagnostic)

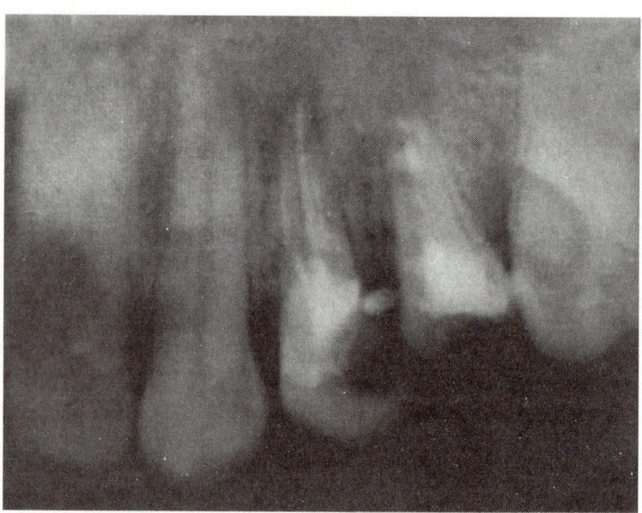

Fig. 13.31b Three canals in maxillary first premolar (obturated)

Maxillary First Premolar					
Length of tooth	*Number of roots*	*Number of root canals*	*Cross-section of root*	*Root curvature*	*Inclination*
21.8 mm (average) 23.8 mm (maximum) 18.8 mm (minimum)	1 Root: 20–30% 2 Roots: 50–75% 3 Roots: 0–6%	1-1: 8–10% 2:1: 1–1.5% 1–2: 72% 3–3: 6%	Coronal (ovoid) Middle (ovoid) Apical (round)	Single root Straight: 38% Distal: 37%	Distal-axial: 10% Buccal-axial: 6% Labial: 15% Lingual: 3% Double root **Buccal** Straight: 28% Distal: 14% Labial: 36% Bayonet curve: 8% **Palatal** Straight: 45% Distal: 14% Labial: 9% Lingual: 9%

- The configuration of tooth roots, root canals, their deviations, curvatures and inclination, etc. are depicted above.

Pecora et al (1991) studied internal anatomy of 240 extracted maxillary first premolars and observed single canal in 17.1%, two canals in 80.4% and three canals in 2.5% cases.

e. Maxillary Second Premolar

- The occlusal pulp chamber is similar to that of the first premolar, but the pulpal canal floor is deeper. Buccal and palatal pulp horns present (buccal pulp horn is larger).
- In majority of cases, a single canal is present. Two canals are also prevalent in 30% cases.
- The pulp chamber is large and is continuous with the canal. At the cervical level, the pulp cavity is elliptical and wide buccolingually (Fig. 13.32).
- As first premolar, the apical third of the root may curve considerably to distal (rarely to buccal).
- Deviations of root canal system of maxillary second premolar are depicted in Fig. 13.33a and b.
- The configuration of tooth roots, root canals, their deviations, curvatures, inclinations, etc. are depicted as follows.

Maxillary Second Premolar					
Length of tooth	*Number of roots*	*Number of root canals*	*Cross-section of root*	*Root curvature*	*Inclination*
21.0 mm (average) 23.0 mm (maximum) 19.0 mm (minimum)	1 Root: 20–30% 2 Roots: 50–75% 3 Roots: 0–6%	1-1: 8–10% 2-1: 5% 1-1: 5% 2-2: 72% 3-3: 6%	Coronal (ovoid) Middle (ovoid) Apical (round)	Straight: 9.5% Distal: 27% Mesial: 16%	Distal-axial: 6% Lingual-axial: 21% Labial: 12.7% Lingual: 4% Bayonet curve: 20.6%

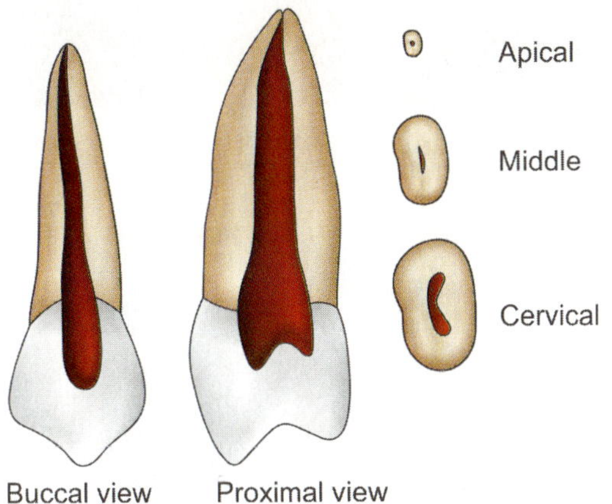

Fig. 13.32 Maxillary second premolar

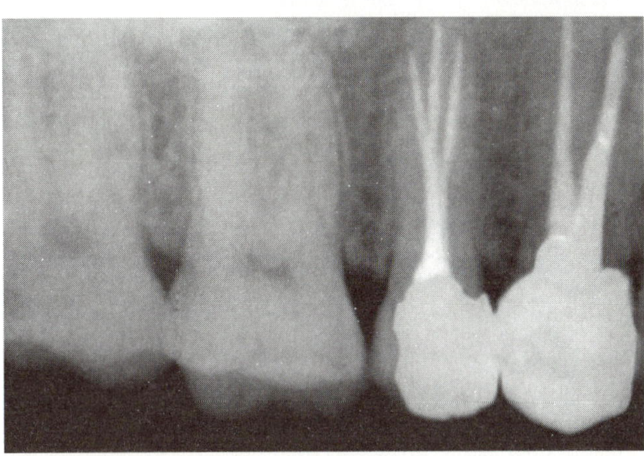

Fig. 13.33b Maxillary second premolar with three canals (obturated)

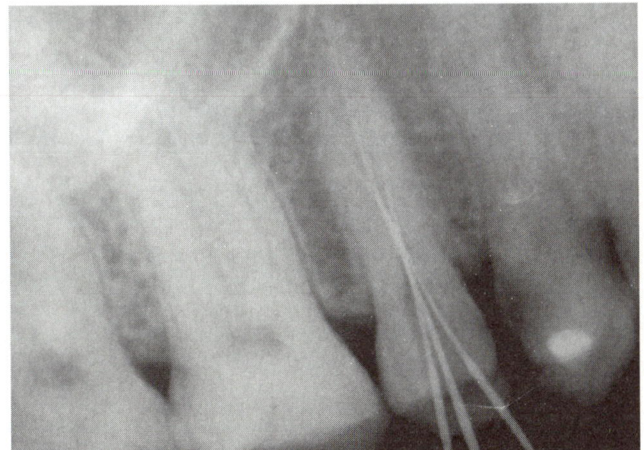

Fig. 13.33a Maxillary second premolar with three canals (diagrammatic)

Pecora et al (1992) studied internal anatomy of 300 maxillary second premolars. They observed one canal in 90.3% cases; two canals in 32.4% and three canals in 0.3% of the samples studied (one root was present in 90.3% and two roots in 9.7%). A predominance of root curvature towards distal was also observed (similar to first).

Udaykumar and Sumitha (2010) studied root canal morphology of 200 maxillary second premolars in an Indian population and observed 1-1 canal configuration in 29.2%; 2-1 in 33.6%; 2-2 in 31.1% and 2-1-2-1 in few cases. They also observed apical deltas in 14% and isthmi in 19% samples studied.

f. Maxillary First Molar

- The maxillary first molar has three separate roots: two buccal and one palatal. The roots may be straight or slightly curved at the apical area (mesiobuccal distally curved; distobuccal, distal/mesial curved and palate curved buccally). Any root can have an extra canal, prevalence is more in the mesiobuccal root. The palatal canal is wider than either of the buccal canals (Fig. 13.34). The palatal orifice is largest, round or oval in shape and is easily accessible for exploration. It lies near the central pit, mesial to oblique ridge. Mesiobuccal orifice lies under mesiobuccal cusp and is longer buccopalatally. The orifice of a fourth canal (extra MB) may be present (Fig. 13.35a to c) mesial-palatal to the main orifice or lie on a line drawn from the main mesiobuccal orifice to the palatal orifice. Distobuccal orifice is located slightly distal and palatal to the mesiobuccal orifice.

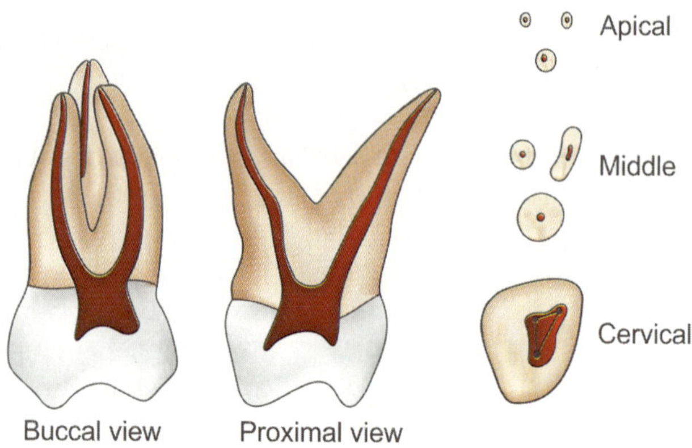

Fig. 13.34 Maxillary first molar

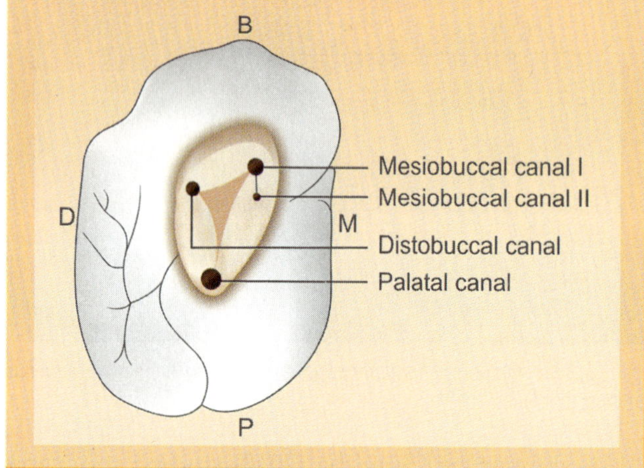

Fig. 13.35a Location of fourth canal (MB2)

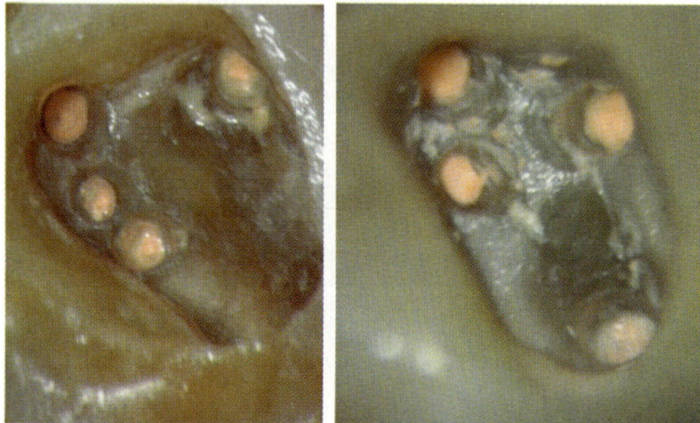

Fig. 13.35b MB2

Fig. 13.35c MB3

- Each root has one canal mostly; the pulp chamber is in mesial half of the tooth.
- Deviations of root canal system of maxillary molars are depicted in Fig. 13.36a to c.
- The incidence of anomalies have been reported by many authors in their case reports.
  - Four rooted maxillary molars (Christie, 1991)

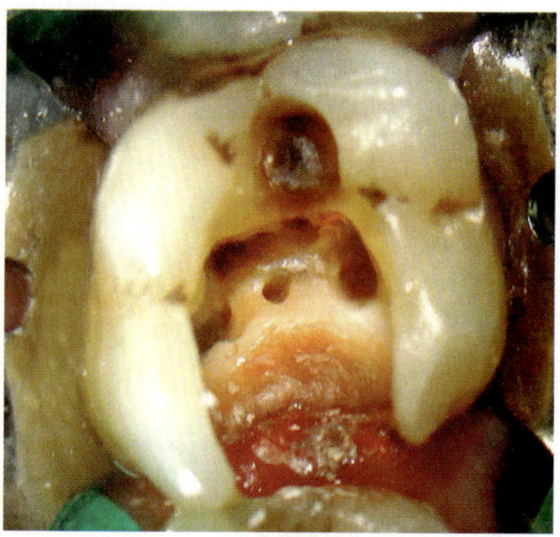

Fig. 13.36a Maxillary first molar with eight canals (*see* canal orifices)

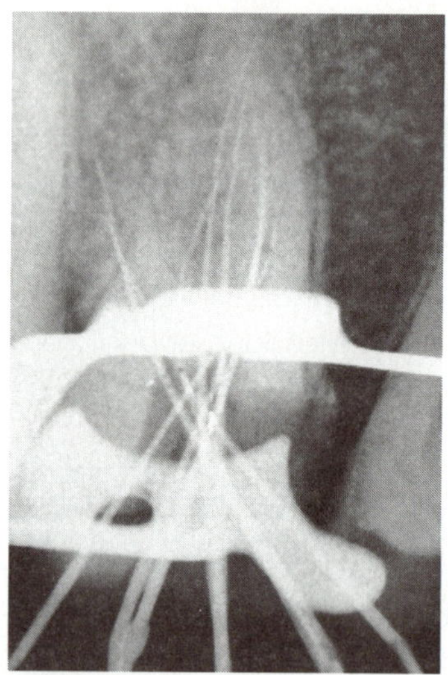

Fig. 13.36b Maxillary first molar with eight canals (diagnostic)

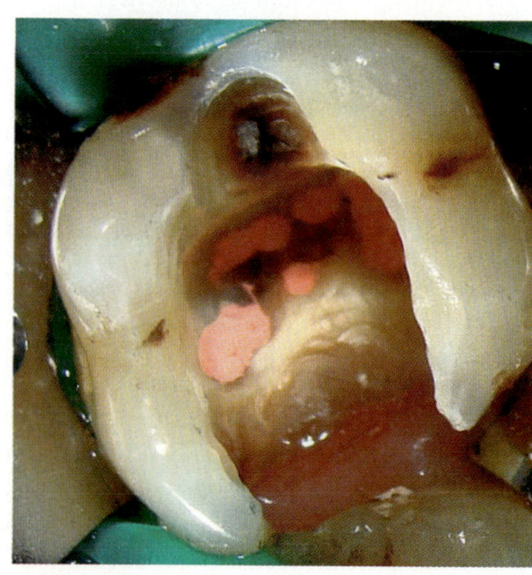

Fig. 13.36c Maxillary first molar with eight canals (obturated)

13

- Two palatal canal in three rooted teeth (Stone 1981, Hartwell, 1982)
- Two palatal canals and two palatal roots (Baratto-Filho, 2002)
- Three palatal canals in one root (Maggiore et al 2002)
- Root fusion
  - Fusion of palatal and distobuccal root (De Moor, 2002)
  - Fusion of mesiobuccal and distobuccal root (Fava, 2001)
- C-shaped canals (Danker et al 1990)
- Two canals in distobuccal root (Hulsmann, 1997)
- 41% maxillary first molars have three root canals; 56% four canals and 3–4% more than four root canals, 6, 7 and 8 canals have also been reported in literature (*pulp chamber is triangular, if three canals present and rhomboidal, if four or more canals present*).
- Mesiobuccal root has concavity on one side (usually distal). Judicious instrumentation is mandatory in the canal along that depression (thin dentin wall along that area).
- The incidence of two canals in mesiobuccal root is 55% and one canal 45%. With the use of microscopes, the studies have reported higher percentage of second mesiobuccal canal.
- In distobuccal root, one canal is prevalent in 94% of teeth and in palatal, it is more than 99%.
- The selected studies as regard root canals in mesiobuccal root of maxillary first molar is summarized in Table 13.1.
- The configuration of tooth, roots, root canals, their deviations and curvatures, etc. are depicted below.

Ahmad and Al-Jadaa (2014) reported three root canals in mesiobuccal root of maxillary first molars (two case reports). They observed 1.3–2.4% maxillary first molar had three canals in mesiobuccal root (3-2 canal configuration is common).

Table 13.1 Mesiobuccal root and root canals (selected studies)

Author (year)	*Type of study*	*Number of teeth studied*	*One canal (%)*	*Two canals (%)*	*One apical opening (%)*	*Two apical openings (%)*
Vertussi (1984)	Vitro	100	45	55	82	18
Pineda and Kutler (1972)	Vitro	262	39.3	60.7	51.50	48.50
Caliskan et al (1995)	Vitro	100	34.4	65.6	75.4	24.60
Imura et al (1998)	Vitro	42	19	80.9	11.80	88.20
Weine et al (1999)	Vitro	293	42.0	58	66.20	33.80
Sert and Bayirli (2004)	Vitro	200	6.5	93.5	60.50	37.50
Neaverth et al (1987)	Clinical	228	19.3	80.3	35.60	64.40
Slowey (1974)	Clinical	103	49.6	50.4	—	—
Wolcott et al (2002)	Clinical	1193	39.0	61.0	—	—
Stropko (1999)	Clinical	1096	26.6	73.2	45.10	54.90
Zactar et al (1997)	Clinical	133	59.4	40.6	85	15

Maxillary First Molar

Length of tooth			*Number of roots*	*Number of root canals*	*Root curvature*		
Mesiobuccal	**Distobuccal**	**Palatal**			**Palatal**	**Mesial**	**Distal**
19.9 mm (average) 21.6 mm (maximum) 18.2 mm (minimum)	19.4 mm (average) 21.2 mm (maximum) 17.6 mm (minimum)	20.6 mm (average) 22.5 mm (maximum) 17.6 mm (minimum)	2 roots: 4–5% 3 roots: 95% Four roots: 2–3% C-shaped: 0.10%	3 Canals: 41% 4 Canals: 56% 5 Canals: 2.5% More than 5 canals: 10% Canals in mesiobuccal root: 1-1: 41% 2-1: 40% 2-2: 19%	Straight: 40% Mesial: 4% Distal: 1% Buccal: 55%	Straight: 21% Distal: 78% Bayonet: 1%	Straight: 54% Mesial: 19% Distal: 17% Buccal : 1%

g. Maxillary Second Molar

- Maxillary second molar is similar to first molar with slight difference, such as short and closer roots with comparatively less curvature. It is usually three rooted; however, four rooted, two rooted and even single rooted are also prevalent. Fusion of root is also common; with or without merging of root canals.
- The root canals can be three as in first molar and two or one depending upon the number of roots. Extra canals can also be present in any root, usually prevalent in mesiobuccal root.
- Pulp chamber is usually triangular (Fig. 13.37). Mesiobuccal canal orifice lies under the mesiobuccal cusp (the orifice is more towards mesiobuccal side as compared to first molar). The distobuccal orifice lies midway between mesiobuccal and palatal orifices. The palatal canal orifice lies on the palatal aspect of the root (Fig. 13.38).
- Taurodontism and C-shaped canals are common.
- Being closer to maxillary sinus (roots almost touching the floor), pulpal diseases may cause sinusitis and sinusitis may lead to discomfort in these teeth.
- The configuration of tooth roots, root canals, their deviations and curvatures, etc. are depicted below.

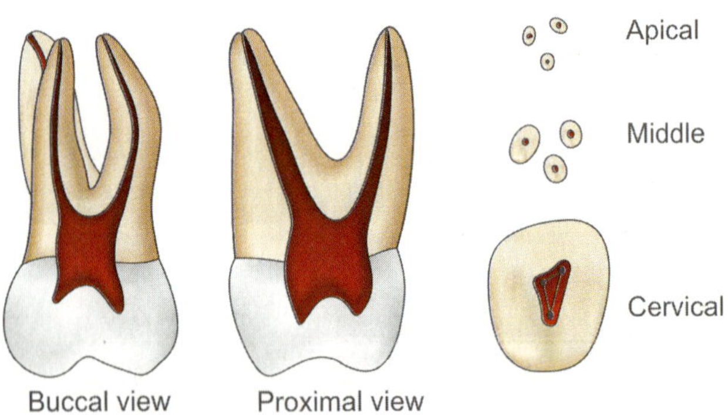

Fig. 13.37 Maxillary second molar

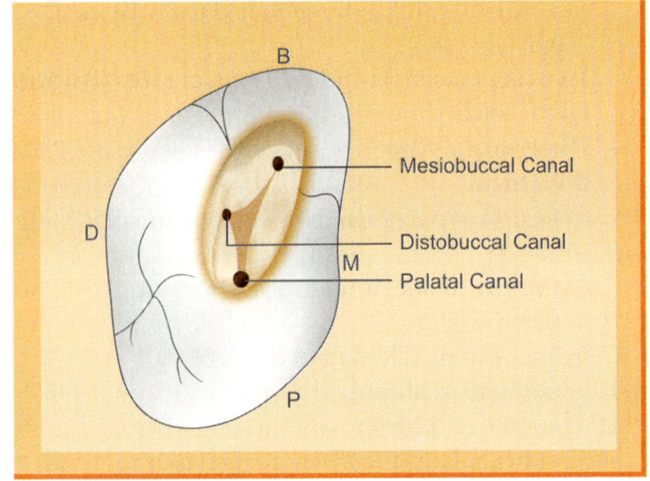

Fig. 13.38 Maxillary second molar (location of canals)

Fontana et al (2012) reported unusual maxillary second molar with four roots and two independent palatal canals (incidence of extrapalatal canal has also been reported in literature).

Badole et al (2012) reported maxillary second molar with four roots and four canals (two independent palatal canals: mesiopalatal and distopalatal).

Zhang Q et al (2014) reported 42.25% maxillary second molars with fused roots; a total of 187 samples studies 22 samples showed partial canal merging and 6 as complete merging of root canals.

h. Maxillary Third Molar

- Anatomically, it resembles second molar (length decreases from first to third molar).
- The number of roots in maxillary third molar ranges from one to five; corresponding canals range from one to six.
- Prevalence of second canal in mesiobuccal root (MB2) in maxillary third molar range from 35–40% (25% MB2 show 2-1 canal configuration and 15% show 2-2 canal configuration).

Maxillary Second Molar

Length of tooth			*Number of roots*	*Number of root canals*	*Root curvature*		
Mesiobuccal	Distobuccal	Palatal	3 Roots: 55%	1 Canal : 2–4%	Palatal	Mesial	Distal
20.2 mm (average)	19.4 mm (average)	20.8 mm (average)	2 Roots: 40–45%	2 Canals: 8–10%	Straight: 63%	Straight: 22%	Straight: 54%
22.2 mm (maximum)	21.3 mm (maximum)	22.6 mm (maximum)	1 Root: 1–2%	3 Canals: 60%	Buccal: 37% curve	Distal: 1% curve	Mesial: 17% curve
18.2 mm (minimum)	17.5 mm (minimum)	19.0 mm (minimum)	Four roots: 1–2%	4 Canals: 30%			
				Canals in mesiobuccal root 1-1: 63% 2-1: 13% 2-2: 24%			

Maxillary Third Molar							
	Length of tooth		*Number of roots*	*Number of root canals*	*Root curvature*		
Mesiobuccal 18.5 mm (average)	Distobuccal 18.10 mm (average)	Palatal 19.2 mm (average)	3 Roots: 50% 2 Roots: 45% 1 Root: 5%	3 Canals: 50% 2 Canals: 38% 1 Canal: 2% [4th canal (MB2) in less than 40%: 2-1: 25% 2-2: 15%	Palatal Straight: 80% Curved: 20%	Mesial Straight: 60% Curved: 40%	Distal Straight: 80% Curved: 20%

- The distobuccal and palatal roots in three rooted maxillary third molar presents single root canal (1-1 type).
- Lateral canals have also been reported in 1.0–15% maxillary third molars.
- The pulp chamber can be triangular with three canal orifices, or rhomboidal with 4 or 5 root canal orifices or a conical chamber with only one root canal (shows great variation in configuration of pulp chamber).
- Usually tipped to distobuccal side; creates problem in access opening.
- The root canal anatomy of maxillary third molar and obturation is depicted in Fig. 13.39a and b.
- The configuration of tooth, roots, root canals, their deviations and curvatures, etc. are depicted above.

Pecora et al (1992) observed MB2 canals in maxillary third molar as: 68% 1-1 canal configuration; 14%, 2-2 and 18%, 2-1 canal configuration. A few authors have reported only 20% MB2 in mesiobuccal root of maxillary third molars.

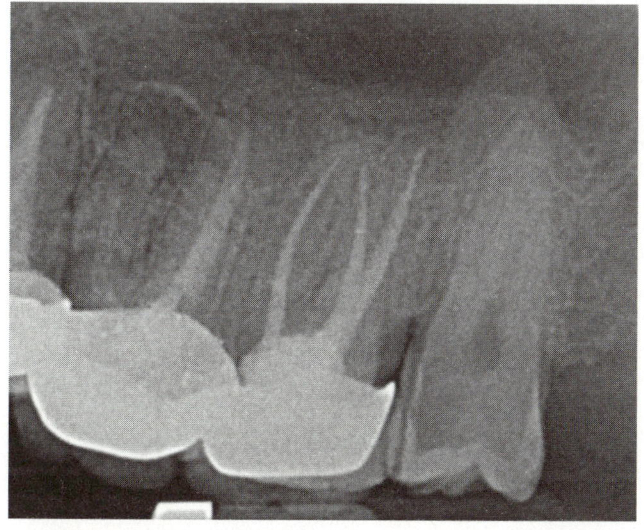

Fig. 13.39a Maxillary third molar (preoperative)

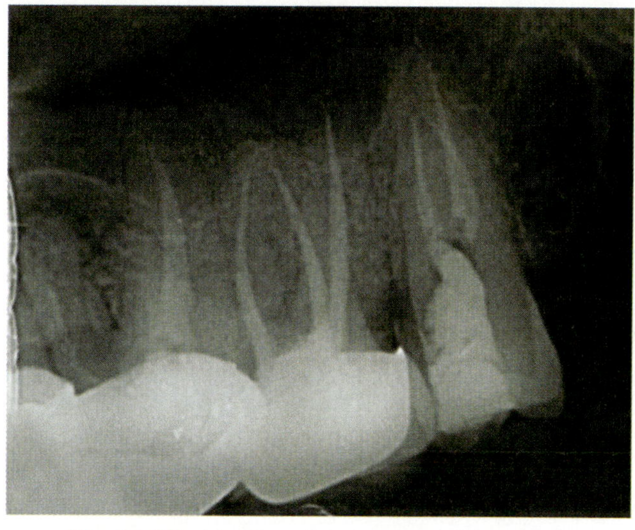

Fig. 13.39b Maxillary third molar (obturated)

B. MANDIBULAR TEETH

a. Mandibular Incisors (Central and Lateral)

- The incisors are mostly single rooted; root may be curved distobuccally.
- The root canal is usually rounded mesiodistally and slightly flat in labiolingual direction (Figs 13.40 and 13.41).

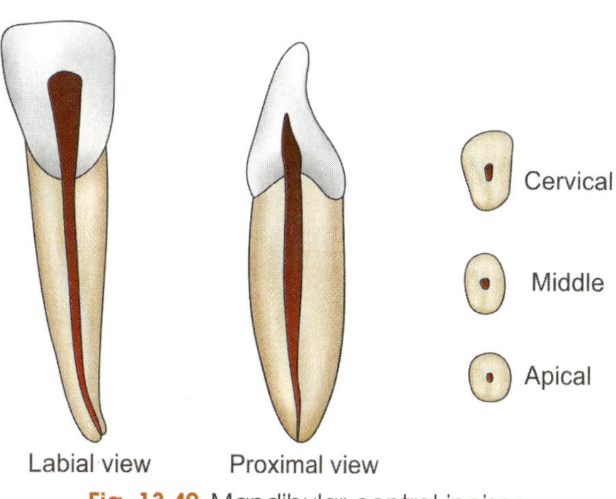

Fig. 13.40 Mandibular central incisor

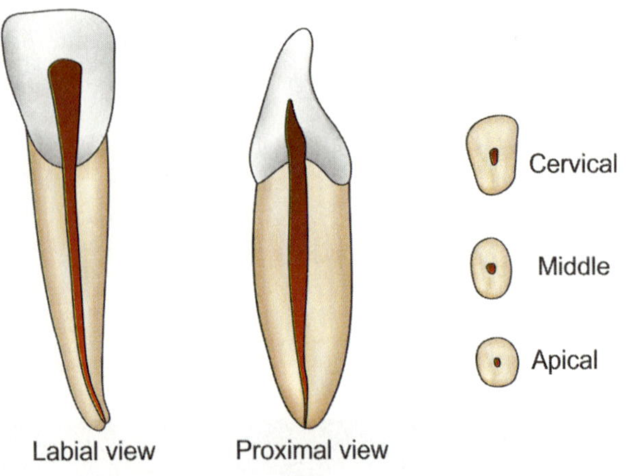

Fig. 13.41 Mandibular lateral incisor

- The mandibular incisors may have second root canal (40% incidence). Mostly two root canals join at apex (2-1 type). Rarely two separate canals (2-2 type).
- Mandibular incisors are lingually tilted (lateral incisors are also distally tilted).
- Cross-section at cervical area is oval; whereas, it is ribbon-shaped in midroot and round in apical third area.
- Deviations of root canal system of mandibular incisors are depicted in Fig. 13.42a and b.
- Fusion, germination and dens invagination are the possible anatomical variations.
- The configuration of tooth roots, root canals, their deviations, curvatures and inclination, etc. are depicted in boxes.

Sikri and Sikri (1992) studied root canal morphology of mandibular incisors by radiographic evaluation and reported that 4.16% central incisors and 5.52% lateral incisors exhibited two root canals. 35.42% root canals in central incisors were curved and 39.13% canals were curved in lateral incisors.

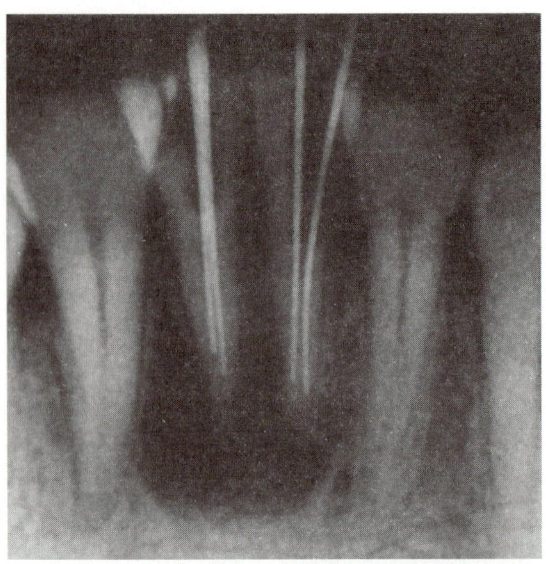

Fig. 13.42a Two root canals in mandibular incisors (diagnostic)

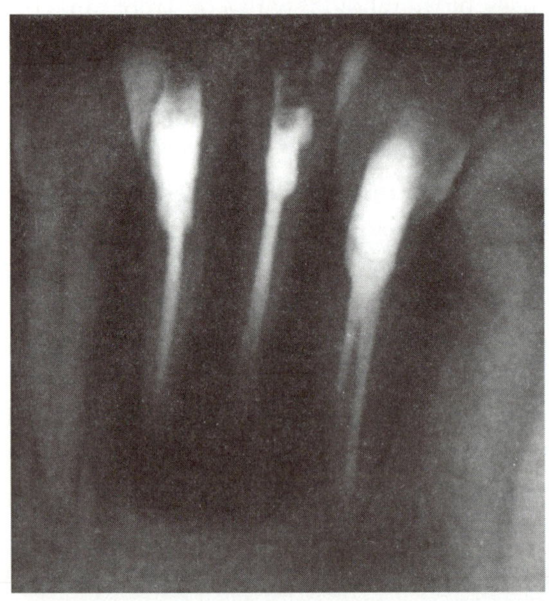

Fig. 13.42b Two root canals in mandibular incisors (obturated)

Mandibular Central Incisor

Length of tooth	*Number of roots*	*Number of root canals*	*Cross-section of root*	*Root curvature*	*Inclination*
21.5 mm (average) 23.4 mm (maximum) 19.6 mm (minimum)	1	1-1: 70% 2-1:40%	**One canal** Coronal (ovoid) Middle (ovoid) Apical (round) **Two canal** Coronal (ovoid) Middle (round) Apical (round and curve toward incisal)	Straight: 60% Distal: 23% Labial: 13%	Mesial-axial: 2% Lingual-axial: 29%

Mandibular Lateral Incisor					
Length of tooth	*Number of roots*	*Number of root canals*	*Cross-section of root*	*Root curvature*	*Inclination*
22.4 mm (average) 24.6 mm (maximum) 20.2 mm (minimum)	1	1-2: 55–60% 2-1: 14–16%	**One Canal** Coronal (ovoid) Middle (round) Apical (round) **Two canal** Coronal (ovoid) Middle (round) Apical: (round and curved toward incisal)	Straight: 60% Distal: 23% Labial: 13%	Mesial-axial: 17% Lingual-axial: 29%

Al-Fourzan et al (2012) studied incidence of two canals in extracted mandibular incisors of Saudi Arabian population and observed 70% teeth showing 1-1 canal configuration and 30%, 2-1 configuration.

Kabak et al (2007) reported a case exhibiting two canals in four mandibular incisors.

b. Mandibular Canine

- Mostly single rooted; root may curve distobuccally. Rarely two roots present.
- Mostly single canal; rarely two canals present (Fig. 13.43a to d).
- Pulpal chamber is narrow mesiodistally; pulp floor is oval (Fig. 13.43e).
- Fusion and dens invagination have been reported.

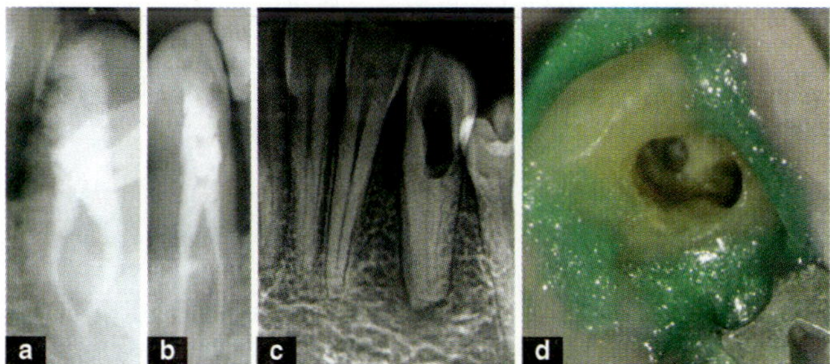

Fig. 13.43a to d Mandibular canine with two root canals

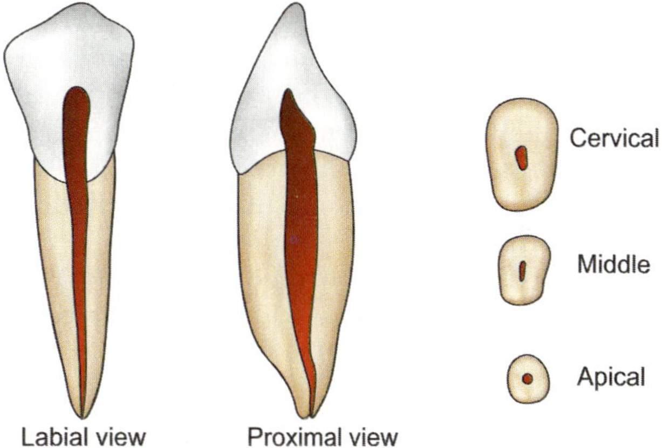

Fig. 13.43e Mandibular canine

- Cross-section at cervical area is ovoid funnel-shaped; whereas, ovoid in midroot and round in apical third area.
- The configuration of roots, root canals, their deviations tooth, curvatures and inclination, etc. are depicted below.

Shemesh et al (2016) evaluated root anatomy and root canal morphology of 1981 mandibular canines in Israeli population using CBCT imaging. They reported 1.9% cases had bifurcated roots and 10.3% bifurcated root canals.

Mandibular Canine						
Length of tooth	*Number of roots*	*Number of root canals*	*Lateral/ accessory canals*	*Cross-section of root*	*Root curvature*	*Inclination*
25.5 mm (average) 27.5 mm (maximum) 22.9 mm (minimum)	1 root: 95–99% 2 roots: 1–5%	1-2: 92–96% 2-2: 4–8%	9.5%	Coronal (ovoid) Middle (ovoid) Apical (round)	Straight: 68% Distal: 20% Mesial: 1% Labial: 7% Bayonet curve: 20%	Mesial-axial: 13% Lingual-axial: 15%

Pecora et al (1993) studied internal anatomy, direction and number of roots and size of human mandibular canines and observed 98.3% as one rooted and 1.7% two rooted canines. 92.2% presented with one canal (1-1); 4.9% with 2-1 type canal and 1.2% with 2-2 type canal configuration.

Nikhita et al (2014) studied root canal morphology of 250 permanent mandibular canines using CBCT imaging. They observed 79.6% teeth exhibited 1-1 canal configuration; 13.6% (1-2-1), 3.2% (2-1), 2% (1-2) and 1.6% (2-1-2-1).

Holtzman (1997) reported a rare case of mandibular permanent canine with three root canals.

c. Mandibular First Premolar

- It is documented that mandibular first premolar is the most difficult tooth to be treated endodontically.
- The mandibular first premolar resembles canine; the cingulum simulates the lingual cusp (Fig. 13.44).
- The mesiolingual developmental groove makes the tooth asymmetrical.
- The crown is lingually tilted by 45°. The distal inclination is approximately 10°. The bifurcated root canals are quite prevalent in first premolar.

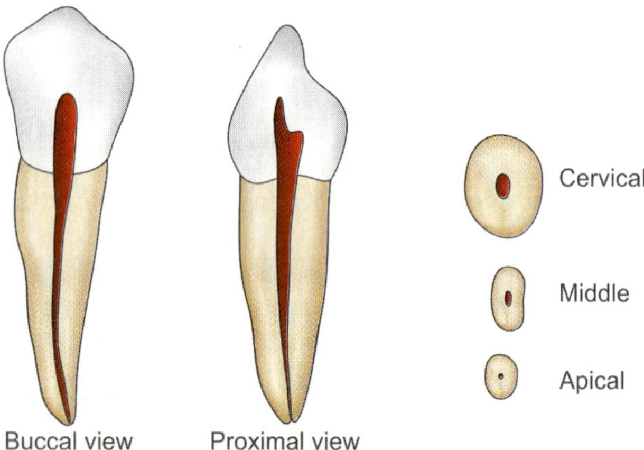

Fig. 13.44 Mandibular first premolar

- Usually one rooted; 2–3 roots may be present (root may be curved distobuccally).
- Incidence of bifurcated canals varies considerably (3–60%).
- Pulp chamber wider buccolingually.
- In single canal, the outline is oval; it is round in two or more root canals.
- Gemination, fusion and dens invagination are common variations.
- Deviations of root canal system of mandibular first premolars are depicted in Fig. 13.45a to e.
- The configuration of tooth, roots, root canals, their deviations, curvatures and inclination, etc. are depicted below.

Slowey (1979) has observed that mandibular first premolar are probably the most difficult teeth to be treated endodontically due to wide variation in root canal morphology. The incidence of two or more root canals in first premolar has been reported to be as low as 2.7% and as high as 62.5%.

Sikri and Sikri (1994) studied mandibular premolars by radiographs and cross-sections and reported that 29.5% of mandibular first premolars and 13.5% mandibular second premolars exhibited second root canal. They also found C-shaped canals in 10% of mandibular first premolar. According to them ovoid shape of canals was most prevalent at cervical third area, while canals became round at middle and apical third area.

Caliskan et al (1995) examined the root canal morphology of 100 mandibular premolars and observed as: 64.15% (1-1), 7.5% (2-1), 3.77% (1-2-1), 7.55% (2-2), 9.43% (1-2), 1.89% (2-1-2), Nil (1-2-1-2), 5.66% (3-3).

They also observed that 52.33% of mandibular first premolars had lateral canals and 16.98% had transverse anastomosis.

Tzu-Yi et al (2006) studied root canal morphology of 82 mandibular first premolars in a Chinese population

Mandibular First Premolar						
Length of tooth	*Number of roots*	*Number of root canals*	*Lateral/ accessory canals*	*Cross-section of root*	*Root curvature*	*Inclination*
22.1 mm (average) 24.1 mm (maximum) 20.1 mm (minimum)	1 Root: 98% 2 Roots: 1–2% 3 Roots: 0–0.5%	1-1: 73–5% 2-1: 6.5% 2-2: 19.5% 3 Canals: 5%	52.33%	Coronal (ovoid) Middle (ovoid) Apical (round)	Straight: 48% Distal: 35% Labial: 2% Lingual: 7% Bayonet curve: 7%	Distal-axial: 14% Lingual-axial: 10%

and observed single canal in 54% samples; 22% having two canals and 18% presented with C-shaped canal configuration.

Parekh et al (2011) studied root canal morphology and variations of 40 mandibular first premolars and observed 20% (1-1), 5% (2-1), 5% (1-2-1), 25% (2-2), 12.5% (1-2) and 2.5% (2-1-2) canal configuration.

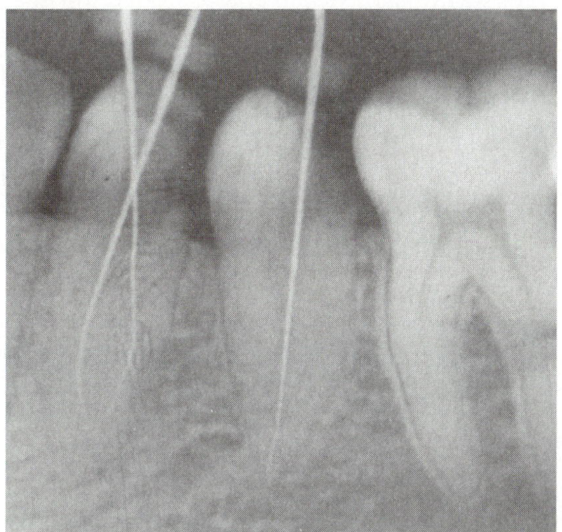

Fig. 13.45a Mandibular first premolar with two canals (diagnostic)

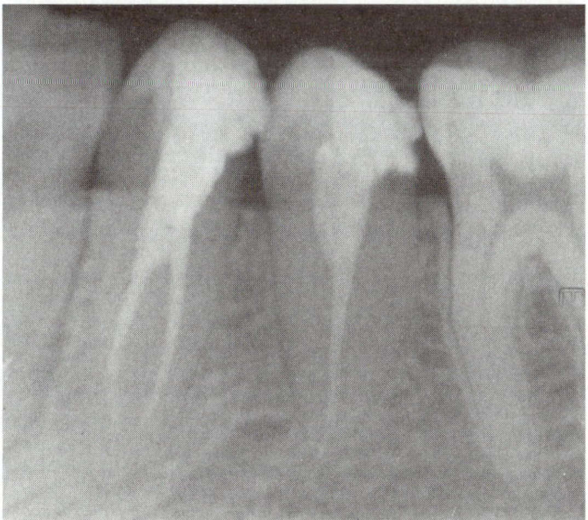

Fig. 13.45b Obturated

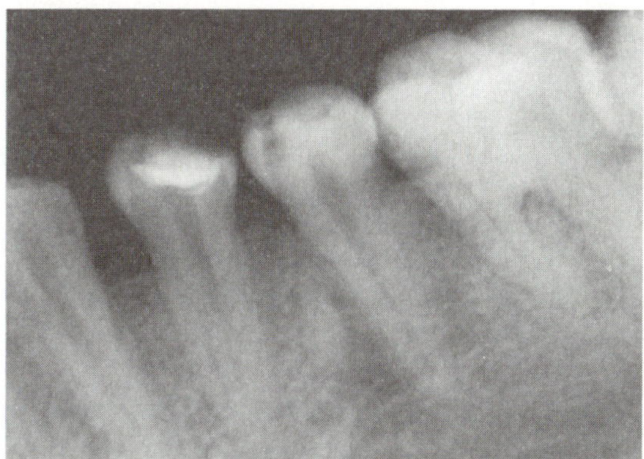

Fig. 13.45c Mandibular first premolar with three canals (preoperative)

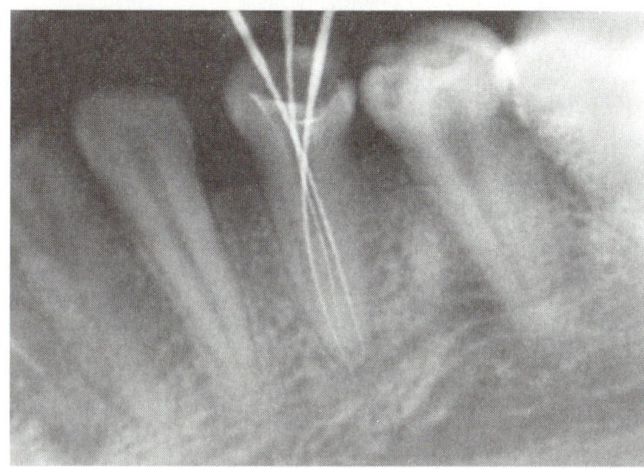

Fig. 13.45d Diagnostic

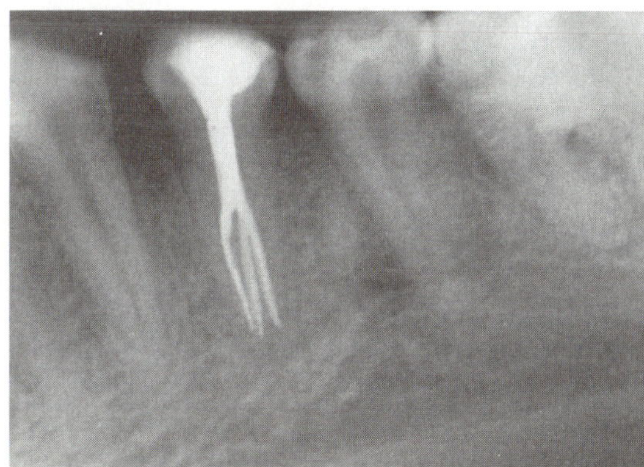

Fig. 13.45e Obturated

d. Mandibular Second Premolar

- The mandibular second premolar can be of three cusp type or two cusp type.
- The crown is distally and lingually inclined, though not as much as the first premolar. Lingual pulp horn is quite prominent.
- Usually single rooted; root may be curved to disto-buccally.
- Incidence of second root canal is 12–15%.
- Pulp chamber wider buccolingual (lingual pulp horn larger than first premolars).
- Cross-section at cervical area is ovoid bucco-lingually; ovoid in midroot and round in apical third area (Fig. 13.46).
- Deviations of root canal system of mandibular second premolar are depicted in Fig. 13.47a to d.

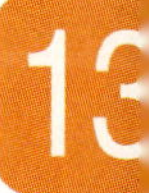

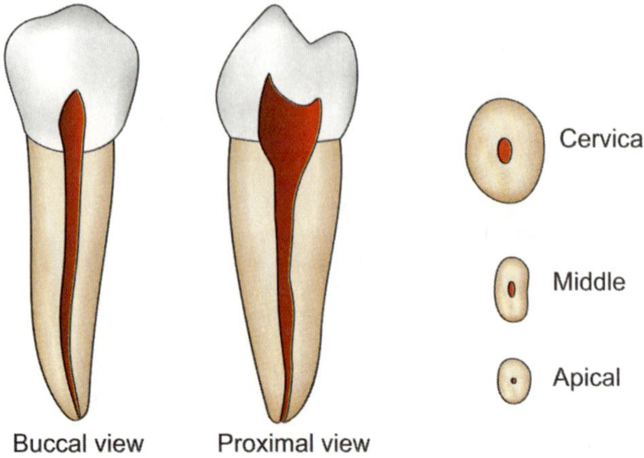

Fig. 13.46 Mandibular second premolar

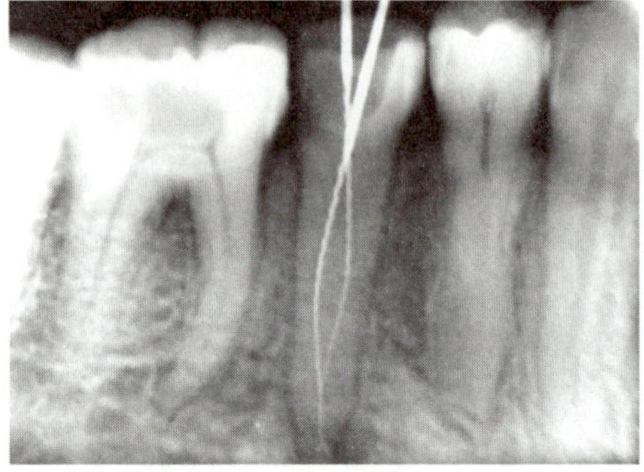

Fig. 13.47a Mandibular second premolar with two canals (diagnostic)

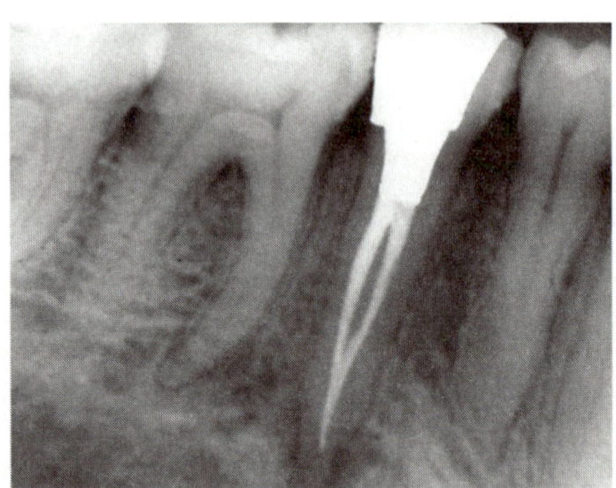

Fig. 13.47b Obturated

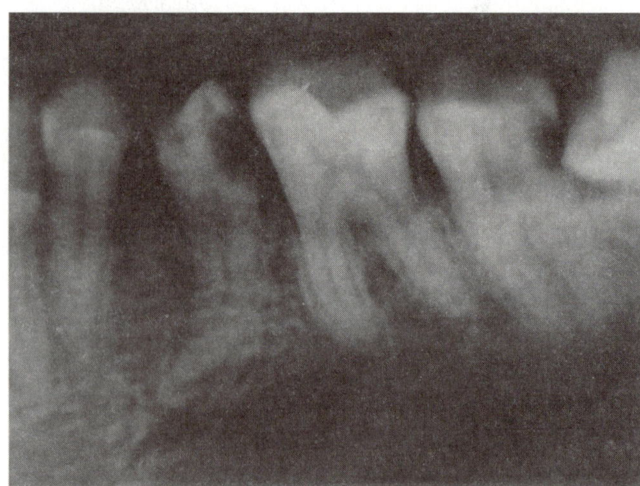

Fig. 13.47c Mandibular second premolar with curved (C-shaped) canal (preoperative)

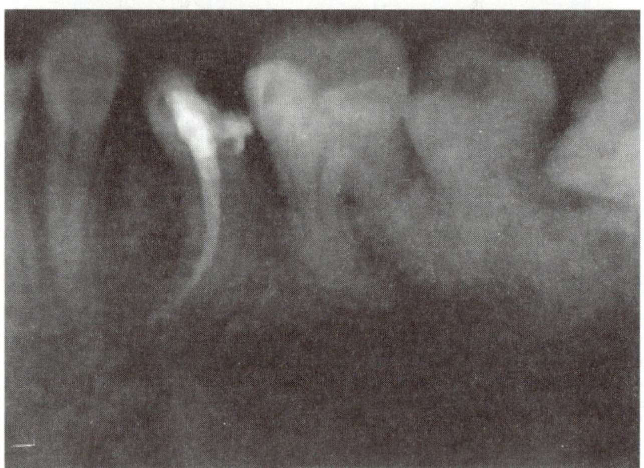

Fig. 13.47d Obturated

- The configuration of tooth, roots, root canals, their deviations, curvatures and inclination, etc. are depicted below.

Parekh et al (2011) studied root canal morphology and variations of 40 mandibular second premolars and observed 80% samples exhibited 1-1 canal configuration, 2.5% (2-2) and 17.5% (1-2). Other types of canal configurations were not observed.

Mandibular Second Premolar

Length of tooth	*Number of roots*	*Number of root canals*	*Lateral/ accessory canals*	*Cross-section of root*	*Root curvature*	*Inclination*
21.4 mm (average) 23.7 mm (maximum) 19.1 mm (minimum)	1 Root: 99% 2 Roots: 0–0.5% 3 Roots: 0–0.1%	1-1: 85–90% 2-1: 1.5–2.5% 2-2:10–12% 3 canals: 0.5%	55%	Coronal (ovoid) Middle (ovoid) Apical (ovoid)	Straight: 39% Distal: 40% Labial: 10% Lingual: 3% Bayonet curve: 7% Trifurcation: 1%	Distal-axial: 14% Lingual-axial: 10%

e. Mandibular First Molar

- Mandibular first molar generally has two distinct roots, one mesial and the other distal. Three canals are usually present: one in distal root and two in mesial root, i.e. mesiobuccal and mesiolingual.
- The buccolingual section reveals that the pulp chamber is in the centre of the crown and that the distal canal is ribbon-shaped; whereas, the mesial canals are rounded and thin (Fig. 13.48).
- The selected studies as regards aberrant root canal anatomy of mandibular first molar is tabulated in Table 13.2.
- Deviations of root canal system of mandibular first molar are depicted in Fig. 13.49a and b.
- A rare case of mandibular first molar with one root canal is depicted in Fig. 13.49c to e.
- The configuration of tooth, roots, root canals, their deviations and curvatures, etc. are depicted below.

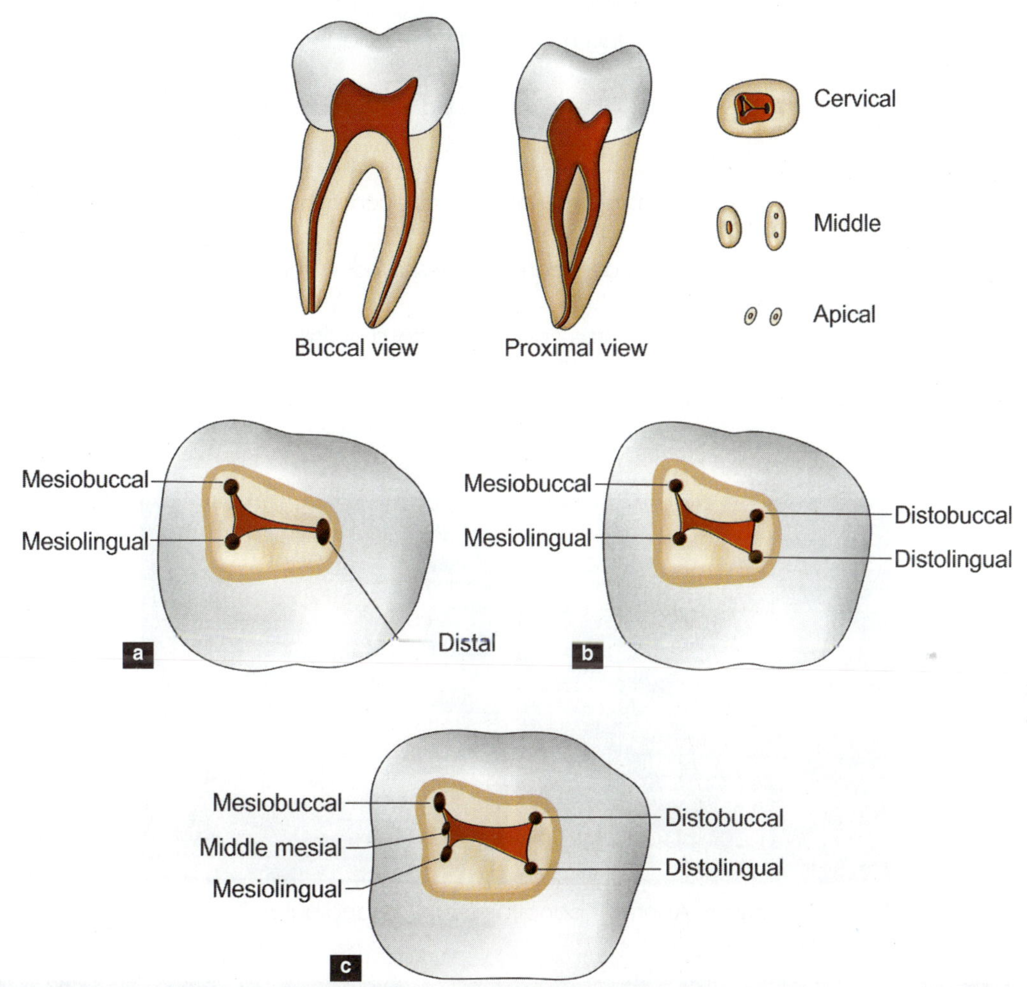

Fig. 13.48 Mandibular first molar: (a) Three canals; (b) Four canals; (c) Five canals

Mandibular First Molar

Length of tooth		*Number of roots*	*Number of root canals*		*Root curvature*	
Mesial	**Distal**		**Mesial**	**Distal**	**Mesial**	**Distal**
20.9 mm (average) 22.7 mm (maximum) 19.1 mm (minimum)	20.9 mm (average) 22.6 mm (maximum) 19.2 mm (minimum)	2 Root: 98% 3 Roots: 2%	2-1: 40.5% 2-2: 59.5%	1-1: 75% 2-2: 30% 2-1: 60%	Straight: 16% Distal: 84%	Straight: 74% Distal: 21% Mesial: 5%

Table 13.2 Aberrant root canal anatomy of mandibular first molar (selected cases)

Author (year) study	*Extra root canals*
Stroner et al (1984) *In vivo* study	3 Roots: 2 canals in mesial root 2 canals in distobuccal root 1 canal in distolingual root (five distinct foramina)
Friedman et al (1986) *In vivo* study	4 roots (one mesial and three distal) Two root canals in mesial root and one each in distal roots (five distinct foramina)
Ricucci (1997) *In vivo* study	5 canals; three separate mesial and two merging distal (four foramina)
Reeh (1998) *In vivo* study	7 canals; four mesial and three distal
Mortman and Singhee (2003) *In vivo* study	6 canals; three in mesial and three in distal root
Lee et al (2006) *In vivo* study	5 canals; two mesial and one each in three distal roots
Lee et al (2010) *In vivo* study	5 independent canals in mesial root with varying configuration
Yesilsoy et al (2009) *In vivo* study	5 canals; three canals in mesial and one each in two distal roots (five distinct foramina)
Faramazi et al (2010) *In vivo* study	Three distinct canals in mesial root

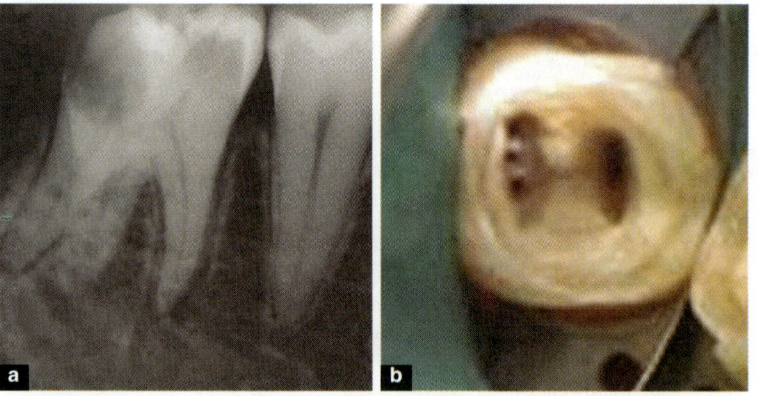

Fig. 13.49a and b Aberrant canal anatomy (mandibular first molar)

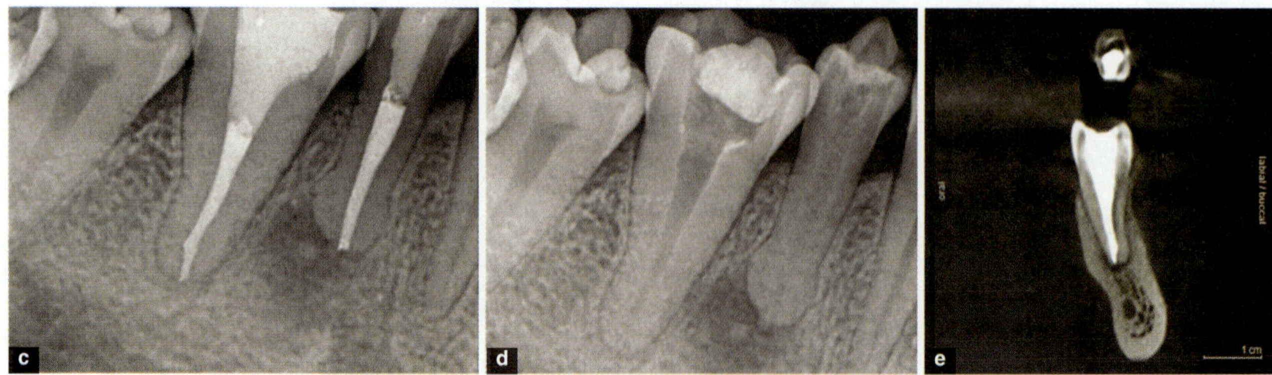

Fig. 13.49c to e Mandibular first molar with one root canal

13

Navarro et al (2007) evaluated third canal in the mesial root of permanent mandibular first molars in his review of literature and three clinical case reports. They reported 13% mesial roots presented third canal. Earlier studies, as reviewed, have observed 1.0–15% third canal in mesial root.

de Pablo et al (2010) in their systematic review of root anatomy and canal configuration of the permanent mandibular first molar comprising 18,781 teeth from 41 studies observed as: 13% of samples showed third root; 61.3% three canals, 35.7% four canals, and 1% showed five canals. Root canal configuration of mesial root revealed two canals in 94.4% and three canals in 2.3% cases; whereas, distal root revealed one canal in 62.7%, and rest two canals (14.5% 2-1 and 12.4% 2-2 canal configuration).

f. Mandibular Second Molar

- The second molar is inclined more lingually than the first molar; therefore, the access preparation should correspond to the tilt of the tooth (Fig. 13.50).
- Intercanal communications more common in distal root than mesial root.
- Maximum variations usually seen in mesial canals.
- 5.0–6.0% mandibular second molars exhibit lateral canals; mostly in middle third of root.
- C-shaped canal configuration has been reported in 1.0–10% cases (a few studies have shown up to 50%).
- Deviations of root canal system of mandibular second molar is depicted in Fig. 13.51a to d.
- The configuration of tooth, roots, root canals and curvatures, etc. are depicted below.

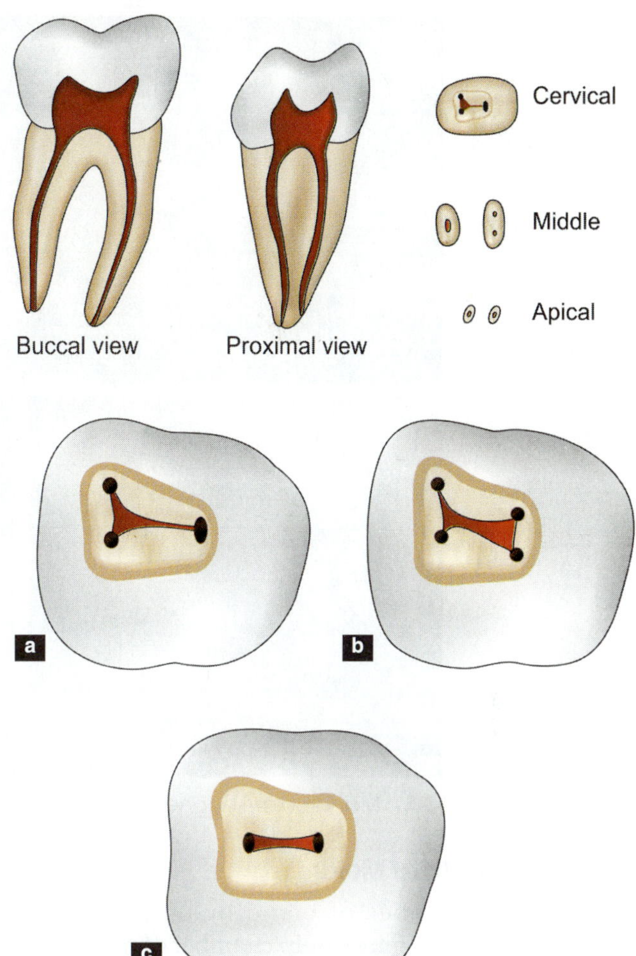

Fig. 13.50 Mandibular second molar: (a) Three canals; (b) Four canals; (c) Two canals

Neelakantan et al (2010) studied root and canal morphology of mandibular second molars in an Indian population and observed as: 87.8% had two roots with three canals, 7.5% had C-shaped canal morphology. 2-2 type canal configuration was common in mesial root and 1-1 in distal root.

Jahromi et al (2013) examined 100 intact human mandibular second molars in Iranian population as regard their roots and root canal morphology. They observed 89% two rooted, 6% one rooted and 3% three rooted teeth. 54% teeth exhibited three canals, 6% two canals, 3% single canal and 34% four canals. Most common canal configuration noted was 2-1 in mesial root and 1-1 in distal root.

Nur et al (2014) evaluated root canal morphology of mandibular permanent molars in a south-eastern Turkish population using cone beam tomography. They reported 0.01% mandibular second molars had three roots. 90% mesial roots had two canals and 10% one canal. 97% distal root had one canal and 3% two canals.

Mandibular Second Molar

	Length of tooth	*Number of roots*	*Number of root canals*		*Root curvature*		
Mesial	**Distal**	One root: 10%	**Mesial**	**Distal**	**Single root**	**Mesial**	**Distal**
20.9 mm (average)	20.8 mm (average)	Two roots: 90%	1-1: 13%	1-1: 92%	Straight: 53%	Straight: 27%	Straight: 58%
22.6 mm (maximum)	22.6 mm (maximum)		2-1: 49%	2-1: 5%	Distal: 26%	Distal: 61%	Distal: 18%
19.2 mm (minimum)	19.0 mm (minimum)		2-2: 38%	2-2: 3%	Lingual: 2%	Buccal: 4%	Buccal: 4%
					Bayonet: 19%	Bayonet: 7%	Bayonet: 6%

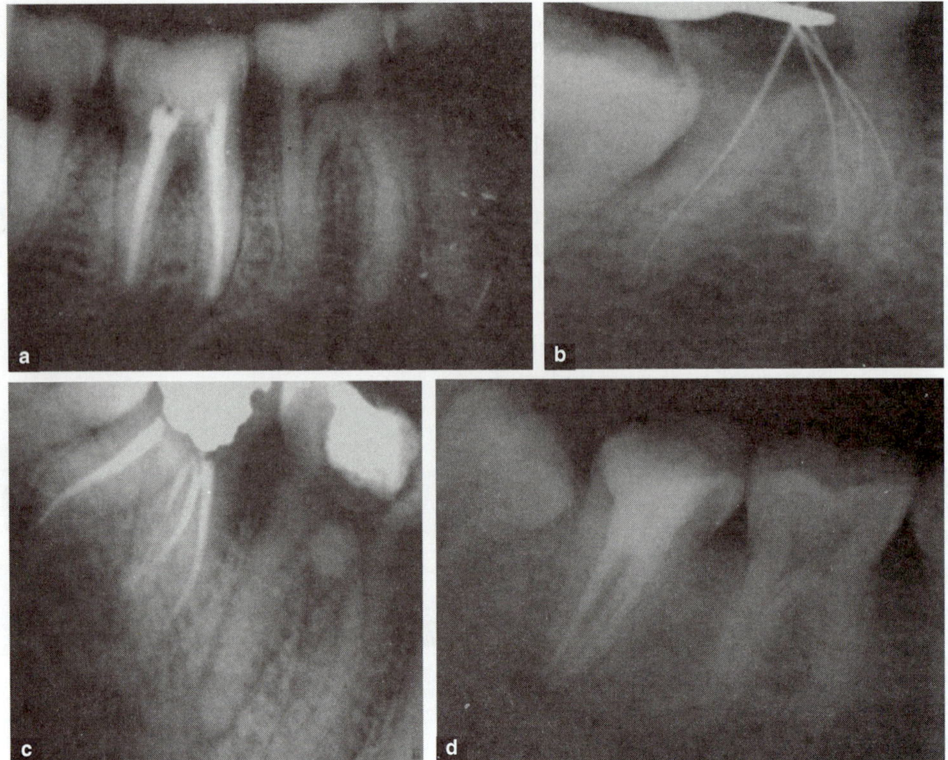

Fig. 13.51 Mandibular second molar: (a) Preoperative; (b) Diagnostic; (c) and (d) Obturated

g. Mandibular Third Molar

- The pulp chamber of mandibular third molar anatomically resembles pulp chamber of mandibular first and second molars. It is large and possesses many anomalous configurations such as C-shaped root canal orifices.
- Displays most irregular canal configuration.
- The mandibular third molar usually has two roots and two canals, but occasionally one root and one canal or three roots and three canals are present (may have one to four roots and one to six root canals).
- The alveolar socket of mandibular third molar may project onto lingual plate of mandible. The apex of root may be in close proximity to mandibular canal.
- Mesial inclination of tooth makes the access easier.
- In double rooted mandibular third molars, mesial root may have canal configuration as 1-1, 2-1, 2-2 and 1-2; whereas, distal root usually exhibit 1-1 canal configuration.
- In single rooted teeth, mesial root canal presented similar canal configuration (1-1, 2-1, 2-2 and 1-2) and distal canal exhibiting 1-1 canal configuration.
- A few authors have reported rare occurrence of 1-2-1 type and even 2-5-1 type canal configuration.
- Mandibular third molar with type II canal anatomy is depicted in Fig. 13.52.
- Treated impacted third molar is depicted in Fig. 13.53.
- The configuration of tooth roots, root canals and curvatures, etc. are depicted below.

Mandibular Third Molar							
	Length of tooth	*Number of roots*	*Number of root canals*		*Root curvature*		
Mesial 18.5 mm	**Distal** 18.2 mm	One root: 21% Two roots: 73% Three roots: 5.5%	**Mesial** 1-1: 59% 2-1: 19% 1-2-1: 15% 2-2: 2% 1-2: 6%	**Distal** 1-1:95% 2-1: 3% 1-2-1: 2% In three root canals 1-1 type most prevalent	**Single root** Straight 80% Curved 20%	**Mesial** Straight 34% Curved 66%	**Distal** Straight 92% Curved 8%

13

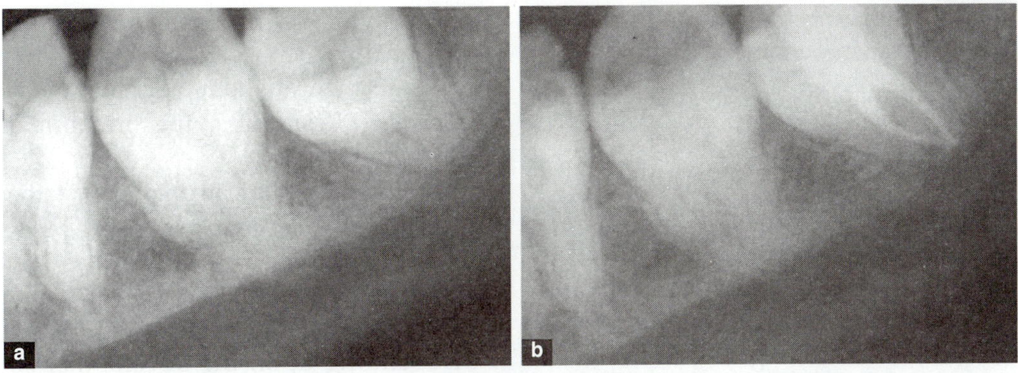

Fig. 13.52 Mandibular third molar (type II canal anatomy): (a) Preoperative; (b) Obturated

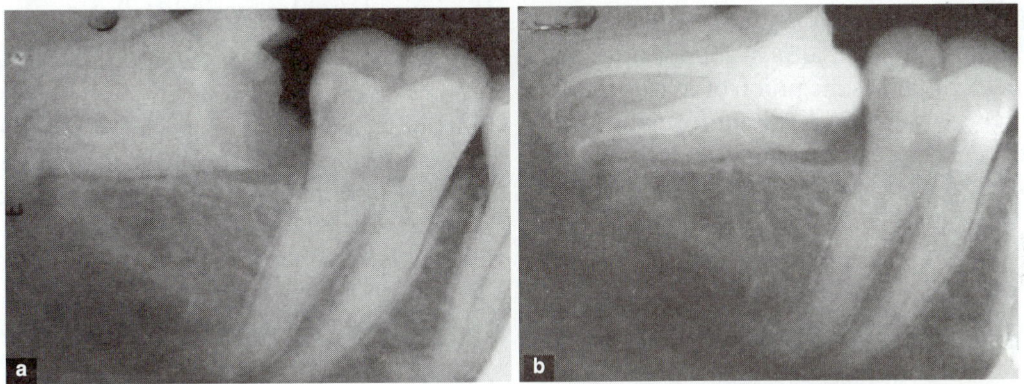

Fig. 13.53 Impacted mandibular third molar: (a) Preoperative; (b) Obturated

Kuzekanani et al (2012) studied root canal morphology of 150 mandibular third molars in an Iranian population and observed as: 73% samples with two roots, 21% had one root and 5.5% had three roots. 60% mesial root and 95% distal root had single canal. Other types 2-1 (19%), 1-2-1 (15%), 2-2 (2%) were reported in mesial root.

Sidow et al (2000) studied root canal morphology of 150 human mandibular third molars and observed as: 77% had two roots (one to six root canals); 17% one root (40% contain two canals); 5% three roots and 1% four roots. 2.2% root canals were C-shaped.

DEVELOPMENTAL ANOMALIES AND ROOT CANAL SYSTEM

The common developmental anomalies affecting root canal system are:

1. ***Dens invaginatus***: Dens invaginatus, also known as dens-in-dente (invaginated odontome) is a developmental anomaly resulting from infolding of the crown before calcification has occurred. Usually anterior teeth are involved; mostly prevalent in maxillary central incisors (Fig. 13.54a to d). Three types of Dens invaginatus have been recognized (Oehler's classification):

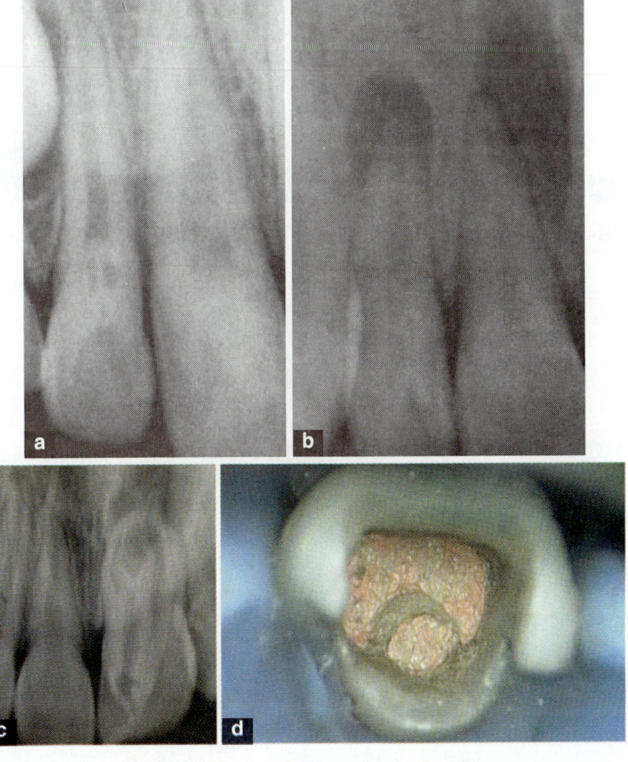

Fig. 13.54a to d Dens invaginatus

Type 1: Lined by enamel that occurs within the crown; not extending beyond cementoenamel junction (CEJ).

Type 2: Enamel lined sac that invades the root and may connect with pulp.

Type 3: Extending up to root and opens in the apical region; no connection with pulp.

2. ***Dens evaginatus***: It appears as an accessory cusp on occlusal surface of premolars; rarely on molars and incisors. Mostly it is located in between buccal and lingual cusps of premolars. This globule of enamel (accessory cusp) may pose difficulties in root canal treatment procedures.

3. ***Fusion and gemination***: Fusion and gemination are two different anomalies with almost identical appearance. Fusion is identified as the union of two normally separated tooth buds with the resultant formation of a joint tooth with confluence of dentin (Fig. 13.55a and b). Gemination is recognized as an attempt of a single tooth bud to divide, with a resultant formation of either a large tooth with a bifid crown or two completely divided teeth throughout the crown and root (Fig. 13.56).

Complete: Resulting in the formation of a wide tooth (crown and root).

Incomplete: Resulting in union only at the crown or root.

Fused teeth may contain separate canals or may share a common canal. The canals may be separated in coronal aspect and then unite into a common canal in radicular area or *vice versa*.

Depending upon the developmental stage of this union; owing to the usual existence of combined pulp chamber in fused teeth, a modified access preparation is required, (wider mesiodistally).

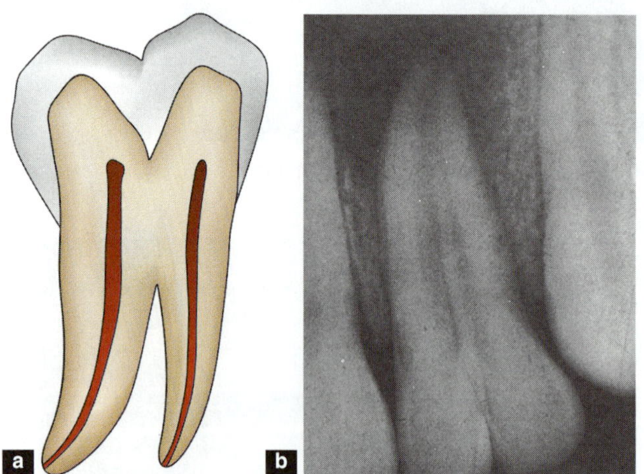

Fig. 13.55 (a) Fusion (diagrammatic); (b) Fusion (radiological)

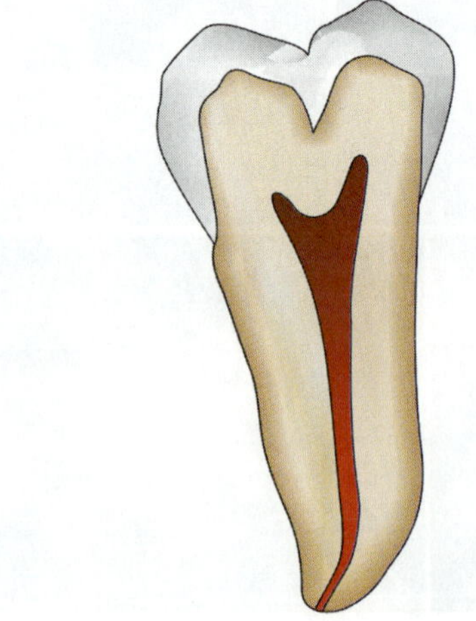

Fig. 13.56 Gemination (diagrammatic)

4. ***Talon cusp (Eagle's talon)***: Talon cusp is a supernumerary structure projecting from the dentinoenamel junction to a variable distance towards the incisal edge of an anterior tooth. It consists of enamel, dentin and variable amount of pulp (there is a deep developmental groove where the Talon's cusp blends with the sloping lingual tooth surface that consists of pulp horns). Mostly present on the palatal aspect but few cases have been reported with talon cusp present on the facial aspect of the teeth. It is commonly found in permanent maxillary lateral incisors and deciduous maxillary central incisors.

5. ***Dilaceration***: The term 'dilaceration' refers to an angulation or a sharp curve of 90° or even more in the root or the crown of a fully grown tooth, mainly caused due to trauma during tooth development. A few authors have opined that other factors, such as hereditary factors and effect of related anatomical structure (maxillary sinus and mandibular canal) are the causative factors than trauma. The curve may occur anywhere along the length of the tooth. Most affected teeth are third molars followed by upper lateral incisors. Roots tend to curve in a distal direction and/or in lingual direction. Root dilacerations may also occur in more than one plane (distolingual direction).

The root canal treatment of dilacerated roots is always challenging. The basic guidelines of unobstructed, straight line access are followed during access preparation. The coronal flaring is also helpful before initiating apical preparations (Fig. 13.57a and b).

The flexible, small files are preferred in narrow canals [stresses exerted on file (not sharp curves) may lead to its separation]. The selected files are precurved and moved slowly along the curvatures.

The curved canals can be obturated with lateral compaction technique using flexible Ni-Ti spreaders, which can penetrate greater depths as compared to stainless steel spreaders.

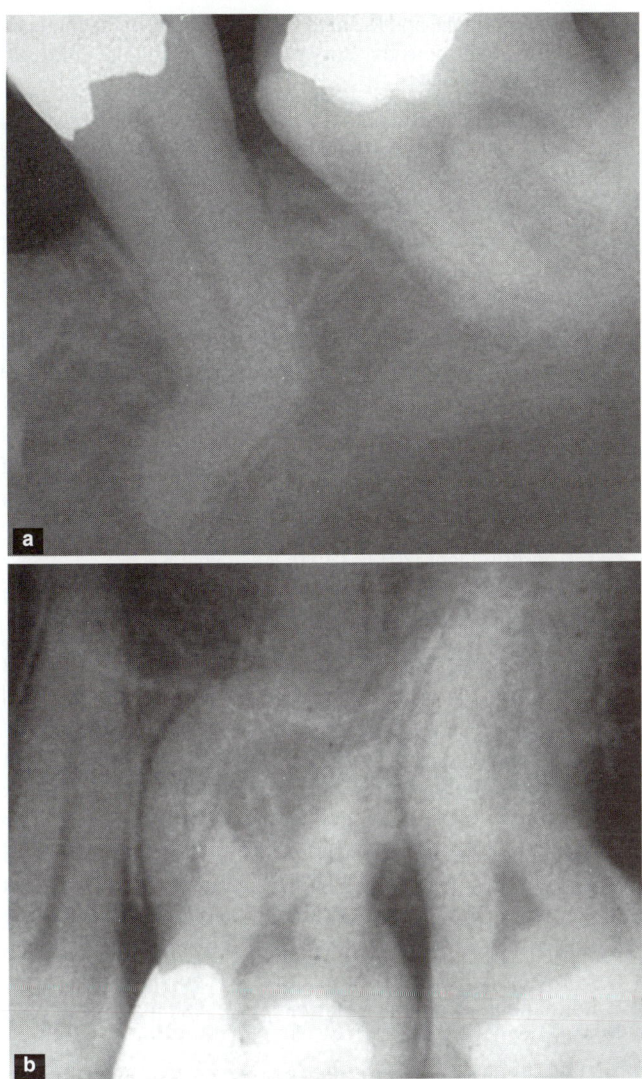

Fig. 13.57a and b Dilaceration

Prevalence of dilacerations have been found to be higher in mandibular third molars ranging from 3.0–30% and in maxillary molars (1.3–8.5%).

6. ***Taurodontism***: A tooth anomaly characterized by the enlargement of the pulp chamber, which may reach the proximity of the root apex. In this condition coronal portion is enlarged at the expense of the roots (Fig. 13.58a to d).

A taurodont may appear as a normal tooth. The tooth is usually rectangular in shape rather than tapering towards the roots. The long rectangular shape of the pulp chamber seems to cause difficulty in locating the orifice of the canal and subsequent difficulties in instrumentation and obturation. Taurodontism may be associated with periodontal problems.

7. ***Palatal developmental groove***: It originates from the cingulum of the maxillary incisors (mostly lateral incisors) and ends apically at various levels of root.

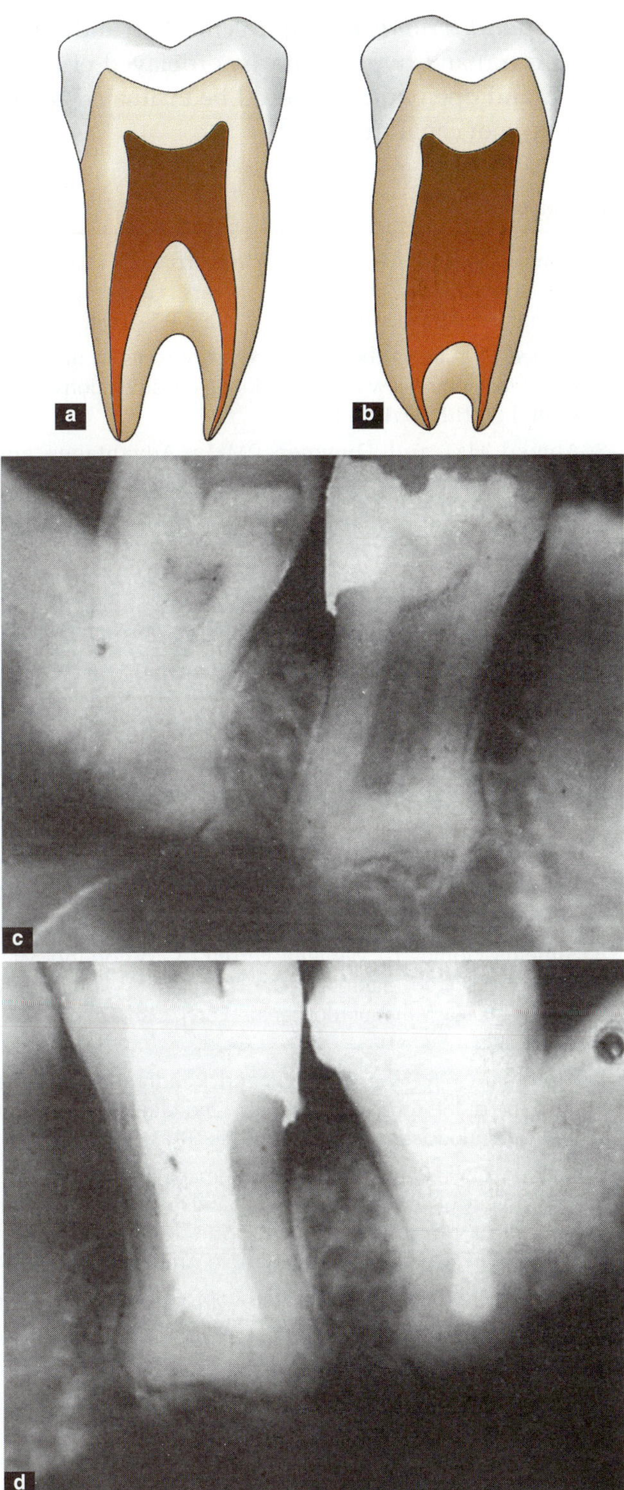

Fig. 13.58 Taurodontism: (a) Normal anatomy; (b) Taurodont (diagrammatic); (c) Preoperative (radiological); (d) Taurodont (obturated)

8. ***Dentinogenesis imperfecta***: Dentinogenesis imperfecta implies partial (type 1) or complete (type 2) obliteration of pulp chamber and root canals by continued formation of dentin.

9. ***Hyperparathyroidism*** (pulp calcification and loss of lamina dura) and **hypopituitarism** (delayed eruption of teeth and open apices) should be evaluated before initiating root canal treatment.

BIBLIOGRAPHY

1. Ahmad IA and Al-Jadaa A. Three root canals in the mesiobuccal root of maxillary molars: case reports and literature review. J. Endod.: 2014; 40:2087–2094.
2. Ahmed HM and Abbott PV. Accessory roots in maxillary molar teeth: a review and endodontic considerations. Aust. Dent. J.: 2012; 57:123–131.
3. Ahmed HM and Dummer PMH.: Advantages and applications of a new system for classifying roots and canal systems in research and clinical practice. Eur. Endod. J.:2017 (in press).
4. Al Qudah AA and Awawdeh IA. Root canal morphology of mandibular first and second molar teeth in a Jordanian population. Int. Endod. J.: 2009; 42:775–784.
5. Al Shalabi RM, Omer OE, Glennon J, Jennings M and Claffey NM. Root canal anatomy of maxillary first and second permanent molrs. Int. Endod. J.: 2000; 33:405–414.
6. Al-Fouzan KS, AlManee A, Jan J and Al-Rejaie M. Incidence of two canals in extracted mandibular incisors teeth of Saudi Arabian samples. Saudi Endod. J.: 2012; 2:65–69.
7. Almedia-Gomes FD, De Sousa BC, De Souza FD, Dos Santos RA and Ferreira RA. Three root canals in maxillary second premolar. Ind. J. Dent. Res.: 2009; 20:241–242.
8. Almeida-Gomes F, Maniglia-Ferreira C, Vitoriano MD, de Sousa BC, dos Santos RA and Durate MA. A maxillary central incisor with four root canals. Eur. J. Gen. Dent.: 2012; 1:201–203.
9. Alothmani OS, Chandler NP and Friedlander LT. The anatomy of the root apex: a review and clinical considerations in endodontics. Saudi Endod. J.: 2013; 3:1–9.
10. Amardeep NS, Raghu S and Natanasabapathy V. Root canal morphology of permanent maxillary and mandibular canines in Indian population using cone beam computed tomography. Anatomy Res. Int.:2014; Article ID 731859.
11. Arora R, Sikri V and Bal CS. Study of root canals and their configuration in maxillary second permanent molar. JCD: 1998; 1:128–138.
12. Arora S and Tewari S. The morphology of the apical foramen in posterior teeth in a North Indian population. Int. Endod. J.:2009; 42:930–939.
13. Aydemir S, Helvacioglu-Yigit D, Sinanoglu A and Ozel E. Retreatment of a maxillary lateral incisor with two separate root canals confirmed with cone beam computed tomography. J. Clin. Med. Res.:2015; 7:560–563.
14. Badole GP, Bahadure RN, Warhadpande MM and Kubde R. A rare root canal configuration of maxillary second molars: A case report. Case Reports in Dent.:2012; Article ID767582.
15. Bal CS, Sikri VK and Arora R. Study of root canals and their configuration in maxillary second premolar. IJDR:1994; 5:3–6.
16. Balani P, Niazi F and Rashid H. A brief review of the methods used to determine the curvature of root canals. J. Restor. Dent.:2015; 3:57–63.
17. Baratto-Filho F, Farinuk LF, Ferreira EL, Pecora JD, Cruz-Filho AM and Sousa-Neto MD. Clinical and macroscopic study of maxillary molars with two palatal roots. Int. Endod. J.:2002; 35:796–801.
18. Barbizam JV, Ribeiro RG and Tanomaru FM. Unusual anatomy of permanent maxillary molars. J. Endod.:2004; 30:668–671.
19. Bertrand T and Kim SG. Endodontic treatment of a c-shaped mandibular second premolar with four root canals and three apical foramina: a case report. Restor. Dent. Endod.:2016; 41:68–73.
20. Blaskovic-Subat V, Maricic B and Sutalo J. Asymmetry of the root canal foramen. Int. Endod. J.:1992; 25:158–164.
21. Bolla N and Kavuri SR. Maxillary canine with two root canals. J. Conserv. Dent.:2011; 14:80–82.
22. Carrotte P. Endodontics: Part 4. Morphology of the root canal system. Br. Dent. J.:2004; 197:379–383.
23. Cleghorn BM, Christie WH and Dong CC. The root and root canal morphology of the human mandibular second premolar: a literature review. J. Endod.:2007; 33:1031–1037.
24. Cleghorn BM, Christie WH and Dong CC. The root and root canal morphology of the human mandibular first premolar: a literature review. J. Endod.:2007; 33:509–516.
25. Cleghorn BM, Christie WH and Dong GC. Root and root canal morphology of the human permanent maxillary first molar: A literature review. J. Endod.:2006; 32:813–821.
26. de Pablo OV, Estevez R, Sanchez MP, Heilborn C and Cohenca N. Root anatomy and canal configuration of the permanent mandibular first molar: A systematic review. J. Endod.:2010; 36:1919–1931.
27. Dong-Ryul S, Jin-Man K, Duck-Su K, Sun-Young K, Abbott PV and Sang-Hyuk P. A maxillary canine with two separated root canals: a case report. JKACD:2011; 36:431–435.
28. Dummer PM, McGinn JH and Rees DG. The position and topography of the apical canal constriction and apical foramen. Int. Endod. J.:1984; 17:192–198.
29. Eskoz N and Weine FS. Canal configuration of the mesiobuccal root of the maxillary second molar. J. Endod.:1995; 21:38–42.
30. Estrela C, Bueno MR, Sousa-Nets MD and Pecora JD. Method for determination of root curvature radius using cone-beam computed tomography images. Braz. Dent. J.:2008; 19:114–118.
31. Fan B, Min Y and Lu G. Negotiation of C-shaped canal systems in mandibular second molars. J. Endod.:2009; 35:1003–1008.
32. Fan B, Pan Y, Gao Y, Fang F, Wu Q and Gutmann JL. Three-dimensional morphologic analysis of isthmuses in the mesial roots of mandibular molars. J. Endod.:2010; 36:1866–1869.
33. Fontana CE, Ibanez, CD, Davini F, De Martin AS, Silveira CF, Rocha DG and Bueno CE. Endodontic therapy of maxillary second molar showing an unusual internal anatomy. RSBO.:2012; 9:213–217.

34. Gandhi B, Majety KK and Gowdra RH. Root canal treatment of bilateral three-rooted maxillary first premolars. J. Orofacial Sci.:2012; 4:56–59.

35. Ghoddusi J, Naghavi N, Zarei M and Rohani E. Mandibular first molar with four distal canals. J. Endod.:2007; 33: 1481–1483.

36. Gu Y, Lu Q, Wang H, Ding Y, Wang P and Ni L. Root canal morphology of permanent three-rooted mandibular first molar: Part I: pulp floor and root canal system. J. Endod.:2010; 36:990–994.

37. Holtzman L. Root canal treatment of a mandibular canine with three root canals - Case report. Int. Endod. J.:1997; 30:291–293.

38. Hsu YY and Kim S. The resected root surface. The issue of canal thymuses. Dent. Clin. North Am.:1997; 41:529–40.

39. Hulsmann M. A maxillary first molar with two disto-buccal root canals. J. Endod.:1997; 23:707–708.

40. Irodi S, Farook AZ. Three rooted mandibular molar; Radix Entomolaris and Radix Paramolaris. Int. J. Dent. Clinics:2011; 3:102.

41. Jacobsen EI, Dick K and Bodell R. Mandibular first molar with multiple mesial canals. J. Endod.:1994; 20:610–613.

42. Jahromi MZ, Golestan FJ, Esmaeil MM, Zahed SHM and Sarami M. Root and canal morphology of mandibular second molar in an Iranian population by clearing method. J. Dent. (Shiraz):2013; 14:78–81.

43. Johal S. Unusual maxillary first molar with 2 palatal canals within a single root: a case report. J. Can. Dent. Assoc.:2001; 67:211–214.

44. Jung M. Endodontic treatment of dens invagination type III with three root canals and open apical foramen. Int. Endod. J.:2004; 37:205–213.

45. Kabak YS and Abbott PV. Endodontic treatment of mandibular incisors with two root canals: Report of two cases. Aust. Endod. J.:2007; 33:27–31.

46. Kartal N, Ozcelik B and Cimilli H. Root canal morphology of maxillary premolars. J. Endod.:1998; 24:417–419.

47. Kasahara E, Yasuda E, Yamamoto A and Anzai M. Root canal system of the maxillary central incisor. J. Endod.:1990; 16:158–161.

48. Keinan D, Nuni E and Slutzky-Goldberg I. Is a C-shaped configuration possible in teeth other than mandibular molars? Quint. Int.:2009; 40:541–543.

49. Kim D, Ha JH, Jin MU, Kim YK and Kim SK. Proximity of the mandibular molar root apex from the buccal bone surface: a cone-beam computed tomographic study. Restor. Dent. Endod.:2016; 41:182–188.

50. Kimura Y and Matsumoto K. Mandibular first molar with three distal root canals. Int. Endod. J.:2000; 33:468–470.

51. Kontakiotis EG and Tzanetakis GN. Four canals in the mesial root of a mandibular first molar: a case report under the operating microscope. Aust. Endod. J.:2007; 33:84–88.

52. Kottoor J, Murugesan R and Albuquerque DV. A maxillary lateral incisor with four root canals. Int. Endod. J.:2012; 45:393–397.

53. Kottoor J, Sudha R and Velmurugan N. Middle distal canal of the mandibular first molar: a case report and literatue review. Int. Endod. J.:2010; 43:714–722.

54. Kuzekanani M, Haghani J and Nosrati H. Root and canal morphology of mandibular third molars in an Iranian population. J. Dent. Res. Dent. Clin. Dent. Prospect.:2012; 6:85–88.

55. Libfeld H and Rotstein I. Incidence of four-rooted maxillary second molar: literature review and radiographic survey of 1,200 teeth. J. Endod.:1989; 15:129–131.

56. Lu TY, Yang SF and Pat SF. Complicated root canal morphology of mandibular first premolar in a Chinese population using the cross section method. J. Endod.:2006; 32:932–936.

57. Maggiore F, Jou YT and Kim S. A six-canal maxillary first molar: case report. Int. Endod. J.:2002; 35:486–491.

58. Maghsoudlou A, Jafarzadeh H and Forghani M. Endodontic treatment of a maxillary central incisor with two roots. J. Contemp. Dent. Pract.:2013; 14:345–347.

59. Manning SA. Root canal anatomy of mandibular secondmolars. Part I. Int.Endod. J.:1990; 23:34.

60. Mannocci F, Peru M and Sherriff M. The isthmuses of the mesial root of mandibular molars: a micro-computed tomographic study. Int. Endod. J.:2005; 38:558–563.

61. Martos J, Ferrer-Luque CM, Gonzalez-Rodriguez MP and de Castro LA. Topographical evaluation of the major apical foramen in permanent human teeth. Int. Endod. J.:2009; 42:329–334.

62. Martos J, Lubian C, Silveira LF, de Castro LA and Ferrer Luque CM. Morphologic analysis of the root apex in human teeth. J. Endod.:2010; 36:664–667.

63. Matherne RP, Angelopoulos C, Kulid JC and Tira D. Use of cone-beam computed tomography to identify root canal systems *in vitro*. J. Endod.:2008; 34:87–89.

64. Mehrvarzfar P, Akhlagi NM, Khodaei F, Shojaee G and Shirazi S. Evaluation of isthmus prevalence, location and types in mesial roots of mandibular molars in the Iranian Population. Dent. Res. J.:2014; 11:251–256.

65. Min K. Clinical management of a mandibular first molar with multiple mesial canals: a case report. J. Contemp. Dent. Pract.:2004; 5:142–149.

66. Mohammadi Z, Jafarzadeh H, Shalavi S, Bandi S and Patil S. Root and root canal morphology of human third molar teeth. J. Contemp. Dent. Pract.:2015; 15:310–313.

67. Mohan AG, Rajesh EA, George L, Josy SA. Maxillary lateral incisors with two canals and two separate curved roots. Contemp. Clin. Dent.:2012; 3:519–521.

68. Moon-Hwan L, Jung-Hong H, Myoung-UK J, Young-Kyung K and Sung-Kyo K. Endodontic treatment of maxillary lateral incisors with anatomical variations. Restor. Dent. Endod.: 2013; 38:253–257.

69. Mounce R. Negotiating challenging mid root curvature: Rounding the bend. Dent. Today:2007; 26:108.

70. Mupaparapu M and Singer SR. A rare presentation of dens invaginatus in a mandibular lateral incisor occurring

concurrently with bilateral maxillary dens invaginatus: Case report and review of literature. Aust. Dent. J.:2004; 49:90–93.

71. Muppalla JN, Kavuda K, Punna R and Vanapatla A. Management of an unusual maxillary canines: A rare entity. Case Report in Dent.:2015; Article ID 780908.
72. Navarro LF, Luzi A, Garcia AA and Garcia AH. Third canal in the mesial root of permanent mandibular first molars: review of literature and presentation of 3 clinical reports and 2 *in vitro* studies. Med. Oral Patol. Oral Circ. Buccal.:2007; 12:e605–9.
73. Nayak G, Aeran H and Singh I. Radix mesiolingualis and radix distolingualis: a case report of a tooth with an unusual morphology. Restor. Dent. Endod.:2016; 41:322–331.
74. Neelakantan P, Subbarao C, Ahuja R, Subbarao CV and Gutmann JL. Cone-beam computed tomography study of root and canal morphology of maxillary first and second molars in an Indian population. J. Endod.:2010; 36:1622–1627.
75. Neelakantan P, Subbarao C, Subbarao CV and Ravindranath M. Root and canal morphology of mandibular second molars in an Indian population. J. Endod.:2010; 36:1319–1322.
76. Nishant J and Bhuyan AC. Maxillary first molar with eight canals: A case report. *i*dentistry-the journal:2011; 7:35–38.
77. Nur BG, Ok E, Altunsoy M, Aglarci OS, Colak M and Gungor E. Evaluation of the root canal morphology of mandibular permanent molars in a south-eastern Turkish population using cone-beam computed tomography. Eur. J. Dent.:2014; 8:154–159.
78. Olson DG, Roberts S, Joyee AP, Collins DE and McPherson JC. Unevenness of the apical constriction in human maxillary central incisors. J. Endod.:2008; 34:157–159.
79. Parekh V, Shah N and Joshi H. Root canal morphology and variations on mandibular premolars by clearing technique: An in vitro study. J. Contemp. Dent.: Pract.:2011; 12:318–321.
80. Pecora JD, Neto MD, Saquy PC and Woelfel JB. In vitro study of root canal anatomy of maxillary second premolars. Braz. Dent. J.:1992; 3:81–85.
81. Pecora JD, Saquy PC, Neto MD and Woelfel JB. Root form and canal anatomy of maxillary first premolars. Braz. Dent. J.:1991; 2:87–94.
82. Pecora JD, Woelfel JB and Sousa Neto MD. Morphologic study of the maxillary molars. I. External anatomy. Braz. Dent.J.:1991; 2:45–50.
83. Pecora JD, Woelfel JB, Sousa Neto MD and Issa EP. Morphologic study of the maxillary molars. Part II: Internal anatomy. Braz. Dent. J.:1992; 3:53–57.
84. Peix-Sanchez M and Minana-Laliga R. A case of unusual anatomy: a maxillary lateral incisor with three canals. Int. Endod. J.:1999; 236–240.
85. Plotino G. A mandibular third molar with three mesial roots: a case report. J. Endod.:2008; 34:224–226.
86. Ponce EH, Vilar Fernandez JA. The cemenodentinocanal junction, the apical foramen, and the apical constriction: evaluation by optical microscopy. J. Endod.:2003; 29: 214–219.
87. Purra AR, Mushtaq M, Robbai I and Farooq R. Spiral computed tomographic evaluation and endodontic management of a mandibular second molar with four roots. A case report and literature review. Iran Endod. J.:2013; 8:69–71.
88. Raj UJ and Mylswamy S. Root canal morphology of maxillary second premolars in an Indian population. J. Conserv. Dent.:2010; 13:148–151.
89. Reeh ES. Seven canals in a lower first molar. J. Endod.:1998; 24:497–499.
90. Ricucci D and Siqueira JF Jr. Fate of the tissue in lateral canals and apical ramifications in response to pathologic conditions and treatment procedures. J. Endod.:2010; 36:1–15.
91. Ricucci D. Apical limit of root canal instrumentation and obturation, part 1:literature review. Int. Endod. J.:1998; 31:384–393.
92. Rodrigues E, Braitt HA, Galvao BF Leal da Silva EJ. Maxillary first molar with 7 root canals diagnosed using cone-beam computed tomography. Rest. Dent. Endod.:2016.
93. Ross IF and Evanchik PA. Root fusion in molars: incidence and sex linkage. J. Periodontol.:1981; 52:663–667.
94. Sadeghi S and Poryousef V. A novel approach in assessment of root canal curvature. I.E.J.:2009; 4:131–134.
95. Sempira HN and Hartwell GR. Frequency of second mesiobuccal canals in maxillary molars as determined by use of an operating microscope: a clinical study. J. Endod.:2000; 26:673–674.
96. Sert S and Bayrl G. Taurodontism in six molars: a case report. J. Endod.:2004; 30:601–602.
97. Sert S, Sahinkesen G, Topen FT, Eroglu SE and Oklay EA. Root canal configuration of third molar teeth. A comparison with first and second molars in the Turkish population. Aust. Endod. J.:2011; 37, 109–117.
98. Sidow SJ, West LA, Liewehr FR and Loushine RJ. Root canal morphology of human maxillary and mandibular third molars. J. Endod.:2000; 26:675–678.
99. Sikri V and Sikri P. Mandibular premolars: Aberrations in pulp space morphology. Ind. J. Dent. Res.:1994; 5:9–14.
100. Sikri VK and Sikri P. Maxillary second premolar: Configuration and root canal deviation. JIDA:1991; 62: 46–49.
101. Sikri VK and Sikri P. Root canal morphology of mandibular incisors. Endodontology:1994; 9–13.
102. Sikri VK. Aberrant root canal anatomy of human permanent teeth. JIDA:1989; 60:51–53.
103. Sikri VK. Root canal anatomy of human permanent maxillary incisors. IJDR:1992; 3:7–12.
104. Silva EJ, Nejaim Y, Silva AV, Haiter-Neto F and Cohenca N. Evaluation of root canal configuration of mandibular molars in a Brazilian population by using cone-beam computed tomography: An *in vivo* study. J. Endod.:2013; 39:849–852.
105. Slowey and Carlos L. Radiographic aids in detection of extra root canals. O. Surg., O. Med., O. Path.:1974; 37:762.
106. Sonntag D, Stachniss-Crap S and Stchniss V. Determination of root canal curvature before and after canal preparation (part I): A literature review. Aust. Endod. J.:2005; 31:89–93.

107. Teixeira FB, Sano CL, Gomes BP, Zaia AA, Ferraz CC and Souza-Filho FJ. A preliminary *in vitro* study of the incidence and position of the root canal isthmus in maxillary and mandibular first molars. Int. Endod. J.:2003; 36:276–280.

108. Velmurugan N. and Sandhya R. Root canal morphology of mandibular first premolars in an Indian population: a laboratory study. Int. Endod. J.:2009; 42:54–58.

109. Venturi M, Prati C, Capelli G, Falconi M and Breschi L. A preliminary analysis of the morphology of lateral canals after root canal filling using a tooth-clearing technique. Int. Endod. J.:2003; 36:54–63.

110. Verma P and Love RM. A Micro CT study of the mesiobuccal root canal morphology of the maxillary first molar teeth. Int. Endod. J.:2010; 44:210–217.

111. Versiani MA, Pecora JD, deSousa-Neto MD. Root and root canal morphology of four rooted maxillary second molars: a micro-computed tomography study. J. Endod 2012; 38, 977–982.

112. Vertucci FJ. Root canal morphology and its relationship to an unusual endodontic procedures. Endod. Topics:2005; 10:3–29.

113. vonArx T. Frequency and type of canal isthmuses in first molars detected by endoscopic inspection during periradicular surgery. Int. Endod. J.:2005; 38:160–168.

114. Weine FS and Buchanan LS. Controversies in clinical endodontics: part 1 - the significance and filling of lateral canals. Compend. Contin. Educ. Dent.:1996; 17:1028–1032, 1035–1036.

115. Wilson RW and Henry P. The bifurcated root canal in lower anterior teeth. JADA:1965; 70:1162.

116. Wong M. Maxillary first molar with three palatal canals. J. Endod.:1991; 17:298–299.

117. Yang H, Tian C, Li G, Yang L, Han X and Wang Y. A cone-beam computed tomography study of the root canal morphology of mandibular first premolars and the location of root canal orifices and apical foramina in a Chinese population. J. Endod.:2013; 39P:435–438.

118. Yesilsoy C, Porras O and Gordon W. Importance of third mesial canals in mandibular molars: report of 2 cases. Oral Surg., Oral Med., Oral Pathol. Oral Radio. Endod.:2009; 108:e55–58.

119. Yoshioka T, Kikuchi I, Fukumoto Y, Kobayashi C and Suda H. Detection of the second mesiobuccal canal in mesiobuccal roots of maxillary molar teeth *ex vivo*. Int. Endod. J.:2005; 38:124–128.

120. Zhang Q, Chen H, Fan B, Fan W and Gutmann JL. Root and root canal morphology in maxillary second molar with fused root from a native Chinese population. J. Endod.:2014; 40:871–875.

121. Zhang Q, Zhang L, Zhou X, Wang Q, Tang L, Song F and Huang D. C-shaped root canal system in mandibular second molars in a Chinese population evaluated by cone-beam computer tomography. Int. Endod. J.:2011; 44:857–862.

Chapter 14

Access Cavity Preparation

Endodontic treatment may help the patient retain a clinically jeopardized tooth that would otherwise be destined for extraction. However, it greatly depends on the ability of operator to achieve successful results thereby maintaining the tooth in its physiological position with form and functions.

The operator must have the knowledge of the internal anatomy of teeth and the possible variations before undertaking endodontic therapy. It has been established that the root with a normal tapering canal and a single apical foramen is an exception. Any tooth may have extra root and any root may have extra root canal, accessory canals, communicating canals, fins, deltas, loops, etc. Thorough knowledge of the complexity of root canal system is mandatory to carry out thorough cleaning and shaping and hermetic obturation; subsequently, the successful outcome of the treatment. Access cavity design and preparation is imperative for successful endodontic treatment and also prevention of iatrogenic problems, which usually leads to failure. Recently, the trend of endodontic access cavity preparation is being shifted from traditional (based on operator needs) to conservative preparation (based on dentin support and structural strength of tooth). It is established that treatment failures are mostly because of structural compromises of the tooth. With the advent of modern endodontic techniques coupled with panoramic viewing with operating microscope and better illumination, the access cavity preparation is dictated by the morphology of individual pulp chamber and the availability of dentin around the pulp spaces of the tooth being treated.

BASIC PRINCIPLES OF ENDODONTIC TREATMENT

Basic principles of endodontic treatment are to be followed before initiating root canal treatment in any tooth. The principles are:

i. Pain Management

Pain and dentistry are considered synonymous. Pain in any form and severity must be dealt with carefully before initiating endodontic procedures. Pain may be due to inflammatory conditions, neurovascular/neuropathic disorders, musculoskeletal and/or odontogenic problems. An effective strategy for pain management is proper diagnosis, drugs, followed by specific treatment. In any case, it is important to determine whether the pain originates from tooth or is referred from another tissue (non-odontogenic). Pain relieving drugs, premedication/sedatives and local anesthesia can be useful in relieving pain. Details of drugs used in endodontics are given in Chapter 4.

ii. Sterilization (Asepsis)

Understanding and following infection control procedures are very important prior to endodontic treatment. Cross-infection (spread of microorganisms from one patient to another) should be managed by proper disinfection and sterilization. Aseptic environment coupled with sterilized instruments is mandatory for successful endodontic treatment. The general guidelines of handwashing, use of gloves, masks and protective glasses, etc. should be followed religiously. Details of sterilization and infection control are given in Chapter 12.

iii. Drainage-Trephination

Incisions and drainage are the most effective way to control pain associated with abscess formation in the apical tissues. The abscess can be drained via root canals or through surrounding soft tissues. Drainage through root canal is preferred, being convenient and it also minimizes patient's anxiety. Drainage lead to ease out the pus and increase in pH of surroundings; and subsequently, lead to reduction in pressure by allowing accumulated gases to escape.

Trephination (fistulation) involves creating a surgical passage in the root apex. It provides a channel for the escape of pus, which subsequently relieves the accumulated pressure. The detailed procedure is described in Chapter 23.

iv. Immobilization

Immobilization implies stabilizing the tooth (teeth) to be endodontically treated so as to minimize trauma to the periodontal ligament. It is established that traumatized teeth are more susceptible to infection and the inflamed tissues yield easily to trauma.

The concerned tooth can be splinted or should be 'hold' with fingers during endodontic procedures. It is good practice to relieve occlusion in all endodontic cases because it lessens the possibility of hurting the periodontal ligament. Before use of burs for access cavity preparation or use of rotary instruments during canal preparation, immobilizing the tooth will certainly lead to better success of endodontic treatment.

v. Isolation (Rubber Dam Application)

Isolation of teeth under treatment is mandatory for successful endodontic outcome. Isolation creates an aseptic field and also protect the patient and the operator from inadvertent mishaps during endodontic procedures. S. Barnum introduced the idea of using rubber dam to keep the teeth dry during operative/ endodontic procedures. The rubber dam as an isolation armamentarium has become indispensable in endodontics (Fig. 14.1).

Over the years the trend of using rubber dam has increased. The simplicity of its placement has encouraged practitioners and endodontists to use rubber dam in routine. Patients are also aware of the advantages and insist on using rubber dam.

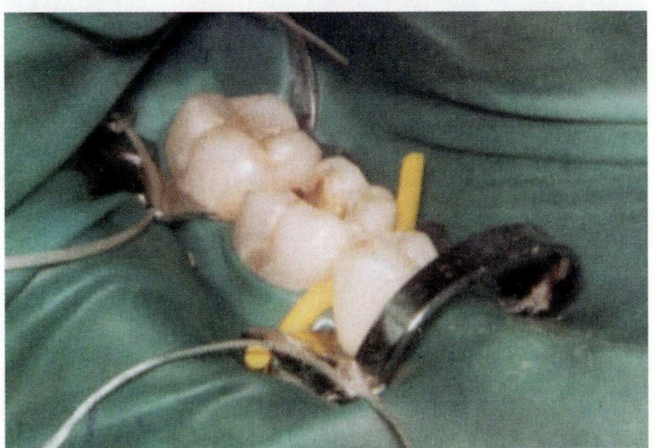

Fig. 14.1 Rubber dam applied over mandibular first molar

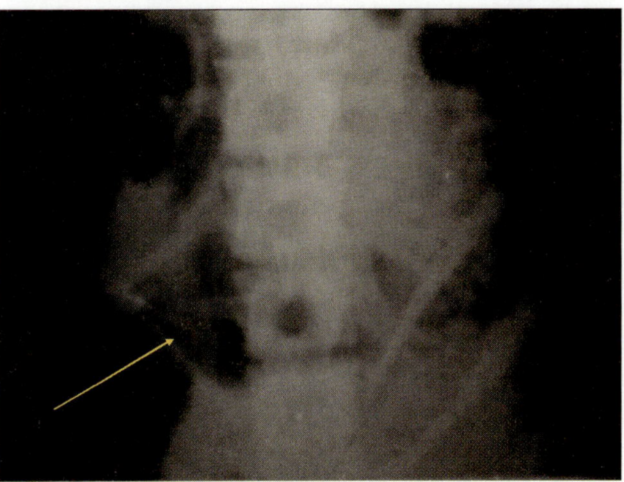

Fig. 14.2 Root canal file aspirated (arrow)

Advantages

- Provide clean surgical field
- Protect patient from ingestion or aspiration of endodontic instruments (Fig. 14.2)
- Facilitate retraction of soft tissues
- Protect tongue, lips and cheeks from cutting action of burs
- Operator and team is protected from splash of saliva; subsequently the infection
- Provides better visibility
- Both patient and the operator feel comfortable
- Reduces risk of cross-infection, significantly reducing the microbial content of aerosols.

Use of rubber dam should be avoided in certain cases, such as:

- Asthmatics and mouth breathers as they may not tolerate the dam
- Partially erupted and malpositioned teeth; difficult to receive a retainer (clamp)
- Patient may not allow placement of a rubber dam because of psychological reasons
- Patients allergic to latex (non-latex rubber dam in also available).

Armamentarium

A rubber dam kit (Fig. 14.3) should have the following items:

a. *Rubber dam sheets*: Available in the form of rolls from which requisite sheets can be cut; individual sheets are also available (Fig. 14.4) with the following characteristics:

Size: 5 × 5″, 6 × 6″, 5 × 6″

14

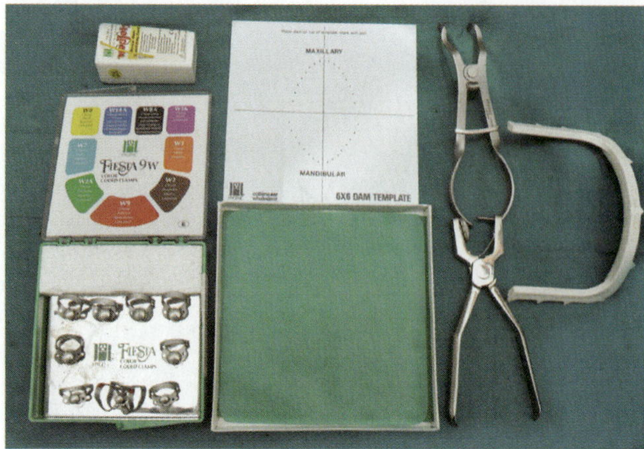

Fig. 14.3 Rubber dam kit

Fig. 14.4 Rubber dam sheet

Thickness

Thin: 0.006″

Medium: 0.008″

Heavy: 0.010″ (provides better retraction of soft tissue and are more resistant to tearing)

Extra heavy: 0.012″

Special heavy: 0.014″

Color: Available in several colors, but green and blue colors are preferred because they provide good contrast with the surroundings. Rubber dam sheet has a shiny side and a dull side. The dull side should face the operator so as to reduce any light reflected from it.

The modified/recently introduced rubber dam sheets are:

- *Hygiene dental dam*: It is a non-latex rubber dam for patients with latex allergy. This is powder-free synthetic material (6 × 6″ size and medium gauge thickness).
- *Derma dam*: It is a non-latex and powder-free rubber dam. It provides sufficient resistance during use in endodontic procedures.
- *Flexi dam*: It is an elastic, non-latex dental dam (can be elongated 1000% before tearing). It is also powder-free, reducing the chances of allergic reaction. It is available in blue and violet colors, providing good contrast to the operating area.

b. *Rubber dam clamps (retainers)*: These are used to secure the dam to the teeth that are to be isolated (Fig. 14.5). A retainer has two jaws connected by a bow. On each jaw, two prongs are present which means that there are four prongs in a clamp. Each prong rests on the mesial/distal line angle of the tooth to be clamped. A prong should not extend beyond the angle of the tooth otherwise it would interfere with the placement of a wedge or matrix band during restoration. Certain retainers have inverted prongs, i.e. directed gingivally; preferred in partially erupted teeth.

Two types of retainers are:

i. *Winged retainers*: These retainers have wing like projections on the outer aspect of their jaws. Hence, they provide extra retraction of the rubber dam from the field of operation. The wings are passed through the punched hole in the dam and then the dam and the retainer placed together onto the concerned tooth. After placement, the dam is slipped carefully over the wings onto the tooth.

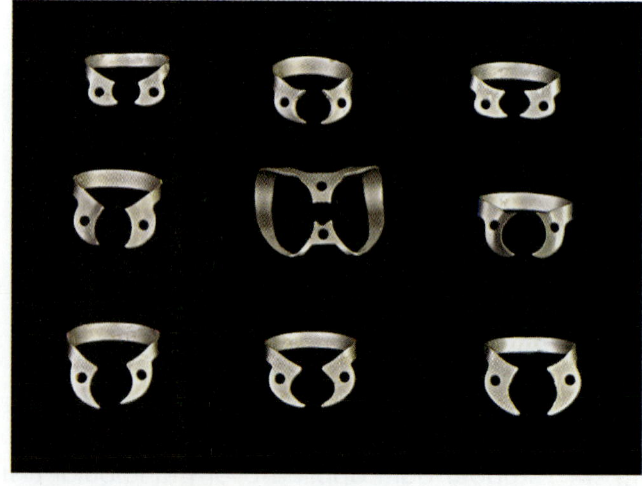

Fig. 14.5 Rubber dam clamps

ii. *Wingless retainers*: These have no wings on their jaws, i.e. they are smooth on their outer aspect. The retainer is first placed on the tooth and then the dam is stretched over the clamp onto the tooth.

Several clamps are available. The larger clamps are used for adult patients and the smaller ones for children. Newer clamps have also been introduced (with modified wings and jaws), such as:

Tiger clamp

- The clamp has serrated jaws
- Used mainly for partially erupted and structurally compromised teeth.

Silker-Glickman clamp (S-G clamp)

- Extended wings facilitate rubber dam placement around teeth with minimal tooth structure.

Haller clamp

- Hold tongue and cheek and improve the impression making.

Cushee clamp

- Increases patient comfort (avoid contact of steel clamp with gingiva and tooth).
- Enhances rubber dam seal to limit leaking from above or below the dam.

c. ***Retainer forceps***: The retainer forceps holds the retainer and facilitates its placement and removal from the tooth (Fig. 14.6).

d. ***Rubber dam frame***: It holds borders of the dam and position the dam as required. The frame is U shaped, usually made of metal or plastic. The metal one is known as the Young's frame. Plastic frame is useful when a radiograph is to be taken without removing the frame (Fig. 14.7). The frame has minute projections on its outer surface where the dam is secured. An additional two hooks may be present on the sides of the frame. The frame is preferably placed beneath the dam rather than above it. The commonly used frames are metal frames with plastic caps on the ends to protect the patient's skin and eyes.

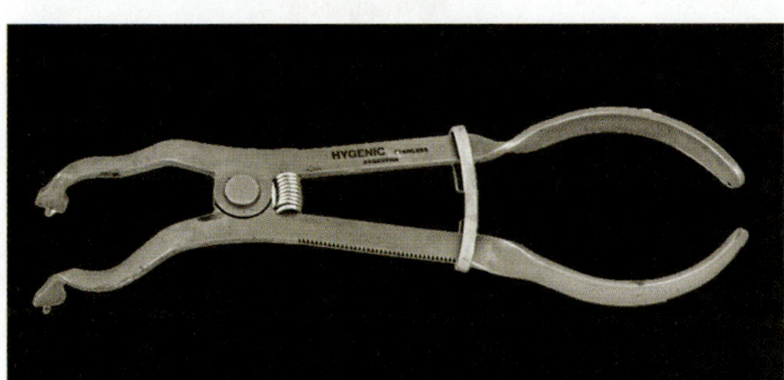

Fig. 14.6 Retainer forceps

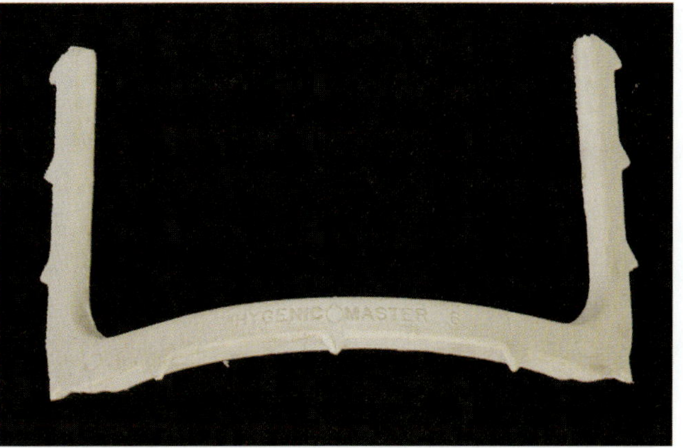

Fig. 14.7 Rubber dam frame

Newer frames, as given below, have been introduced providing improved functioning.

Nygaard Ostby frame (Shark mouth frame)

- Radiolucent nylon frame; polygonal in shape.

Articulated frame

- Foldable plastic frame (polysulfone), facilitate endodontic radiography (a double hinge in the vertical axis of the frame facilitates its folding).

Derma frame

- Pliable metal frame; can be bent to take radiographs.

Safe-T frame

- Two piece frame design; provides secure fit without stretching the rubber dam sheet. The raised edges of the frame provide barrier, preventing fluids from escaping onto the patient.

e. ***Rubber dam punch***: It is a punch for making holes in the dam and is characterized by a rotating metal disc, which bears five or six holes of different sizes, and a sharp pointed plunger (Fig. 14.8). When the handle of the punch is pressed, the plunger should rest in the center of the hole. If not, the plunger tip would get

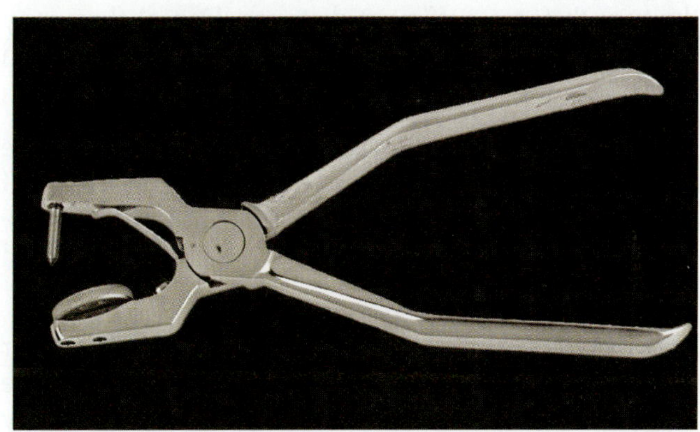

Fig. 14.8 Rubber dam punch

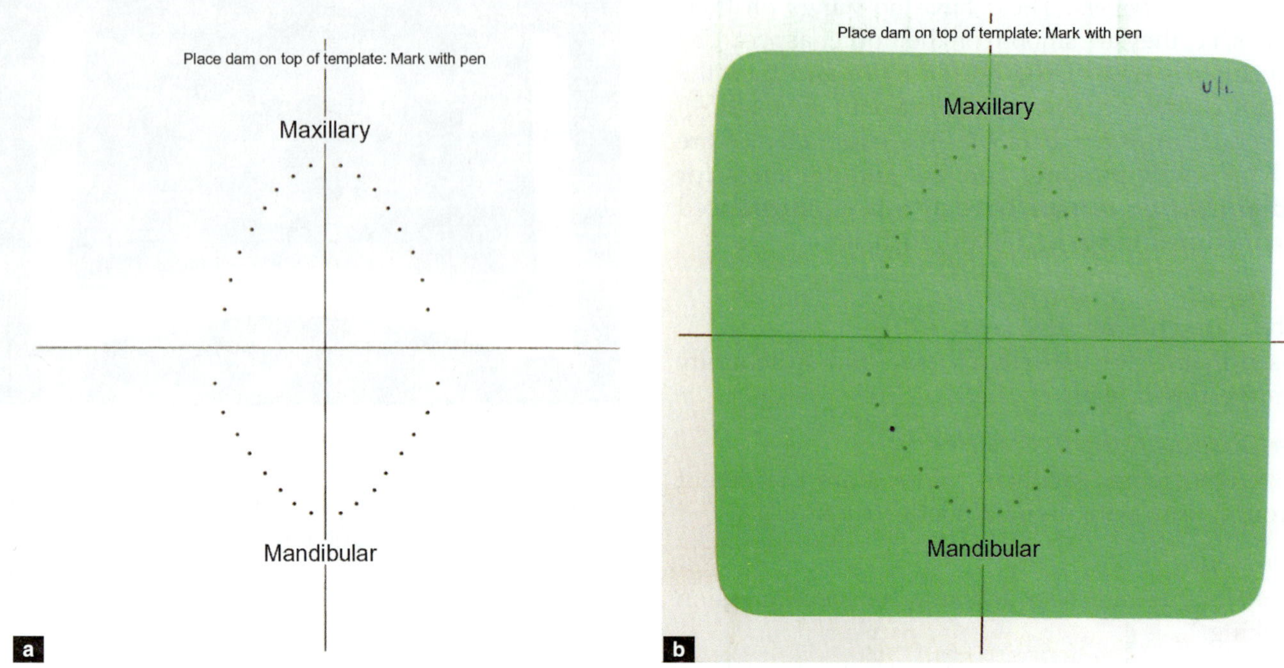

Fig. 14.9a and b Rubber dam template

damaged compromising its cutting ability. The holes are of different sizes according to the size of different teeth. Appropriate hole should be used for particular tooth, otherwise the dam may tear during its placement.

e. *Rubber dam template*: The positions of the teeth are marked and are used to transfer these markings to the rubber dam sheet for the holes to be punched (Fig. 14.9a and b).

f. *Dental floss*: A strand of dental floss (Fig. 14.10) should be tied around the retainer before it is carried into the oral cavity. This is a safety measure to prevent accidental aspiration of the clamp. Floss should be passed through both the holes in the jaws and around the bow of the clamp. The floss should be adequately long, say twelve inches, so that the strand hangs out of the mouth for a sufficient distance. Dental floss may also be used for passing the rubber dam sheet through interproximal contact.

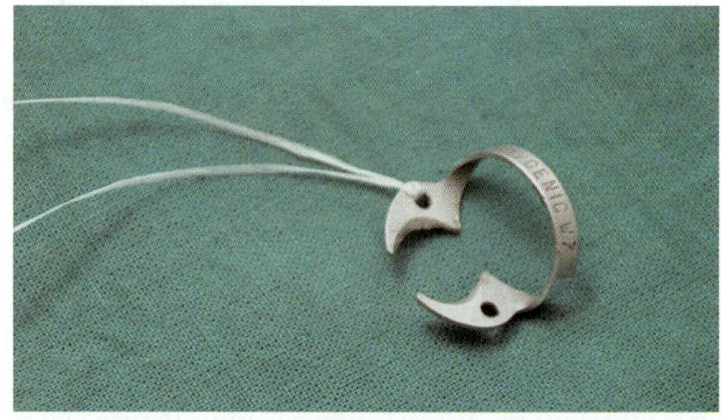

Fig. 14.10 Dental floss tied with the retainer

g. *Wedjet*: An elastic cord generally used to secure the dam around teeth away from the clamp (Fig. 14.11). It can also be used to push the dam through the interproximal contact. Rarely, it is used as a retainer instead of a clamp.

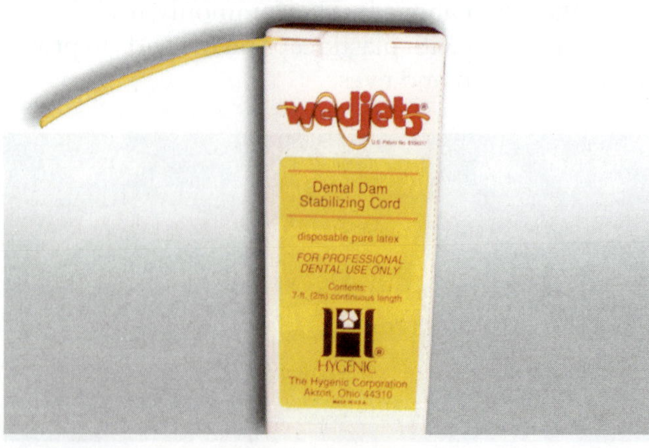

Fig. 14.11 Wedjet elastic cord

h. *Lubricant*: A lubricant aids in passing the dam over the tooth. It is applied on both sides of the dam in the area of punched holes. Lubricants may be commercially available; alternatively soap, vaseline, shaving cream, etc. can also be employed. Vaseline or petroleum jelly should also be applied on the patient's lips and corners of the mouth to avoid constant irritation from the rubber dam.

New Rubber Dam

a. *Instidam*

- Made of translucent natural latex that is very stretchable, tear resistant and provides easy visibility.
- Compact design fits outside the patient's mouth. Comfortable to the patient.
- Built in flexible frame, with prepunched hole off-center by half an inch. (Prepunched hole helps eliminate tearing and additional holes may be punched if necessary.)
- Radiographs may be taken without removing the dam by bending the Instidam to one side.
- Produces minimal pull on clamp.
- Single use only.

b. *Handidam*: Handidam is a preframed rubber dam; easy to place on the patient and saves time.

c. *Optra dam* (Fig. 14.12)

- Available in two sizes: Regular and small.
- Anatomical shape and integrated frame make placement fast and easy.
- Flexible in all directions; comfortable for patient for long duration procedures.
- Both arches are fully exposed and provide easier access to the treatment field.
- Metal clamps are not required.
- Can be kept in place during radiography.

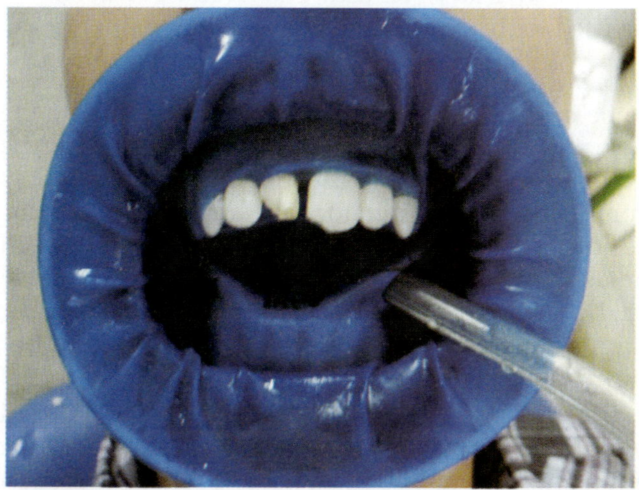

Fig. 14.12 Optra dam

d. *Optidam*

- Available in anterior and posterior versions.
- 3-D anatomically contoured design; allows easy placement and accommodates anatomical variations in the oral cavity. Very comfortable for the patient.
- Can be autoclaved in routine.
- Minimal tension on the clamp due to its design.
- Powder free dam; reduces the chance of air borne particles that can cause an allergic reaction.

e. *Dry dam*

- An alternative type of rubber dam, which does not require a frame
- Fits like a face mask
- Absorbent lining provides comfort to the patient
- Non-allergic
- Useful in anterior teeth; not good for posterior teeth
- Not useful during bleaching.

f. *Flexi dam* (Fig. 14.13)

- It is non-latex flexi dam available with built-in frame
- Good tear resistance and is odorless
- Plastic frame provides requisite comfort to the patient.

Alternative Rubber Dams

a. *Kool dam*: It is a light cured material applied on gingiva and adjacent teeth prior to power bleaching and sand blasting providing the requisite isolation. This is also known as liquid rubber dam. It is flexible, showing good tear resistance and is easy to remove. It is user friendly rubber dam substitute (Fig. 14.14). Opal dam, a resin based product, is not used these days because the heat produced during curing of resin cause discomfort/pain to the patient.

b. *Fast dam*: Fast dam can be anatomically shaped providing requisite dry field for the operator. All saliva ejectors can be adjusted with the suction holes provided along the perimeter. It effectively retracts

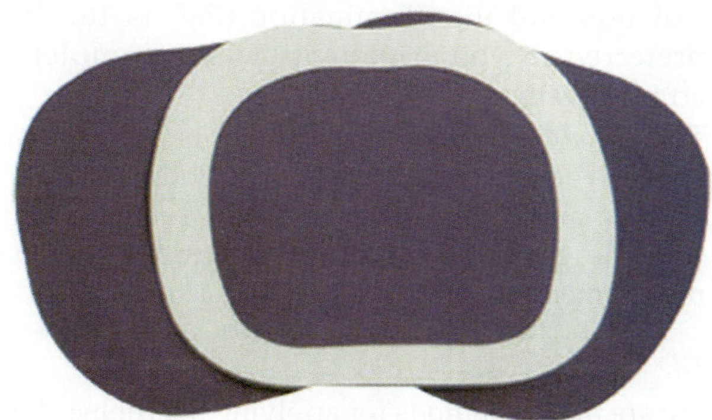

Fig. 14.13 Flexi dam

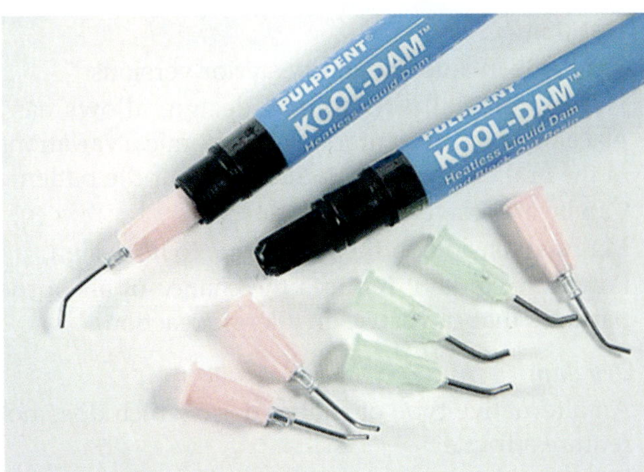

Fig. 14.14 Kool dam

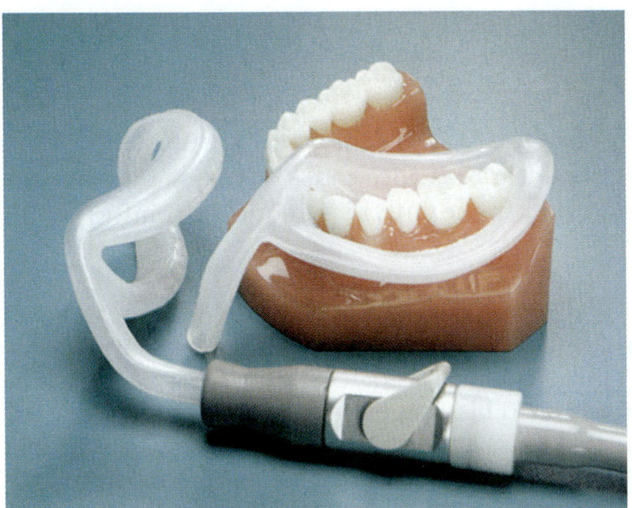

Fig. 14.15 Fast dam

the tongue and the cheeks, maintaining a continuous dry field (Fig. 14.15).

c. *Isolite*: A new device, provides illumination, retraction, isolation and throat protection. It has soft and flexible mouthpiece, which isolates maxillary and mandibular quadrants simultaneously, providing isolation and the illumination (Fig. 14.16). It is preferred in young patients with incompletely erupted teeth.

The *disadvantage* of this device is being more expensive than rubber dam, not providing the color contrast and may damage gingiva (isolite does not seal the gingiva from irrigants and intracanal medicaments).

14

Rubber Dam Application

There are many methods for applying the rubber dam. The important features are:

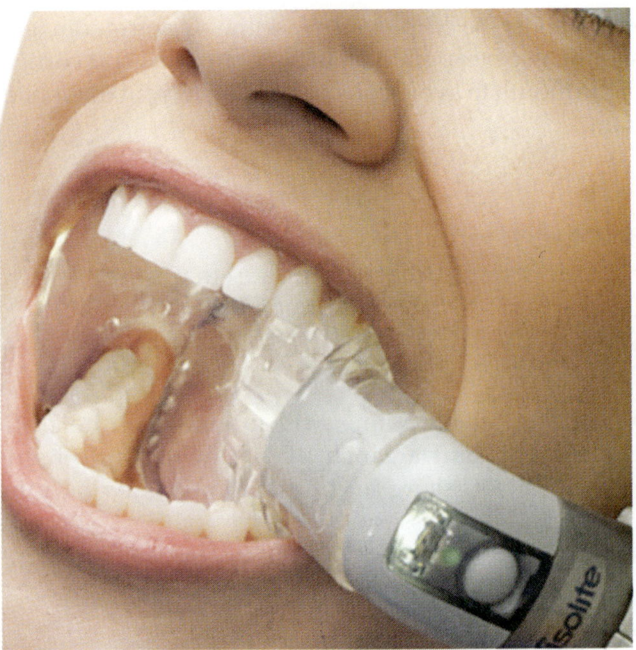

Fig. 14.16 Isolite

- If the clamp is attached to the rubber sheet before it is carried to the oral cavity, ligation with dental floss to prevent the clamp from being swallowed is not necessary.
- Having the rubber already stretched over the frame makes it easier to mount it symmetrically and reduces the application time.

The routinely used techniques for rubber dam application are:

a. ***Bow technique***: The bow technique can be employed without an assistant. It provides a good view of the oral cavity as the clamp is being placed. A *disadvantage* is that the rubber must be stretched over the wings, which may lead to its tear. The largest punch should be used for making the hole to avoid tearing.

b. ***Wing technique***: In this technique the rubber dam is to be inserted along both wings of the clamp into the hole punched in the dam. The preliminary steps can be accomplished by the assistant and the placement is completed by the operator. The assistant inserts the selected clamp into the hole in the rubber sheet at an angle of 45° with the bow towards the distal, relative to the dental arch. Then the attachment to the rubber dam frame is carried out stretching the rubber diagonally.

The *disadvantage* of this technique is the reduced visibility, especially on the more distal teeth. In addition, care must be taken not to pinch or injure soft tissues, such as tongue, lips, or cheeks. As the clamp is carefully placed into undercut areas of the tooth, the patient is instructed to signal if there is any discomfort in the gingiva. Once the rubber dam is released from the wings of the clamp, the placement is completed.

c. *Rubber sheet first technique*: The rubber dam clamp and forceps should be kept ready and the rubber sheet is stretched over the frame. A special rubber dam is provided with frame, which has guiding grooves for a saliva ejector at the lower right and left borders. The next step is fitting of the clamp. If it fits well, the rubber dam attached to frame is carried to the oral cavity. The hole may be spread wider with the fingers, and the rubber is pulled down around the tooth. The clamp is then placed over the isolated tooth (Fig. 14.17a and b).

The *advantage* of this procedure is that all types of clamps can be used and the visibility is better.

d. *Clamp first technique*: The clamp is placed first on the tooth. The clamp-forceps and rubber sheet-frame should be kept ready (Fig. 14.18a to e). The order in which they are brought into the oral cavity is reversed. It is essential that the clamp be secured against the possibility of its slipping into the pharyngeal cavity.

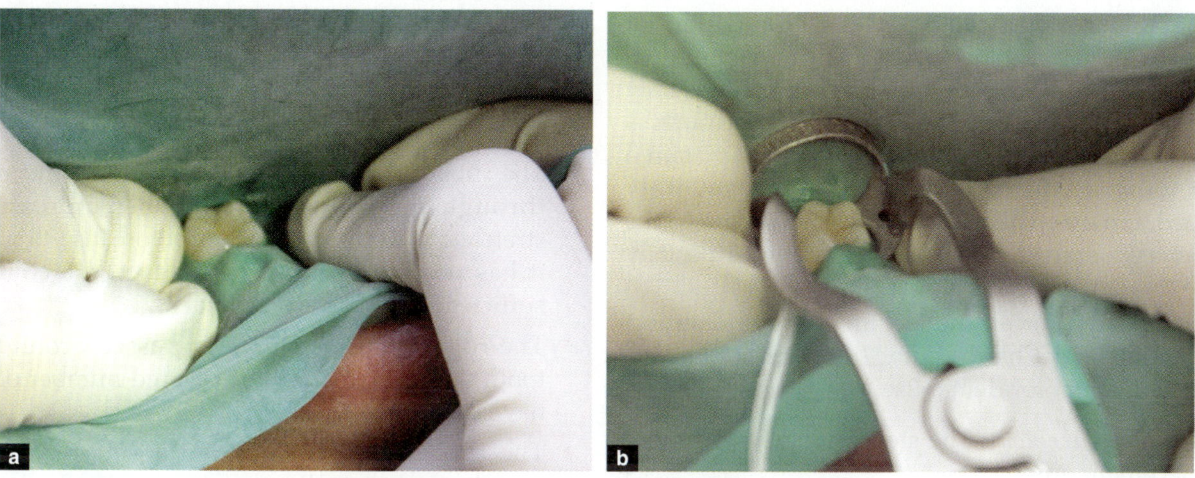

Fig. 14.17a and b Rubber sheet first technique

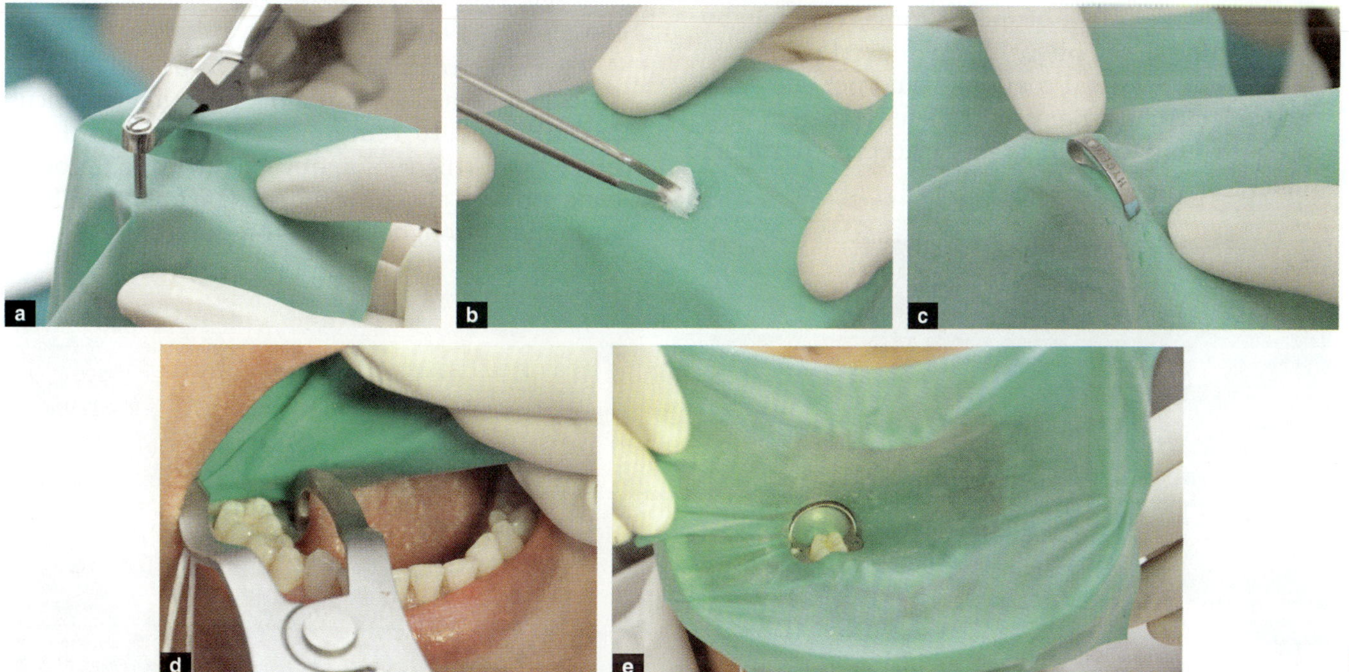

Fig. 14.18 Placing rubber dam: (a) Punching hold in rubber dam sheet; (b) Application of lubricant; (c) Placement of rubber dam sheet over the clamp; (d) Evaluation of rubber dam placement; (e) Completion of rubber dam placement

This is accomplished by looping a long piece of dental floss over the bow of the clamp and letting it hang out of the mouth where it can be quickly grasped in case of emergency. The problem generally, faced during placement of the rubber dam in that the hole must be stretched wide to pass over the selected clamp. Therefore, the use of wingless clamps is recommended because the smaller width makes it less susceptible to tear. The *advantage* is the unobstructed view as the clamp is being applied.

In a few cases, the techniques described above will have to be modified in order to achieve a well-placed, tightly fitting rubber dam. Patients with fixed orthodontic appliances pose problems. In such situations, it is possible to place a rubber dam by using dental floss ligatures (Fig. 14.19). Teeth with fixed prostheses may need endodontic treatment. If only single tooth is involved, it is better to remove the crown to obtain a better view. If the underlying tooth is severely damaged, it may be necessary to attach the dam to the adjacent teeth or to employ a clamp designed especially for deeply damaged teeth.

The final step for all the techniques is to disinfect the operating field. Chlorhexidine/betadine are suitable disinfecting agent for dental use.

***Rubber dam placement*:** The steps involved in rubber dam placement are:

- Attain a comfortable patient position. Remove calculus, overhanging restorations, etc.
- Check for tightness of the proximal contacts by passing the floss obliquely from buccal or lingual side. Tight proximal contacts would not allow the passage of rubber dam; immediate separation may be carried out to facilitate easy placement of rubber dam.
- Select a rubber dam clamp depending on the type of the tooth to be isolated. A clamp forcep is used to seat the clamp onto the tooth first on the lingual cervical region then onto the buccal cervical region. Before trying the clamp onto the tooth, dental floss is tied around it. The length of the floss should be such that it hangs outside the mouth for a sufficient distance.
- Take a rubber dam sheet. Punch a hole on its upper right corner or mark it with 'R' for identifying the patient's right side. The sheet is then placed on a template and the position of the holes are marked with a pen.
- A lubricant is then applied on both sides of the punched hole to facilitate the passage of dam over the tooth. The patient's lips and corners of the mouth are also coated with a lubricant (Fig. 14.20).
- The rubber dam is placed on the tooth and passed through the contact. The rubber dam sheet is stretched at the lips of the hole before insertion. Once it has passed through the contact, the contact is sufficient to hold the sheet back.
- The rubber dam is similarly passed around each tooth one by one, until the desired number of teeth have been isolated.
- The rubber dam is unfolded and spread neatly. Slowly and steadily the dam is hooked to the projections on the frame while making sure there are minimal folds in the dam. The frame should be placed beneath the dam.
- A low volume evacuator tip may be passed through an extra hole made in the dam into the lingual sulcus and allowed to remain there throughout the procedure. A high volume evacuator tip on the other hand is placed above the rubber dam for intermittent suctioning throughout the procedure.

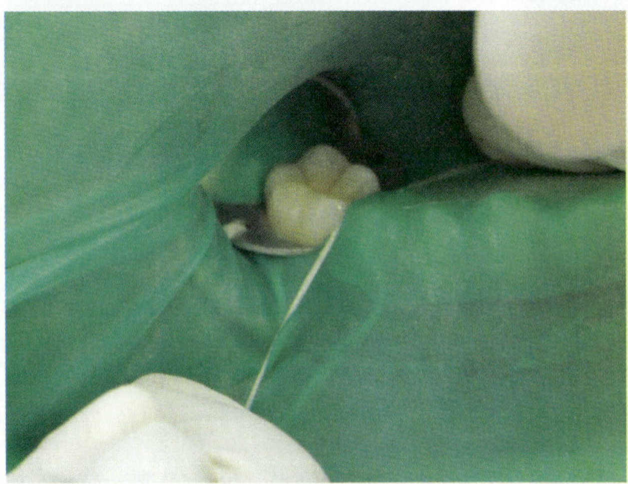

Fig. 14.19 Crossing contact with dental floss

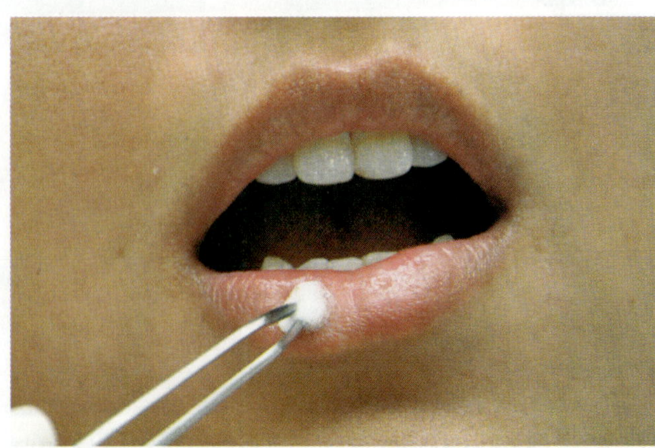

Fig. 14.20 Applying vaseline to patient's lips

ACCESS CAVITY PREPARATION

The main objective of preparing an access cavity is to detect the root canal orifices for further penetration into the canal system. This will in turn avoid potential complications, which are likely to confront in the way of successful treatment.

Before considering root canal treatment in any tooth, the accessibility of that tooth needs to be ascertained. An extremely malpositioned tooth, very limited mouth opening and uncooperative patients may compromise the outcome of treatment.

The main aim of the design of the cavity, 'access cavity', is to provide straight-line approach to the apical foramen. Access cavity preparation implies the creation of a space from occlusal table to canal orifice(s) so as to facilitate instrumentation, irrigation and obturation of the root canals. This is so significant in root canal therapy that it is described as 'gateway to success'. The access preparation should allow proper débridement of the pulp chamber and introduction of the root canal instruments without any obstruction.

Objectives of Access Cavity Preparation

- To gain direct access to the apical foramen (not merely to the canal orifices).
- To facilitate removal of pulp tissue from coronal as well as radicular spaces.
- To facilitate instrumentation of the canal spaces, subsequently preparing and obturating the canals.
- To maintain structural integrity of the tooth (conserve as much tooth structure as possible).

Points to Remember

- The rubber dam should be placed onto the concerned tooth and the adjacent tooth for better visibility.
- The initial entry should be made either through occlusal or lingual surface but never through proximal surface [approaching the pulp chamber and the canals through the proximal surface may lead to ledge formation and/or even breakage of the instruments. And also, by doing so, the pulp tissue in the coronal aspect remains untouched, which leads to failure (Fig. 14.21)].
- The radiograph should be evaluated for overall configuration of the pulp chamber and the root canals and also the inclination of the roots in the jaws (Fig. 14.22).
- During 'reading' the radiograph, if the radiolucency abruptly vanishes or diminishes in size, a bifurcation of the canal is suspected (Fig. 14.23). Another radiograph at an angle of 20–30° mesial/distal can help confirming the bifurcation.

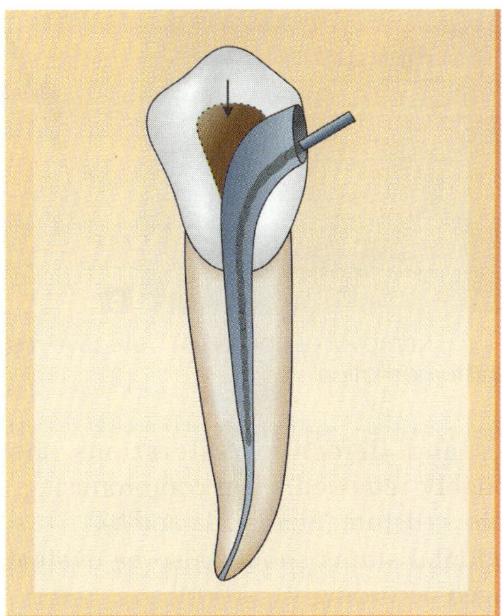

Fig. 14.21 Avoid access from proximal surface

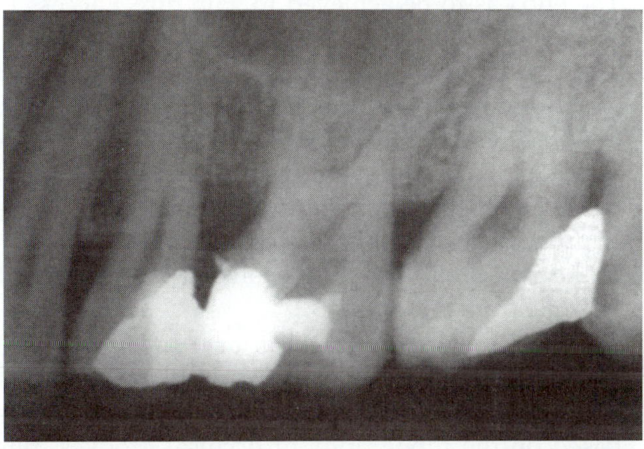

Fig. 14.22 Evaluation of radiograph (*see* pulp chamber, roots and periodontal condition)

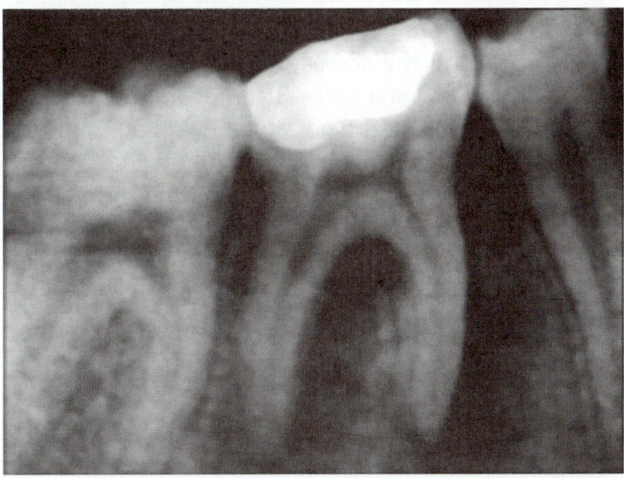

Fig. 14.23 Abrupt diminishing the root canal indicates bifurcation of the canal

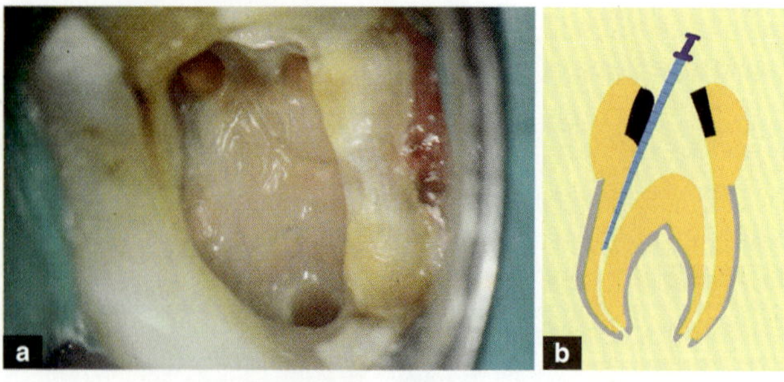

Fig. 14.24 (a) Removal of caries; (b) Defective restoration, prior to instrumentation

- Caries and defective restorations should be thoroughly removed, even compromising the loss of tooth structure (Fig. 14.24a and b).
- Periodontal status should also be evaluated and managed accordingly.

Rules for Access Cavity Preparation

- The entry is to be achieved to gain direct access to the apical foramina, not merely to the canal orifices. The cavity is widened so as to remove remnant of the coronal pulp, which can be source of infection even after the treatment. Straight line access is important for better instrumentation, irrigation and subsequently obturating the canals. No conservative approach is followed at the cost of non-negotiation of the root canal. The pulp chamber must be free of necrotic pulp remnants.
- Access cavity preparations are different from occlusal cavity preparation used in operative dentistry. The principle of occlusal preparation is based on the topography of occlusal grooves, pits and fissures. The access cavity preparations are designed for uncovering the roof of the pulp chamber and providing direct access to the apical foramina through root canals.
- Before starting the access preparation, radiographs taken from at least two different angles must be evaluated to know the possible deviation of internal anatomy. After thorough evaluation, the operator will be able to accurately ascertain the pulp spaces present in the tooth under treatment.
- When the canal orifices are difficult to locate, rubber dam should not be placed until correct location has been confirmed. Isolating multiple teeth with rubber dam improves visibility and accessibility.
- Endodontic entries are prepared through occlusal or lingual surface and never through proximal or gingival surface. When proximal or gingival tooth destruction occurs, affected areas should be excavated and restored with either a temporary or permanent filling material (preendodontic build-up). Then the normal access cavity is prepared through the occlusal or lingual surface.
- All unsupported cusps must be reduced to obtain a definite clearance in occlusal and lateral movement. This decreases the chances of cuspal fracture or even the vertical fracture of root.
- The access cavity should have a certain amount of resistance form to ensure that the tooth does not fracture during treatment as well as retention form to allow a proper coronal seal of the restorations (both interim and permanent).

Armamentarium for Access Cavity Preparation

The following armamentarium is usually required for access cavity preparation of any tooth:

a. Magnification and Illumination

The preparation of an ideal access cavity preparation requires the use of magnification and an appropriate light source. A number of adjuncts, like the microscope, dental loupes, endoscopes and orascopes, etc. can aid the clinician to locate canal orifices and also the calcified and additional canals. Transilluminating devices are preferred to visualize floor of the pulp chamber.

b. Handpieces

A high-speed handpiece can be used for most phases of access cavity preparation. A slow-speed handpiece can be used in cases where increased tactile awareness is required like in teeth with calcified and receded pulp chambers.

c. Burs and Diamond Points

i. *Endo access kit* is provided by different companies, containing set of burs required to initiate, open and prepare access cavity in any tooth. Inverted cone bur is used for initial nick followed by round burs for the initial entry into the pulp chamber of anterior teeth.

ii. *Diamond round burs* (No. 2 for anterior teeth and No. 4 for posterior teeth) are commonly used to initiate entry in old restorations. Once the 'drop' into the pulp chamber is attained, the overhanging dentin is removed from the roof of the chamber using tapered burs. Diamond points can also be used for axial wall extensions of the access cavity preparation. But they need to be used with caution as gouging of the pulpal floor and axial walls can occur. Using burs and diamond points with safe ended tips (non-cutting tips) have the advantage of not damaging the pulpal floor and avoiding perforations. They can also be used to level off cusp tips and incisal edges, which are used as reference points for working length determination.

iii. *Transmetal burs* will help in preparing access cavity preparations through amalgams, all-metal cast restorations, or metal copings of porcelain fused to metal crowns. The saw-tooth blade configuration is efficient in reducing vibrations [preferred when entering a tooth with pulpitis (hot tooth)].

iv. *Extended-shank round burs,* such as the Mueller bur and Munce Discovery burs, can be used in teeth with receded pulp chamber and calcified orifices. The extra-long shank of these burs moves the head of the handpiece away from the tooth, improving the clinician's visibility during access preparation.

v. *Gates-Glidden burs (X-Gates)* can be used to enlarge canal orifices of the access cavity starting with smaller sizes and progressing to larger sizes. This facilitates canal instrumentation during endodontic procedures; X-Gates also facilitate removal of internal flanges of dentin, if any, from the canal openings.

d. Hand Instruments

The DG-16 and the JW-17 endodontic explorers are used to identify canal orifices and to determine canal angulation. The endodontic spoon excavator can be used to assist in removing coronal pulp and carious dentin.

e. Ultrasonic Instruments

Pulp stones, calcifications present in the pulp chamber act as hindrances in accessing the canal orifices. Ultrasonically driven procedures remove bulky head of traditional handpiece, facilitating better view of operating field. Ultrasonic tips can be used to trough and remove these obstructions. Fine ultrasonic tips are smaller than conventional round burs, and their abrasive coatings allow clinicians to remove dentin conservatively. Ultrasonic procedures are utilized to refine and finish the access preparation.

Phases of Access Cavity Preparation

The preparation of access cavity (initiating process of cleaning pulp spaces) is to be carried out in phases; starting from pre-access analysis, preparation of tooth, removal of pulp chamber roof and coronal pulp, identification of canal orifices and preparing radicular portion.

a. Pre-access Analysis

The anatomy of the tooth to be treated along with surrounding tissues are evaluated before initiating access cavity preparation. Clinical and radiological examination is carried out to analyze the position, size, depth and shape of pulp chamber and also the number and curvature of the radicular pulp. The dimensions of pulp chamber and canal orifices may be influenced by the amount of tertiary dentin deposition and also presence of dystrophic calcifications/pulp stones, etc. The law of centrality (pulp chamber of every tooth is in the centre of tooth and at the level of the cementoenamel junction) should be used as a guide for initiating access. The coronal pulp chamber is usually mesially placed, which should not be confused with law of centrality. The initial penetrating bur should be directed towards centre of circumference of cementoenamel junction.

- The position of cementoenamel junction is identified by using periodontal probes, noting the complete circumference.
- The complete visualization of anatomy of pulp chamber is also guided by law of concentricity (the walls of pulp chamber are concentric to the external outline of the tooth at the level of cementoenamel junction). In case the operator finds deviated wall at cementoenamel junction, the pulp chamber will also follow that deviation (e.g. if the tooth is narrow buccolingually, the pulp chamber will also be narrow buccolingually).
- Angulation of tooth is also to be determined. Conventional radiography or CBCT imaging are helpful in ascertaining the angulation.
- The distance from the cusp tip to furcation area is to be measured (shank of bur for access preparation should be selected short of this length to avoid mishaps at the furcation area).

b. Preparation of Tooth

Caries and defective restorations must be completely removed prior to preparation of access cavity enabling the operator to assess the remaining tooth structure for future restoration. The removal of existing restorations may reveal hairline cracks on any axial wall, which may influence the prognosis of endodontic treatment and require immediate attention.

The remaining caries and defective restorations must be removed for the following reasons:

- To mechanically eradicate microorganisms from the inner side of the tooth.
- If caries removal lead to perforation, the perforation site is sealed from the inside, thus minimizing the chances of saliva leaking into the prepared cavity and contaminating it.
- To remove any discolored tooth structure, that may ultimately lead to staining of the crown.

Unsupported cusps should also be removed; or can be covered by orthodontic bands to prevent eventual tooth fracture. In some cases, undercuts are filled with glass-ionomers or composites, which facilitate rubber dam placement as well as access cavity preparation.

c. Removal of Pulp Chamber Roof and Coronal Pulp

The type and shape of burs are to be finalized keeping in mind the pre-access factors (circumference of cementoenamel junction, angulation of tooth and distance of cusp tip to furcation area).

The principles involved are by and large the same as Black's principle for cavity preparation. The main principles are:

i. Outline form
ii. Convenience form
iii. Cleaning the cavity

i. *Outline form*: The outline form should be so shaped as it must establish complete freedom for instrumentation during endodontic procedures. The external outline form is dictated by the internal anatomy of pulp. Because of this internal-external relationship, endodontic preparations must be carried out in reverse manner, from inside of the tooth to the outside.

To achieve optimal preparation, three factors of internal anatomy must be considered:

- *Size of pulp chamber*: The outline form is influenced by the size of pulp chamber. In young patients, the preparations must be more extensive than in older patients (pulp chamber is reduced three dimensionally in older patients).
- *Shape of pulp chamber*: The outline form should accurately reflect the shape of the pulp chamber. For example, teeth with three canals, reflect a triangular shaped cavity outline; four canal anatomy will result in a square, rectangular or rhomboid cavity outline.
- *Configuration of root canals*: To prepare each canal efficiently and without any interference, the cavity walls are extended accordingly to allow for unrestricted instrument approach to the apical foramen.

The roof of pulp chamber is continually shaved off following the sequence as:

- *Penetration phase*: Round diamond point is used to drill through the roof of the pulp chamber to make a way into the pulp chamber.
- *Enlargement phase*: A long shank diamond point is used to widen the pulp chamber and remove any overhangs and obstructions to the canal orifices.
- *Finishing and flaring phase*: A tapered non- end cutting bur is used to smoothen the walls of the cavity and make them slightly divergent towards the occlusal.

The law of color change (the color of floor of pulp chamber is always darker than the surrounding walls) provides guidance to know whether the access outline is complete or not. The walls being lighter than floor, the junction of wall-floor is easily recognized (if operator can see wall-floor junction, the access outline is considered as 'complete').

ii. *Convenience form*: Convenience form implies modifying the cavity design so as to facilitate easy instrumentation during root canal procedures. It provides:

- *Unobstructed view of pulpal floor and the canal orifices*: During access cavity preparations, enough tooth structure must be removed to enable a clear view of the pulpal floor and possibly all the canal orifices. The canal orifice may appear partially on the axial wall giving a 'mouse hole' effect, if axial walls extension is incomplete.
- *Unhindered access to the canal orifice*: The root canal instruments should be freely introduced into the orifice of each canal without interference from side walls.
- *Direct access to the apical foramen*: Endodontic instruments can gain direct access to the canal in an unstrained position, even if the canal is severely curved.
- *Outline extension to accommodate root canal filling techniques*: Rarely, the outline form may be appropriately widened to carry out certain root canal filling modalities.
- *Control over the instruments*: The factors controlling the root canal instruments are: (i) The clinician's fingers on the handle of the instrument and (ii) the walls of the canal at the tip of the instrument. Any dentinal overhangs coming in between these two points would result in binding instrument in the canal; subsequently leading to mishaps, such as root perforation, ledge formation, instrument breakage, zipping or apical transportation.

iii. *Cleaning the cavity*: The feature, cleaning of cavity is important, since loose debris invites bacterial growth and stain the tooth as well. After removing all the hard and soft necrotic material, remnants of previous restorations and debris are removed from the chamber with copious irrigation with a suitable irrigant. The chamber may finally be wiped out with cotton, and gently air dried to eliminate any remaining loose debris. Air, if used, should not be directed towards the canal orifices; it may cause emphysema.

d. Identification of Canal Orifices

It is always difficult to know the number of root canals prior to commencement of treatment. Radiographs do assess roots and canals, but may not be able to capture all anatomical aberrations. The effective way is to analyse full view of pulp chamber floor and use different anatomic landmarks.

As the floor-wall junction is clearly visible, the laws of symmetry and the laws of orifice location are used to identify the number and location of the orifices (law of symmetry 1: Except for maxillary molars, the orifices of canals are equidistant from a line drawn in mesio-distal direction through the centre of the pulp chamber; Law of symmetry 2: Except for the maxillary molars, the orifices of the canals lie on a line perpendicular to a line drawn in a mesial-distal direction through the centre of the pulp chamber flow; law of color change: The color of the pulp chamber floor is always darker than walls; Law of orifice location 1: The orifices of the root canals are always located at the junction of the walls and the floor; Law of orifice location 2: The orifices of the root canals are located at the vertices of the floor-wall junction).

The laws of orifice location 1 and 2 are very useful in identifying third/fourth root canal in premolars and also to negotiate second mesiobuccal root canal (MB2) in maxillary first molars.

e. Preparation of Radicular Portion

After achieving unhindered access to the canal orifices, the coronal end of the root canal is enlarged for better instrumentation during root canal treatment; a specific shape is to be developed to receive a root canal filling that is going to completely obturate the space previously occupied by the pulp.

Except for calcified teeth, most orifices accommodate the head of X-Gates, which on activation serve to open, expand and flare the orifice. The lateral cutting with X-Gates is used to intentionally relocate the coronal-most aspect of the canal away from the furcal danger (cross-sections through coronal one-third of furcated roots reveal that canals are not exactly centred within the root; generally displaced towards the furcal side concavities). The preflared orifices produce smooth flowing funnel to facilitate subsequent instrumentation. Ni-Ti orifice shapers (different sizes available) are preferred to flare the canal orifices. Many authors do not favour use of gates-glidden burs, as they believe, lead to excessive dentin damage.

PRE-ENDODONTIC BUILD-UP TECHNIQUE

One of the requisite of access cavity preparation is to provide 'field of operation' completely dry and isolated. Another important feature is to provide adequate retention for the interim restorations. Availability of sufficient tooth structure facilitates adequate isolation and also the feasibility of proper interim restoration. In case, sufficient tooth structure is not available (excessive loss of tooth structure, may be because of caries or trauma), the placement of rubber dam is difficult; so as placing the interim restorative material.

The pre-endodontic build-up of the lost tooth structure, commonly refer to as *'Donut technique'*, implies building walls of the tooth around the access cavity, enabling retention of rubber dam and facilitating endodontic procedures (Fig. 14.25). The build-up procedure is performed with an adhesive composite, which can last during the root canal treatment and provide support for temporization. Earlier authors tried several techniques, viz. placing clamp on gingiva, clamping adjacent multiple teeth, copper bands, build-up with amalgam and so on.

Procedure

- After removing the caries and the soft tissues, astringent solution is applied to achieve hemostasis and to clean the area.
- Gingival retraction cord is applied around the tooth below the gingival margin (provide hemostasis and better visualization of any subgingival tooth margins).
- Place cotton pellets or appropriate sized rubber wheel over the pre assumed access cavity.
- Around this area, flowable composite is applied initially, followed by curing composites in layers. Incremental curing provides better adaptation of composites.
- A football-shaped diamond point is used to reduce the occlusal surface and contour the restoration.

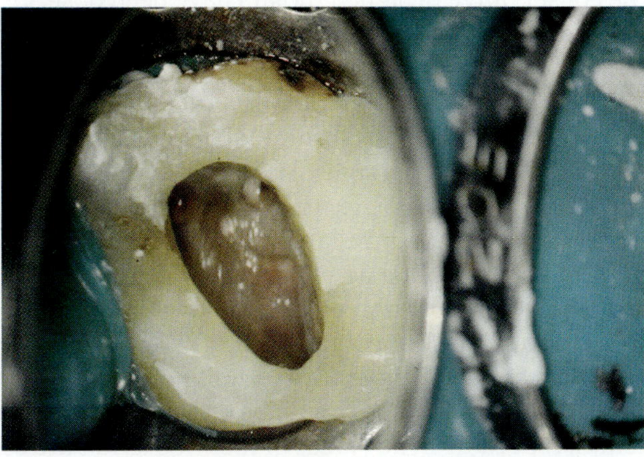

Fig. 14.25 Pre-endodontic build-up

14

- The build-up should mimic the natural anatomical structure, which can be used as guide for access cavity and further endodontic procedures.

The techniques of pre-access endodontic build-up has been modified by various authors.

After negotiating canal orifices and removing caries/ old restorations, etc. a canal projector cone is inserted into each canal. After stabilizing the cones, adhesive composite is built around the cones. Once, completely set and finished, the cones are removed to facilitate routine endodontic procedure.

A few authors have placed gutta-percha points and even 'posts' into the canal orifices, followed by building the lost walls in routine with adhesive composites. The rubber dam is sealed with Oraseal, if any leakage of saliva is suspected after build-up procedure. The technique is effective in maintaining dry field during the endodontic procedures, improving visualization and instrumentation as well.

CONSERVATIVE ACCESS CAVITY PREPARATIONS

Conservative access cavity preparation, also known as 'Minimal invasive endodontics' or even 'Micro-endodontics', implies preparing smaller access cavities and using smaller tapered files to conserve more of dentin around pulp spaces (Fig. 14.26a and b).

The rationale of conservative endodontic preparation is to preserve pericervical dentin [*Dentin 4.0 mm above and 6.0 mm below the cementoenamel junction of all teeth is pericervical dentin (PCD)*]. It is not all about making 'small' preparations, but about designing cavity in such a way so as to preserve maximum dentin and also fulfilling the treatment objectives. Pericervical dentin is considered as crucial for tooth strength and for long-lasting restorations.

It has been established that greater the amount of dentin conserved, the greater the increase in strength. The conservative designed molars have been observed to be 2.5 times stronger than traditionally designed molars.

Conservative cavity preparation involves reducing the excessive widening of pulp chamber, eliminating the convenience form and also using instruments of smaller flute diameter, especially at the coronal ends of the root canals. It disregards the traditional requirement of a straight line access and complete unroofing of the pulp chamber and emphasize the importance of preserving crucial pericervical dentin as far as possible. Since no restorative material or technique can overcome the lost dentin, the steps should be directed to conserve dentin, especially in key areas of tooth, so as to buttress the endodontically treated teeth.

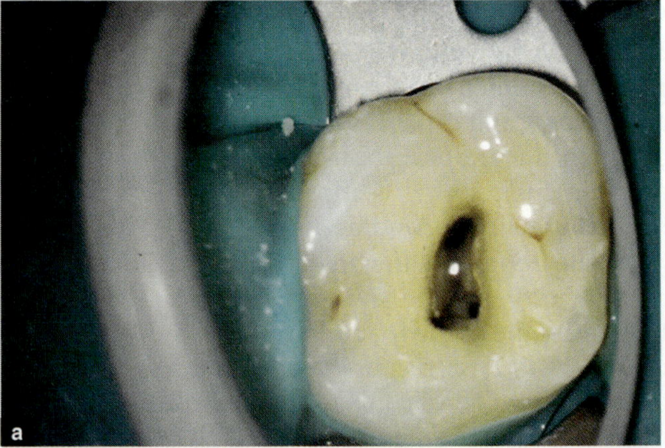

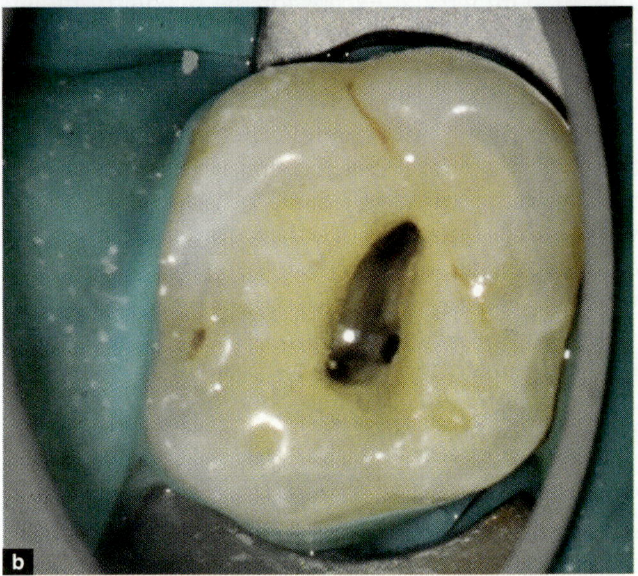

Fig. 14.26a and b Conservative access cavity

Clarke and Khademi, credited with the idea of conservative cavity preparation, encourages the use of endoguide burs (instead of round burs and gates-glidden burs) for access and orifice enlargement along with orifice openers. They prefer use of V-taper rotary Ni-Ti variable taper files (diameter less than 1.0 mm as midcanal shaft size).

Maintaining pericervical dentin is considered a key factor in reducing fractures in endodontically treated teeth. Smaller tapers are also preferred in calcified and severely curved canals. However, it is opined that the conservative preparations should not take precedence over traditional preparations, which are necessary to locate, negotiate and prepare the root canals.

Clinical Tips

The operator should have the knowledge of different variations in canal anatomy and also the possibility of extracanals to achieve successful root canal treatment.

The important clinical tips are:

- Two or more radiographs taken at 30° mesial/distal angulation must be thoroughly evaluated before initiating endodontic procedures (SLOB: same lingual, opposite buccal rule be applied to visualize location of canals).
- Sudden disappearance or narrowing of radiolucency of root canal in-between the root indicates bifurcation of root canal (fast-break phenomenon of Slowey).
- If the outline of root has unusual contour or not very clear, one should suspect extracanal.
- Proper 'reading' the radiograph may reveal lateral canals; a knob-like eversion of apex reveal curved apex towards/away from X-ray beam.
- Canal/root curvatures should be evaluated on 'angled radiographs'; palatal root of maxillary molars usually have sharp apical curvatures towards the buccal.
- Canal located in the centre of pulpal floor indicate presence of one canal only.
- When two canals join to form one canal, lingual/palatal canal has direct access to apex.
- When the first file inserted into distal canal of mandibular molar shows buccal/lingual direction; possibility of second distal canal.
- Pulp floor should be analysed with the possible magnification. Fiberoptic illumination can reveal orifices location, calcifications, fracture lines, etc.

CAVITY DESIGNS FOR INDIVIDUAL TEETH

Maxillary Anterior Teeth

Maxillary anterior teeth are mostly single rooted with 1-1 canal configuration (rarely two roots and extra-canals present).

Steps of Access Cavity Preparation (Applicable for all Anterior Teeth)

- The first step is to give a "nick" just below the cingulum in the center of the lingual surface with the help of an inverted cone bur, keeping the bur perpendicular to the tooth surface. The nick prevents slipping of the bur into the gingival sulcus (Fig. 14.27a).
- Through this 'nick', penetrate into dentin with the help of appropriate round bur, keeping it perpendicular to the tooth surface (Fig. 14.27b).
- Once dentin is reached, the bur is held parallel to the long-axis of the tooth until the pulp chamber is reached (Fig. 14.27c).
- Now using tapering fissure bur, the walls of the pulp chamber is removed from inside to outside and extended according to need. Pulp tissue remnants should not be left in the pulp chamber, which may get infected/re-infected, subsequently leading to failure of the root canal therapy (Fig. 14.28a). Such residual pulp remnants may also discolor the remaining tooth structure.
- The access is enlarged both labiolingually and mesiodistally. In the labiolingual direction, labial and lingual triangles should be removed. In the mesiodistal direction, pulp horns should be uncovered (Fig. 14.28b and c).
- Small round bur can be used to eliminate remnants of caries and attached debris, if any.
- The root of maxillary central incisor is inclined 5–10° palatally. Therefore, the bur should be angled accordingly, to be parallel to the long-axis of the tooth. This angle is known as *'access angle'*. The

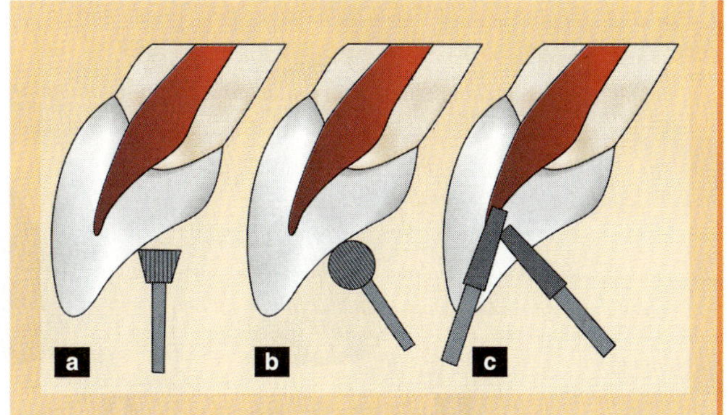

Fig. 14.27 (a) Creating nick using inverted cone bur; (b) Angulation of round bur during access cavity preparation; (c) Change in angulation of fissure bur during access cavity preparation

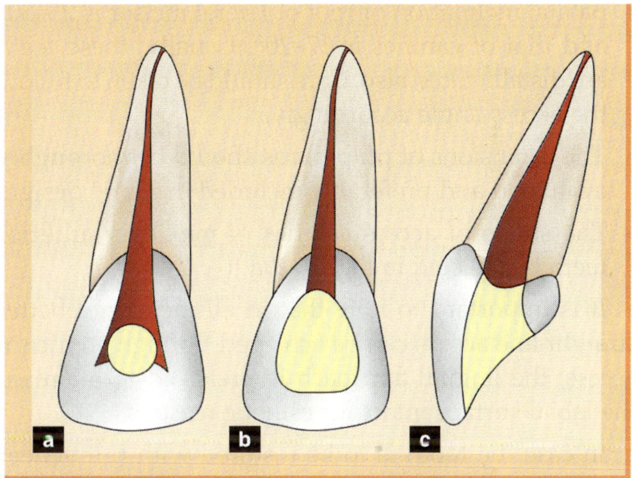

Fig. 14.28 (a) Improper access cavity (pulp remnants left in coronal half); (b) Proper access cavity (mesiodistal view); (c) Proper access cavity (labiolingual view)

14

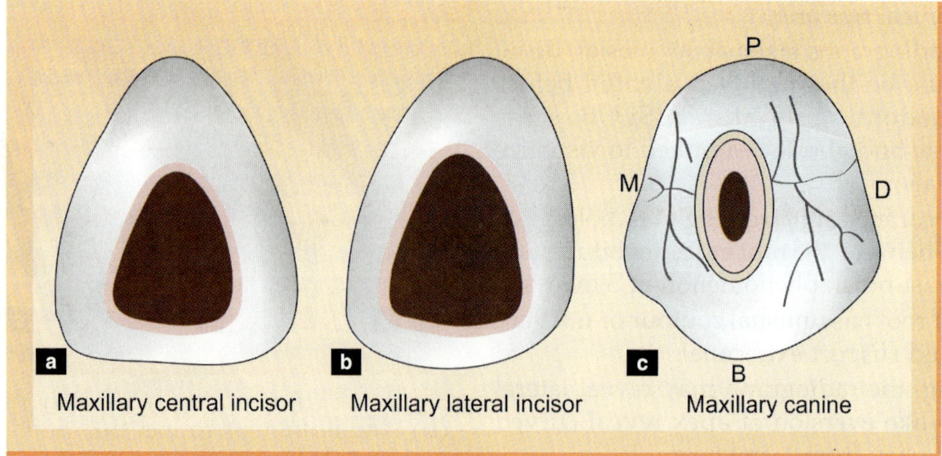

Fig. 14.29a to c Access cavities of maxillary anterior teeth

palatal inclination of root of lateral incisor is 25–30° and that of canines is 17–20°. Usually, these teeth are distally tilted also. Care should be taken to follow the access angle accordingly.

- The extensions of pulp horns should be thoroughly evaluated and preferably included in cavity design.
- The shape of access cavities of maxillary anterior teeth is depicted in Fig. 14.29a to c.

It is important to note that in all incisors, a better straight line access can be achieved through an incisal access; the lingual approach is preferred to maintain the labial surface intact for esthetic reasons.

In case the tooth is to be restored with full veneer crown, the endodontic access may be achieved through incisal surface.

Errors in Access Cavity Preparation of Maxillary Anterior Teeth

- Gouging of labial wall-caused by failure to recognize the linguoaxial inclination of tooth (most important is maxillary lateral incisors).
- Gouging of distal wall-caused by failure to recognize mesioaxial inclination of tooth.
- Pear-shaped preparation of apical area caused by failure to achieve proper convenience form.
- Discoloration of crown caused by failure to remove pulp debris. The access cavity is too far gingivally with minimum incisal extension.
- Ledge formation at apical-labial/apical-distal curve caused by failure to achieve the proper convenience form.
- Mishaps during access cavity preparations (anterior teeth) are depicted in Fig. 14.30a to c.

14

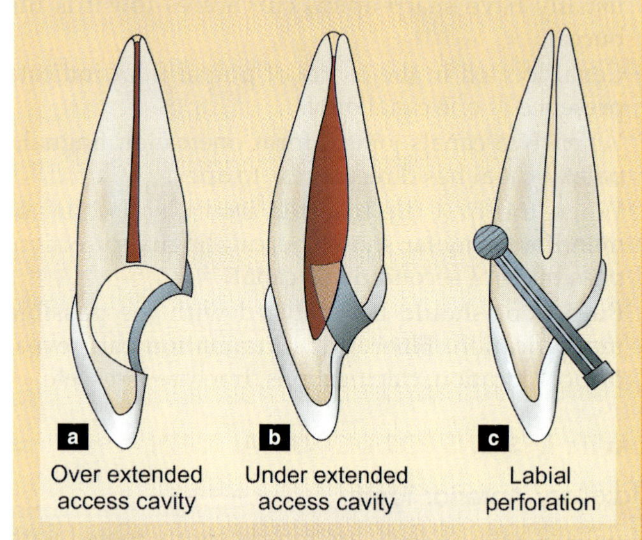

Fig. 14.30a to c Mishaps during access cavity preparation (anterior teeth)

Maxillary First Premolar

Maxillary premolars account for 15–20% of the total root canal treated teeth. The maxillary first premolar is predominantly two rooted teeth with two canals (variety of canal aberrations have been reported). The operator should be familiar with the possible variations of these teeth before initiating root canal treatment.

Steps of Access Cavity Preparation

- The access cavity is prepared using tapered fissure bur keeping parallel to the long-axis of the tooth, starting from center of the fossa and moving to buccal and palatal sides. The oval shape is achieved.
- An appropriate round bur is used to open into the pulp chamber. The tactile sense will feel 'dropping the bur' when the pulp chamber is reached. In chronic

cases and also where the pulp is calcified, such a 'drop' is not felt. (Minimum of 2.0 mm of pulp is necessary to feed the 'drop'). The bur can be penetrated deep clearing the pulp chamber. Care must be exercised not to injure the furcation area (Fig. 14.31a to c).

- After penetrating the pulp chamber, the orifices can be located using fine instruments and follow the laws of orifice location as described earlier.
- The buccal canal lies beneath the buccal cusp and the palatal canal lies beneath the palatal cusp.
- The lumen of the palatal canal is larger than that of buccal canal. The buccal canal is generally more difficult to negotiate.
- One should explore the possibility of third canal, which is usually in mesiobuccal direction.
- The shape of the access cavity is depicted in Fig. 14.32.

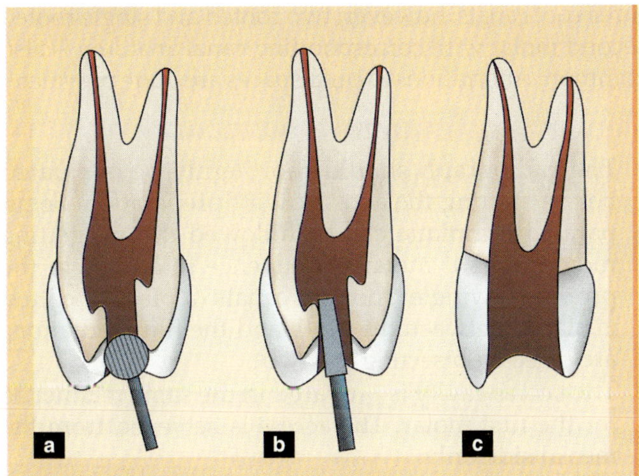

Fig. 14.31 Access cavity preparation in maxillary premolars (a) Initiation of access cavity preparation; (b) Removal of root with tapered fissure bur; (c) Completed access cavity

Maxillary Second Premolar

Maxillary premolars account for 15–20% of the total root canal treated teeth. The maxillary second premolars are predominantly one rooted teeth with 1 or 2 canals (canal aberrations are quite common). The operator should keep in mind the anatomical variations of these teeth before root canal treatment.

Steps of Access Cavity Preparation

- The access cavity preparation is same as for maxillary first premolar.
- Usually one canal is present in the center; however, if the canal is not negotiated at the center, there is possibility of a second root canal.
- The two canals, if present, are palatal and buccal.
- Very rarely third canal can also be present.
- The shape of the access cavity is depicted in Fig. 14.33.

Errors in Access Cavity Preparation of Maxillary Premolars

- Under-extended preparation (the white color of roof of chamber is a clue to shallow cavity).
- Over-extended preparation (undermining of enamel walls).
- Failure to observe the distal-axial inclination of tooth may lead to perforation (maxillary first premolar is the most susceptible tooth to be perforated).
- Failure to explore the third canal in first premolar.
- Failure to explore second canal in second premolar.

Maxillary First Molar

The maxillary first molar has three separate roots: two buccal and one palatal with one canal in each root. The palatal canal is wider than either of the buccal canals. The palatal orifice is largest and is easily accessible. It

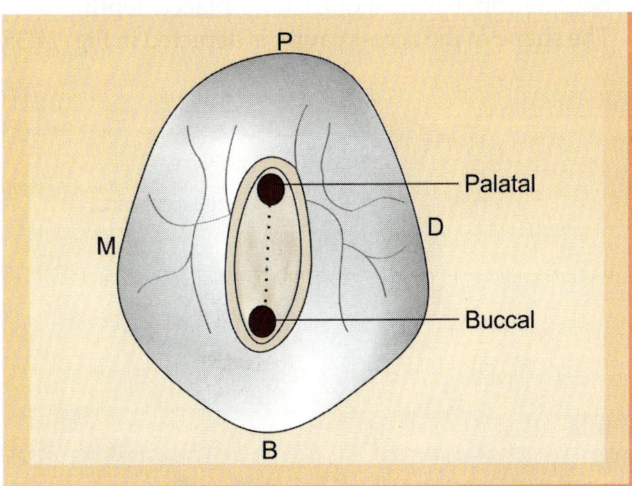

Fig. 14.32 Maxillary first premolar (diagrammatic)

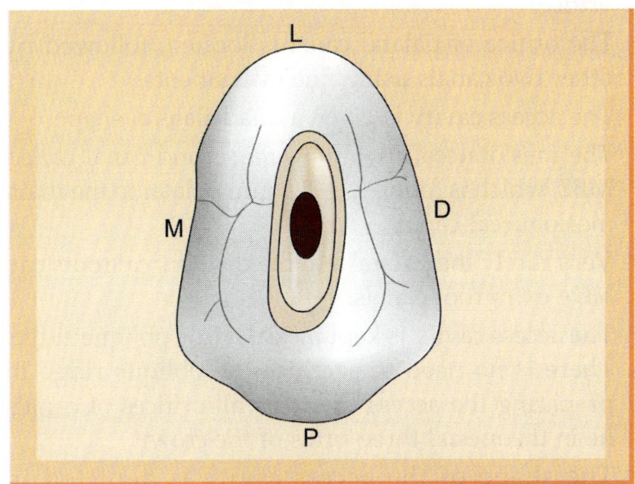

Fig. 14.33 Maxillary second premolar (diagrammatic)

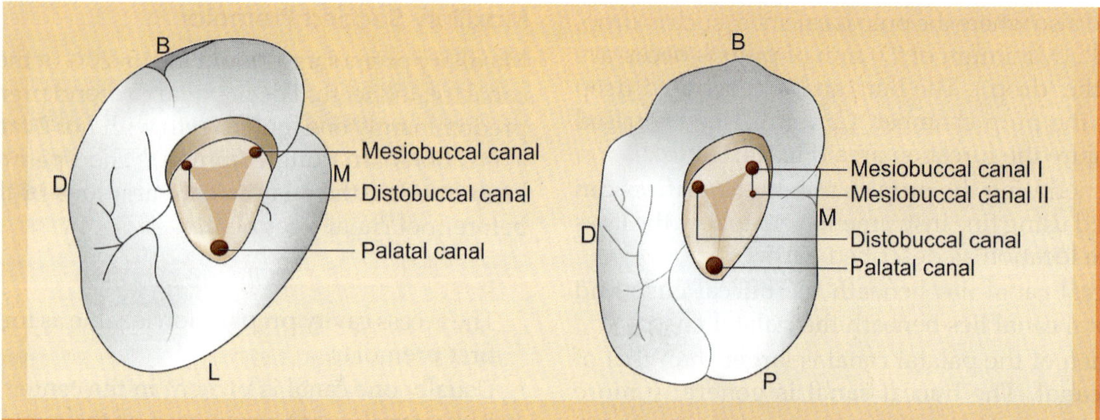

Fig. 14.34 Shape of access cavity preparation: (a) Maxillary first molar (diagrammatic: three canals); (b) Maxillary first molar (diagrammatic: four canals)

lies near the central pit, mesial to oblique ridge. Mesiobuccal orifice lies under mesiobuccal cusp and is longer buccopalatally; may have a depression at palatal end in which the orifice of a fourth canal may be present (MB2). Distobuccal orifice is located slightly distal and palatal to the mesiobuccal orifice.

Steps of Access Cavity Preparation

- Access cavity preparation should be initiated in the mesial fossa using an appropriate size of round bur followed by fissure bur.
- The fissure bur is extended towards the mesiopalatal cusp as the orifice of palatal canal is present beneath the mesiopalatal cusp.
- The orifice of mesiobuccal canal is located beneath the mesiobuccal cusp but the distobuccal canal orifice does not relate to its cusp. It is usually located by means of its relation to the mesiobuccal orifice and is found approximately 2.0 to 3.0 mm to the distal and slightly to the palatal aspect of the mesiobuccal orifice.
- The orifice of palatal canal is located, followed by other two canals using fine instruments.
- The access cavity is given a quadrilateral shape.
- The mesiobuccal root shows a second canal called MB2, which is found 1.0– 2.0 mm palatal to the main mesiobuccal canal.
- Very rarely the palatal and the distobuccal roots can have extra root canals.
- The access cavity is kept mesial to the oblique ridge. There is no need to sacrifice the oblique ridge in preparing the access cavity as all orifices of canals lie in the mesial three-fifths of the crown.
- The shape of the access cavity is depicted in Fig. 14.34a and b.

Maxillary Second Molar

The maxillary second molar is mostly three rooted with three root canals; however, two rooted and single rooted second molar with corresponding canal anatomy is also common. Aberrations in pulp spaces are quite prevalent.

Steps of Access Cavity Preparation

- The radiograph should thoroughly be evaluated before starting the access cavity preparation. Semi-parallel technique can be followed during getting radiographs if molar prominence interferes in the proper viewing of the root canals (a piece of cotton is placed between the tooth and the film; radiations are directed bisecting the two).
- The access cavity is prepared in the same manner as for the first molar. The access is achieved from the mesial side only.
- The floor of the access cavity is more dome-shaped.
- The mesiobuccal canal and root are not as long as those of the first molar.
- The mesiobuccal canal if present, pose difficulties in negotiation, because of distally placed tooth.
- The shape of the access cavity is depicted in Fig. 14.35.

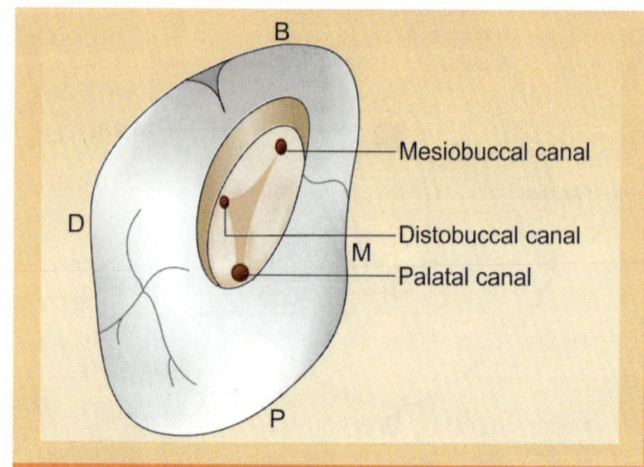

Fig. 14.35 Maxillary second molar (diagrammatic)

Maxillary Third Molar

Maxillary third molars are commonly three rooted; number of roots may range from one to five. The number of root canals also vary accordingly. Presence of MB2 in mesiobuccal root is also prevalent.

Steps of Access Cavity Preparation

- Since, the tooth is placed in the most posterior location with minimum opening space, certain guidelines should be followed, such as:
  - Use of short head handpiece
  - Use of short files; short shank drills
  - Mouth prop to facilitate mouth opening.
- Radiograph of these teeth needs extra cautions. Placement of film may lead to gag-reflex, which get worse while placing rubber dam. It can be controlled by:
  - Semi-parallel radiographic technique is preferred
  - Patient is asked to breathe through nose only; tongue is to be relaxed
  - Minimize patient apprehension by suitable drugs
  - In extreme cases, tongue and palate can be anesthetized.
- Opening and negotiation of canals is same as for maxillary second molars.
- The association of roots of maxillary third molar with maxillary sinus is to be evaluated thoroughly and managed accordingly.

Errors in Access Cavity Preparation in Maxillary Molar Teeth

- Under-extended preparation (entire roof of pulp chamber remains).
- Over-extended preparation (undermining enamel walls).
- Furcation perforation, especially using a long shank bur (failure to realize the distance from cusp tip to furcation area).
- Improper outline from exposing only the palatal canal.

Mandibular Anterior Teeth

Mandibular anterior teeth are usually single rooted with slight distobuccal curvature. One root canal is prevalent; however, two or more canals may also be present.

Wilson and Henry (1965) have cautioned that during treatment of mandibular incisors, due to anatomical inaccessibility, organic debris may remain in the lingual aspect of the canal as the instrument always passes along the labial aspect of canal.

Steps of Access Cavity Preparation

- A small 'nick' is given just above the cingulum using inverted cone bur perpendicular to the tooth surface (Fig. 14.36a). Initially, only enamel is penetrated (as in maxillary incisors).
- Through the nick, the access cavity is deepened up to dentin using round bur, keeping bur perpendicular to the tooth surface (Fig. 14.36b).
- With appropriate fissure bur, directing parallel to the tooth surface, the cavity is extended mesiodistally to include the pulp chamber. The enamel and dentin are beveled towards the incisal surface (Fig. 14.36c).
- Final access cavity shape is ovoid and funnel-shaped, which is wider labiolingually (access cavity must be wider labiolingually and inciso-gingivally to locate extracanals, if any).
- The preparation is similar for lateral incisors and canines.
- The possibility of extracanals should be explored thoroughly.
- The shape of access cavity is depicted in Fig. 14.37a to c.

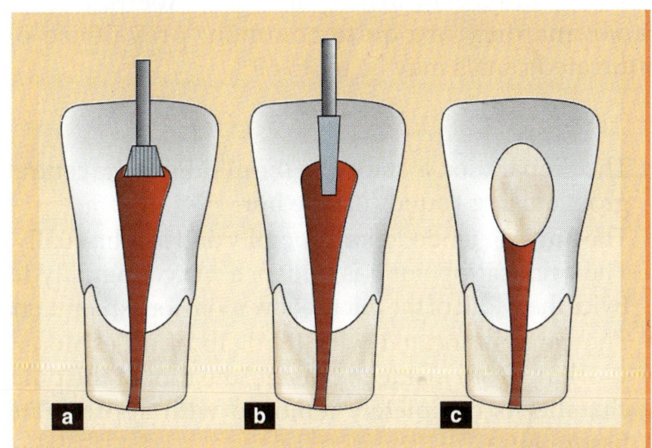

Fig. 14.36 Access cavity preparation in mandibular anterior teeth: (a) Creating a 'nick' using inverted cone bur; (b) Extending access cavity using fissure bur; (c) Completed access cavity

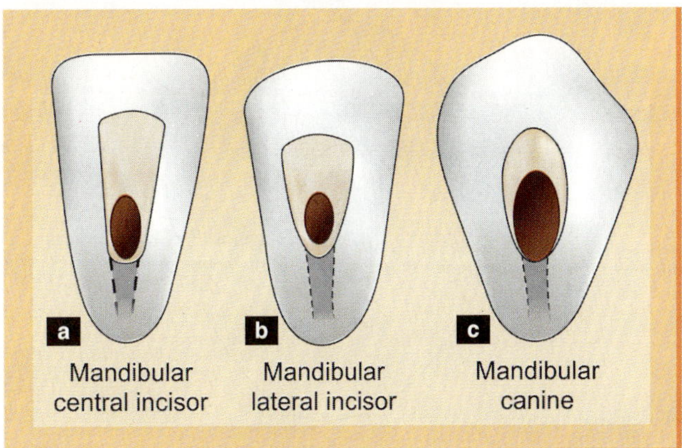

Fig. 14.37a to c Access cavities in mandibular anterior teeth (diagrammatic)

Errors in Access Cavity Preparation of Mandibular Anterior Teeth

- Gouging of labial wall-caused by failure to recognize the linguoaxial inclination of the tooth.
- Gouging of distal wall-caused by failure to recognize the mesioaxial inclination of the tooth.
- Failure to explore the extracanal (inadequate inciso-gingival extension of access cavity).
- Discoloration of crown caused by failure to remove pulp remnants (the access cavity may be too far gingivally with minimum incisal extension).
- Ledge formation caused by complete loss of control of instrument, especially if access cavity prepared through proximal surfaces.

Mandibular First Premolar

Mandibular first premolar is usually single rooted; more than one root may be present. The crown is lingually tilted and distally inclined. Aberrations in canal anatomy are quite common; prevalence of bifurcated canals may be up to 60%.

Steps of Access Cavity Preparation

- The preparation is started in the middle of the central groove using round/fissure bur.
- The bur is extended more buccally and less lingually. The occlusal opening is widened buccolingually to twice the width of the bur to allow room for exploration.
- The canal is located with the help of an explorer. Working from inside to outside, the roof of the pulp chamber is completely removed with appropriate fissure burs.
- Final preparation is ovoid and tapered towards cementoenamel junction, providing a straight line access to the canal(s) (Fig. 14.38).

Mandibular Second Premolar

Mandibular second premolars are usually single rooted; roots may be curved distobuccally. The crown is tilted slightly to lingual side (much less than first premolar) and also distally. Extraroot canals are common and should be explored thoroughly.

Steps of Access Cavity Preparation

- Access cavity is prepared in the same manner as the first premolar. (Usually has one root and one well-centered canal; but may have bifurcated canals.)
- Access is made ovoid, wider in the buccolingual dimensions (Fig. 14.39).

Errors in Access Cavity Preparation in Mandibular Premolars

- Perforation at distogingival area (failure to recognize the distal tilt of premolar)
- Incomplete preparation may lead to loss of instrument control.

Mandibular First Molar

Mandibular first molar generally is two rooted with three distinct root canals. The pulp chamber is mesially placed, so access is directed within from central pit to mesial pit. Extra root canals, especially in distal root should be explored thoroughly (40% may have two root canals; distobuccal and distolingual). A few molars may have extradistal root with separate canal.

Steps of Access Cavity Preparation

- General outline of the access cavity is trapezoidal. The buccal and lingual sides are of approximately the same configuration and taper towards each other distally.

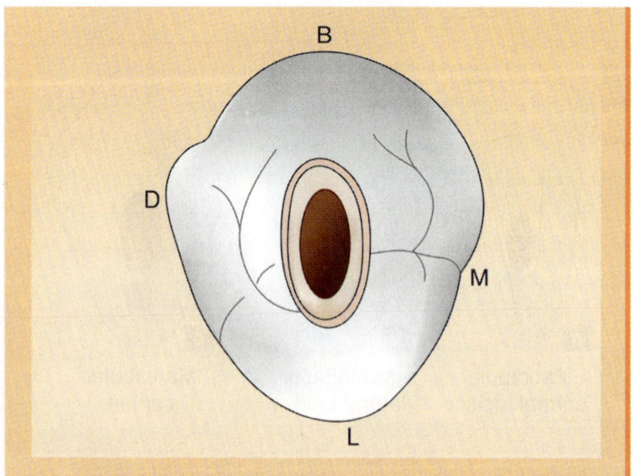

Fig. 14.38 Mandibular first premolar (diagrammatic)

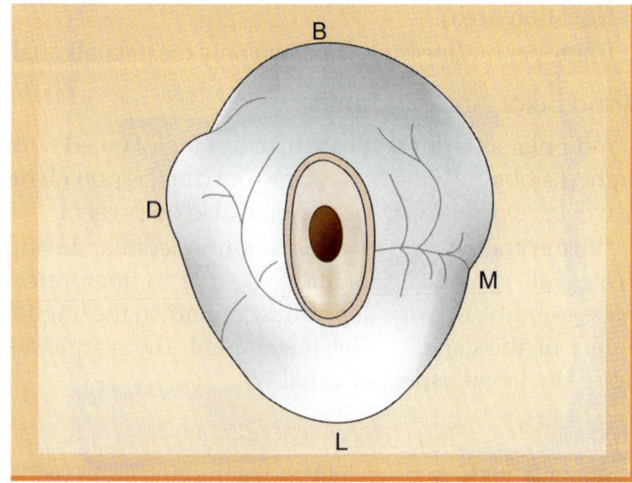

Fig. 14.39 Mandibular second premolar (diagrammatic)

- The access cavity is confined to mesial half of the crown.
- The access cavity preparation is started just mesial to the central pit. Since, the tooth is lingually and mesially inclined, the bur should mimic these angulations.
- The orifice of the distal canal lies beneath the central pit. It is generally large and slightly elliptical.
- The mesiolingual canal lies beneath the mesial pit. The mesiobuccal canal lies beneath the mesiobuccal cusp. The orifices are often connected by a groove which helps to locate both canals (5% mandibular molars have three mesial canals; middle mesial canal is usually located between mesiobuccal and mesiolingual canal).
- An appropriate bur is used to remove the roof of pulp chamber guiding the bur from inside to outside.
- A wider access cavity to locate extracanals is considered better than ignoring these canals for the sake of a 'conservative' preparation, which may lead to failure.
- The shape of the access cavity is depicted in Fig. 14.40.

Mandibular Second Molar

Mandibular second molar is similar to first molar and is more compact; mostly two rooted with three canals (two mesial and one distal). Two roots and two canals are also prevalent. The mesial canals are usually close to each other and the incidence of second canal in distal root is rare. The volume of the pulp chamber and canal entrances are smaller than in first molars.

Steps of Access Cavity Preparation

- Access cavity is prepared in the same way as in the case of a first molar.
- C-shape canal configuration is common.
- The shape of the access cavity is depicted in Fig. 14.41.

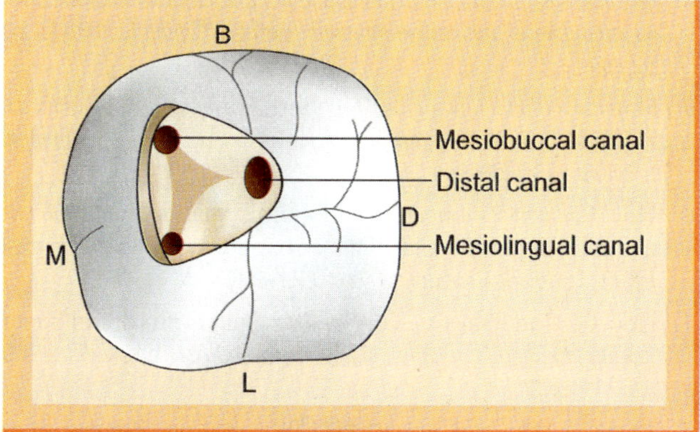

Fig. 14.40 Mandibular first molar

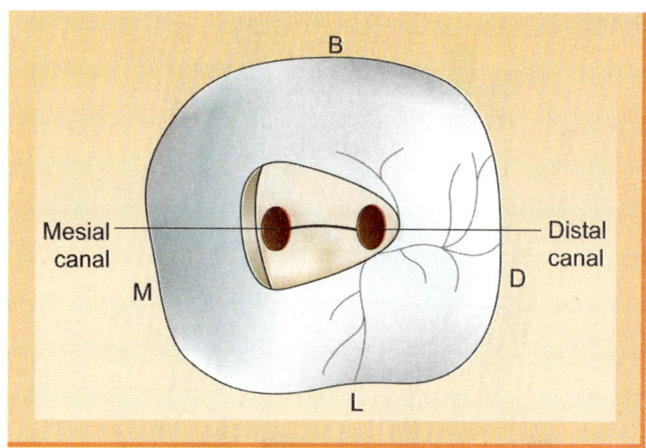

Fig. 14.41 Mandibular second molar

Mandibular Third Molar

Mandibular third molars usually have two roots and two root canals. The tooth is mostly mesially inclined, which facilitate access cavity preparation. Isolation is usually difficult in third molars.

Steps of Access Cavity Preparation

- The access cavity preparation for mandibular third molar is almost same as for mandibular first and second molars, with the variation as the anatomic structures may dictate.
- Roots lie close to mandibular canal; operator should be careful during endodontic procedures. Following features are important:
  - Avoid mechanical trauma (over-instrumentation)
  - Use of side vented needles and less concentration of irrigant solution.
  - Avoid pressure irrigation (extrusion of toxic chemicals cause damage and even delay healing).
  - Avoid using thermal techniques, such as thermoplasticized gutta-percha for obturation.
- In case the access is unmanageable, autotransplantation can be considered (third molars are considered reliable to replace missing first/second molars).

Errors in Access Cavity Preparation of Mandibular Molar Teeth

- Overextended preparation (undermining enamel walls).
- Furcation perforation by using long shank bur (failing to realize that the narrow pulp chamber had passed).
- Perforation at mesial cervical area (failure to orient bur in severely tipped molars).
- Improper outline form exposing only mesiobuccal canal.

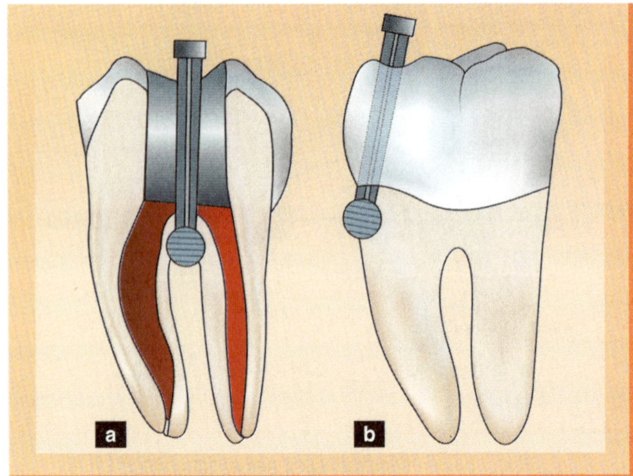

Fig. 14.42 Mishaps during access cavity preparation (mandibular molars). (a) Furcation perforation; (b) Lateral (cervical) perforation

- Mishaps during access cavity preparations (mandibular molars) are depicted in Fig. 14.42a and b.

ACCESS CAVITY PREPARATION IN DIFFICULT CASES

a. Teeth with Limited Mouth Opening

Limited mouth openings or unfavourable position of tooth in the arch result in difficulty in aligning the bur and the handpiece along the long-axis of the tooth. Location of canals and their preparation always pose problems. Use of mouth prop and pediatric handpiece can be helpful to some extent. The shank of burs can be shortened by 3.0–4.0 mm; or the cusp tips are reduced so as to improve the visibility and accessibility prior to negotiating and preparing the canals.

b. Teeth with Calcified Canals

Pulp calcifications pose a problem in locating canals. Localized deposition of tertiary dentin as a result of caries or leakage, will reduce the volume of pulp chamber. The pulp chamber floor becomes flatter with narrow canal entrances. Careful use of magnification, and tests like 'champagne bubble' test, can help the clinician to locate these canals. Long shank burs or ultrasonics should be used to remove tertiary dentin. Pulp stones and calcifications are also removed with long shank excavation and ultrasonic tips. Once canal entrance is identified, a small file (K1 size 06 or K2 size 08) should be used in slow progressive motion to negotiate the canal. Rigid C-Pilot files having cutting tips are considered ideal to negotiate sclerosed canals (these files are less likely to distort during canal negotiations). In all such cases, periodic radiographs should be taken to confirm the orientation of file in the canal.

14

c. Rotated Teeth

Rotated teeth have an altered crown-root relationship posing difficulties like difficulty in canal location and débridement. Access cavity preparation may also lead to perforation. Similar problems can occur in the case of crowded teeth; buccal access preparation is preferred in such cases.

d. Access Cavity in Restored Teeth

Preparation of access cavities through crowns or extensive restorations is very challenging because of the altered shape of the clinical crown (crowns usually mask the orientation of tooth). If the canals are not identified by cutting through the crown, it is necessary to remove the crown to avoid further damage. Removing crown will reduce the likelihood of removing sound dentin unnecessary and also minimizes chances of perforation.

BIBLIOGRAPHY

1. Ahmed HM. Management of third molar teeth from an endodontic perspective. Eur. J. Gen. Dent.: 2012; 1:48–60.
2. Beaudry RJ. Prevention of rubber dam hypersensitivity. J. Endod.: 1984; 10:544–545.
3. Buhrley IJ, Barrows MJ, BeGole EA and Wenckus CS. Effect of magnification on locating the MB-2 canal in maxillary molars. J. Endod.: 2002; 28:324–327.
4. Calberson, FI., De Moor, RJ and Deroose, CA: The radix entomolaris and paramolaris: clinical approach in endodontics. J. Endod : 2007; 33, 58–63.
5. Carrotte P. Endodontics: Part 6 Rubber dam and access cavities. Br. Dent. J.: 2004; 197:527–534.
6. Clark D and Khademi J. Modern molar endodontic and directed dentin conservation. Dent. Clin. N. Am.: 2010; 54:249–273.
7. Dias de Andrade E, Ranali J, Volpato MC, Motta Maia de Oliveira M. Allergic reaction after rubber dam placement. J. Endod.: 2000; 26:182–183.
8. Greene RR, Sikora FA and House JR. Rubber dam application to crownless and cone-shaped teeth. J. Endod.: 1984; 10: 82–84.
9. Hauman CH, Chandler NP and Tong DC. Endodontic implications of the maxillary sinus: A review. Int. Endod. J.:2002; 35:127–141.
10. Hilu RE and Zmener O. Endodontic management of two mandibular third molar with c-shaped root canals: A case report. Endod. Pract.: 2007; 10:21–24.
11. Hou GL and Tsai CC. Fusion of maxillary third and supernumerary fourth molars: Case report. Aust. Dent. J.: 1989; 34:219–222.
12. Jafarzadeh H and Abbott PV. Dilaceration: Review of an endodontic challenge. J. Endod.: 2007; 33:1025–1030.

13. Kilic C, Kamburoglu K, Yuksel SP and Ozen T. An assessment of the relationship between the maxillary sinus floor and the maxillary posterior teeth root tips using dental cone-beam computerized tomography. Eur. J. Dent.: 2010; 4:462–467.
14. Krasner P and Rankow HJ. Anatomy of the pulp chamber floor. J. Endod.: 2004; 30:5–16.
15. Moreinis SA. Avoiding perforation during endodontic access. J. Am. Dent. Assoc.:1979; 98:707–712.
16. Patel S and Rhodes S. A practical guide to endodontic access cavity preparation in molar teeth. Br. Dent. J.: 2007; 203: 133–140.
17. Patterson CJ. Polydam-polythene sheet, a practical alternative to rubber dam for patients allergic to rubber compounds. Int. Endod. J.: 1989; 22:252–253.
18. Rankow HJ and Krasner P. The access box: An Ah-Ha phenomenon. J. Endod.: 1995; 21:212–214.
19. Riccuci D. Apical limit of root canal instrumentation and obturation, part 1: literature review. Int. Endod. J.: 1998; 31:384–393.
20. Ricucci D, Siqueira JF. Fate of the tissue in lateral canals and apical ramifications in response to pathologic conditions and treatment procedures. J. Endod.: 2010; 36:1–15.
21. Schilder H. Cleaning and shaping the root canal. Dent. Clin. North Am.: 1974; 18:269–296.
22. Turell IL and Zmener O. Endodontic therapy in a fused mandibular molar. J. Endod.: 1999; 25:208–209.
23. Weine FS and Buchanan LS. Controversies in clinical endodontics: Part I- the significance and filling of lateral canals. Compend. Contin. Educ. Dent.:1996; 17:1028–1032.
24. Weine FS. The enigma of the lateral canal. Dent. Clin. North Am.:1984; 28:833–852.
25. Weller RN and Hartwell G. The impact of improved access and searching techniques on detection of the mesiolingual canal in maxillary molars. J. Endod.: 1989; 15:82–83.
26. Yoshioka T, Kobayshi C and Suda H. Detection rate of root canal entrances with a microscope. J. Endod.: 2002; 28:452–453.
27. Zeylabi A, Shirani F, Heidari F and Farhad AR. Endodontic management of a fused mandibular third molar and distomolar: A case report. Aust. Endod. J.: 2010; 36:29–31.

Chapter 15

Working Length and Working Width

The root canal preparation is carried out with the aim to preserve the biological integrity of the periapical tissues so as to provide conducive environment for healing. The nature has provided an apical constriction area inside the root canal, which acts as a natural barrier. It is imperative that the operator should restrict intra-canal treatment procedures to the apical constriction or cementodentinal junction. Instrumentation beyond this junction can cause inflammation in the periapical tissues, subsequently failure of the treatment. The length of the canal from the coronal access to the apical constriction is the 'working length'.

Before proceeding to know the modalities of working length measurement, it is mandatory to understand the anatomy of root apex.

ANATOMY OF THE ROOT APEX

The root apex visualizes the junction where dentin ends and the cementum/periodontal tissue begins (Fig. 15.1).

The cementum portion is usually in the form of an inverted cone with its shortest or narrowest diameter near the cementodentinal junction and base at the apical foramen. The configuration of cementodentinal junction may vary in different teeth. Cementum may be at edge to edge with dentin at the apex or may extend for a considerable distance into the root canal, lining the dentin. Such an extension of cementum onto dentin is usually unorganized and irregular. This is more prevalent in periodontally involved teeth.

The apical pulp tissue differs structurally from the coronal pulp tissue. The coronal pulp tissue consists mainly of cellular connective tissue and fewer collagen fibers; whereas, the apical pulp tissue is more fibrous and contains fewer cells.

The fibrous tissue of the apical pulp is identical to that of the periodontal ligament. This fibrous tissue acts as a barrier against the apical progression of pulp inflammation.

It is established that the tissue beyond the cementodentinal junction is not pulpal. The apical constriction is the junction where the pulpal tissue terminates and the periodontal tissue begins.

The distance from the radiographic apex to the apical constriction generally varies considerably from root to root. Histologically, cementodentinal junction being highly irregular, did not coincide with the apical constriction. It may be up to 3.0 mm higher on one wall than the opposite wall. Thus, it is difficult to accept any distances from the radiographic apex as an accurate indicator for the termination of the endodontic instrumentation and obturation.

Very rarely the root canal ends at the radiographic apex, it frequently ends at a distance short of the apex.

The apical foramen does not always lie at the exact apex of the tooth. Usually, it exits laterally short of the radiographic apex.

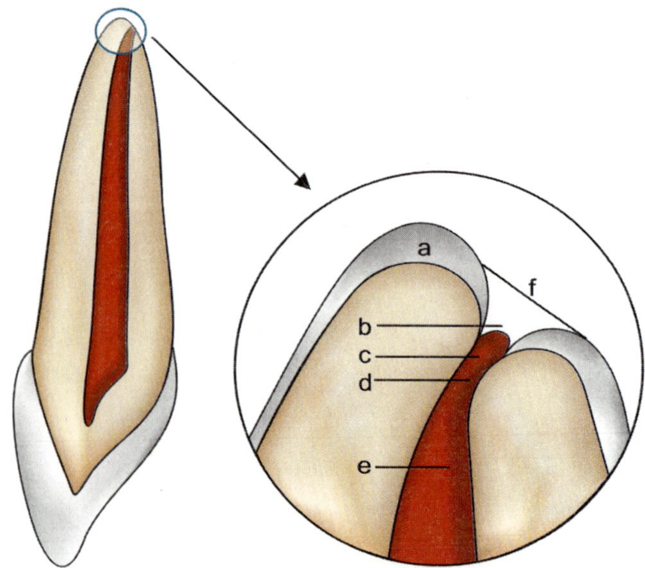

Fig. 15.1 Root end anatomy diagrammatic: (a) Cementum, (b) apical formation, (c) cementodentinal junction, (d) minor constriction, (e) root canal, (f) major opening

The root canals usually deviate from the long-axis of their roots and the openings may be 0.2 to 3.8 mm short of apex. When the foramen ends on the buccal or the lingual aspect, it is not possible to recognize it radiographically.

In such situations, the apex locators can be of great help in accurately locating the apex as an adjunct to conventional radiography. This is because they actually locate the apical constriction or the vital periodontal ligament tissue.

It is demonstrated that the apical foramen deviates from the tip in at least 2/3 rd of the teeth. Furthermore, the deviation occurs towards the buccal or lingual aspects twice as often as it does towards the mesial or distal aspect.

The following features govern the configuration of the foramen:

- As age increases, the center of the foramen deviates more and more from the vertex of apical center because of increase in thickness of the apical cementum.
- The diameter of the foramen increases with age because of apposition of new layers of cementum. The average diameter is somewhat larger buccolingually than mesiodistally.
- The minor diameter of the root canal is found usually in the dentin just before the canal penetrates the cementum. From this point onwards, the canal gradually increases in size to form a funnel shape. This funnel shape is accentuated in the older teeth because of widening of the foramen and narrowing of the canal.
- The average thickness of the apical cementum is 0.5 mm in the younger age group and 0.67 mm in the older age group.
- Since the diameter of the foramen is uneven and because of its shape, this portion cannot be sealed hermetically unless it is overfilled with cement.

The components of root apex

- Apical center
- Center of the foramen
- Distance between vertex and apical foramen
- Diameter of the foramen (major diameter of the canal)
- Diameter of the foramen perpendicular to the axis of the canal
- Diameter of the canal at cementodentinal junction (minor diameter of the canal).

Apical termination of Root Canal Preparation and Obturation

The exact point/area up to which level the root canal is prepared and subsequently filled, remains debatable. Various authors are of different opinion; however, following four views are discussed.

a. Short of the radiographic apex
b. At the radiographic apex
c. Beyond the radiographic apex
d. At the cementodentinal junction

a. Short of the Radiographic Apex

This working length can be calculated by generally identifying the radiographic apex and then subtracting a specific measurement from this length. Earlier, the specific measurement was considered to be 0.5 mm; but later, 1.0 mm was considered adequate, since cementodentinal junction was usually more than 0.5 mm from the root apex.

Disadvantages

- When the canal exits more than 1.0 mm short of the radiographic apex, this length could result in tear-drop apical preparations and, subsequently lead to overfilling.
- If the working length is kept 1.0 mm short of the apex, a large number of lateral and accessory canals may remain unsealed.

b. At the Radiographic Apex

It is believed that it might be difficult to determine the location of the cementodentinal junction clinically and that the radiographic apex is the only reproducible site in this area. It is also demonstrated that calculating working length to the radiographic apex and using larger files a bit shorter in the body of the canal; the preparation achieved is ideal.

Disadvantages

- The position of radiographic apex may not be exactly reproducible because of:
  - Angulation of the tooth
  - Position of the film
  - Holding agent for the film
  - Length of the X-ray cone and the technique used
  - Anatomic structures adjacent to the tooth.
- When the canals exit short of the radiographic apex, filling to this point could result in 'tear-drop' shape preparations, which are very difficult to seal.
- A root canal filling that generally extends to the apex radiographically is extruding in actuality. This causes impingement onto the vital tissues.

- Complete regeneration of cementum and bone does not usually occur around teeth with overfilled root canals.
- The epithelium may grow around the filling material. The possibility of radicular cyst formation is enhanced. Even if repair occurs, a fibrous encapsulation usually remains around the excess filling material.

c. Beyond the Radiographic Apex

A few operators prefer to fill the canal beyond the radiographic apex. They are of the view that the puff or button formed at the apex is designed to compensate for the shrinkage of the gutta-percha and hence pulls the filling closely down the apex. However, these reasonings are not authentic.

Overfilled canals may lead to more incidence of discomfort.

The inflammatory response persists regardless of the type of filling material. No foreign material implanted in living tissue is inert. If the material is toxic, the surrounding tissue gets necrotic. If the material is nontoxic, three types of responses can occur:

i. If the material is dissolved, the area is replaced by surrounding tissue.
ii. If the material is biologically inactive, a fibrous encapsulation of varying thickness forms.
iii. If the material is biologically active, an interfacial bond forms.

Many clinical studies have shown that with this technique, clinical success is poor and chances of failure are increased.

d. At the Cementodentinal Junction

It has been established that narrowest diameter of the canal was not at its site of exit, but in the dentin just before the cementum. This site is referred as the 'minor diameter', also known as 'apical constriction'. Beyond that the canal widens as it joins the periapical areas. This is known as 'major diameter'. The major diameter is almost twice as that of the minor diameter. The distance between the two is approximately 0.5 mm for 18–25 years of age group and 0.65 mm for 55 years of age group. The apical terminus is preferred at the apical constriction.

From a biological standpoint, the apical constriction has the minimum blood supply. As the canal widens, it develops broad blood supply. Extending the filling material beyond the apical constriction would induce an inflammatory reaction.

15

Advantages

- Prevents impingement of periapical tissues (minimum postoperative discomfort).
- Minor errors (0.5–1.0 mm) on either side, i.e. long or short will not be much harmful.
- Allows the development of an apical dentinal matrix against which filling material can be easily condensed. It helps to retain the filling material within the canal.
- Prevents obturating material and the sealer from escaping through the foramen.
- Anatomically and histologically, the constriction area is ideal.

Disadvantages

- Difficult to recognize the constriction area
- Time consuming
- May need costly gadgets.

In case of periapical radiolucencies, the preparation may need to be terminated all the more coronally. If a definite periapical radiolucency is seen with an indication of root resorption, then reduce working length by further 0.5 mm. If root resorption is extensive, then working length may need to be reduced by even 2.0 mm.

It is established that the most clinically relevant working landmark is the apical constriction, regardless of whether it is in dentin or cementum. The constriction is the narrowest point of the canal and therefore minimum of blood supply. The cleaning and shaping up to the apical constriction completely eliminates pathogenic canal contents and provides conducive environment for healing.

ASSESSING APICAL CONSTRICTION AREA

Various methods and techniques are being employed to exactly assess the apical constriction area. The routinely used methods are:

1. Tactile Method

This method utilizes tactile sense of the operator, i.e. ability of the fingers to perceive the presence of an apical constriction. After access cavity preparation and establishing patency of the canals, an appropriate file is introduced into the canal slowly. The area where the operator feels resistance is considered as the apical constriction.

The tactile method can be confirmed or reinforced with paper point evaluation. After drying the canal, a paper point of appropriate size is inserted into the root canal. It is kept in the root canal for ten seconds and withdrawn. If the tip of paper point is wet or covered with blood, it indicates over extension of the working length. The point of touch of blood is often taken as the working length.

Advantages

- No need for expensive gadgets
- Easy manipulation.

Disadvantages

- Any obstruction in the canal can be perceived as apical constriction
- Gloves may reduce tactile perception
- Not suitable for open apices and narrow canals
- Bifurcated canals also pose difficulties.

2. Radiographic Method

The radiographic method is the most commonly used method for determining the working length.

Advantages

- Easy manipulation
- Comparatively cheap.

Disadvantages

- Exposing patient to radiation
- Superimposition of anatomic structure (common in bisecting technique)
- Three-dimensional objects are projected onto a two dimensional radiograph
- Time consuming.

Various authors have described different methods of calculating tooth length using radiographs.

a. ***Coolidge and Kesel method:*** In this method, a suitable diagnostic wire was inserted into the canal as accurately as possible and a radiograph taken. After the radiograph, the wire was removed and preserved. An estimate of the tooth length can be obtained by the following formula:

$$\frac{\text{length of wire image}}{\text{length of tooth image}} = \frac{\text{length of wire in actual}}{\text{length of tooth in actual}}$$

Earlier, best fixed 10 mm wire on the labial surface and took radiograph to measure tooth length. The method was discarded soon, as angulation and other radiographic features gave incorrect results.

b. ***Grossman method:*** Grossman utilizes comparatively easy method with reasonable accuracy. The steps followed are:

- The length of the tooth is measured from the reference point to the apex of the tooth on the radiograph.
- Establish the length on the diagnostic instrument, i.e. K-file with a silicon stop. The instrument is placed in the root canal and a radiograph is taken.
- The canal length is the length/distance from the apical exit of the canal to the reference point on the tooth crown. The working length should be established 0.5–1.0 mm shorter than the measured canal length (because the actual length of the tooth is 1.2 mm less than the radiographic image and the apical foramen is approximately 0.3 mm short of the actual root tip).

In case the K-file is 1.0 mm shorter or longer than the actual working length, the necessary adjustments are made. If the difference is more than 1.0 mm, radiograph is repeated with the adjusted length.

c. ***Ingle's method:*** Ingle's method is the most accepted, easy to understand and accurate radiographic method.

The steps followed are:

- Measure the tooth length on the preoperative radiograph (Fig. 15.2a).
- Select an instrument with stop at that length (small size files are preferred).
- Place the instrument in the canal until the stop is at the plane of reference point (incisal edge of anterior teeth and cusp tips of posterior teeth are preferred).
- Insert the selected file into the root canal with proper length stopper. Get another radiograph (Fig. 15.2b).
- Three possibilities can be evident. One, the tip of the instrument is up to the apical end of the root. Second, the instrument goes beyond the apical end (Fig. 15.2c) and third, the instrument is falling short of the apical end. In case of first possibility, the length remains the same; in case of second possibility, the length of the instrument extending beyond the apical end is to be subtracted from the premeasured length. In case of third possibility, the length of the instrument falling short is to be added to that length.

The length so achieved is the length of the tooth. Another 1.0–1.5 mm is to be subtracted to achieve the working length (Fig. 15.2d).

In curved canals, as preparation proceeds, the curvature gets straighten out and approximately 1.0 mm of the length may be lost further. Therefore, the length should be reaffirmed in cases with curved canals.

When two canals superimpose in one radiograph, two individual radiographs may be taken.

d. ***Radiovisiography (RVG):*** RVG system consists of four main components: An X-ray generator with special timer, an intraoral sensor, a display processing unit and a printer.

The X-ray generator is of the conventional type; however, a special electronic timer provides accurately controlled and short exposure times, as required.

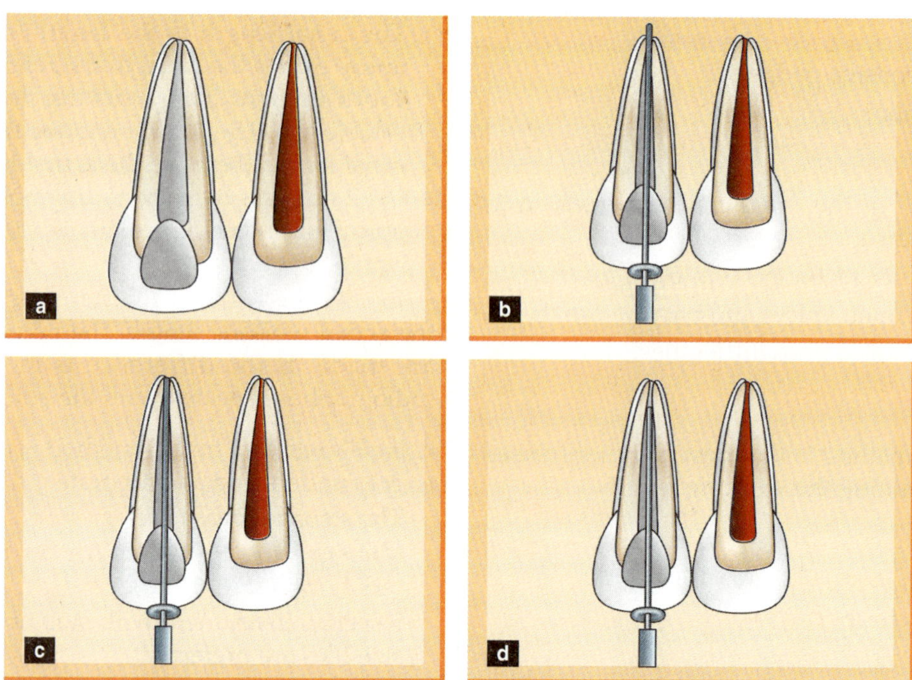

Fig. 15.2 **Ingle's method:** (a) Measuring tooth length on preoperative radiograph; (b) File at predetermined length; (c) File extending beyond the apical end; (d) File short of apical end

The intraoral sensor is the primary image receptor. The intensifying screen fluoresces when X-rays fall upon it and the light is then conducted by the optical fibers to a charge-couple device (CCD). The CCD detects the pattern of light and translates it into an electrical signal, which is received by the display processing unit.

The display processing unit consists of the electronic equipment, which digitizes, processes and stores the analog signal from the CCD.

The display unit carries a number of controls, which allow manipulation of the image. The brightness and the contrast controls permit adjustment of the images as with any TV set. The image can then be changed in two ways:

- Reversal of gray scale
- Image enhancement by increasing the contrast and decreasing the latitude.

The original image remains stored and can be returned to the screen at any time or can be printed out using a thermal paper. A zoom feature can be used to produce an enlarged image.

The minimal inherent distortion of the RVG image is a clear advantage over conventional radiography.

e. ***Digital image processing***: The development of this type of image analysis enables radiographs to be digitized and manipulated electronically. A high quality video camera, an analog to digital converter and a computer form the basis of the hardware needed for this type of image. Radiographs are taken using conventional techniques. They are then digitized and the images are converted to 256 gray scales. Traditionally, additional radiographs, taken over time, are digitized and a gray level value of 32 is added to the subsequent image to give the subtraction image a gray value in the middle of the dynamic range. As the subtraction image can be manipulated electronically, it is possible to remove bony trabeculae and enhance the remaining image, typically the tooth. This enables the clinician to visualize the tooth anatomy that would be difficult to capture by conventional radiographic means. Subsequently, diagnostic and working films can be manipulated by this system and then stored electronically.

3. Electronic Method

The electronic devices provide quite accurate information and also diminish the radiation exposure to the patient. These devices are useful for the pregnant, the handicapped and such patients where placement of radiographs is extremely difficult.

Generally all electronic apex locators are identical in function; however, they vary in their mode of action.

TYPES OF APEX LOCATORS

Various types of apex locators are available depending upon their principle of action. For convenience they are classified as 'generations' (first generation, second generation and so on).

a. First generation (resistance type, e.g. Dentometer, Sono explorer Mark I, Endo Radar)
b. Second generation (impedance type, e.g. Sono explorer Mark II and III, Endocator, Formatron IV, Digipex, Exact-A-Pex)
c. Third generation (frequency type, e.g. Root ZX, Endex, Formatron D10, NovApex)
d. Fourth generation (modified frequency type, e.g. Raypex 4, ProPex, ipex)
e. Fifth generation (blue tooth technology, e.g. Apex NRG-Blue, Medic-NRG, ProPex 2, Raypexe 5)
f. Sixth generation (adaptive type, e.g. DenApex).

a. First Generation (Resistance Type)

The basic principle of these apex locators is: '*The resistance between the periodontal membrane and the oral mucosa is a constant value*'. [The resistance between periodontium and oral mucous membrane in humans was constant at 6.5 kilo-ohms (current 40 mA). It measures opposition to the flow of direct current or resistance.]

Advantages

The advantages of these apex locators are:

- Perforations, either as a result of instrumentation or iatrogenic can be detected with these units.
- Can operate with RC Prep.
- Provides audible indication.

Disadvantages

The disadvantages of these apex locators are:

- The root canal should be reasonably dry (excessive moisture or vital pulp tissues must be removed before accurate readings can be obtained). In case of even minor amount of fluid in the canal, the device may indicate that the apex has been reached. However, the units can operate in the presence of RC Prep because it has a carbo-wax base that provides sufficient electrical insulation for obtaining correct readings.
- The file contacting a metal restoration and the presence of defective restoration may also pose problems. (The problem of the file touching a metal restoration has been solved by the use of insulating sleeves, which can be placed on the file to prevent short circuits. The defective restoration should be removed prior to the use of these gadgets.)
- Most of the units provide a digital measurement of the distance from the endpoint of the current position of the file tip in millimeters. (In case the file do not touch periodontal tissue apically as in a tooth with an open apex, it is not possible to detect endpoint. A similar situation can occur in a tooth with a large periapical lesion.)
- These devices generate a current flow, which can be detected by patients as a tingling sensation even under profound local anesthesia. This reaction seems to be patient dependent and does not affect the accuracy of the unit. Because of the current flow, the use of these devices is contraindicated in patients with cardiac pacemakers.

Many resistance type apex locators are available with a built-in pulp tester. Some of the units are required to be switched and calibrated for use with the pulp testing probe, which is connected to the unit in place of the apex locator leads. Other units are calibrated automatically with the connection of the pulp testing probe.

b. Second Generation (Impedance Type)

These units operate on the principle that '*there is electric impedance across the walls of the root canal due to presence of transparent dentin*'. It measures opposite to the flow of alternating current or impedance. It is assumed that the tooth is a long, hollow tube closed over at the end (apex). The tooth also exhibits increase in electrical impedance across the walls of the root canal, which is greater apically than coronally. This phenomenon is caused by the presence of transparent dentin that begins to form at approximately 17 years of age and continues throughout life. At the dentinocementum junction, there is a constriction in the canal as well as an abrupt increase in the impedance across the root canal wall, which the apex locator can detect. The unit indicates this constriction as the end position of the root canal on an analog meter dial.

Impedance type apex locators do overcome some of the disadvantages of the resistance-based units (Fig. 15.3).

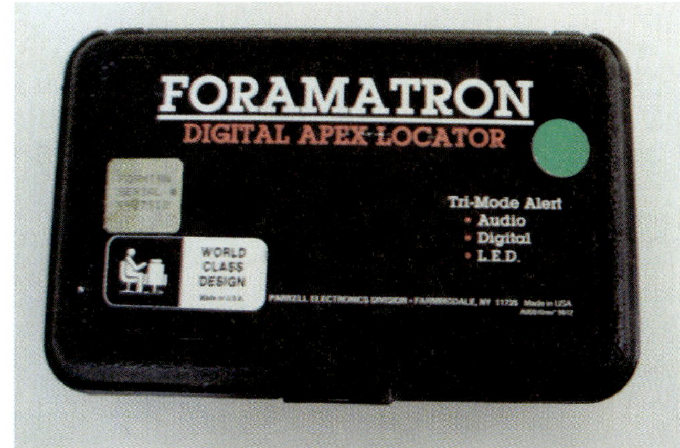

Fig. 15.3 Foramatron (impedance type apex locator)

The use of insulated canal probe eliminates the need of having a reasonably dry canal. Although this system enables the machine to operate in a fluid environment, the additional thickness that the insulation adds to the probe diameter can restrict the passage of the probe to the apex. Apart from locating the apical constriction, this type of device is able to detect bifurcated canals, lateral canals and perforations. The ability of the unit to function in young teeth without transparent dentin and in teeth with open apices, is however variable.

c. Third Generation (Frequency Type)

The frequency type apex locator operates on the principle that '*there is a maximum difference of impedance between electrodes depending on the frequencies used (measures the impedance of tooth at two different frequencies)*'.

The unit uses a lip clip and is calibrated by insertion of a file into the coronal position of the canal (Fig. 15.4). At the coronal portion, the impedance difference between the two frequencies is almost constant. As the file is advanced apically, the difference between the impedance values begins to differ greatly and is maximally different at the apical constriction.

The unit can operate in an electroconductive environment using K-files, which is a major advantage over all other types of apex locators. Secondly, the unit can operate in the presence of pus and pulpal tissues. As this type of unit uses conventional files, the problems of coated probes in the impedance type of device are overcome. Accurate calibration of the unit is important, and the file must touch the coronal portion of the canal when this step is being performed. Failure to ensure these steps results in measurement errors.

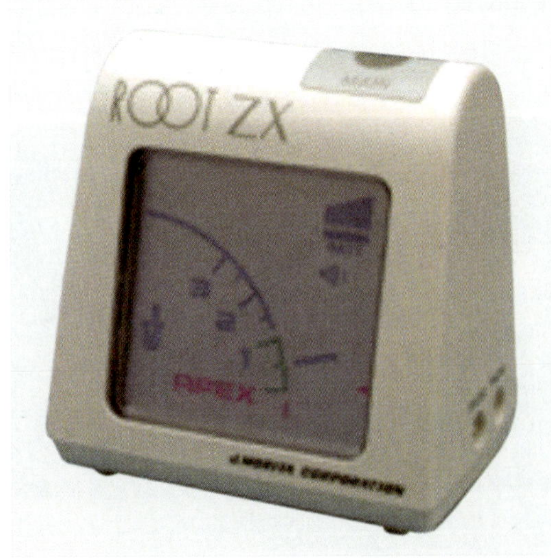

Fig. 15.4 Root ZX (frequency type apex locator)

The file should fit the size of the canal snugly. If a canal is being retreated then it is important to remove all the existing gutta-percha as it has insulating properties that may cause inaccurate readings.

Technique

The technique for using a frequency based apex locator is as follows:

- Turn on the device and attach the lip-clip near the arch being treated. Place a size 15 file into the reamer/file holder. A 25 mm long plastic file is used so that enough metal should protrude through the tooth to attach the file clip. Insert the tip of the file approximately 0.5 mm into the tooth being treated. Adjust the control knob until the reference needle is centered on the meter scale and produces audible beeps. Set the holder aside until needed to record the measurement.
- Access cavity is prepared and the canals are thoroughly irrigated. Irrigate the canal and remove any pulp tissue and debris.
- The length can be estimated provisionally from the preoperative radiographs. The canals should be slightly wet with irrigant. Hydrogen peroxide can be used instead of sodium hypochlorite, as it is a non-ionic liquid. If bleeding from a vital pulp extirpation is excessive, dry with paper points until it recedes.
- Insert the file slowly into the canal until the reference needle moves from the extreme left to the center of the scale and the alarm beep sounds.
- A radiograph with the file placed at the length indicated by the apex locator can be taken to reassure the findings. If the suggested length is considerably shorter or longer, it is possible that the preoperative films and/or the apex locator would be inaccurate. The process is repeated till accuracy is achieved.

d. Fourth Generation (Modified Frequency Type)

The fourth generation devices measure and compare the complex electrical characteristic feature of the root canal through two or more frequencies of electrical impulses (Fig. 15.5).

The *disadvantage* of these devices is that they need to perform in relatively dry or in partially dried canals. In the presence of exudates or blood this method becomes inapplicable.

e. Fifth Generation (Bluetooth Technology)

To overcome disadvantages of fourth generation apex locators, a measuring method based on comparison of the data taken from the electrical characteristics of the canal and additional mathematical processing, was developed. Apex locators of this type are fifth generation

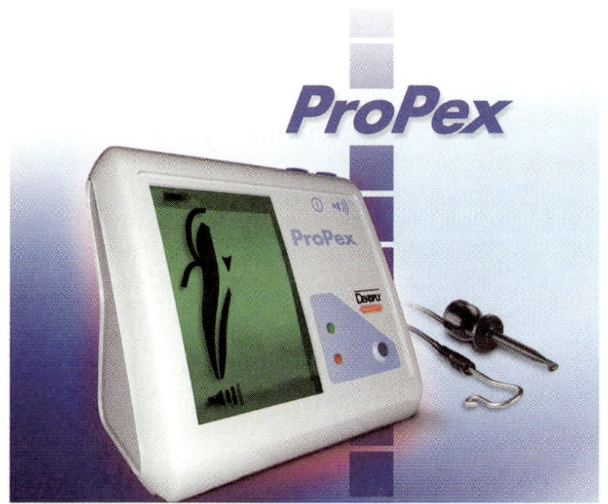

Fig. 15.5 ProPex (modified frequency type apex locator)

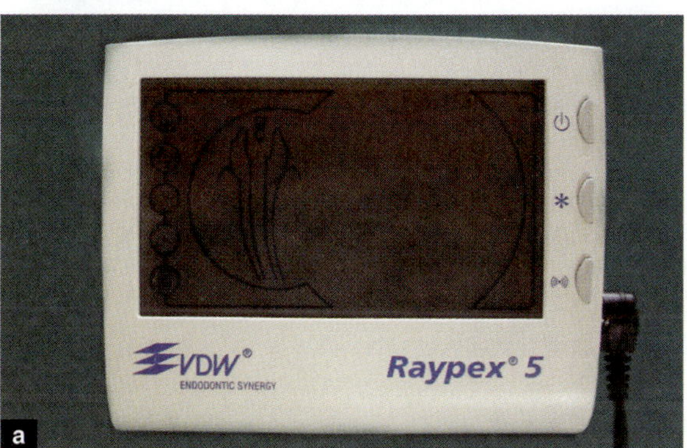

a

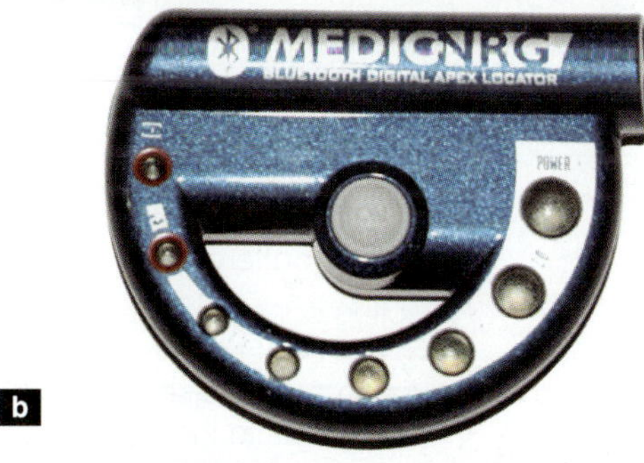

b

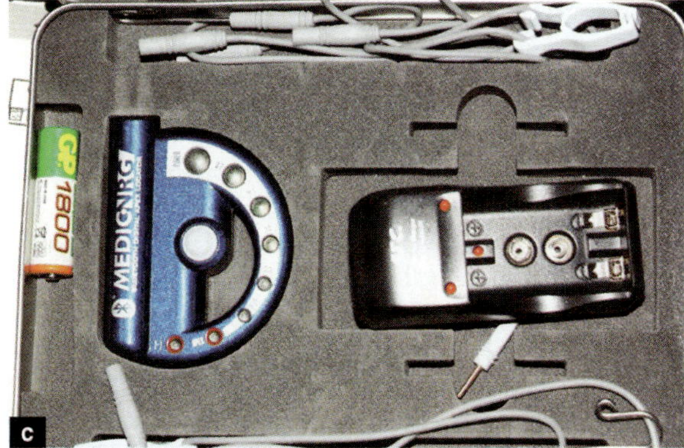

c

Fig. 15.6 Bluetooth technology apex locators: (a) Raypex 5; (b) and (c) MedicNRG

devices (Fig. 15.6a to c). These devices perform well in the presence of blood and exudates; however, it is difficult to operate in dry canals. Addition of liquid is required for accurate performance.

f. Sixth Generation (Adaptive Type)

A steady algorithm for adapting the difference of frequencies in the root canal is created to determine the canal length depending on the moisture characteristics (the device adapts the measuring method for either a dry or a wet canal).

The measuring mode provides for graphic information to be displayed on the monitor. The adaptive apex locator can retrieve audio information through beep or speech massage.

The device can measure moisture in the canal. The message 'apex' signifies the tip of the instrument is touching the physiological narrow part and the message 'over' means the tip has passed the anatomical foramen.

DenApex, a sixth generation multi-frequency operating system, that gives accurate readings in both dry and wet conditions has been introduced (Fig. 15.7). It has large LCD display with time graphic and adjustable angle of view. The moving trace of file in the canal can also be viewed.

The advantages and disadvantages of different types of apex locator are summarized in Table 15.1.

The problems faced during use of apex locators, the causes of said problems and their solutions are tabulated in Table 15.2.

Advantages of Apex Locators

- The major advantage is that it provides an objective information with a high degree of accuracy about the location of the apex and the point where the apical termination should end.

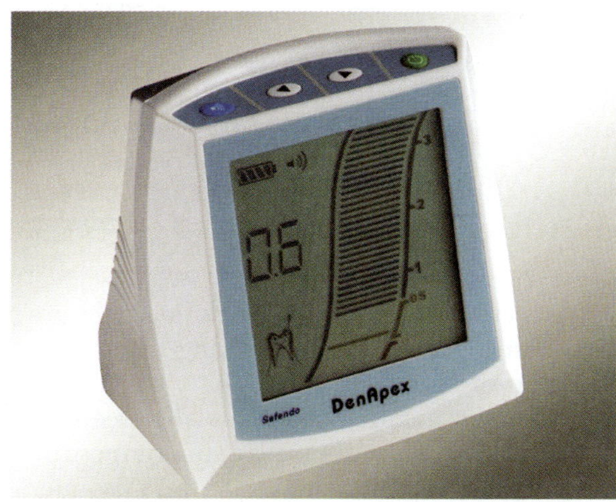

Fig. 15.7 DenApex (adaptive type apex locator)

Table 15.1 Advantages and disadvantages of different types of apex locators

Apex locator	*Advantages*	*Disadvantages*
First generation (Resistance type)	• Easy to operate • Digital read-out • Audible indication • Uses K-type files • May incorporate pulp tester • Perforations can be detected • Operates with RC Prep	• Requires dry environment • Defective restorations may pose problems • Patient sensitivity • Requires calibration • Requires a lip-clip with good contact • Perforation near apex may give false reading • Not indicated in patient with cardiac pacemaker
Second generation (Impedance type)	• Operates in a fluid environment • Analog meter • No patient sensitivity • No lip-clip required • Operates with RC Prep	• Difficult to operate • No digital read-out • Requires coated probes
Third generation (Frequency type)	• Easy to operate • Operates in a fluid environment • Uses K-type files • Analog readout • Audible indication • Rechargeable	• May be short circuited • Requires a lip-clip with good lip contact • Each canal is to be calibrated • Sensitive to extra fluid in the canal (irrigant should be in the canal and not in the chamber)
Fourth generation (Modified frequency type)	• Multiple frequencies employed	• Need to perform in relatively dry canal
Fifth generation (Bluetooth technology)	• Additional mathematical processing comparing electrical characteristics • Perform better in presence of blood and/or exudate	• Difficult to perform in dry canals
Sixth generation (Adaptive type)	• Useful in both dry and wet canals • Small size is easy to operate • Movement of the instrument displayed on the monitor	• Clinical accuracy is yet to be established

Table 15.2 Problems, causes and solution with the use of apex locators

Problem	*Possible cause*	*Solution*
Apex locator has continuous high pitched whining sound	• Machine remained 'on' overnight. • Battery is running low	• Turn off and let rest • Replace battery
When the file is introduced, the indicator moves erratically	• Too much tissue in the canal • Too much moisture in the canal • Perforation • File is too far from foramen	• Débride canal and the instrument • Dry with paper points • X-ray to evaluate/seal perforation • Put file closer to the tip of the tooth
File is in but indicator does not move	• Blockage is present or canal is calcified apically • Instrumentation finished, but apical plug present • Lip-clip not properly placed • Connection to file holder faulty	• Bypass blockage with EDTA/file • Clear apical plug (area) • Readjust lip-clip • Buy new wire leads

- It is especially important where radiographs are not sufficient to interpret the working length. Such a situation often exists in maxillary molars where radiopaque structures of the molar process or the floor of the maxillary sinus may superimpose on the apices of the teeth or mandibular tori may interfere in mandibular bicuspids.
- Useful in patients who gag easily.
- Useful in handicapped patients.
- Excellent for detecting apical and chamber perforations.
- Can verify the level at which the root is resorbed.
- Can determine if two canals join apically. Insert one file using the apex locator to determine the working

length. Then place a second file in the adjacent canal and if the files contact each other along the root, the apex locator will read as if the second file has reached the apex. This will indicate that the two canals lead into a single foramen.

- Useful to determine whether the apical bridge formation is complete in apexification procedures.
- The exact location of horizontal root fracture can also be detected.

Disadvantages of Apex Locators

- The overall accuracy is 90%.
- Most apex locators utilize a 9V battery. If the 9V battery drops below approximately 7V, inaccurate readings will result.
- All apex locators do not work in the presence of sodium hypochlorite, anesthetic solution or any other ionized solution.

Table 15.3 Working length determination: Comparison of apex locators with other modalities

Author (year)	*Study sample*	*Apex locator used*	*Aim of study (type)*	*Inference*
Busch et al (1976)	77 (46 vital + 26 necrotic)	Sono-Explorer	Evaluated accuracy of the device in working length measurement (*in vitro* study)	Accurate reading for both vital and necrotic teeth
Berman et al (1984)	29 (24 mature + 5 immature teeth)	Nesono-D	Evaluated accuracy of the device in working length measurement (*in vitro* study)	Accurate in mature teeth (doubtful in immature teeth)
Wu et al (1992)	20 (single rooted)	Sono-Explorer Type III	Evaluated accuracy of the device in working length measurement (*in vitro* study)	Clinically acceptable accuracy
Himel et al (1993)	96	Formatron-IV	Compared the accuracy of apex locators with radiography (*in vivo* study)	Apex locators were not accurate
Frank et al (1993)	185	Endex	Compared the accuracy of apex locators with radiography (*in vivo* study)	Apex locator was comparable with radiographic method
Shabahang et al (1996)	26	Root ZX	Evaluated accuracy of the device in working length measurement (*in vitro* study)	Clinically acceptable accuracy
Stavrianos et al (2007)	85	Raypex-5	Evaluated accuracy of the device in working length measurement (*in vitro* study)	Apex locator was accurate
Ounsi et al (1999)	39 (single rooted)	Root ZX	Evaluated accuracy of the device in working length measurement (*in vitro* study)	Could not detect apical constriction, accurate for apical foramen
Martinez Lozano et al (2001)	70	Apit	Comparison of apex locator and radiography in working length determination (*in vitro* study)	No significant difference
Subramanian et al (2005)	20	Formatron D10	Comparison of apex locator and radiography in working length determination (*in vitro* study)	No significant difference
Smadi, L (2006)	151	Tri Auto2X	Comparison of apex locator and radiography in working length determination (*in vitro* study)	Apex locator was effective; no need of radiography
Krajezar et al (2008)	70	ProPex	Comparison of apex locator and radiography in working length determination (*in vitro* study)	Apex locator was more accurate

(*Contd...*)

Table 15.3 Working length determination: Comparison of apex locators with other modalities (*Contd.*)

Author (year)	*Study sample*	*Apex locator used*	*Aim of study (type)*	*Inference*
Cianconi et al (2010)	101	Endex Propex II	Comparison of apex locator and radiography in working length determination (*in vitro* study)	Apex locator was more accurate
Zand et al (2011)	75	Root ZX	Comparison of apex locator and radiography in working length determination (*in vitro* study)	No significant difference
Chougute et al (2012)	13 (primary)	Dentaport ZX	Comparison of apex locator and radiography in working length determination (*in vitro* study)	Apex locator was more accurate
Sivadas et al (2013)	30 (primary molars)	Root ZX	Comparative evaluation of Root ZX and conventional radiography to measure working length in deciduous molars (*in vitro* study)	No significant difference. Both are comparable
Lucena et al (2014)	150	RayPex-6	Comparative evaluation of RayPex-6 and CBCT to measure accurate working length (*in vitro* study)	Apex locator was more accurate than CBCT
Singh et al (2015)	153 (single canal)	RayPex-5	Comparative evaluation of RayPex-5 and conventional radiography to determine working length (*in vitro* study)	Apex locator was comparable to radiography
Carneiro et al (2016)	40 (single rooted)	JoyPex-5	Comparison of JoyPex-5 and manual method to determine working length (*ex vivo* study)	Apex locator was more accurate
Jafarzadeh et al (2017)	22 canals (C-shaped)	Root ZX (Mini)	Comparison of apex locator and radiography (CBCT) in working length determination of c-shaped canals (*in vitro* study)	Apex locator was more accurate
Bhat et al (2017)	30 (primary teeth)	iPex	Comparison of iPex and conventional radiography to determine working length in primary teeth (*in vitro* study)	Both are comparable

Various authors have evaluated apex locators and many others have compared apex locators with other means to determine accurate working length, both in deciduous and permanent teeth. The selected few studies are summarized in Table 15.3.

ENDODONTIC WORKING WIDTH

The extent of apical enlargement is typically based on an estimate of initial canal size as determined by the size of hand file that 'binds' at the working length. The tactile detection of apical constriction and apical file size determination depend on the assumption that the canal is narrowest in the apical region. However, this may not be true in all cases. The configuration and diameter at the constriction as well as other areas of the root canal are important for proper cleaning and obturating the pulp spaces (Fig. 15.8a and b).

Apical enlargement at working length referred to the sequential widening of apical constriction area without its destruction.

The horizontal dimensions of the root canal system at apical constriction and other levels of root canal are designated as *'working width'*.

In a relatively round canal, the horizontal dimensions are usually, the same but in oval, flat and other canals, these dimensions vary.

The working width is important at apical constriction (working length), 1.0 to 3.0 m short of working length, at the centre of canal and also the coronal aspects.

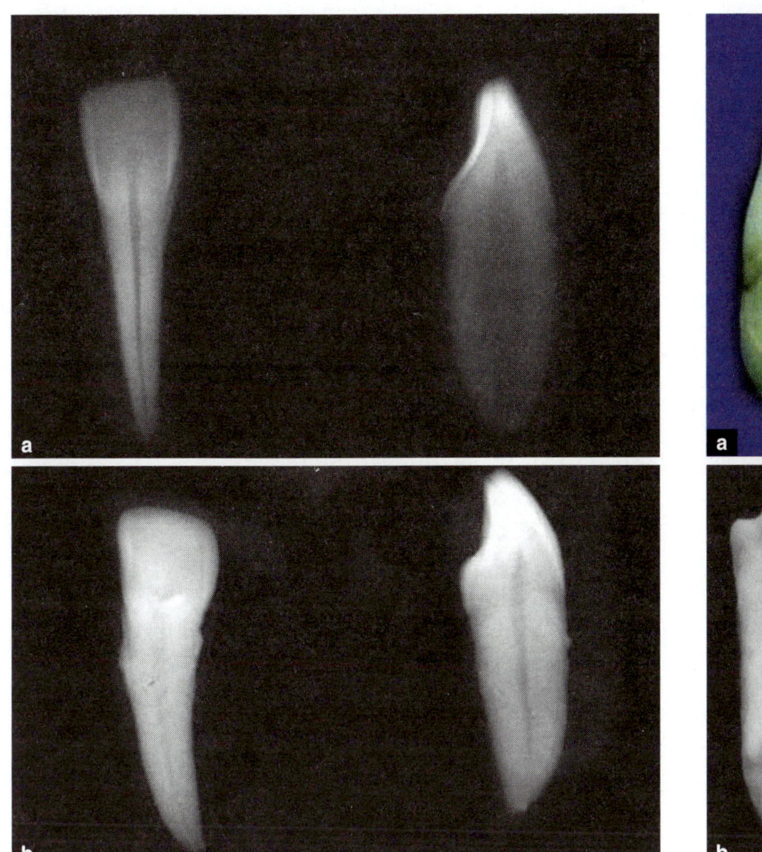

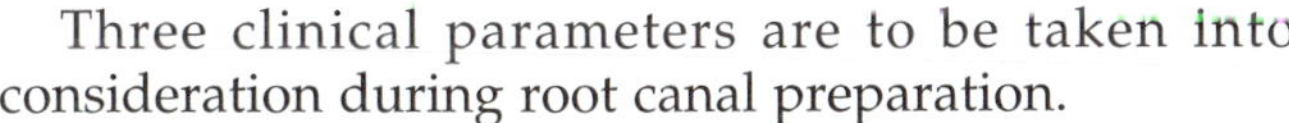

Fig. 15.8a and b Variation in root canal configuration in mesiodistal and labiolingual view

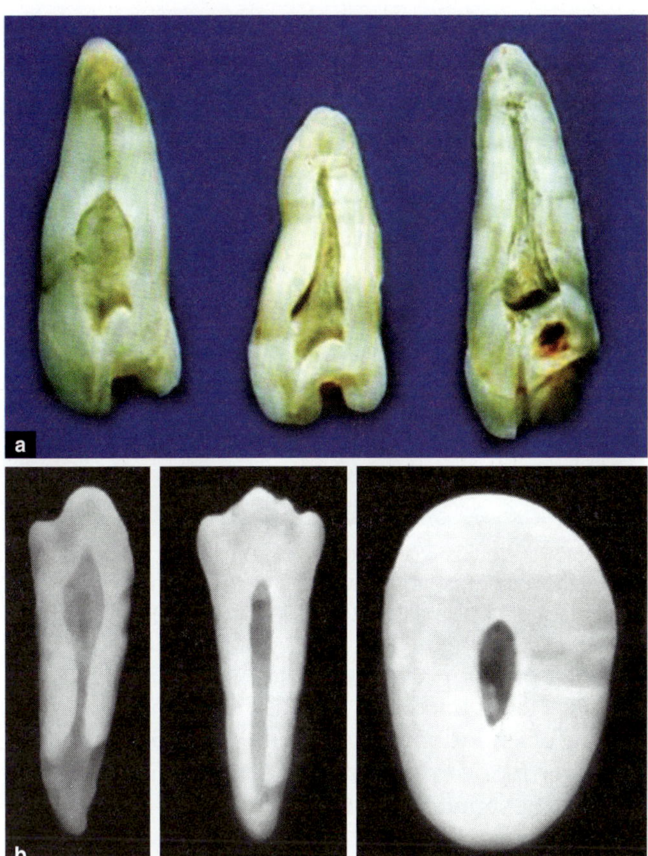

Fig. 15.9a and b Root canal width (different sections)

Three clinical parameters are to be taken into consideration during root canal preparation.

a. Length of canal
b. Taper of preparation
c. Horizontal dimension of the preparation, especially at its most apical extent.

The apical enlargement depends on this first file that binds at the apical constriction. However, it is established that the first file that bound at working length did not accurately reflect the diameter of the canal at the apex. Such inaccuracy and discrepancy can be due to various morphologic and procedural factors such as canal shape, canal length, curvature of canal, coronal interference, etc.

Factors Affecting Determination of Initial Working Width

The rigidity, flexibility and taper of the instrument used for determining initial working width can affect accuracy. The discrepancy between taper of canal and gauging instrument can alter the tactile sensation and may lead to wrong judgment. The factors affecting determination of working width are:

a. *Canal shape*: Oval/flat canals pose clinical difficulty in estimating initial working width; however, in round canals it is easy to assess (Fig. 15.9a and b).
b. *Canal length*: Longer the canal, greater is the frictional resistance which may affect the clinician's tactile sense for measuring the initial working width.
c. *Canal taper*: The discrepancy of taper between the gauging instrument and the canal may lead to an early instrument engagement in the canal, assuming the same as apical binding.
d. *Canal curvature*: The gauging instrument may feel the frictional resistance while intercepting curvatures, which can lead to false estimation of working width.
e. *Canal obstructions*: The pulp stones, denticles and reparative dentin, etc. may create problems in assessing the initial working width.

Clinical Suggestions

- Before working width determination, it is suggested to widen the orifices and achieve coronal flaring so that the interferences with tactile sensation are minimized.
- The adequate instrument having maximum flexibility and minimal taper may be selected to avoid interference.

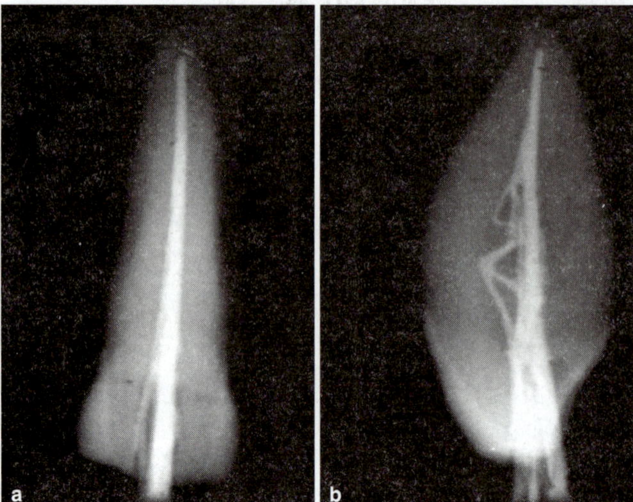

Fig. 15.10a and b Root canal obturation: a. Satisfactory obturation in mesiodistal view, b. part of root canal not prepared and obturated (labiolingual view)

If any part of root canal remains unprepared, it can harbor a lot of microbes, which will ultimately lead to failure of endodontic treatment (Fig. 15.10a and b). However, the overpreparation of canal may unnecessarily remove the sound tooth structure, hence weakening the root. It increases the risk of fracture and also increases chances of procedure errors, such as perforation, ledging, transportation, etc.

The reduction in intracanal bacteria during root canal preparation with and without apical enlargement has been compared. It is established that the bacterial reduction in both is insignificant.

Need to enlarge Apical Constriction Area

The apical constriction or the cementodentinal junction has long been advocated as the terminal end of instrumentation and obturation. Theoretically, it is the narrowest part of the canal and a junction where the pulp ends and periodontium begins.

The apical constriction may not be round. Generally, it is either oval or irregular in shape. When débriding and preparing this area with root canal instruments, extra care is exercised not to disturb the configuration of this area.

The apical portion of the root canal system can retain microorganisms that play a significant role in endodontic treatment failures.

The earlier authors advocated enlarging the apical constriction area of the root canal to three sizes larger than the first file bound. However, other authors were of the view that the three sizes larger preparation is not relevant in all the clinical cases. Certain cases may warrant the enlargement more than three sizes, because of the presence of necrosed dentin, while other cases may not require the enlargement at all.

A few authors have advocated minimal apical preparation (size 20 or 25) to prevent apical transportation or zips. Another author tried to standardize the apical preparation, by advocating fixed criteria for the given teeth. For example, maxillary central incisor is to be prepared up to size 80 and mesiobuccal and mesiolingual canals of mandibular molars to be prepared up to size 25. This school of thought was also not acceptable since unnecessary enlargement of the canal is never advisable; secondly each case warrants the enlargement depending upon the amount of necrosed dentin present coupled with chronicity of the disease. If necrosed dentin is present even after enlarging to size 80 or so in maxillary central incisors, there is need to enlarge the same till the necrosed dentin is comprehensively removed. And also, if the tooth is vital with no sign of necrosed dentin, there is no need to enlarge the canal three times even.

Summarily, the root canal is to be enlarged depending upon the amount of substrate present, i.e. necrosed dentin. It is established that the apical preparation be kept minimum, which minimizes the potential for creating procedural errors and provide better control of obturating material. However, larger apical preparation aid in better elimination of bacteria and cleaner canals due to better penetration of the irrigant into this region.

BIBLIOGRAPHY

1. Ahmad IA. Rubber dam usage for endodontic treatment: a review. Int. Endod. J.:2009; 42:963–972.
2. Alothmani OS, Friedlander LT and Chandler NP. Radiogrpahic assessment of endodontic working length. Saudi Endod. J.:2013; 3:57–64.
3. Anthony W and Robert H. The influence of Sodium Hypochlorite irrigation on the accuracy of the root ZX electronic apex locator. J. Endod.: 2002; 28:595–598.
4. Asako O, Takamoto Y, Chihiro K and Hideaki S. Electronic detection of root canal constrictions. J. Endod.: 2002; 28: 361–364.
5. Ballal NV, Khandelwal D and Saraswathi MV. Rubber dam in endodontics – an overview of recent advances. Int. J. Clin. Dent.:2015; 6:319–330.
6. Bhat KV, Shetty P and Anandkrishna L. A comparative evaluation of accuracy of new generation electronic apex locator with conventional radiography to determine working length in primary teeth (An *in vitro* study). Int. J. Clin. Pediat. Dent.:2017; 10:34–37.
7. Busch LR, Chiat LR, Goldstein LG, Held SA and Rosenberg PA. Determination of the accuracy of the Sono-Explorer for establishing endodontic measurement control. J. Endod.: 1976; 2:295–297.

15

8. Caldwell JL. Changes in working length following instruments of molar canals. O. Surg., O. Med., O. Path.:1976; 41:114–118.
9. Carneiro JA, deCarvalho FM, Marques AF, Sponchiado Jr EC, Garcio FR and Gonclaves LCU. Comparison of working length determination using apex locator and manual method – *ex vivo* study. Dentistry and Medical Research:2016; 4: 39–43.
10. Chai WL and Thong YL. Cross-sectional morphology and minimum canal walls widths in c-shaped roots of mandibular molars. J. Endod.:2004; 30:502–512.
11. Chougule RB, Padmanabhan MY and Mandal MS. A comparative evaluation of root canal length measurement techniques in primary teeth. Pediatr. Dent.: 2012; 34:56.
12. Cianconi L, Angotti V, Felici R, Conte G and Mancini M. Accuracy of three electronic apex locators compared with digital radiography: An ex vivo study. J. Endod.:2010; 36:2003–2007.
13. Farber JP and Bernstein M. The effect of instrumentation on root canal length as measured by an electronic device. J. Endod.:1983; 9:114–115.
14. Frank AL and Torabinejad M. An *in vivo* evaluation of Endex electronic apex locators. J. Endod.:1993; 19:177–179.
15. Gordon MPJ and Chandler NP. Electronic apex locators. Int. Endod. J.:2004; 37:425–437.
16. Herrera M, Abalos C, Planas AJ and Liamas R. Influence of apical constriction diameter on root ZX apex locator precision. J. Endod.: 2007; 33:998.
17. Hoer D and Attin, T. The accuracy of electronic working length determination. Int. Endod. J.: 2004; 37:125–131.
18. Jou YT, Karabucak B, Levin J and Liu D. Endodontic working width: current concepts and techniques. Dent Clinic North Am.: 2004; 48:323–335.
19. Lucena C, Lopez JM, Martin JA, Robles V and Gonzalez-Rodriguez MD. Accuracy of working length measurement: electronic apex locator versus cone beam computed tomography. Int. Endod. J.:2014; 47:246–256.
20. Lucena C, Lopez JM, Martin JA, Robles V and Gonzalez-Rodriguez MP. Accuracy of working with measurement: electronoc apex locator versus cone beam computed tomography. Int. End. J. 2014; 47:245–256.
21. McDonald NJ. The electronic determination of working length. Dent. Cl. North Am.: 1992; 36:293–307.
22. Morroquin BB, Frajlich S, Goldberg F and Willershausen B. Influence of instrument size on the accuracy of different apex locators: An *in vitro* study. J. Endod.: 2008; 34:698–702.
23. Mosleh H, Khazaei S, Razavian H, Vali A and Ziaei F. Electronic apex locator: A comprehensive literature review-Part I: Different generations, comparison with other techniques and different usages. Dent. Hypothesis:2014; 5:84–97.
24. Nekoofar MH, Chandi MM, Hayes SJ and Dummer PM. The fundamental operating principles of electronic root canal length measurement devices. Int. Endod. J.: 2006; 39:595–609.
25. Ounsi HF and Naaman A. *In vitro* evaluation of the reliability of the Root ZX electronic apex locator. Int. Endod. J.:1999; 32:120–123.
26. Singh D, Tyagi SP, Gupta S and Jain A. Comparative evaluation of adequacy of final working length after using RayPex-5 or Radiography – An *in vivo* study. J. Indian Soc. Paedo. Prev. Dent.:2015; 33:208–212.
27. Sivadas G, Sudha P, Shenoy R, Rao A and Suprabha BS. Accuracy of apex locator for root canal length determination of deciduous molars compared to conventional radiography. J. Interdiscip. Dent.:2013; 3:163–166.
28. Smadi L. Comparison between two methods of working length determination and its effect on radiographic extent of root canal filling: A clinical study. BMC Oral Health:2006; 6:4.
29. Stein TJ, Corcoran JF and Zillich RM. The influence of the major and minor foramen diameters on apical electronic probe measurements. J. Endo.: 1990; 16:520–522.
30. Tilk MA, Lommel TJ and Gerstein H. A study of mandibular and maxillary root widths to determine dowel size. J. Endod.: 1979; 5:79–82.
31. Wiggler R, Huber R, Lin S and Kaufman AY. Accuracy and reliability of working length determination by gold reciproc motor in reciprocating movement. J. Endod.:2014; 40:694–697.
32. Wrbas KT, Zeigler AA, Altenburger MJ and Schirrmeister JF. *In vivo* comparison of working length determination with the electronic apex locators. Int. Endod. J.: 2007; 40:133–138.
33. Wu YN, Shi JN, Huang LZ and Xu YY. Variables effecting elec-tronic root canal measurement. Int. Endod. J.:1992; 25:88–92.
34. Zafarzadeh H, Beyrami M and Forghani M. Evaluation of conventional radiography of an apex locator in determining the working length in C-shaped canals. Iran. Endod. J.:2017; 12:60–63.
35. Zand V, Mokhtari H, Lotfi M, Reyhani MF, Sohrab A and Tehranchi P. Accuracy of working length determination with root ZX apex locator and radiography: An *in vivo* and ex vivo study. Afr. J. Biotechnol.:2013; 10:7088–7091.

Chapter 16

Cleaning and Shaping of Root Canals

The earlier concept of preparation of root canals as envisaged by Grossman and others is being modified as cleaning and shaping in the past couple of years. The basic idea of preparation of root canal is to remove all organic and inorganic debris and microorganisms from the root canal system along with the substrate which harbors the microorganisms. The preparation also shape the root canal walls, facilitating placement of medicament/obturating material into the root canal spaces.

The term *'biomechanical preparation'* as described by Schilder, involves biological and mechanical objectives in preparation of root canals.

It has been emphasized that tooth root rarely contains a simple canal that can be cleaned in a hollow tube manner; rather, it is a complex system containing accessory/lateral canals, fins/apical delta and other anatomical variations. A few of these anatomical intricacies may not be accessible to instrumentation and hence some chemical agent is necessary to clean these areas (concept of chemomechanical preparation). The penetration of the chemical agent deep into the canal system to aid in flushing and dissolving organic debris requires prior mechanical preparation. The shaping is achieved prior to cleaning. Therefore, the term *'shaping and cleaning'* is gaining popularity instead of *'cleaning and shaping'*; however, the conventional term *'root canal preparation'* is used in routine.

Complete removal of organic contents of the entire root canal space followed by abundant irrigation has always been emphasized. The axiom 'what comes out is more important than what goes in' forms the basis for successful endodontics. It is established that shaping must not only be carried out according to anatomy of each canal but also in relation to the technique and material for final obturation. The basic shape of the prepared canal should be a continuously tapering funnel simulating the shape of the root canal. This was termed 'concept of flow', facilitating placement of obturating materials and also their removal, if need be.

OBJECTIVES OF ROOT CANAL PREPARATION

The objective features of root canal preparation can be mechanical and biological.

Mechanical objectives

- Continuously tapering funnel from the apex to the access cavity.
- Cross-sectional diameter should be narrowest apically.
- Preparation should flow with shape of the original canal.
- Position of the apical foramen should not change; maintaining the original position of the foramen.
- The apical opening should be maintained as small as practically possible.

Biologic objectives

- All instrumentation to be confined within the root canal.
- Necrotic debris is not to be forced beyond the foramen.
- Removal of substrate harboring microorganisms from the root canal space.
- Creation of sufficient space for intracanal medicaments.

Goals to Achieve

The goals of root canal preparation, which the clinician should achieve are:

- Removal of vital and necrotic tissue from the main root canal(s).
- Creation of sufficient space for irrigation and medication.
- Preservation of the integrity and location of the apical canal anatomy.

- Avoidance of iatrogenic damage to the root structure.
- Preservation of sound root dentin to allow long-term function of the tooth.
- Facilitation of root canal filling.
- Avoidance of irritation and/or infection of the periradicular tissues.

All these features aid in promotion of healing and prevention of periradicular disease.

Before preparing the root canal, the concept of 'working length' and 'working width' should be understood (Chapter 15).

Instrument Motions during Root Canal Preparation

Root canal instruments utilize various motions during root canal preparation. The commonly used motions are:

a. ***Watch-winding motion***: This motion is used to explore the canal at the beginning before carrying out the coronal flaring. In this motion, a small K file, referred to as path finders (number 06 or 08) is used to negotiate the working length with quarter-turn rotational movement (Fig. 16.1).

b. ***Reaming***: Reaming is carried out to produce a round tapered preparation and is preferred in straight canals. The purpose of reaming is to enlarge or taper pre-existing spaces. The reamers perform the action of cutting dentin by being inserted into the canal, twisted clockwise 1/4th to ½ turn, engaged their blades into dentin and finally withdrawn, i.e. penetration, rotation, retraction (cutting is achieved during retraction) (Fig. 16.2).

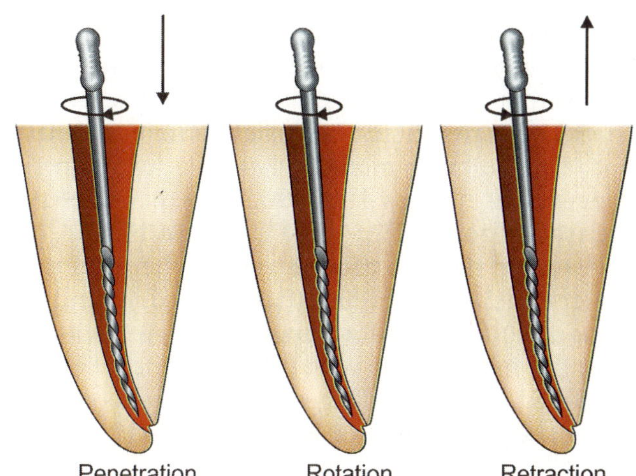

Fig. 16.2 Reaming motion (cutting achieved during retraction)

c. ***Filing***: In this motion, the instrument is placed to the desired length applying pressure against the walls of the canal. The instrument is withdrawn while maintaining the pressure and without turning; the cutting is achieved during withdrawing. K-files are more popular; however, H-files perform filing efficiently (Fig. 16.3).

d. ***Circumferential filing***: In case the file cannot contact all walls of canal simultaneously (large diameter canals), circumferential filing is carried out; i.e. filing motion performed around all the walls circumferentially (Fig. 16.4). Circumferential filing facilitate removal of infected dentin thoroughly from the root canal walls.

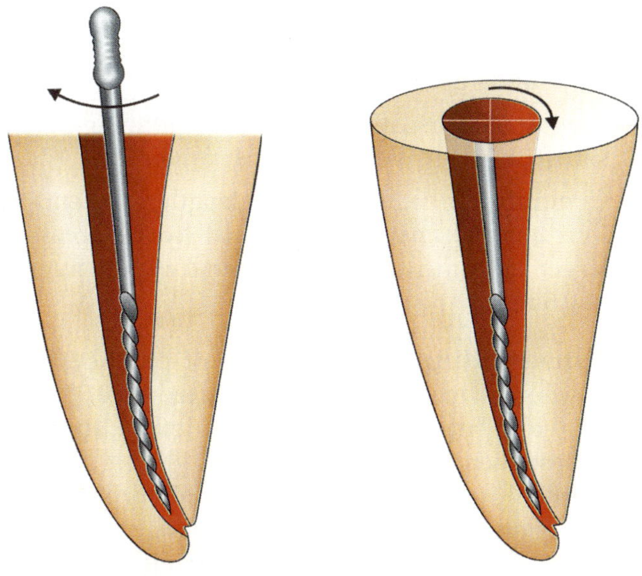
Fig.16.1 Watch winding motion

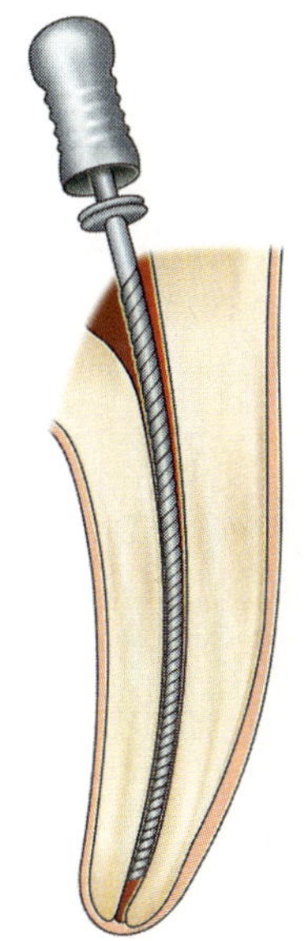
Fig. 16.3 Filing motion

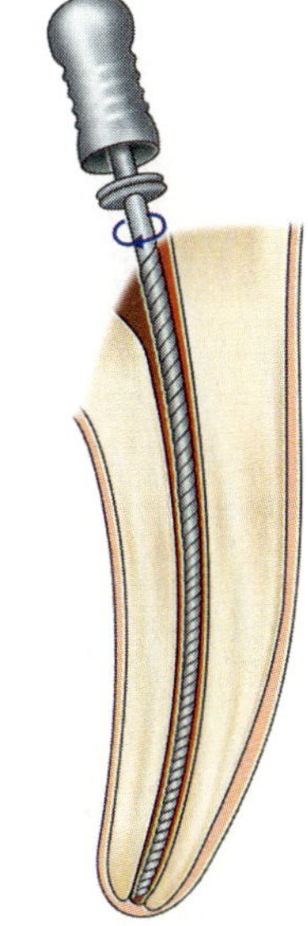
Fig. 16.4 Circumferential filing

e. ***Anticurvature filing***: Anticurvature filing motion is used to prevent the excessive removal of dentin from thinner root sections in curved canals, thus reducing the risk of perforation. The basic example is a mesial root of mandibular molars where the furcation side (danger zone) has less dentin thickness than the mesial side (safety zone) (Fig. 16.5). In this technique, pre-curved hand files are used to prepare the canal at the danger zone. Safety H-files (flattened edges and dull at one side) are used for filing the danger zone area. Recently, instruments with advanced flexibility are developed to prepare danger zones of the root canals, without any possibility of strip perforation.

f. ***Rotary***: Different rotary files are available; files are continuously rotated in the root canal (not more than 5 seconds at one time) to achieve requisite preparation. Rotary instrumentation have revolutionized the root canal preparation protocol.

Root Canal Preparation: Concepts/Terms

a. ***Apical gauging***: Apical gauging implies measuring/assessing the apical diameter of the canal, where the instrument fits snuggly and resist further apical movements. This ensures apical terminus of the prepared canal (Fig. 16.6).

- Ni-Ti instruments are preferred for gauging because of their flexibility (especially in curved canals).

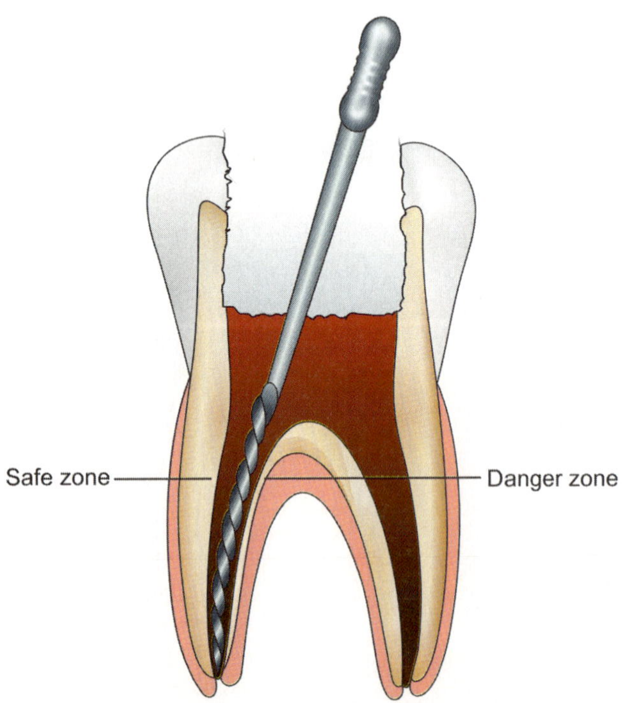

Fig. 16.5 Depiction of safe zone and danger zone (anticurvature filing: Mandibular molar)

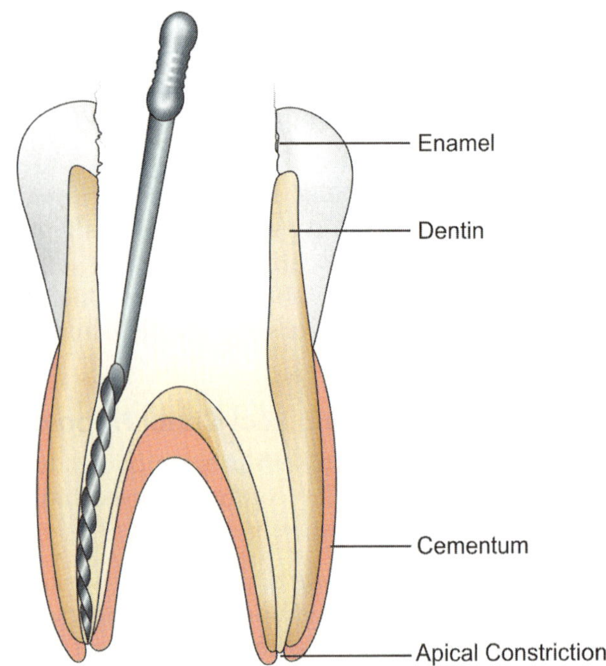

Fig. 16.6 Apical gauging (assessing apical diameter)

- The gauging instrument is inserted straight in and straight out, without any rotation.
- 17% EDTA as irrigant is used to remove the smear layer, facilitating better gauging.
- Endogauge, a gadget, is available with holes of different diameters for confirming the diameter of the instrument and the gutta-percha as well.
- Gauging is carried out after root canal preparation; master apical file is preferred.

b. ***Apical tuning***: Apical tuning implies a confirming parameter, whereby the apical diameter of the master apical file represents the true diameter of the apical configuration of the root canal.

- Tuning is a clinical activity of recapitulating using series of successively larger instruments.
- Clinically, the file that goes full length represents the '*true apical diameter*' of the canal (each successive larger instrument backs out of canal with an interval of 0.5 mm).

c. ***Patency filing***: The technique of patency filing involves passively inserting a small sized (size 08 or 10) file, 2.0 mm beyond the apical constriction. Buchanan first described the concept of patency filing; defined as '*small K-file, which passively moves through the apical constriction without widening the apical constriction*' (Fig. 16.7). No preparation is carried out at this stage.

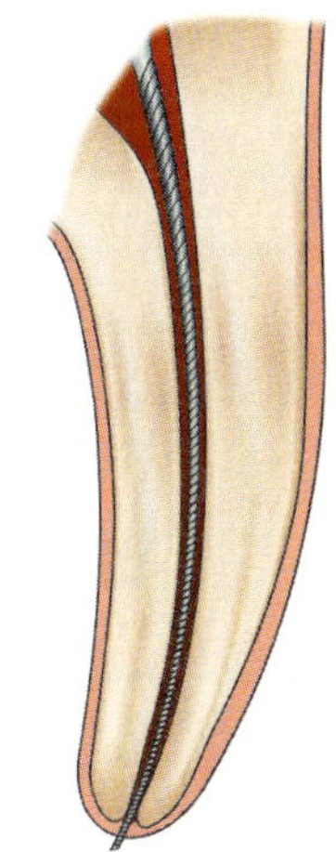
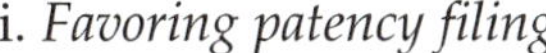

Fig.16.7 Patency filing

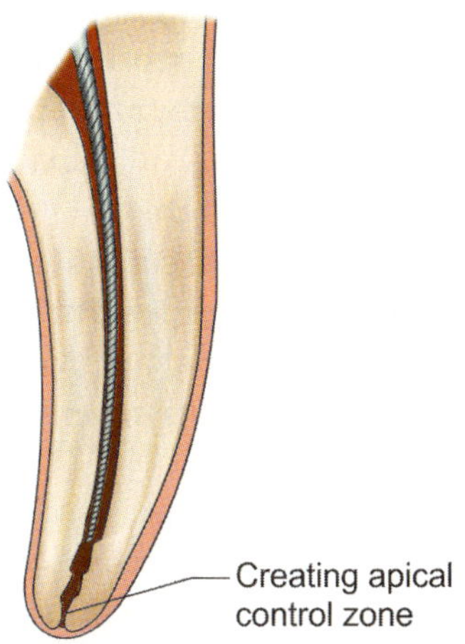

Fig. 16.8 Apical control zone

i. *Favoring patency filing*

- Cleans apical constriction/foramen area
- Maintains working length
- Prevents packing of debris at the apical constriction end
- Help keeping apical zone area free of microorganisms.

ii. *Disfavoring patency filing*

- May push debris into periapical areas
- May push microorganisms into periapical area
- May injure the configuration of apical constriction.

d. *Apical scouting*: Apical scouting, similar to apical gauging, implies determining the cross-section diameter of the apical third of the root canal. Smaller sized instruments are used to assess the diameter at the apical end.

e. *Coronal scouting*: The process of determining the cross-sectional diameter of coronal 2/3rd of the root canal. Appropriate size of the file is used to assess the diameter of the root canal at the coronal orifices and also within the coronal 2/3rd area.

Scouting files also analyze the site of curvature in the root canal (how far the canal is straight from coronal opening and from where the curvature begins).

f. *Apical stop/apical seat*: A matrix of dentin or other material at the apical end of root canal preparation. Apical seat implies lack of complete barrier, but presence of constriction; whereas, apical stop means complete barrier at the preparation end.

g. *Apical control zone*: The 'apical control zone' is the mechanical alteration created in the apical third of the root canal. This area (around 1.5 mm from the apical constriction) affects the rheology of gutta-percha and provides resistance form against the condensation pressure of obturation (coronal to constriction, exaggerated taper is given, which provides resistance against condensation pressure and also prevent extrusion of debris out of periapex). It facilitates 'apical cleaning' (maximize débridement of apical one-third area, especially in curved canals) (Fig. 16.8).

This area, initially proposed by Roane for balanced force technique, should be evaluated with smaller files (glide path) prior to instrumentation.

Points to remember

- *75% of the instrument that bound in the canal at working length, contact only one wall; the other 25% do not contact; Inference is 'The first file that bind may not reflect the diameter at working length'.*
- *The major foramen of all teeth are deviated from the anatomic apex (average distance between anatomic apex and foramen is 0.59 mm).*
- *Average distance from apical foramen (major diameter) to cementodentinal junction (apical constriction) is 0.72 mm; whereas, width of cementodentinal junction is 0.189 mm (size increases with age).*

TECHNIQUES OF ROOT CANAL PREPARATION

The techniques of root canal preparation can be divided into two groups:

A. Apical-coronal Techniques

In apical-coronal techniques, the canal is prepared starting from apical end and sequentially increasing in size coronally, until the final shape is achieved. The shape is refined from apically up to coronally.

16

Root canal preparation: Key points

- Visualize and analyze the tooth to be treated
- Customize the access cavity preparation
- Analyze pulp anatomy of root canals
- 'Read' radiograph thoroughly
- Concentrate on each canal separately
- Proceed with delicacy; go slow, have patience
- Anticipate preparation of shape required
- Use sterilized, new instruments; discard old instruments
- Do not force instruments; use gentle pressure
- Use ample and continuous irrigation
- Carry out preparation in one sitting.

The routinely used apical-coronal preparation techniques are:

a. Standardized technique
b. Step-back technique
c. Modified step-back technique
d. Balanced force technique.

a. Standardized Technique

The standardized technique, introduced by Ingle, involves determining working length followed by placement of smallest size file/reamer to the full working length. The instrument is rotated clockwise to engage dentin and then withdrawn. The instrument is wiped clean and then reinserted till it became loose.

The canal is enlarged three times the size of first instrument that binds at apex or until clean white dentin shavings are seen in the apical few millimeters of the instrument.

The canal shape so produced matches the last instrument used. This technique works well in straight canals; however, it is unsuitable for curved canals.

The technique cannot débride canals with complex shapes; the obturation of such areas relies on the sealers only. The technique is also associated with procedural errors (Fig. 16.9) like ledging, zipping, perforation, loss of working length especially in case of curved canals (as the instrument size increases it becomes more rigid). The technique is no longer followed, since the three times enlargement is not sufficient in some case, and in other cases, it might not be necessary. The presence of clean dentin shavings is also not a confirmative parameter of root canal preparation.

b. Step-back Technique

16

The step-back technique is also known as telescopic or serial root canal preparation. This technique was devised to overcome the shortcomings of the standardized technique, especially for the preparation of curved canals; however, the technique remained suitable for straight canals.

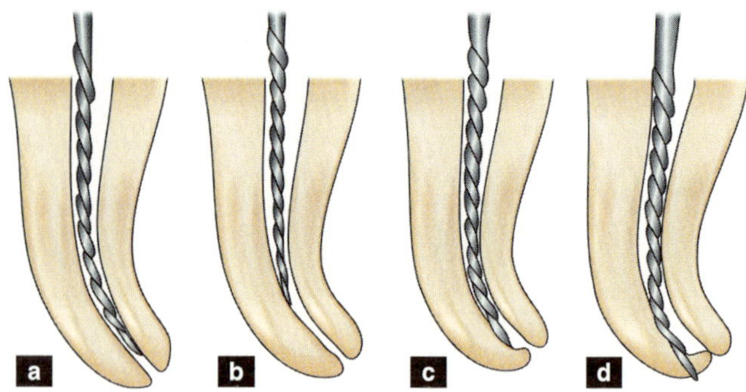

Fig. 16.9 Procedural errors: (a) Non-uniform force in curved canal (b) Ledge formation (loss of working length); (c) Apical transportation; (d) Perforation

The technique prepares the canal using files with a push-pull/watch-winding motion leading to a wider taper than that produced in the standardized technique. The wider taper facilitates the obturation, precisely with lateral condensation technique.

Step wise procedure

The steps are described for straight canals; the modifications for curved canals are described subsequently:

i. Determine the working length.
ii. Insert the file that precisely fits to the full working length. File circumferentially until the next size file reaches the full working length. Simultaneous irrigation with suitable irrigants is mandatory.
iii. The process is repeated until two sizes large file can reach the working length. Each next size file should be introduced only when the previous file is just loose at the working length (Fig. 16.10a). This completes the preparation of apical area. (*First three steps are also designated as phase I of the preparation*) (Fig. 16.10b).
iv. The preparation is now flared by using the next size file 1.0 mm shorter than the previous file until it is loose. After each filing, it is paramount to recapitulate, i.e. the smaller file is introduced again to full working length under copious irrigation. The process of recapitulation ensures canal patency till the preparation continues. Recapitulation is beneficial as:
    - Prevent blocking the canal with dentinal debris
    - Smoothen the walls of the canal
    - Facilitate subsequent insertion of larger instrument as the preparation proceeds.
v. Again the next size file is introduced 1.0 mm shorter than the file used at step iv. The recapitulation is

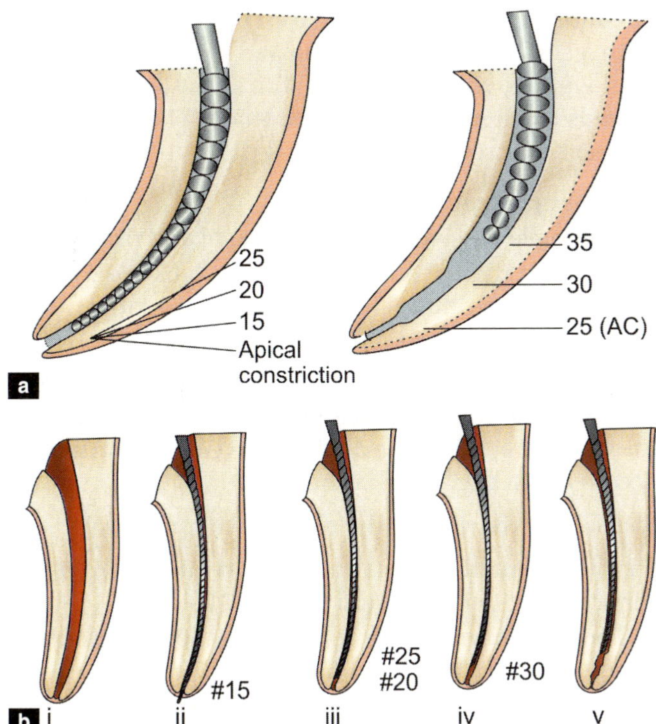

Fig. 16.10 Step-back technique: (a) Apical preparation; (b) Root canal preparation (Phases I and II)

also repeated. This process is repeated and the preparation is completed in steps from apical end to coronal end.

(The steps iv and v are designated as phase II of the preparation).

vi. The coronal portion is then refined with Gates Glidden drills and the apical portion is refined with the same size file as used for apical preparation (master apical file). Usually a file of the same number as the master apical file is used for this purpose to remove the irregular surface created by the step-back procedure as well as to produce a smooth tapering canal preparation (Fig. 16.11a and b).

[This step is phase III, the refining phase; a few authors have further modified as refining phase A (coronal refining) and refining phase B (apical refining)].

Modification for curved root canals

i. Smaller files are precurved as per the curvature; instrument step is adjusted accordingly.

ii. In narrow canals, sequential enlarging is modified by cutting 1.0 mm tip of the file (file 10 can be made file 12, 13 and so on). These intermediate filing help negotiating narrow canals more effectively (Fig. 16.12).

iii. The files should not bind at any stages during canal preparation.

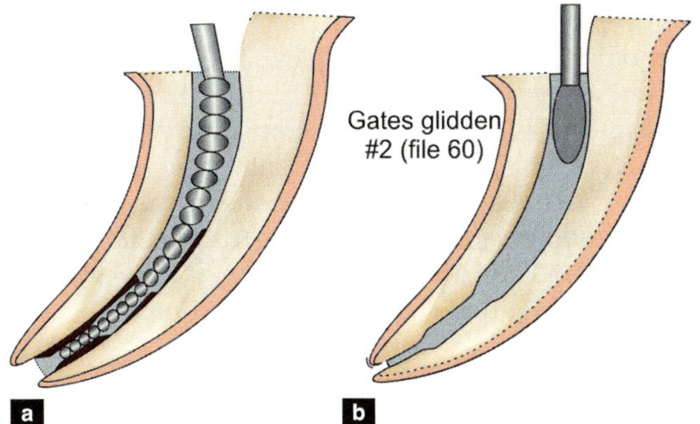

Fig. 16.11 Step-back technique: (a) Apical refining, (b) Coronal refining (Phase III)

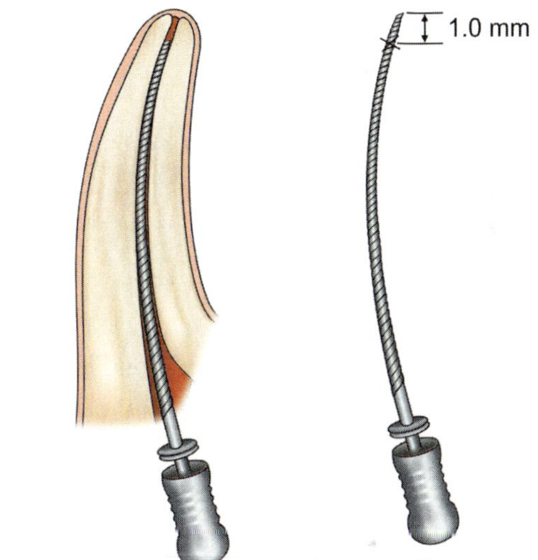

Fig. 16.12 Step-back technique (modification of instrument for curved canals)

Advantages

- Greater flare facilitate dense obturation
- Less chances of trauma to periapical tissues
- Allows effective removal of debris
- Apical matrix at apical area minimizes chances of over instrumentation and subsequently overfiling. *(This technique is likely to achieve cleaner canals and allows better control over the apical preparation than the standardized technique.)*

Disadvantages

- May lead to apical blockage (debris collected below the apical constriction area)
- Alteration of working length
- Tendency for canal deviation when using the larger inflexible instruments (Hour-glass preparation)
- The H-file may cause overflaring or strip-perforation.

c. Modified Step-back Technique

In modified technique, the apical area is prepared in routine using circumferential filing. After the apical preparation is complete, the step-back procedure is initiated 2.0 to 3.0 mm coronal to the apical end. This gives a parallel and round form in the apical area. Such a preparation provides tight fitting gutta-percha in the apical 2.0–3.0 mm of the prepared canal. The rest of the canal is flared and is obturated conventionally.

Advantages

- Minimal chances of apical transportation
- Better adaptation of gutta-percha at the apical area.

Disadvantages

- Debris may accumulate at apical-third area
- Irrigating the apical area is difficult.

d. Balanced Force Technique

Balanced force technique, popularly known as Roane's technique, was introduced in 1985 by Roane. The objectives of the technique are:

- Reduce instrument breakage
- Minimize canal straightening
- Eliminate apical zipping.

The balanced force technique utilizes Flex-R file (a file made from diamond shaped wire with a non-cutting tip), a modified version of K-file (conventional K-file can also be used).

The Flex-R is a triangular cross-section file which is ground in a helical position rather than in a vertical orientation and twisted to create the helical spiral. The triangular cross-section is more flexible, has more flute space and less cross-sectional area than either a diamond or square one.

All K-files function much like wood screws. If you turn a wood screw clockwise, it goes into the wood. If you turn the same screw counter-clockwise, it comes out of the wood, but if you place a screw into the wood with a slight clockwise motion and then turn counter-clockwise as you push down, the screw will strip the threads it originally cut into the wood. The same thing happens in a root canal.

Stepwise procedure (Fig. 16.13)

Place the file passively in the root canal and proceed as:

Step I. Turn the file one quarter turn clockwise, which seats the file with a slight screwing in motion. This motion should be as limited as possible.

Step II. Move the file three-quarter turn counter-clockwise; hold it in place with inward pressure. As the shear strength of the dentin is exceeded, a stripping occurs and a slight click is heard.

Step III. Advance apically (light apical pressure).

Step IV. After the file is free, it is removed from the canal in clockwise rotation (Fig. 16.14).

- These movements are repeated as the instrument is advanced up to the working length.
- Continuous irrigation with suitable irrigant is mandatory.
- Coronal access can be flared with Gates Glidden drills.

Roane initially proposed an 'Apical control zone' in balanced forced technique; wherein, the canals are prepared to a predesigned dimension. The three sizes are recognized, i.e. 45, 60 and 80 according to the size of the apical preparation. These dimensions refer to the size of the file used at the third step-back and not the size of the master apical file.

Each step back from the master apical file at the constriction area is 0.5 mm shorter than the previous one. This combined area is known as the apical control zone, recognizing three different diameters in the apical control zone area.

- The first diameter is at 0.5 mm short of the working length.

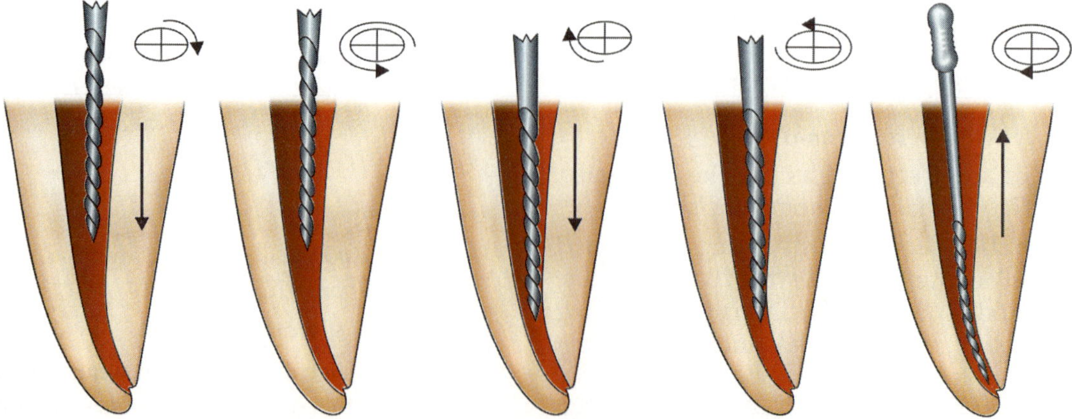

Fig. 16.13 Balanced force technique (procedure)

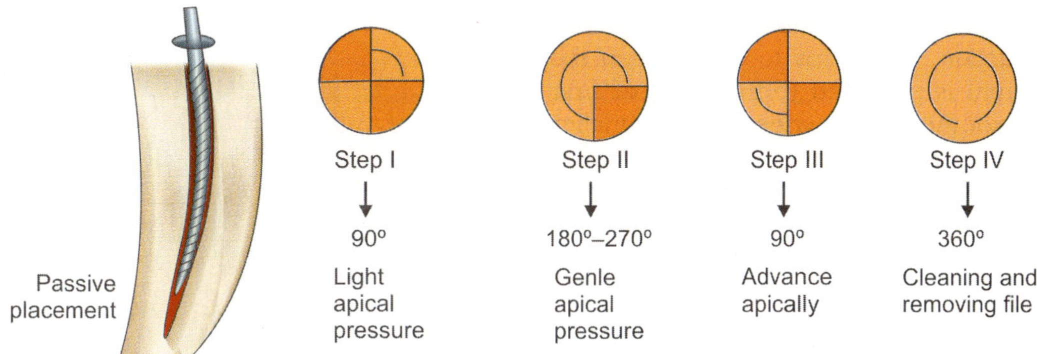

Fig. 16.14 Balanced force technique (Steps)

- The next diameter is 1.0 mm coronal to the first one.
- The third is 1.5 mm short of the working length (0.5 mm short of the second one).

This type of preparation creates an apical stop, which facilitates three-dimensional obturation.

Conventionally, the apical zone is prepared using size 20 file to radiographic length; stepback 0.5 mm with size 25 and size 30 followed by size 35 and size 40 at 1.0 mm back. Finally, prepare with size 45 at 1.5 mm short (Fig. 16.8).

Advantages

- Minimum chances of extrusion of debris beyond the apical foramen
- Less chances of canal transportation
- Provide excellent canal centering ability.

Disadvantage

- Sensitive and meticulous technique.

B. Coronal-apical Techniques

In coronal-apical techniques, the coronal part of the root canal is prepared first followed by preparation of the canal moving from coronal end to the apical end.

Advantages of coronal-apical over apical-coronal technique

- Allows early débridement of the coronal part of the canal which may contain the bulk of organic and microbial debris; thus minimizing the chances of apical extrusion of the material through the foramen.
- Better and deeper penetration of the irrigant aids in better cleaning and disinfection of the root canal system along with decreasing the risk of apical blockage.
- Cares for shortening of the working length, which occurs after preparation of the root canals due to the straightening of the canals in apical-coronal technique.
- Better control over apical instrumentation; hence, reduction in the chances of procedural errors like transportation, ledging and perforation, etc.

The routinely used coronal-apical preparation techniques are:

a. Step-down technique
b. Crown-down pressureless technique
c. Double flare technique
d. Rotary techniques

a. Step-down Technique

This is a combination of crown-down/step-back technique. It is also known as modified step-back technique.

Step wise procedure

- The coronal portion of the canal to a depth of 6.0–8.0 mm or at the beginning of the canal curvature is prepared using Gates Glidden drills or appropriate sized K-files.
- Use appropriate Gates Glidden drills to refine the coronal preparation.
- Determine the working length.
- Use step-back technique from apical area to merge with the coronal preparation.
- The canal is recapitulated conventionally.

This technique offers all the advantages of the coronal-apical preparation and partially overcome the disadvantages of the conventional step-back preparation.

b. Crown-down Pressureless Technique

Crown-down pressureless technique was introduced by Marshall and Pappin with the aim to prepare curved canals without causing any deviation. The technique mostly utilizes rotary action to prepare the canal; hand instruments can also be used.

Stepwise procedure

- Determine radicular access length (the depth to which no. 35 file penetrates to its point of first resistance). If it is more than 16 mm, the coronal portion of the canal should be prepared to this length. If it is less than 16 mm, a radiograph should be used

16

to determine whether it is because of canal curvature or any obstruction. If it is due to curvature of the canal, the canal is prepared to the point of first resistance; if not the canal is widened with smaller file until #35 file penetrates to 16 mm depth (Fig. 16.15).

- Establish provisional working length to 3.0 mm short of the radiographic apex.
- Place #35 file into the canal until it encounters resistance. At this point give two full revolutions without apical pressure. Repeat this sequence with the next smaller file till the provisional working length is reached.
- Establish a definite working length with the help of radiograph.
- Again start preparing with #40 file till the apical portion of the canal is prepared to desired diameter (Fig. 16.16).

This technique maintains the canal shape but tends to prepare it in a circular fashion. Without the use of appropriate irrigants, the canals may not be as clean as the one prepared using circumferential filing.

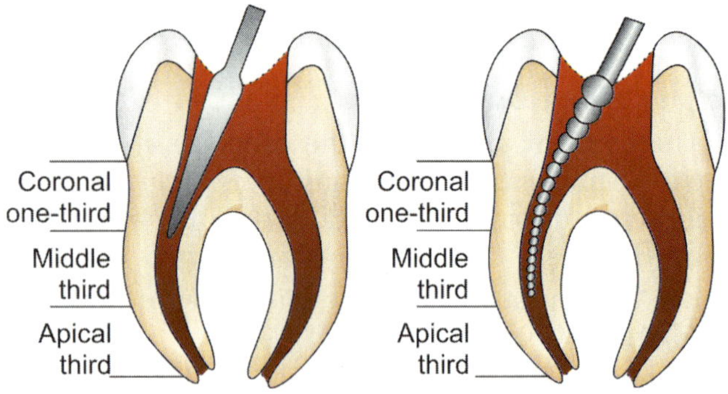

Fig. 16.15 Crown-down technique (coronal and middle preparation)

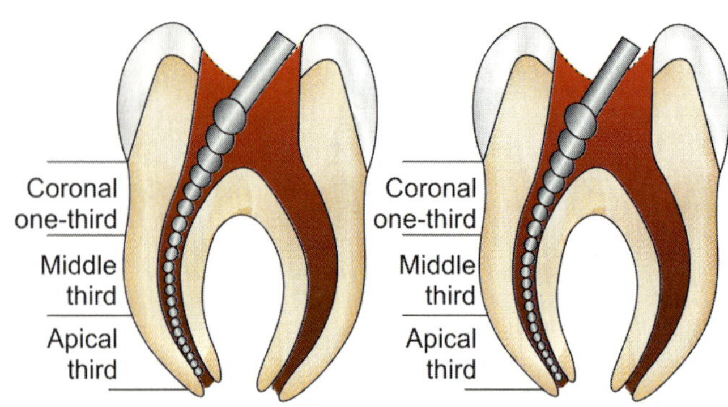

Fig. 16.16 Crown-down technique (apical preparation)

Advantages

- Less periapical extrusion of debris
- Less apical zip formation
- Less chances of ledge formation
- Straight access to the apical region
- Better penetration of the irrigant.

Disadvantage

- Apical cleanliness is doubtful.

The differences of step-back and crown-down technique are summarized in Table 16.1.

c. Double Flare Technique

Double flare technique, introduced by Fava, involves preparing the canal in crown-down manner using K-files, followed by step-back manner. Conventional recapitulation along with copious irrigation is mandatory. This technique is indicated for straight canals/straight portion of the curved canals and is contraindicated for calcified canals/canals with open apices.

Table 16.1 Differences of step-back technique and crown-down technique

Step-back technique	*Crown-down technique*
• Also known as telescopic, serial root canal preparation	• Also known as pressureless crown-down, step-down preparation
• Use hand instruments	• Use both hand and rotary instruments
• Small file is used at apex, followed by sequentially increasing the size to the coronal	• Large file is used at coronal end followed by sequential decreasing the size to the apex
• Narrow coronal portion prevents adequate irrigation	• Wider coronal preparation allow deeper penetration of irrigant
• Instrumentation difficult because of narrow coronal preparation	• Easy instrumentation
• Less tactile control	• Adequate tactile control
• Debris accumulation at apical third area; liable to be pushed out of apex	• Minimum debris accumulation at apical third area because of better irrigation; less debris extrusion
• Obstruction in coronal portion pose difficulties in managing apical control zone	• Apical control zone is managed properly
• Not frequently used; clinicians do not prefer	• Most frequently used; clinician's preference

Stepwise procedure
- Introduce the irrigant into the canal using a small file in a push and pull motion (without binding). The file is pushed only up to the length estimated from the preoperative radiograph.
- Take a new radiograph to redetermine the working length.
- The canal is prepared in crown-down manner.
- Introduce a large instrument (size 70 or 80) into the canal to a depth of about 14 mm or up to the start of the canal curvature. Prepare the canal to this length with a filing motion.
- Again introduce the next size smaller instrument 1.0 mm deeper into the canal and file gently.
- Repeat till the working length is reached and apical area is prepared.
- The root canal is again prepared in a step-back manner using recapitulation in between.

Advantages
- Effectively remove the canal contents
- Necrotic root dentin is effectively removed
- Minimum iatrogenic errors
- Facilitate compact obturation

Double flare technique was modified, whereby after preparing the coronal half, balanced force technique was used to prepare the middle and apical half. The preparation was followed by step-back technique to provide double flare in the preparation.

The preparation techniques are summarized in Table 16.2.

d. Rotary techniques

Various rotary instruments (files) of different designs have been utilized for root canal preparation. The details of rotary instrumentation are described in Chapter 11.

Table 16.2 Summary of the preparation techniques

Technique	*Key features*	*Advantages*	*Disadvantages*
Standardized technique	The file is inserted to the full working length cleaning the canal	Easy to prepare straight canals	Not suitable for curved canals (ledge formation, zipping, and perforation in curved canals)
Balanced forced technique	• Placement of file with a clockwise motion, gentle apical advancement • Counterclockwise rotation with gentle apical pressure • Clockwise rotation with coronal movement of file	• Better apical control of file • Less amount of extrusion of debris from canal • Good centering of instrument in the canal	• High incidence of procedural errors such as instrumental breakage and canal stripping • Time consuming
Step-back technique	Apical preparation is carried out with smaller files and sequentially the canal is prepared with increase in file size	• Greater flare facilitate dense obturation • Less chances of trauma to periapical tissues • Allows effective removal of debris • Apical matrix at apical area minimizes chances of over instrumentation and subsequently overfiling	• May lead to apical blockage (debris collected below the apical constriction area) • Alteration of working length • Tendency for canal deviation when using the larger inflexible instruments (Hour-glass preparation) • The H-file may cause overflaring or strip-perforation
Crown-down technique	The coronal portion of the canal is prepared first followed by the apical portion prepared with smaller files	• Less periapical extrusion of debris • Less apical zip formation • Less chances of ledge formation • Straight access to the apical region • Better penetration of the irrigant	Apical cleanliness is doubtful
Double flare technique	Involves preparing the canal in crown-down manner using K-files, followed by step-back manner	• Effectively remove the canal contents • Necrotic root dentin is effectively removed • Minimum iatrogenic errors • Facilitate compact obturation	Not suitable in canals with open apices

16

BIBLIOGRAPHY

1. Abou-Rass M, Frank A and Glick D. The anticurvature filling method to prepare the curved root canal. J. Am. Dent. Assoc.: 1980; 101:792–794.
2. Ahmad M, Pittford T and Crum L. Ultrasonic debridement of root canals: an insight into the mechanisms involved. J. Endod.: 1987; 13:93–101.
3. Ansari I and Maria R. Managing curved canal. Contemp. Clin. Dent.: 2012; 3:237–241.
4. Baugh D and Wallace J. The role of apical instrumentation in root canal treatment: a review of the literature. J. Endod.: 2005; 31:333–340.
5. Buchanan LS. The predefined preparation comes of age. Endod. Pract.: 2001; 4:6–18.
6. Buchanan LS. The standardized-taper root canal preparation. Part 1: concepts for variably tapered shaping instruments. Int. Endod. J.: 2000; 33:516–529.
7. Buchanan LS. The standardized-taper root canal preparation. Part 2: GT file selection and safe handpiece driven file use. Int. Endod. J.: 2001; 34:63–71.
8. Burklein S and Schafer E. Critical evaluation of root canal transportation by instrumentation. Endod. Topics: 2013; 29:110–124.
9. Carrotte P. Endodontics: Part 7. Preparing the root canal. Br. Dent. J.: 2004; 197:603–613.
10. Cassim I and Van der Vyver PJ. The importance of glide path preparation in endodontics: a consideration of instruments and literature. SADJ: 2013; 68:322, 324–327.
11. Charles TJ and Charles JE. The 'balanced force' concept for instrumentation of curved canals revisited. Int. Endod. J.: 1998; 31:166–172.
12. Dummer PM, McGinn JH and Rees DG. The position and topography of the apical root canal constriction and apical foramen. Int. Endod. J.: 1984; 17:192–198.
13. Fava LR. The double flared technique: an alternative for biomechanical preparation. J. Endod.: 1983; 9:76–80.
14. Habib AA, Taha MI and Farah EM. Methologies used in quality assessment of root canal preparation techniques: Review of the literature. J. Taibah Univ. Med. Sci.: 2015; 10:123–131.
15. Hulsman M, Peters OA and Dummer PMH. Mechanical preparation of root canals: Shaping of goals, techniques and means. Endod. Topic: 2005; 10:30–76.
16. Hung-Hong H, Sang WK, Sung-Kyo K and Hyeon-Cheol K. Screw-in forces during instrumentation by various file systems. Restor. Dent. Endod.: 2016; 41:304–309.
17. Ja JH, Cheung GS, Vrsluis S, Lee CJ, Kwak SW, and Kim HC. "Screw-in" tendency of rotary nickel-titanium files due to design geometry. Int. Endod. J.: 2015; 48:666–672.
18. Jafarzadeh H and Abbott PV. Dilaceration: review of an endodontic challenge. J. Endod.: 2007; 33:1025–1030.
19. Jafarzadeh H and Abbott PV. Ledge formation: Review of a great challenge in endodontics. J. Endod.: 2007; 33:1155–1162.
20. Juric IB and Anic I. The use of lasers in disinfection and cleaning of root canals: a review. Acta. Stomatol. Croat.: 2014; 48:6–15.
21. Kesler G, Gal R, Kesler A and Koren R. Histological and scanning electron microscope examination of root canal after preparation with Er: YAG laser microprobe: a preliminary in vitro study. J. Clin. Laser Med. Surg.: 2002; 20:269–277.
22. Kim HC, Sung SY, Ha JH, Solomonov M, Lee JM, Lee CJ and Kim BM. Stress generation during self-adjusting file movement: minimally invasive instrumentation. J. Endod.: 2013; 39:1572–1575.
23. Kyomen SM, Caputo AA and White SN. Critical analysis of the balanced force technique in endodontics. J. Endod.: 1994; 20:332–337.
24. Lambrianidis T. Ledging and blockage of root canals during canal preparation: Causes, recognition, prevention, management and outcomes. Endod. Topics: 2006; 15:56–74.
25. Lopez FU, Travessas JAC, Fachin E, Fontanella V and Grecca F. Apical transportation: two assessment methods. Aust. Endod. J.: 2009; 35:85–88.
26. Micket AK. The role of apical size determination and enlargement in reduction of intracanal bacteria. J. Endod.: 2007; 33:21–23.
27. Morgan LF and Montgomery S. An evaluation of the crown-down pressureless technique. J. Endod.: 1984; 10:491–498.
28. Mounce RE. New possibilities for managing severe curvature: the twisted file. Endod. Turbine: 2008; 9–12.
29. Olson DG, Roberts S, Joyce AP, Collins DE and McPherson JC. Unevenness of the apical constriction in human maxillary central incisors. J. Endod.: 2008; 34:157–159.
30. Peters OA, Bahia MG and Pereira ESJ. Contemporary root canal preparation: Innovation in biomechanics. Dent. Clinic. N. Am.: 2017; 61:37–58.
31. Peters OA. Current challenges and concepts in the preparation of root canal systems: a review. J. Endod.: 2004; 30:559–567.
32. Plotino G, Ahmed HM and Grande NM. Current assessment of reciprocation in endodontic preparation: a comprehensive review-part II: properties and effectiveness. J. Endod.: 2015; 41:1939–1950.
33. Plotino G, Pameijer CH, Grande NM and Somma F. Ultrasonics in endodontics: a review of literature. J. Endod.: 2007; 33:81–95.
34. Roane JB, Sabala CL and Duncanson MG. The 'balanced force' concept for instrumentation of curved canals. J. Endod.: 1987; 13:93–101.
35. Ruddle CJ. Current concepts for preparing the root canal system. Dent. Today: 2001; 1–9.
36. Ruddle CJ. Endodontic canal preparation: new innovations in glide path management and shaping canals. Dentistry: 2014; 33:1–7.
37. Sakkir N, Thaha KA, Nair MG, Joseph S and Christlin R. Management of dilacerated and S-shaped root canals – An endodontic challenge. J. Clin. Diagn. Res. 2014;8: ZD22–24.
38. Simon JHS. The apex: how critical is it? Gen. Dent.: 1994; 42:330–334.
39. Usman W, Baumgartner JC and Marshall JG. Influence of instrument size on root canal debridement. J. Endod.: 2004; 30:110–112.
40. West JD. The endodontic glidepath: "secret to rotary safety". Dent. Today: 2010; 29:86, 88, 90–93.
41. Wu MK, Barkis D, Roris A and Wasselink PR. Does the first file to bind correspond to the diameter of the canal in apical region? Int. Endod J.: 2002; 35:264–267.
42. Wu MK, Wesselink PR and Walton RE. Apical terminus location of root canal treatment procedures. O. Surg., O. Med., O. Path. 2000, 89, 99–103.

Chapter 17

Endodontic Smear Layer

Successful endodontic treatment depends upon thorough cleaning, shaping, disinfecting and obturation of root canals so as to achieve three-dimensional hermetic sealing of the pulp spaces. During mechanical preparation or whenever dentin is cut using hand or rotary instruments, the mineralized tissues are scattered producing considerable amount of debris. The debris so produced in the form of small particles of collagen matrix (composed of organic and inorganic material) is spread as an amorphous, irregular layer over dentinal surface, is known as *'smear layer'*. This layer primarily contains ground dentin, remnants of pulp tissue, odontoblastic processes and bacteria.

American Association of Endodontists defined smear layer as *'a surface film of debris retained on dentin or other surfaces after instrumentation with either rotary instruments or endodontic files; consists of dentin particles, remnants of vital or necrotic pulp tissue, bacterial components and retained irrigants'*. A few authors have described smear layer as 'organic matter trapped in translocated inorganic dentin'. McComb and Smith (1975) were the first researchers who described the presence of smear layer on surfaces of instrumented root canals in their Scanning Electron Microscopic study (Fig. 17.1a and b). The smear layer formed in cavities (coronal) and in the root canals is different. The instrumentation tools and procedures are different in coronal cavities; the dentinal tubules in root dentin show great variation and also the root canal contains pulp remnants and bacteria (odontoblastic processes, remnants of pulp tissue and bacteria present in root canal smear layer).

The thickness of smear layer depends on the type and sharpness of cutting instrument and also whether the cutting was carried out on dry or wet dentin.

The smear layer contents are described in two parts; the superficial smear layer and the smear layer where contents are packed into dentinal tubules. The superficial smear layer is estimated to be 1.0–2.5 µm in thickness; whereas, the smear layer contents may get packed into the dentinal tubules to a depth of 40 µm. The penetration of smear layer components into dentinal tubules could be caused by capillary action as a result of adhesive forces between the dentinal tubules and the smear contents, known as *'smear plugs'*.

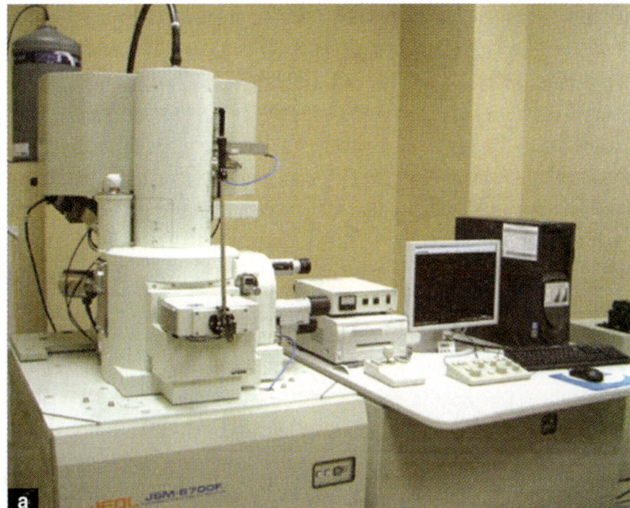

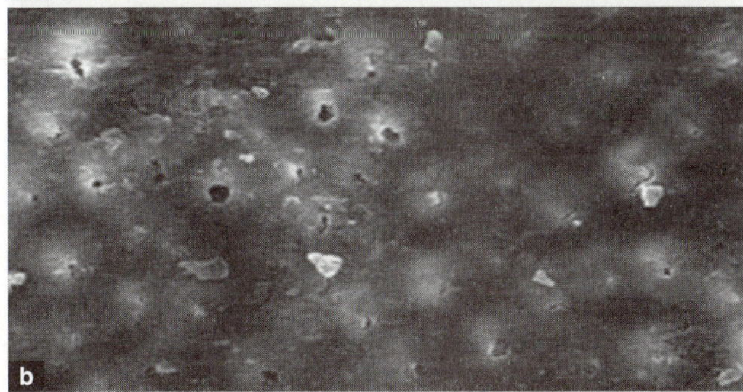

Fig. 17.1 (a) Scanning electron microscope; (b) Heavy smear layer

It has been established that the amount of smear layer produced during rotary instrumentation is far greater as compared to hand filing.

FACTORS INFLUENCING FORMATION OF SMEAR LAYER

The complexity of root canal system usually limits the efficacy of thorough cleaning the pulp spaces. The deviated root canal anatomy may pose difficulties in instrumentation, subsequently leading to unevenly prepared zones on root canal walls. These uneven zones may contribute to produce more of smear layer.

During instrumentation of root canal, dentin is cut by rotational and filing movements. Efficacy of cutting is dependent upon working dynamics, applied force, shape and size of the blade, instrument's axis configuration, etc. When dentinal chips are accumulated in flutes of the instrument, working effect is impaired and friction between instrument and canal walls is increased. The cutting effect is decreased, consequently larger amount of smear layer is formed (Fig. 17.2a and b).

A few studies have confirmed that manual instrumentation produced less smear layer as compared to the use of rotary instruments. Rotary preparation of root canal provide more effective instrumentation; however, higher speed may compact smear layer on the canal surface and into the dentinal tubules (Fig. 17.3a and b). It is established that sonic and ultrasonic preparation of root canal are the most efficient methods leading to only minor formation of smear layer. Massive irrigation directed towards working part on the instrument facilitates removal of dentin and prevents debris binding on the root canal walls. Preparation of root canal without irrigation causes up to 70% more stagnation of smear layer.

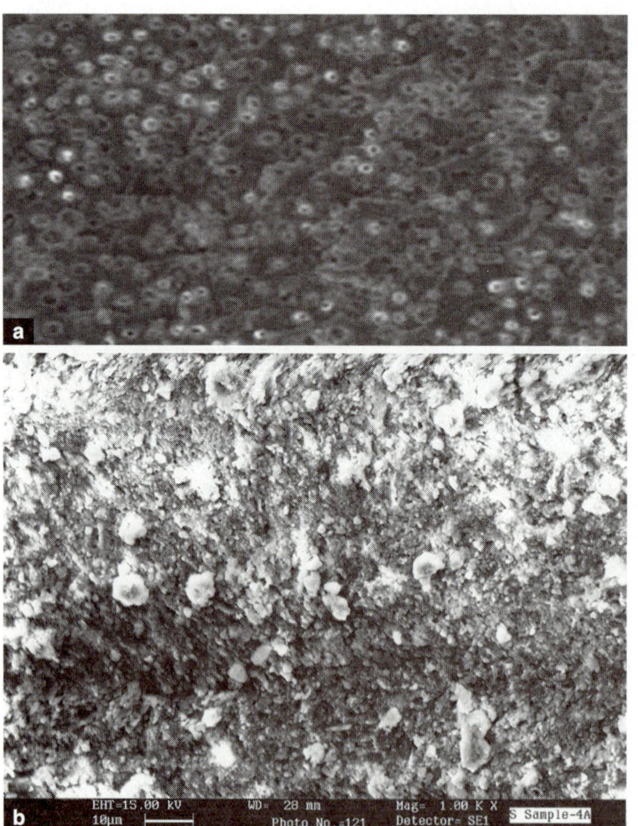

Fig. 17.2 (a) Smear layer in apical third area; (b) Generalized smear layer after instrumentation

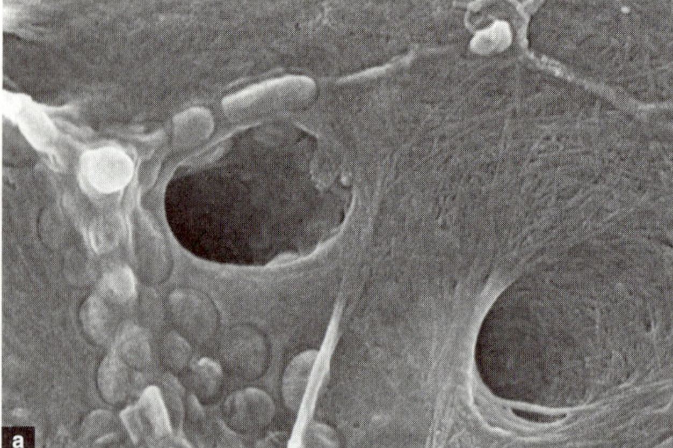

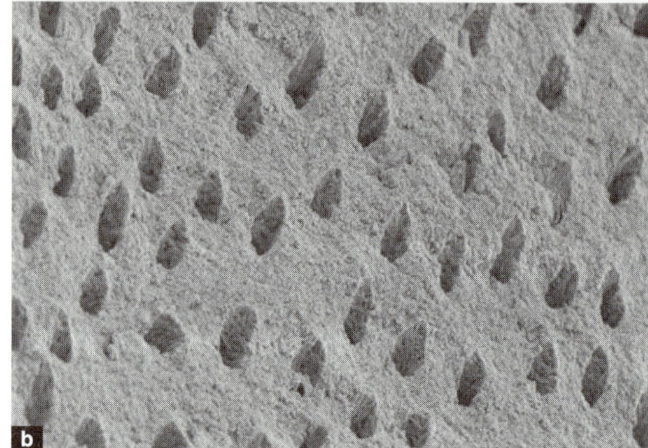

Fig. 17.3 (a) Smear layer after hand filing; (b) Smear layer after rotary instrumentation

It is demonstrated that significant stagnation of smear layer was observed following irrigation with standard needle; whereas,vent needle enable detaching of smear layer from root canal walls under pressure, thus making débridement more efficient. Most of irrigation solutions have physical (removal of smear layer) and chemical (dilute and demineralize) properties, subsequently enhancing permeability of radicular dentin.

The non-instrumentation technique of canal preparation may prepare the canal without producing smear layer. A hydrodynamic technique with sonically driven polymer instruments can disrupt the smear layer, the process known as *'hydrodynamic disinfection'*.

MANAGEMENT OF SMEAR LAYER

The management of smear layer in endodontics has always been controversial. Various investigators are of the view that maintaining the smear layer may block the dentinal tubules and limit bacterial or toxin penetration by altering dentinal permeability. Another school of belief is that the smear layer, being a loosely adherent structure, should be completely removed from the surface of root canal walls because it can harbor bacteria and provide an avenue for leakage. Further, it may also limit the effective disinfection of dentinal tubules by preventing intracanal medicaments from penetrating the dentinal tubules. Earlier studies have observed that the smear layer was not a complete barrier and could only delay bacterial penetration.

Majority of investigators favor removal of smear layer. The smear layer is non-homogenous and easily get dislodged from the underlying tubules. It slowly disintegrates and dissolves leaving a void between canal wall and the sealer.

It has been established that removing the smear layer enhanced the adaptation of gutta-percha in both cold and heat compacted obturation without a sealer. It is also confirmed that removal of smear layer improved the fluid-tight seal of the root canals; whereas, even modified obturating techniques might not be able to achieve effective results.

A few authors have observed that removal of smear layer did not prevent bacterial penetration along the root canal fillings.

Should the smear layer be removed or retained has always been a matter of concern amongst the investigators.

Features warrant the removal of smear layer are:

- Unpredictable thickness and volume.
- Mainly contains bacteria, their by-products and necrotic tissue.
- Act as a substrate for bacteria and may allow bacteria penetrating deeper in the dentinal tubules.
- May limit the penetration of disinfecting agents into the dentinal tubules. Bacteria present deep within dentinal tubules may not be disinfected because of smear layer. It is established that following the removal of the smear layer, bacteria in dentinal tubules can easily be destroyed.
- Act as a barrier between filling materials and the canal wall, compromising achieving the hermetic seal. The sealers can penetrate dentinal tubules only if the smear layer is removed. It is documented that coronal leakage of root canal fillings was less in smear-free cases than those with smear layer.
- Being loosely adherent structure, it is a potential avenue for leakage between root canal obturated material and the dentinal walls.

Features warrant the retention of smear layer are:

- Smear layer block the dentinal tubules, preventing the exchange of bacteria and other irritants by altering their permeability.
- It serves as a barrier to prevent bacterial migration into dentinal tubules.
- A few authors have observed that bacteria remaining after root canal preparation were sealed into dentinal tubules by smear layer and subsequent filling materials.

Removal of the Smear Layer

It is established that the smear layer may be infected and also protect the bacteria already present in the dentinal tubules. It is wiser to remove the initially created smear layer in infected root canals and to allow penetration of intracanal medicaments into the dentinal tubules. The smear layer can be removed using mechanical, chemical, ultrasonic and by means of laser.

a. Mechanical Removal

The smear layer removal has been tried using mechanical means. The mechanical removal of smear layer includes:

i. *Microbrush (canal brush)*: A microbrush (canal brush), has been specifically fabricated for root canal cleaning. The brush is available in three sizes, small, medium and large, corresponding to apical diameter of 25, 30 and 40 respectively. The brush is used along with the irrigating solution, being revolved at a slow speed. However, it did not provide any added advantage as regard removal of smear layer. The appropriate size of the brush is the main parameter, which is difficult to coincide with the canal configuration. Studies have confirmed that smear layer removal would be because of the 'irrigant' used in the root canal, rather than the action of brush. However, various investigators have confirmed that the use of flexible microbrushes can reduce debris and remove smear layer from the root canal walls.

ii. *XP-endo finisher*: It is established that rotary Ni-Ti files during instrumentation come into contact with only 40–50% of the canal walls; therefore, large portion of the root canal wall remain untreated. XP-endo finisher is a modified Ni-Ti file without taper and of small diameter (25/.00). Due to its specific design, it can reach the inaccessible areas of the canal wall and efficiently remove the smear layer. The file has added advantage of changing the shape during rotation in the root canal, which effectively remove dentin debris and smear layer.

b. Chemical Removal

A number of chemicals used as irrigants have been tried to remove the smear layer. Various irrigating solutions have the potential to remove the debris and smear layer created by the instrumentation process. The solution commonly used to remove smear layer are:

i. *Sodium hypochlorite/chlorhexidine*: Sodium hypochlorite is known for its potential to dissolve organic tissues; however, it cannot effectively remove smear layer from the instrumented root canal walls. The combination of sodium hypochlorite and hydrogen peroxide was also ineffective; however, alternating use of sodium hypochlorite with EDTA was effective in smear layer removal. Chlorhexidine, has antibacterial effect, but not dissolve organic debris and is also ineffective in smear layer removal.

ii. *Ethylenediaminetetra-acetic acid (EDTA)*: The most common chelating solutions are EDTA based, which reacts with calcium ions in the dentin and forms soluble calcium chelates. EDTA can decalcify dentin to a depth of 20–30 µ in five minutes (Fig. 17.4a to d). The timings of EDTA application is important, otherwise EDTA remains ineffective, especially in apical third area of root canals. The alternate use of 17% EDTA and 5.25% sodium hypochlorite removes smear layer completely from coronal and middle thirds; however, less effective in apical third areas (EDTA removes the inorganic component and sodium hypochlorite removes the organic part). As regard smear layer removal, ethylene-glycol tetra-acetic acid (EGTA) was comparable to EDTA.

A quaternary ammonium bromide (cetavlon) has been added to EDTA solutions to reduce surface tension and increase penetrability of the solution; the solution is called EDTAC. EDTA and cetavlon (EDTAC) solution has been effective in removing smear layer (to be kept in root canals for 15 minutes for effective results). However, chelating/penetrating effect remained negligible in apical third area. It has been established that paste-type chelating agents, having lubricating effect, do not remove smear layer effectively as compared to liquid EDTA.

A combination of bis-dequalinium-acetate and EDTA (Solvidont) has shown effective potential to remove the smear layer, even in the apical third area.

iii. *Tetracyclines*: Tetracyclines including doxycycline and minocycline are effective against a wide range of microorganisms. They have low pH in concentrated solution and act as a calcium chelator; may cause root surface demineralization. They are effective in removing smear layer from the surface of instrumented canals

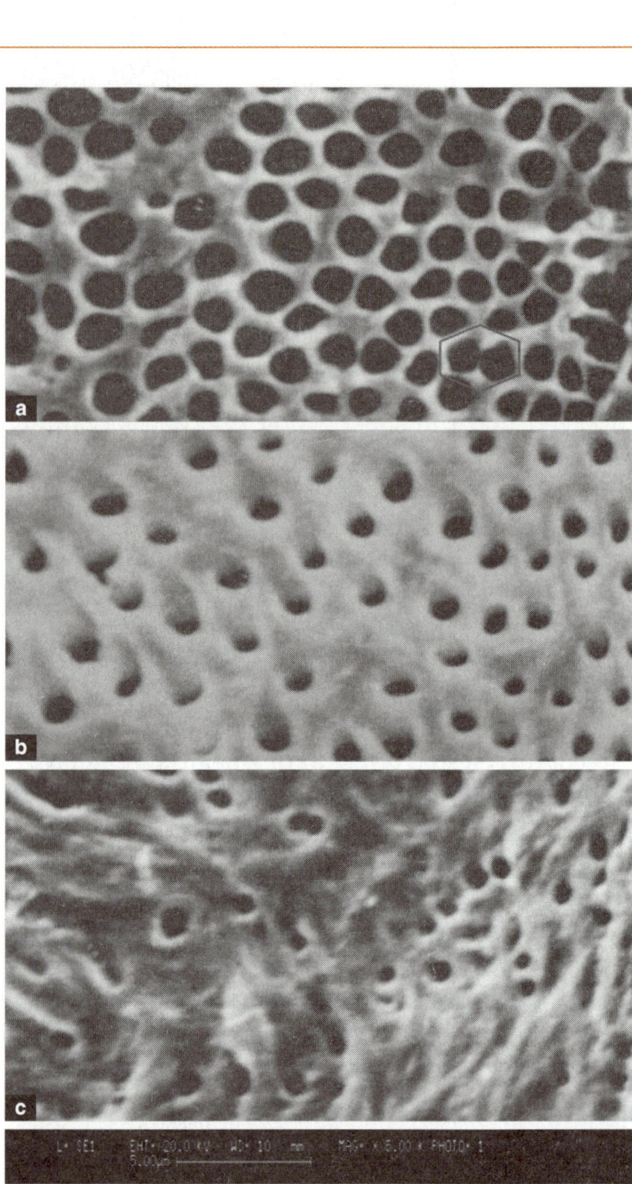

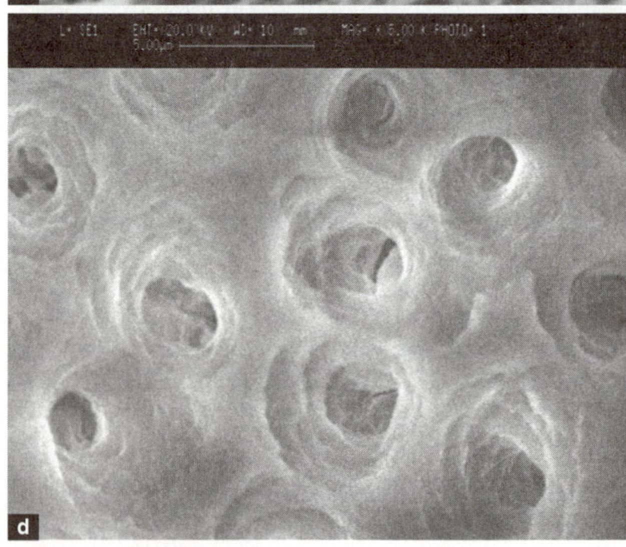

Fig. 17.4 (a) Absence of smear layer in coronal third after using EDTA; (b) Absence of smear layer in middle third after using EDTA; (c) Presence of smear layer in apical third after using EDTA; (d) Erosion of peritubular and intertubular dentin caused by EDTA

and root-end cavity preparations. It is speculated that a reservoir of active antibacterial solution might remain sticking to root canal walls because doxycycline readily attaches to root dentin and is released subsequently.

iv. *MTAD*: MTAD, an irrigating solution, containing mixture of tetracyclines, a detergent and an acid (3.0% doxycycline hyclate, 4.25% citric acid and 0.5% polysorbate detergent) was developed having potential of removing smear layer and also disinfecting the root canals. Various studies have observed that MTAD demineralized dentin faster than 17% EDTA (Fig. 17.5a to c).

v. *QMix*: QMix 2 in 1 is a new irrigation solution that facilitates smear layer removal and also provides disinfection. The solution contains a mixture of bisguanide (antimicrobial agent), polyaminocarboxylic acid (a calcium chelating agent) and a surfactant. The use of QMix 2 in 1 saves time as compared to sequential use of 17% EDTA and 2.0% chlorhexidine. The solution provides fair activity against bacteria and also an effective irrigation in 60 to 90 seconds. The manufacturers advocate its use as the final rinse before obturation. Various studies have confirmed the superior effect of QMix as compared to 17% EDTA (Fig. 17.6a to c).

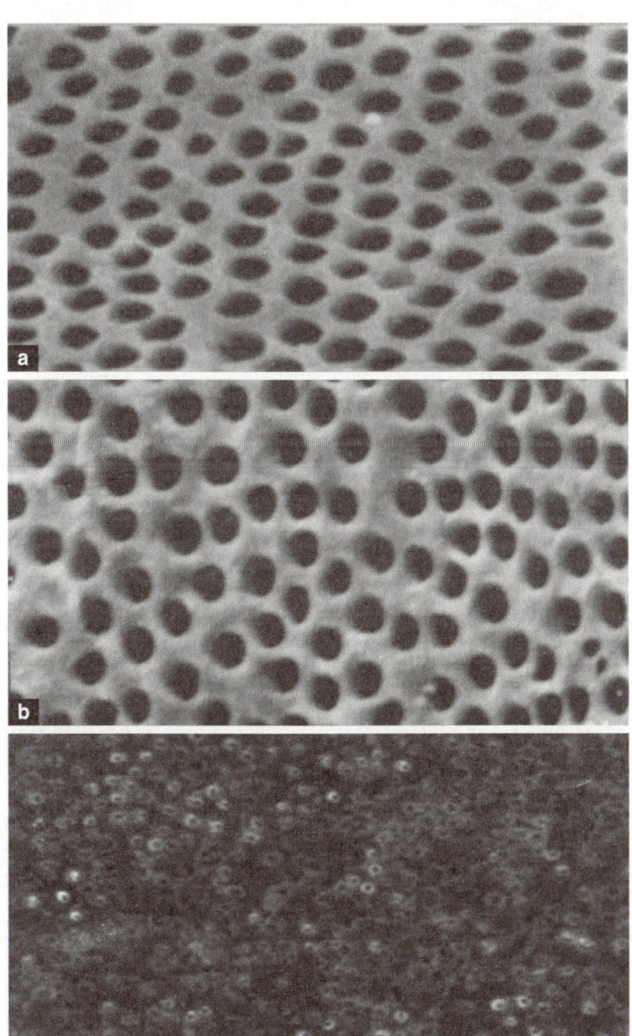

Fig. 17.5 (a) Absence of smear layer in coronal third after using MTAD; (b) Absence of smear layer in middle third after using MTAD; (c) Presence of smear layer in apical third after using MTAD

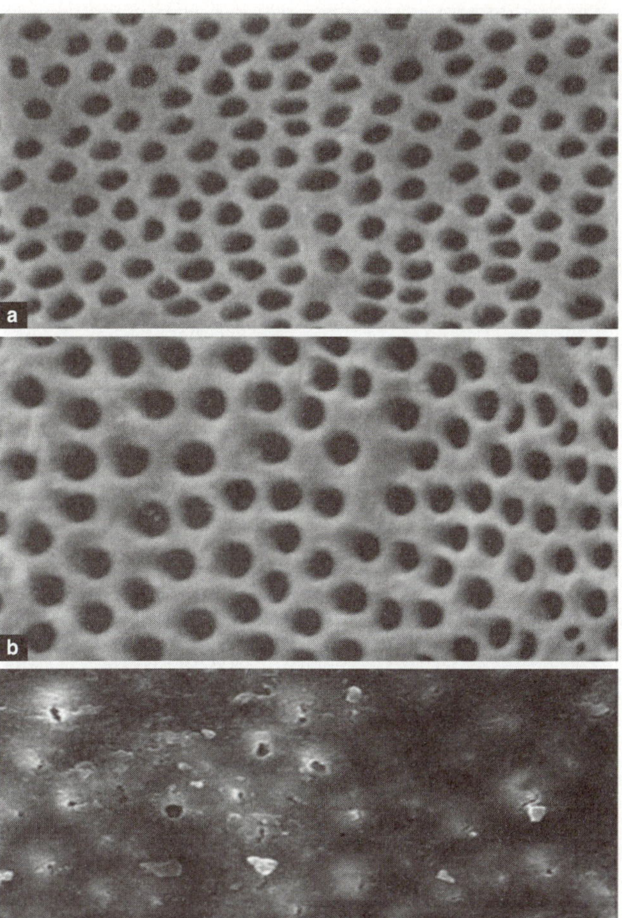

Fig. 17.6 (a) Absence of smear layer in coronal third after using QMix; (b) Absence of smear layer in middle third after using QMix; (c) Presence of smear layer in apical third after using QMix

A few authors observed that the smear layer removal and antimicrobial effects of QMix was comparable to EDTA. QMix is considered effective against *Enterococcus faecalis* (QMix has low surface tension; wettability of dentin is effectively achieved with QMix).

vi. *Organic acids*: The effectiveness of mild acids as a root canal irrigant has been demonstrated. Citric acid, polyacrylic acid, lactic acid and phosphoric acid are being used to remove smear layer. Citric acid is considered better than the other acids used (Fig. 17.7a and b).

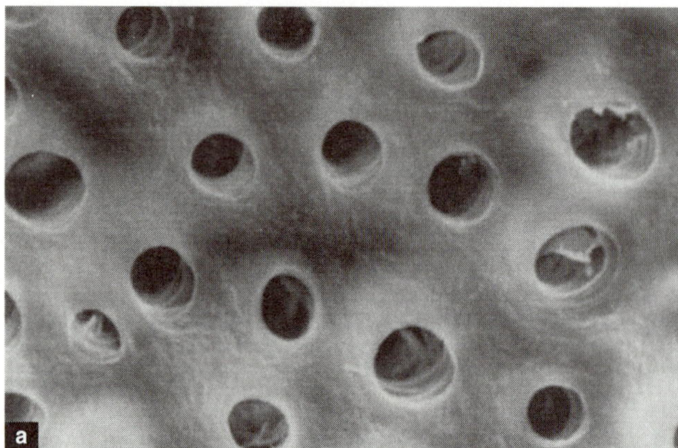

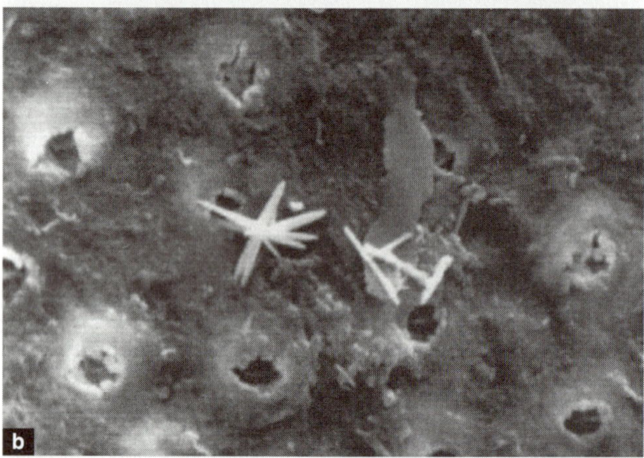

Fig. 17.7 (a) Root canal dentin treated with citric acid demonstrating open dentinal tubules; (b) Precipitate of citric acid formed on the root canal dentin

Sequential use of 10% citric acid and 2.5% sodium hypochlorite solution is considered as a better combination. A few authors have observed that citric acid-sodium hypochlorite combination was not as effective as citric acid-EDTA combination. It is emphasized that the quality of smear layer removal is related to pH and time of exposure of the acids.

Five to ten percent polyacrylic acid as an irrigant is effective in removing smear layer in accessible regions. 40% polyacrylic acid has been reported to be very effective; however, it is advised to use it for 30 seconds only. 50% lactic acid was less effective than 50% citric acid for removal of smear layer (attributed to viscosity of lactic acid). 25% tannic acid has also been used successfully in eradicating smear layer (Fig. 17.8).

vii. *Super-oxide water (oxum)*: Super-oxide water is a powerful antimicrobial agent against bacteria, fungi and viruses. It is rich in reactive oxygen and has neutral pH. Super-oxidized water, commercially available as oxum, is stable and has longer shelf-life. The free radicals (oxygen anion) of this solution rapidly damage the cell wall protein of the microorganisms.

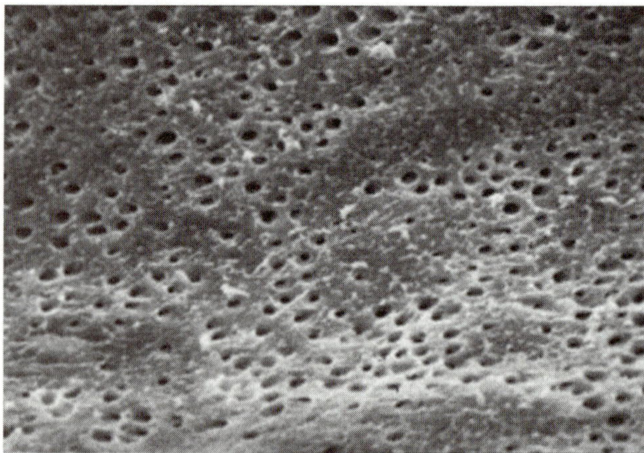

Fig. 17.8 Partial removal of smear layer in the apical third of the root canal by tannic acid

It effectively removes the smear layer when used as root canal irrigant. Various studies have observed that the efficacy of super-oxidised water was comparable to 17% EDTA, with significantly less erosion of dentinal surface.

viii. *Chitosan*: Chitosan, a natural polysaccharide, has broad-spectrum of antimicrobial properties and also has chelating characteristics. It shows excellent biocompatibility, high bioactivity, biodegradability, absorption capacity and low toxicity. Chitosan compounds (chitosan nitrate and chitosan acetate) alone and in combination with chlorhexidine have effectively removed smear layer from the root canal walls. 0.6% chitosan has also been used as dentin conditioning agent, producing smooth, wide open dentinal tubules.

Various studies have confirmed the use of 0.2 to 0.6% chitosan when irrigated for three minutes, adequately removed the smear layer. It has also been reported that it caused less erosion of dentin as compared to EDTA. A few studies showed that chitosan and their derivatives interacted with metalloproteinase matrix, improving the resistance of dentin to degradation.

ix. *Smear clear*: A recently introduced chelating agent, smear clear contains 17% EDTA and two surfactants (polyoxyethylene and isobutyl cyclohexyl phthalate ether).

A few studies comparing efficacy of smear clear and 17% EDTA in removing smear layer have observed similar performance in smear layer removal from coronal and middle third of the root canals; however, in apical third, smear clear showed significantly better results as compared to 17% EDTA. Smear clear has low surface tension and improved dentin-wettability, facilitating easy flow into narrow canals. This property

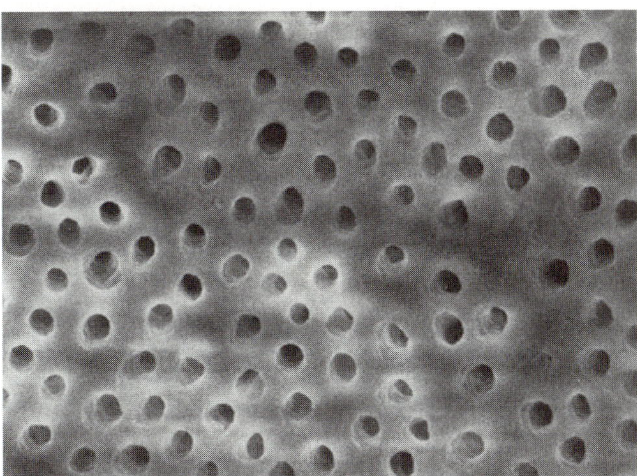

Fig. 17.9 Root canal dentin treated with smear clear demonstrating clean open dentinal tubules devoid of smear layer and debris

might be the probable reason for better removal of smear layer from the apical third area of root canals (Fig. 17.9).

As regards timings, most of the irrigants are effective only at longer duration time (5.25% sodium hypochlorite and 17% EDTA need minimum of 3–5 minute to be effective); whereas, smear clear is effective in one minute application. Ankur Dua et al (2015) in their SEM study, evaluating the effect of duration of application of smear clear in removing intracanal smear layer, observed that final irrigation with smear clear or 17% EDTA followed by 1.0% sodium hypochlorite were effective in removing smear layer for all duration of applications (one minute, 3 minutes and 5 minutes).

c. Ultrasonic

Sodium hypochlorite activated by the ultrasonic delivery system when used as an irrigant provided smear-free root canal surfaces. Varying concentration of sodium hypochlorite (1.0–5.0%) when used with ultrasonic energy, has been effective in removing smear layer.

Studies comparing the effect of different ultrasonic irrigation periods on removing smear layer, observed that smear layer removal was effective in 3–5 minute timings, whereas, one minute was ineffective. A few authors have even reported no effect of ultrasonics on smear layer removal (ultrasonically energized sodium hypochlorite, even at full concentration was ineffective in smear layer removal). It is advised to use EDTA/EDTAC with sodium hypochlorite using ultrasonic streaming to achieve desired results.

d. Lasers

Lasers are being used to vaporize necrotic tissues and debris in the root canals. The effectiveness of laser depends on many factors; viz. wavelength of laser, the duration of exposure and absorption in the tissue, the geometry of root canal and the conductors. Almost all types of lasers effectively remove the smear layer.

The most commonly used laser in endodontics is Neodium: Yttrium-Aluminium-Garnet (Nd:YAG) having wavelength of 1064 nm. The wavelength, being in the near-infrared range, the flexible conductor can effectively be used in narrow and curved canals, providing bactericidal effect and removing the smear layer.

Erbium-Yttrium-Aluminium-Garnet (Er:YAG) having wavelength of 2940 nm is used for cleaning and shaping of root canals. When applied in the canal, the water of the hard tissue inside evaporates and ablates the surrounding tissues. The increase in temperature on the root surface is within the acceptable limits.

Various studies have observed that the removal of smear layer with Er:YAG laser is greater as compared to removal with Nd:YAG laser (energy of Er:YAG laser is absorbed by water, the water evaporates and ablates the molecules of dentinal surface; whereas, Nd:YAG laser is poorly absorbed by water and is absorbed by proteins of the tissues).

The main difficulty with laser removal is access to narrow canals (root canal intricacies) with the availability of relatively large probes for delivery of laser beam. A few authors have also observed destruction of peritubular dentin along with removal of smear layer.

The main difficulty with laser is the access to small root canal areas. Laser probe is relatively large; however, flexible conductors are now available with a tip of 300 μm for inaccessible areas.

BIBLIOGRAPHY

1. Amaral P, Forner L and Llena C. Smear layer removal in canals shaped with reciprocating rotary systems. J. Clin. Exp. Dent.: 2013; 5:227–230.
2. Andrabi SM, Kumar A, Mishra SK, Tewari RK, Alam S and Siddiqui S. Effect of manual dynamic activation on smear layer removal efficacy of ethylene diamine tetra-acetic acid and smear clear: an *in vitro* scanning electron microscopic study. Aust. Endod. J.: 2013; 39:131–136.
3. Calt S and Serper A. Smear layer removal by EGTA. J. Endod.: 2000; 26:459–461.
4. Cameron JA. The use of ultrasound for the removal of the smear layer. The effect of sodium hypochlorite concentration: SEM study. Aust. Dent. J.: 1988; 33:193–200.
5. Card SJ, Sigurdsson S, Orstavik D and Trope M. The effectiveness of increased apical enlargement in reducing intracanal bacteria. J. Endod.: 2002; 28:779–783.

6. Caron G, Nham K, Bronnec F and Machtou P. Effectiveness of different final irrigant activation protocols on smear layer removal in curved canals. J. Endod.: 2010; 36:1361–1366.
7. da Silva LA, Sanguino AC, Rocha CT, Leonardo MR and Silva RA. Scanning electron microscopic preliminary study of the efficacy of smear clear and EDTA for smear layer removal after root canal instrumentation in permanent teeth. J. Endod.: 2008; 34:1541–1544.
8. Dechichi P and Moura CCG. Smear layer: a brief review of general concepts. Part I. Characteristics, compounds, structure, bacteria and sealing. RFO UPF: 2006; 11:96–99.
9. De-Deus G, Reis C, Fiedel S, Fiedel R and Paciornik S. Dentin demineralization when subjected to BioPure MTAD: a longitudinal and quantitative assessment. J. Endod.: 2007; 33:1364–1368.
10. Del Carpio-Perochena A, Bramante C, Duarte M, de Moura M, Aouada F and Kishen A. Chelating and antibacterial properties of chitosan nanoparticles on dentin. Restor. Dent. Endod.: 2015; 40:195–201.
11. Divito E, Peters OA and Olivi G. Effectiveness of the Erbium: YAG laser and new design radial and stripped tips in removing the smear layer after root canal instrumentation. Lasers Med. Sci.: 2012; 27:273–280.
12. Dotto SR, Travassos RM, de Oliveira MP, de Lima Machado E and Martins L. Evaluation of ethylendiaminetetraacetic acid (EDTA) solution and gel for smear layer removal. Aust. Endod. J.: 2007; 33:1–4.
13. Dua A, Dua D and Uppin VM. Evaluation of the effect of duration of application of smear clear in removing intracanal smear layer: SEM study. Saudi Endod. J.: 2015; 5:26–32.
14. Eliot C, Hatton JF, Stewart GP, Hildebolt CF, Jane GM and Gutmann JL. The effect of the irrigantQMix on removal of canal wall smear layer: An *ex vivo* study. Odontology: 2014; 102:232–240.
15. Fachin EVF, Scarparo RK and Massoni LIS. Influence of smear layer removal on the obturation of root canal ramifications. J. Appl. Oral Sci.: 2009; 17:240–243.
16. Garip Y, Sazak H and Hatipoglu GM. Evaluation of smear layer removal after use of a canal brush: an SEM study. Oral Surg., Oral Med., Oral Pathol., Oral Radiol. Endod.: 2010; 110:62–66.
17. Gusiyska A, Dyulgerova E, Vassileva R and Gyulbenkiyan E. The effectiveness of a Chitosna-Citrate solution to remove the smear layer in root canal treatment—an *in vitro* study. Int. J. Sci. Resch.: 2016; 5:1169–1174.
18. Kamel WH and Kataia EM. Comparison of the efficacy of smear clear with and without a canal brush in smear layer and debris removal from instrumented root canal using WaveOne versus Pro Taper: a scanning electron microscopic study. J. Endod.: 2014; 40:446–450.
19. Keles A, Kamalak A, Keskin C, Akcay M and Uzun I. The efficacy of laser, ultrasound and self-adjustable file in removing smear layer debris from oval root canals following retreatment: a scanning electron microscopy study. Aust. Endod. J.: 2016; 1–8.
20. Khedmat S and Shokouhinejad N. Comparison of the efficacy of three chelating agents in smear layer removal. J. Endod.: 2008; 34:599–602.
21. Lui JN, Kuah HG and Chen NN. Effect of EDTA with and without surfactants or ultrasonics on removal of smear layer. J. Endod.: 2007; 33:472–475.
22. Mancini M, Armellin E, Casaglia A, Cerroni L and Cianconi L. A comparative study of smear layer removal and erosion in apical intraradicular dentine with three irrigating solutions: a scanning electron microscopy evaluation. J. Endod.: 2009; 35:900–903.
23. Mandorah A. Effect of irrigating needle depth in smear layer removal: Scanning electron microscope study. Saudi Endod. J.: 2013; 3:114–119.
24. Mello I, Coil J and Antoniazzi JH. Does a final rinse to remove smear layer interfere on dentin permeability of root canals? Oral Surg., Oral Med., Oral Pathol., Oral Radiol. Endod.: 2009; 107:e47–51.
25. O'Connell M, Morgan L, Beeler W and Baumgartner C. A comparative study of smear layer removal using different salts of EDTA. J. Endod.: 2000; 26:739–743.
26. Perez-Heredia M, Ferrer-Luque CM, Gonzalez-Rodriguez MP, Martin-Peinado FJ and Gonzalez-Lopez S. Decalcifying effect of 15% EDTA, 15% citric acid, 5% phosphoric acid and 2.5% sodium hypochlorite on root canal dentin. Int. Endod. J.: 2008; 41:418–423.
27. Periera RS, Miranda PF, Pereira GS, Barroso JM, Bortolotti MGL and Junqueira JLC. Effectiveness of 17% EDTA in the removal of smear layer and calcium hydroxide dressing from the root canal walls. Rev. Gaucha Odontol.: 2013; 61:313–317.
28. Pimento J, Zaparolli D, Pecora J and Cruz-Filho A. Chitosan: effect of a new chelating agent on the microhardness of root dentin. Braz. Dent. J.: 2012; 23:212–217.
29. Protogerou E, Arvaniti I, Vlachos I and Khabbaz MG. Effectiveness of a canal brush on removing smear layer: a scanning electron microscopy study. Braz. Dent. J.: 2013; 24:580–584.
30. Rathakrishnan M, Sukumaran VG and Subbiya A. To evaluate the efficacy of an innovative irrigant on smear layer removal – SEM analysis. J. Clin. Diagn. Res.: 2016; 10:104–106.
31. Reza B, Mohsen HS, Elham F, Mina N and Sara N. Evaluation of root canal smear layer removal by two types of lasers: A scanning electron microscopy study. Eur. J. Gen. Dent.: 2013; 2:151–157.
32. Schoop U, Moritz A, Kluger W, Patruta S, Goharkhay K and Sperr W. The Er:YAG laser in endodontics: Results of an *in vitro* study. Lasers Surg. Med.: 2002; 30:360–364.
33. Silva P, Guedes D, Nakadi F, Pecora J and Cruz-Filho A. Chitosan: a new solution for removal of smear layer after root canal instrumentation. Int. Endod.: 2013; 46:332–338.
34. Spano JC, Silva RG, Guedes DF, Sousa-Neto MD, Estrela C and Pecora JD. Atomic absorption spectrometry and scanning electron microscopy evaluation of calcium ions and smear layer removal with root canal chelators. J. Endod.: 2009; 35:727–730.

35. Stojicic S, Shen Y, Qian W, Johnson B and Haapasalo M. Antibacterial and smear layer removal ability of a novel irrigant, QMix. Int. Endod. J.: 2012; 45:363–371.

36. Timpawat S, Vongsavan N and Messer HH. Effect of removal of the smear layer on apical microleakage. J. Endod.: 2001; 27:351–353.

37. Torabinejad M, Handysides R, Khademi AA and Bakland LK. Clinical implications of the smear layer in endodontics: a review. Oral Surg., Oral Med., Oral Pathol., Oral Radiol. Endod.: 2002; 94:658–666.

38. Torbabinejad M, Khademi AA and Babgoli J. A new solution for the removal of smear layer. J. Endod.: 2003; 29:170–175.

39. Uroz-Torres D, Gonzalez-Rodriguez MP and Ferrer-Luque CM. Effectiveness of the EndoActivator System in removing the smear layer after root canal instrumentation. J. Endod.: 2010; 36:308–311.

40. Vemuri S, Kolanu SK, Varri S, Pabbati RK, Penumaka R and Bolla N. Effect of different final irrigating solutions on smear layer removal in apical third of root canal: A scanning electron microscope study. J. Conserv. Dent.: 2016; 19:87–90.

41. Violich DR and Chandler NP. The smear layer in endodontics – a review. Int. Endod. J.: 2010; 43:2–15.

42. Vlad R, Kovacs M, Sita D and Pop M. Comparison between different endodontic irrigating protocols in smear layer removal from radicular dentin. Eur. Sci. J.: 2016; 12:38–43.

43. Zargar N, Dianat O, Asnaashan M, Ganjali M and Zadsirjan S. The effect of smear layer on antimicrobial efficacy of three root canal irrigants. Iran. Endod. J.: 2015; 10:179–183.

44. Zivkovic S, Neskovic J, Jovanovic-Medojevic M, Popovic-Bajic M and Zivkovic-Sandic M. XP-Endo Finisher: A new solution for smear layer removal. Serbian Dent. J.: 2015; 62:122–126.

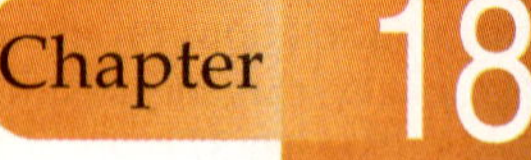

Chapter 18

Root Canal Irrigants and Medicaments

Microorganisms and their toxic products are the main etiological factors in pulpal and periapical pathology. The main aim of endodontic treatment is the elimination of bacteria and their by-products from the infected root canal. Instrumentation and irrigation are important procedures involved in the physical removal of microorganisms from the root canal system, subsequently controlling endodontic infection. Irrigation is defined as *'to wash out body cavity or wound with saline or medicated solutions'*.

The morphology of pulp cavity is of the most complex nature. It is unrealistic to assume that a linear streamlined instrument can reach out into the delicate intricacies of the pulp spaces to effectively débride its contents. The effective use of an irrigant can clean areas of the webs, deltas, fins and anastomoses in the root canal.

Irrigants are used during root canal preparation to help lubricate canal walls, soften dentin, remove debris and smear layer, dissolve organic matter, flush out microorganisms and their by-products, and clean areas inaccessible to endodontic instruments.

Over the years, a variety of solutions have been used during root canal treatment. These include hot water, coconut water, physiologic saline, local anesthetic solution, urea and urea peroxide in glycerine, hydrogen peroxide, chlorhexidine sodium hypochlorite, ethylenediaminetetra-acetic acid (EDTA), BioPure/MTAD and various plant extracts. Recently, ozonated water, bioactive glasses, nanosilver and various acids are also being used as irrigating agents.

Objectives

The primary objectives of root canal irrigation are:

- Reduction of intraradicular microorganisms and neutralization of endotoxins in an infected canal.
- Dissolution of vital or necrotic pulp tissue, to remove pulpal remnants from accessory canals and other irregularities where the instruments cannot reach.
- Lubrication of canal walls and instruments.
- Removal of dentin debris and smear layer produced by instrumentation, by physical flushing action.

Requisites for an Ideal Irrigant

Based on the objectives, the ideal irrigant should have the following requisites:

- Should be non-toxic and non-carcinogenic to tissues (should not induce cell-mediated immune response)
- Broad antimicrobial spectrum and high efficacy against anaerobic and facultative microorganisms organized in necrotic pulp spaces
- Tissue dissolving ability; should dissolve remaining pulp/organic tissues
- Biocompatible
- Low surface tension (better wetting potential)
- Low neutralizability (should not get nullified by canal components)
- Non-irritating to periapical tissues (should not interfere with periapical healing)
- Able to remove the smear layer
- Should not affect the sealing ability of obturating materials
- Should not damage the root canal dentin
- Easy availability
- Cost-effective
- Convenient for usage
- Good shelf-life and easy storage.

Currently, there is no single irrigant that can fulfill all the required criteria. Therefore, combinations of various irrigants are suggested for getting the desired results.

Classification

There is no definite classification of irrigating solutions. Various authors have classified irrigating solutions; the accepted ones are:

a. Tagger's Classification

Tagger's classification is based on functions, as:

i. *Working solutions* (solutions having certain specific function, such as tissue dissolution/chelation; used in smaller quantities and for a longer time).

ii. *Irrigants* (solutions mainly meant for physically flushing out the debris; used in larger quantities).

b. Stock's Classification

Stock's classification is based on chemical activity of the irrigants, as:

i. *Chemically inactive solutions,* viz. water, saline and local anesthetic solution

ii. *Chemically active solutions,* viz. alkalis, acids, chelators, oxidisers, antibacterials, detergents and enzymes.

c. Walton's Classification

Walton's classification is based on functions of irrigants, as:

i. Irrigants

ii. Dentin softners
- Chelators
- Decalcifiers

iii. Lubricants

iv. Desiccants.

d. Sikri's Classification

The classification of irrigants as proposed by the author is described in Flowchart 18.1.

COMMONLY USED IRRIGANTS

1. Normal Saline

Normal saline is a chemically inactive irrigant. Its main action is to physically flush out debris from the root canal. It also provides minor lubrication. Since, it is very mild in action, it can be used as an adjunct to chemical irrigants. It is preferably used as final rinse to remove any chemical agent left after root canal preparation and irrigation.

Advantages
- Biocompatible
- No adverse reaction, even if extruded periapically, because of its isotonicity to blood.

Disadvantage
- Does not perform other desired functions of an irrigant, like disinfection, tissue dissolution, removal of smear layer, etc.

2. Sodium Hypochlorite

Sodium hypochlorite is a clear, pale, green-yellow liquid with strong odor of chlorine. Sodium hypochlorite

Flowchart 18.1: Classification of irrigants

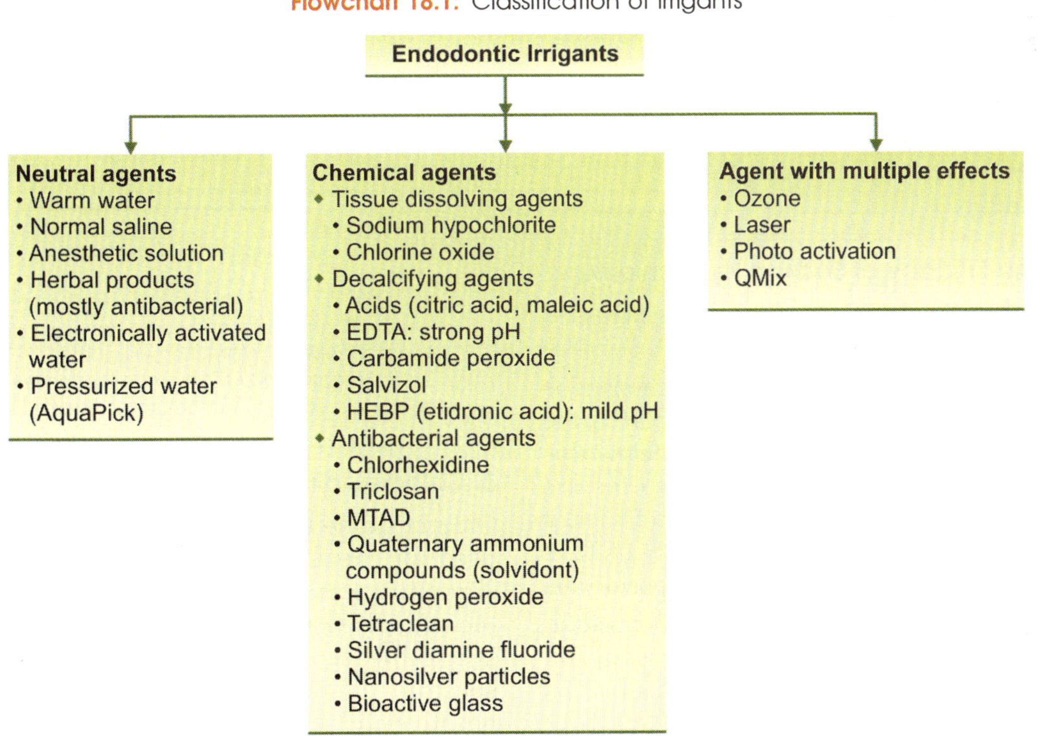

solutions have been used as wound irrigants since long and also as an endodontic irrigant. 1.0–5.25% sodium hypochlorite solutions are being used as irrigant depending upon the requirements.

Sodium hypochlorite is a reducing agent having 5.0% available chlorine. It is highly alkaline with a pH of 11–11.5.

Properties

i. *Proteolytic action*: It is a hydrolyzing agent and can dissolve pulp within 20 minutes to two hours. The removal of organic tissue by sodium hypochlorite is by the release of hypochlorous acid, which reacts with insoluble proteins to form soluble polypeptides, amino acids and other by-products.
ii. *Bactericidal and virucidal*: When sodium hypochlorite comes in contact with organic debris/pulp tissue, hypochlorous acid is formed. The latter is able to penetrate the bacterial cell, oxidizes the sulfhydryl groups of the bacterial enzymes and disrupts the metabolism, which eventually leads to their death.
iii. *Alkalinity*: Sodium hypochlorite has a high pH of 11–11.5, which is effective in eliminating anaerobes.

Disadvantages

- Causes mild to severe cellular damage
- Toxic if extruded beyond the apex (severity depends upon the concentration and volume)
- High surface tension, which decreases its dentin wetting capacity
- Caustic and can cause inflammation of gingival tissue and skin, when in contact
- Unpleasant taste and odor
- Vapors can irritate the eyes
- May corrode root canal instruments
- Not effective against *Enterococcus faecalis*
- Not substantive.

Increasing the Efficacy of Sodium Hypochlorite

The efficacy of sodium hypochlorite can be increased by any of the following methods:

i. *Altering the pH*: The state of available chlorine is dependent on pH of the solution; above pH 7.6, the predominant form is hypochlorite and below this value, it is hypochlorous acid. Both forms are extremely reactive oxidizing agents. The efficiency of pure hypochlorite solution having pH of 12 is better than the routinely used sodium hypochlorite.
ii. *Heating (increase in temperature)*: The increase in temperature of sodium hypochlorite solution improves its efficiency, mainly the tissue-dissolution capacity. Further, the heated hypochlorite solutions remove organic debris more efficiently as compared to cold solution. It is established that the tissue dissolving efficacy of 1.0% sodium hypochlorite at 45°C is as good as 5.25% sodium hypochlorite at 20°C.
iii. *Use of ultrasonics*: The use of ultrasonic agitation increases the effectiveness of sodium hypochlorite especially in the apical third of the root canal. Passive ultrasonic activation with a Ni-Ti tip has shown to produce superior tissue-dissolving effects as compared to sonic activation.
iv. *Volume and concentration*: It is established that higher concentration of sodium hypochlorite (5.25%) has more tissue dissolving activity than lower concentration (0.5–1.0%). Volume of solution is considered more critical for disinfection than its concentration. The lower and higher concentration are equally effective in reducing number of bacteria in infected root canals.
v. *Use of fresh solution*: Sodium hypochlorite decomposes quickly. The solution should be fresh before use. Fresh solution has better antibacterial and tissue dissolving effects. The solution should be stored in opaque containers.

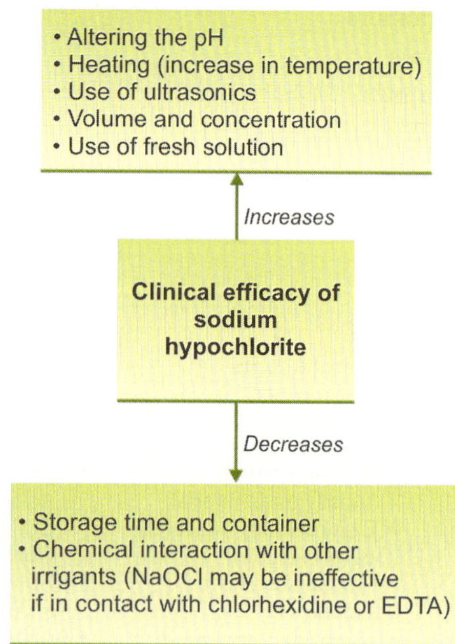

3. Chlorhexidine

Chlorhexidine is a potent antiseptic, which is widely used for chemical plaque control in the oral cavity. Aqueous solutions of 0.1 to 0.2% are generally recommended for plaque control. 2.0% concentration is effective as an irrigant. Chlorhexidine is a broad-spectrum antimicrobial agent, effective against gram-negative and gram-positive bacteria.

18

Chlorhexidine antimicrobial activity is pH dependant; the optimal range being 5.5–7.0. It is a strong base and is most stable in the form of its salts, i.e. chlorhexidine gluconate. At low concentration, it acts as a bacteriostatic; whereas, at higher concentrations it causes coagulation and precipitation of cytoplasm and therefore acts as bactericidal. The cationic properties of chlorhexidine allow them to bind electrostatically to root dentin surface. Heating of chlorhexidine solution also improves its efficiency.

0.1% *octenidine* has the same potential as chlorhexidine.

Cetrehexidin (combination of 0.2% chlorhexidine and 0.2% cetrimide) has also been tried as irrigant. The solution provides better penetration of chlorhexidine into the dentinal tubules and has better antimicrobial efficacy.

The combined use of chlorhexidine and sodium hypochlorite is controversial. Many studies indicate that the reaction product of chlorhexidine and sodium hypochlorite, i.e. Parachloroaniline has carcinogenic and mutagenic potential. Further, the combination may discolor the tooth. However, a few authors found the combination more effective as root canal irrigant.

Properties

i. Substantivity (the continuous/residual effect of chlorhexidine): 2.0% chlorhexidine can cause residual antimicrobial activity for 72 hours when used as an endodontic irrigant.
ii. Chlorhexidine is more effective than sodium hypochlorite against resistant *Enterococcus faecalis*, which are commonly found in failed endodontic cases.

Advantages

- Broad-spectrum antimicrobial (effective even against *Enterococcus faecalis* and *Eubacterium nucleatum* associated with endodontic failures)
- Bacteriostatic at a concentration of 0.12–2.0% (causing increased cell permeability and leakage of important intracellular components)
- Bactericidal at a concentration above 2.0% (causing precipitation of bacterial cytoplasm and ultimately cell death)
- Effective antifungal agent
- Better absorption
- Substantivity (binds to dentin and enamel; sustained release)
- Effective in infected canals and retreatment cases
- Because of its inhibitory effect on the enzyme MMP2, it can significantly improve the stability of resin-dentin bond.

Disadvantages

- Unable to dissolve necrotic tissue remnants
- Reduced action in the presence of exudates
- Does not inactivate lipopolysaccharide, which is a structural component of the gram-negative bacteria's outer cell wall
- Less effective against gram-negative bacteria
- Does not remove smear layer
- Antimicrobial effect of chlorhexidine is reduced by the presence of inflammatory exudates, serum albumin and dentin matrix, etc.
- May cause hypersensitivity reactions like contact dermatitis (2.0% concentration may irritate skin).

4. QMix

QMix is a mixture of EDTA, chlorhexidine and a detergent, available as a clear solution. The low surface tension of the solution is good characteristic to be used as an irrigant. It is equally effective in smear layer removal. It is also considered effective disinfectant against the root canal biofilm (penetrate dentinal tubules).

5. Hydrogen Peroxide

Hydrogen peroxide is being used in dentistry in various forms. 3.0% concentration is preferred as root canal irrigant.

Properties

i. Various concentrations of hydrogen peroxide are chemically stable. 3.0% H_2O_2 is considered active against bacteria, yeasts, and viruses due to the production of hydroxyl free radicals, which attack several cell components.
ii. The antimicrobial efficiency and the tissue-dissolving capacity of hydrogen peroxide are poor in comparison with sodium hypochlorite. The alternate use of sodium hypochlorite and hydrogen peroxide would be beneficial in reducing intraradicular microorganisms, could not be substantiated.
iii. The combination of chlorhexidine and hydrogen peroxide at low concentrations was found to have greater antimicrobial activity.

6. Iodophors (Iodine Potassium Iodide)

Iodophors are complexes of iodine and a solubilizing agent potassium iodide, which acts as a reservoir of the active 'free' iodine. The iodophors are strongly germicidal; however, they are considered less active against fungi and spores. The action of iodine is rapid, even at low concentrations. Iodine penetrates into microorganisms and attacks key groups of cell molecules, such as proteins, nucleotides, etc. resulting in cell death.

Combinations of iodine potassium iodide and chlorhexidine kill resistant bacteria more efficiently.

Advantages

- Active against a wide spectrum of microbes
- Low tissue toxicity
- Effective disinfectant for infected dentin surface
- An effective irrigant; especially against *enterococci*
- Biocompatible (iodine compounds are less cytotoxic and irritating to vital tissues than other commonly used irrigants).

7. Chlorine Dioxide

Chlorine dioxide is familiar household bleach, commonly used to eliminate contaminants from drinking water. Chemically, it is similar to chlorine/hypochlorite. Its disinfectant properties have been established. It is used in routine as surface disinfection and in dental waterline treatment. Its powerful oxidizing properties kill bacteria by disrupting the transport of nutrients across the cell wall. This strong antibacterial activity makes it a potentially useful endodontic irrigant. Chlorine dioxide is very efficient in dissolving organic tissues; as good as sodium hypochlorite.

Advantages

- Strong antimicrobial properties
- Effective tissue dissolving ability
- Ease of use
- Easy availability.

8. Carbamide Peroxide (Glyoxide)

Carbamide peroxide is available in an anhydrous glycerol base; 10% concentration is used as irrigant. It is more germicidal than hydrogen peroxide. It has strong lubricating effect, facilitating negotiation of narrow and/or curved canals. Sodium hypochlorite when mixed with glyoxide, release (O), which effectively kills microorganisms in the root canals.

9. Maleic Acid

Maleic acid, a mild organic acid, is an effective irrigant when used in concentration of 5–7%. It effectively removes smear layer from the root canal walls; considered better than 17% EDTA and QMix. It is less toxic as compared to 17% EDTA. It has also shown to improve the bond strength of resin sealer to root canal dentin when compared to 17% EDTA.

10. Chelating Agents

18

Sodium hypochlorite is considered to be the most desirable endodontic irrigant, effectively removing the organic contents from the root canals; however, the limitation of not removing the smear layer especially the inorganic material, is a matter of concern. Demineralizing agents, such as ethylenediaminetetra-acetic acid (EDTA) and citric acid have been used as adjuvants in root canal therapy to effectively remove the inorganic content of the smear layer. The removal of the smear layer is a crucial step to facilitate disinfection of the root canal system. First, the micro-organisms embedded in the smear layer are eliminated and canal cleanliness is improved. Secondly, it has been shown that the removal of smear layer improves the antimicrobial effect of intraradicular medicaments in the deeper layer of dentin. The commonly used chelating agents as root canal irrigants are:

a. EDTA

It is the most commonly used chelating agent. It helps in negotiation of narrow and calcified canals. It forms complexes with calcium. EDTA decalcify dentin up to the depth of 20–30 µm; however, the action of EDTA is self-limiting because the chelator gets used up. For optimal cleaning of root canals, EDTA should be used at neutral pH and with lower concentrations (15–17% accepted). EDTA has almost no antibacterial activity, is highly biocompatible, can demineralize intertubular dentin and reduces the surface hardness of root dentin. EDTA should be used with caution inside root canals because prolonged exposure to EDTA may weaken root dentin and may increase the risk of creating a perforation during mechanical root canal instrumentation.

Properties

The properties of 17% EDTA are:

i. Chelates the inorganic components of the dentin
ii. Soften dentin effectively (KHN of dentin is reduced almost 5–10 times); Demineralizes 20–30 µ of dentin when used for five minutes
iii. Good cleaning efficacy between 1–5 minute working time
iv. Removal of smear layer when used alternatively with sodium hypochlorite (sodium hypochlorite removes organic contents; whereas, EDTA removes inorganic material)
v. Help in detaching biofilm from root canal walls
vi. Relative non-toxic (may cause irritation)
vii. Effective lubricant
viii. Reduces time necessary for débridement and disinfection
ix. Aids in negotiating narrow/calcified canals
x. Biocompatible.

Functions

- Increased depth of penetration.
- Better débridement caused by foaming action.

- Facilitate emulsification of organic tissue (collagen in the pulp is quite elastic and difficult to remove; resists repeated attempts of removal by getting stretched and then collapsing back to its original position). EDTA helps to emulsify the pulpal tissue and thus aids in its easy removal.
- Holds the debris in suspension by encouraging floatation of pulpal remnant, which can be effectively removed by a subsequent sodium hypochlorite irrigation.

Different forms of EDTA

Different forms (mainly paste and liquid) of EDTA chelators are:

Paste chelators

- Calcinase slide (15% EDTA + 58–64% water)
- RC Prep [15% EDTA + 10% urea peroxide + glycol (ointment based)]
- Glyde file/file care EDTA (15% EDTA + 10% urea peroxide in aqueous solution)
- File EZE (19% EDTA).

Liquid chelators

- Calcinase: (17% sodium edetate, sodium hydroxide and purified water)
- REDTA: (17% EDTA + 0.84 gm cetrimide + sodium hydroxide and distilled water)
- EDTAC: (15% EDTA + 0.75 gm cetavalon)
- DTPAC: (Diethyl-triamine-penta acetic acid + Cetavalon)
- EDTA-T: [17% EDTA + tergentol (sodium lauryl ether sulphate)]
- EGTA: (Ethylene glycol + tetra acetic acid)
- CDTA: (1% solution of cyclohexane-1, 2-diaminetetra acetic acid)
- Tublicid plus: (Disodium EDTA dehydrate, benzalkonium chloride, citric acid and phosphate buffer, distilled water)
- Hypaque: (5% sodium hypochlorite + 17% EDTA + a high contrast injectable dye hypaque).

b. Citric Acid

Citric acid in varying concentrations has been used to remove the smear layer after root canal preparation. 10% citric acid has been established as a cheaper alternative to 17% EDTA. It acts by demineralizing the intertubular dentin around the opening of the tubules; subsequently, enlarging the tubules. It has proven to be more biocompatible than 17% EDTA.

The use of 10% citric acid as final irrigant has shown good results, especially in smear layer removal; however, even higher concentration (25%) was found ineffective in eradication of biofilm (especially, *Enterococcus faecalis*). It can be used alone or in combination with other irrigants; however, EDTA or citric acid should never be mixed with sodium hypochlorite because they strongly interact with sodium hypochlorite. This reduces the available chlorine in the combined solution, thus making it ineffective against root canal microorganisms.

c. Hydroxy-ethylidene Bisphosphonate (HEBP)

Hydroxy-ethylidene Bisphosphonate (HEBP) in varying concentrations (9–18%) has chelating properties and can be used as an irrigating solution. The demineralization induced by HEBP was significantly slower as compared to 17% EDTA. The advantageous property of HEBP as chelating agent is that it shows only short-term interference with sodium hypochlorite. HEBP has been used to prevent bone resorption in patients suffering from osteoporosis or Paget's disease. The overall effects of HEBP are considered equivalent to citric acid.

d. Salvizol

Salvizol, a quaternary ammonium (detergent) material has been tried as an irrigant. It is established that salvizol, with a neutral pH, has a broad-spectrum bactericidal activity and also the ability to chelate calcium. Salvizol has effective cleaning potential and is biologically compatible. Its low-surface tension and chelating effect aids in biomechanical cleaning of the root canal spaces. Salvizol induces irritation of tissue similar to those of iodophors, but less as compared to sodium hypochlorite or other quaternary ammonium compounds.

e. Solvidont

Solvidont is bis-dequalinium acetate, used mainly as a disinfectant. It provides lubrication and is non-toxic. It is recommended as substitute for sodium hypochlorite, especially in those patients who are allergic to the latter. The chelation properties of solvidont in removing the smear layer coupled with low surface tension allowing the solution to penetrate into the inaccessible areas, make it an excellent irrigant.

11. MTAD

MTAD is a mixture of a tetracycline isomer (doxycycline: 3.0%, citric acid 4.25% and a detergent: Tween 80). It is mainly used as a final rinse before obturation. Doxycycline with its low pH acts as a calcium chelator and cause root surface demineralization. Citric acid also has demineralising potential. Doxycycline primarily inhibit protein synthesis by binding to bacterial ribosomes. Doxycycline is active against wide range of gram-positive and gram-negative organisms, but it is not effective against fungi. Citric acid has antibacterial properties but not effective against *C. albicans*. Clinically, 1.3% sodium hypochlorite is used for 20 minutes followed by five minutes of MTAD to effectively remove smear layer. The solubilizing effects of MTAD on pulp and dentin are somewhat similar to those of EDTA. The major difference between the actions of these solutions is a high binding affinity of the doxycycline present in MTAD for the dentin. The three constituents of MTAD act synergistically against bacteria. The combination of sodium hypochlorite and MTAD has been advocated to remove the smear layer and also to achieve substantial antimicrobial efficacy. MTAD is effective against *E. faecalis* and is less toxic than other agents, viz. 3.0% H_2O_2, EDTA and calcium hydroxide. MTAD is found to be as effective as 5.25% sodium hypochlorite and significantly more effective than EDTA. A final rinse with MTAD might have a negative effect on the bonding ability of both resin-based and calcium hydroxide-based sealers. Its effectiveness in apical third area is controversial; a few studies observed not efficient (Maneini et al. 2009); whereas, other studies consider it efficient (Torabinejad et al 2003).

12. Tetraclean

Tetraclean, a modified form of MTAD, is also used as an irrigant. MTAD and tetraclean differ in the concentration of antibiotics (doxycycline 150 mg/5.0 ml for MTAD and 50 mg/5.0 ml for tetraclean) and the kind of detergent (tween 80 for MTAD, polypropylene glycol for tetraclean). Tetraclean has the lower surface tension values as compared to MTAD and sodium hypochlorite. It effectively disengages biofilm from the root canal walls.

13. Bioactive Glass

Bioactive glasses are a group of surface reactive glass-ceramics ($SiO_2 - Na_2O - CaO - P_2O_5$), exhibit antimicrobial activity by their ability to increase the pH environment. The commercially available bioactive glass (S53P4) when used in root canals, effectively kill root canal microorganisms. Various studies have confirmed significant antibacterial activity against almost all organisms when used in 50–100 mg/ml concentration. The mechanism of action is not pH dependent and does not alter dentin.

18

14. Electrochemically Activated Solutions

Electrochemically activated solutions are produced from natural water and low concentration of salt. The principle of electrochemical activation is transferring water into a metastable state via an electrochemical anode or cathode through the use of a reactor (Fig. 18.1). Electrochemical solution in anode and cathode chambers result in synthesis of two forms of solution: that produced in anode chamber is termed anolyte and that produced in cathode chamber is catholyte.

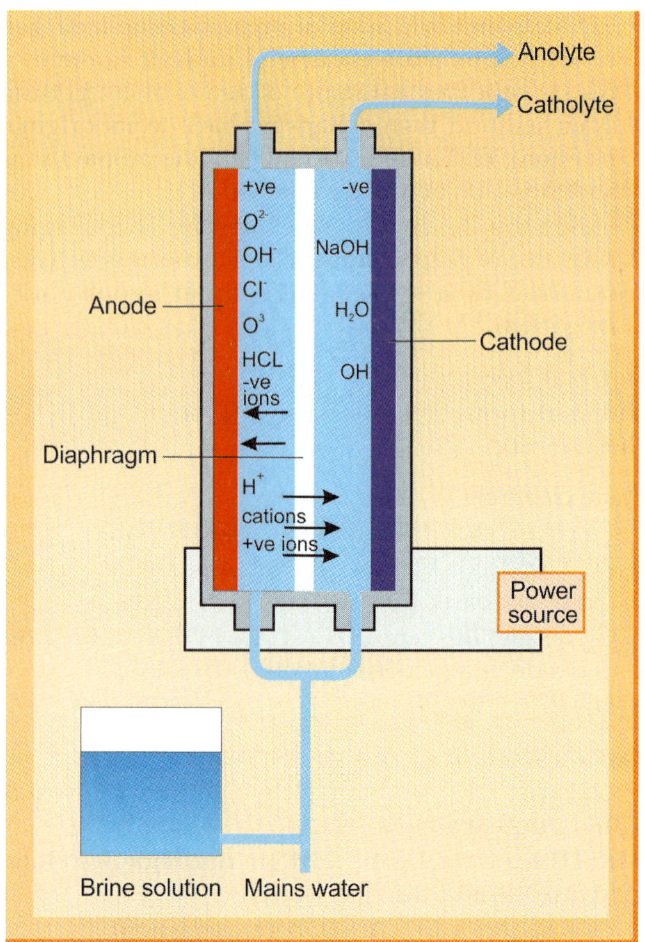

Fig. 18.1 Electrochemically activated water

i. An 'analytic' solution has high oxidation potential, which makes it highly antibacterial
ii. A 'catholytic' solution with a high reducing potential, used as a detergent.

The electrochemically activated solutions are nontoxic and their action is comparable to sodium hypochlorite. Anolytic solutions are superoxidized water and/or oxidative potential water.

a. ***Superoxidized water (Sterilox)*:** The saline water is electrolyzed to form superoxidized water, which contains hypocholorus acid and free chlorine radicals. Commercially, the solution is supplied as sterilox. The solution is nontoxic; however, effectively kill microorganisms.

b. *Oxidative potential water*: Oxidative potential water is produced by electrolyzing sodium hypochlorite in a special machine, called 'aquacida'. This is effective against bacteria as well as viruses. The oxidative potential water is biocompatible and can remove smear layer as well.

15. Ozonated Water

Ozonated water is a powerful antimicrobial agent against bacteria, fungi, protozoa, and viruses. Ozone, a chemical compound consisting of three oxygen atoms (O_3), is produced naturally by the following methods:

i. Ozone is created when an oxygen molecule receives an electrical discharge (from thunderstorm) breaking it into two oxygen atoms. The individual atom combines with another oxygen molecule to form O_3 (ozone).
ii. Ultraviolet rays from sun help electric discharge over natural oxygen of environment, creating ozone layer.

It is established that ozone at low concentration (0.1 ppm) is sufficient to inactivate bacterial cells including spores. It is considered effective against microorganisms; however, its role in eradicating *E. faecalis* has not been established. Various studies have confirmed that ozonated water is not effective against *Candida albicans, E. faecalis* and lipopolysaccharides in root canal biofilms.

It is used as a solution to soak surgical instruments. The *advantages* of ozone are its potency, ease of handling, lack of mutagenicity and rapid microbicidal effects. Ozonated water has nearly the same antimicrobial activity as 2.5% sodium hypochlorite during irrigation and is less toxic (Fig. 18.2).

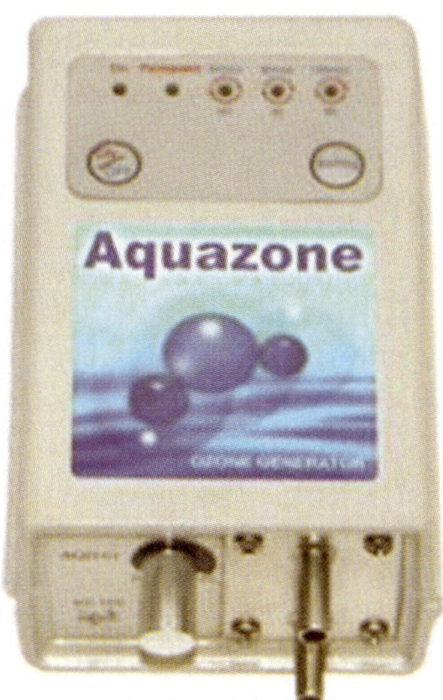

Fig. 18.2 Ozonated water

16. Carisolv

Carisolv is used for chemomechanical removal of caries. It may have same potential as an irrigant as it is antibacterial and has collagen dissolving potential. Its use has not been established.

17. Photon-activated Disinfection (Photodynamic Therapy)

The word 'photodynamic' implies applying dynamics of photons of light on the biological molecules. It is also known as photon-radiations or phototherapy, which employs the photochemical interaction of three components: light, photosensitizer and oxygen. It is based upon the principle that when photosensitizer is excited by light source of suitable wavelength, it is activated and produce free radicals, which have site-specific toxic effect on the cells. Two basic mechanisms by which cell damage can occur are:

i. DNA damage
ii. Damage to cytoplasmic membrane allowing leakage of cellular contents or inactivation of membrane transport system and enzymes.

The commonly used photosensitizers are:

- Methylene blue
- Toluidine blue
- Tolonium chloride
- Aluminium disulphonated phthalocyanine.

Methylene blue is established photosensitizer that is used in photodynamic therapy for targeting various gram-positive and gram-negative oral bacteria. A few studies have shown incomplete destruction of oral biofilms to photodynamic therapy using methylene blue. The reduced susceptibility has been attributed to reduced penetration of the photosensitizer. To improve upon this deficiency, drug delivery system was developed, which significantly improved the clinical efficacy of methylene blue.

Recently, polymer-based nanoparticles for photosensitizer delivery and release system is being studied. The *advantages* of nanoparticles containing photosensitizers are:

- Larger concentrated mass for production of reactive oxygen
- Limiting the target cell's ability to pump the drug molecule back, thus reducing the possibility of multiple drug resistance
- Nanoparticles matrix is non-immunogenic (nanoparticles showed time dependent release of photosensitizer).

18. Herbal Irrigants

The routinely used antimicrobial irrigants may lose the effectiveness because of increased bacterial resistance and other side effects. The alternative antimicrobial agents are being tried to overcome these limitations. Herbal products are gaining popularity because of their high antimicrobial potential, biocompatibility and anti-inflammatory properties.

The commonly used herbal products as irrigants are:

i. *Turmeric (Curcumin longa)*: Turmeric (curcumin) is an established anti-inflammatory and antimicrobial agent. Various authors have confirmed the antibacterial potential of turmeric against *Enterococcus faecalis*. It is used as root canal irrigant as an alternative to sodium hypochlorite. It is an effective irrigant, especially in failed root canal cases.

ii. *Babool (Acacia nilotica)*: Babool (Acacia nilotica) is an excellent antimicrobial agent, used in routine as a root canal irrigant. It is also effective against fungi and viruses. Various studies have confirmed its chemical efficacy, especially against *Enterococcus faecalis*. In comparative studies, 50% concentration has been found to have best antimicrobial potential.

iii. *Neem (Azadirachta indica)*: Neem extract has been widely used to minimize dental plaque. It is potent antibacterial and anti-inflammatory agent and is also biocompatible. Studies have confirmed its effectiveness against *E. faecalis* and found Neem to be superior to sodium hypochlorite.

iv. *Propolis*: Propolis has been used as pulp capping agent and also as mouth rinse in the treatment of periodontitis. Propolis is also used as intracanal medicament and also as a storage media for avulsed teeth to maintain vitality of periodontal ligament. Extract of propolis (natural substance collected by honeybees from trees) induces hard tissue formation in pulp capping and pulpotomy. Its effectiveness as root canal irrigant has been found to be comparable to sodium hypochlorite.

v. *Green Tea (Camellia sinensis)*: Green tea has significant anti-inflammatory, antimicrobial and probiotic properties. It is a potent root canal irrigant having scavenging properties. Studies have confirmed the antimicrobial potential of green tea against *E. faecalis*. It is considered as a better irrigant as compared to sodium hypochlorite.

vi. *Triphala*: Triphala extract is rich in citric acid, which is effective chelator to remove smear layer from root canal walls. Its efficacy is considered equivalent to sodium hypochlorite.

18

vii. *Aloevera*: Aloevera extract, especially the chloroform extracts, possesses good antibacterial and anti-inflammatory potential. Various studies have confirmed significant antimicrobial affect against *E. faecalis*.

viii. *Tea tree oil*: Tea tree oil has significant anti-inflammatory and antimicrobial properties. Tea tree oil when compared with 3.0% sodium hypochlorite and 2.0% chlorhexidine, was found to be better than sodium hypochlorite and less effective than chlorhexidine against *E. faecalis*.

ix. *Miswak-Siwak (Salvadora persica)*: It is established that 15% extract of Miswak-Siwak has significant effect against both aerobic and anaerobic bacteria. Its effect was found to be comparable with 5.25% sodium hypochlorite and 0.2% chlorhexidine.

x. *Lemon grass (Cymbopogon citratus)*: Lemon grass was found to have a significant antimicrobial efficacy against *Candida albicans* when compared to 2.0% chlorhexidine gluconate when used as an endodontic irrigant.

xi. *Cashew*: The leaf extract of *Anacardium occidentale* when used as an endodontic irrigant, had antibacterial activity against *E. faecalis* which was equivalent to 2.0% chlorhexidine gluconate. However, its antifungal activity against *C. albicans* was poor as compared to 2.0% chlorhexidine gluconate.

xii. *The following herbs have also been tried as root canal irrigant, establishing their antibacterial potential*:

- Garlic (Allium sativum)
- German chamomile
- Casearia sylvestris
- Carvacrol
- Acacia nilotica
- Psoralea corylifolia

19. NanoCare Plus

NanoCare plus is a nanosilver and nanogold based root canal irrigant. It is available both in liquid form (as irrigant) and paste form (as intracanal medicament). NanoCare plus is preferably used as final rinse. The main characteristic of NanoCare plus is that it leaves a layer of nanosilver and nanogold particles on the canal surface, which has a strong bacteriostatic effect. Low surface tension of 'NanoCare+' allows nanoparticles to get into the smallest intricacies and even dentinal tubules. It is established that it helps in preventing bacterial colonization, especially *Enterococcus faecalis* (Fig. 18.3).

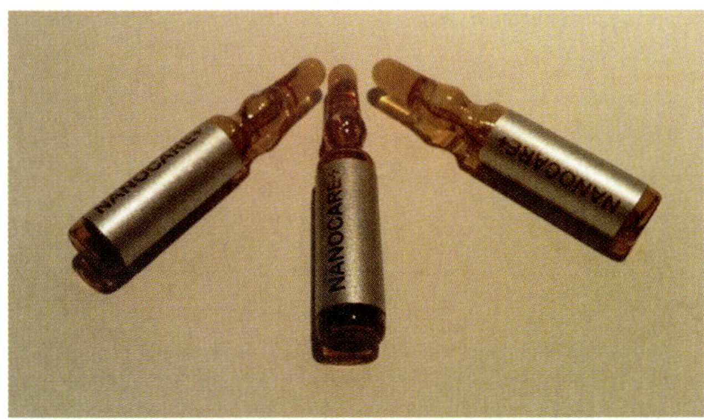

Fig. 18.3 NanoCare plus

Nanosilver particles exhibit properties such as high catalytic capabilities and ability to generate reactive oxygen species. Nanosilver particles react with three main components of the bacterial cell to produce the bactericidal effect; the cell wall (plasma membrane), cytoplasmic DNA and bacterial proteins. Application of nanosilver particles prevents the biofilm formation and inhibit bacterial growth. Various studies have confirmed its efficacy as root canal irrigant. Its non-cytotoxic affects to both mouse fibroblasts and periodontal ligament cells have also been established.

A new irrigation solution has also been tried (Moghadas et al 2012), containing silver nanoparticles and two other components, ethanol and sodium hydroxide. The combination provides essential capabilities of an ideal root canal irrigant.

Silver ions have been established as an antimicrobial agents. Ethanol, being good disinfectant, reduces surface tension of the solution facilitating penetration of nanosilver containing solution into accessory canals and dentinal tubules.

Sodium hydroxide dissolves and neutralizes soft pulpal tissues, remove the organic portion of smear layer, facilitating nanosilver particles to penetrate deeper into dentinal tubules and other intricacies of pulp spaces. The authors have observed the effectiveness of this combination as good as 5.25% sodium hypochlorite.

The comparative evaluation of commonly used irrigants are summarized in Table 18.1.

Efficacy of Irrigants

The efficacy of irrigants depends upon various factors. The cleaning efficacy of the irrigant is directly proportional to the volume and the frequency of the irrigant used. It is important that canal should be irrigated copiously during mechanical preparation after using each instrument in sequence. The change of irrigants may enhance the efficacy. The lower the surface tension of the irrigant more will be its wettability and more will be its penetration into narrow/inaccessible areas and better will be the débridement. The temperature of the irrigant is also important as it has been shown that if sodium hypochlorite is warmed (60–70°C) before irrigation, it is much more effective as a tissue solvent. The irrigant should properly contact the canal substrate to be able to dissolve/flush out the debris. So, it is critical that the canals should be mechanically enlarged to carry the solution to the apical extent of canal preparation.

Choosing the Right Irrigant

The choice of irrigant should depend upon the clinical situation; the clinical case may warrant the use of combination of irrigants. Choosing the right combination of irrigant is essential to prevent its misuse. The chemicals used to clean infected canals should be combined in such a manner so that they can be effective as irrigant rather than act on each other.

Sodium hypochlorite appears to be the most desirable endodontic irrigant solution fulfilling the maximum requirements of an ideal irrigant. It can be employed practically for all cases, except when there are chances of periapical extrusion/presence of active pus drainage. It has excellent ability to dissolve necrotic tissue and the organic components of the smear layer. However, it cannot dissolve the inorganic dentin particles. In addition, calcifications hindering mechanical preparation are frequently encountered in the canal system. Demineralizing agents such as ethylene-diamine-tetra acetic acid (EDTA) and citric acid are recommended as adjuvants in root canal therapy.

Once the cleaning and shaping procedure is completed, canals can be thoroughly rinsed using aqueous EDTA or citric acid (chelators) for removal of smear layer. Generally each canal is rinsed for at least one minute using 5.0 to 10 ml of the chelator agent. Prolonged exposure to chelators such as EDTA may weaken root dentin.

A final rinse with an antiseptic solution is always beneficial. The choice of the final irrigant depends on the next treatment step, i.e. whether an intervisit dressing is planned or not. If calcium hydroxide is used as intracanal medicament, the final rinse should be with sodium hypochlorite, as these two chemicals are complementary.

If the canal walls are perceived to be clean of debris/necrotic tissue, chlorhexidine would be the most promising agent as a final irrigant. It has the property of substantivity (affinity to bind dental hard tissues, slow release and prolonged antimicrobial activity). Hence, a final irrigation using a chlorhexidine solution

Table 18.1 Comparative evaluation of commonly used endodontic irrigants

Irrigant agent	*Concentrations (normally used)*	*Antimicrobial activity*	*Tissue solvent potential*	*Biofilm/smear layer removal potential*	*Toxicity/ cytotoxicity*	*Miscellaneous (additional characteristics)*
Sodium hypochlorite	0.5–5.25%	Antibacterial and antifungal	Dissolves only organic matter	Higher concentration is effective	Tissue irritation	• With chlorhexidine, forms parachloranaline • EDTA reduces tissues dissolving property of sodium hypochloride • Forms calcium chlorite (antibacterial) with calcium hydroxide
Chlorhexidine	0.2–2.0%	Antibacterial and antifungal	Nil	May not disrupt smear layer	Mild to moderate cytotoxicity	Sodium hypochlorite and EDTA in combination with chlorhexidine form precipitate
Octenidine	0.1%	Antimicrobial	Nil	Biofilm disruption	Mild to moderate cytotoxicity	Not established (tried as alternative to chlorhexidine)
EDTA (chelating agent)	15–17%	No antimicrobial activity	Pulp and dentin	Removes smear layer	Nil	Chlorhexidine and EDTA form white precipitate
MTAD	NA	Antimicrobial (superior to chlorhexidine) No antifungal activity	Pulp and dentin	Removes smear layer	Biocompatible	Effectively removes smear layer
Iodophors	N/A	Effective antimicrobial	Mild effect	Disrupts biofilm	Biocompatible	Effective disinfectant; attack cell molecules resulting in cell death
Ozonated water	N/A	Antimicrobial	Mild	Not effective	Biocompatible	Not effective against *Candida albicans* and *E. faecalis*
Herbal irrigants	N/A (concentration varies)	Antimicrobial	Mild	Not effective	Biocompatible	As effective as sodium hypochlorite; few are antifungal also
Tetraclean	NA	Antimicrobial (superior to chlorhexidine) No antifungal activity	Pulp and dentin	Removes smear layer	Biocompatible	Effective irrigant
Q mix	NA	Antimicrobial	No	Removes biofilm	Nil	Forms precipitate with sodium hypochlorite
Maleic acid	5.0–7.0%	Antimicrobial	Mild effect	Effective in removing smear layer	Mild	Improves bond strength of resin sealers to root dentin
Bioactive glass	N/A	Antimicrobial	Mild effect	May not disrupt smear layer	Nil	Long-term evaluation still to be documented
NanoCare Plus	N/A	Antimicrobial	Mild effect	Effective in removing smear layer	Nil	Long-term evaluation still to be documented

Table 18.2 Protocol for use of irrigants

Condition	*Irrigant*
Necrotic pulp	• Sodium hypochlorite • Final rinse with chlorhexidine
Vital pulp exposure	• Sodium hypochlorite • Final rinse with EDTA
Calcified/sclerotic canal	• EDTA • Sodium hypochlorite
Infected canal (exudate present)	• Sodium hypochlorite • Chlorhexidine
Periapical abscess (to establish drainage)	• Hot water/saline • Sodium hypochlorite
Open apex/apical perforation	• Chlorhexidine
Curved canals	• Glyoxide • Sodium hypochlorite
Canals left open for drainage	• 3% hydrogen peroxide • Saline
Retreatment cases	• Chlorhexidine • Sodium hypochlorite
Removing smear layer in noninfected cases	• EDTA/citric acid • Sodium hypochlorite

appears advantageous, especially in retreatment cases. The common protocol for use of irrigants is tabulated in Table 18.2.

(If residual hypochlorite is still present in the canal, irrigation with chlorhexidine will precipitate in the form of a brownish-reddish mass. The precipitates hinder the action of chlorhexidine and may discolor the tooth. The canal should be dried using paper points before the final chlorhexidine rinse.)

IRRIGATING TECHNIQUES

Efficacy of root canal irrigation depends upon many factors, such as diameter of the prepared canal, canal curvatures, depth of needle insertion into root canal and volume/concentration of the solution used. Various techniques have been tried to achieve effective irrigation. The techniques are:

1. Conventional Technique

A small gauge needle (27 or 28 gauge) is used in routine to irrigate root canals. The irrigation needle gauge and the amount of root canal widened affect the cleaning efficacy. The 'gauge' unit is separate entity and is not related to the size of the endodontic instruments. According to ISO 9626 standards, the diameter of the needle according to gauge is: 21 (0.8 mm), 23 (0.6 mm), 25 (0.5 mm), 27 (0.4 mm), 30 (0.3 mm) and 31 (0.25 mm). The needle may have one opening on top or one/two/many openings on the sides (Fig. 18.4). In case the needle has opening on top, the same should be inserted half-way into the canal. The irrigant when pushed with pressure will not extrude into the periapical areas. In case the needle is closed on top and has side openings, the same can be inserted up to the apical third area of the root canal. The irrigant when pushed will be circulated along the canal walls, without disturbing the periapical areas (Fig. 18.5). Slight agitation can be achieved by moving the needle up and down in the root canal. Gutta-percha point can also be used to agitate the irrigation solution. The modified needles used in irrigation are:

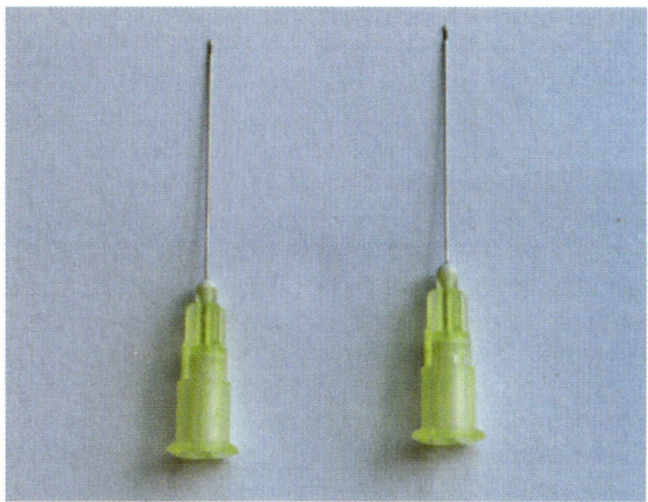

Fig. 18.4 Irrigation needles with side opening

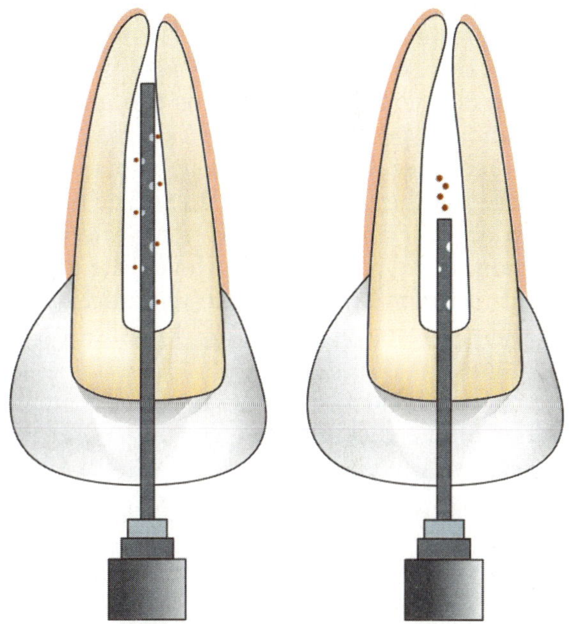

Fig. 18.5 Irrigation using side vent needle (left) and conventional (right)

i. ***Max-i probe***: The max-i-probe irrigation needle provides effective patient comfort and safety in irrigating root canals. It is also used for irrigating periodontal pockets. It has rounded end and one side/open port. It is available in five sizes; 23 gauge (light blue), 24 gauge (violet), 25 gauge (orange), 28 gauge (red) and 30 gauge (blue) (Fig. 18.6).

ii. ***Cala-sept needle***: The needle provides excellent irrigation with its double side ports. It is available in two sizes, 27 gauge (gray) and 31 gauge (violet).

iii. ***Vista-probe irrigating tips***: These are bendable, one inch needle tip, designed to irrigate subgingival surgical sites and sulcus. It has universal luer-lock design with closed end and side port delivery. It is available in 23, 27 and 30 gauges.

iv. ***Ni-Ti superflex***: Ni-Ti superflex has 2.5 times more flexible tip. It has adjustable needle angle for longer life and produces less clogging. It is available in 30 gauge with luer-lock system.

v. ***NaviTip and NaviTip Fx***: Flexible irrigating tips, available in different lengths (17 mm, 21 mm, 25 mm and 27 mm) and in two sizes (gauge 29 and gauge 30) (Fig. 18.7). The tips are effective in irrigation, especially at the apical areas. NaviTip Fx is modified version, wherein a small brush is attached at the opening (Fig. 18.8). The brush has been observed to effectively clean the occlusal portion of the root canal; however, the dislodgement of brush bristles inside the apical aspects of the root canal may lead to difficulties for the operator.

The conventional techniques may utilize manual agitation with needles, gutta-percha or brushes.

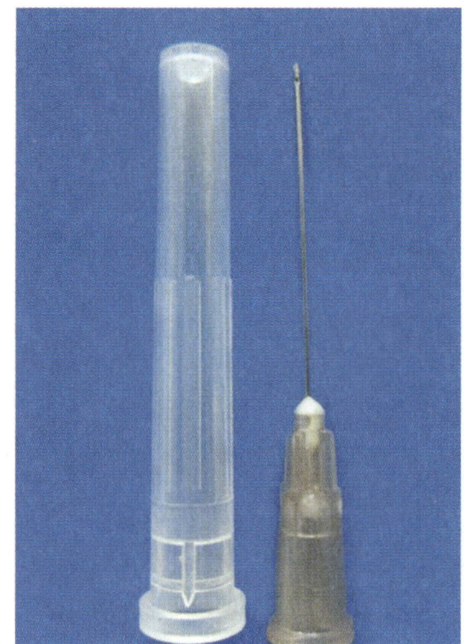

Fig. 18.6 Maxi-i probe

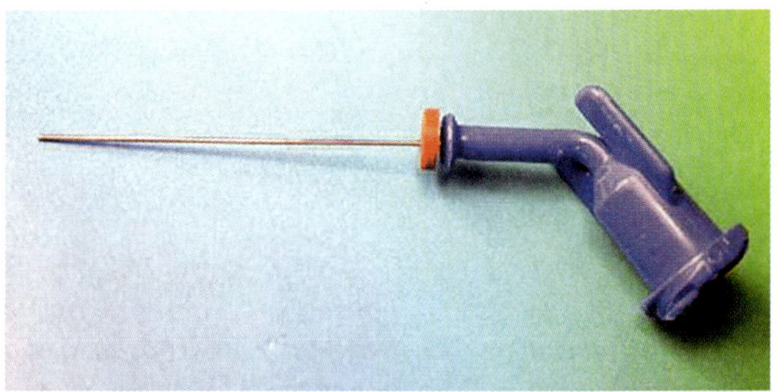

Fig. 18.7 NaviTip

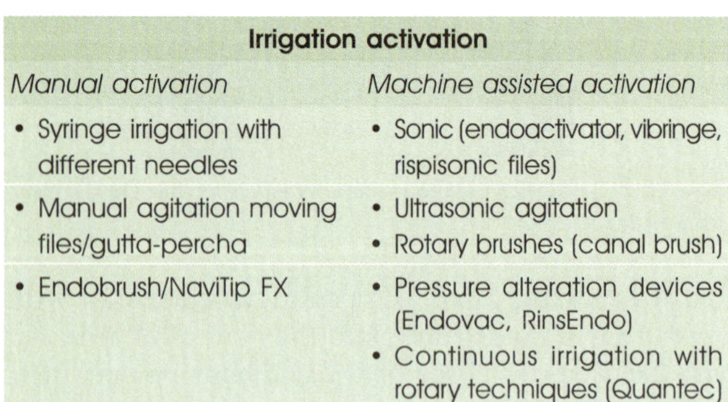

Irrigation activation	
Manual activation	*Machine assisted activation*
• Syringe irrigation with different needles	• Sonic (endoactivator, vibringe, rispisonic files)
• Manual agitation moving files/gutta-percha	• Ultrasonic agitation • Rotary brushes (canal brush)
• Endobrush/NaviTip FX	• Pressure alteration devices (Endovac, RinsEndo) • Continuous irrigation with rotary techniques (Quantec)

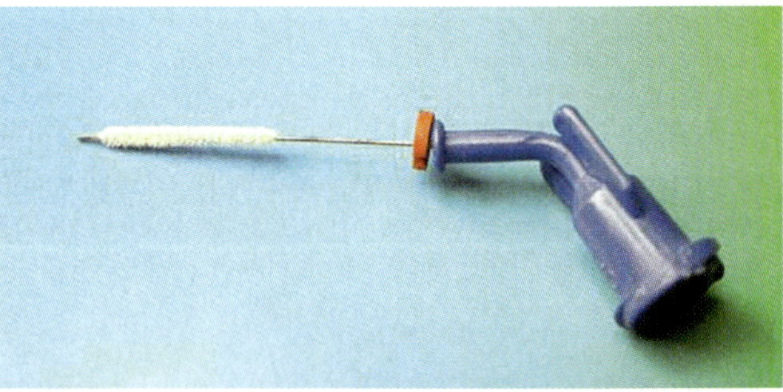

Fig. 18.8 NaviTip Fx

2. Sonic Irrigation

Sonic irrigation operates at lower frequency (less than 6 kHz) and is as effective as ultrasonic agitation of irrigant solution. The devices used are:

a. EndoActivator System

The EndoActivator system is comprised of cordless, battery operated handpiece along with three different sized polymer tips (Fig. 18.9). The tips are color coded according to their sizes; 15/02 – yellow, 25/04 – red and 35/04 – blue. The handpiece provides three-speed motor option, viz. high, medium and low. The operator is to decide the speed settings depending upon the clinical experience. The activation tips are preferably to be used for once only. Re-using the tips may lead to cross-contamination. Vibrating the tips and their up and

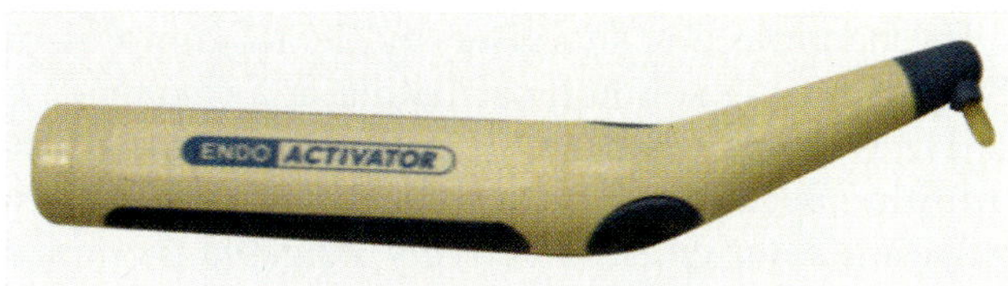

Fig. 18.9 Endoactivator

down movement produces a hydrodynamic phenomenon (active irrigation). Such a fluid activation help in cleaning all aspects of the root canal system.

The EndoActivator system provides safe and effective method to clean the canal. The hydrodynamic activation facilitates penetration and flow of irrigant into inaccessible areas of the root canal spaces.

Recently, pressurized water irrigation technique (AquaPick device), when compared with sonic irrigation device (Endoactivator), has shown promising results, especially irrigation of apical third area.

b. Vibringe System (Sonic Activation)

It is an irrigation device that combines manual delivery and sonic activation of the solution. The vibringe is a cordless handpiece that fits in a special disposable 10 ml luer-lock syringe (Fig. 18.10) that is compatible with any irrigation needle. The ergonomic designed vibringe system features single-button operation, battery charge indicator, auto shut off and white LED light for user feedback. The battery sonically activates the irrigating solution. Vibringe system is significantly better than manual irrigation; however, not as effective as passive ultrasonic irrigation.

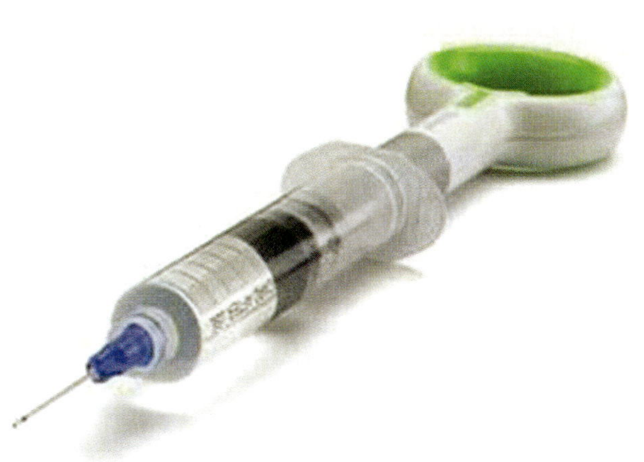

Fig. 18.10 Vibringe system syringe

3. Ultrasonic Irrigation

In ultrasonic irrigation system, the irrigant is delivered to the root canal by a syringe needle (Fig. 18.11a to c). The piezoflow irrigation needles are used in conjunction with a piezoelectric ultrasonic energy generating unit

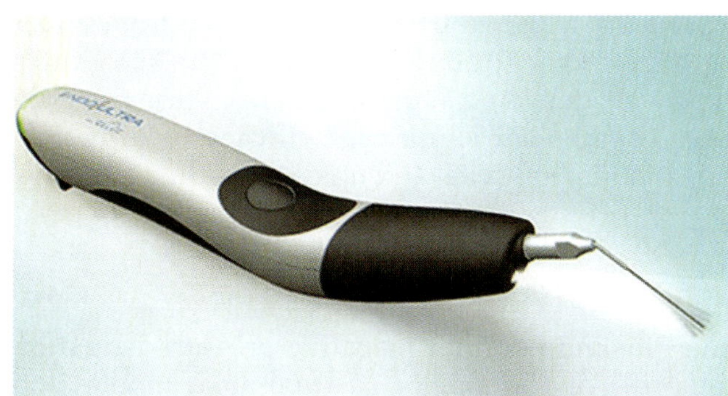

Fig. 18.11a Ultrasonic device

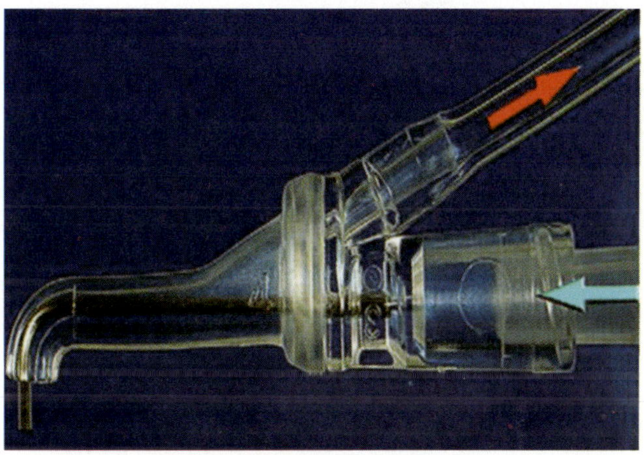

Fig. 18.11b Ultrasonic needle

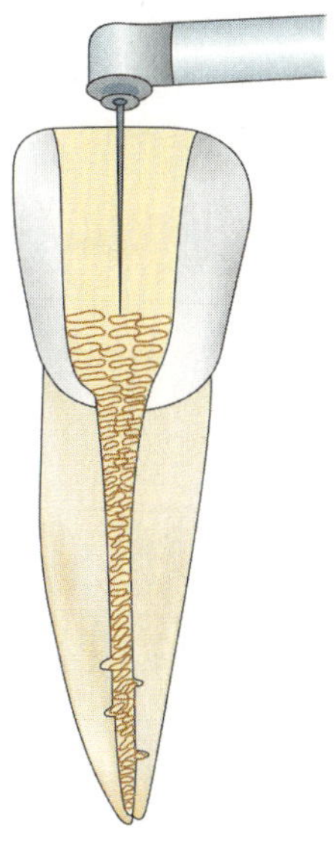

Fig. 18.11c Ultrasonic activation of irrigant solution

to provide the energy for tip oscillation. A syringe or other irrigation source is attached to the luer-lock connection on the ultrasonic needle. Removal of irrigant is through the conventional suction. During ultrasonic activation, a 25 gauge irrigation needle is used. The needle is simultaneously activated by the ultrasonic handpiece, while an irrigant is delivered from a luer-lock irrigation delivery syringe. The irrigant is effectively delivered at the apical area. Various studies have established significant efficacy of ultrasonic irrigation in both vital and nonvital teeth.

4. Negative Pressure Irrigation

a. RinsEndo system

The RinsEndo system (negative pressure irrigation) comprises of a handpiece, 20 disposable cannulas with 7.0 mm aperture and three 5.0 ml syringes carrying irrigant (Fig. 18.12). RinsEndo can be autoclaved.

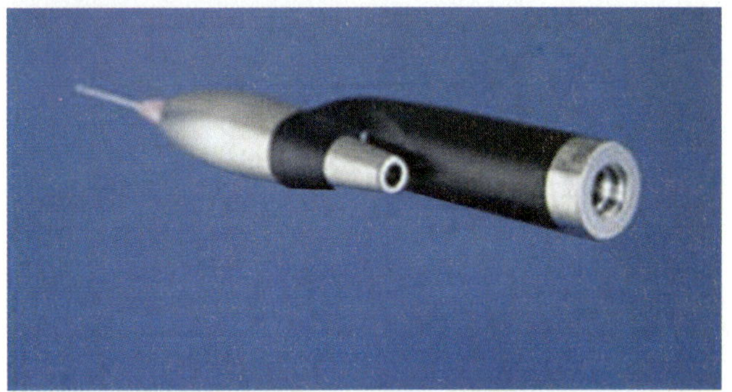

Fig. 18.12 RinsEndo system

The handpiece is energised by dental compressor. 65 ml of rinsing solution oscillating at a frequency of 1.6 Hz is transported to the root canal through the cannula. Because of the pulsating nature of the irrigating solution, it effectively irrigates the apical areas. During suction, the solution is aspirated back from the root canals.

It is established that the pressure created by RinsEndo irrigation is lower than the pressure created by a syringe during manual irrigation. RinsEndo is compatible with all types of irrigating solutions. It is considered as an effective irrigating modality.

b. Endovac System

The Endovac system (apical negative pressure irrigation) utilizes three components: the masters tip, microcannula and the macrocannula. The masters tip delivers and evacuates the irrigant simultaneously. The tip is connected to the irrigation syringe and the evacuation hood is connected to the high speed suction, preferably macrocannula is connected via tubing to high speed suction. The plastic macrocannula has an open end that measures ISO size 55 with a 0.02 taper. The stainless steel microcannula has 12 small, laterally positioned, offset holes in 4 rows of 3, with a closed end measuring ISO size 32. The microcannula can be used at working length in a canal enlarged to ISO size 35 or larger (Fig. 18.13).

During irrigation, the tip delivers irrigation solution to the pulp chamber and also evacuates the excess irrigant. The cannulas in the root canal exerts negative

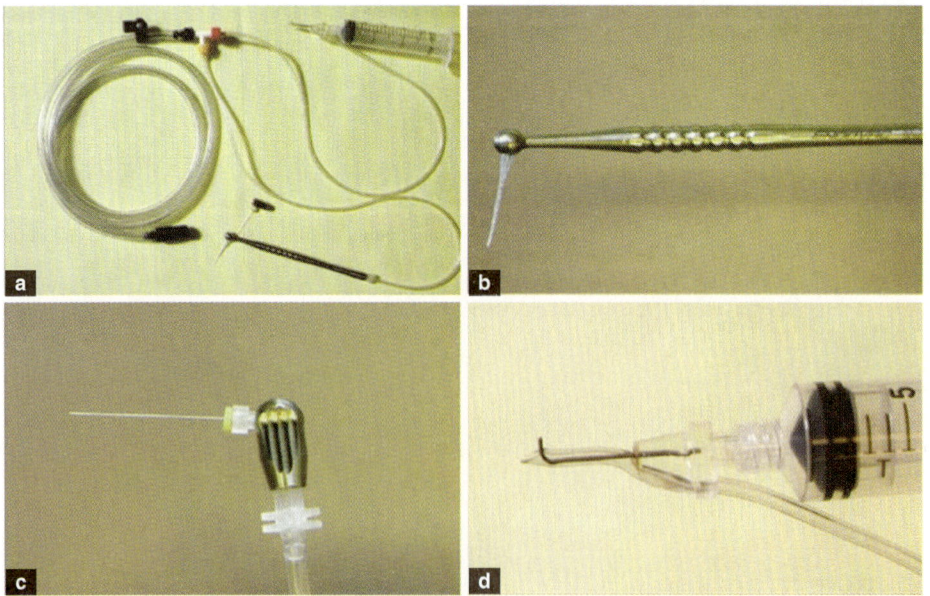

Fig. 18.13 Endovac system: (a) Endovac tubing and vacuum attachment; (b) Macrocannula; (c) Microcannula; (d) Evacuation tip

pressure that pulls irrigant from the canals to the suction unit. Various studies comparing Endovac system with other irrigation modules have confirmed its ability of thorough irrigating/cleaning the root canals.

Advantages

- Ability to safely deliver irrigant up to the working length.
- Avoids sodium hypochlorite accidents (by keeping the irrigating needle short of working length).
- Volume of irrigant delivered is more as compared to needle irrigation.

Disadvantage

Possibility of blockage of microcannula.

5. Irrivac Needle Pressure System

The Irrivac is available in both positive needle pressure version and a negative pressure version; the positive pressure Irrivac for dispensing sodium hypochlorite for removing gross material and the negative pressure for final irrigation with sodium hypochlorite (Fig. 18.14a and b).

This system includes titanium handpiece, solution reservoir and a specialized tubing, which is inert to caustic irrigants.

The negative needle pressure dispenses solution through the tubing funnel onto the needle, then flows down the canal and finally suctioned up and removed.

The positive needle pressure dispenses solution through the needle while the suction funnel sucks off the irrigant solution from top of the canal.

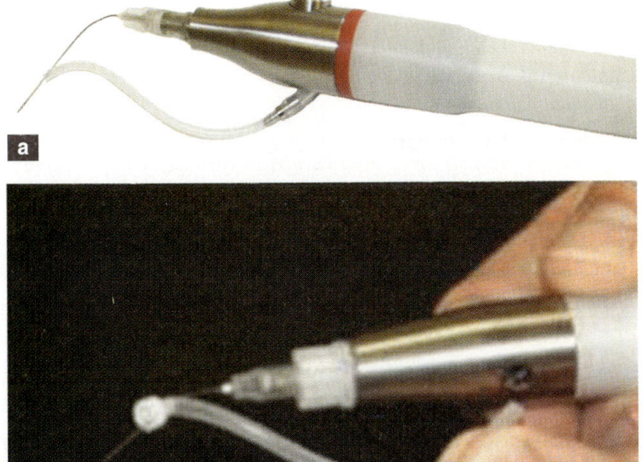

Fig. 18.14a and b Irrivac needle

6. VATEA Self-adjusting file (SAF) system

The VATEA irrigation system is an integral part of the self-adjusting file (SAF) rotary system. The irrigation delivery unit is attached to the handpiece during root canal treatment procedure. The irrigant is delivered via silicone tube to the endodontic file. The system is effective in irrigating root canals and is considered superior to the manual needle irrigation.

Quantum irrigation system containing two irrigation reservoirs, provides continuous irrigation during rotary instrumentation.

7. Intracanal Aspiration Technique

It has been established that the effectiveness of irrigation regimen depends upon the ability of irrigating agent to contact the entire canal system. It is usually difficult to contact the canal walls along apical constriction area; even smaller diameter needles are not effective. A new irrigation system is designed with an aim to inject irrigation solution up to apical area with injection needle and at the same time the solution is aspirated using aspiration needle to minimize extrusion through apical foramen (Fig. 18.15).

The aspiration technique has shown promising results in removing smear layer even from the apical region of the canal, without extrusion of debris/irrigant solution out of apical foramen. It is recommended to use Root ZX to monitor the activity of irrigant at the apical-end area.

COMPLICATIONS DURING ROOT CANAL IRRIGATION

Irrigation techniques mainly tend to maintain balance between cleaning efficacy and the patient safety. Usually irrigation techniques are either delivery system or activation or combination of both. Syringe irrigation is common delivery system; whereas, sonic, ultrasonic

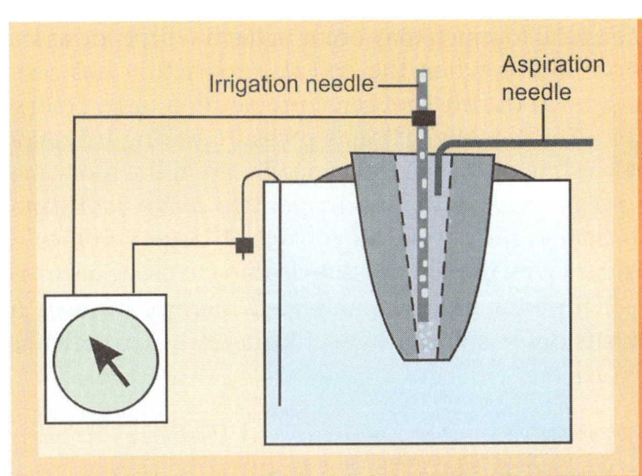

Fig. 18.15 Intracanal aspiration technique

18

and laser are the activation systems. A few systems such as RinsEndo follow both the protocol.

The common complications during irrigation are:

1. Apical Extrusion

Inadvertent extrusion of irrigant during root canal irrigation is a rare incident, though many studies have been reported.

Apical extrusion of debris caused by revolving instruments in an apical direction is a common feature during endodontic treatment. The extrusion is facilitated by instruments acting as a plunger, or by irrigation. The only way to prevent such extrusion would be an iatrogenic blockage of the apical foramen, which is not feasible practically. Endodontic treatment will always be a balance between blockage and some degree of extrusion of debris including irrigant. The extrusion of irrigant solution may lead to:

A. Involvement of Surrounding Anatomical Structures

a. ***Maxillary sinus***: Inflammation and infection may spread from the root canal to the maxillary sinus. Maxillary sinus is in close proximity to root tips of the maxillary posterior teeth. Periapical pathosis may result in destruction of the bone between root tip and sinus floor. The symptoms of maxillary sinusitis are similar to an acute pulpitis.

b. ***Nerve injury***: Apical extrusion of root canal filling materials may result in severe damage to the mandibular nerve, such as paresthesia, or in rare cases a hyperesthesia. The highest risk of iatrogenic nerve damage exists during endodontic treatment of second mandibular molars.

B. Effect of Extrusion of Sodium Hypochlorite

Inadvertent extrusion of sodium hypochlorite beyond the apical foramen may occur in teeth with wide apical foramina or when the apical constriction has been destroyed during root canal preparation or by resorption. Additionally, extreme pressure during irrigation or binding of the irrigation needle tip in the root canal with no release for the irrigant to leave root canal coronally, may result in contact of large volumes of irrigant with the apical tissues leading to tissue necrosis.

Symptoms and recommended therapy in cases of extrusion of sodium hypochlorite into periradicular tissues are:

Symptoms

- Immediate severe pain
- Edema of neighboring soft tissues
- Edema may extend over the injured side of the face, upper lip, infraorbital region
- Profuse bleeding from the root canal
- Profuse interstitial bleeding with hemorrhage of the skin and mucosa (ecchymosis)
- Chlorine taste and irritation of the throat
- Possibility of reversible anesthesia or paresthesia.

Therapy

- Patient should be informed as regard kind and severity of complication
- Local anesthesia for immediate relief of pain (analgesics in due course)
- Extraoral cold compression for reduction of swelling (after 24 hours warm mouth rinses for stimulation of local systemic circulation)
- Antibiotics are prescribed only in case of high-risk or evidence of secondary infection
- Antihistamines can be prescribed
- In severe cases, patient may be referred to a hospital.

C. Effect of Extrusion of Hydrogen Peroxide

The symptoms of such type of incident may be similar to that of sodium hypochlorite: sudden and severe pain, swelling and emphysema, and crepitus. It is recommended that analgesics and antibiotics be prescribed. In most cases, further intervention seems unnecessary and swelling subsides in a few days.

D. Effect of Extrusion of EDTA

Extrusion of even a low concentration of EDTA solution through the apical foramen results not only in an irreversible decalcification of periapical bone, but can also have consequences for neuroimmunological regulatory mechanisms.

3. Allergic Reaction

a. Sodium Hypochlorite

Allergic reactions to sodium hypochlorite are unlikely, since both sodium and chlorine are essential elements in the physiology of human body. Nevertheless, hypersensitivity and contact dermatitis may occur in rare cases.

In case of hypersensitivity against sodium hypochlorite, chlorhexidine should not be used. Alternatively, iodine-potassium-iodide should be considered. Before use, any type of allergy against iodine must be ruled out.

b. Chlorhexidine

It is relatively safe solution; rarely may induce allergic reaction. Allergic reactions such as anaphylaxis, contact dermatitis, and urticaria have been reported following direct contact to mucosal tissue or open wounds; however, allergic reactions following root canal irrigation with chlorhexidine have not been reported.

c. Iodine-potassium Iodide

Although the irritating potential of solution containing iodine is well known, there is no evidence on allergic reactions to iodine-potassium iodide. However, the irrigant should not be used in patients with known or suspected allergies to other iodine preparations.

4. Inadvertent use of Sodium Hypochlorite as Anesthetic Solution

Owing to the excellent tissue-dissolving ability of sodium hypochlorite, severe tissue and bone necrosis may occur if sodium hypochlorite is inadvertently used as anesthetic solution.

Correct labelling and use of different colored tips are safe and easy techniques to prevent such incidents.

5. Damage to Eyes and Skin

Damage to the patient's eyes may occur when needle and syringe are not connected tightly and get separated during irrigation. This may be facilitated by inadequate irrigation pressure. When using irrigation needles with small diameter, it may be kept in mind that much more pressure is necessary to apply the same amount of the solution in the same time, compared with tips with large diameter. When using such small needles, blockage of the tips may occur by deposition of sodium chlorite crystals.

Skin injuries may occur following inadequate isolation, leakage of the rubber dam, or splashing of the irrigant. In order to prevent such mishaps, the patient's eyes may be protected with glasses. Additionally, patients should be asked to close their eyes during irrigation. Luer-lock syringes should preferably be used to avoid separation from the irrigation needles.

6. Airway Obstruction

Although root canal treatment needs to be performed using a rubber dam, irrigant inadvertently may come into contact with the airways.

Sodium hypochlorite in contact with airway tissues may result in obstruction of the airways.

Exposure of airways to citric acid may provoke bronchoconstriction.

7. Damage to Clothing

The most common incident during root canal irrigation concerns damage to the patient's clothing. As sodium hypochlorite is a common household bleaching agent, even small amounts may cause severe damage. These mishaps should be prevented by proper protection of the patient's clothing. When using hand irrigation, one should ensure that the irrigation needle and syringe are securely attached and will not separate during transfer or irrigation in order to prevent leakage on clothing.

8. Air Emphysema

Air emphysema is defined as *'the abnormal presence of air under pressure where it is not normally present'*, such as neck and face.

Such incident may occur while drying root canals with compressed air or when large amount of hydrogen peroxide injected beyond the apical foramen, releases oxygen and causes edema. The spread of air is rapid and extensive, resulting in immediate edema that may cross the facial midline. Intensity of pain varies but mostly last for a short duration.

The emphysema caused by endodontic therapy does not require any treatment and mostly resolve within one week.

9. Postoperative and Inter-appointment Pain

Postoperative pain may occur due to several reasons; apical extrusion of the irrigant may be one of the reasons. It is difficult to distinguish clinically, whether postoperative discomfort is due to over instrumentation, extrusion of infected debris, extrusion of the irrigant, or a combination of these factors.

10. Staining and Discoloration

The subsequent use of chlorhexidine and sodium hypochlorite may result in discoloration of dentin. The brownish flocculate will occur with different concentrations of the two solutions. The subsequent use of sodium hypochlorite and MTAD has been reported to result in a red-purple discoloration of the root and crown dentin.

Iodine-potassium-iodide has also been reported to stain dentin.

11. Other Side Effects of Irrigants

Corrosion of rubber dam clamps and endodontic instruments may occur as a result of long-time contact with sodium hypochlorite.

Mercury release from amalgam fillings has been reported with the use of sodium hypochlorite.

Air contamination of the dental office with increased concentrations of chlorine may affect skin, eyes and airways of the office personnel and the patient, especially when used with an ultrasonic unit.

Ultrasonic activation results in a fine fog of sodium hypochlorite that may affect the eyes and skin of the patient, the operator and the supporting staff.

INTRACANAL MEDICAMENTS

Intracanal medicaments have traditionally been considered hand-in-glove with Endodontics. They are undoubtedly an integral part of treatment and important to the success of root canal therapy. The placement of a specific chemical agent during the inter-appointment period of a multi-visit procedure, forms part of the chemical preparation of the root canal system; eradicating microorganisms prior to permanent obturation.

Rationale

The main rationale for using such medicaments is to help degrade residual microbial biofilm/organic tissue and to kill remaining bacteria. The medicament should prevent bacterial recolonization of the root canal system, from either bacteria left after preparation or new invaders through lateral communications/coronal access. It also suppresses pain and facilitates apical healing.

Ideal Requirements

The ideal requirements of a root canal medicament are:
- Able to kill root canal bacteria
- Have long-duration of action
- Help degrade residual organic tissue and microbial biofilm
- Easily placed and removed
- Radiopaque
- Should not stain the tooth
- Able to induce regeneration of periapical tissue
- Not get inactivated in the presence of organic material
- Be inexpensive and easily available
- Should not irritate periapical tissue or have systemic toxicity
- Have anodyne properties
- Induce hard tissue formation.

Functions

The functions of intracanal medicaments are categorized as:
1. Primary
   - Antisepsis
   - Disinfection
2. Secondary
   - Pain control
   - Exudation control
   - Resorption control
   - Hard tissue formation.

18

Limitations and Contraindications

- The chemical or therapeutic action of medicaments depends on direct contact of the agent with microbes or tissue.
- To be effective, the agents should remain chemically active between appointments.
- The allergic manifestations are common with phenolics and aldehydes.
- Patients may also object disagreeable taste and pungent odor associated with phenolics.

Classification

The intracanal medicaments are classified as:
1. Essential oils
   i. Eugenol
2. Phenol based agents (phenolic compounds)
   i. Phenol/methylphenol (Cresol)/thymol
   ii. Camphorated monochlorophenol (CMCP)
   iii. Parachlorophenol (PCP)/camphorated parachlorophenol (CPC)
   iv. Metacresyl acetate (cresatin)
   v. Creosote (beechwood creosote)
3. Aldehydes
   i. Formocresol (formaldehyde)
   ii. Glutaraldehyde
4. Halides
   i. Sodium hypochlorite (chlorine)
   ii. Iodine-potassium iodide (iodine)
5. Calcium hydroxide
6. Antibiotics, steroids and their combinations
7. Bioactive glass
8. Phytomedicines.

1. Essential Oils

i. ***Eugenol:*** This is the chemical essence of oil of clove with mild antiseptic and anodyne properties. It is used as pulp cavity dressing after removal of non-infected vital pulp and also aids in anesthetising severed pulp remnants (Fig. 18.16).

2. Phenol Based Agents

i. ***Phenol/Methylphenol (cresol)/thymol:*** This is a protoplasm poison and a potent antimicrobial agent. Liquefied phenol is made by addition of one part of water to 109 parts of phenol crystals. It is indicated where sensitive tissue remains in the canal during instrumentation. Both cresol and thymol (derivatives of phenol) are equally effective intracanal medicament.

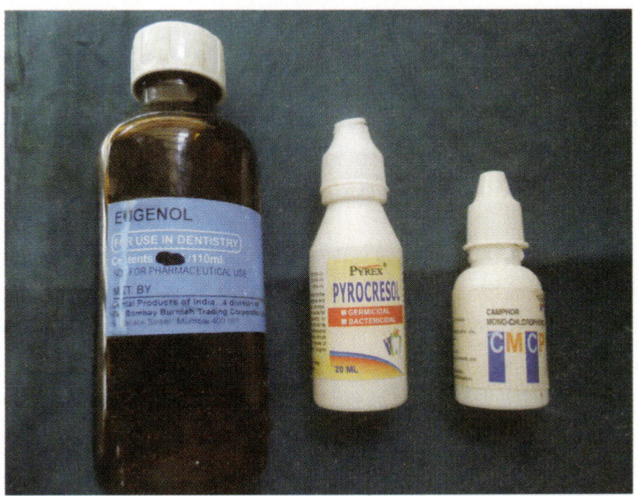

Fig. 18.16 Eugenol/pyrocresol

ii. ***Camphorated monochlorophenol (CMCP)*:** CMCP is prepared by mixing 2 parts PCP and 3 parts of camphor. Camphor is added to reduce irritating effect of parachlorophenol and to prolong the antibacterial action. It is more powerful bactericidal agent than phenol and is most toxic.

iii. ***Parachlorophenol (PCP)*:** One percent aqueous form of PCP is most commonly used and is found to be more penetrating into dentinal tubules than camphorated parachlorophenol (CPC).

iv. ***Metacresyl acetate (cresatin)*:** This is a clear liquid derivative of metacresol with low surface tension. It is non-irritating and exhibits anodyne and sedative properties.

v. ***Creosote (Beechwood Creosote):*** Beechwood creosote is a potent antibacterial and antifungal agent. The allergic reactions to beechwood creosote, though rare, should also be taken care of during its endodontic use. The use of beechwood creosote is not preferred in pregnant/breastfeeding women.

3. Aldehydes

Formaldehyde, paraformaldehyde and glutaraldehyde have been widely used in dentistry including endodontics. These are water soluble, protein denaturing agents and are most potent disinfectants.

i. ***Formocresol*:** Formocresol contains 19% formaldehyde and 35% cresol, dissolved in 46% water and glycerine. It is mainly used in pulpotomy procedures. The *main disadvantages* include toxicity, mutagenicity and carcinogenicity.

Paraformaldehyde is the polymer form of formaldehyde, a constituent of N2 and endomethasone.

ii. ***Glutaraldehyde*:** Glutaraldehyde is also a strong disinfectant and fixative. 2.0% is most commonly used.

4. Halides

Halides consist of chlorine and iodine which are used in various formulations in endodontics. They are potent oxidising agents with rapid bactericidal effects.

i. ***Sodium hypochlorite*:** Chlorine, an active component of sodium hypochlorite is used as antiseptic.

ii. ***Iodine-potassium iodide:*** Iodine is used as iodine-potassium iodide and iodophors that release iodine continuously. This medicament is made by mixing 4.0 gm potassium iodide with 2.0 gm iodine and 94 ml water. The main *disadvantages* are allergic responses and tooth staining.

5. Calcium Hydroxide

Calcium hydroxide has gained wide popularity and acceptance as intracanal medicament (Fig. 18.17). It is effective against most root canal pathogens and has the ability to degrade residual organic tissue. Its use in endodontics relates mainly to its antibacterial property, ability to induce repair and stimulate hard tissue formation. The bactericidal nature of calcium hydroxide is attributed to its high pH (range of 10–12). Calcium hydroxide acts by releasing hydroxyl ions, which destroy bacteria by damaging cytoplasmic membrane and bacterial DNA.

Calcium hydroxide, to be used as intracanal medicament, can be either in powder or paste forms. Powder form is mixed with distilled water, saline, polyethylene glycol, propylene glycol, etc. The vehicle used to mix calcium hydroxide and the manner in which it is dispensed plays a vital role in achieving maximum antibacterial effects. The paste form (hypocal, multical, reogan, etc.) can be easily dispensed in the root canal space and can be retrieved during obturation.

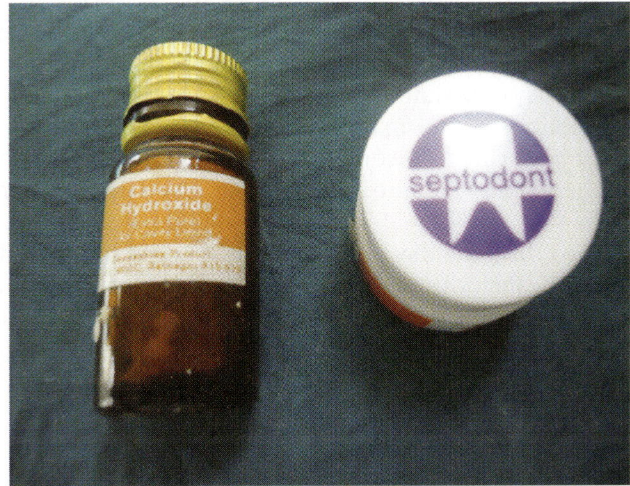

Fig. 18.17 Calcium hydroxide: Powder and paste form

Calcium hydroxide has been shown to be ineffective against *Candida* spp. and *Enterococcus faecalis*, commonly associated with root canal failures. To improve the ability to disinfect and to penetrate more deep into dentinal tubules against these organisms, Calcium hydroxide is combined with CMCP, corticosteroids and antibiotics.

Calcium hydroxide is mainly used for closure of root apex, root perforations, resorptions, management of large periapical lesions and weeping canals.

The placement of calcium hydroxide is usually a matter of personal preference. The commercially available pastes may be applied with files or paper points, but the material is unlikely to reach all aspects of root canal system. Spiral fillers or ultrasonically activated files are the most effective means of placement of calcium hydroxide in root canal.

***Removal and replacement*:** Calcium hydroxide is easily removed by washing and irrigating with water or sodium hypochlorite. Ultrasonically activated file is also used to remove calcium hydroxide dressings. Calcium hydroxide mixed with oil-based vehicle can be removed by using a chelating agent or acid (EDTA or maleic acid).

The duration of dressing is dependent upon the objective of dressing. A week is sufficient if routine antibacterial dressing is used. In cases of weeping canals dressing with stiff paste or only powder is necessary for a period of 2 weeks. To induce calcific repair at the periapex, dressing is changed every 2 weeks to evaluate for the loss or contamination of calcium hydroxide. The dressing may then be left in place and healing is assessed at 3–4 month interval.

6. Antibiotics, Corticosteroids and their Combinations

Topical application of antibiotics in the root canal therapy has been popular as they are active in the presence of tissue fluids; do not stain the tooth and virtually non-irritant to tissue cells. As there is no single antibiotic effective against all microorganisms present in the root canals, a combination of antibiotics is used in the form of paste. The earlier used intracanal antibiotics, sulphonamides, are no longer in use, as they tend to discolor the teeth. The most commonly used antibiotic includes combination of penicillin, bacitracin, sodium caprylate and nystatin (PBSC/PBSCN).

The combination of antibiotics and steroids are being widely used as intracanal medicament in a paste form; the commonly used are:

- *Ledermix paste*: Ledermix paste contains demeclocycline HCl, corticosteroid and triamcinolone in a polyethylene glycol base. The ingredients are capable of diffusing through dentinal tubules to reach cementum and periradicular tissues. Ledermix is water soluble and can be rinsed off easily.
- *Septomixine forte paste*: Septomixine forte paste contains neomycin sulphate, dexamethasone polymyxin B and tyrothricin. It is not recommended because of inactivity of ingredients against endodontic microorganisms.
- *Odontopaste*: Odontopaste contains clindamycin hydrochloride, triamcinolone in zinc oxide base. The paste is effective against most of the endodontic microorganisms and also alleviate inflammation. Addition of calcium hydroxide led to poor quality paste as steroid present gets destroyed by high alkalinity of calcium hydroxide.
- *Doxypaste*: Doxypaste contains doxycycline hyclate and triamcinolone in polyethylene glycol base (doxycycline is more active and effective than demeclocycline).
- *Triple antibiotic paste*: A combination of antibiotics decreases the likelihood of developing resistant strains. The most promising and commonly used combination of intracanal medicament consist of metronidazole, ciprofloxacin and minocycline. A few authors have added rifampicin to improve upon the antibacterial effect. The antibiotic paste in combination is effective in eradicating microorganisms from the root canals; whereas, none of single antibiotic result in complete elimination of endodontic microbes. Similar combination of erythromycin, metronidazole and ciprofloxacin has also been tried.
- *Double antibiotic paste*: A combination of clindamycin and metronidazole in ethylene acetate base has also shown promising results, significantly reducing bacterial load inside the root canal system including dentinal tubules.

The development of bacterial resistant strains, allergic reactions and possible sensitization make the antibiotic paste to be used with caution as intracanal medicament.

Steroids have been used during root canal therapy mainly for pain relief. The *main disadvantage* of steroids is their depressive effect on the defence mechanism.

7. Bioactive Glass (BAG)

Bioactive glass contains oxides of calcium, sodium, phosphorous and silicone in a proportion that provides the material with surface activity and with a property to form a bond with mineralized hard tissues such as bone or dentin. BAG decreases bacterial viability of several gram-positive facultative bacteria, such as *E. faecalis, S. sanguis, S. mutans, P. aeruginon* and

C. albicans; also act against gram-negative species, such as, *Actinobacillus, Actinomycetemcomitans* and *P. gingivalis*.

8. Phytomedicines

The cytotoxic reactions of most of the intracanal medicaments and their inability to eliminate bacteria from dentinal tubules, lead to use of biologic medicament extracted from natural plants. A wide variety of herbal products, viz. *Morinda citrifolia*, propolis, green tea, lemon solution, aloevera gel, turmeric, etc. are being used as intracanal medicaments. Further studies are needed to investigate the safety, toxicity and drug interactions of these plant extracts for application as intracanal medicaments.

BIBLIOGRAPHY

1. Aksel H, Askerbeyli S, Canbazoglu C and Serper A. Effect of needle insertion depth and apical diameter on irrigant extrusion in simulated immature permanent teeth. Braz. Oral Res.: 2014; 28:1–6.
2. Allaker RP. The use of nanoparticles to control oral biofilm formation. J. Dent. Res.: 2010; 89:1175–1186.
3. Arias-Moliz MT, Ferrer-Luque CM, Espigares-Garcia M and Baca P. *Enterococcus faecalis* biofilms eradication by root canal irrigants. J. Endod.: 2009; 35:711–714.
4. Bahador A, Khaledi A and Ghorbanzadeh R. Evaluation of antibacterial properties of nano silver Iranian MTA against *Fusobacterium nucleatum*. Eur. J. Experi. Biol.: 2013; 3:88–94.
5. Bednarski M, Soska-Czop A, Zarycka B, Ebert J and Pawlicka H. NanoCare Plus Silver Gold can eliminate *Enterococcus faecalis* from dentinal tubules. Dent. Med. Probl.: 2013; 50:418–423.
6. Behrents KT, Speer ML and Noujeim M. Sodium hypochlorite accident with evaluation by cone beam computed tomography. Int. Endod. J.: 2012; 45:492–498.
7. Beltz RE, Torabinejad M and Pouresmail M. Quantitative analysis of the solubilizing action of MTAD, sodium hypochlorite, and EDTA on bovine pulp and EDTA on bovine pulp and dentin. J. Endod.: 2003; 29:334–337.
8. Besinis A, De Peralta T and Handy RD. Inhibition of biofilm formation and antibacterial properties of a silver nano-coating on human dentine. Nanotoxicology: 2013; 1–10.
9. Boutsioukis C, Gogos C, Verhaagen B, Versluis M, Kastrinakis E and Van der sluis, LW. The effect of root canal taper on the irrigant flow:evaluation using an unsteady Computational fluid dynamics model. Int. Endod. J.: 2010; 43:909–916.
10. Boutsioukis C, Psmiaa Z and van der Sluis LWM. Factors affecting irrigant extrusion during root canal irrigation: a systematic review. Int. Endod. J.: 2013; 46:599–618.
11. Boutsioukis C, Verhaagen B, Versluis M, Kastrinakis E, Wesselink PR and van der Sluis LWM. Evaluation of irrigant flow in the root canal using different needle types by an unsteady computational fluid dynamics model. J. Endod. 2010; 36:875–879.
12. Calt S and Serper A. Time-dependent effects of EDTA on dentin structures. J. Endod.: 2002; 28:17–19.
13. Chan LK, Zhang C and Cheung SP. Cytotoxicity of a novel nano-silver particle endodontic irrigant. Clin. Cosmet. Investig. Dent.: 2015; 7:65–74.
14. Chandrasekhar V, Amulya V, Rani VS, Prakash TJ, Ranjani AS and Gayathri C. Evaluation of biocompatibility of a new root canal irrigant Q MixTM 2 in 1- An *in vivo* study. J. Conserv. Dent.: 2013; 16:36–40.
15. Desai P and Himel V. Comparatively safety of various intracanal irrigation systems. J. Endod.: 2009; 35:545–549.
16. El karim I, Kennedy J and Hussey D. The antimicrobial effects of root canal irrigation and medication. Orag Surg., Oral Med., Oral Path. Oral Radiol.: 2007; 103:560–569.
17. Elumalai D, Kumar A, Tewari RK, Mishra SK, Iftekhar H, Alam S and Andrabi A. Newer endodontic irrigation devices: an update. IOSR J. Dent. Med. Sci.:2014; 13:4–8.
18. Esterla C, Cyntia RA and Barbin EL. Mechanism of action of sodium hypochlorite. Braz. Dent. J.: 2002; 13:13–17.
19. Ghisi AC, Kopper PMP, Baldasso FER, Sturmer CP, Rossi-Fedele G, Steier L, Poli de Figueiredo JAP, Morgental RD and Vier-Pelisser FV. Effect of super-oxidized water, sodium hypochlorite and EDTA on dentin microhardness. Braz. Dent. J. 2014; 25:420–424.
20. Giardino L, Ambu E and Savoldi E. Comparative evaluation of antimicrobial efficacy of sodium hypochlorite, MTAD, and Tetraclean against *Enterococcus faecalis* biofilm. J. Endod.: 2007; 33:852–855.
21. Gomes PFA. Chlorhexidine in Endodontics. Braz. Dent. J.: 2013; 24:89–102.
22. Gomes-Filho JE, Silva FO, Watanabe S, Cintra LT, Tendoro KV, Dalto LG, Pacanaro SV, Lodi CS and De Melo FF. Tissue reaction to silver nanoparticles dispersion as an alternative irrigating solution. J. Endod.: 2010; 36:1698–1702.
23. Gu LS, Kim JR, Ling J, Choi KK, Pashley DH and Tay ER. Review of contemporary irrigant agitation techniques and device. J. Endod.: 2009; 35:791–804.
24. Guerreiro-Tanomaru JM, Loiola LE, Morgental RD, Leonardo RT, Tanomaru-Filho, M. Efficacy of four irrigation needles in cleaning the apical third of root canals. Braz. Dent. J.: 2013; 24:21–24.
25. Gusiyska A, Gyulbenkiyan E, Vassileva R, Dyulgerova E and Mironova J. Effective root canal irrigation - A key factor of endodontic treatment - Review of the literature. Int. J. Recent Sci. Resch.: 2016; 7:9962–9970.
26. Gutierrez JH, Jofre A and Villena F. Scanning electron microscope study on the action of endodontic irrigants on bacteria invading the dentinal tubules. O. Surg., O. Med., O. Path.: 1990; 69:491–501.
27. Haapasalo M, Endal U, Zandi H and Coil J. Eradication of endodontic infection by instrumentation and irrigation solutions. Endodontic Topics: 2005; 10:77–102.

28. Haapasalo M, Qian W, Portenier I and Waltimo J. Effect of dentin on antimicrobial properties of endodontic medicaments. J. Endod.: 2007; 33:917–925.
29. Haapasalo M, Shen Y and Qian W. Irrigation in Endodontics. Dent. Clin. North Am.: 2010; 54:291–312.
30. Hulsmann M and Hahn W. Complications during root canal irrigation – literature review and case reports. Int. Endod. J.: 2000; 33:186–193.
31. Hülsmann M, Heckendorff M and Lennon A. Chelating agents in root canal treatment: mode of action and indications for their use. Int. Endod. J.: 2003; 36:810–830.
32. Hulsmann M, Rodig T and Nordmeyer S. Complications during root canal irrigation. Endo. Topics: 2009; 16:27–63.
33. Huth KC, Quirling S, Maier S and Kamereck K. Effectiveness of ozone against endodontopathogenic microorganisms in a root canal biofilm model. Int. Endod. J.: 2009; 42:3–13.
34. Jain P and Ranjan M. Role of herbs in root canal irrigation – a review. IOSR J. Pharm. Biol. Sci.: 2014; 9:6–10.
35. Jaju S and Jaju PP. Newer root canal irrigants in horizon: a review. Int. J. Dent.: 2011; Article ID 851359:1–9.
36. Jawad S, Taylor C, Roudsari RV and Hunter M. Modern endodontic principles Part 4 : Irrigation. Dent. Update: 2016; 43:20–33.
37. Johnson M, Sidow SJ, Looney SW, Lindsey K, Niu LN and Tay FR. Canal and isthmus debridement efficacy using a sonic irrigation technique in a closed-canal system. J. Endod.: 2012; 38:1265–1268.
38. Kishan A and Shrestha A. Emerging technologies in root canal disinfection. Pocket dentistry: 2016; 1–6.
39. Kishen, A, Shi Z, Shrestha A and Neoh KG. An investigation on the antibacterial and antibiofilm efficacy of cationic nanoparticulates for root canal disinfection. J. Endod.: 2008; 34:1515–1520.
40. Kishor N. Oral tissue complications during endodontic irrigation: a literature review. NY. State Dent. J.: 2013; 37–42.
41. Lee J, Lorenzo D, Rawlins T and Cardo VA. Sodium hypochlorite extrusion: an atypical case of massive soft tissue necrosis. J. Oral Maxillo. Surg.: 2011; 69:1776–1781.
42. Lim Z, Cheng JL and Lim TW. Light activated disinfection: an alternative endodontic disinfection strategy. Aust. Dent. J.: 2009; 54:108–114.
43. Lotfi M, Vosoughhosseini S, Ranjkesh B, Khani S, Saghiri M and Zand V. Antimicrobial efficacy of nanosilver, sodium hypochlorite and chlorhexidine gluconate against *Enterococcus faecalis*. Afr. J. Biotech.: 2011; 10:6799–6803.
44. Mahmoud Torabinejad DM, Shahrokh Shabahang M, Aprecio O, James DK. The antimicrobial effect of MTAD: An *in vitro* investigation. J. Endod.: 2003; 29:400–403.
45. Mancini M, Armellin E, Casaglia A, Cerroni L and Cianconi L. A comparative study of smear layer removal and erosion in apical intraradicular dentine with three irrigating solutions: a scanning electron microscopy evaluation. J. Endod.: 2009; 35:900–903.
46. Marais JT. Cleaning efficacy of a new Root Canal Irrigation Solution: A preliminary evaluation. Int. Endod. J.: 2000; 33:320–325.
47. McDonnell G and Russell AD. Antiseptics and disinfectants: activity, action and resistance. Clin. Microbiol. Rev.: 1999; 12:147–179.
48. McGill S, Gulabivala K, Mordan N and Ng YL. The efficacy of dynamic irrigation using a commercially available system (RisEndo) determined by removal of a collagen 'bio-molecular film' from an *ex vivo* model. Int. Endod. J.: 2008;41: 602–608.
49. Mehrvazfar P, Akhavan H, Rasgarian H, Akhlage NM, Soleymanpour R and Ahmad A. An *in vitro* comparative study on the antimicrobial effects of bioglass 4555 vs calcium hydroxide on *Enterococcus faecalis*. Iranian Endod. J.: 2011; 6:29–33.
50. Mello I, Kammerer BA and Yoshimoto D. Influence of Final Rinse Technique on Ability of Ethylenediaminetetraacetic acid of removing smear layer. J. Endod.: 2010; 36:512–514.
51. Mensudar R. Photodynamic therapy – a review. World J. Med. Sci.: 2014; 10:139–142.
52. Miller TA and Baumgartner JC. Comparison of the antimicrobial efficacy of irrigation using the EndoVac to endodontic needle delivery. J. Endod.: 2010; 36:509–511.
53. Moghadas L, Shahmoradi M and Narimani T. Antimicrobial activity of a new nanobased endodontic irrigation solution: *In vitro* study. Dent. Hypotheses: 2012; 3:142–146.
54. Mohammadi Z and Abbott PV. The properties and applications of chlorhexidine in endodontics. Int. Endod. J.: 2009; 42:288–302.
55. Mohammadi Z, Soltani MK and Shalavi S. An update on the management of endodontic biofilms using root canal irrigants and medicaments. Iran. Endod. J.: 2014; 9:89–97.
56. Mohammadi Z, Soltani MK, Shalavi S and Asgary S. A review of the properties and applications of ozone in endodontics: an update. Iran. Endod. J.: 2013; 8:40–43.
57. Mohammadi Z. An update on the antibiotic-based root canal irrigation solutions. Iran. Endod. J.: 2008; 3:1–7.
58. Moliz MT, Luque CM, Garcia ME and Baca P. *Enterococcus faecalis* Biofilms eradication by root canal irrigants. J. Endod.: 2009; 35:711–714.
59. Motta MV, Chaves MA and Stirton CG Sodium hypochlorite: Accidental injection with report of a case. Int. Endod. J.: 2009; 42:175–182.
60. Mujoo T and Ballal V. Novel root canal irrigants: an endodontic experience. Int. J. Dent. Health Sci.: 2014; 1:356–366.
61. Murray PE, Farber RM, Namerow KM, Kuttler S and Godoy FG. Evaluation of Morindacitrifolia as an endodontic irrigant. J. Endod.: 2008; 34:66–70.
62. Orstavik D. Root canal disinfection: A review of concepts and recent developments. Aust Endod J.: 2003; 29:70–74.
63. Pagonis TC, Chen J, Fontana CR, Devalapally H, Ruggiero K, Song X, Foschi F, Dunham J, Skobe Z, Yamazaki H, Kent R, Tanner ACR, Amiji MM and Soukos NS. Nanoparticle-based endodontic antimicrobial photodynamic therapy. J. Endod.: 2010; 36:322–328.
64. Pasricha SK, Makkar S and Gupta P. Pressure alteration techniques in endodontics: a review of literature. J. Clin. Diag. Res.: 2015; 9:1–6.

65. Paul J. Recent trends in irrigation in endodontics. Int. J. Curr. Microbiol. App. Sci.: 2014; 3:941–952.
66. Peters LB, Wesselink PR and Moorer WR. The fate and the role of bacteria left in root dentinal tubules. Int. Endod. J.: 1995; 28:95–99.
67. Pitt WG. Removal of oral biofilm by sonic phenomena. Am. J. Dent.: 2005; 18:345–352.
68. Plotino G, Cortese T, Grande NM, Leonardi DP, Giorgio G, Testarelli L and Gambarini G. New technologies to improve root canal disinfection. Braz. Dent. J.: 2016; 27:3–8.
69. Rahimi S, Janani M, Lotfi M, Shahi S, Aghbali A, Pakdel MV, Milani AS and Ghasemi N. A review of antibacterial agents in endodontic treatment. Iran. Endod. J.: 2014; 9:161–168.
70. Rekha P, Abdullah A and Safavi K. Influence of an apical negative pressure irrigation system von bacterial elimination during endodontic therapy: a prospective randomized clinical study. J. Endod.: 2012; 38:1177–1181.
71. Ruddle CJ. Endodontic disinfection: tsunami irrigation. Endod. Practice: Feb. 2008; 7–15.
72. Russell S, Eddy AP, Joyce Steven Roberts, Thomas, BB and Frederick L. An *in vitro* evaluation of the antibacterial efficacy of chlorine dioxide on *E. faecalis* in Bovine Incisors. J. Endod.: 2005; 31:672–675.
73. Sarno MU, Sidow SJ, Looney SW, Lindsey KW, Niu LN and Tay FR. Canal and isthmus debridement efficacy of the VPro Endo Safe Negative-pressure irrigation technique. J. Endod.: 2012; 38:1631–1634.
74. Sathorn C, Parashos P and Messer II. Antibacterial efficacy of calcium hydroxide intracanal dressing: a systematic review and meta-analysis. Int. Endod. J.: 2007; 40:2–10.
75. Schoeffel GJ. The EndoVac Method of endodontic irrigation Part 2 – Efficacy. Dent. Today: 2008; 27:48–52.
76. Schoeffel GJ. The EndoVac Method of endodontic irrigation Part 3 – System Components and their interaction. Dent. Today: 2008; 27:108–111.
77. Sedgley CM, Nagel AC, Hall D and Applegate B. Influence of irrigant needle depth in removing bioluminescent bacteria inoculated into instrumental root canals using real-time imaging *in vitro*. Int. Endod. J.: 2005; 38:97–104.
78. Shalan LA and Al-huwaizi HF.: Cleaning efficiency of root canal after irrigation with new irrigation technique: A scanning electron microscopic study. Iran. J. Endod.: 2018; 13:102–107.
79. Shen Y, Gao Y and Qian W. Three-dimensional numeric stimulation of root canal irrigant flow with different irrigation needles. J. Endod.: 2010; 36:884–889.
80. Sikri V and Baljeet S. Irrigating root canals: Techniques, complications and management. BFUDJ: 2010; 1:22–26.
81. Silveira CFM, Cunha RS, Fontana CE, Martin AS, Gomes BPFA, Motta RHL and Bueno CES. Assessment of antibacterial activity of calcium hydroxide combined with chlorhexidine paste and other intracanal medications against bacterial pathogen. European J. Dent.: 2001; 5:1.
82. Siqueira JF Jr and Lopes HP. Mechanisms of antimicrobial activity of calcium hydroxide: A critical review. Int Endod J: 1991; 32:361–369.
83. Solovyeva AM and Dummer PMH. Cleaning effectiveness of root canal irrigation with electrochemically activated anolyte and catholyte solutions: a pilot study. Int. Endod. J.: 2000; 33:494–504.
84. Soukos NS, Chen PSY, Morris JT. Photodynamic therapy for endodontic disinfection. J. Endod.: 2006; 32:979–984.
85. Srikumar GPV, Sekhar KS and Nischith KG. Mixture tetracycline citric acid and detergent – a root canal irrigant. A review. J. Oral Biol. Craniofac. Res.: 2013; 3:31–35.
86. Steinberg D, Heling I, Daniel I and Ginsburg I. Antibacterial synergistic effect of chlorhexidine and hydrogen peroxide against *Streptococcus sobrinus, Streptococcus faecalis* and *Staphylococcus aureus*. J. Oral Rehab.: 1999; 26:151–156.
87. Stuart CH, Schwartz SA, Besson TJ and Owatz CB. *Enterococcus*: its role in root canal treatment failure and current concepts in retreatment. J. Endod.: 2006; 32:93–98.
88. Tanalp J and Gunger T. Apical extrusion of debris: a literature review of an inherent occurrence during root canal treatment. Int. Endod. J.: 2014; 47:211–221.
89. Tay FR, Gu L, Schoeffel GJ, Wimmer C, Susin L, Zhang K, Arun SN, Kim J, Looney SW and Pashley DH. Effect of vapour lock on root canal debridement by using a side-vented needle for positive-pressure irrigant delivery. J. Endod.: 2010; 36: 745–750.
90. Torabinejad M, Cho Y, Khademi AA, Bakland LK and Shabahang S. The effect of various concentrations of sodium hypochorite on the ability of MTAD to remove the smear layer. J. Endod.: 2003; 29:233–239.
91. Vander SLM, Versluis M, Wu MK and Wasselink PR. Passive ultrasonic irrigation of the root canals: a review of the literature. Int. Endod. J.: 2007; 40:415–426.
92. Vemuri S, Kolanu SK, Pabbati RK, Penumaka R and Bolla N. Effect of different final irrigating solutions on smear layer removal in apical third of root canal: a scanning electron microscope study. J. Conserv. Dent.: 2016; 19:87–90.
93. Vineet AS, Rajesh M, Kapoor S and Mukesh P. A contemporary overview of endodontic irrigants - a review. J. Dent. Appl.: 2014; 1:105–115.
94. Yaduka P and Sharma S. Novel intracanal medicaments and its future scope. IJPBS: 2014; 4:65–69.
95. Zehnder M, Grawehr M, Hasselgren G and Waltimo T. Tissue-dissolution capacity and dentin-disinfecting potential of calcium hydroxide mixed with irrigating solutions. O. Surg., O. Med., O. Path.: 2003; 96:608–613.
96. Zehnder M. Root canal irrigants. J. Endod.: 2006; 32: 389–398.

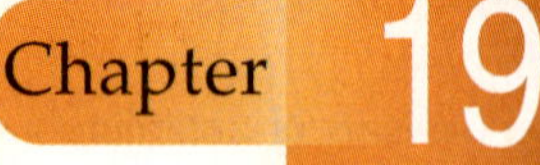

Root Canal Sealers

Three-dimensional sealing of root canal spaces has always been the main goal of endodontic treatment. Such hermetic sealing ensures healing of periapical tissues and also prevent re-infection of the root canal spaces. Root canal sealers along with core material plays a major role in achieving the three-dimensional sealing both apically and coronally.

The accepted method of obturation of prepared canals employs a solid or semisolid core and a root canal sealer. Gutta-percha and other routinely used materials have no adhesives qualities to dentin regardless of the obturation techniques used.

Root canal sealers facilitate filling the accessory root canals, voids and irregularities of the root canal spaces; subsequently minimizing leakage/percolation. The hermetic sealing so achieved reduces the chances of failure of root canal treatment.

Sealers are defined as *'the binding agents used to fill up the gap between root canal and the obturating material'*. They also fill up the irregularities, discrepancies, lateral canals and accessory canals. Conventional sealers are non-bonding (do not bind with the root dentin); whereas, bonded sealers have also been introduced with the desired effect of creating monoblock within the root canal. Bioceramic-based sealers are also being used with the aim of achieving monoblock effect and also to strengthen the root structure. The quest for 'perfect sealer' is still continuing.

Requisite Characteristics of Root Canal Sealer

The requirements of an ideal root canal sealer are as follows:

- Should provide an excellent seal apically and laterally
- Should have adequate flow
- Should produce adequate adhesion between filling material and canal walls
- Radiopaque (should be distinct in radiograph)
- Non-staining (should not discolor tooth)
- Dimensionally stable
- Should be easily mixed and introduced into the root canal
- Should be easily removed, if necessary
- Insoluble in tissue fluids
- Bacteriostatic
- Non-irritating to periapical tissues
- Slow setting to ensure sufficient working time
- Preferably be absorbable when extruded into periapical tissues
- Film thickness should be as minimum as possible
- Should not be mutagenic or carcinogenic (should not provoke any immune response).

Functions

- *Antimicrobial*: Almost all sealers contain antibacterial agent; provide germicidal quality.
- *Binding agent*: The sealer is able to form a bond between the filling material and the dentinal walls.
- *Filler*: Facilitates filling the discrepancies between obturating material and the canal walls.
- *Lubricant*: Act as lubricant when used in conjunction with semisolid material.
- *Radiopacity*: Most of the sealers are radiopaque. Radiopacity helps identifying presence of auxiliary canals, resorptive areas, root fractures and shape of apical foramen.
- *Obturating material*: Sealers can be used as obturating materials, especially in deciduous teeth and in techniques, which use chemically plasticized gutta-percha.

BIOPHYSICAL PROPERTIES OF ROOT CANAL SEALERS

The biophysical properties of root canal sealers are:

i. *Biocompatibility*: The root canal sealer components usually come in contact with vital tissues of apical area and also lateral foramina of the root canals, may be directly or indirectly. The sealer should be conducive to the tissues, should not evoke any inflammatory or immunological response (be biocompatible). Biocompatibility is defined as *'the ability of a material to achieve a positive host response during and after specific applications'*. In simple words, the material should not trigger any adverse reactions, such as toxicity, allergic, inflammatory or carcinogenicity.

Cytotoxicity of sealers has been evaluated using human osteoblast cells and human periodontal ligament cells. Presence of chemical agents, such as iodoform in certain sealers, evoke cytotoxic response. Even zinc oxide eugenol has been observed to evoke mild cytotoxic effect. Such toxicities are usually not of clinical significance; might be of short duration or mild in action. Bioceramic-based sealers have been established as biocompatible. X-ray microanalysis of root canal sealers has confirmed that calcium containing sealers exhibited less toxicity than lead/ magnesium containing sealers (N2, RCB sealer). Calcium enriched mixture (CEM) cement has shown excellent biocompatibility (ability to release calcium ions during setting and subsequent binding of calcium and phosphorous to form hydroxyapatite).

ii. *Flow*: The sealer should fill the irregularities of dentin, accessory canals, voids and difficult-to-access areas; the property of flow facilitates this filling. Factors that influence flow include particle size, temperature, shear rate and mixing time/ technique. Most of bioceramic-based sealers exhibit less flow rate as compared to the zinc oxide-based sealers and even cement sealers. Flow of Apexit is comparable to AH26 and Tubliseal.

iii. *Solubility*: ADA and other such institutions have suggested that the solubility of a root canal sealer should not exceed 3.0% by mass. Solubility is defined as *'the mass's loss of a material during a period of immersion in water or tissue fluids'*. The soluble sealer allows formation of gaps within core and the dentin; facilitating leakage from the periapical tissues. MTA-Fillapex and Root SP show solubility much above the accepted values (15 to 20%). The presence of crystalline silica in Endosequence BC and MTA-Angelus make these sealers less soluble; meat ADA specifications.

iv. *Adhesion/Bonding*: The capacity of the root canal sealer to adhere to the root dentin and create bonding is the desirable property of a sealer [bond strength is the force per unit area required to debond the material from the substrate (dentin)]. Sealing ability has been evaluated using leakage studies. Various sealers have comparable sealing abilities. Bioceramic-based sealers have exhibited better bonding and adaptability as compared to other sealers. Recently introduced EndoCPM has significantly better bond strength as compared to MTA-Fillapex and AH Plus.

v. *Antimicrobial property*: Antimicrobial activity of root canal sealer helps eliminating residual infection that might have survived the canal spaces through leakage. Two properties of root canal sealers, (i) hydrophilicity and (ii) calcium diffusion, contribute to the antimicrobial activity (hydrophilicity reduces the contact angle of the sealer and facilitate penetration of the sealer into the fine areas of root canal system, enhancing antimicrobial activity; Diffusion of active calcium ions, creating alkaline pH also enhances antimicrobial activity). Most of the studies have been conducted observing antibacterial effect on *Enterococcus faecalis*. Other microbes have also been tested by various investigators. Endo CPM, MTA-Angelus and MTA-Fillapex have shown effective antimicrobial activity against almost all the microorganisms inhabiting in the root canals. Calcium enriched mixture (CEM) cement has good antimicrobial and antifungal effect; however, it is ineffective against *E. faecalis*.

Sealapex, Dycal and Apexit sealers are mildly antibacterial (ineffective against *Enterococcus faecalis*). Calcium hydroxide based sealers have been found ineffective against candida (limited antibacterial action might be due to limited diffusibility of calcium hydroxide into dentinal tubules and also the possible buffering ions present in tubules). Zinc oxide eugenol when exposed to aqueous medium releases free eugenol by hydrolysis of zinc eugenolate; capable of inhibiting cell respiration even at low concentration, which accounts for high antibacterial effect of zinc oxide eugenol as compared to calcium hydroxide.

vi. *Setting time*: The setting time of root canal sealers should be within limits and permit adequate working time. Slow-setting sealers may produce mild inflammatory and toxic reactions. The complete setting time of root canal sealers varies considerably from four hours to four days. The setting time is usually affected by the presence of moisture in the root dentin, which might get affected by absorption with paper points, smear plugs or even sclerosis of tubules. Sealapex sets in

2–3 weeks in 100% relative humidity and does not set in dry environment. Calcium hydroxide containing sealers have complex setting reaction; outer mass becomes harder (set), and inner mass remains soft (unset) for an extended period. Manufacturer's claim that MTA-Fillapex sets within two hours; whereas, MTA preparation sets in 24 hours. Most of the root canal sealers have prolonged setting time.

vii. *Radiopacity*: The root canal sealers should be sufficiently radiopaque so as to ascertain its extension in the periapical and other inaccessible areas (radiopacity is generally achieved by adding metal salts). The minimum radiopacity for a root canal sealer is based on a reference standard of 3.0 mm aluminium. Sealers, especially those containing bismuth sulphate and bismuth trioxide, exhibit good radiopacity. Zinc oxide based sealers and also the bioceramic-based sealers exhibit superior radiopacity as compared to others (Sealapex is less radiopaque).

viii. *Ease of removal*: The complete removal of sealer is important during retreatment of any tooth. It has been observed in many studies that during retreatment, most of the material left in root canals is the sealer. Bonded sealers usually pose difficulty in their removal from the canal. Endosequence BC sealer has been reported to be the most difficult to be removed from the root canals. Bioceramic-based sealers usually are not easily removed even with the use of solvents. It has been established that removability of all sealers is almost comparable. Various investigators have suggested that the removal should be accomplished with ultrasonics in the coronal half, followed by rotary instruments and hand files in the apical half area (judicious use of traces of chloroform has also been suggested).

CLASSIFICATION

Definite classification of sealers has not been established; however, for convenience, the sealers are divided into following groups:

I. Zinc oxide based sealers (Kerr pulp canal sealer-Rickert's sealer, Procosol silver cement, Procosol non-staining cement, Grossman's sealer, Tubliseal, Wach's sealer)
II. Medicated zinc oxide eugenol based (Endomethasone, Riebler's paste, Mynol, N2, Endoflas FS)
III. Resin-based sealers (AH 26, AH Plus, Diaket, Hydron, EndoREZ, Fiberfill, ADSeal)
IV. Gutta-percha in organic solvents (Chloropercha, Eucapercha)
V. Cements as sealers (Glass ionomer cement Polycarboxylate cement)
VI. Silicone-based sealers (GuttaFlow, RoekoSeal)
VII. Calcium hydroxide-based sealers (Apexit, Apexit-plus, Sealapex, Biocalex, CRCS)
VIII. Bioceramic-based sealers (Endosequence BC/i Root SP, Proroot, EndoCPM, Fillapex).

INDIVIDUAL SEALERS

I. Zinc Oxide-based Sealers

a. Kerr Pulp Canal Sealer (Rickert's Sealer)

Kerr pulp canal sealer (Rickert's sealer) is available in powder and liquid form (powder contained in a pellet and liquid in a proper bottle). One drop of liquid is added to one pellet of powder (1:1 ratio) and mixed with a heavy spatula until relative homogeneity is obtained (precipitated silver gives a granular appearance).

The cement sets within 15–30 minutes and remain inert; thus decreased inflammatory responses, compared to other cements that may take 24–36 hours to set.

Composition

Powder	*Liquid*
Zinc oxide (34–41%)	Oil of cloves (78–80%)
Precipitated silver (25–30%)	Canada balsam (20–22%)
Oleo resins (30–16%)	
Thymol iodide (11–22%)	

Advantages

- Excellent lubricating properties
- Allows working time of around 30 minutes when mixed in 1:1 ratio
- Germicidal
- Biocompatible
- Greater bulk than any sealer (ideal for condensation techniques to fill voids, auxiliary canals and irregularities)
- Prostaglandin inhibition property (zinc oxide and eugenol form zinc eugenolate, which is prostaglandin inhibitor).

Disadvantage

- Silver present in sealer usually stain the teeth.

b. Procosol Silver Cement

The amount of precipitated silver was reduced and the eugenol increased. The characteristics are same as Kerr sealer; only working time is increased.

19

Composition

Powder	Liquid
Zinc oxide (45%)	Eugenol (90%)
Precipitated silver (17%)	Canada balsam (10%)
Hydrogenated resin (36%)	
Magnesium oxide (2.0%)	

c. Procosol Non-staining (non-silver) Cement

Silver was removed from the sealer and Barium sulfate was added for radiopacity.

Composition

Powder	Liquid
Zinc oxide (40%)	Eugenol (80%)
Staybelite resin (27%)	Oil of almond (20%)
Bismuth subcarbonate (15%)	
Barium sulfate (16%)	

d. Grossman Sealer (Endoseal, Roth 801)

This sealer is widely used and satisfies most of the requirements for an ideal sealer. The root canal sealer is mixed on sterile glass slab with spatula. Two or three drops of liquid is taken on a sterilized glass slab and small increments of cement powder is added slowly to the liquid; mix is spatulated to a smooth creamy consistency (Fig. 19.1a and b).

Composition

Powder	Liquid
Zinc oxide (40%)	Eugenol (5%)
Staybelite resin (30%)	
Bismuth subcarbonate (15%)	
Barium sulfate (15%)	
Sodium borate anhydrous (1.0%)	

The consistency of mix can be tested by two methods, (i) Drop test and (ii) String out test.

In drop test, the mass of the cement is collected on the spatula and held edgewise. The cement should not drop off the spatula edge in less than 10–12 seconds.

In string out test, the mass of the cement is touched with flat surface of the spatula and is raised up slowly from the glass slab. The cement should string out for at least one inch without breaking.

Advantages

- Plasticity and low setting time.
- Good sealing potential and small volumetric change on setting.

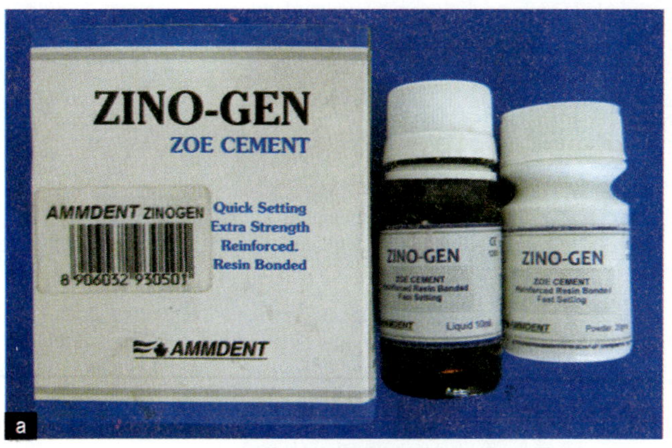

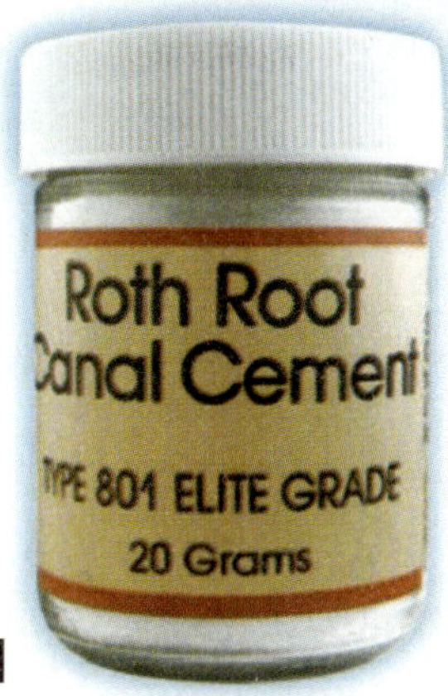

Fig. 19.1a and b Zinc oxide eugenol (Roth 801) sealer

- Zinc eugenolate is decomposed by water through continuous loss of eugenol—thus a weak unstable compound.
- Setting time (hardens in two hours at 37°C).

Disadvantage

- The coarse particle size of resin may lodge on the walls of the canal and obstruct the root canal filling from seating at correct level.

e. Tubli-Seal

It is a modification of Rickert's formula to eliminate the staining. It is available as a two paste system; base and catalyst. The setting time is five minutes. It has good lubricating property (Fig. 19.2).

Composition

Base	Catalyst
Zinc oxide (57–59%)	Eugenol
Bismuth trioxide (18–21%)	Polymerized resin
Thymol iodide (3.5–5.0%)	Annidalin
Oil + waxes (10%)	
Barium sulfate (3.0–5.0%)	

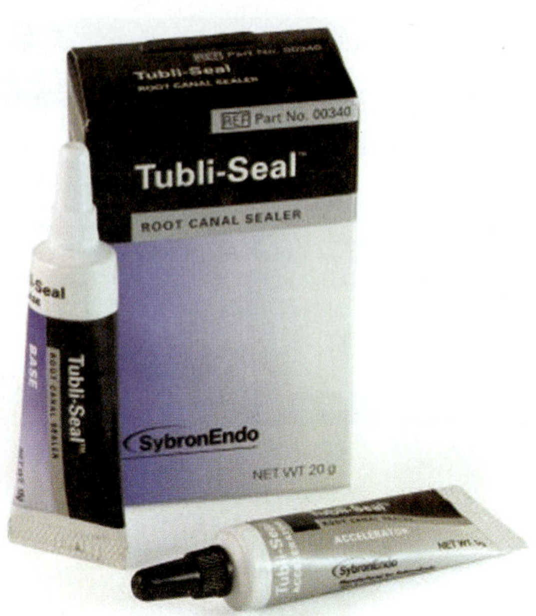

Fig. 19.2 Tubli-Seal (zinc oxide eugenol sealer in paste form)

Advantages

- Easy to mix
- Effective lubricant
- Does not stain tooth structure
- Expands after setting.

Disadvantages

- Irritant to periapical tissues
- Working time is less than 30 minutes; even shorter in presence of moisture
- Tendency to extrude out of root canal.

f. Wach's Sealer

Composition

Powder	Liquid
Zinc oxide (10 gm)	Canada balsam (20 ml)
Tricalcium phosphate (2.0 gm)	Oil of cloves (6.0 ml)
Bismuth subnitrate (3.5 gm)	
Bismuth iodide (0.3 gm)	
Magnesium oxide (0.5 gm)	

Properties

- Medium working time.
- Minimum lubricating quality.
- Minimal periapical irritation.
- Sticky, due to the presence of Canada balsam.
- Increasing the thickness of the sealer lessens its lubricating effect (indicated when there is a possibility of over extension).

Advantages

- Germicidal
- Less periapical irritation
- Light body.

Disadvantage

- Odor of liquid.

g. EndoFill

EndoFill is an improved version of Tubli-Seal. It has been successfully tried as root canal sealer.

Composition

Powder	Liquid
Zinc oxide	Eugenol
Bismuth subcarbonate	Hydrogenated resin
Barium sulfate	Oil of almonds
Sodium borate	

Advantages

- Ample working time
- Easy manipulation
- Good sealability
- Radiopaque.

Disadvantages

- Slight shrinkage upon setting
- Complete removal is difficult.

h. Nogenol

Nogenol was developed to overcome the irritating quality of eugenol. It is considerably less irritating than other sealers. Nogenol expands on setting and improves its sealing efficacy with time (Fig. 19.3).

Composition

Base	Catalyst
Zinc oxide	Resin methyl
Barium sulfate	Salicylic acid

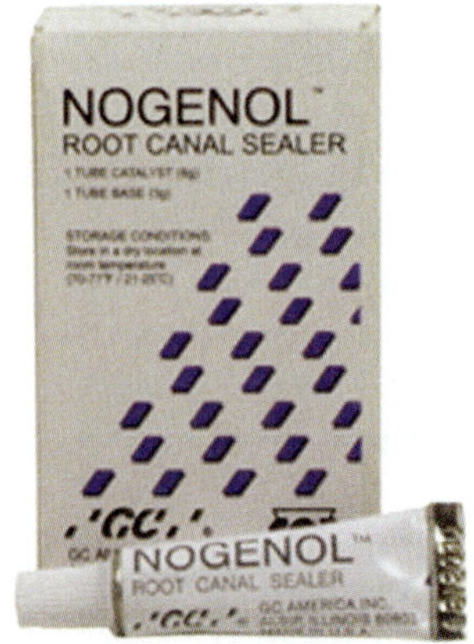

Fig. 19.3 Nogenol sealer

II. Medicated Zinc Oxide Eugenol Sealers

a. Riebler's Paste

Composition

Powder	Liquid
Zinc oxide	Formaldehyde
Formaldehyde	Sulfuric acid
Barium sulfate	Ammonia
Phenol	Glycerine

b. Mynol Cement

Composition

Powder	Liquid
Zinc oxide	Eugenol
Iodoform	Creosol
Resin	Thymol
Bismuth subnitrate	

Both these sealers are usually used without core materials; introduced into the root canal by means of either a lentulospiral or some injection device.

c. N2

Two different types of N2 sealers are available: N2-normal (used for root filling) and N2-apical (used for antiseptic medication of canal).

N2-'universal', a sealer containing the features of both N2-normal and N2-apical has been tried as root canal sealer. This is no longer used because of severe irritation of periapical tissues and may lead to paresthesia.

Composition

Property	Powder	Liquid
Radiopacifiers	Zinc oxide (68.51 gm) Lead tetroxide (12 gm) Paraformaldehyde (4.7 gm) Bismuth subcarbonate (2.60 gm) Bismuth subnitrate (3.7 gm)	Eugenol Cleumrosea Cleum Lavandula
Pigments	Titanium dioxide (8.4 gm)	—
Antiseptic	Phenyl mercuric borate (0.09 gm)	—

d. Endomethasone

Endomethasone has been successfully tried as obturating material in deciduous teeth. It is very effective as root canal sealer. Endomethasone root canal sealers may give rise to pain or discomfort after 6–8 weeks of insertion (Fig. 19.4).

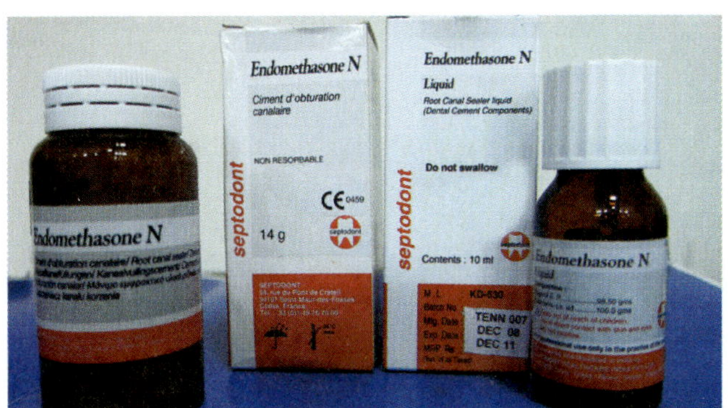

Fig. 19.4 Endomethasone

Composition

Powder	Liquid
Zinc oxide (100 gm)	Eugenol
Bismuth subnitrate (100 gm)	
Dexamethasone (0.019 gm)	
Hydrocortisone (1.6 gm)	
Thymol iodide (25 gm)	
Paraformaldehyde (2.20 gm)	

Advantages

- Radiopaque
- Antibacterial
- Good sealing ability.

e. Endoflas FS

Endoflas FS is one of the most commonly used sealers in clinical practice. It is zinc oxide based medicated sealer marketed as powder and liquid (Fig. 19.5).

Composition

Powder	Liquid
Zinc oxide	Eugenol
Iodoform	Para chlorophenol
Calcium hydroxide	
Barium sulfate (radiopacifier)	

Various studies have confirmed that Endoflas is an effective sealing material, especially in cases of periapical lesions, due to its medicinal properties. It is resorbed periapically in case of extrusion with no side effects; however, it does not resorb intraradicularly.

Advantages

- Ample setting time (35–40 minutes)
- Good sealing ability
- Antibacterial.

Disadvantage

- May irritate periapical tissues.

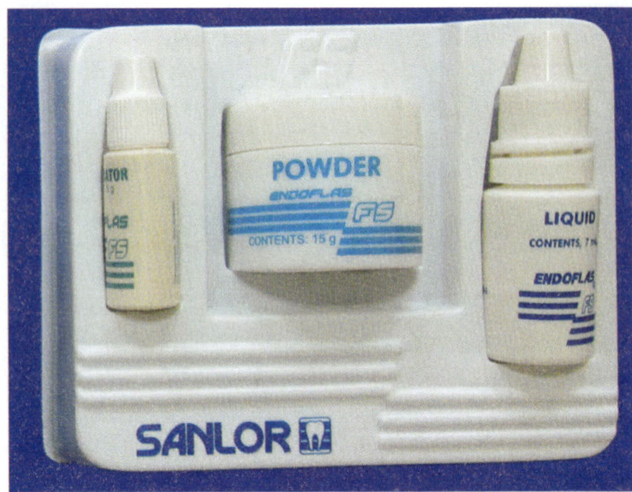

Fig. 19.5 Endoflas FS (powder-liquid)

f. SPAD

SPAD is being used as a one visit obturating material. It is a resorcinol formaldehyde resin supplied as a powder and two liquids. The mix has also been used as root canal sealer.

Equal parts of two liquids are mixed with the powder. The essential reaction to form the resin is between the resorcinol and the formaldehyde. The sealer is used in pulpotomies of deciduous and permanent teeth.

Setting time of SPAD is 24 hours.

Composition

Powder	Liquid (Clear)
Zinc oxide (72.9 gm)	Formaldehyde (57 gm)
Barium sulfate (13 gm)	Glycerine (13 gm)
Titanium dioxide (6.30 gm)	
Paraformaldehyde (4.70 gm)	Liquid (red)
Hydrocortisone acetate (2.0 gm)	Glycerine (55 gm)
Calcium hydroxide (0.44 gm)	Resorcinol (25 gm)
Phenyl mercuric borate (0.16 gm)	Hydrochloric acid (20 gm)

Advantages

- Radiopaque
- Good sealing ability.

Disadvantage

- May irritate periapical tissues.

III. Resin-based Sealers

After the successful use of self-adhesive material in restorative dentistry, low viscosity resin based materials are being tried as root canal sealers. These bondable root canal sealers facilitate creating monoblock (root canal spaces filled with gap-free mass of core and sealer; act as one unit with root dentin, improving the seal and fracture resistance of the root). The resin-based sealers can be applied easily and uniformly along the root canal walls. All these sealers possess acceptable physical and biological properties. Resin-based sealers (Fig. 19.6) are either epoxy resin based or methacrylate resin based (Diaket is a polyvinyl resin sealer).

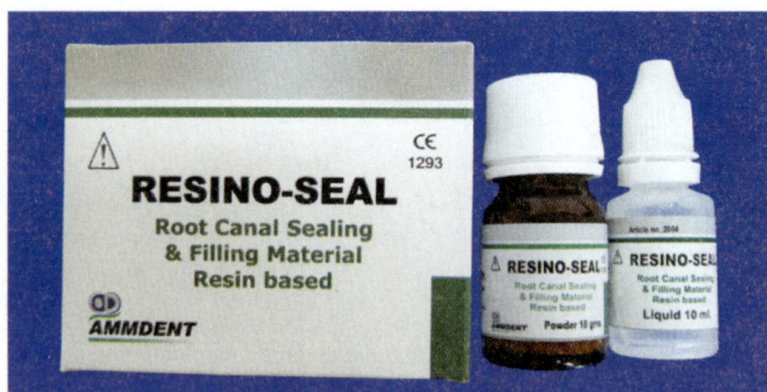

Fig. 19.6 Resin-based sealer (Resino-seal)

Monoblock Concept

The term monoblock literally means a single unit. Franklin Tay first described the concept of monoblock in Endodontics. Monoblocks created in root canal spaces are classified as primary monoblock, secondary monoblock, and tertiary monoblock depending on the number of interfaces present between the bonding substrate and the core material (Fig. 19.7).

i. *Primary monoblock*: Primary monoblock has only one interface that extends circumferentially between the material and the root canal wall (examples of primary monoblock are obturating the root canals with gutta-percha, without using the sealer and use of hydron sealer alone). However, lack of sufficient strength and stiffness as major drawback led to the development of secondary monoblock.

ii. *Secondary monoblock*: Secondary monoblocks are having two circumferential interfaces, such as one between the cement and dentin and the other between the cement and the core material (common example is

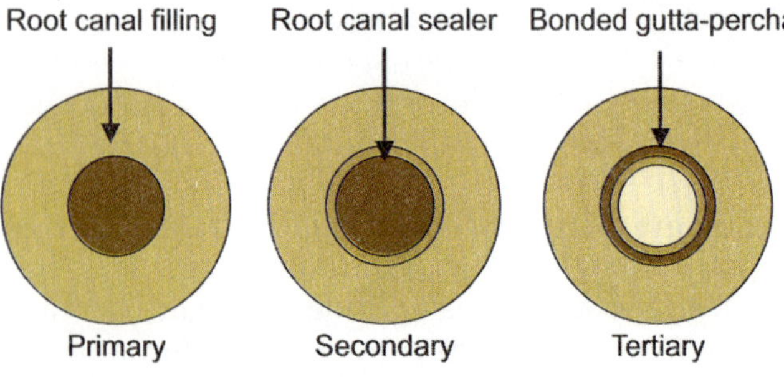

Fig. 19.7 Monoblock concept

obturation with gutta-percha and sealer, where one interface is between gutta-percha point and sealer and the second one between the sealer and root canal wall).

Resilon, a bondable root filling material also falls in this category. As resilon is applied using a methacrylate based sealer to self-etching primer treated root dentin, it contains two interfaces, one between the sealer and primed dentin and the other between the sealer and resilon; hence, categorized as secondary monoblock.

iii. *Tertiary monoblock*: Tertiary monoblocks are having an additional third circumferential interface between the bonding substrate and the abutment material. Fiber posts that contain either an external silicate coating or unpolymerized resin composite for relining root canals that are too wide or not perfectly round for the fitting of conventional fiber posts may be considered as tertiary monoblocks (example: EndoRez system), in which the conventional gutta-percha cones are coated with a proprietary resin coating).

These monoblocks created by adhesive sealers and post systems have the potential to improve the quality of seal and also to reinforce teeth. The treatment protocol consists of extirpating diseased pulp, disinfecting the root canal system and filling it with inert obturating materials. However, the rigidity of root canal treated teeth is compromised by both endodontic instrumentation and restorative intervention. In such cases, the tooth strengthening potential of monoblocks assumes significant value.

Resin-based sealers are either epoxy resin-based or methacrylate-based sealers.

a. Epoxy Resin-based Sealers

Epoxy resin-based sealers are:

i. *AH 26*: AH 26 is a slow setting epoxy resin, available in powder/resin paste system. The sealer releases formaldehyde on setting (freshly mixed sealer releases maximum, which may continue up to 48 hours). The setting time varies from 36 to 48 hours. AH 26 sealer offers good adhesion to dentin, especially when smear layer is removed.

Composition

Powder	*Resin paste*
Bismuth oxide (60%)	Bisphenol A
Hexamethylene tetra-amine (25%)	Diglycidyl ether
Silver powder (10%)	
Titanium dioxide and calcium hydroxide (5.0%)	

The formulation has been altered recently with the removal of silver as one of the constituent to prevent tooth discoloration (Fig. 19.8). ThermaSeal, based on similar formulations has also been tried as root canal sealer.

Advantages

- Well-tolerated by periapical tissues (low toxicity).
- Excess material in the periodontal ligament tends to become encapsulated.
- Effective sealing agent (good adhesive property).
- Antibacterial.

Disadvantages

- Overfilling may lead to paresthesia; partial recovery within 1–2 years.
- Releases formaldehyde, which can be toxic.
- Exceptionally slow setting cement (setting time is 36–48 hours at body temperature and 5–7 days at room temperature).
- Contracts slightly while hardening.

ii. *AH Plus*: AH Plus is a modified form of AH 26, available as two paste system (Fig. 19.9). The sealer offers easy manipulations and color stability. The setting time of the sealer is 8 hours. Film thickness and solubility properties are also improved (film thickness of AH 26 is 39 µm and AH Plus is 22 µm; solubility in AH 26 is 0.5% and in AH Plus is 0.3%). Addition of calcium hydroxide in AH plus make the sealer less viscous and increases pH. The increase in alkalinity improves antimicrobial abilities. Calcium may also enhance deposition of mineralized tissues.

TOPSeal was also introduced having similar formulation.

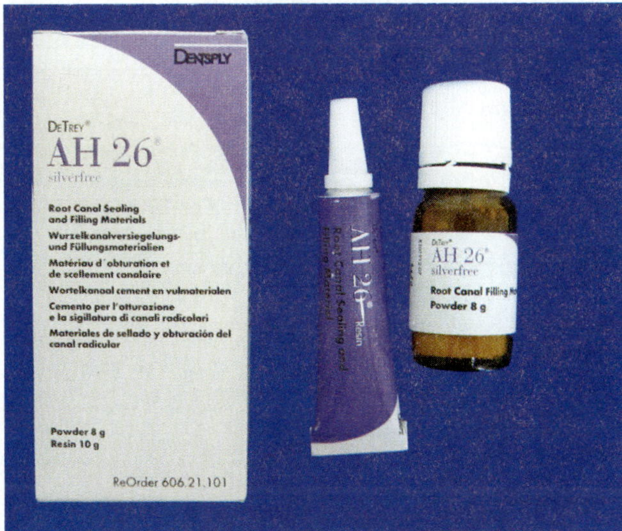

Fig. 19.8 AH 26 (epoxy resin-based) sealer

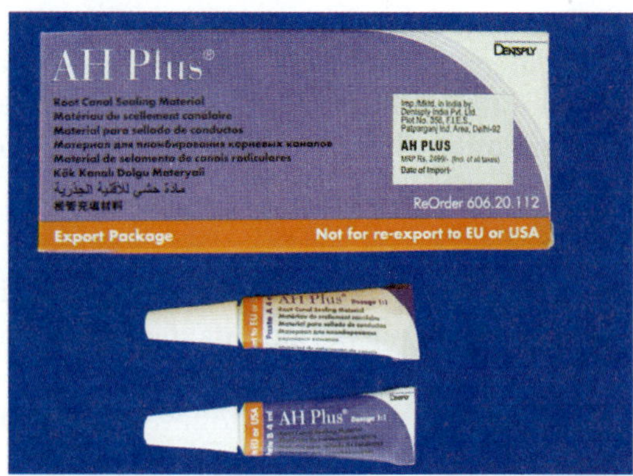

Fig. 19.9 AH Plus (epoxy resin-based) sealer

Composition

Paste A	*Paste B*
Epoxy resin	Adamantane amine
Calcium tungstate	n, n-dibenzoyl-5-oxanonane-diamine
Zirconium oxide	tcd-diamine
Iron oxide	Silicone oil
Aerosil fumed silica	
Calcium hydroxide	

Advantages

- High radiopacity
- Low solubility
- Little shrinkage
- Good tissue compatibility
- No tendency to discolor
- No release of formaldehyde
- Can be removed easily from the root canal.

iii. *Diaket*: Diaket (polyvinyl resin) consists of a fine, pure white powder and a viscous, honey colored liquid. Diaket is one of the few medicated cements, which does not contain paraformaldehyde. Diaket sealer is frequently used to cement endosseous implant. Diaket is known for its resistance to absorption.

Composition

Powder	*Liquid*
Zinc oxide	Polyvinyl resin (copolymer of acetate, vinyl chloride, triethanolamine)
Bismuth phosphate	Propionyl acetophenone

Advantages

- Hardens rapidly
- Setting time is 6–8 minutes
- Antibacterial
- Good sealability.

Disadvantage

- Produce inflammatory reaction, when in contact with periapex.

A modified form of Diaket is, Diaket A, which is similar to Diaket but also contains the disinfectant hexachlorophene.

iv. *Sealer Plus*: Sealer Plus is a recent addition to epoxy-resin based sealer; considered superior to AH Plus. Main ingredients are: Base paste (Bisphenol A/Bisphenol F epoxy resin) and Catalyst paste (Hexmethylenetetramine).

b. Methacrylate Resin-based Sealers

Five generations of methacrylate resin-based sealers have been introduced.

The **first generation** sealer is hydron.

i. *Hydron*: Hydron is a rapid setting, hydrophilic plastic material, used as a root canal sealer without the use of a core.

It is a polymer of hydroxy ethyl methacrylate (poly HEMA), available as injectable root canal sealing material; polymerized *in situ* and act as en-mass filling of root canal.

Hydron conforms to the shape of the root canal because of its plasticity. When the material comes in contact with moisture, the gel absorbs water and swells.

Advantages

- Biocompatible
- Non-irritating
- Early adaptability to root canals
- Do not encourage bacterial growth
- Easy insertion in root canal.

Disadvantages

- Cause severe inflammatory reaction
- Severe leakage
- Water sorption and swelling
- Less radiopaque (complicates radiographic observations).

The use of hydron is obsolete because of the above mentioned disadvantages.

The **second generation** of these sealers are hydrophilic and do not require dentin adhesive.

ii. *EndoREZ*: EndoREZ (ultradent) is a dual cured, radiopaque sealer. EndoREZ has been used with either conventional gutta-percha cones or with specific resin-coated gutta-percha. An accelerator is now available, which facilitate rapid cure of the sealer.

Composition

Paste 1	*Paste 2*
Zinc oxide	Urethane methacrylate resin
Barium sulfate pigments	

Advantages

- Penetrate dentinal walls and adapt closely to root canal walls
- Effectively seals the canal without any leakage.

The **third generation** of these sealers contain self-etching primer and dual-cure composite root canal sealer. Self-etching primer favours incorporating smear layer along sealer-dentin interface.

iii. *FiberFill*: FiberFill root canal sealer (pentron) is an example of third generation sealers. The sealer is used along with primer (FibreFill Primer A and B). Equal drops of primer A and primer B are mixed and coated onto the root dentin. Effective bonding is achieved with penetration of monomer into conditioned dentin surface.

Composition

Paste 1	*Paste 2*
Barium borosilicate glasses	BisGMA
Barium sulfate	Urethane dimethyl/methacrylate
Calcium hydroxide	Benzoyl peroxide
Silica	

FiberFill Primer A	Mixture of acetone and NTG-glymethacrylate
FiberFill Primer B	Mixture of acetone and poly-methyl glycidyl dimethacrylate

The **fourth generation** of these sealers have eliminated the separate etching/bonding step.

iv. *MetaSeal and RealSeal*: MetaSeal and RealSeal are the commercially available fourth generation sealers. The inclusion of 4-methacryloyloxyethyl trimellitate anhydride (4-META) makes the sealer self-etching and hydrophilic. The sealer monomer promotes diffusion into dentinal tubules and produces hybrid layer after polymerization. These sealers are used with resilon cones/pellets by using lateral condensation technique or with a carrier based resilon obturation system.

- **MetaSeal**

Composition

Powder	*Liquid*
Silica nanofillers	4-META (methacrylate monomer)
Zirconium oxide	HEMA
Hydrophilic initiators	

- **RealSeal:** Earlier, RealSeal was named as Epiphany sealer (now discontinued).

Composition

Powder	*Liquid*
Calcium hydroxide	4-META (methacrylate monomer)
Bismuth oxychloride	BisGMA
Silica, borosilicate glass	UDMA
Barium sulfate	Tertiary amine photoinitiators

The **fifth generation** of these sealers (ADSeal and Dia-Proseal) are the improved version of the fourth generation technology. These sealers possess excellent physical properties, good biocompatibility and effectively seals the root canals. The sealers are available in two paste system.

i. ADSeal (Fig. 19.10)

Composition

Paste A	*Paste B*
Epoxy resin	Polyaminobenzoate
Ethylene glycol salicylate	Calcium phosphate
Calcium phosphate	Bismuth subcarbonate
Zirconium oxide	Zirconium oxide
Bismuth subcarbonate	Calcium oxide triethanolamine

ii. Dia-Proseal

Composition

Paste A	*Paste B*
Epoxy resin	Calcium tungstate
Zirconium oxide	Zirconium oxide
Calcium hydroxide	Calcium hydroxide

Both the sealers offer advantages such as:

Advantages

- Effectively seals the canals
- Good flow
- Excellent biocompatibility
- Radiopaque
- Easy to mix and manipulate
- Insoluble in tissue fluids
- Non-staining.

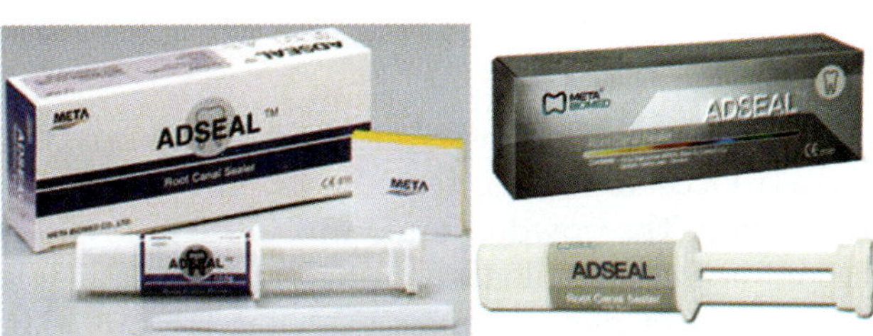

Fig. 19.10 ADSeal (methacrylate resin-based) sealer

19

IV. Gutta-percha in Organic Solvents

Gutta-percha dissolved in organic solvents (mainly chloroform) has been used as root canal sealers. These sealers are no longer used because of the carcinogenic property of the chloroform used as solvent. Further, these sealers proved ineffective in sealing the root canal.

a. Kloroperka N-O Sealer

Composition

Powder		Liquid
Canada balsam	19.6%	Chloroform
Resin	11.8%	
Gutta-percha	19.6%	
Zinc oxide	49%	

The powder is mixed with liquid chloroform. The chloroform evaporates and may leave voids. Greater degree of leakage is associated with this sealer.

b. Chloropercha

This is a mixture of gutta-percha and chloroform. The excessive shrinkage of the filling after evaporation of the chloroform may lead to leakage and voids.

Chloropercha sealer is useful in unusually curved canals or canals with ledge formations. It is used in conjunction with well-fitted primary cone. Chloropercha can fill accessory canals and the root canals spaces.

c. Modified Chloropercha Methods

- *Johnson Callahan method*: The root canal is flooded with 95% alcohol and dried with absorbent points. Callahan resin chloroform solution is applied for two to three minutes.

  A suitable gutta-percha cone is inserted and compressed laterally and apically with a stirring matrix of the plugger until the gutta-percha is dissolved completely in the chloroform solution in the root canal.
- *Nygaard-Ostby method*: The root canal walls are coated with kloroperka; the primary cone is dipped in sealer and inserted apically into the root canal.

V. Cements as Sealers

a. Glass-Ionomer Cement

Glass-ionomer because of its adhesive quality has been used as root canal sealers. Ketac-Endo is the commercial preparation. The powder-liquid mix in 1:2 ratio can be injected in the root canal. Active GP is also available, wherein gutta-percha cones are coated with glass ionomer cement.

19

Advantages
- Better physical qualities
- Bonding to dentin
- Low surface tension.

Disadvantages
- Cannot be removed from the root canal is case of retreatment.
- May create voids.

b. Polycarboxylate Cements

Polycarboxylate cement consists of modified zinc oxide powder and an aqueous solution of polyacrylic acid.

The cement has chelating action and can bond both to enamel and dentin. Because of its adhesive and antibacterial properties, the cement has been tried as a root canal sealer. The modified form of polycarboxylate cement, adding calcium hydroxide and sodium fluoride has been effectively used as sealers.

Advantages
- Bonds well to dentin
- Antibacterial property.

Disadvantages
- Lack of viscosity of the material does not allow proper placement.
- Special plastic plugger is required for insertion since it has great adhesiveness to steel instruments.
- Produce inferior apical seal.

c. Cyanoacrylate Cements

Cyanoacrylate cements are composite type polymers containing fillers that can be polymerized to hard products. They have been tried as root canal sealers.

Advantage
- Biocompatible.

Disadvantages
- Placement difficult
- Non-uniform sealing (produce voids).

VI. Silicone-based Sealers

Silicone-based sealers are mostly used as pastes in obturating the root canals. Examples of these sealers, RoekoSeal, GuttaFlow, etc. have been used as obturating materials as well as sealers.

a. RoekoSeal

RoekoSeal is supplied in two-barrel syringe (base and catalyst). Equal quantity of base and catalyst is squeezed out through a removable tip. The pastes are

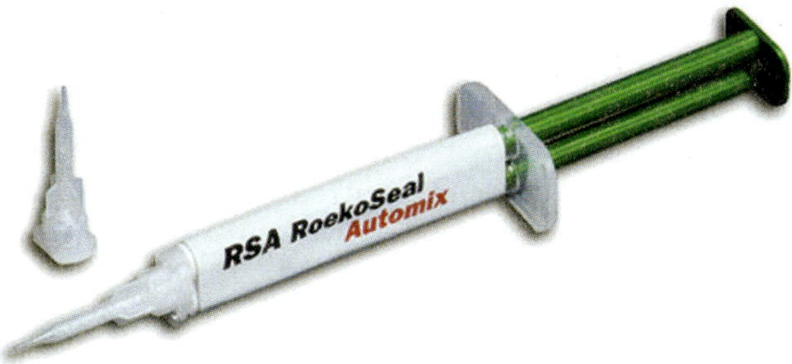

Fig. 19.11 RoekoSeal (silicone-based sealer)

mixed automatically as the base and catalyst are extruded and folded over each other (Fig. 19.11). Silicone-based impression materials and liners are preferred because of low dimensional changes. Silicone-based implants have also shown biocompatibility.

Composition

Paste 1	*Paste 2*
Polydimethyl siloxane	Hexachloroplastinic acid (catalyst)
Silicone oil	Zirconium dioxide (radiopacity)
Paraffin base oil	

Advantages

- Biocompatible
- Radiopaque
- Slight expansion on setting.

Disadvantages

- Average flow
- Manipulation/insertion is difficult.

b. GuttaFlow

GuttaFlow is a free flowing injectable gutta-percha obturation system. It contains gutta-percha in powder form (particle size less than 30 µm), polyvinyl siloxane (polydimethyl siloxane), silicone oil, paraffin oil, zirconium dioxide, nanosilver particles and coloring agents. It is eugenol free and radiopaque. It is a self-polymerizing system, which combines the properties of sealer and gutta-percha. The two components are homogeneously mixed in a mixing capsule and then injected into root canal (Fig. 19.12). It may also fill lateral canals and dentinal tubules. This new filling system does not shrink on setting. Two variants are available: the routine GuttaFlow (working time 10–15 minutes and setting time 25–30 minutes); and GuttaFlow-fast (working time 4–5 minutes and setting time 8–10 minutes).

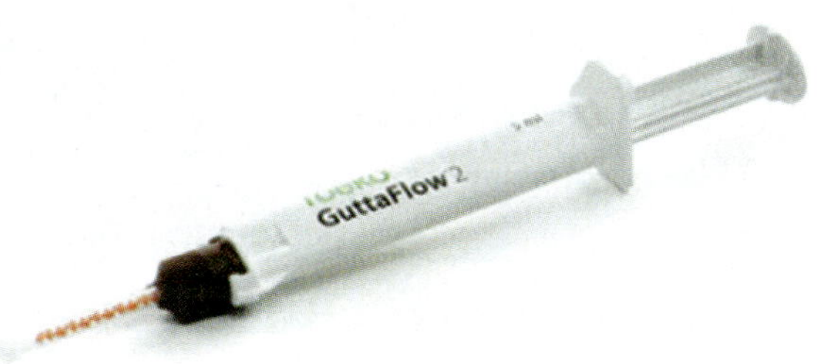

Fig. 19.12 GuttaFlow (silicone-based sealer)

Advantages

- Easy and quick
- Excellent flow properties, which allow optimum distribution in the root canal
- Biocompatible
- Can be removed easily during retreatment
- Provides a good seal
- Radiopaque.

VII. Calcium Hydroxide-based Sealers

Calcium hydroxide has been used as a root canal filling material, or as a sealer in conjunction with solid core materials.

Calcium hydroxide powder can be mixed with normal saline solution and used as sealer. The alkalinity of calcium hydroxide (pH 12.3–12.5) stimulates the induction of mineralized tissue.

The use of calcium hydroxide is based on the assumption that a hard structure or tissue would be created at the apical foramen. Exact mechanism of action is not known; however, following hypothesis is proposed:

- Free hydroxyl ion (H) provide high alkalinity, act as antibacterial and encourages repair.
- Alkaline pH of calcium hydroxide neutralizes lactic acid from osteoclasts and prevents dissolution of mineralized components of teeth.
- Calcium hydroxide denatures protein in bacterial cell walls and makes them less toxic.
- Calcium hydroxide activates alkaline phosphatase and adenosine triphosphatase, which play important role in hard tissue formation.
- Calcium hydroxide makes the environment conducive for healing.

a. Sealapex

It is calcium hydroxide polymeric resin root canal sealer; available in two paste system in collapsible tubes. In 100% humidity, it takes three weeks to reach a final set. It easily sets in dry atmosphere and expands while setting (Fig. 19.13).

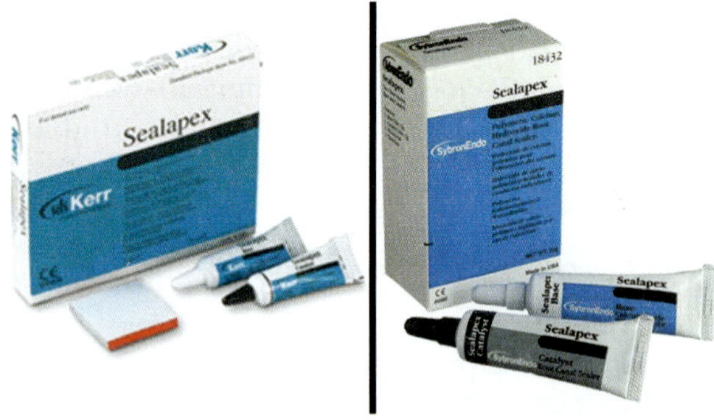

Fig. 19.13 Sealapex (calcium hydroxide-based sealer)

Composition

Base	*Catalyst*
Zinc oxide	Barium sulfate
Calcium hydroxide	Titanium dioxide
Butyl benzene	Resin
Sulfonamide	Isobutyl salicylate
Zinc stearate	Aerosil R 972

b. Calcibiotic Root Canal Sealer (CRCS)

The calcibiotic root canal sealer (CRCS) is the first calcium hydroxide-based sealer.

CRCS is a zinc oxide eugenol eucalyptol sealer to which calcium hydroxide has been added for its osteogenic effect. CRCS takes three days to set fully either in dry or humid environment.

Composition

Powder	*Liquid*
Zinc oxide	Eugenol
Hydrogenated resin	Eucalyptol
Barium sulfate	
Calcium hydroxide	
Bismuth subcarbonate	

The difference between CRCS and Sealapex is that CRCS consists of a powder-liquid combination; whereas, Sealapex is in the form of two paste preparation.

c. Biocalex

Composition

Powder	*Liquid*
Calcium oxide	Glycol
Zinc oxide	Water

Powder and liquid are mixed to form a paste. The sealer can expand to more than 6 times its original volume. Manufacturers advocate that it is not necessary to prepare the root canal prior to root canal filling. Calcium oxide and water react within the tooth to form calcium hydroxide, which ionizes to release OH ions. These OH ions decompose necrotic pulpal tissue to form water and carbon dioxide.

d. Iodoform Paste

Iodoform alone or in combination with zinc oxide/calcium hydroxide has been used as a root canal sealer with core materials (Fig. 19.14). It is available in two paste formulation. Iodoform paste stimulates the periapical tissues and accelerates bone formation.

Composition

Paste 1	*Paste 2*
Iodoform (60 parts)	Solution (40 parts) • Parachlorophenol • Camphor • Menthol

Disadvantages

- Periapical irritation.
- Discoloration.
- Aqueous parachlorophenol solution may evoke mild connective tissue inflammatory response (camphorated parachlorophenol is highly toxic; capable of causing tissue necrosis).

e. Endoflas

Composition

Powder	*Liquid*
Zinc oxide	Eugenol
Calcium hydroxide	Para-monochlorophenol
Iodoform (radiopacifier)	Barium sulfate

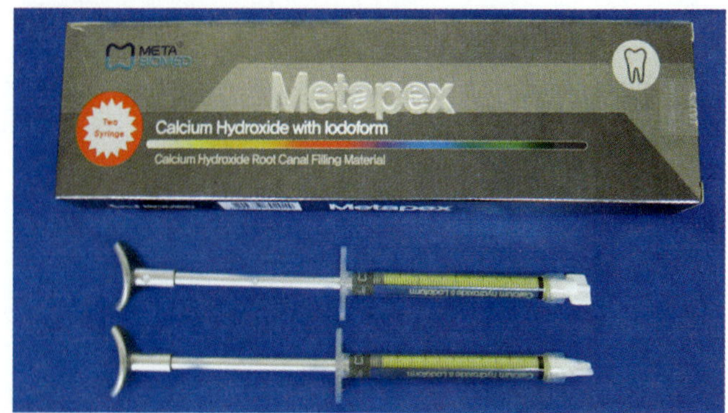

Fig. 19.14 Metapex (calcium hydroxide iodoform) sealer

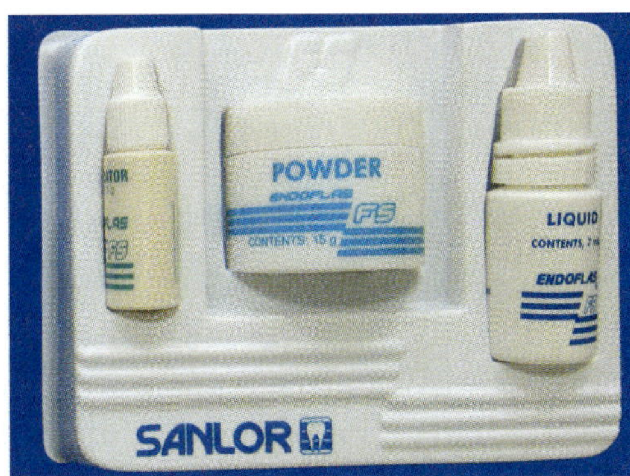

Fig. 19.15 Endoflas

Root canal cement may be placed in the canal either by lentulospiral or reamer. The spiral is turned clockwise by either fingers or the handpiece, placing the cement apically (Fig. 19.15).

An overview of conventional sealers is tabulated in Table 19.1. The advantages and disadvantages of conventional sealers are summarized in Table 19.2.

VIII. Bioceramic-based Root Canal Sealers

Bioceramic are the ceramic materials, which have compatibility with biological tissues; name 'Bioceramics'. Their focus is mainly on apatite agent (calcium phosphate), especially the hydroxyapatite. Bioceramic material includes bioactive glass, zirconia, alumina, calcium phosphate and hydroxyapatite. On the basis of their interaction with the surrounding living tissues, these materials are categorized as *'bioactive'* and *'bioinert'*. Bioactive materials (glass and calcium phosphate) encourages growth of tissues; whereas, bioinert materials (zirconia and alumina) produce no or little biological effect. The bioactive materials have also been classified as (i) degradable and (ii) non-degradable.

The use of bioceramics as root canal sealers provide two advantages; (i) biocompatibility with the surrounding tissues and (ii) chemical component enhance stimulation of crystalline structure simulating tooth and bone. However, one major disadvantage is the difficulty in removing these sealers after setting for retreatment purpose or post-preparation.

It is established that bioceramic root canal sealers have excellent bonding to root dentin. The exact mechanism is not clear; however, suggested hypothesis are:

- Sealer particles diffuse into the dentinal tubules producing mechanical interlocking bonds.
- The mineral contents of the sealers infiltrate into intertubular dentin after denaturing their collagen fibers, resulting in mineralized zone at the interface.
- Calcium silicate of the sealers reacts with dentin's moisture and result in formation of hydroxyapatite along the interface.

Table 19.1 Overview of conventional sealers

Type	*Brand*	*Principle components*
Zinc oxide eugenol based	Kerr Pulp canal sealer (Rickert's sealer) ProcoSol Tubli-seal Wach's sealer	Zinc oxide-eugenol, colophony, bismuth salts, barium salts Zinc oxide-eugenol, thymol, silver Zinc oxide-eugenol, colophony, bismuth salts, barium salts
Medicated zinc oxide eugenol based	Endomethasone Riebler's paste EndoFlas FS	Zinc oxide-eugenol, paraformaldehyde
Resin based sealers	AH 26, AH Plus Epiphany EndoRez Acroseal RealSeal Diaket	Expoxy-bis-phenol resin, adamantine BisGMA, UDMA and hydrophilic methacrylates Epoxy-bis-phenol resin, methenamine, enoxolone, calcium hydroxide
Cements as sealers	Ketac-Endo ActivGP	Polyalkeonate cement, modified zinc oxide, polyacrylic acid
Silicone based	RoekoSeal GuttaFlow	Polydimethylsiloxane, silicone oil, zirconium oxide Polydimethylsiloxane, silicone oil, zirconium oxide, gutta-percha
Calcium hydroxide based	Sealapex Apexit, Apexit Plus	Toluene salicylate, calcium oxide Salicylates, calcium hydroxide

Table 19.2 Advantages and disadvantages of conventional sealers

Type	*Brand*	*Advantages*	*Disadvantages*
Zinc oxide eugenol based	Kerr Pulp canal sealer (Rickert's sealer) ProcoSol Tubli-seal Wach's sealer	• Radiopaque • Slow setting time • Good sealability • Will absorb if extruded	• Shrink on setting • May stain tooth structure • No bonding to core material
Medicated zinc oxide eugenol based	Endomethasone Riebler's paste EndoFlas FS	• Radiopaque • Slow setting time • Good sealability • Antibacterial	• Shrink on setting • May stain tooth structure • No bonding to core material
Resin based	AH 26, AH Plus Epiphany EndoRez Acroseal RealSeal Diaket	• Radiopaque • Slow setting time • Good sealability • Adhesive to dentin; may be to core material	• May release formaldehyde when setting
Cements as sealers	Ketac-Endo ActivGP	• Radiopaque • Bond to dentin	• Not antibacterial • Difficult to remove
Silicone based	RoekoSeal GuttaFlow	• Radiopaque • Long working time • Good sealability • Biocompatible	• Expand on setting • Inconsistent setting time
Calcium hydroxide based	Sealapex Apexit, Apexit Plus	• Radiopaque • Good sealability • Antibacterial	• Soluble • May weaken dentin

The bioceramic root canal sealers are classified according to their major constituent as (a) calcium phosphate-based, (b) calcium silicate based, (c) MTA-based sealers and (d) calcium enriched mixture (CEM) cement.

The bioceramic-based sealers and their chemical components are tabulated in Table 19.3. The advantages and disadvantages of bioceramic-based sealers are summarized in Table 19.4.

Table 19.3 Overview of bioceramic-based sealers

Type	*Brand name*	*Chemical Components*
Calcium phosphate-based sealer	• Sankin apatite root canal sealer (I, II and III)	*Powder*: Tricalcium phosphate and hydroxyl-apatite (in Sankin type I), iodoform added to powder in Type II (30%) and type III (5%) *Liquid*: Polyacrylic acid and water
	• CapSeal (I and II)	*Powder*: Tetracalcium phosphate and anhydrous dicalcium phosphate, portland cement (gray cement in type I and white cement in type II), zirconium oxide, etc. *Liquid*: Solution of Hydroxypropyl methyl cellulose in sodium phosphate
Calcium silicate-based sealer	iRootSP/endosequence BC sealer, biodentine	Zirconium oxide, dicalcium silicates, tricalcium silicate, calcium carbonate, fillers (metal oxide) Calcium chloride and water
MTA-based sealer	• MTA-Fillapex	Salicylate resin, natural resin, bismuth trioxide, nanoparticulate silica, mineral trioxide aggregate, pigments, etc.
	• Endo CPM sealer	Silicon dioxide, calcium carbonate, bismuth trioxide, barium sulfate, propylene glycol alginate, sodium citrate, calcium chloride, etc.

(contd...)

Table 19.3 Overview of bioceramic-based sealers (*contd.*)

Type	*Brand name*	*Chemical Components*
	• MTA-Angelus	Tricalcium silicate, dicalcium silicate, tricalcium aluminate, aluminium oxide, bismuth oxide, calcium carbonate, magnesium oxide, crystalline silica, and traces of calcium oxide, magnesium oxide, potassium/sodium sulfate compounds
	• ProRoot Endo Sealer	*Powder*: Tricalcium silicate, dicalcium silicate, calcium sulfate, bismuth oxide, traces of tricalcium aluminate *Liquid*: Aqueous solution of a water-soluble polymer
Calcium enriched mixture (CEM) cement		Calcium oxide, sulfur trioxide, phosphorus pentoxide, silicone dioxide, traces of aluminium trioxide, sodium oxide, magnesium oxide and water-based solution

Table 19.4 Advantages and disadvantages of bioceramic-based sealers

Type	*Brand name*	*Advantages*	*Disadvantages*
Calcium phosphate-based sealer	• Sankin apatite root canal sealer (I, II and III) • CapSeal (I and II)	• Biocompatible • Radiopaque • Hydrophilic • Antibacterial • Do not shrink on setting	• Difficult to remove
Calcium silicate-based sealer	iRootSP/Endosequence BC sealer, biodentine	• Biocompatible • Radiopaque • Hydrophilic • Antibacterial • Do not shrink on setting • Excellent sealability	• Difficult to remove
MTA-based sealer	• MTA-Fillapex • Endo CPM sealer • MTA-angelus • ProRoot Endo Sealer	• Exhibits an alkaline pH (mild antimicrobial) • Good flow rate • Ideal working time (35 minutes) • Good sealability • Easily penetrates into accessory canals	• Removal is difficult • Slight toxicity reported
Calcium enriched mixture (CEM) cement		• Biocompatible • Short setting time • Easy manipulation • Radiopaque • Do not stain tooth • Antibacterial (ineffective against *E. faecalis*) • Excellent sealability • Ability to induce cemento-genesis • Slight expansion on setting	• Film thickness is inadequate ($175 \pm 25\ \mu$) • Removal is difficult

a. Calcium Phosphate-based Sealers

Calcium phosphate-based sealers are:

i. Sankin Apatite Type I (Vital pulpectomy)

Composition

Powder	Liquid
80% Tricalcium phosphate	25% Polyacrylic acid
20% Hydroxyapatite	75% Water

ii. Sankin Apatite Type II (Infected root canals)

Composition

Powder	Liquid
56% Tricalcium phosphate	25% Polyacrylic acid
14% Hydroxyapatite	75% Water
30% Iodoform	

iii. Sankin Apatite Type III (Partially vital)

Composition

Powder	Liquid
80% Tricalcium phosphate	25% Polyacrylic acid
10 % Hydroxyapatite	75% Water
5.0% Iodoform	
1.0% Bismuth subcarbonate	

Studies revealed that Type II and Type III were more biocompatible probably due to the presence of iodoform.

b. Calcium Silicate-based Sealers

Calcium silicate-based sealers are:

i. ***Endosequence BC Sealer/iRoot SP***: Endosequence BC, also known as iRoot SP, is a non-toxic calcium silicate cement sealer. It is available as a premixed paste in a syringe with intraoral tips for dispensing.

Endosequence BC sealer is hydrophilic and does not set until it comes in contact with water.

When the sealer is placed in the root canal, the material absorbs water from the dentinal tubules, causing a hydration reaction of the dicalcium silicate and tricalcium silicate.

Calcium phosphate reacts with calcium hydroxide at the same time to precipitate hydroxyapatite and water.

Hydration of the calcium silicates continues due to absorption of water and led to the formation of a composite network of gel-like calcium silicate hydrate, which mixes with the hydroxyapatite bioceramics and provides an impervious seal. The pH during the setting process is alkaline (pH 12.9).

The biocompatible, osseoconductive hydroxyapatite has the ability to expand and harden inside the canal, which helps to create a clinically excellent obturation.

Composition

Powder	Liquid
Tricalcium silicate	Water free-vehicle (for flow in paste)
Dicalcium silicate	
Calcium phosphates	
Colloidal silica	
Calcium hydroxide	
Zirconium oxide (radiopacifier)	

Advantages

- Biocompatible
- Excellent sealability
- Non-toxic
- Radiopaque.

ii. ***Biodentine***: Biodentine is calcium silicate-based material, especially marketed as 'dentin replacement' material. It has been successfully used in root perforations, root resorption, retrograde filling material and as an obturating material (Fig. 19.16). Biodentine is also being tried as root canal sealer. Compared to other calcium based cements, this material offers two advantages, (i) faster setting time (12 minutes) and (ii) better mechanical properties. Tricalcium silicate based materials are a source of forming hydroxyapatite when they come in contact with tissue fluids.

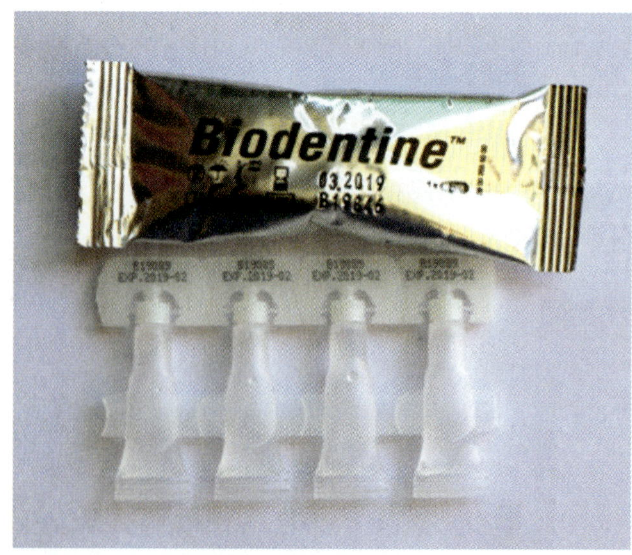

Fig. 19.16 Biodentine

19

Composition

Powder	Liquid
Tricalcium silicate (regulates setting reaction and time)	Calcium chloride (accelerators)
Dicalcium silicate (regulates setting reaction and time)	Water hydrosoluble polymer (water reducing agent – plasticizer)
Calcium carbonate (filler)	
Zirconium oxide (radiopacity)	

Advantages

- Reduced setting time
- Better/easy manipulation
- Biocompatible
- Significantly antibacterial
- Radiopaque
- Good sealability.

c. Mineral Trioxide (MTA)-based Sealers

Mineral trioxide (MTA)-based sealers (Fig. 19.17) are:

i. ***ProRoot Endo Sealer***: ProRoot Endo sealer is an MTA-based endodontic sealer, available in powder and liquid form (Fig. 19.18).

Composition

Powder	Liquid
Tricalcium silicate	Water soluble polymer to improve the workability and flow
Dicalcium silicate	
Calcium sulfate (as a retarder to increase the setting time)	
Bismuth oxide (radiopacifier)	
Tricalcium aluminate (traces)	

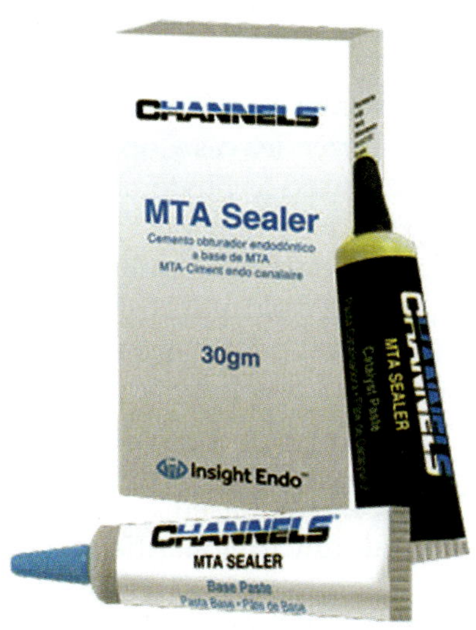

Fig. 19.17 MTA-sealer

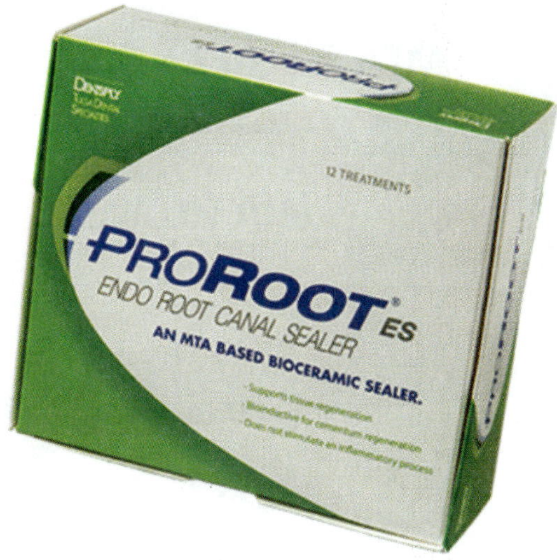

Fig. 19.18 ProRoot (MTA-based) sealer

When placed in the root canal, calcium and hydroxyl ions are produced from the set sealer, giving rise to hydroxyapatite, which aids in the formation of a physical bond between sealer and MTA.

ii. ***Endo CPM Sealer***: Endo CPM sealer effectively incorporates the physiochemical properties of root canal sealer with the biological characteristics of MTA.

Composition

Powder	Liquid
Tricalcium silicate	Saline solution
Tricalcium oxide	Calcium chloride
Tricalcium aluminate	

The powder consists of fine hydrophilic particles that form a gel in the presence of moisture.

The material solidifies and forms a hard mass within one hour.

The added *advantage* of Endo CPM sealer, making it superior to other bioceramic sealers, is that it contains calcium carbonate, which increases the release of calcium ions and improve adhesion to the dentinal walls.

iii. ***Fillapex***: Fillapex, (an MTA-based sealer), is marketed as a two paste system (Fig. 19.19).

Composition

Paste 1	Paste 2
MTA-based salicylate resin	Fumed silica
Bismuth trioxide	Titanium dioxide
Fumed silica	MTA (40%) and base resin

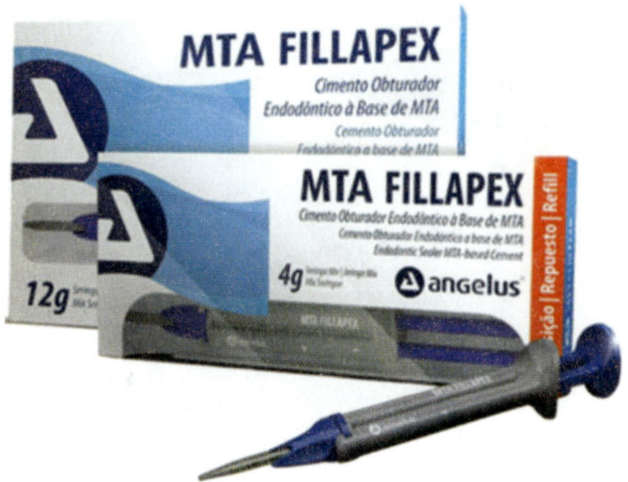

Fig. 19.19 MTA Fillapex (MTA-based) sealer

It exhibits excellent handling characteristics and an improved setting time.

The salicylate reacts with calcium hydroxide and MTA within the mixture reacts with water from the dentinal fluid. The two pastes are mixed homogeneously to form a rigid but semipermeable structure.

Advantages

- Exhibits an alkaline pH (mild antimicrobial)
- Good flow rate
- Ideal working time (35 minutes)
- Good sealability
- Easily penetrates into the accessory canals.

iv. ***Fluoride-doped MTA cements***: Fluoride-doped MTA cements are recently introduced sealers.

Composition

Powder	Liquid
White Portland cement	Alphacaine SP
Bismuth oxide anhydrite	Sodium fluoride (retarder)
Sodium fluoride	

The main *advantage* is that fluoride ions can penetrate into the dentin and enhance the mineralization of the dentin.

d. ***Calcium enriched mixture (CEM) cement***: Calcium enriched mixture (CEM) cement is considered as an improved version of mineral trioxide. This is available in powder and liquid form. When powder is mixed with water-based solution, it forms bioactive calcium and phosphate enriched mixture. The cement releases hydroxyl ions (OH^-), which are used in the process of hydroxyapatite production. CEM differs from MTA; phosphorous is the major component of CEM, whereas in MTA, it may be in traces (most of the physical properties are similar).

Calcium enriched mixture (CEM) cement has been tried successfully in furcation region, root resorption, root-end fillings, pulp capping, vital pulp therapy and in regenerative endodontics.

Composition

Powder	Liquid
Calcium oxide	Water-based solutions
Sulfur trioxide	
Phosphorus pentoxide	
Silicone dioxide	
Traces of aluminium trioxide, magnesium oxide and sodium oxide	

Advantages

- Biocompatible
- Short setting time
- Easy manipulation
- Radiopaque
- Do not stain tooth
- Antibacterial (ineffective against *E. faecalis*)
- Excellent sealability
- Ability to induce cementogenesis
- Slight expansion on setting.

Disadvantages

- Film thickness is inadequate (175 ± 25 µ)
- Removal is difficult.

IX. Miscellaneous Sealers

a. Herbal Sealer (Biosealer)

Trees belonging to the genus Copaifera are present mainly in the Amazon Rainforest of South America. The extract of the tree leaves Copaifera langsdorffii oleoresin is widely used as phytomedicines in Brazil.

The resin extract as liquid along with powder (composed of zinc oxide, calcium hydroxide, bismuth subcarbonate, natural resin and borax) is being tried as endodontic sealer. The effectiveness of the sealer has not been documented properly.

b. Nanoseal Plus Sealer

Nanoseal Plus sealer is based on nanotechnology, which actively seals tiny irregularities in the root canal. It is made of calcium phosphate hydroxyapatite nanoparticles ranging from 40 to 60 µm. These particles can penetrate the dentinal tubules and enter accessory

19

canals to ensure that all the spaces are effectively sealed. The biophysical properties are comparable to bioceramic-based sealers.

Advantages

- Biocompatible
- Antibacterial
- Provides a good hermetic apical seal
- Prevents leakage by increasing adhesiveness.

BIBLIOGRAPHY

1. Abdulkader A, Duguid R and Saunders EM. The antimicrobial activity of endodontic sealers to anaerobic bacteria. Int. Endod. J. 1996; 29:280–283.
2. Al-Haddad A, Zeti A. Bioceramic-based root canal sealers: a review. Int. J. Biomater.: 2016; 1–10.
3. Belli S, Eraslan O, Eskitascioglu G and Karbhari V. Monoblocks in root canals: a finite elemental stress analysis study. Int. Endod. J.: 2011; 44:817–826.
4. Best SM, Porter AE, Thian ES and Huang J. Bioceramics: past, present and for the future. J. Er. Ceramic Soc.: 2008; 28:1319–1327.
5. Bidar M, Disfani R, Asgary S, Forghani M, Gharagozlo S and Rouhani A. Effect of calcium hydroxide premedication on the marginal adaptation of calcium-enriched mixture cement apical plug. Dent. Res. J. (Isfahan): 2012; 9:706–709.
6. Bodrumulu E, Parlak E and Bodrumulu EH. The effect of irrigation solutions on the apical sealing ability in different root canal sealers. Braz. Oral Res.: 2010; 24:165–169.
7. Bouillaguet S, Bertossa B, Krejci I, Wataha JC, Tay FR and Pashley DH. Alternative adhesive strategies to optimize bonding to radicular dentin. J. Endod.: 2007; 33:1227–1230.
8. Boutsioukis C, Noula G and Lambrianidis T. *Ex vivo* study of the efficiency of two techniques for the removal of mineral trioxide aggregate used as a root canal filling material. J. Endod.: 2008; 34:1239–1242.
9. Bsali P, Shivekshith AK, Allamaprabhu CR and Vivek HP. Calcium enriched mixture cement: a review. Int. J. Contemp. Dent. Med. Rev.: 2014; Article ID 061214.
10. Buck RA. Glass ionomer endodontic sealers—a literature review. Gen. Dent.: 2002; 50:365–368.
11. Camilleri J, Gandolfi MG, Siboni F and Prati C. Dynamic sealing ability of MTA root canal sealer. Int. Endod. J.: 2011; 44:9–20.
12. Camps J, Pommel L, Bukiet F. and About I. Influence of the power/liquid ratio on the properties of zinc oxide-eugenol-based root canal sealers. Dent. Mater. 2004: 20, 915–919.
13. Chandra SS, Shankar P and Indira R. Depth of penetration of four resin sealers into radicular dentinal tubules: a confocal microscopic study. J. Endod.: 2012; 38:1412–1416.
14. Chang SW, Lee YK, Zhu Q, Shon WJ, Lee WC, Kum KY, Baek SH, Lee IB, Lim BS and Bae KS. Comparison of the rheological properties of four root canal sealers. Int. J. Oral Sci.: 2015; 23:56–61.
15. Cherng A, Chow I and Takagi S. *In vitro* evaluation of a calcium phosphate cement root canal filler/sealer. J. Endod.: 2001; 27:613–615.
16. Costa JA, Rached-Junior FA, Souza-Gabriel AE, Silva-Sousa YTC and Sousa-Neto MD. Push-out strength of methacrylate resin-based sealers to root canal walls. Int. Endod. J.: 2010; 43:698–706.
17. Desai S and Chandler N. Calcium hydroxide-based root canal sealers: a review. J. Endod.: 2009; 35:475–480.
18. Donnelly A, Sword J, Nishitani Y, Yoshiyama M, Agee K, Tay FR and Pashley DH. Water sorption and solubility of methacrylate resin-based root canal sealers. J. Endod.: 2007; 33:990–994.
19. Gandolfi MG and Prati C. MTA and F-doped MTA cements used as sealers with warm gutta-percha. Long-term study of sealing ability. Int. Endod. J.: 2010; 43:889–901.
20. Gencoglu N, Turkmen C and Ahiskali R. A new silicon-based root canal sealer (Roekoseal-Automix). J. Oral Rehab.: 2003; 30:753–757.
21. Gomes-Filho JE, Moreira JV, Watanabe S, Lodi CS, Cintra LT and Dezan EJ. Sealability of MTA and calcium hydroxide containing sealers. J. Appl. Oral Sci.: 2012; 20:347–351.
22. Grech L, Mallia B and Camilleri J. Characterization of set Intermediate Restorative Material, Biodentine, Bioaggregate and a prototype calcium silicate cement for use as root-end filling materials. Int. Endod. J.: 2013; 46:632–641.
23. Hammad M, Aualtrough A and Silikas N. Extended setting shrinkage behavior of endodontic sealers. J. Endod.: 2008; 34:90–93.
24. Han L and Okiji T. Bioactivity evaluation of three calcium silicate-based endodontic materials. Int. Endod. J.: 2013; 46:808–814.
25. Hess D, Solomon E, Spears R and He J. Retreatability of a bioceramic root canal sealing material. J. Endod.: 2011; 37:1547–1549.
26. Heyder M, Kranz S, Vlpel A, Pfister W, Watts DC and Jandt KD. Antibacterial effect of different root canal sealers on three bacterial species. Dent. Mater.: 2013; 29:542–549.
27. Holland R and de Souza V. Ability of a new calcium hydroxide root canal filling material to induce hard tissue formation. J. Endod.: 1985; 11:535–543.
28. Ioannidis K, Mistakidis I, Beltes P and Karagiannis V. Spectophotometric analysis of crown discoloration induced by MTA- and ZOE- based sealers. J. Appl. Oral Sci.: 2013; 21:138–144.
29. Kangarlou A, Sofiabadi S, Yadegari Z and Asgary S. Antifungal effect of calcium enriched mixture cement against Candida albicans. Iran Endod. J.: 2009; 4:101–105.
30. Kim YK, Grandini S and Ames JM. Critical review on methacrylate resin-based root canal sealers. J. Endod.: 2010; 36:383–399.
31. Kokorikos I, Kolokouris I, Economides N, Gogos C and Helvatjoglu-Antoniades M. Long-term evaluation of the sealing ability of two root canal sealers in combination with self-etching bonding agents. J. Adhes. Dent.: 2009; 11:239–246.

32. Kossev D and Stefanov V. Ceramics-based sealers as new alternative to currently used endodontic sealers. Roots: 2009; 42–48.
33. Lacey S, Pitt Ford TR, Watson TF and Sherriff M. A study of the rheological properties of endodontic sealers. Int. Endod. J. 2005: 38, 499.
34. Lodiene G, Morisbak E, Bruzell E and Orstavik D. Toxicity evaluation of root canal sealers *in vitro*. Int. Endod. J.: 2008; 41:72–77.
35. Lucena-Martin C, Ferrer-Luque CM, Gonzalez-Rodriguez MP, Robles-Gijon V, Navajas-Rodriguez de Mondelo JM. A comparative study of apical leakage of endomethasone, topseal and roeko seal cements. J. Endod.: 2002; 28:423–426.
36. Malkondu O, Kazandag MK and Kazazoglu E. A review on biodentine, a contemporary dentine replacement and repair material. BioMed. Resch. Int.: 2014; 1–10.
37. Marciano MA, Guimaraes BM, Ordinola-Zapata R, Bramante CM, Cavenago BC, Garcia RB, Bernardineli N, Andrade FB, Moraes IG and Durate MA. Physical properties and interfacial adaptation of three epoxy resin-based sealers. J. Endod.: 2011; 37:1417–1421.
38. Mohammadi Z, Giardino L, Palazzi F and Shalavi S. Antibacterial activity of a new mineral trioxide aggregate-based root canal sealer. Int. Dent. J.: 2012; 62:70–73.
39. Monea M, Beresescu G, Stoica A and Stefanescu T. Biocompatibility of calcium hydroxide-based root canal sealers: a histological study. Key Engg. Mater. 2016; 695:243–246.
40. Nagas E, Uyanik MO and Eymirli A. Dentin moisture conditions after the adhesion of root canal sealers. J. Endod.: 2012; 38:240–244.
41. Nagas E, Uyanik MO, Eymirli A, Cehreli ZC, Vallittu PK and Lassila LV. Dentin moisture conditions affect the adhesion of root canal sealers. Int. Endod. J.: 2011; 44:126–135.
42. Nielsen BA, Beeler WJ, Vy C and Baumgartner JC. Setting times of Resilon and other seals in aerobic and anaerobic environments. J. Endod.: 2006; 32:130–132.
43. Orstavik D, Nordahl I and Tibballs JE. Dimensional change following setting of root canal sealer materials. Dent. Mater.: 2001; 17:512–519.
44. Ozcan E, Capar I, Cetin AR, Tuncdemir AR and Aydinbelge HA. The effect of calcium silicate-based sealer on the push-out bond strength of fiber posts. Aust. Dent. J.: 2012; 57:166–170.
45. Patel DV, Sherriff M, Ford TR, Watson TF and Mannocci F. The penetration of RealSeal primer and Tubilseal into root canal dentinal tubules: a confocal microscopic study. Int. Endod. J.: 2007; 40:67–71.
46. Pumarola J, Berastegui E, Brau E, Canalda C and Anta TJU. Antimicrobial activity of seven root canal sealers. Oral Surg., Oral Med., Oral Pathol.1992; 74:216–220.
47. Schafer E and Zandbiglari T. Solubility of root-canal sealers in water and artificial saliva. Int. Endod. J. 2003: 36, 660–669.
48. Silva EJ, Rosa TP, Herrera DR, Jacinto RC, Gomes, BP and Zaia AA. Evaluation of cytotoxicity and physico-chemical properties of calcium silicate-based endodontic sealer MTA fillapex. J. Endod.: 2013; 39:274–277.
49. Silva EJ, Santos CC and Zaia AA. Long-term cytotoxic effect of contemporary root canal sealers. J. Appl. Oral Sci.: 2013; 21:43–47.
50. Singh H, Kaur M, Markan S and Kapoor P. Biodentine: A promising dentin substitute. J. Interdiscipl. Med. Dent. Sci.: 2014; 2:1–5.
51. Siqueira JF, Favieri A, Gahyva SM, Moraes SR, Lima KC and Lopes HP. Antimicrobial activity and flow rate of newer and established root canal sealers. J. Endod.: 2000; 26:274–277.
52. Siqueira JJ and Lopes H. Mechanisms of antimicrobial activity of calcium hydroxide: a critical review. Int. Endod. J.: 1999; 32:361–369.
53. Song YS, Choi Y, Lim MJ, Yu MK, Hong CU, Lee KW and Min KS. *In vitro* evaluation of a newly produced resin-based endodontic sealer. Restor. Dent. Endod.: 2016; 41:189–195.
54. Stoll R, Thull P, Hobeck C, Yuksel S, Jablonski-Momeni A, Roggendorf MJ and Frankenberger R. Adhesion of self-adhesive root canal sealers on gutta-percha and Resilon. J. Endod.: 2010; 36:890–893.
55. Tay FR and Pashley DH. Monoblocks in root canals: a hypothetical or a tangible goal. J. Endod.: 2007; 33:391–398.
56. Tay FR, Hiraishi N, Pashley DH, Loushine RJ and Weller N. Bondability of Resilon to a methacrylate-based root canal sealer. J. Endod.: 2006; 32:133–137.
57. Teixeira FB, Teixeira EC, Thompson J, Leinfelder KF and Trope M. Dentinal bonding reaches the root canal system. J. Esthet. Rest. Dent.: 2004; 16:348–354.
58. Utneja S, Nawal RR, Talwar S and Verma M. Current perspectives of bioceramic technology in endodontics: calcium enriched mixture cement - review of its composition, properties and applications. Restor. Dent. Endod.: 2015; 40:1–13.
59. Vertuan GC, Duarte MAH, de Moraes IG, Piazza B, Vasconcelos BC, Alcade MP and Vivan RR.: Evaluation of physiochemical properties of a new root canal sealer. J. Endod.:2017; 1-5.
60. Vouzara T, Dimosiari G, Koulauzidou EA and Economides N.: Cytotoxicity of a new calcium silicate endodontic sealer. J. Endod.:2018; 44:849-852.
61. Yigit DH and Gencoglu N. Evaluation of resin/silicone based root canal sealers. Part I : Physical properties. Digest J. Nanomater. Biostruc.: 2012; 7:107–115.
62. Zhang H, Shen Y, Ruse ND and Haapasalo M. Antibacterial activity of endodontic sealers by modified direct contact test against *Enterococcus faecalis*. J. Endod.: 2009; 35: 1051–1055.
63. Zhou HM, Shen Y, Zheng W, Li L, Zheng YF and Haapasalo M. Physical properties of 5 root canal sealers. J. Endod.: 2013; 39:1281–1286.
64. Zmener O and Pameijer CH. Clinical and radiographic evaluation of a resin-based root canal sealer. Am. J. Dent.: 2004; 17:19–22.
65. Zmener O and Pameijer CH. Clinical and radiographic evaluation of a resin-based root canal sealer: an eight-year update. J. Endod.: 2010; 36:1311–1314.
66. Zoufan K, Jiang J, Komabayashi T, Wang YH, Safavi KE and Zhu Q. Cytotoxicity evaluation of Gutta Flow and EndoSequence BC sealers. Oral Surg., Oral Med., Oral Pathol., Oral Radiol. Endod.: 2011; 112:657–661.

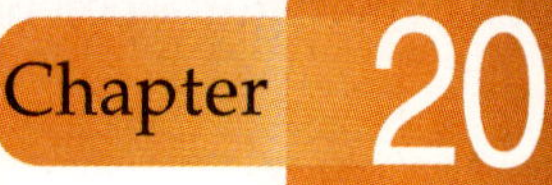

Chapter 20

Obturation of Root Canal Spaces

Success of root canal treatment depends on meticulous cleaning and shaping of the canal system, three-dimensional sealing, and a well-fitting, 'fluid-tight' coronal restoration. The substitution of inert material in the space previously occupied by the pulp tissue is technically known as obturation. Over the years, pitfalls with one technique have led to the development of newer methods of obturation; also recognizing the fact that no one method of obturation could satisfy all clinical situations. It is also emphasized that no obturating technique and/or material can compensate for inadequate disinfection protocol.

Root canal obturation is defined as *'the three-dimensional filling of the entire root canal system as close to the cementodentinal junction as possible. Minimal amounts of root canal sealer, which have been demonstrated to be biologically compatible, are used in conjunction with the core filling material to establish an adequate seal'.*

Aims and Objectives

The aim of filling the root canal system is to prevent recontamination by microorganism, either from those microbes left in the canal after preparation or from new invaders from the coronal access or lateral communications. The root filling should be able to destroy residual microorganisms and adapt adequately to root canal walls to prevent their seepage and growth. The degree of seal required is dictated by the smallest molecule capable of initiating and sustaining periapical inflammation. Since, the pathogenesis of periapical lesions is a diverse phenomenon, it is wiser to achieve maximum seal without leaving any space between root dentin and the obturating material.

The main objectives of obturation are to prevent percolation of periapical exudates into the root canal, minimizing chances of reinfection and creating a favourable biological environment for the process of tissue healing.

When to Obturate

- Asymptomatic tooth (no pain, no tenderness)
- No exudate/seepage (dry canal)
- No sign of apical periodontitis
- No sinus tract
- No foul odor (suggests residual infection/re-infection due to anaerobes)
- Intact temporary filling (broken/leaking fillings cause re-contamination of the canal)
- A negative culture (preferably).

Requirements of an Ideal Obturating Material

The requirements of an ideal obturating material are:
- Can be easily introduced into the root canal
- Should seal the canal laterally as well as apically
- Dimensionally stable
- Should be impervious to moisture
- Bacteriostatic
- Radiopaque
- Should not stain tooth structure
- Should not irritate periradicular tissues
- Should be easily and quickly sterilized
- Should be removed easily from the root canal, if necessary.

APICAL TERMINATION OF OBTURATION

It has been established that the position/extent of root canal obturation is inconsistent because of unpredictable anatomy at the root apex. Kutler, an early investigator, has cautioned that the cemental funnel beyond the minor diameter would present difficulties when attempting to create hermetic sealing at that area.

Microanalysis of root apices have observed varied shapes and irregularities in the shape of cementodentinal junction. The apical constriction area is never uniform at all points in a canal. The shape and contour of foramen also varies with age, occlusal stresses and inflammatory influences. The variation in position of these three locations (CDJ/constriction/foramen) have been the cause of controversy in endodontics as regard where to finish the preparation and also the extension of obturation.

The accepted hypothesis is that the root canals should be filled up to the dentinocemental junction, anatomically demarcating periodontal tissue with the pulpal tissues. It has been established that the dentinocemental junction is at an average of about 0.5 to 0.7 mm from the external surface of the apical foramen. A few authors prefer to fill up to the radiographic external surface of the root. They seek to develop a small 'puff' or 'button' of overfilling. The 'puff' or 'button' is designed to compensate for shrinkage of the gutta-percha by pulling down tightly against the apex. It also facilitates dense packing of gutta-percha in the apical area along with lateral/accessory canals, if any.

With the use of electronic technology, the clinician can determine the required position of the cemento-dentinal junction and plan their preparation and obturation.

Overfilling and Overextension

Overextension and underextension of a root canal filling is a matter of its vertical dimensions; beyond or short of apex. Overextension implies gutta-percha extending beyond the apex (say the working length is 22 mm and the gutta-percha filling at 25 mm). The retrieval of overextended gutta-percha is difficult.

Overfilled canal implies well-filled root canal, but exhibiting surplus filling material past the apex (gutta-percha is well-condensed, but radiographically beyond the apex). Overjealous preparation of the apical constriction area may lead to overfilling.

Underfilling/underextension is where gutta-percha is short of apex.

Difference between overfilling and overextension

- *Overfilling denotes total obturation of the root canal space with excess material extruding beyond the apical foramen.*
- *Overextension may also denote extrusion of the filling material beyond the apical foramen but with the impression that the canal has not been adequately filled and the apex has not been sealed.*

Preventing Overextension

- Meticulous working length control
- Avoid over preparation at the apical constriction
- Rotary instruments should be used with caution
- In case of discrepancy with gutta-percha fit and working length, confirm again
- Plasticized gutta-percha should be used judiciously
- Obturation of 2-1 canal anatomy should be thoroughly analysed; gutta-percha in second canal may need be adjusted.

MATERIALS USED FOR OBTURATION: CLASSIFICATION

A large variety of root canal filling materials have been advocated, ranging from plaster of paris, asbestos and bamboo to precious metals, such as gold and platinum, etc. However, none of the materials satisfied the requirements of an ideal root canal filling material.

The root canal obturating materials can be classified as depicted in Flowchart 20.1.

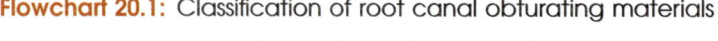

Flowchart 20.1: Classification of root canal obturating materials

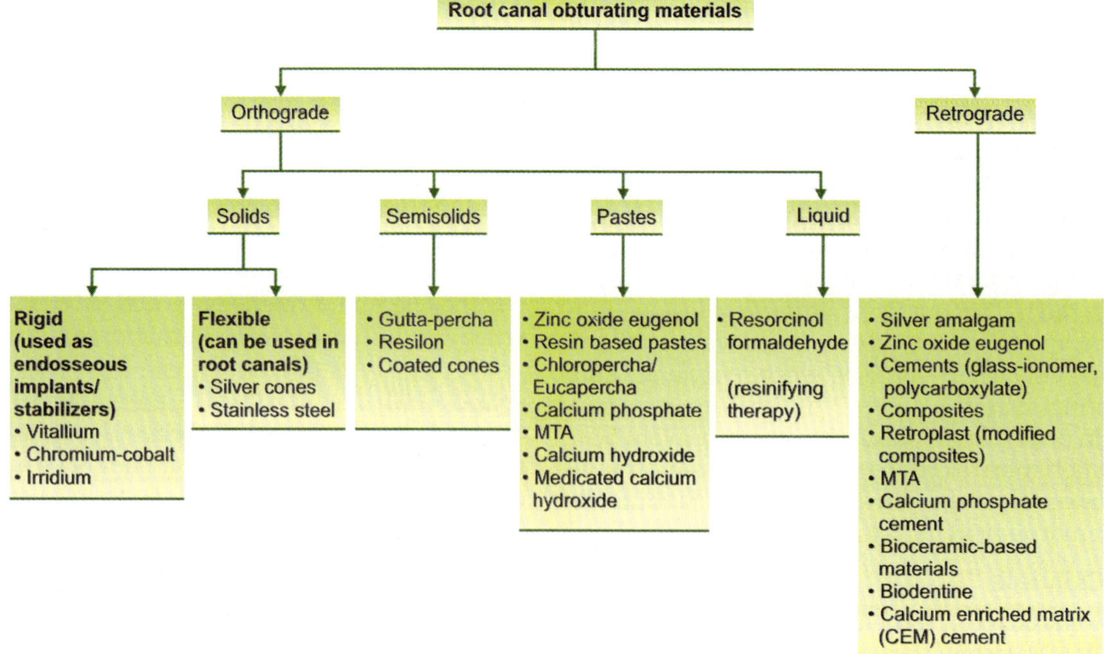

MATERIALS/TECHNIQUES OF OBTURATION

1. Gutta-percha
A. Cold gutta-percha
   a. Lateral compaction method
   b. Modifications of lateral compaction method
      i. For curved canals
      ii. For immature apices/tubular canals
         - Inverted point technique
         - Roll-cone technique (tailor made gutta-percha roll).
B. Chemically softened gutta-percha.
C. Heat softened gutta-percha.
   a. Intraradicular (gutta-percha is heated within the canal) techniques
      i. Warm vertical condensation
         - Touch 'n' heat
         - System B
         - Elements system
      ii. Warm lateral condensation
         - Endotec/Endotec II
         - DownPak
         - Thermapact
      iii. Thermocompaction
         - McSpadden compactor
         - Modified McSpadden (microseal system)
         - Maillefer guttacondenser
         - Zipperer thermocompactor/engine plugger
         - Quickfill compactor
      iv. Ultrasonic plasticizing.
   b. Extra-radicular (gutta-percha is heated outside the oral cavity and then placed in the root canal) techniques
      i. Injectable gutta-percha
         - Obtura II/Obtura III Max
         - Calamus dual 3D system
         - Ultrafil
         - PAC-160
      ii. Solid core carrier
         - Successfil
         - Thermafil
         - Densfil
         - Trifecta system.
2. Silver cones.
3. Miscellaneous obturating techniques
   a. GuttaFlow/GuttaFlow 2
   b. Guttacore system
   c. Resilon
      - RealSeal/Realseal SE
      - RealSeal one
   d. EZfill system
   e. SmartSeal
      - Propoint
      - Smart paste/Smart paste Bio
   f. Coated cones
      - EndoREZ
      - Activ GP Precision.
4. Obturation of apical third area
   a. Warm/sectional gutta-percha
   b. Dentin chips
   c. Mineral trioxide aggregate
   d. Carrier based systems
      i. SimpliFill system
      ii. FiberFill system
      iii. EZFill system.
5. Pastes as obturating materials
   a. N2 (Sargenti paste)
   b. Mineral trioxide aggregate
   c. Calcium phosphate cement
   d. Calcium enriched matrix (CEM) cement
   e. Biodentine.
6. Retrograde (root-end) filling materials
   a. Amalgam
   b. Gutta-percha
   c. Zinc oxide eugenol/reinforced zinc oxide eugenol compounds
   d. Cements
      i. Polycarboxylate cement
      ii. Glass ionomer cement
   e. Composite resins
   f. Mineral trioxide aggregate
   g. Calcium phosphate cement
   h. Bioceramic-based materials
   i. Biodentine.

1. GUTTA-PERCHA

Gutta-percha was obtained from sap of the Indian rubber trees, indigenous to Malaysia. Now, it is extracted from Palaquium trees of South America. Gutta-percha is white in color as squeezed from the trees. It is dyed to red and pink color to match the color of the pulp.

Gutta-percha exists in two distinct crystalline forms, (α and β). Raw gutta-percha, as it comes directly from the tree, is in the α-form. Once purified, as available commercially, gutta-percha is in the β-crystalline form.

When β-form of gutta-percha is heated, a crystalline phase transition to the α-form takes place between 42 to 49°C.

Composition

Matrix	:	Gutta-percha (18–22%)
Filler	:	Zinc oxide (59–67%)
Radiopacifiers	:	Heavy metal sulfate (1–18%)
Plasticizers	:	Waxes/resins/rosins (1–4%)
Trace elements	:	(0–1.0%)

Gutta-percha is available in following forms:

i. Standardized cones correspond to ISO sizes and 0.02 taper
ii. Standardized cones with non ISO taper: 0.04, 0.06, 0.08, etc.
iii. Non-standardized cones: Available in sizes extra-fine, fine-fine, medium-fine, fine, fine-medium, medium, medium-large, large
iv. Gutta-percha pellets/bars (for use in injectable thermoplasticized gutta-percha systems, e.g. Obtura)
v. Gutta-percha coated on carriers, e.g. Thermafil
vi. Medicated gutta-percha, e.g. gutta-percha containing calcium hydroxide, iodoform, chlorhexidine, etc.
vii. Gutta-percha powder in combination with resin, e.g. GuttaFlow.

Disinfection of Gutta-percha

Though commercialized gutta-percha cones are pre-sterilized, it is advisable to disinfect them before use. gutta-percha cannot be sterilized by heat. It is disinfected by immersing in 5.25% sodium hypochlorite for one minute and then rinsing in hydrogen peroxide/ethyl alcohol. Lower concentration of sodium hypochlorite has also been tried; however, higher concentration is preferred.

2.0% digluconate chlorhexidine is also effective in decontaminating gutta-percha cones within five minutes. It is documented that 10% polyvinylpyrrolidone-iodine aqueous solution (30 seconds to one minute) and paraformaldehyde vapors (one hour) are equally effective in decontaminating gutta-percha cones.

Advantages

- Compactible and compressible
- Excellent adaptability to the irregularities of the canal
- Inert
- Dimensionally stable
- Excellent tissue tolerance
- Radiopaque
- Can be easily removed from the canal, if necessary
- Elongability when fresh; however, turns brittle over time.

Disadvantages

- Lacks rigidity (smallest standardized gutta-percha cones are difficult to use unless canals are enlarged to size 25)
- Lacks adhesive quality (sealer has to be used)
- Can easily be displaced under pressure (may lead to overextension during condensation).

A. Cold Gutta-percha

a. Lateral Compaction Method

The lateral compaction method is the most accepted and widely used method of obturation. This technique requires the introduction of a gutta-percha cone that fits well to the apical preparation (master cone), together with a small amount of sealer. The appropriate spreader is used to compact the cone against the canal wall. Subsequently additional cones are inserted.

Technique

- A gutta-percha cone, referred to as the 'master cone' is selected, consistent with the size of master apical file (Fig. 20.1).
- It is checked clinically for a snug fit and 'tug-back'.
- The apical fit of the master cone is verified by radiographs.
- Check for the length of the master cone; if less or more, adjust accordingly (Fig. 20.2).
- Gutta-percha is notched at the level of coronal reference point (Fig. 20.3a), and dipped in 5.0% sodium hypochlorite (Fig. 20.3b).
- Canal is dried with absorbent paper points.

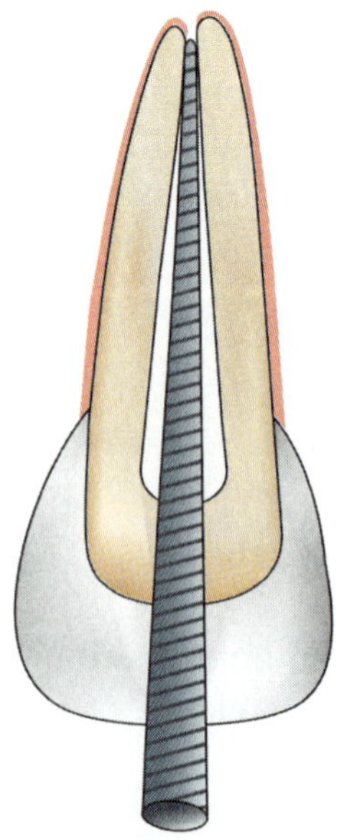

Fig. 20.1 Master cone (selected according to master apical file)

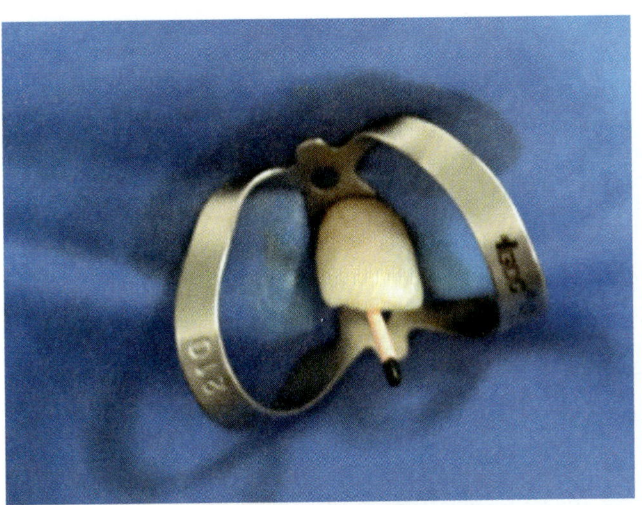

Fig. 20.2 Checking master cone

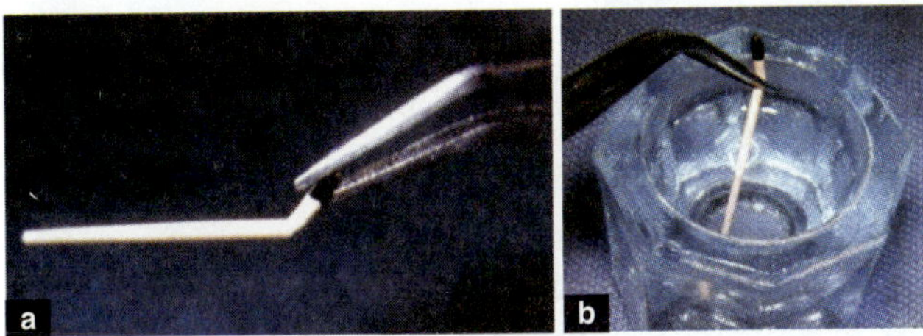

Fig. 20.3 (a) Notching of gutta-percha at coronal reference; (b) Notched gutta-percha dipped in 5.0% sodium hypochlorite

- The walls of the canal are coated with a thin layer of sealer.
- The selected master cone is coated with sealer. The apical 2.0 mm of sealer (Fig. 20.4a) is wiped out (apical sealer may be pushed into the periapical area during lateral compaction, as little vertical pressure is also created). The cone is then placed in the canal (Fig. 20.4b).
- A spreader is selected that reaches 1.0–2.0 mm apical of the working length (Fig. 20.5).
- The selected spreader is kept there for at least 20 seconds (time needed to compact the gutta-percha).
- The spreader is disengaged from the cone by rotating it between fingertips or when using a long handled spreader, by rotating the handle in an arc.
- An accessory cone is inserted in the space previously occupied by the spreader. Cones are placed parallel to the spreader blade into the space created by the removal of the spreader (Fig. 20.6).
- This process is repeated until the entire canal is filled with a well-compacted gutta-percha (Fig. 20.7).
- Verify the obturation of the canal by radiograph.

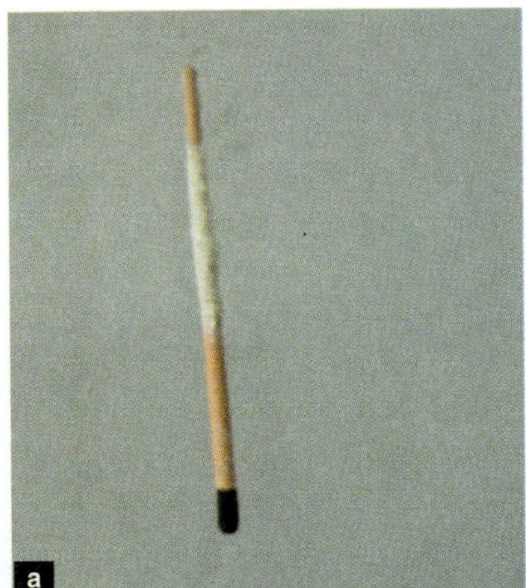

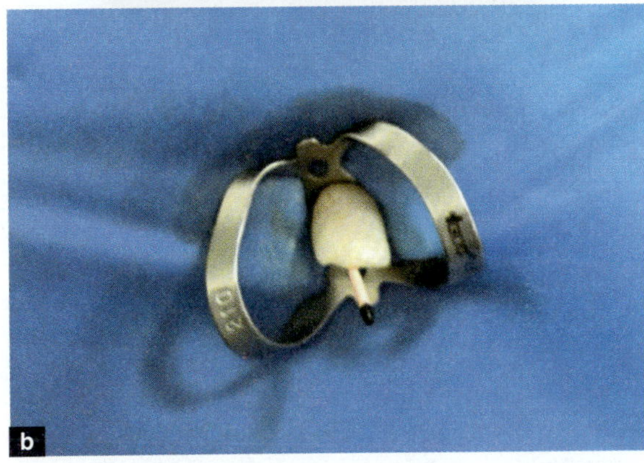

Fig. 20.4 (a) Gutta-percha coated with sealer, except at the apical end; (b) Cone in the canal

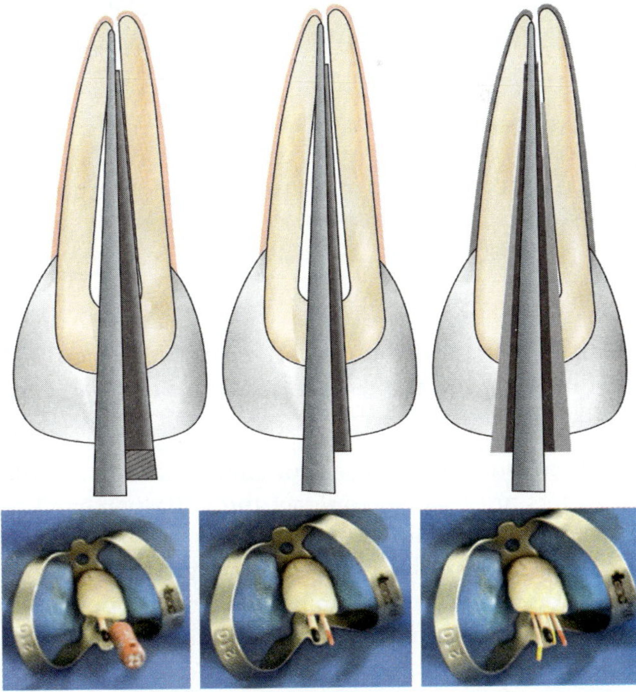

Fig. 20.5 Selection of spreader (2.0 mm short of apex)

Fig. 20.6 Placement of accessory cones

Fig. 20.7 Gutta-percha adequately condensed

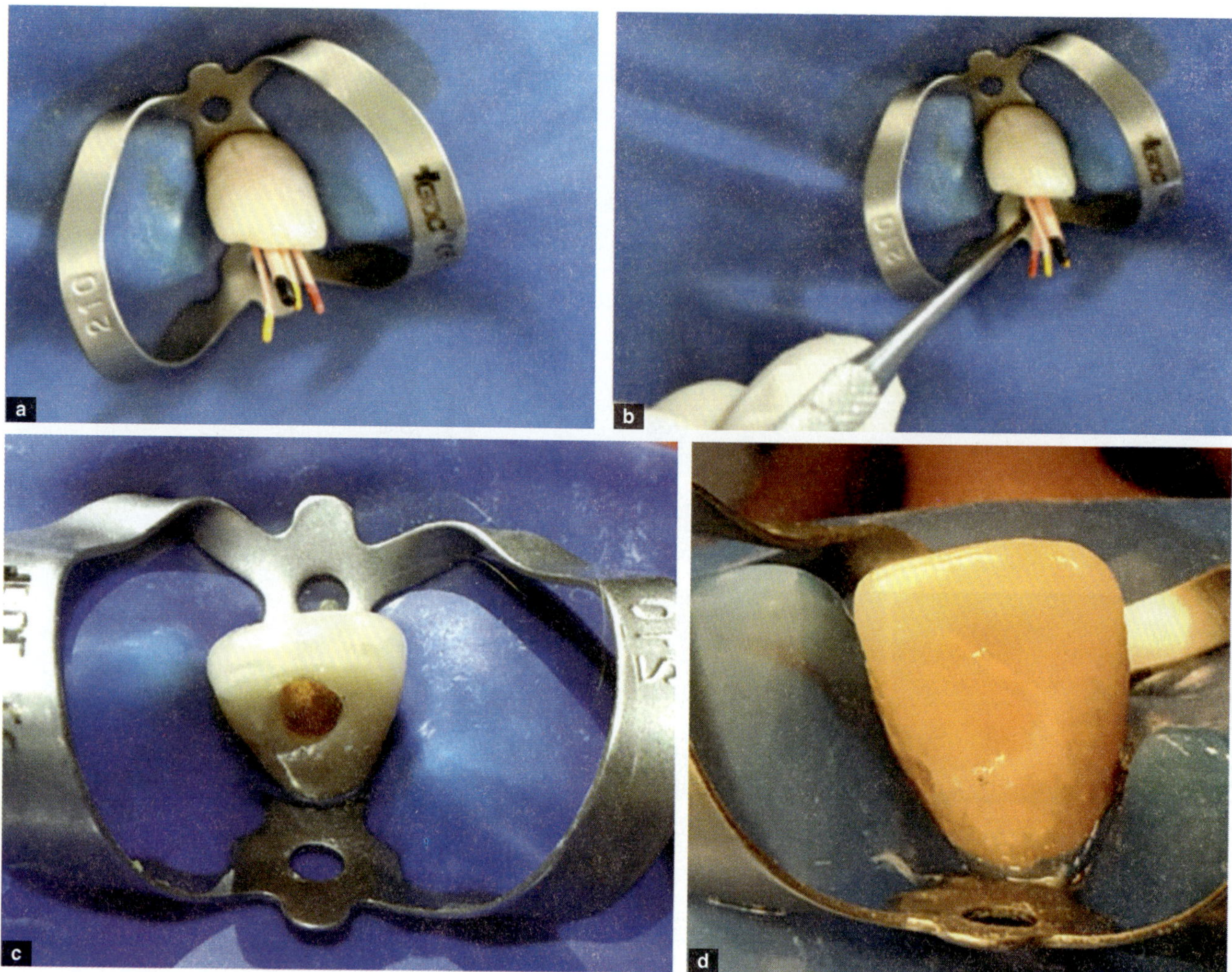

Fig. 20.8a to d Removal of excess gutta-percha and filling the access cavity

- Excess gutta-percha is removed from the pulp chamber with an instrument and temporary restoration is placed in the access cavity (Fig. 20.8a to d).

b. Modifications of Lateral Compaction Method

The routinely used compaction technique is modified for filling curved canals and immature open apices/ tubular canals.

i. *For curved canals*: In case of curved canals, flexible spreaders are used to compact the gutta-percha. The other features remain the same, except the master point is placed 2.0 mm short of apical terminus; since more vertical force is exerted against the primary points, as the spreader tend to compact the gutta-percha, it may push the gutta-percha apically.

In case of severe curvatures, dilacerations, etc. lateral compaction is not feasible; thermoplasticized gutta-percha technique should be preferred.

ii. *For immature open apices/tubular canals*: The immature teeth, where root is not fully developed, exhibit tubular canal and open/wide foramen. The apical opening is either a flaring foramen of a 'blunder buss' shape. Apexification should be tried, for apical closure. If it fails then special methods have to be employed for obturation; e.g. inverted point technique and roll-cone technique (tailor-made gutta-percha roll).

- *Inverted point technique*
  - 'Coarse' gutta-percha cone is selected as a primary point and the serrated butt end of the point is cut with the scissors/scalpel.
  - Point is inverted and tried in the canal; should reach up to the working length and exhibit the requisite 'tug back'.
  - Radiograph is taken to confirm its position (Fig. 20.9 a and b).

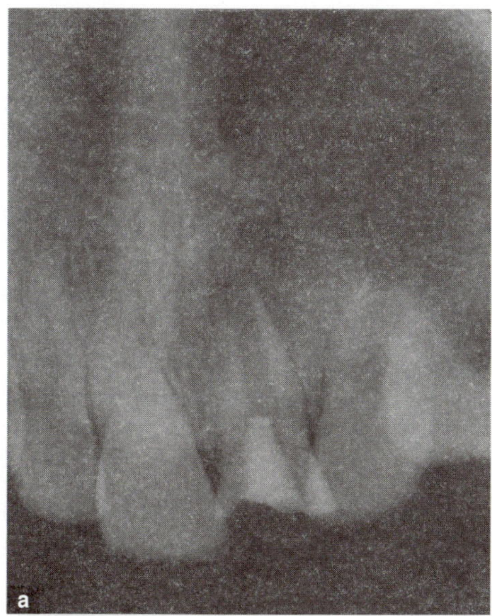

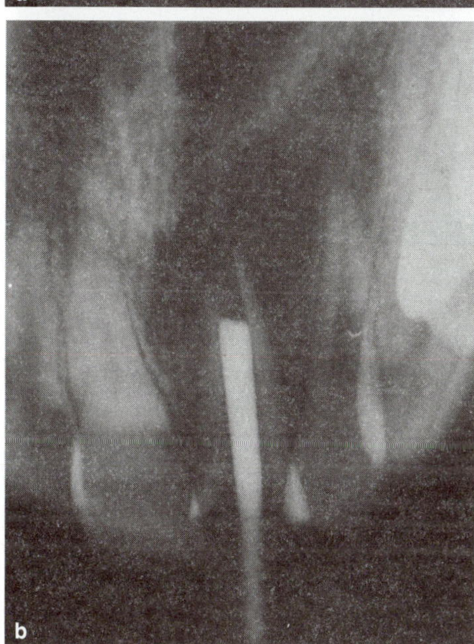

Fig. 20.9 (a) Preoperative (open apex); (b) Confirming position of inverted gutta-percha cone

– Canal is obturated like in lateral compaction technique with freshly prepared cone as the primary cone (Fig. 20.10).

> ***Points to remember***
> *Proper and balanced/uniform pressure is mandatory during lateral compaction. Insufficient pressure may result in poorly condensed obturation and over pressure may lead to overfilling.*

- *Tailor-Made Gutta-percha Roll/Roll-Cone technique*
  - If the apical opening is so wide that even the largest inverted gutta-percha point is still loose in the canal, a tailor made point must be used as a primary point.

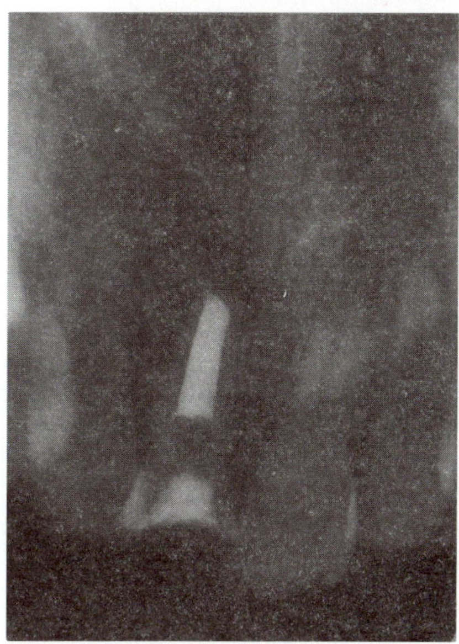

Fig. 20.10 Inverted cone gutta-percha (obturated)

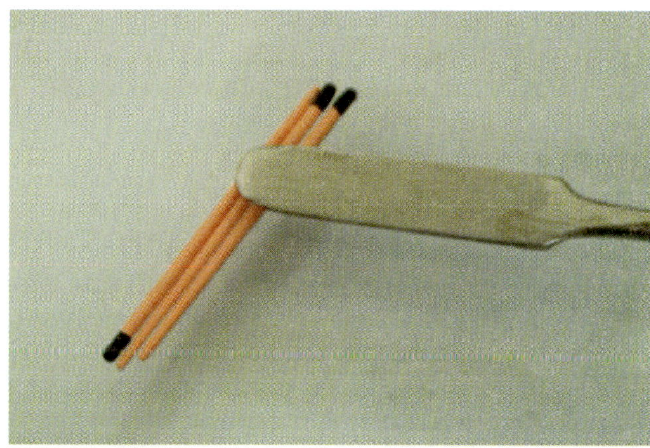

Fig. 20.11 Preparing gutta-percha for Roll-cone technique

  - The master gutta-percha point is prepared by heating a number of gutta-percha points and combining them, butt to tip, until a roll has been developed to match the size and shape of the canal (Fig. 20. 11).
  - Roll is chilled with a spray of ethyl chloride or ice water to stiffen it.
  - This cone is tried in the canal; if still loose, more gutta-percha can be added.
  - Gutta-percha cone so prepared is referred to as 'master gutta-percha'.
  - Rest of the procedure is same as for lateral compaction method.

B. Chemically Softened Gutta-percha

The primary gutta-percha point is chemically softened, which facilitate better conformation to the aberrations in apical canal anatomy. Chloroform, halothane and Eucalyptol are the routinely used chemical softeners. Earlier it was thought that chloroform is carcinogenic; however, it has been approved by FDA and ADA for clinical use. This is a variation of an old obturation method called '*Callahan-Johnston technique*', in which too much chloroform was used (on evaporation, there was 24% decrease in volume). Now, only the tip of the point is dipped in the solvent for one second. Sealers are prepared by dissolving gutta-percha in these solvents, and also resin and balsam. Such mixtures are called 'chloropercha' and 'eucapercha'.

Technique

- Primary cone is blunted and fitted 2.0 mm short of the working length.
- It is dipped in solvent for one second and kept aside for partial evaporation of the solvent.
- Meanwhile sealer is placed in the canal. Primary cone is inserted to the working length.
- Spreader placed for one minute to allow softened gutta-percha to flow.
- Rest of the canal can be filled conventionally.

C. Heat Softened Gutta-percha

a. Intraradicular Techniques (Gutta-percha is Heated within the Canal)

i. *Warm vertical condensation*: Schilder (1967) advocated vertical condensation technique as an alternative to lateral condensation. The root canals are obturated with a maximum amount of gutta-percha and a minimum amount of sealer. The main advantage of vertical condensation is its ability to adapt the gutta-percha to the irregularities of the root canal, as well as accessory and lateral canals.

Technique

- The canal is prepared, irrigated and dried (Fig. 20.12).
- A master cone is selected according to canal size and the working length. The snuggly fit of the cone is checked radiographically. Once checked, the cone is coated with sealer and placed in the root canal (Fig. 20.13).
- Cut-off the butt end of the cone at the incisal/occlusal reference point.
- Remove the cone and cut back 0.5 to 1.0 mm of tip, reinsert and check the length and tug back. The cone's apical diameter should be same as the diameter of last apical instrument. Remove the cone, keep it aside.
- Three pluggers are used, that are slightly smaller than the diameter of the root canal at different depths (Fig. 20.14a to c). The smallest plugger should extend to 4.0–5.0 mm coronal to the apical foramen. In the coronal third, the broadest plugger is used which does not touch the canal walls; a narrower plugger is used for the middle third of the canal. The pluggers are selected before try-in of the master point. The length is marked on these pluggers.
- Lightly coat all the walls with sealer.
- Insert the cone in the canal to the working length.
- Using a hot spoon excavator remove gutta-percha cone from pulp chamber to cervical level. This transfers the heat to the coronal third of the

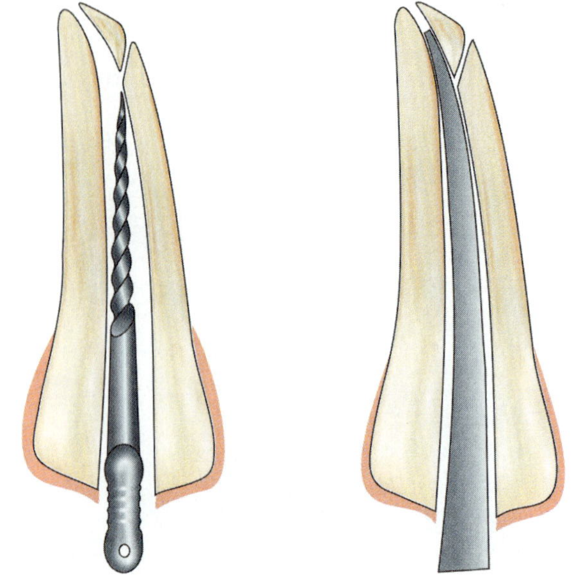

Fig. 20.12 Preparation of root canal

Fig. 20.13 Master apical cone

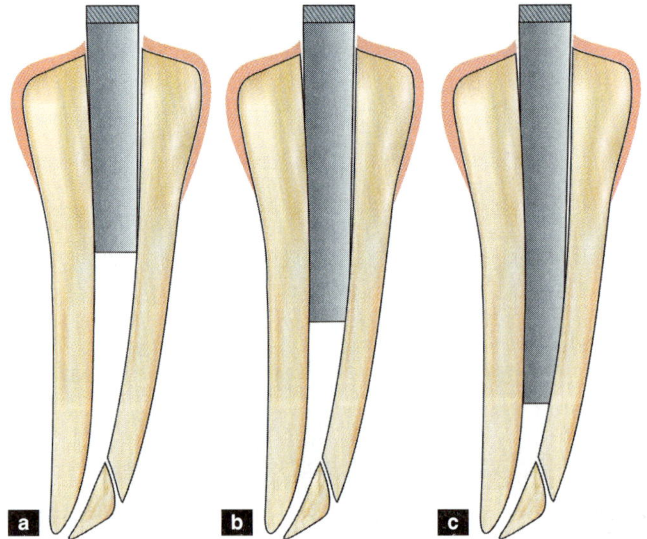

Fig. 20.14 Selection of pluggers (a) Coronal; (b) Middle; (c) Apical third

20

gutta-percha cone. This softened gutta-percha is folded into a mass and compacted in an apical direction with sustained pressure with the largest cold plugger.

- The second heat wave begins with the introduction of heated carrier into the gutta-percha, for 2 to 3 seconds and when retrieved, carries with it the first selective gutta-percha removal (Fig. 20.15).
- Immediately, the mid-sized plugger is pushed into the warm gutta-percha. The vertical pressure also exerts lateral pressure. The filling mass is compacted apically in 3.0 to 4.0 mm, created by repeated heat and compaction cycles (Fig. 20.16).
- When apical 4.0–5.0 mm of gutta-percha is left, it is again softened with heat. The narrowest plugger is immediately inserted in the canal and the surplus material along the walls is folded centrally into the apical mass. Warmed gutta-percha is then compacted vertically sealing portals of exit (Fig. 20.17).
- The apical filling is over. If post is to be placed, no more gutta-percha need be used.
- 'Back packing' the remainder of the canal completes the obturation. The classic method consists of packing 5.0 mm precut segments of gutta-percha, cold welding them to apical segment. Procedure is continued until the entire canal is obturated (Fig. 20.18).
- Remove excess gutta-percha and sealer from the chamber and place temporary filling.

Advantage

Dense, homogenous obturation is achieved.

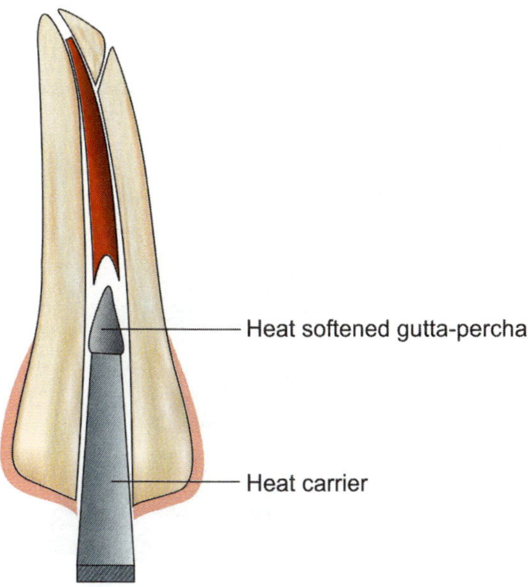

Fig. 20.15 Heat carrier removing selective gutta-percha

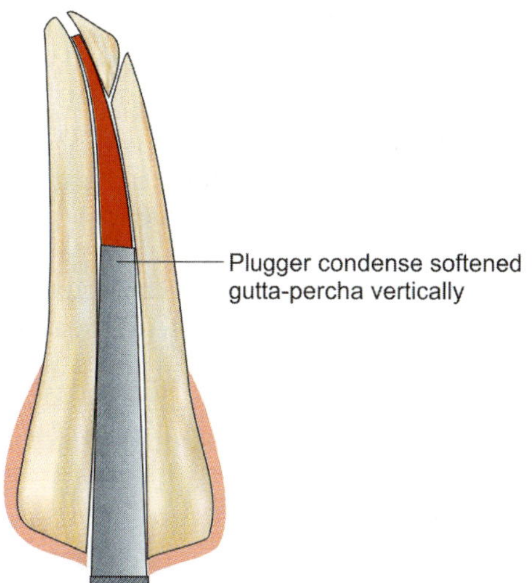

Fig. 20.16 Vertically compacting gutta-percha

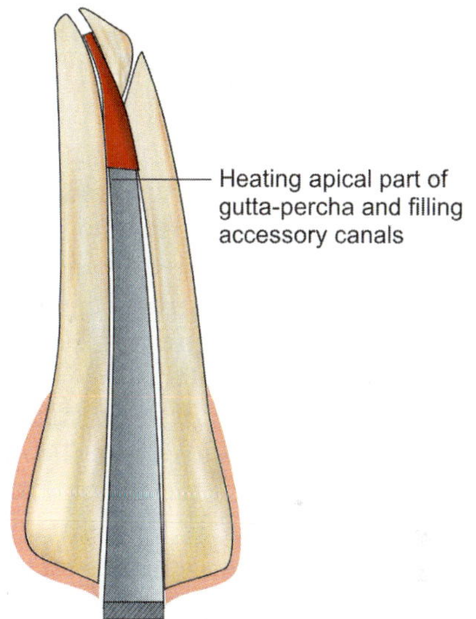

Fig. 20.17 Compacting the gutta-percha

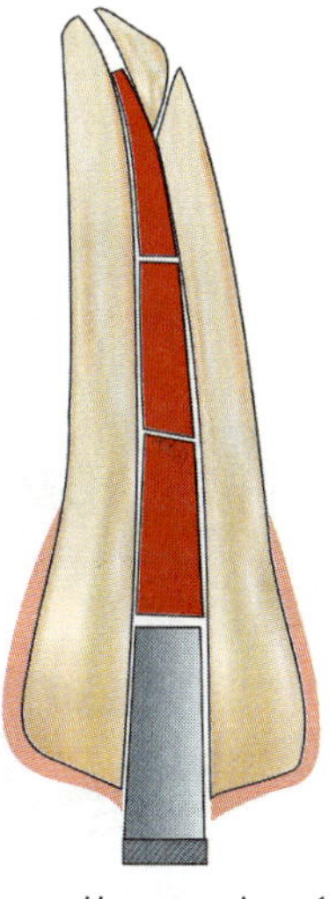

Fig. 20.18 Back filling gutta-percha (either in smart parts or with thermoplasticized technique)

Disadvantages

- Technique is difficult to master.
- Time consuming.
- Difficult to use in curved canals where the straight, rigid pluggers are unable to penetrate to the necessary depth. To allow the rigid carriers to contact the gutta-percha within 4.0 or 5.0 mm of the apex, the canals must be prepared larger and more tapered than in the lateral compaction technique, requiring the removal of additional dentin, which weakens the root.
- Risk of vertical root fracture because of compaction forces.
- Length control is less than lateral compaction.
- Potential for extrusion of material into the periradicular tissues.

A slight modification of Schilder's technique, the continuous wave compaction technique, utilizes commercial heating devices.

The heating devices are as follows.

1. Touch 'n' heat

The Touch 'n' heat (model 5003 and 5004) is an electronic device, especially developed for the warm vertical condensation of gutta-percha. It works with battery and alternating current as well (Fig. 20.19).

It exhibits the same thermal properties as the original heat carrier used by Schilder but has the advantage of generating heat automatically at the tip of the instrument. The instrument is capable of providing a range of high temperatures instantly, ranging from 0 to 700°C. The device may also be used for pulp testing/bleaching by changing the tips and adjusting the heat level.

The heat is applied alongside the master gutta-percha using appropriate pluggers/spreaders. The canal is then back filled using obtura gun.

Advantages

- Fill accessory canal
- Homogenous filling

Disadvantages

- Voids (inadequate control of the depth of insertion)
- Small plugger is ineffective
- Plugger binding apically may split root.

Precautions

- There should be a continuous tapering canal preparation (diameter is narrowed apically).
- Master cone is fitted correctly.
- Temperature of Touch 'n' heat instrument should not exceed 45°C.
- Heated plugger should not be placed closer than 4.0 to 5.0 mm of canal terminus.

2. System B

'System B' (model 100) utilizes a digital temperature display and a variable resistance control that allows the clinician to attain a desired temperature (Fig. 20.20).

These heat carriers are designed as pluggers that concentrate the heat at the tip of the carrier. The system B is also based on the Schilder technique. The tip of the plugger can be heated to 200°C; this softens the gutta-percha in half a second.

A wave of heat (250–300°C) is produced as the plugger is forced through the already fitted cone and is used to drive the gutta-percha into the canal.

As the plugger approaches the apex, the heat button is released and apical pressure is maintained with the plugger for 10 seconds. It sustains push to take up the shrinkage that occurs on cooling. The heat button is pushed again while maintaining pressure. A wave of heat is produced (300°C in 5 seconds) that immediately separates the plugger from apical mass of gutta-percha, facilitating rapid withdrawal of the instrument. The canal is then backfilled with obtura.

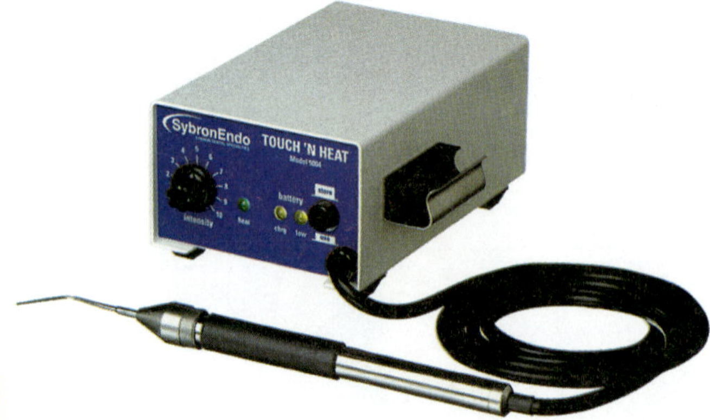

Fig. 20.19 Touch 'n' heat

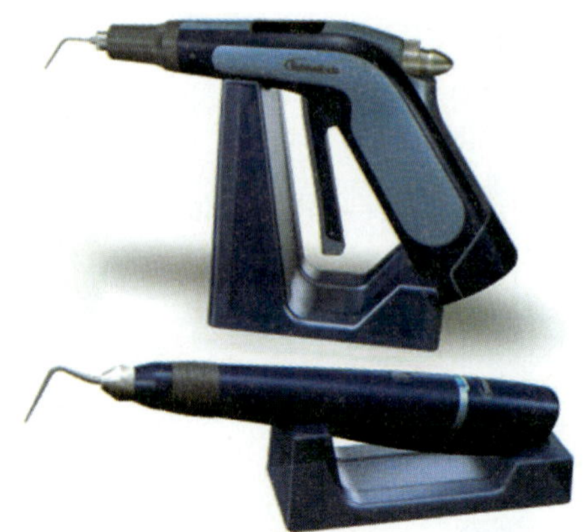

Fig. 20.20 System B (cordless)

Advantages
- Eliminates voids created during normal lateral condensation of warm gutta-percha.
- Produces less heat than Touch 'n' heat.

Disadvantages
- Easy breakage
- Kinking of spreaders.

3. Elements system

The elements system utilizes motorized handpiece, combining system B device and the gutta-percha extruder. System B provides control for temperature and duration. The tip temperature is continuously maintained and displayed, and the system has a time-out option that prevents overheating.

The elements obturation technique combines two separate machines that usually used for down pack and backfill into one device.

The extruder (tips available in sizes 20, 23 and 25 gauge) facilitate flow of gutta-percha.

The handpieces are fitted with silicon insulator to avoid excessive heat transferring to the clinician's hands during its usage (Fig. 20.21).

A case of mandibular second molar obturated with element system is depicted in Fig. 20.22a to c.

ii. *Warm lateral condensation*: Warm lateral condensation offer advantage over vertical condensation, being able to control the obturation up to the working length. A master cone corresponding to the working length is coated with sealer and inserted into the canal. Various

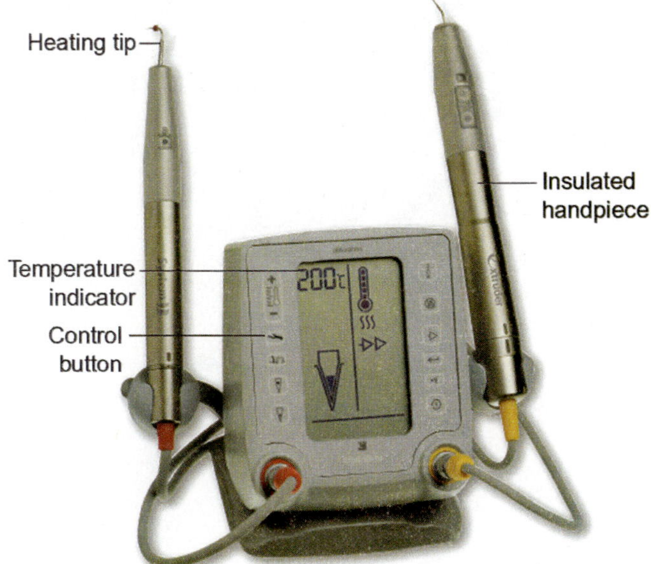

Fig. 20.21 Elements obturation unit

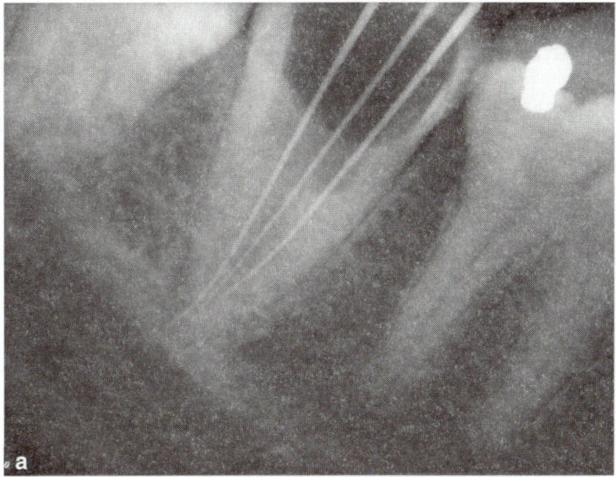

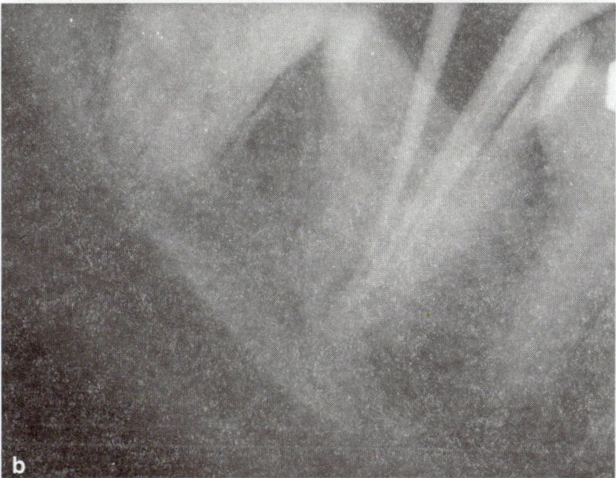

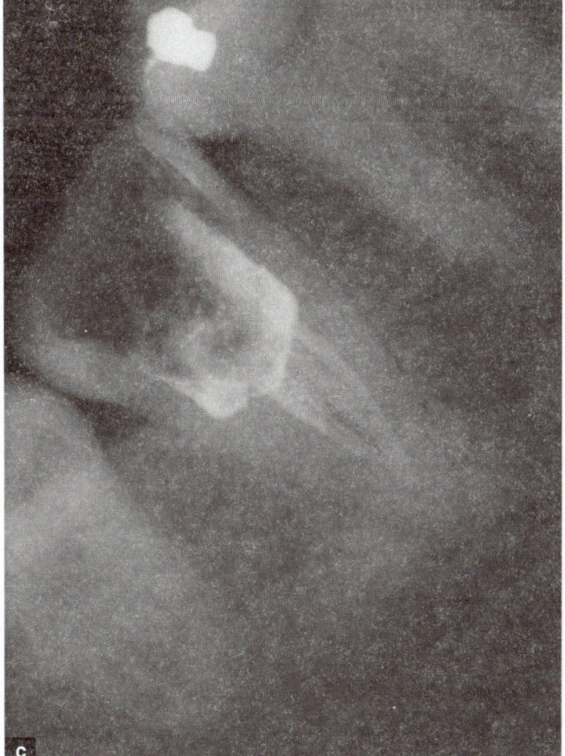

Fig. 20.22 (a) Elements working length; (b) Elements master cone; (c) Elements obturation

devices are used to warm and condense the core material laterally. The devices used are:

4. Endotec

The 'Endotec' is a thermal compactor, consisting of a cordless handpiece fitted with battery that supplies requisite heat to the attached spreader/plugger tips. When not in use, the handpiece is kept in a battery charger base.

Two tips are used; smaller one equivalent to size 30 file (for curved canals) and larger one equivalent to size 45 file (for routine use). The device can achieve temperatures up to 350°C.

Procedure

- Dry the canal and apply sealer.
- Adapt master cone in the canal.
- Endotec is placed in the canal to full length alongside the gutta-percha.
- Activator button is pressed and the device is moved in clockwise direction.
- Release the button; the plugger cools immediately.
- Remove the device in anticlockwise direction.
- Space is created for additional gutta-percha point.
- Additional gutta-percha can be inserted if required.
- Cold plugger can be used to compact the softened gutta-percha.

The gutta-percha compaction can be improved by using the Endotec in a *ZAP* and *TAP method*, especially in C-shaped canals of molars.

ZAP: The 'Endotec' is preheated for 4 to 5 seconds before insertion along the gutta-percha point.

TAP: The instrument is moved in and out in short continuous strokes 10–15 times. The tip is removed from the canal when it is still hot. Later, cold spreader is used and accessory points are placed.

Endotec may lead to overheating and/or development of stresses.

The internal temperature may reach up to 102°C; since gutta-percha and dentin are poor conductors of heat, the temperature may not cause any damage to periodontium.

Advantages

- The obturation is superior to cold lateral compaction method.
- Provide three-dimensional obturation.

Disadvantages

- Time consuming relative to other methods of lateral compaction.
- Device tips are primarily used for heating; do not compact the gutta-percha.

5. Endotec II

It is established that warm lateral compaction with the Endotec II increased the gutta-percha mass when compared with traditional cold lateral compaction.

The instrument consists of a cordless handpiece with a heat/temperature control button to deliver optimum heat through its microheating tip, which can soften the gutta-percha (Fig. 20.23). After placing the master gutta-percha in the root canal, Endotec II tip is inserted 2.0–4.0 mm short of working length.

The tip is heat activated outside the canal for 3 to 4 seconds and inserted to the marked length in a circumferential rotation manner for 5 to 8 seconds; the tip cools down and is withdrawn slowly. The procedure is repeated till the entire canal is completely filled.

6. DownPak

DownPak obturation device, also popular as EndoTwinn and Root Buddy, utilizes warm lateral condensation technique, using a combination of ultrasonic vibration and heat.

The cordless unit has a heating and vibrating device; can be used for both vertical and lateral obturation (temperature and vibrations are both adjustable within limits).

DownPak can be used with different materials like gutta-percha, resilon and hybrid resin filling materials having variable softening temperatures (Fig. 20.24).

A master cone is placed in the root canal in the same manner as with lateral compaction.

The spreader is selected, keeping 2.0 mm short of the working length. The system is vibrated and activated

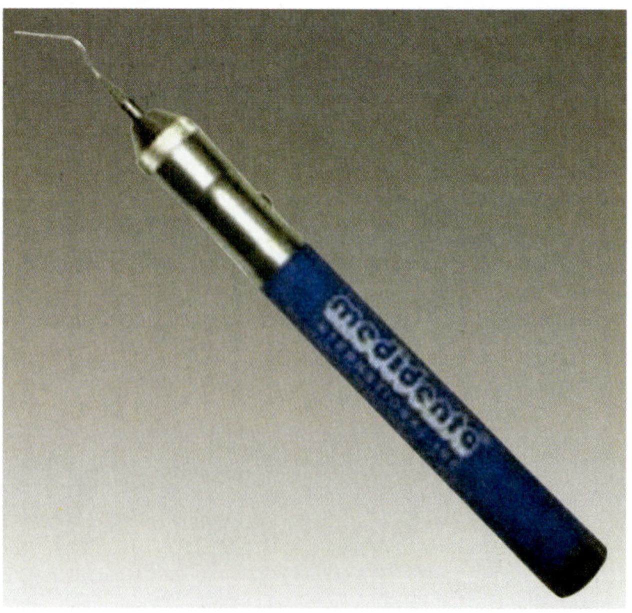

Fig. 20.23 Endotec II

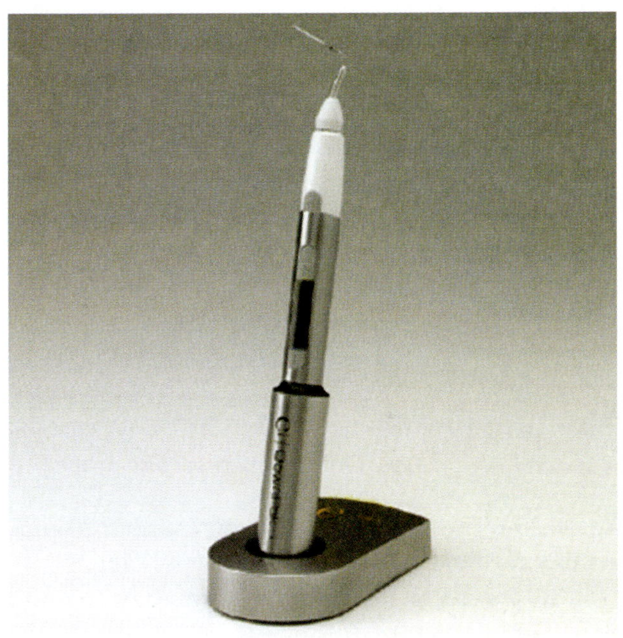

Fig. 20.24 DownPak

with heat for two seconds and subsequently inserted till it reaches the predetermined working length. A spreader is then used to condense the filling material.

Accessory cones are inserted as per need. Heat is transferred to the canal after the placement of each accessory gutta-percha cone. The vibration and heat cause softening of the entire mass of the gutta-percha, which can be condensed properly. The procedure is repeated till the final obturation.

The combined use of heat and vibration by this system provide dense and more compact fillings than heat alone.

7. Thermapact

Thermapact unit consists of a transformer and an electronically controlled circuit for heat generation. The unit provides a handpiece adapted with different sized spreaders and a heat carrier. The temperature can be regulated and maintained at any desired level from 40 to 70°C.

It is suggested that 'Thermapact' must be maintained at 42°C for warm lateral condensation and at about 59° C for warm vertical condensation. The operating temperature should be set precisely and constantly maintained.

Advantages

- Warm lateral condensation effectively provides a dense and more compact obturation with a maximum amount of gutta-percha and a minimum amount of sealer.
- Minimal condensing pressure is required to obtain a compact filling.

iii. ***Thermocompaction***: In this technique friction between gutta-percha and the rotating "reverse file" generates heat to soften the gutta-percha and forces it apically. Different designs of thermocompactors are available; the main are:

- McSpadden compactor
- Modified McSpadden (microseal system)
- Maillefer guttacondenser
- Zipperer thermocompactor/engine plugger
- Quick fill compactor

8. McSpadden compactor

McSpadden (1979) introduced an instrument, 'McSpadden compactor', for heat softening gutta-percha.

It resembles the reverse H-file which fits into a latch type handpiece and rotates at 8,000–20,000 rpm. It generates frictional heat that softens gutta-percha and forces the material apically and laterally. As canal is filled, the compactor is forced out coronally.

Disadvantages

- Fragility of the instrument; prone to fracture.
- Cannot be used in curved canals.
- Likely to overfill the canals.
- Difficulty in mastering the technique; manipulation difficult.
- Frequent overheating may lead to resorption and ankylosis.

9. Modified McSpadden (MicroSeal system)

The modified McSpadden utilizes Ni-Ti condensers, which rotates at slower speed (1000–4000). This is also known as MicroSeal system. It is used mainly in curved canals. (Being flexible, it is advantageous in curved canals.) It can be used both with α-phase heat softened gutta-percha and normal gutta-percha.

The master gutta-percha cone is placed in root canal.

The appropriate size condenser is selected and coated with gutta-percha (heat softened); gutta-percha I (α) or gutta-percha II (β).

The condenser is then spun in the canal at 1000–4000 rpm, which fills the gutta-percha laterally and vertically.

10. Maillefer Guttacondenser

The Headstrom instrument is modified and used as guttacondenser. The instrument has less number of compacting blades with deeper grooves and increased sharpness. Guttacondenser is mainly used for back filling of canals already filled at apical third.

11. Zipperer thermocompactor/Engine plugger

Zipperer thermocompactor resembles an inverted K-file with increased number of flutes (also quoted as

Engine plugger). It is used for backfilling canals already filled at apical third and also for hybrid technique.

12. Quickfill compactor

Quickfill compactor has titanium core device resembling latch type drills. The core is coated with α-phase gutta-percha. The sealer is applied to the core and is fitted to the prepared root canal. As the instrument spins in the canal with regular low speed, frictional heat is liberated. This heat plasticizes the gutta-percha and it is also compacted.

After compaction, the instrument is removed and final compaction is carried out with hand plugger. A few authors prefer leaving the titanium core in place, which can be separated by appropriate burs.

iv. *Ultrasonic plasticizing*: Ultrasonic plasticizing can be used only in anterior teeth. A cavitron scaler with a PR (pull out resistant) is used for the purpose.

Technique

- Master gutta-percha is selected and placed in the root canal
- The ultrasonic unit with the rheostat is activated for 3–4 seconds
- The energy released by vibrating motion of the ultrasonic file plasticizes the gutta-percha
- The file is removed and the spreader is immediately inserted to make space for new cones
- The process is repeated till obturation is completed. The heat produced (63.0°C) by this method is not harmful.

The *Enac Ultrasonic unit*, wherein a spreader is attached is a modified version of ultrasonic plasticizing unit. The spreader can penetrate the gutta-percha more easily producing the requisite heat, which can plasticize the gutta-percha. The heat generated by the unit is 191°C, more than the required heat.

b. Extraradicular Techniques (Gutta-percha is heated outside the Canal and then placed in the Canal)

i. *Injectable gutta-percha*: The commonly employed injectable gutta-percha techniques are Obtura II and III, Calamus 3D, Ultrafil and PAC –160.

13. Obtura II

Martin (1977) introduced Obtura and later modified it to presently available Obtura II. The unit consists of an electrical control unit, which is equipped with a digital display of temperature and a safe circuit for controlling the temperature. Regular α-phase gutta-percha is used with this system. A flexible silver needle is used for delivery of plasticized gutta-percha into the root canal (Fig. 20.25). The size of silver needle is either 20 gauge (number 60 file) or 23 gauge (number 40 file).

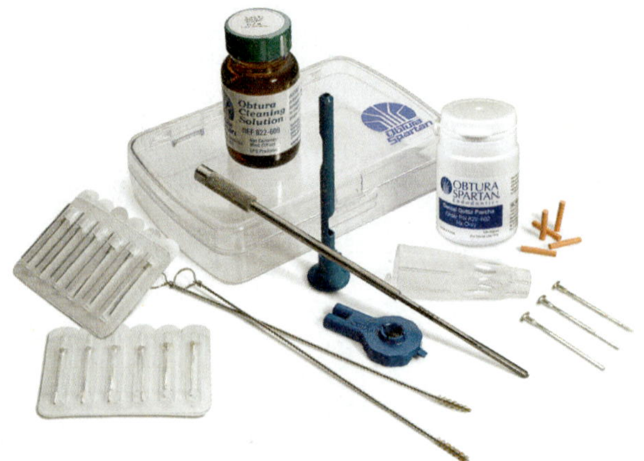

Fig. 20.25 Obtura accessories

Gutta-percha is heated approximately to 160 to 200°C. The thermoplasticized gutta-percha (temperature ranging from 62 to 65°C) extrudes from the 'needle tip' and filled in the root canals.

The technique is indicated mainly for curved canals and other canal irregularities, such as root canal webbings, internal resorption, C-shaped canals and accessory/lateral canals. It is also preferred for backfilling of gutta-percha.

Technique

Sealer is necessary for this method, which facilitates filling the microscopic interface between the dentin and gutta-percha and also act as a lubricant. The irregularities of the canal surface are also filled with sealer, which effectively compensates for shrinkage as the gutta-percha cools.

Gutta-percha is preheated in the gun. The needle is positioned in the canal within 3.0 to 5.0 mm of the apical preparation. The gutta-percha is passively injected into the root canal, avoiding apical pressure. The needle is withdrawn slowly out of the canal as the apical portion is filled. Plugger dipped in alcohol is used to compact the gutta-percha.

A segmental technique may also be used, wherein 3.0 to 4.0 mm segments of gutta-percha are sequentially injected and compacted. In either case, compaction should continue until the gutta-percha cools and solidifies to compensate for the contraction that takes place on cooling.

Advantages

- The compaction of gutta-percha adaptation is significantly better than lateral compaction method.
- If the smear layer has been removed, this system may push gutta-percha and sealer into the dentinal tubules.

Disadvantages

- Potential for extrusion of gutta-percha and sealer beyond the apical foramen.
- Heat may damage the periodontium.

14. Obtura III Max

The Obtura III Max is the modified version of Obtura II that provides better tactile sense, ergonomics and handling (Fig. 20.26).

A specially designed handpiece along the unit provide the thermoplasticized gutta-percha.

An enhanced thermal protector in the system can protect patient from thermal shocks during treatment.

The cartridge-free operation eliminates mid-procedure filling problems.

15. Calamus dual 3D system

The Calamus dual 3D system provide Calamus 'Pack' and Calamus 'Flow' handpieces. The Calamus Pack handpiece, an electric heat plugger, is used to thermo-soften, remove, and condense gutta-percha during the downpacking phase of obturation. The handpiece (electrical plugger) is available in three sizes; size-based on apical configuration (sizes 40/03, 50/05 and 60/06 and color coded as black, yellow and blue respectively).

The Calamus Pack handpiece, with its 'thermal response tip' is also used for conducting 'heat test' on the pulps (Fig. 20.27).

The Calamus Flow handpiece is used along with disposable gutta-percha cartridge and integrated cannula (cartridges of 20 and 23 gauge size), to dispense warm gutta-percha into the canal during the back-packing phase of obturation. The cannula can be bent depending upon the curvature of root canal.

The bent cannula can pass through the coronal two-thirds and compact the previously placed master cone.

The temperature of the thermoplasticized gutta-percha dispensed for use is around 38 to 44°C.

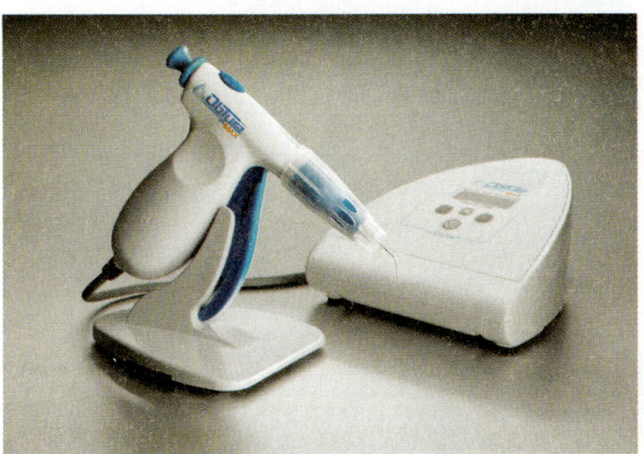

Fig. 20.26 Obtura III Max

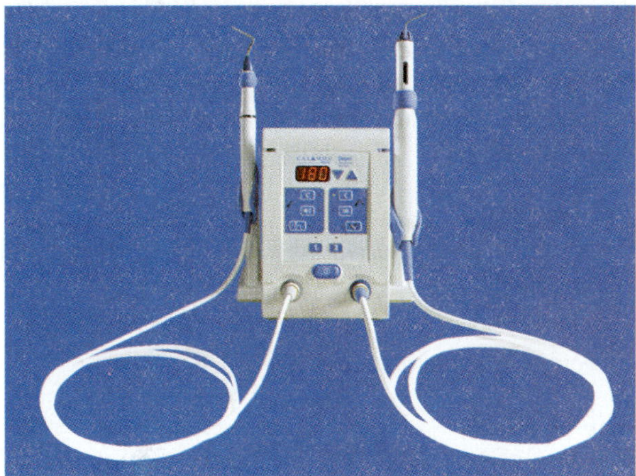

Fig. 20.27 Calamus dual 3D system

The gutta-percha has the ability to flow for 45 to 60 seconds, depending on the viscosity.

The downpacking phase implies searing off the gutta-percha at coronal orifice with an appropriate heat plugger. The plugger is used to vertically condense the warm gutta-percha for 5 seconds.

The condensation provides a three-dimensional distribution of sealer; the hydraulic forces help in compacting the gutta-percha laterally as well as vertically.

The plugger is then allowed to cool, and is removed. The process is repeated till the canals are filled with condensed gutta-percha. The coronal portion is also filled thereafter.

16. Ultrafil system

Ultrafil system utilizes α-phase gutta-percha prepacked in cannulas with attached 22 gauge needle. Gutta-percha softens at a temperature of approximately 70–90°C in a special heater. The warm cannula is placed in a special sterilizable syringe for delivery to the prepared canal.

The gutta-percha is available in three consistencies based on its viscosity; i.e.

Regular (low viscosity)	: White cannula
Firm set (moderate viscosity)	: Blue cannula
Endoset (high viscosity)	: Green cannula

Placement of the needle and sealer are almost similar as in Obtura II technique. Needle placement is usually further from the apical matrix (8–10 mm). Working time is approximately 60–70 seconds.

For the delivery of low viscosity gutta-percha (regular set—white cannula), the syringe trigger is squeezed pushing a bolus of gutta-percha towards the apical preparation. The needle is not withdrawn but is left in place until the mass of softened gutta-percha is felt to lift the needle (backflow) from the canal. The material is completely set within 30 minutes.

Firmset (blue cannula) gutta-percha controlled compaction can follow the injection delivery of the material; whereas, Endoset (green cannula) gutta-percha has less flow and can be compacted with plugger and spreader.

Advantages

- Better flow characteristic; broken instruments may be bypassed.
- Internal resorption defects can be filled properly.
- Effective compaction is achieved.

Disadvantages

- Because of low viscosity, the material may extrude out of apical foramen.
- Cannot be compacted; possibility of shrinkage (sealers cannot compensate the shrinkage).
- Restricted to cases with a substantial apical matrix and minimal apical foramina opening.

17. PAC-160

The device denotes '*Precision apical control at 160°C*'. PAC-160 unit uses standardized gutta-percha. Definite apical constriction and coronal flare is preferred in root canal preparation.

Advantages

- Fills accessory/lateral canal
- Irregular configurations of the root canal can be obturated
- Temperature is maintained at 160°C.

ii. *Solid core carrier*: The development of gutta-percha in different isomeric forms, such as α- and β-phase led to creation of Thermafil, Successfil and Sensfil (α-phase gutta-percha can be heated, placed on a carrier and delivered into the canal without an injection system).

18. Successfil

Successfil consists of a solid core carrier (titanium/radiopaque plastic) coated with α-phase gutta-percha. Gutta-percha in a warm plasticized state is added to the carrier just before it is inserted in the canal. The successfil syringes contain high viscosity gutta-percha that sets in two minutes.

Technique

- The root canal is dried and the sealer is applied.
- A successfil core of the same number as the last apical file is selected and placed up to the working length without binding; placement checked by radiograph.
- With a plugger dipped in alcohol, the gutta-percha is compacted around the carrier.
- The core coated with gutta-percha is immediately inserted to full depth without twisting.
- Core is severed at the coronal orifice with appropriate bur.
- The placement is confirmed by radiographs.

19. Thermafil

Thermafil, an endodontic obturator, consists of a flexible steel/titanium/plastic central carrier coated with uniform α-phase gutta-percha. The size and taper of the carrier correspond to standard endodontic files. Plastic carriers, being flexible, are preferred. If metal carrier is used, it is notched with suitable burs before applying gutta-percha.

The carrier should preferably be heated in the oven at 115°C for 3–7 minutes depending on the size, which ranges from 20–140. The gutta-percha coating extends beyond the carrier by 1.0–2.0 mm.

The coronal portion of the carrier has markings at 18, 19 and 20 mm and a rubber stop.

A plugger is used to apically compress the gutta-percha.

Technique

- The step back technique of canal preparation is effective for obturation with Thermafil.
- A Thermafil obturator is selected which corresponds to the master apical file.
- The canal is coated with a suitable sealer.
- The Thermafil obturator is heated in the oven (Oven's uniform heat effectively plasticize the gutta-percha).
- Once the gutta-percha attains a surface shine, it is introduced into the canal with gentle pressure up to the working length (Fig. 20.28).
- The carrier shaft is severed at the coronal orifice while applying firm pressure to the obturator handle. The handle is removed and discarded.
- Placement is verified by radiographs.

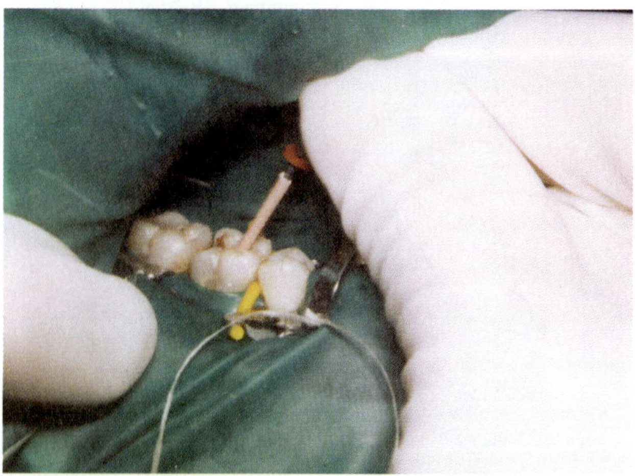

Fig. 20.28 Obturation with Thermafil

> *Remember*
> *While obturating posterior teeth (obturating one canal), the other canal orifices must be sealed with damp cotton otherwise gutta-percha may block these orifices.*

Advantages

- Quick and easy.
- Can be curved to fill curved canals (with newer flexible carriers, precurving is not required).
- Internal resorptive defects, fins, lateral canals, etc. can be filled.
- Can be used effectively in open apices.
- Less stresses in the root because of minimal condensation forces.

Disadvantages

- Chances of extrusion
- Post space preparation is difficult
- Removal of carriers may be difficult during retreatment.

20. Densfil

Densfil carriers are of two variants; plastic and titanium. The plastic carrier are available in size 20 to 140 and titanium carrier in size 20 to 60. Both the carriers are 25 mm long. The heating is carried out in propriety DensHeat oven. The techniques of placement are same as in Thermafil. Removal is comparatively easy in case of retreatment.

21. Trifecta system

Trifecta system is the combination of both approaches, Successfil and Ultrafil. A small amount (1.0–2.0 mm) of α-phase Successfil gutta-percha is coated on the tip of a carrier, placed to the required depth of the canal and is slowly rotated counter-clockwise and withdrawn from the canal. This is followed by compaction of the small mass of gutta-percha in the canal. The coronal position of the canal is backfilled with Ultrafil gutta-percha.

2. SILVER CONES

Silver cones have been used as obturating material despite its disadvantages. Other solid materials are used only as endodontic stabilizers. The use of silver cones is preferred in teeth with fine and tortuous canals that are difficult to be filled with gutta-percha (Fig. 20.29).

Silver cones are machined to correspond to the instruments used for canal preparation. Sealer is used along with silver cones. Gutta-percha may be laterally condensed around the cone to ensure a proper lateral seal.

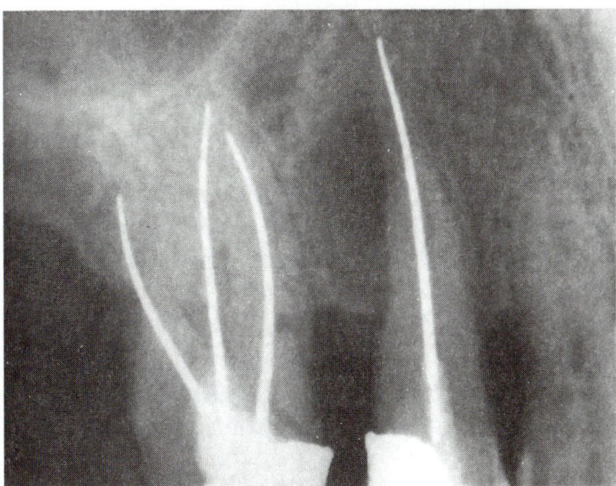

Fig. 20.29 Obturation with silver cones

Technique

- Select a cone corresponding in size to the last instrument used in the preparation of the root canal.
- Sterilize the cone by passing through the open flame, at least 2–3 times.
- Insert the cone in the canal using silver cone pliers or stieglitz forceps and press it apically (the cone should fit snugly and should bind at the apical foramen because it corresponds to the diameter and taper of the prepared canal).
- Take a radiograph to check the fit of the cone in the canal. If it protrudes beyond the apex, cut-off the excess at the tip, so that final fit will terminate 0.5 mm short of the root apex. If the silver cone is too short, either select another one that fits or re-prepare the canal so that the selected cone seats properly.
- Coat the canal with sealer and insert the sterilized silver cone with slight pressure to the working length.
- Verify placement by radiographs.
- Laterally condense gutta-percha cones around the primary silver cone, if need be.
- Excess is removed and the access cavity is filled with temporary restoration.

Disadvantages

- Corrosion
- Difficult to remove in retreatment
- Poor sealing as they cannot be compacted to root canal walls (sealing is because of sealers only).

Improved Silver Points

The silver points were improved, which have a color plastic handle attached at 25 mm from the tip and has a standardized taper (equivalent to that of the enlarging instrument).

Advantages over conventional silver points

- Conventional silver points are inserted with pliers or a hemostat held in the operator's hand. When these points encounter an obstruction/curvature/any irregularity, forceful apical pressure will often cause a buckling or bending of the point. With improved silver points, the fingers can feel the tactile sense; and a slight back and forth movement along the long-axis of point facilitate by-passing the obstruction.
- With improved silver points, same angle of insertion is utilized for point placement; whereas, the angle may differ with use of pliers. This is important factor in treating molars, in which the angle of insertion is important.
- Since, the handles of the improved silver points are color coded; the size is recognized easily.

Sectional or 'Twist Off' Silver Cone Technique

The sectional technique is indicated wherever post and core restoration is planned. In case of multiple rooted teeth, one canal should be filled with sectional technique, which is planned for post placement. Usually, the largest canal is selected (palatal canal in maxillary molars and distal canal in mandibular molars).

Technique

- The selection and verification of apical fit are carried out as in conventional points.
- Silver point pliers or hemostat is used to hold the points for twisting off. But in case of posterior teeth, either improved silver points or measurement control handles, should be used (also known as test handles).
- After determining the apical fit, the handle is attached to the point.
- Point notcher is used to partially cut and weaken the silver point at the desired position.
- The sealer is placed in the canal.
- Silver point is seated with gentle apical pressure. Once the correct depth is reached, the handle is rotated until a decrease in resistance is felt. This indicates that the apical portion has separated.
- The apical fit is verified by radiographs.
- The post preparation can be started in same visit as the operator is familiar with the angulation and width of the canal.

The advantages and disadvantages of different obturating materials are summarized in Table 20.1.

Table 20.1 Advantages and disadvantages of different obturation methods

Method	*Advantages*	*Disadvantages*
Single point gutta-percha/ Silver cones	• Simple • Fast • Inexpensive	• Inadequate fill • Rely on sealers
Lateral compaction (cold)	• Good for canals with irregular tapers • Good control of gutta-percha • Fair compact obturation	• Sealer may create voids • Not good for irregular-shaped canals • Technique sensitive
Chemically softened gutta-percha	• Good flow; fills intricacies of canals	• Shrinkage; lead to leakage
Warm vertical condensation	• Three-dimensional obturation achieved (Hermetic seal)	• Technique sensitive • Risk of vertical root fracture • Risk of apical extrusion
Warm lateral condensation	• Three-dimensional obturation achieved • Minimum condensation pressure required	• Tips used for heating do not compact gutta-percha
Thermocompaction techniques	• Three-dimensional obturation achieved	• Risk of apical extrusion • Difficulty in curved canals • Frequent heating may lead to resorption • Manipulation difficult
Injectable gutta-percha techniques	• Compaction is better than lateral condensation • Fill intricacies of root canal	• Heat may damage periosteum • Potential for extrusion
Solid core carriers	• Less stresses in root canal • Effective in open apex • Simple and fast	• Gutta-percha may strip from carrier • Technique sensitive • Difficult to remove; post space preparation difficult • Risk of apical extrusion
Apical barrier	• Good apical control of material • Bioactive • Stimulate hard tissue formation	• Difficult to remove • Technique sensitive

3. MISCELLANEOUS OBTURATING TECHNIQUES

a. GuttaFlow/GuttaFlow 2

GuttaFlow is a cold free-flowing injectable gutta-percha obturation system. It contains gutta-percha in powder form (particle size less than 30 µm), polyvinylsiloxane (polydimethyl siloxane), silicone oil, paraffin oil, zirconium dioxide, nanosilver particles and coloring agents (Fig. 20.30a and b). Triturated gutta-percha is mixed with resin sealer (polyvinylsiloxane) in an amalgamator to form a cold flowable matrix. The matrix is injected into the canal (Fig. 20.30 a and b). A few authors prefer using single master cone along with guttaFlow. It is eugenol free, radiopaque and does not shrink. It is a self polymerizing system, which combines the properties of sealer and gutta-percha. It may also fill lateral canals and dentinal tubules. Two variants are available: the routine GuttaFlow has working time 10–15 minutes and setting time, 25–30 minutes; whereas, GuttaFlow (fast) has working time, 4–5 minutes and setting time, 8–10 minutes.

Advantages

- Easy and quick
- Excellent flow properties
- Biocompatible
- Do not shrink
- Can be removed easily during retreatment
- Good sealability
- Radiopaque.

Guttaflow 2

GuttaFlow 2, an improved version of GuttaFlow, contains microsilver particles (Fig. 20.31a and b).

The microsilver particles provide optimum protection against re-infection of the root canal. The chemical form of silver ions does not lead to any corrosion or discoloration under clinical conditions.

It is flowable, non-heated gutta-percha that does not shrink, but expands slightly (0.2%).

The syringe dispenses just the quantity required, which is homogeneously mixed (working time is 10–15 minutes).

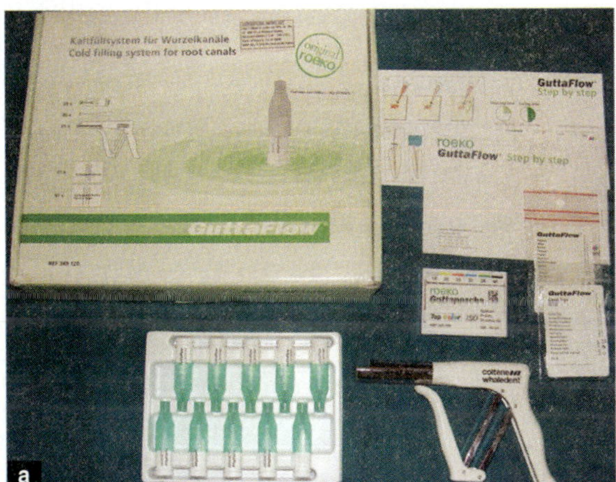

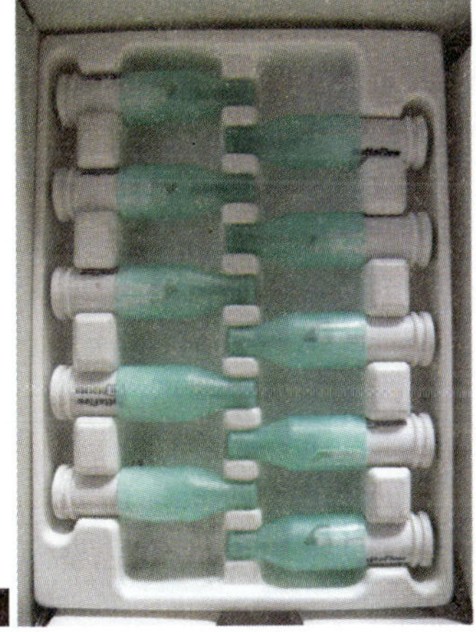

Fig. 20.30a and b GuttaFlow

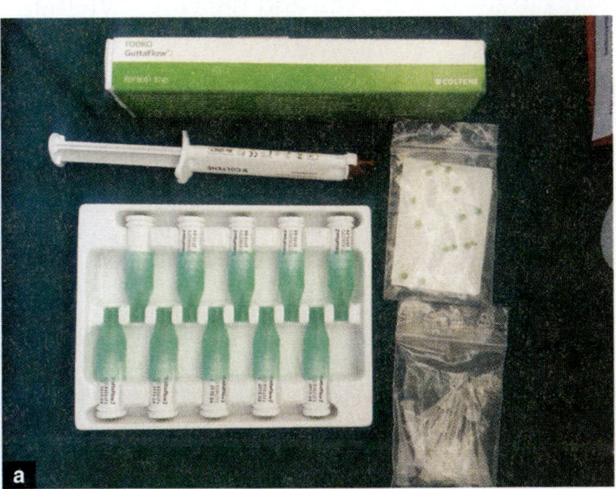

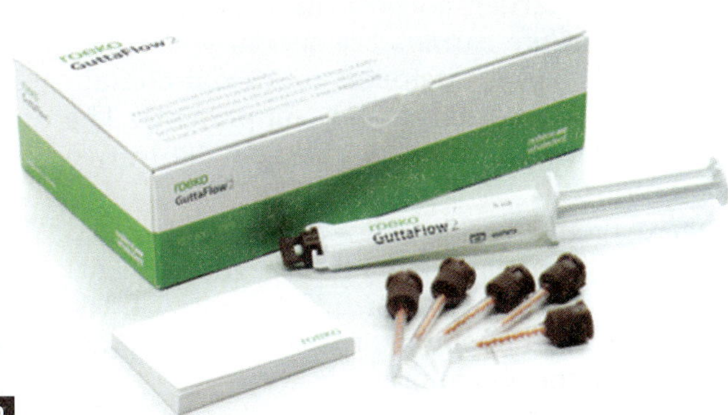

Fig. 20.31a and b GuttaFlow 2

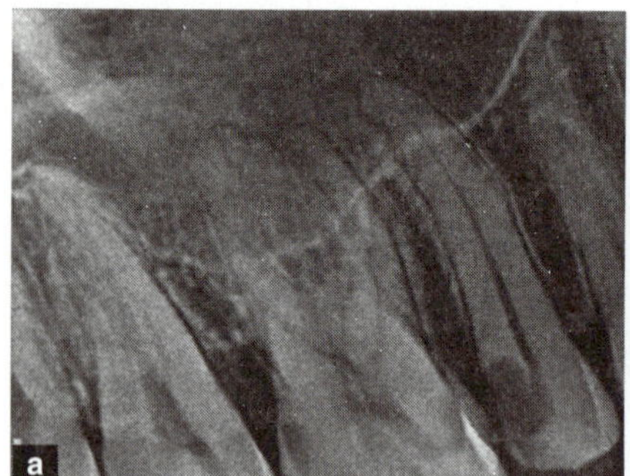
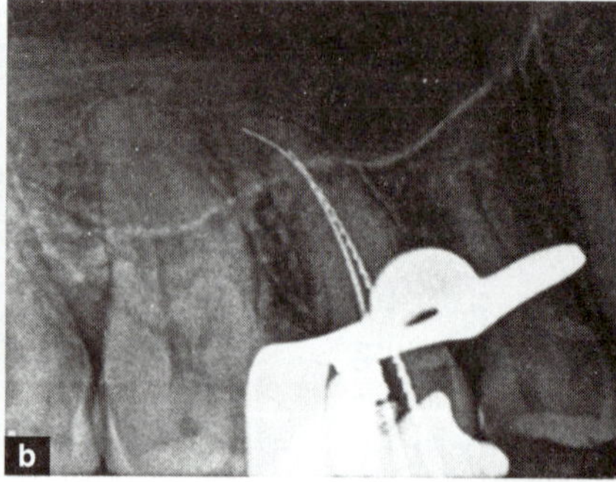
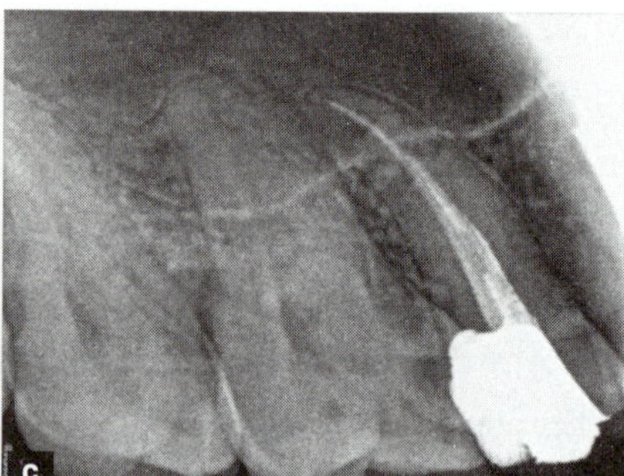

Fig. 20.32 (a) Preoperative (maxillary second premolar); (b) Working length determination; (c) GuttaFlow obturation

GuttaFlow 2 provides good adhesion to gutta-percha points and dentin walls. The combination of expansion and adhesion creates an excellent seal.

It is thixotropic (viscosity diminishes under pressure); flows into the smallest canal spaces during placement of master cone.

Mostly root canal sealers are soluble in tissue fluid, to a varying degree; however, the solubility of GuttaFlow 2 is virtually zero, resulting in impervious root canal filling.

GuttaFlow is extremely biocompatible.

A clinical case depicting obturation with GuttaFlow is exhibited in Fig. 20.32a to c.

Advantages

- Adhesion to gutta-percha point and dentin wall
- Easy to remove during retreatment and post preparation
- Radiopaque
- Excellent sealing
- Antibacterial
- Ease of handling
- Biocompatible.

b. GuttaCore System

The GuttaCore is a carrier-based gutta-percha obturating system.

The obturator carriers are normally made of plastic; whereas, GuttaCore carriers are specially designed from a gutta-percha elastomer (does not contain polysulfone—a routinely used component). The obturator is made entirely of gutta-percha in two different forms.

The core comprises of cross-linked gutta-percha and the outer surface has alpha gutta-percha. The root canal should be widened to at least size 20/06 or 25/04. The right sized GuttaCore obturator is selected (working length is set on the obturator).

A thin layer of sealer is applied in the prepared root canal.

The selected obturator with working length marking is placed into a holder in the oven for heating (20 to 25°C heat is sufficient).

ThermaPrep ovens are available providing three-dimensional heating of obturators.

The obturator is inserted into the root canal to the working length slowly without rotation.

The heated gutta-percha can be condensed with a plugger in the coronal part of the root canal.

The carrier is cut-off at the orifice using appropriate burs.

Advantages

- Three-dimensional obturation can be achieved
- Easy to remove during retreatment.

c. Resilon

The Resilon obturating system (Fig. 20.33) consists of the following components:

i. *Resilon*: A thermoplastic synthetic polymer (polycaprolactone) filling material (the major component); contains polymers of polyester, bioactive glass and radiopaque filler (bismuth, oxychloride and bismuth sulfate).

ii. *Sealer*: A dual-cure resin-based sealer that forms a bond to the dentin wall and the core material.

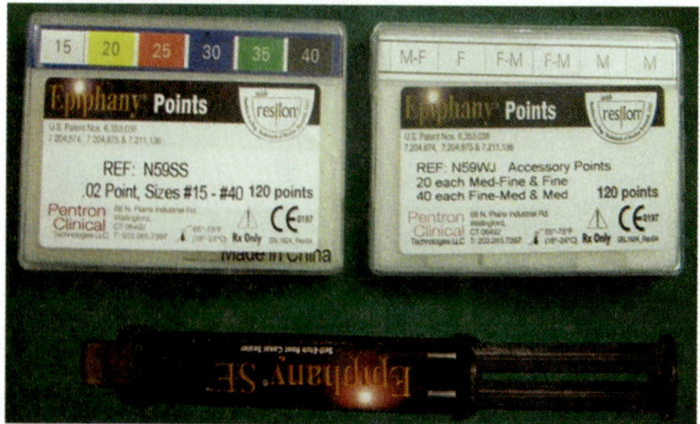

Fig. 20.33 Resilon obturating system

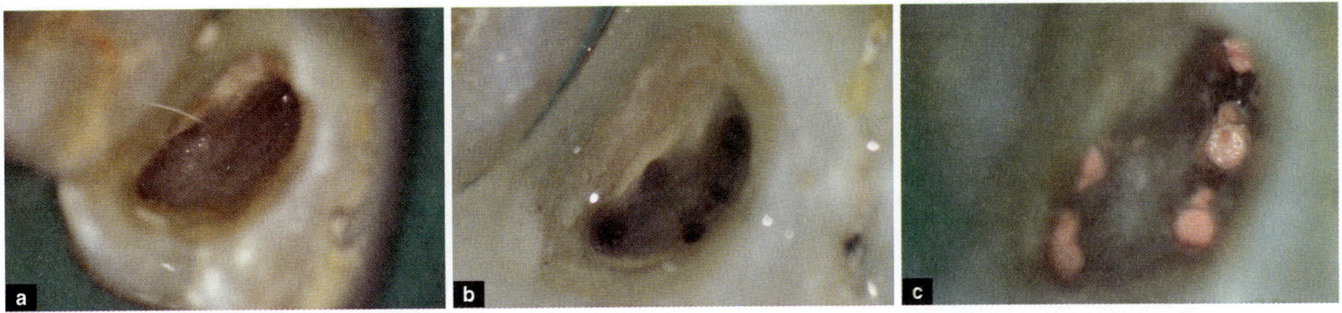

Fig. 20.34 (a) Initial access preparation; (b) Prepared root canals; (c) Postoperative (obturation)

iii. *Primer*: Prepares the canal wall to get in contact with Resilon and the sealer; contains HEMA, sulfonic acid and water.

Resilon resembles gutta-percha and is available in standardized (2.0% taper) and non-standardized cones; and also in pellet form for use in 'obtura' gun (thermal injection technique). It is also known as 'resin-percha', because of accompanying sealer and the primer.

Various techniques (single-cone method, cold lateral condensation and thermoplastic techniques) can be employed to place Resilon in the canal, with the same instruments and devices that are used for gutta-percha condensation (Fig. 20.34a to c). The coronal portion of the filling is light cured for 40 seconds.

This system facilitates formation of 'mono-block', comprising of root dentin, sealer and resin-percha.

Advantages

- Radiopacity better than gutta-percha
- Less irritant than zinc oxide sealers
- Biocompatible (non-mutagenic)
- Creates monoblock effect; better sealability.

RealSeal/RealSeal SE

The RealSeal system is available in two variants: the RealSeal system and the RealSeal Self-Etch (SE) system (Fig. 20.35).

RealSeal points are identical to Resilon obturating points (standardized/non-standardized pellets).

RealSeal sealer contains conventional resin matrix, silane-treated barium borosilicate glasses, barium sulfate, silica, calcium hydroxide, bismuth oxychloride, photo initiator and pigment.

The primer is an acidic monomer solution in water.

The root canals are obturated with lateral or vertical condensation technique.

RealSeal can be used in an Obtura gun as injectable filling material and also with the elements obturation system.

Real seal system show less microleakage than other resin-based obturating systems due to better bonding to canal walls.

RealSeal 1

RealSeal 1 is carrier-based obturating material containing a core of polysulfone coated with RealSeal Resilon material (Fig. 20.36).

The routinely used carrier-based obturation systems use gutta-percha coating, which may not be uniform (the gutta-percha coating can be stripped off in constricted area of the root canal).

However, the RealSeal 1 obturator is covered with Resilon, which does not get distorted easily (when the obturator encounters constriction in the canal, only the surface portion of the Resilon is affected. A thin layer of Resilon still remains adhered to the carrier).

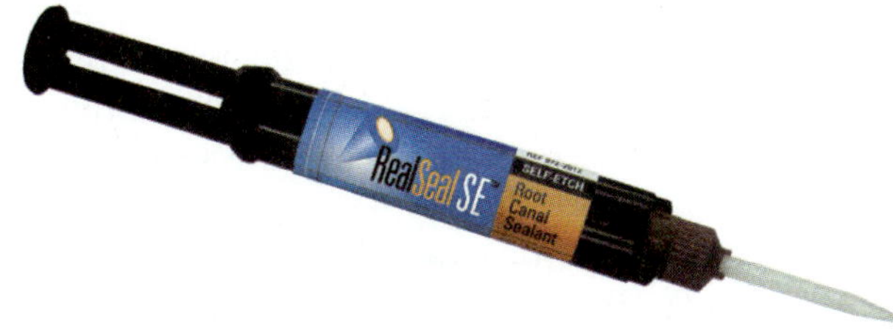

Fig. 20.35 RealSeal SE

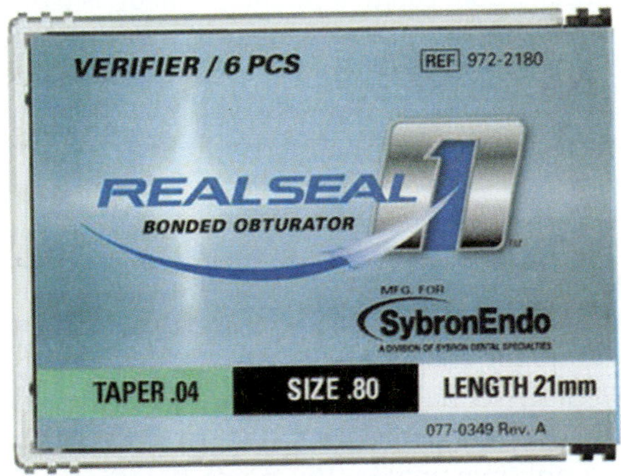

Fig. 20.36 RealSeal 1

20

Only methacrylate resin-based sealers are preferred with the system.

Advantages

- Reduced microleakage
- Provide monoblock effect; better sealability
- Easily removed during retreatment and post space preparation.

d. EZ Fill System

EZ-Fill system consists of a bi-directional spiral filler and epoxy resin based root canal cement. The bi-directional spiral ensures uniform distribution of cement in the root canal, minimizing chances of cement crossing the periapex. This controlled distribution is achieved because the spirals at the coronal end spin the cement toward the apex while the spirals at the apical end spin the cement toward the coronal end. The area where they meet (about 3.0–4.0 mm from the apical end of the shaft), the cement is thrown out laterally. A prefitted single gutta-percha point is placed to the working length. The tapered shape of the canal facilitates escape of excess cement coronally. The cement seals the apex and also the lateral and accessory canals. The excess gutta-percha is seared off and the access cavity is filled with temporary restorative materials.

Advantages

- Three-dimensional filling is achieved, without any lateral stress on the root
- Obturation is at room temperature (unlike thermoplastic techniques, there is no shrinkage upon cooling)
- Radiopaque
- Flow is superior to thermoplastic gutta-percha
- Adhesive to both dentin and gutta-percha.

e. SmartSeal

SmartSeal, a root canal obturating system, is based on the hydrophilic nature of the obturating points (polymer technology), which can absorb surrounding moisture and expand resulting in three-dimensional filling of root canals.

SmartSeal is a two-part system consisting of Propoint and Smartpaste/Smartpaste Bio.

Propoint

- Propoint, also known as C Point, consists of premade hydrophilic endodontic points.
- The inner core of C Point is a mix of two nylon polymers: Trogamid T and Trogamid CX.
- The polymer makes the point flexible enough, facilitating easy insertion into the curved spaces; while being rigid enough to pass into narrower canals.
- The outer coating is a cross-linked copolymer, which has been polymerized using thermal initiator. The coating allows the point to swell laterally by absorbing residual water from the instrumented canal space and from naturally occurring intra-radicular moisture. It does not swell axially, so there is no change in length.
- The lateral expansion does not cause any stress and is well within tensile strength of dentin. The expansion occurs within the first 4 hours of obturation facilitating the sealer and the polymer to produce three-dimensional sealing.

Smartpaste/Smartpaste Bio

Smartpaste is a resin-based sealer containing an active polymer that swells and fills all irregularities in the root canal. The degree of swelling is proportional to the amount of active polymer used.

Smartpaste Bio is a resin-based sealer integrated with bioceramics to make the obturation, non resorbable, antibacterial and biocompatible.

The setting time is 4–10 hours allowing sufficient time for the Propoint to expand and seal the canal hermetically. The sealer is delivered in a syringe and can be applied directly into the canal using an intracanal tip.

A Propoint that matches the last file used to prepare the canal is selected, tried and inserted into the canal up to the working length. The adequate insertion can be confirmed by the use of radiographs. The sealer is applied inside the canal using syringe tips. The Propoint is then introduced gently into the canal with the help of tweezers.

The extra Propoint is trimmed at the canal orifice and the coronal cavity is filled with suitable material.

f. Coated Cones

The coated cones have been developed in an attempt to achieve similar results as those claimed by Resilon, a bond between the canal wall, the core and the sealer. A bond is formed when the resin sealer contacts the resin-coated gutta-percha cone. This bonding minimizes the leakage between the solid core and the sealer.

Two versions of coated gutta-percha are available; one is EndoREZ resin-coated gutta-percha points and the second is ActiV GP precision, which is gutta-percha cones coated with glass-ionomer and is used with glass-ionomer sealer.

EndoREZ

EndoREZ is dual-cured radiopaque sealer. The sealer is coated over gutta-percha cones (sealer contains urethane methacrylate resin, zinc oxide and barium sulfate). The coated points along with sealer adapt closely to the dentinal walls, providing three-dimensional obturation.

ActiV GP Precision

ActiV GP is a coated obturation material; conventional gutta-percha cones are coated with glass ionomer sealer (Fig. 20.37).

The working time of the glass ionomer sealer is improved by modifying its particle size to the nanoparticle level (2.0 µm). Glass-ionomer coating facilitates dentin adhesiveness.

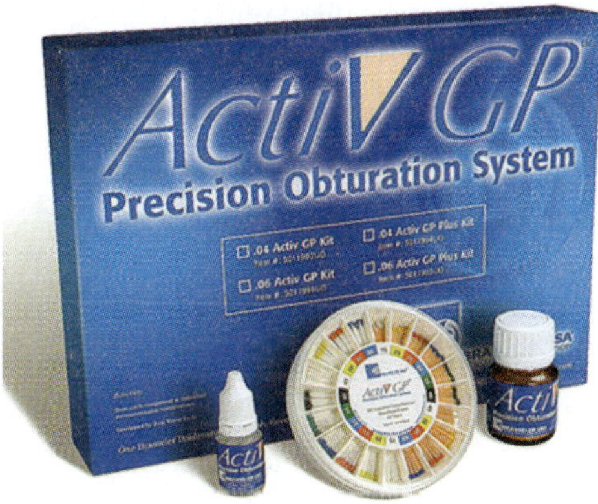

Fig. 20.37 ActiV GP (obturation system)

The cones are available in ISO sizes 15 to 60 in either a 0.04 or 0.06 taper.

The ActiV GP Plus, a modified version has calibration rings for easy depth measurement and a barrel handle for easier insertion into the canal.

The fit of the ActiV GP cone in the root canal is verified using radiographs. The sealer is applied inside the canal. The ActiV GP cone is also coated with the sealer and slowly inserted into the canal to the working length. After the ActiV GP cone has been seated, the extra cone is seated off at the coronal orifice. The coronal cavity is filled with suitable material.

The advantages and disadvantages of core materials are summarized in Table 20.2.

4. OBTURATION OF APICAL THIRD AREA

The obturation of apical third area need special attention, because of the interface formed between root canal walls, obturating material/sealer on one side and periodontium and body fluids on the other side. The microspaces in this interface is a potential source of microbial growth. To avoid microbial growth, a long-term hermetic sealing is required in constantly wet environment of the apical area. Another important feature required is the osteoconductivity of the obturating material and/or the sealer so as to fill the apical area physiologically. Bioceramic-based sealers (features as osteoconductivity, hydrophilicity, adhesiveness and bonding to root dentin) appears to provide effective physiological seal eliminating possible growth of microorganisms.

Table 20.2 Advantages and disadvantages of core materials

Core material	*Advantages*	*Disadvantages*
Gutta-percha	• Plasticity, adapts well • Easy manipulation • Non-toxic • Radiopaque • Ease of removal	• Lack of adhesion to dentin • Shrinkage, may lead to microgaps
Coated cones	• Good adaptability • Radiopaque • Non-toxic • Adhesion to canal wall • Minimizes leakage	• Life of coating, may not last longer
Resilon	• Good adaptability • Radiopaque • Biocompatible • Adhesion to canal wall • May form a monoblock	• Gutta-percha coating may be stripped off in constricted areas of the root canal
Pro-Points	• Expand to fill intricacies of root canal • Expansion does not cause any lateral stress on root dentin	• Limited documentation

A few authors have coined the term **'Endodontic grafting'** for filling apical third areas. Obturating material/sealer is being 'grafted' at the apical 3.0 mm area to achieve the requisite sealing.

The obturation of only apical third area is indicated in certain cases, which are simultaneously restored with post and core. The routinely used modalities are:

a. Warm/Sectional Gutta-percha

A small section of gutta-percha is packed into apical area to achieve apical obturation. The size of the sectioned gutta-percha depends upon the length of root canal and configuration of apical foramen (Fig. 20.38 a and b).

Technique

- A plugger is selected which fit loosely in the root canal and extend to within 3.0 mm of the working length. A stopper is placed to mark the length.
- Primary gutta-percha point is blunted and carried to place 1.0 mm short of working length and confirmed radiographically.
- Upon removal, 3.0 mm of the tip (size can vary) is excised with scalpel.
- Sealer is placed in the canal. Gutta-percha tip is warmed by passing through alcohol flame and carried into the canal.
- The plugger is pressed apically and rotated counter clockwise to separate the gutta-percha from the plugger.
- Gutta-percha is thoroughly packed in the predetermined apical area.
- Radiograph is taken to confirm the placement.
- The rest of space is left to be prepared for post (paper point placed in the canal covered with interim filling material in the coronal cavity).
- Backfilling may be carried out with thermoplasticized gutta-percha, if need be.

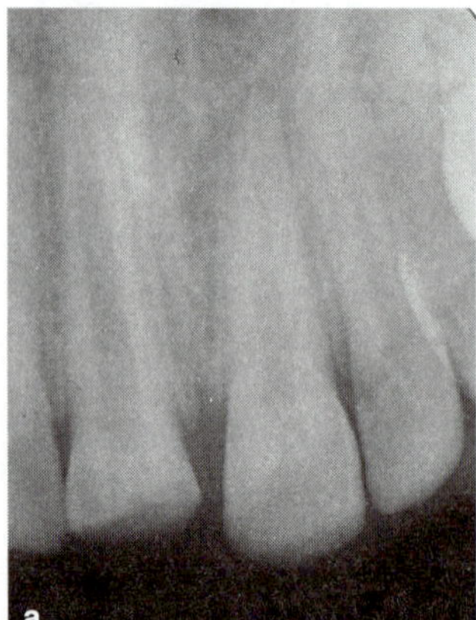

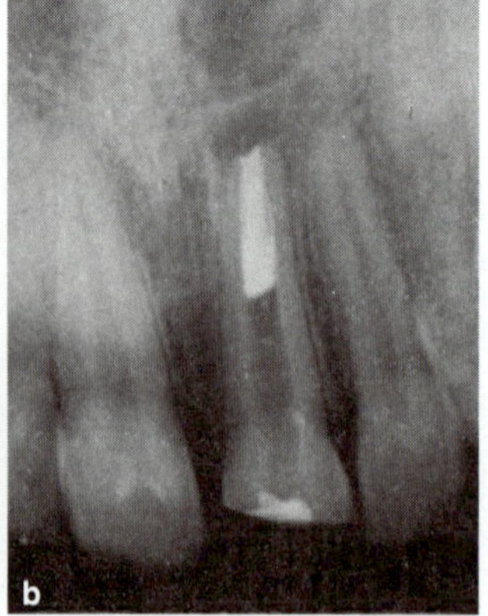

Fig. 20.38 Sectional gutta-percha technique: (a) Preoperative; (b) Gutta-percha obturation in apical half only

b. Dentin Chips

Dentin chips are compacted in apical third area and act as 'apical plug' against which other materials can be obturated. Dentin chips create a 'biologic seal' rather than a mechanical-chemical seal. It has been established that dentin chips stimulate osteogenesis/cementogenesis.

Technique

- Débride and prepare the canal thoroughly.
- Gates glidden drill/Hedstrom file is used to produce dentin chips in central portion of the canal.
- Dentin chips so produced are pushed apically with butt end of the paper point.
- 1.0–2.0 mm of chips are usually sufficient to block the foramen (blockage checked with small size file).
- Apical leakage can be reduced by injecting small amount of dentin adhesive into the coronal half of the dentinal apical plug.
- Rest of the canal can be filled with routine gutta-percha.

Advantages

- Prevents overfilling
- Confines the filling materials to the canal space
- Stimulate healing
- Minimal inflammation
- Apical cementum deposition, even when the apex is perforated.

Disadvantage

Dentin chips, if infected may irritate and hinder repair.

c. Mineral Trioxide Aggregate

The placement of 4.0–5.0 mm apical barrier of mineral trioxide aggregate (MTA) has been a preferred material, especially in a canal with apical transportation. The material offers biological compatibility, stimulating the growth of cementum like tissue on the apical end area (Fig. 20.39 a to d).

Technique

- A dense mix of MTA is pushed into the apical area of the root canal with an appropriate plugger.
- Placement of material is confirmed by radiographs.
- A cotton pellet moistened in saline is placed against the coronal aspect of the material within the canal (periapical fluids of periapical area provide sufficient moisture to the material).
- Rest of the canal is temporarily filled with paper points and interim material.
- In a subsequent visit; a file is used to confirm the hardness of the material.
- Once the setting of material is confirmed, the remaining canal is managed according to the need.

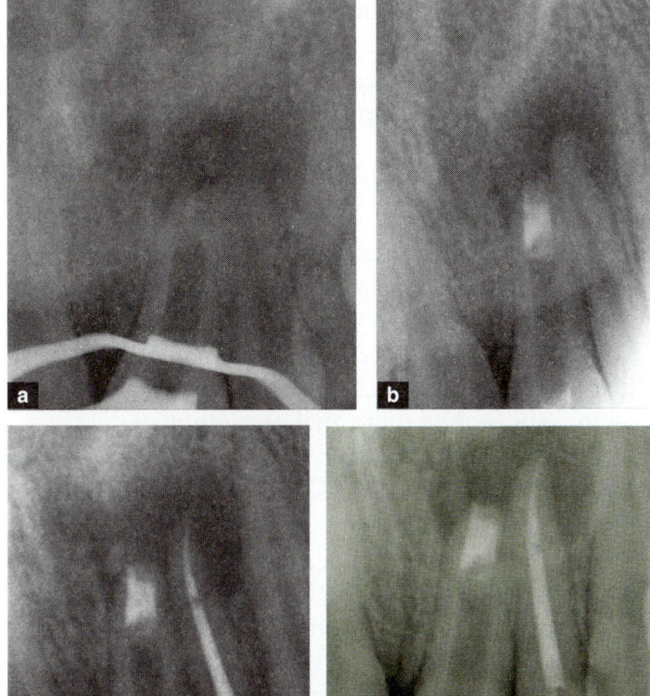

Fig. 20.39 (a) Preoperative; (b) MTA filled in apical area; (c) Adjacent tooth obturated; (d) MTA filling after six weeks

d. Carrier-based Systems

i. SimpliFill System

The SimpliFill system is designed to be compatible with the LightSpeed instrumentation system used for cleaning and shaping the root canal.

The SimpliFill system utilizes a solid piece of gutta-percha (ISO size: 5.0 mm length and 0.02 mm taper) for an apical plug. The carrier for the apical gutta-percha plug is made of stainless steel, which is flexible enough to negotiate curves and rigid enough to push the tight-fitting plug to the working length. A 1.0 mm threaded tip holds the gutta-percha plug on the carrier, and the carrier has a plugger-like surface, which pushed the plug to working length.

Technique

- Check the fit of the apical gutta-percha plug to the working length.
- Place sealer in the apical part of the canal.
- After inserting the plug into the canal, slowly advance it apically without rotating the handle.
- With the plug at working length, leave it thereby turning the carrier handle counter-clockwise and removing the carrier from the canal.
- If a post is not required, fill the remainder of the canal by backfilling.
- If post is required, leave the apical plug intact and prepare the post space.

Advantages

- Quick and easy
- Manipulation simple
- Does not require special equipment
- Does not require heat (no guttapercha shrinkage upon cooling)

ii. FiberFill System

The FiberFill system utilizes glass fiber post with a terminal gutta-percha tip. The gutta-percha is available either in 5.0 or 8.0 mm lengths. The diameter of the post is available in sizes 30, 40, 50, 60, 70 and 80.

Technique

- An obturator is selected that matches the final diameter of the canal.
- A drop of primer is applied in the apical area with the spiral brush provided in the kit.
- The sealer is introduced into the canal with FiberFill syringe.
- The obturator is gently seated to working length allowing excess sealer to be expressed coronally.
- The dual cure FiberFill sealer is light cured to stabilize the obturator.
- Additional primer is applied on the protruding portion of the obturator post and over any dentin and enamel that will be in contact with the core build-up material.
- A resin core build-up material in then injected around the post, filling the coronal portion of the tooth.
- The material is light cured and ready for final restoration.

Advantage

- Provides a durable restoration with a resin/fiber reinforced root that is optimally sealed apically and coronally.

iii. EZ Fill System

The technique has already been explained.

5. PASTES AS OBTURATING MATERIALS

Virtually all types of sealers have been tried as 'pastes' in obturating root canal spaces. The purpose of the paste is to provide volumetrically stable filling which will adapt to the variable configuration of the root canals. The paste, should not remain soft overtime and must set within the root canal in stipulated time so as to provide adequate sealing. The obturating paste should be dimensionally stable, insoluble and also biocompatible.

In the past, numerous obturating pastes with varying chemical composition have been developed and tried. The initially tried pastes are: zinc oxide eugenol paste, reinforced zinc oxide eugenol paste, medicated (with paraformaldehyde and/or corticosteroids), zinc oxide eugenol paste, calcium hydroxide alone and calcium hydroxide-based pastes, resin-based pastes and bioceramic-based pastes. Gutta-percha in paste form and double/triple antibiotic pastes have also been used.

The pastes are usually not preferred, because most of the pastes are toxic when extruded out of apex. The problems of porosities, inadvertent extension and difficulty in removing during retreatment are the other disadvantages quoted in literature.

The obturating paste, commonly used in the past, though no longer used, is N2 (sargenti paste).

a. N2 (Sargenti Paste)

The term N2 was coined by Sargenti to describe the material as the second nerve. N2 filling material has red color to match the color of pulp it replaces. The composition is as follows:

Powder

i. Radiopacifiers
- Zinc oxide (68.51 g)
- Lead tetra oxide (12 g)
- Paraformaldehyde (4.7 g)
- Bismuth subcarbonate (2.60 g)
- Bismuth subnitrate (3.7 g)

ii. Pigments
- Titanium dioxide (8.4 g)

iii. Antiseptic component
- Phenyl mercuric borate (0.09 g)

Liquid

i. Eugenol
ii. Cleum Rosea
iii. Cleum Lavandula.

20

The technique employed canal preparation with no intracanal irrigant and filling with a N2 paste. The whole treatment is carried out in single sitting. Artificial fistulation was recommended in certain cases but without raising the flap. Sargenti called it apical fenestration.

It is no longer used because of following drawbacks:
- Paraformaldehyde cause toxicity, severe periapical inflammation.
- May result in overextension, underextension and voids.
- May lead to paresthesia of the nerve particularly in case of mandibular posterior teeth.
- May lead to ankylosis, root resorption.

Presently, MTA and MTA-based cements, biodentine, calcium enriched matrix (CEM) cements are being tried and investigated as root canal obturation.

b. Mineral Trioxide Aggregate (MTA)

Mineral trioxide aggregate (MTA) has a profound advantage when used as canal obturation material because of its superior physiochemical and bioactive properties. In addition to being sterile, radiopaque and non-shrinking, the material is not sensitive to moisture and blood contamination. MTA is not only bacteriostatic, but has potential bactericidal properties. MTA also provides an effective seal against dentin and cementum and promotes biologic repair and regeneration of the periodontal ligament. Its unique sealing property, combined with an initially high pH that increases to 12.5 after setting, might provide a suitable environment for repair and healing. MTA in paste form has been tried as obturating the total pulp space.

Technique

- The root canal is prepared in routine and dried.
- Smear layer does not affect the sealability of MTA materials, and its presence may improve the seal over time. It has been speculated that the smear layer might act as a 'coupling agent' that might enhance MTA bonding to root canal dentin.
- White MTA has better handling characteristics and compactibility, attributed to smaller particle sizes, but grey MTA appears to have superior sealing properties.
- MTA can be mixed with 0.12% chlorhexidine (rather than sterile water or anesthetic solution), which may increase its antibacterial properties.
- The mixed MTA is placed in the canal with a carrier gun and advanced apically with an endodontic plugger.
- A radiograph is taken to assess the presence of voids.
- When the requisite density is achieved at the periapex, fresh MTA is placed in the canal and compacted from the apical to coronal area by using appropriate pluggers.

Advantages

- Not sensitive to moisture and blood contamination.
- Antibacterial (prevents growth of bacteria)
- Does not shrink
- Biocompatible.

Disadvantages

- Gray MTA can discolor teeth if the material is placed near the cementoenamel junction, especially in anterior teeth.
- Removal is difficult after setting.
- Slow setting time (the material can take 2.5–4.0 hours for an initial set and 21 days for complete setting).

c. Calcium Phosphate Cement

Earlier, decalcified allogenic bone matrix (DABM) and tricalcium phosphate (TCP) have been tried as obturating materials. Calcium phosphate cement (CPC) when used as a root canal filling material has shown positive results.

Tetracalcium phosphate is the basic constituent; the acidic component is either dicalcium phosphate dihydrate or anhydrous dicalcium phosphate. Setting time may be extended by adding glycerine (glycerin also helps improve its extrudability from a 19 gauge needle). It is radiopaque (radiopacity is equal to bone density).

Cement is mild irritant to periapical tissue for some time; however, well-tolerated by tissues with passage of time. Calcium phosphate cement stimulate cementogenesis and osteogenesis within the canal.

d. Calcium Enriched Matrix (CEM) Cement and Biodentine

Calcium enriched matrix (CEM) cement and Biodentine are being tried as root canal obturating materials. Bioceramic-based sealers are also being used in root canal obturation.

Capillary Condensation Method

Dr Kosser Deyan (2009) devised a technique of filling bioceramic materials in root canal and named it as *'Capillary condensation method'*.

The steps followed in this method are:

- The coronal third of root canal is conically widened to form a 'coronal reservoir', which is to be filled with bioceramic materials.
- The bioceramic-based material mixes are either directly placed in the reservoir or with the use of guns. The material is distributed evenly in the reservoir using wet plastic carrier.
- A specially designed instrument/plugger is used to condense the material apically. The plugger is pushed gently up and down; the end should remain in the reservoir.
- The placement of the material is kept 1.0 mm short of the working length.
- The tactile feeling of 'tightening' of plugger is the stage where the plugger is removed from the canal.
- A correct sized gutta-percha is inserted midway into the root canal (the gentle pressure will move the material evenly along the root canal walls).
- Excessive gutta-percha and the bioceramic materials are wiped out of the coronal end.
- After setting of the material (may be 24 hours), the coronal cavity is filled.
- The additional gutta-percha along with bioceramic material facilitates removal during post and core placement and also during retreatment.

6. RETROGRADE (ROOT END) FILLING MATERIALS

Surgical intervention in root canal therapy usually involves resecting a portion of the root apex and filling the root-end cavity with appropriate material. These root-end filling materials or retrograde filling materials are placed in direct contact with vital periapical tissues. The purpose of retrograde filling is to prevent leakage of microorganisms and their byproducts from periradicular tissues to root canals and from root canals to periradicular tissues. The materials, which stimulate deposition of cementum on the cut root end are being preferred as retro-filling materials. The deposition of cementum or tissues simulating cementum/dentin provides the best biological seal.

The retrograde (root-end) filling materials are either of rigid or plastic material (Table 20.3).

Requisite characteristics of root-end filling materials

The ideal requirements of root end filling materials are:

- Non-toxic
- Non-carcinogenic

Table 20.3 Root-end filling materials

Rigid materials	*Plastic materials*
• Gold foil • Gallium alloy • Titanium inserts • Ceramic inserts • Metal inlays • Gutta-percha	• Amalgam • Zinc oxide eugenol/reinforced zinc oxide eugenol compounds • Cements (glass-ionomer, polycarboxylate) • Mineral trioxide aggregate • Composite resin • Calcium phosphate cement • Bioceramic-based materials • Biodentine

- Biocompatible
- Dimensionally stable (presence of moisture should not affect its sealing ability)
- Easy to use
- Radiopaque
- Should stimulate hard-tissue formation
- Should not be electrochemically active
- Non-resorbable
- Antibacterial.

Various materials have been tried in root-end fillings, viz. Gold foil, silver, gallium alloys, zinc oxide eugenol, modified zinc oxide eugenol, polycarboxylate cement, glass-ionomer cements, mineral trioxide aggregate and calcium phosphate cement. Composite resin, bioceramics and a few herbal products have also been tried.

The commonly used retrograde filling materials are as follows.

a. Amalgam

Amalgam has extensively been used as retro-filling material. High copper zinc-free amalgam is preferred. It is established that use of varnish and amalgambond (4-META bonding agent) with amalgam significantly improves the sealing. It is easy to manipulate and has good radiopacity. It is non-soluble in tissue fluids. The sealing improves as amalgam ages due to formation of corrosion products.

Disadvantages

- Initial marginal leakage
- Corrosion
- Scattered silver particles are difficult to remove; not get resorbed
- Tin and mercury contamination of periapical tissues
- Moisture sensitivity of some alloys
- Cytotoxic, especially at initial stages
- Paresthesia has also been reported
- Need for retentive undercut preparation
- Staining of hard and soft tissues
- Technique sensitivity.

b. Gutta-percha

Gutta-percha filled tooth when resected at the apical end, the visible gutta-percha is condensed in the root-end cavity, either by cold or hot burnisher. Thermoplasticized gutta-percha has also been filled at root end cavities. Gutta-percha may absorb moisture initially and expand; however, as the time passes, it contracts. Gutta-percha fillings offer better sealing than amalgam. It is also non-resorbable and biocompatible.

Disadvantages

- Apical seal may get disturbed with time
- Moisture sensitive
- Condensation is difficult from apical end.

c. Zinc Oxide Eugenol/Reinforced Zinc Oxide Eugenol Compounds

Zinc oxide eugenol and reinforced zinc oxide eugenol compounds (IRM, Super EBA Kalzinol, Cavit, etc.) have been effectively used as root-end fillings. Super EBA and IRM show less leakage as compared to silver amalgam.

Cavit is a reinforced zinc oxide based temporary filling material. Cavit is soft when placed in the tooth and subsequently undergoes a hygroscopic set after permeation with water, giving a higher linear expansion (18%). This rationalizes its use as a root-end filling material. These materials have excellent sealing ability and are significantly biocompatible.

Disadvantages

- Moisture sensitive
- Initial tissue irritation
- Eugenol may exhibit mild toxicity
- Solubility and quick disintegration in tissue fluids.

d. Cements

i. Polycarboxylate Cement

Apical leakage studies have indicated that polycarboxylates, when used as root-end fillings, leak significantly greater than amalgam or gutta-percha. Based on their poor sealing ability and uncertain periradicular tissue response, the use of polycarboxylate as root-end filling material is highly questionable.

ii. Glass-ionomer Cement

Glass-ionomer cement has been successfully tried as root-end filling material. It is easy to handle and does not cause any adverse histological reaction in the periapical tissue. Sealing ability of glass-ionomer is adversely affected when the root-end cavities are contaminated with moisture at the time of placement of cement. Light cure glass-ionomer cement show least leakage due to less moisture sensitivity, less curing shrinkage and better penetration into dentinal surface. Metal reinforced glass-ionomer have also shown better results.

Disadvantages

- Moisture sensitive (cavity should be dry)
- Initially cytotoxic.

e. Composite Resin

Composite resins due to their cytotoxic or irritating effects on pulp tissue have received minimal attention as root-end filling materials. However, a few authors opined that when composite resins are properly used, the cytotoxic effects are substantially decreased or eliminated. The proper use of dentin bonding agents and composite resin may play a significant role as root-end filling.

Newer composites, Retroplast and Geristore are being tried as retrograde filling material. 30% colloidal silica/silver provided radiopacity in the materials. Since, colloidal silver had some disadvantages; it was replaced with ytterbium trifluoride. The new combination is successful as retrofilling material.

Disadvantages

- Sensitive to moisture/blood contamination
- Mild cytotoxicity.

f. Mineral Trioxide Aggregate

Mineral trioxide aggregate (MTA) primarily contain tricalcium silicate, tricalcium aluminate, tricalcium oxide and silicate oxide. The material has been successfully used as root-end filling material, offering advantages of being radiopaque, not affected by blood contamination, biocompatible and stimulates formation of cementoid tissue at the resected end.

Disadvantages

- Handling is difficult
- Toxic potential
- Long-setting time
- Discoloration potential
- Difficult to remove after setting.

The modified form of MTA (light cure MTA, MTA-Angelus, fast endodontic cement, bioaggregate, etc.) have been tried. All these materials are biocompatible and well-tolerated by the apical tissues.

The radiopacity of mineral trioxide aggregate is much better than EBA and IRM. It provides superior seal when compared with amalgam, IRM and super EBA. It has been established that osteoblasts have favorable response to MTA as compared to IRM and amalgam.

g. Calcium Phosphate Cement

Calcium phosphate cement (CPC), also referred to as hydroxyapatite cement, is composed of tetracalcium phosphate and dicalcium phosphate reactants. It demonstrates excellent biocompatibility, does not cause inflammatory response/toxic reaction. CPC seems to be quite promising as a retrograde filling material.

h. Bioceramic-based Materials

Bioceramic-based materials having nano-sized particles achieve excellent adhesion to the canal's dentinal walls and, more importantly, form a chemical bond with dentin. They are claimed to promote cementogenesis and form a hermetic seal at the root end. These materials are biocompatible and do not induce any cytotoxic effects. Calcium aluminate silicate-based materials (Endo binder, Generex A, etc.) have shown better results (calcium oxide/magnesium oxide was removed from the powder minimizing expansion and also the staining). The commonly used bioceramic-based materials are:

- Capasio
- Iron-free partially stabilized cement
- Endosequence/iRoot BP
- Root end cement
- Endobinder
- Generex A
- Quickset.

i. Biodentine

Biodentine is also being tried as root-end filling material. Compared to other calcium based cements, this material offers two advantages, (i) faster setting time (12 minutes) and (ii) better mechanical properties. Biodentine has the potential of forming hydroxyapatite when in contact with tissue fluids. Biodentine is biocompatible and easily manipulated in the root-end cavities.

BIBLIOGRAPHY

1. Aguilar FG, Robertl Garcia LF and Panzeri Pires-de-Souza FC. Biocompatibility of new calcium aluminate cement (EndoBinder). J. Endod.: 2012; 38:367–371.
2. Al-Hiyasat AS, Al-Sa'ed OR and Darmahi H. Quality of cellular attachment to various root-end filling materials. J. Appl. Oral Sci.: 2012; 20:82–88.
3. Asrari M and Lobner D. *In vitro* neurotoxic evaluation of root-end filling materials. J. Endod.: 2003; 29:743–746.
4. Bishop D, Griggs J and He J. Effect of dynamic loading on the integrity of the interface between root canal and obturation materials. J. Endod.: 2008; 34:470–473.
5. Blum JY, Machtou P and Micallef JP. Analysis of forces developed during obtruation. Wedging effect: Part II. J. Endod.: 1998; 24:223–228.
6. Bodrumulu E and Alacam T. The antimicrobial and antifungal activity of a root canal core material. J. Am. Dent. Assoc.: 2007; 9:1228–1232.
7. Bodrumulu E and Gungor K. Radiopacity of an endodontic core material. Am. J. Dent.: 2009; 22:157–159.
8. Bodrumulu E and Tunga U. Coronal sealing ability of a new root canal filling material. J. Can. Dent. Assoc.: 2007; 7: 623–628.
9. Borisova-Papancheva T, Panov V, Peev S and Papanchev G. Root-end fillilng materials – Review. Scripta Sic. Med. Dent.: 2015; 1:7–13.

10. Buchanan LS. Filling root canal systems with centered condensation: concepts, instrument and techniques. Endod. Prac.: 2005; 8:9–15.
11. Caron G, Azerad J, Faure MO, Machtou P and Boucher Y. Use of a new retrograde filling material (Biodentine) for endodontic surgery: two case reports. Int. J. Oral Sci.: 2014; 6:250–253.
12. Chong BS and Pittford TR. Root-end filling materials: rationale and tissue response. Endod. Topics: 2005; 11:114–130.
13. Damas BA, Wheater MA, Bringas JS and Hoen MM. Cytotoxicity comparison of mineral trioxide aggregates and EndoSequence bioceramic root repair materials. J. Endod.: 2011; 37:372–375.
14. De-Deus G. Research that matters – root canal filling and leakage studies. Int. Endod. J.: 2012; 45:1063–1064.
15. Deshpande PM and Naik RR. Comprehensive review on recent root canal filling materials and techniques – an update. Int. J. Appl. Dent. Sci.: 2015; 1:30–34.
16. Dimitrova I and Kuzmanova Y. Mineral trioxide aggregate (MTA): Clinical application. Part II – ortograde and retrograde obturation of root canals, injuries and resorptive processes. Dent. Med.: 2011; 93:56–68.
17. Ezzie E, Fleury A, Solomon E, Spears R and He J. Efficacy of retreatment techniques for a resin-based root canal obturation material. J. Endod.: 2006; 32:341–344.
18. Gandolfi MG, Taddei P, Tinti A and Prati C. Apatite-forming ability (bioactivity) of ProRoot MTA. Int. Endod. J.; 2010; 43:917–920.
19. Ghoneim AG, Lutfy RA, Sabet NE and Fayyad DM. Resistance to fracture of roots obturated wit novel canal-filling systems. J. Endod.: 2011; 37:1590–1592.
20. Glassman G. Bioactive endodontic obturation: combining the new with the tried and true. MTA fillapex and continuous wave of condensation. Roots The J. Endod.: 2013; 4:16–24.
21. Glassman G. Three dimensional obtuation of the root-canal system: continuous wave of condensation. Roots The J. Endod.: 2012; 3:20–26.
22. Gluskin AH. Anatomy of an overfill: a reflection on the process. Endod. Topics: 2009; 16:64–81.
23. Gluskin AH. Mishaps and serious complications in endodontic obturation. Endod. Topics: 2005; 12:52–70.
24. Goon WWY. The apical push: hermatic seal enhancement using lateral condensation into warm GP. Compend. Contin. Educ. Dent.: 1985; 6:499.
25. Gorgiev T, Peev S, Papanchev G, Borisova-Papancheva TS and Aleksieva E. A clinical case of paresthesia due to amalgam retrograde filling disseminated in the upper jaw and soft tissues. Scripta Sci. Med.: 2012; 44:97–101.
26. Grech L, Mallia B and Camilleri J. Investigation of the physical properties of tricalcium silicate cement-based root-end filling materials. Dent. Mater.: 2013; 29:e20–e28.
27. Guo-hua L, Li-na N, Zhang W, Olsen M, De-Deus G, Eid AA, Chen J, Pashley DH and Tay FR. Ability of new obturation materials to improve the seal of the root canal system – a review. Acta Biomater.: 2014; 10:1050–1063.
28. Hale R, Gatti R, Glickman GN and Opperman LA. Comparative analysis of carrier-based obturation and lateral compaction: a retrospective clinical outcomes study. Int. J. Dent.: 2012; 2012:954–975.
29. Hammad M, Qualtrough A and Silikas N. Evaluation of root canal obtruation: a three-dimensional *in vitro* study. J. Endod.: 2009; 35:541–544.
30. Handa T, Quevedo CGA, Motoko O, Iwasaki N, Takahashi H and Suda H. Effects of new adhesive resin root canal filling materials on vertical root fractures. Aust.
31. Heeren TJ and Levitan ME. Effect of canal preparation to fill length in straight root canals obturated with RealSeal1 and Thermafil Plus. J. Endod.: 2012; 38:1380–1382.
32. Hemasathya B, Mony CM and Prakash V. Recent advances in root end filling materials: a review. Biomed. and Pharmaco. J.: 2015; 8:219–224.
33. Jamleh A, Awawdeh L, Albanyan H, Masuadi E and Alfouzan K. Apical guttapercha cone adaptation and degree of tug-back sensation after canal preparation. Saudi Endod. J.: 2016; 6:131–135.
34. Kangarlou A, Dianat O, Esfahrood ZR, Asharaf H, Zandi B and Eslami G. Bacterial leakage of guttaflow-filled root canals compared with Resilon/Epiphany and Gutta-percha/AH26-filled root canals. Aust. Endod. J.: 2012; 38:10–13.
35. Kratchman S. Warm gutta-percha revisited: Classic technique meets new technology. Oral Health Dent. J.: 2011, 73–80.
36. Lee JH, Shon WJ, Lee W and Baek SH. The effect of several root-end filling materials on MG63 osteoblast-like cells. J. Korean Acad. Conserv. Dent.: 2010; 35:222–228.
37. Lotfi M, Ghasemi N, Rahimi S, Vosoughhosseini S, Saghiri M and Shahidi A. Resilon: A Comprehensive literature review. J. Dent. Res. Dent. Clin. Dent. Prospects.: 2013; 7:119–130.
38. Lui JN, Sae-Lim V, Song KP and Chen NN. *In vitro* anti-microbial effect of chlorhexidine-impregnated gutta-percha points on *Enterococcus faecalis*. Int. Endod. J. : 2004; 37, 105–113.
39. Maltezos C, Glickman GN, Ezzo P and He J. Comparison of the sealing of Resilon, Pro Root MTA, and Super-EBA as Root-End filling materials: a bacterial leakage study. J. Endod.: 2006; 32:324–327.
40. Mandke L. Importance of coronal seal: Preventing coronal leakage in endodontics. J. Res. Dent.: 2016; 4:71–75.
41. Melker K, Vertucci F, Rojas F and Belanger M. Antimicrobial efficacy of medicated root canal filling materials. J. Endod.: 2006; 32:148–151.
42. Michaud RA, Burgess J, Barfield RD, Cakir D, McNeal SF and Eleazer PD. Volumetric expansion of gutta-percha in contact with eugenol. J. Endod.: 2008; 34:1528–1532.
43. Miner MR, Berzins DW and Bahcall JK. A comparison of thermal properties between Gutta-percha and a synthetic polymer based root canal filling material (Resilon). J. Endod.: 2006; 32:683–686.
44. Monticelli F, Sword J, Martin RL, Schuster GS, Weller RN and Ferrari M. Sealing properties of two contemporary single-cone obturation systems. Int. Endod. J.: 2007; 40: 374–385.

45. Naval RR, Parnande M and Sehgal R. A comparative evaluation of 3 root canal filling systems. Oral Surg., Oral Med., Oral Path., Oral Radiol. Endod.: 2011; 111:387–393.

46. Ndong F, Sadhasivam S, Lin FH, Savitha S, Wen-His W and Lin CP. The development of iron-free partially stabilized cement for use as dental root-end filling material. Int. Endod. J.: 2012; 45:557–564.

47. Orstavik D. Materials used for root canal obturation: technical, biological and clinical testing. Endod. Topics: 2005; 12:25–38.

48. Parrirokh M and Torabinejad M. Mineral trioxide aggregate: a comprehensive literature review – Part III: clinical applications, drawbacks, and mechanism of action. J. Endod.: 2010; 36:400–413.

49. Pawinska M, Kierklo A and Marczuk-Kolada G. New technology in endodontics – the Resilon-Epiphany system for obturation of root canals. Adv. In Med. Sci.: 2006; 1:154–157.

50. Reader CM, Himel VT, Germain LP and Hoen MM. Effect of three obturation techniques on the filling of lateral canals and the main canal. J. Endod.: 1993; 19:404–408.

51. Roudsari RV, Jawad S, Taylor C and Hunter M. Modern endodontic principles part 5: Obturation. Dent. Update: 2016; 43:114–129.

52. Sagsen B, Kahraman Y and Akdogan G. Resistance to fracture of roots filled with three different techniques. Int. Endod. J.: 2007; 1:31–35.

53. Sakkal S, Weine FS and Lemian L. Lateral condensation: inside view. Compend. Contin. Educ. Dent.: 1991; 12:796–802.

54. Samuel E, Hartwell J and Cicalesee C. Completeness of root canal obturations: Epiphany techniques versus Gutta-percha techniques. J. Endod.: 2006; 32:541–544.

55. Santos J, Tjaderhane L, Ferraz C, Zaia A, Alves M, De Goes M and Carrilho MR. Long-term sealing ability of resin-based root canal fillings. Int. Endod. J.: 2010; 43:455–460.

56. Saxena P, Gutpa SK and Newaskar V. Biocompatibility of root-end filling materials: recent update. Restor. Dent. Endod.: 2013; 38:119–127.

57. Schwartz RS. Adhesive dentistry and endodontics, part 2: bonding in the root canal system—the promise and the problems: a review. J. Endod.: 2008; 32:1125–1134.

58. Seabra Pereira OL and Siqueira JF. Contamination of gutta-percha and Resilon cones taken directly from the manufacturer. Clin. Oral Investig.: 2010; 3:327–330.

59. Shanahan DJ and Duncan HF. Root canal filling using Resilon: a review. Br. Dent. J.: 2011; 211:81–88.

60. Shrestha D, Wei X, Wu WC and Ling JQ. Resilon: a methacrylate resin-based obturation system. J. Dent. Sci.: 2010; 5:47–52.

61. Stuart C, Schwartz S and Beeson T. Reinforcement of immature roots with a new resin filling material. J. Endod.: 2006; 32:350–353.

62. Tanomaru-Filho M, Silveira GF, Tanomaru JM and Bjer CA. Evaluation of the thermoplasticity of different gutta-percha cones and Resilon. Aust. Endod. J.: 2007; 33:23–26.

63. Tay FR, Pashley DH, Loushine RJ, Kuttler S, Garcia-Goday F, King NM and Ferrari M. Susceptibility of a polycarpolactone-based root canal filling material to degradation. Evidence of biodegradation from a simulated field test. Am. J. Dent.: 2007; 20:365–369.

64. Teixeira FB. Ideal obturation using synthetic root-filling systems: coronal sealing and fracture resistance. Pract. Proc. and Aesthet. Dent.: 2006; 18:7–11.

65. Testarelli L, Milana V, Rizzo F, Gagliani M and Gambarini G. Sealing ability of a new carrier-based obturating material. Minerva Stomatologica: 2009; 58:217–224.

66. Torabinejad M, Parirokh M and Dummer PMH.: Mineral trioxide aggregate and other bioactive endodontic cements: an updated overview-part II: other clinical applications and complications. Int. Endod. J. 2018; 51:284–317.

67. Tunga U and Bodrumulu E. Assessment of the sealing ability of a new root canal obturation material. J. Endod.: 2006; 32:876–878.

68. Venture M, Di Lenarda R and Breschi L. An *ex vivo* comparison of three different gutta-percha cones when compared at different temperatures: rheological considerations in relation to the filling of lateral canals. Int. Endod. J.: 2006; 39:648–656.

69. Von Fraunhofer JA, Kurtzman GM and Norby CE. Resin-based sealing of root canals in endodontic therapy. Gen. Dent. J.: 2006; 54:243–246.

70. Walivaara DA, Abrahamsson P, Isaksson S, Salata LA, Sennerby L and Dahlin C. Periapical tissue response after use of intermediate restorative material, gutta-percha, reinforced zinc oxide cement, and mineral trioxide aggregate as retrograde root-end filling materials: a histologic study in dogs. J. Oral Maxillofac. Surg.: 2012; 70:2041–2047.

71. Whitworth J. Methods of filling root canals: principles and practices. Endod. Topics: 2005; 12:2–24.

72. Williams C, Loushine RJ, Weller RN, Pashley DH and Tay FR. A comparison of cohesive strength and stiffness of Resilon and Gutta-percha. J. Endod.: 2006; 32:553–555.

Chapter 21

Single-visit Endodontics

The endodontic therapy as a treatment modality to save teeth is gaining importance day-by-day. Over the years the evolution in Ni-Ti instruments coupled with improved techniques of root canal preparation and precision obturation has helped the operator perform endodontic procedures more effectively and efficiently. The endodontic procedure is to be completed in how many visits is not clearly documented. Even the rationale of multiple visits is also not established. The long-term outcome is the standard by which treatment methods are judged in medicine and dentistry. However, even long-term studies could not establish the protocol of time/visits to be successful in endodontic treatment.

What do we achieve in endodontic treatment? Simply, it is the elimination of microorganisms and their substrate from the pulp spaces, followed by three-dimensional obturation so as to avoid subsequent infections.

Can this goal be achieved in single visit? Or, the operator needs multiple visits to get rid of the microorganisms along with substrate from the root canal. If multiple visits are required to completely eliminate the microorganisms and this is the only reason that vital root canal treatment should always be carried out in one visit. But, this is not true always. It seems there might be other factors playing role in successful outcome of the endodontic treatment.

The authors favoring single visit endodontics opine that the rationale for this treatment regime is less stressful for the patients, well-accepted, time saving and reducing the risk of inter-appointment infections. Single visit endodontics is considered more productive and less expensive. However, certain questions have been raised regarding validity of single visit endodontics.

i. Is the same outcome achieved using single visit regime *vis-à-vis* multiple visit?
ii. Is the postoperative healing same for single visit endodontics?
iii. Is the failure/sequelae of treatment same with single visit endodontics?
iv. Is the psychological acceptability same in single visit endodontics as for multiple visit endodontics?
v. The commercial aspects should also be considered (can the operator charge same fee in single visit endodontics as in for multiple visits?)

Traditionally, the root canal treatment is performed in multiple visits, using intracanal medicaments along with irrigating solutions to eliminate microorganisms and toxins from the root canal system. The most commonly used and widely accepted intracanal medicament is calcium hydroxide. It is hypothesized that the alkalinity (pH 11–12) of calcium hydroxide will kill the bacteria in the root canal and also dissolve the endotoxins. However, calcium hydroxide is not capable of eliminating all bacteria; may help in bacterial reduction.

Similarly, use of various irrigants and intracanal medicaments could not fully eradicate the microorganisms present in the root canal.

A plenty of surveys have been conducted to analyze the reasons why not to complete root canal treatment in one visit.

The possible reasons are:

- The mechanical irritation of the instrumentation and extrusion of debris may cause postoperative pain and discomfort. However, with the advent of better techniques and gadgets, coupled with experience of the operator, this irritation and extrusion can be minimized, subsequently, the postoperative pain. The fear of this pain warrants the operator to follow multiple-visit protocol.
- Most of the operators feel that chances of failure are much more with single visit root canal treatment. However, it is not true. If the basic parameters are achieved in single visit without disturbing the surrounding periodontium, the success can be

achieved. The simple parameter is whether the cleaning and shaping of the pulpal space can be achieved in one visit without disturbing the periodontium or the operator needs more time for the same. The chances of failure will be minimal if the operator has the confidence of achieving the goal in one visit.

- Many operators make excuse of lack of time in their clinical practice. Usually, the operator does 'access opening' on day one, 'cleaning and shaping' on day two and 'obturation' in third visit. In between, if the patient is not comfortable, 'dressing' can be repeated. The inter-appointment change of dressing only kills bacteria for the time being. It does not necessarily prepare the canal or in any form achieve the objectives. In case the patient has sufficient time, the root canal treatment objectives can be achieved in single visit. Multiple visits might waste more time in adjusting the patient on the chair, isolation, removal of existing temporary filling and irrigation, etc. Single visit treatment makes sense in busy practice to save overall time.
- Another important issue is economical viability. The commercial aspect of any treatment modality is as good as any other factor for the success of the treatment. A few operators believe that in case of single visit modalities, the charges cannot be the same as for multiple visits. However, this notion is purely on assumptions. The charges can be fixed and vary according to the operator and the surroundings. Secondly, one should not underestimate the patients. The patients are willing to pay more if it saves their time.

The concept of single visit root canal treatment is based on the theory of obscure or inhume; which implies that majority of microorganisms are removed during preparing and irrigating the canals and the remaining bacteria get obscured or inhumed in the dentinal tubules after the root canal obturation. Such bacteria do not survive long because of lack of nutrition and spacing. The antimicrobial activities of sealers during obturation and also the zinc of gutta-percha may kill the residual bacteria.

The persistence and reinfection in the root canal can be minimized by either dressing the canal with antimicrobial agents in multiple visits or immediately obturate the canal to reduce the space for bacterial colonization in a single visit protocol. The success of root canal treatment is based on careful case selection. There should be no compromise with the judicious preparation of root canal without injuring the periodontium.

COMPARATIVE CLINICAL FEATURES

The single visit and multiple visit endodontic procedures are compared clinically. The features considered important for the success of the treatment are:

i. ***Endodontic flare-up and pain***: The intraoperative flare-up and postoperative pain are correlated as measure of success and failure with single visit root canal treatment. The mild pain during the treatment procedure, is however, considered normal and has no effect on the final outcome of the treatment. Postoperative pain can be due to over instrumentation, pushing of debris or irritating the periodontium by any means. It is established that there is no significant difference in postoperative pain when single visit is compared with multiple visit root canal treatment (Table 21.1).

ii. ***Postoperative healing***: The postoperative healing is considered as the main feature of success and failure of endodontic treatment. The short- and long-term follow-up of the radiograph is the commonly used technique to evaluate bony pattern/healing. Numerous studies have established and reported no significant difference in healing process between the single and multiple visit treatment protocol (Table 21.1). A few authors opine that the clinical criteria for success should not be dependent only on pain and flare-ups. The clearly defined clinical criteria should be followed in studies comparing single visit and multiple visit endodontic procedures.

iii. ***Elimination of bacteria and bacterial toxins***: The main objective of root canal treatment is to eradicate bacteria and bacterial toxins, so as to provide bacteria free environments for healing. The lipopolysaccharide (LPS) is considered as the most powerful endotoxin capable of having strong toxic effect on periapical tissues. The accumulation of bacterial components in any area along with endotoxins can stimulate the release of pro-inflammatory cytotoxins.

The irrigating solutions have been found to be ineffective against most of the endotoxins; whereas, intracanal medication with calcium hydroxide inactivates the cytotoxic effects of endotoxins. It is established, however, that root canal preparation followed by sodium hypochlorite irrigation render 33% of the root canal bacteria-free in first appointment. An irrigant could attain complete eradication of bacteria; even calcium hydroxide and other intercanal medicaments fail to obtain the total elimination of bacterial organisms.

Table 21.1 Studies on postoperative complications with single-visit endodontic treatment

Authors (year)	*Method (samples)*	*Clinical complications*	*Success rate (healing)*
Rudner and Oliet (1981)	283 cases Single visit: 98 teeth Multiple visits: 185 teeth	No significant difference in the incidence and severity of postoperative pain between the two groups	No significant difference
Mulhern et al (1982)	60 teeth treated by 2 operators Single visit: 30 single-root teeth Multiple visits: 30 single-root teeth Evaluation period: 2 days	No significant difference in the incidence of pain existed between the single and multiple-visit groups	No significant difference
Roane et al (1983)	359 patients Single visit: 250 teeth Multiple visits: 109 teeth	Multiple-visit treatment had a greater incidence of post-operative pain	—
Pekruhn et al (1986)	925 teeth treated by one operator for single-visit treatment Evaluation period: 1 year	No clinical difference	The overall success rate was 95% (the incidence of failure was higher with retreatment and presence of apical periodontitis)
Trope (1991)	226 teeth for single-visit treatment (treated by one operator)	No flare-up in cases without pre-existing symptoms Higher flare-up rate in retreatment cases with pre-existing symptoms	—
Trope et al (1999)	102 teeth with apical periodontitis Single visit: 45 teeth Multiple visits: 57 teeth Evaluation period: 1 year	—	Both groups had a similar success rate
Peters and Wesselink (2002)	39 patients treated by one operator Single visit: 21 teeth Multiple visits: 18 teeth Evaluation period: 4.5 years	No significant difference	No significant difference in success rate between the two groups
DiRenzo et al (2002)	72 molars treated by two operators Single visit: 39 teeth Multiple visits: 33 teeth Evaluation period: 2 days	No difference in postoperative pain between the two groups One patient (1.3%) in the multiple-visit group with pre-existing apical periodontitis experienced flare-up	No significant difference
Field et al (2004)	223 teeth single visit (both anterior and posterior)	No clinical complication	The overall success rate was 89.2%. No significant difference based on sex and age Anterior teeth were more successful than posterior teeth
Kvist et al (2004)	96 teeth with apical periodontitis Single visit: 48 teeth Multiple visits: 48 teeth	—	No significant difference between the two groups
Yoldas et al (2004)	218 retreatment cases Single visit: 106 teeth Multiple visits: 112 teeth Evaluation period: 1 week	Multiple-visit root canal treatment was more effective in completely eliminating pain that was due to single-visit treatment of previously symptomatic teeth	—

(Contd...)

Table 21.1 Studies on postoperative complications with single-visit endodontic treatment (*Contd...*)

Authors (year)	*Method (samples)*	*Clinical complications*	*Success rate (healing)*
Waltimo et al (2005)	50 teeth with apical periodontitis Single visit: 48 teeth Multiple visits: 30 teeth Evaluation period: 52 weeks	No clinical complication	No significant difference in healing between the two groups
Molander et al (2007)	101 teeth Single visit: 53 teeth Multiple visits: 48 teeth Evaluation period: 24 months	No clinical complication	No significant difference in healing between the two groups
Penesis et al (2008)	63 patients Single visit: 33 Multiple visits: 30 Evaluation period: 12 months	No clinical complication	No significant difference in healing between the two groups
Risso et al (2008)	118 molars with necrotic pulp Single visit: 57 teeth Multiple visits: 61 teeth Evaluation period: 10 days	The frequencies of postoperative pain were 10.5% and 23% for the single-visit and multiple-visit group, respectively	—
Kalhoro and Mirza (2009)	100 patients for single-visit treatment Evaluation period: 1 month	No flare-ups in 1 month (safe in both vital and nonvital teeth, and even in teeth with periapical pathosis)	No significant difference
Ince et al (2009)	306 patients treated by two clinicians Single visit: 153 teeth Multiple visits: 153 teeth Evaluation period: 3 days	No significant difference between vital and nonvital teeth	No significant difference between the two groups
Wang et al (2010)	89 treated incisors by two endodontists Single visit: 43 teeth Multiple visits: 46 teeth Evaluation period: 7 days	No significant difference on the incidence and severity of postoperative pain between the two groups	No significant difference
El Mubarak et al (2010)	234 teeth Single visit: 32 teeth Multiple visits: 202 teeth Evaluation period: 1 day	Overall incidence of postoperative pain was 9% after 1 day	No significant difference between the two groups
Prashanth et al (2011)	32 cases Single visit: 16 teeth Multiple visits: 16 teeth Evaluation period: 6 weeks	No significant difference in post-operative pain, or tenderness with either single-visit or multiple-visit therapy	No significant difference in success between the two groups
Paredes-Vieyra and Enriquez (2012)	282 teeth with apical periodontitis Single visit: 146 teeth Multiple visit: 136 teeth Evaluation period: 2 years	No clinical difference	No significant difference in healing between the two groups
Dorasani et al (2013)	64 single root teeth Single visit: 34 teeth Multiple visits: 30 teeth	No clinical difference	No significant differences in healing between the two groups
Akbar et al (2013)	100 molars Single visit: 50 teeth Multiple visit: 50 teeth	No clinical difference	No significant difference in the flare-up rate between two groups

(*Contd...*)

Table 21.1 Studies on postoperative complications with single-visit endodontic treatment (*Contd...*)

Authors (year)	*Method (samples)*	*Clinical complications*	*Success rate (healing)*
Xavier et al (2013)	48 nonvital teeth Single visit: 24 teeth Multiple visits: 24 teeth Evaluation period: 2 weeks	Two visits were more effective than one visit in reducing endotoxins	No difference in eradicating micro-organisms
Bhagwat and Mehta (2013)	60 patients in single-visit treatments Evaluation period: 2 weeks	No difference of pain in vital and nonvital teeth without apical radiolucency. (Teeth with periapical radiolucency exhibited less pain than teeth without periapical radiolucency)	No significant difference
Rao et al (2014)	140 patients in single visit and multiple visit	No difference of postoperative pain	No significant difference

It is argued that single visit root canal treatment is more effective in entombing the bacteria in dentinal tubules, which later die because of lack of nutrition and the overall healing is effected by the immune mechanisms of the individual. A few authors opine, depending upon their studies, that the obturation should be carried out after completely eradicating the bacteria. This feature could not be achieved in one visit treatment because it is not possible to eradicate all infections from root canal without the support of inter-appointment dressing using various medicaments (Fig. 21.1a and b).

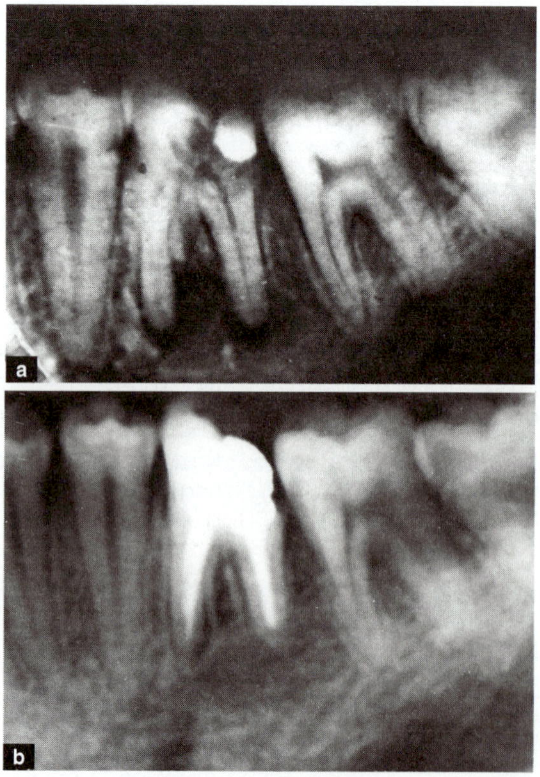

Fig. 21.1 Single visit root canal treatment (mandibular first molar): (a) Preoperative; (b) Postoperative

21

Single visit treatment should be avoided in vital teeth (collagen pulp tissue at the apical constriction area may create problem in later stages).

Indications

- Fractured teeth, especially anteriors, which need immediate restorations
- Apprehensive but cooperative patient
- Physically compromised patients who cannot visit dental office too often
- Uncomplicated nonvital teeth
- Teeth having sinus tract.

Contraindications

- Patients having acute periodontium with severe pain
- Teeth with limited access
- Patients with temporomandibular joint disorders (cannot open the mouth for long)
- Chronic periapical lesions of long-duration
- Teeth with aberrant canal anatomy.

Advantages

- The operator is aware of the intricacies of canal anatomy immediately following preparation. No risk of losing important landmark.
- The canal is always cleaner immediately after preparation. Root canal dressings and medicaments may hamper with the cleanliness.
- The risk of flare-up induced by temporary fillings and inter-appointment period is minimal.
- The risk of fracture of endodontically treated teeth is reduced, since, the final restoration can be placed immediately (most of such teeth fracture during endodontic treatment).
- Patient's preappointment anxiety and post-operative discomfort are limited to one day only.

- Time is saved; both for the patient and the operator.
- The working length remains constant, which might deviate during multiple visits because of change of reference point.
- Minimizes incomplete treatment. Many patients do not turn for final restoration if the pain has subsided and the tooth is functioning reasonably well.
- Esthetically acceptable since, the tooth is restored in the same appointment (especially anterior teeth).

Disadvantages

- Longer working time might be tiring for the patient, especially the older adults and the patients suffering from heart diseases. The longer time may affect temporomandibular joint musculature and increase psychological stress of the patients.
- In case of flare-ups, the removal of filling material might be tedious and time consuming.
- Weeping canals and also difficult/aberrant canal anatomy may require multivisits.
- Operator at the beginning of their career should not follow single visit modality, since experience of not damaging the periodontium is mandatory for successful endodontic treatment.
- Chronic periapical lesions should not be treated in single visit. Even the teeth with chronic periapical lesions, which remained open to environment for long-time, single visit treatment should be avoided.

CRITERIA FOR SINGLE VISIT ENDODONTICS

a. ***Patient cooperation***: Single visit endodontics is not preferred in non-cooperative patients including patient with temporomandibular joint problems, gaggers and limited mouth openings. At least the beginners must not try on these patients.

b. ***Clinical experience***: The clinical competence of the operator is most important in performing root canal treatment in single visit. The operator should know the probable factors which can damage the apical periodontium and ways to minimize the same. Unforeseen errors if encountered during the treatment should be tackled judiciously. This is possible only, if the operator is competent and experienced to handle such errors.

c. ***Easy accessibility***: The single visit root canal treatment can be performed on teeth with easy accessibility. The teeth where access is difficult may need more time, preferably multiple visits to complete the endodontic procedure.

d. ***Clinical symptoms***: The patients with severe pain and tenderness should preferably be treated in multiple visits. Patients with alveolar abscess/swelling should also be treated in multiple visits.

e. ***Vitality of teeth***: Whether vital teeth should be root canal treated in a single visit remained controversial. Majority of authors believe that vital teeth are easy to be treated in single visit; however, a couple of authors claim that the complete pulp extirpation is difficult in apical area, which can later cause problems. Any pulp remnant left at the apical constriction area, which can happen generally in posterior teeth will harbor microorganisms in few weeks leading to failure of root canal treatment. Multiple visits will be preferred so as to completely clean the area of any pulp tissue.

BIBLIOGRAPHY

1. Akbar I, Iqbal A and Al-Omiri MK. Flare-up rate in molars with periapical radiolucency in one-visit vs two-visit endodontic treatment. J. Contemp. Dent. Pract.: 2013; 14:414–418.
2. Al-Rahabi M and Abdulkhayum AM. Single visit root canal treatment: a review. Saudi Endod. J.: 2016; 2:80–84.
3. Amy WY, Zhang C and Chu C. A systematic review of non-surgical single-visit versus multiple-visit endodontic treatment. Clin. Cosm. and Invest. Dent.: 2014; 6:46–55.
4. Ashkenaz PJ. One-visit endodontics. Dent. Clin. North Am.: 1984; 28:853–863.
5. Bhagwat S and Mehta D. Incidence of postoperative pain following single visit endodontics in vital and non-vital teeth: An *in vivo* study. Contemp. Clin. Dent.: 2013; 4:295–302.
6. DiRenzo A, Gresla T, Johnson BR, Rogers M, Tucker D and BeGole EA. Postoperative pain after 1 and 2 visit root canal therapy. Oral Surg., Oral Med., Oral Path. Oral Radiol. Endod.: 2002; 93:605–610.
7. Dorasani G, Madhusudhana K and Chinni SK. Clinical and radiographic evaluation of single-visit and multi-visit endodontic treatment of teeth with periapical pathology: An *in vivo* study. J. Conserv. Dent.: 2013; 16:484–488.
8. El Mubarak AH, Abu-bakr NH and Ibrahim YE. Postoperative pain in multiple-visit and single-visit root canal treatment. J. Endod.: 2010; 36:36–39.
9. Field JW, Gutmann JL, Solomon ES and Rakusin H. A clinical radiographic retrospective assessment of the success rate of single-visit root canal treatment. Int. Endod. J.: 2004; 37:70–82.
10. Figini L, Lodi G, Gorni F and Gagliani M. Single versus multiple visits for endodontic treatment of permanent teeth: a Cochrane systematic review. J. Endod.: 2008; 34:1041–1047.
11. Garcez AS, Nunez SC, Hamblim MR, Suzuki H and Ribeiro MS. Photodynamic therapy associated with conventional endodontic treatment in patient with antibiotic-resistant microflora: a preliminary report. J. Endod.: 2010; 36:1463–1466.
12. Ince B, Ercan E, Dalli, Dulgergil CT, Zorba YO and Colak H. Incidence of postoperative pain after single- and multiple-visit endodontic treatment in teeth with vital and non-vital pulp. Eur. J. Dent.: 2009; 3:273–279.

13. Jorge V, Siqueira JF, Rieneei D, Loghin S, Fernez N and Flores B. One-versus Two-visit endodontic treatment of teeth with apical periodontitis:a histobacteriologic study. J. Endod.: 2012; 38:1040–1052.
14. Kalhoro FA and Mirza AJ. A study of flare-ups following single-visit root canal treatment in endodontic patients. J. Coll. Physic. Surg. Pak.: 2009; 19:410–412.
15. Kenrick S. Endodontics: a multiple-visit or single-visit approach. Aust. Endod.: J.: 2000; 26:82–85.
16. Kvist T, Molander A, Dahlen G and Reit C. Microbiological evaluation of one- and two-visit endodotic treatment of teeth with apical periodontitis: a randomized, clinical trial. J. Endod.: 2004; 30:572–576.
17. Mohammadi Z, Farhad A and Tabrizizadeh M. One-visit versus multiple-visit endodontic therapy—a review. Int. Dent. J.: 2006; 56:289–293.
18. Molander A, Warfvinge J, Reit C and Kvist T. Clinical and radiographic evaluation of one- and two-visit endodontic treatment of asymptomatic necrotic teeth with apical periodontitis: a randomized clinical trial. J. Endod.: 2007; 33:1145–1148.
19. Mulhern JM, Patterson SS, Newton CW and Ringel AM. Incidence of postoperative pain after one-appointment endodontic treatment of asymptomatic pulpal necross in single-rooted teeth. J. Endod.: 1982; 8:370–375.
20. Paredes-Vieyra J and Enriquez FJ. Success rate of single-versus two-visit root canal treatment of teeth with apical peridontitis: a randomized controlled trial. J. Endod.: 2012; 38:1164–1169.
21. Pekruhn RB. Single-visit therapy: a preliminary clinical study. J. Am. Dent. Assoc.: 1981; 103:875–877.
22. Pekruhn RB. The incidence of failure following single-visit endodontic therapy. J. Endod.: 1986; 12:68–72.
23. Penesis VA, Fitzgerald PI, Fayad MI, Wenckus CS, BeGole EA and Johnson BR. Outcome of one-visit and two-visit endodontic treatment of necrotic teeth with apical periodontitis: a randomized controlled trial with one-year evaluation. J. Endod.: 2008; 34:251–257.
24. Peters LB and Wesselink PR. Periapical healing of endodontically treated teeth in one and two visits obturated in the presence or absence of detectable microorganisms. Int. Endod. J.: 2002; 35:660–667.
25. Prashanth MB, Tavane PN, Abraham S and Chacko L. Comparative evaluation of pain, tenderness and swelling followed by radiographic evaluation of periapical changes at various intervals of time following single and multiple visit endodontic therapy: as *in vivo* study. J. Contemp. Dent. Pract.: 2011; 12:187–191.
26. Raveenthiraraja T and Solete P. Flare up in endodontics: A review. Int. J. Pharma. Clin. Res.: 2015; 1–7.
27. Roane JB, Dryden JA and Grimes EW. Incidence of post-operative pain after single- and multiple-visit endodontic procedures. Oral Surg., Oral Med., Oral Path.: 1983; 55:68–72.
28. Sathorn C, Parashos P and Messer HH. Effectiveness of single-versus multiple- visit endodontic treatment of teeth with apical periodontitis: a systematic review and meta-analysis. Int. Endod. J.: 2005; 38:347–355.
29. Siqueira JF and Rocas IN. Optimising single-visit disinfection with supplementary approaches: a quest for predictability. Aust. Endod. J.: 2011; 37:92–98.
30. Spangberg L. Evidence-based endodontics: The one-visit treatment idea. Oral Surg., Oral Med., Oral Path., Oral Radiol. Endod.: 2001; 91:617–618.
31. Trope M and Bergenholtz G. Microbiological basis for endodontic treatment : can a maximal outcome be achieved in one visit? Endod. Topics: 2002; 1:40–60.
32. Trope M, Delano EO and Orstavik D. Endodontic treatment of teeth with apical periodontitis: single vs multivisit treatment. J. Endod.: 1999; 25:345–350.
33. Trope M. Flare-up rate of single-visit endodontics. Int. Endod. J.: 1991; 24:24–26.
34. Vera J, Siqueira J, Ricucci D, Loghin S, Fernandez N, Flores B and Cruz AG. One-versus two-visit endodontic treatment of teeth with apical periodontitis: a histobacteriologic study. J. Endod.: 2012; 1–13.
35. Waltimo T, Trope M, Haapasalo M and Orstavik D. Clinical efficacy of treatment procedures in endodontic infection control and one year follow-up of periapical healing. J. Endod.: 2005; 31:863–866.
36. Wang C, Xu P, Ren L, Dong G and Ye. Comparison of post-obturation pain experience following one-visit and two-visit root canal treatment on teeth with vital pulps: a randomized controlled trial. Int. Endod. J.: 2010; 43:692–697.
37. Xavier AC, Martinho FC and Chung A. One-visit versus two-visit root canal treatement: effectiveness in the removal of endotoxins and cultivable bacteria. J. Endod.: 2013; 39: 959–964.
38. Yilmaz Z, Ozdemir HO and Gorduysus O. Evaluation of single and multiple visit root canal therapy: a randomized clinical cases. Clin. Dent. Res.: 2012; 36:59–63.
39. Yoldas O, Topuz A, Isci AS and Oztune, H. Postoperative pain after endodontic retreatment: single-versus two-visit retreatment. Oral Surg., Oral Med., Oral Path., Oral Radiol. Endod.: 2004; 98:483–487.

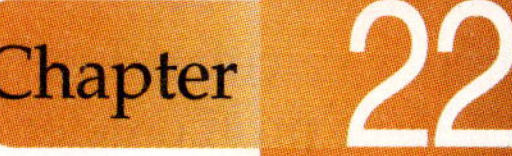

Postendodontic Restorations

The endodontically treated teeth usually undergo a considerable loss of tooth structure because of caries, iatrogenic loss and also the access cavity preparation. The fracture resistance of these teeth is also affected by the amount of substance loss.

The restoration of endodontically treated tooth involves replacement of missing tooth structure along with protection of the remaining tooth. The remaining tooth structure is important in planning and executing the restoration of endodontically treated teeth. The factors, which should be considered by the operator are; the strategic position of the tooth in the arch, the occlusal load, which the tooth will be bearing, overall occlusal pattern and also the oral hygiene of the patient. To replace the missing tooth structure, the operator should decide whether the retention is to be achieved through root canals or the remaining tooth structure. Achieving adequate retention and resistance features for final restoration is always challenging. Over the years, various materials and techniques have been developed to ensure retention, resistance and esthetics of postendodontic restorations.

Effect of root canal treatment on the tooth

After the root canal treatment, the tooth exhibits certain morphological and physical changes, such as:

i. *Loss of tooth structure*: The tooth structure might have been lost prior to the treatment because of caries and fracture, etc. The endodontic procedures, such as access cavity preparation or involuntary cutting during negotiating root canals also lead to loss of tooth structure. The bulk of remaining dentin is important since, the strength of tooth is proportional to it. As the bulk of dentin is decreased, the stiffness of the tooth is decreased. It is established that even the conservative access cavity preparation decreases the stiffness of the tooth by 5%; whereas, in class II preparation there is 40% loss of stiffness and in mesio-occluso-distal preparation, the loss of stiffness is 60%.

ii. *Physical changes*: It is believed that root canal treatment leads to dehydration, consequently weakening the tooth. A few authors, however, do not favour this notion, claiming that dentin hardness is not altered after endodontic treatment. The loss of moisture content from the dentin may lead to loss of translucency of the tooth.

iii. *Altered appearance*: The root canal treated tooth may show altered appearance because of presence of residual pulp remnants and even medicaments. The chemically altered dentin reflects light differently, which modifies the overall appearance of tooth.

iv. *Proprioception*: Sense of proprioception is lost in root canal treated teeth. Neurosensory feedback mechanism is impaired because of loss of pulpal tissues. Decrease in mechanoreceptive feature may lead to inadvertent biting on nonvital teeth, subsequently fracture of the tooth.

Postendodontic changes

- 10% reduction of collagen bonded water
- Aging of collagen (changes in cross-linking)

Not much change in

- Modulus of elasticity (young modulus)
- Dentin hardness
- Fracture resistance

PLANNING POSTENDODONTIC RESTORATIONS

The restoration of endodontically treated teeth is planned following the guidelines as:

- The root canal treatment should be of good quality. Only clinical asymptomatic feature will not be sufficient. Radiological assessment is mandatory; however, computer aided radiography is preferred in evaluating the quality of obturation.

- The common notion that endodontically treated teeth fracture easily because of increased brittleness may not be correct; the amount of remaining tooth structure controls the fracture resistance of the tooth. The operator should take extra care so that the loss of tooth structure during root canal preparation and tooth preparation, be minimized. The root canal treated tooth with sufficient amount of dentin can be restored without the need of extra retentive devices.
- The reinforcement of remaining tooth structure with bonded materials can also be planned. The long-term validity of this reinforcement with time is questionable; however, the treatment is effective in teeth with less surface area remaining (e.g. premolars).
- The operator should analyze all factors before placing post, especially in the posterior teeth. The post in posterior teeth is avoided as far as possible. The post is placed only to retain core. A few authors are of the view that the post and core should be of the same material. It minimizes the vertical stresses and is also time saving.
- Length of the postdepends on the configuration of the core required and the length of the root. The amount of stresses, which destabilize the restorations, should also be considered.
- The removal of gutta-percha always disturbs the apical seal. Early or delayed removal of gutta-percha might not be significant in disturbing the apical seal; however, early removal is preferred. Quick removal of gutta-percha at the predetermined length with heated instruments is considered a better method.

SELECTION OF RESTORATION FOR ENDODONTICALLY TREATED TEETH

The primary aim of postendodontic restoration is to protect the remaining tooth tissue, maintaining the occlusal function and esthetics of the replaced tooth tissue. The amount of remaining tooth structure before and after tooth preparation is important for the long-term success/failure of the restoration. The remaining coronal tooth structure after tooth preparation must be analyzed thoroughly and recorded. Prior to restoration of these teeth, a decision is to be taken whether the support from root is required or not.

Aims of postendodontic restorations
- Replacement of missing tooth structure
- Protection of remaining tooth structure
- Maintenance of occlusal functions
- Esthetics

The salient features of this record are:

i. The remaining dentin volume is calculated either by scanning the cast using a laser profilometer or weighing the remaining die stone and calculating the equivalent dentin volume.
ii. Since, the volume of remaining dentin may not reflect the strategic contribution of dentin, it became apparent that an index assessing the remaining dentin would be useful.

Tooth Restorability Index (TRI)

Tooth Restorability Index (TRI) was developed to provide a structured assessment using defined parameters to evaluate remaining coronal tissue (Fig. 22.1).

- The tooth is divided into six equal sextants: 2 proximal, 2 buccal and 2 lingual areas.
- TRI allowed scores of 0–3 in each tooth sextant with a maximum score of 18 per tooth.
- The contribution of each tooth sextant (remaining dentin) to retention and resistance form can be recorded following the score.
- Experienced clinicians (three or more) can evaluate the casts regarding the remaining dentin.

A scoring system of 0–3 was allocated to each section.

'0'—None: Throughout two-thirds or more of the tooth sextant under consideration; there is no axial wall of dentin (i.e. a box or missing cusp) or any dentin present above the finishing line is so lacking in height that may not be able to contribute to retention and resistance form. The score is appropriate where a margin is visible just apical to the limit of a missing wall, but there is only a small bevel or chamfer comprising the preparation dentin.

'1'—Inadequate: Coronal dentin is present in the tooth sextant but in terms of thickness, height or configuration

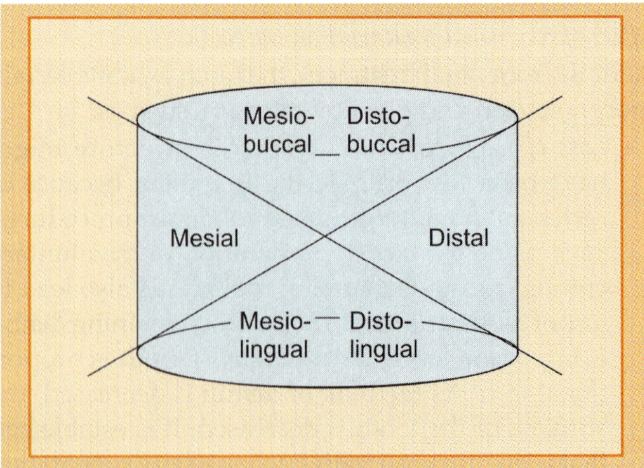

Fig. 22.1 Tooth restorability index (TRI): Scoring sextants (diagrammatic)

(e.g. an undercut) that is insufficient to make any predictable contribution to retention and resistance form as opined by the operator. Dentin walls less than 1.5 mm thick or more than twice as high as their thinnest part would be included in this category.

'2'—Questionable: More dentin is present than in '1', but clinically, it will not make predictable contribution to retention and resistance. This score should only be assigned where the operator finds it difficult to determine whether a score of '1' or '3' is more appropriate.

'3'—Adequate: There is sufficient coronal dentin in terms of height, thickness and the operator is confident that the distribution of forces would provide the requisite resistance and retention form to the final restoration.

Although tooth restorability index helps deciding the type of restoration for endodontically treated teeth, there is no definite consensus regarding the choice of the final restoration. The brittle nature of endodontically treated teeth and also the lack of moisture in these teeth have been disproved. It is established that the thickness of the residual dentinal walls and cusps are the key factors. As cavity size increases and the marginal ridges are lost, the structure durability decreases. For this reason only the full coverage crowns are preferred in such teeth (Fig. 22.2a and b); otherwise, if the structural durability is sufficient, alternatives such as covering functional cusps (Fig. 22.3), bonded restorations (Fig. 22.4) and pinlays can be planned. Composite crowns, which need less tooth reduction, are also used these days. Cusp covering with indirect composite restorations is also effective.

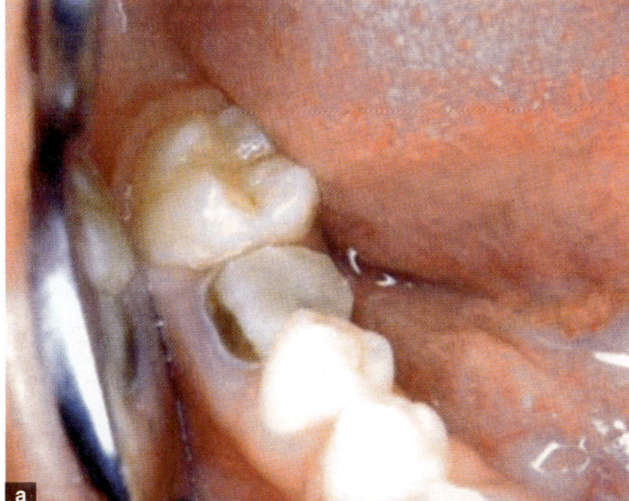

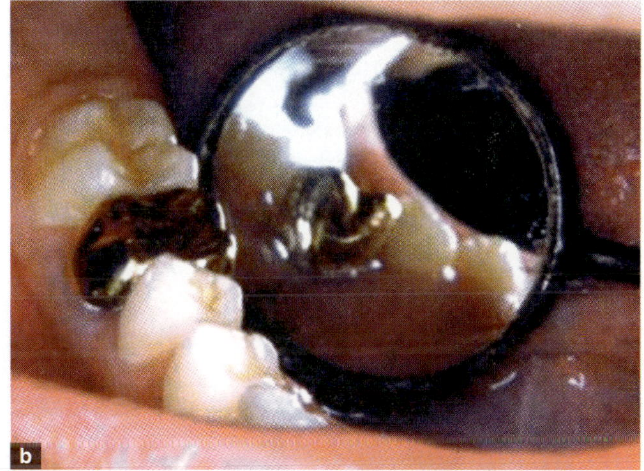

Fig. 22.2 Full veneer crown

Key features in decision-making
- Consider structural durability and esthetics
- Amount of available dentin thickness after removing caries, restorative materials, etc.
- The remaining tooth structure's ability to retain the core
- For full coverage crowns, make balance between esthetics and occlusal load
- Patient's consent before finalizing the restoration

A classification is proposed, which guides the choice of restoration in endodontically treated teeth (Flowchart 22.1)

Type I: More than half the tooth structure is present (Fig. 22.5a)

Type II: Less than half the tooth structure present (Fig. 22.5b)

Type III: Coronal tooth structure absent or minimum (Fig. 22.5c)

Type IV: Root embedded (Fig. 22.5d)

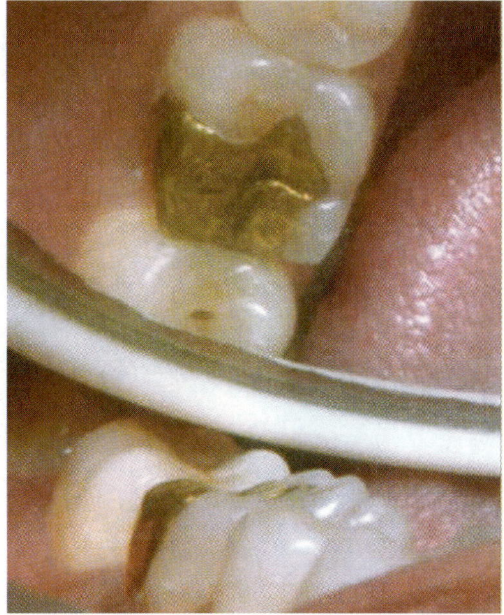

Fig. 22.3 Covering functional cusps with cast metal

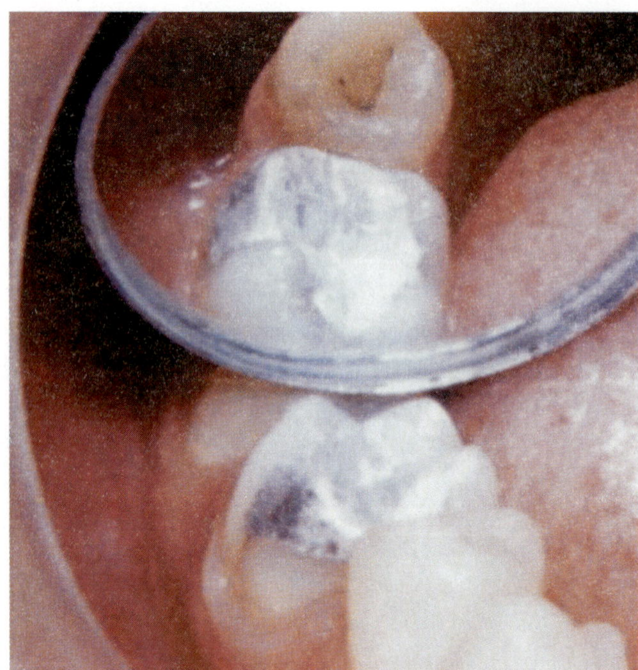

Fig. 22.4 Bonded restoration

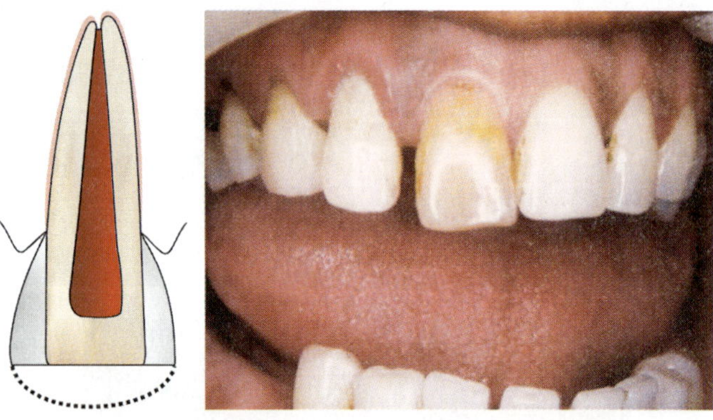

Fig. 22.5a More than half the tooth structure present

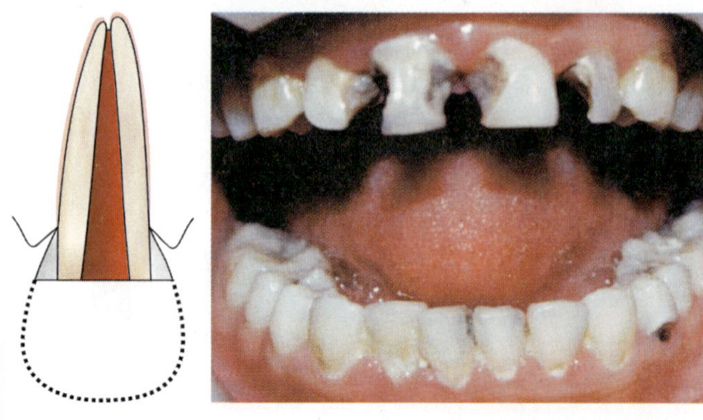

Fig. 22.5b Less than half the tooth structure present

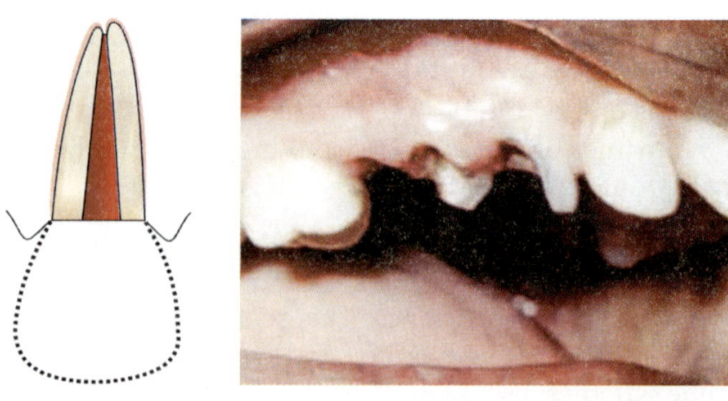

Fig. 22.5c Coronal tooth structure absent or minimum

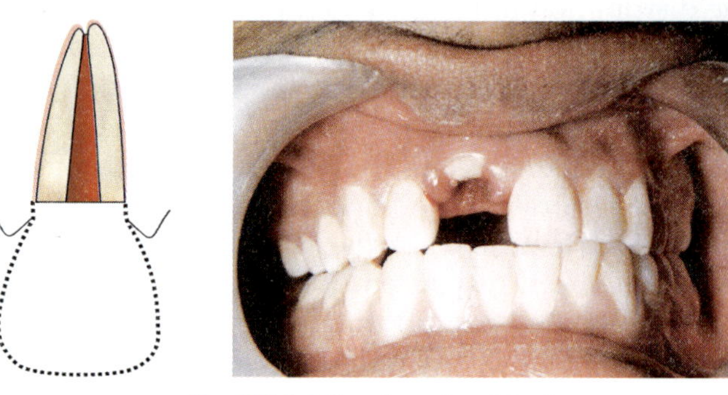

Fig. 22.5d Root embedded

Flowchart 22.2 depicts protocol of selecting restoration for endodontically treated teeth.

The selection of post-core restoration or only coronal filling depends upon the remaining walls (tooth is considered to have five walls; buccal, lingual, mesial, distal and occlusal).

The tooth to receive restoration should be evaluated thoroughly before initiating restorative procedures. The features evaluated are:

a. *Endodontic*: The tooth should be asymptomatic; properly root canal treated and filled with appropriate coronal restorative material. Partially filled root canals, may and may not be symptom-free, should not be restored with permanent restorations (Fig. 22.6a and b).
b. *Periodontal*: The tooth should be stable in the arch and also able to withstand masticatory/functional forces. The crown-root ratio should be favorable (Fig. 22.7a and b).
c. *Restorative*: The position of the tooth in the arch and also the strategic value should be evaluated before initiating definitive restoration (Fig. 22.8a and b).

Flowchart 22.1: Classification guiding the choice of restoration

Root canal treated teeth

Type I (total or more than half tooth structure remaining)
- Restore only access cavity
- Internal bleaching, if need be
- Full crown for esthetics
- Full crown for function

Type II (less than half tooth structure remaining)
- Bonded restorations
- Amalgam/composite core and full crown
- Onlays, covering weakened or functional cusps
- Post, if remaining tooth structure is weak

Type III (coronal portion missing or bare minimum)
- Post and core followed by full crown

Type IV (embedded roots)
- Crown lengthening or orthodontic extrusion
- Post-core followed by full crown

Flowchart 22.2: Protocol of selecting restoration for endodontically treated teeth

Condition of remaining walls	*Photo representation*		*Treatment option*
One wall missing (only access cavity)	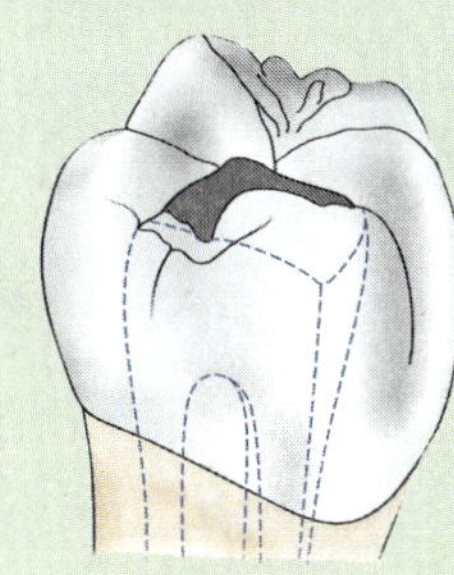	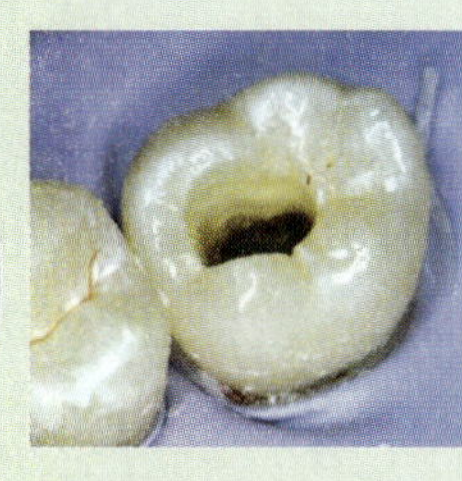	• Fill access cavity/missing wall • No need of post
Two walls missing	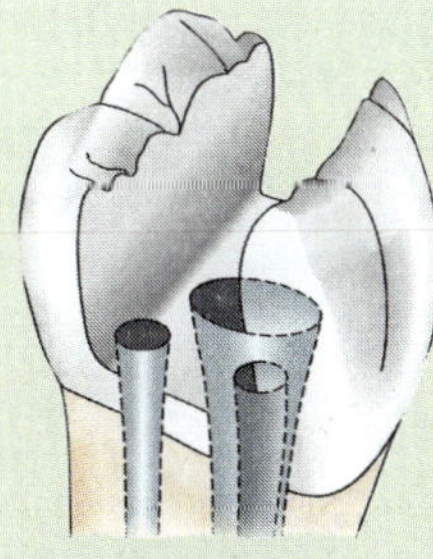	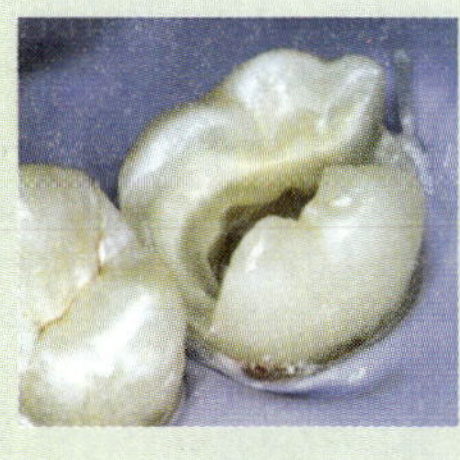	• Fill the coronal cavity/core preparation • Full crown coverage
Three walls missing	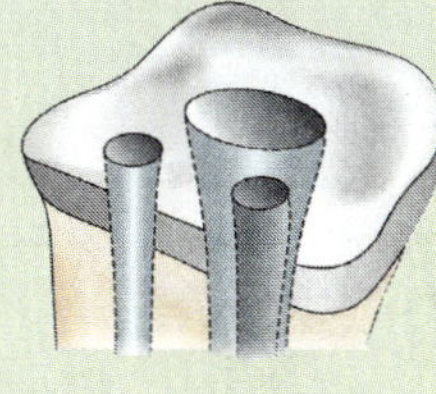	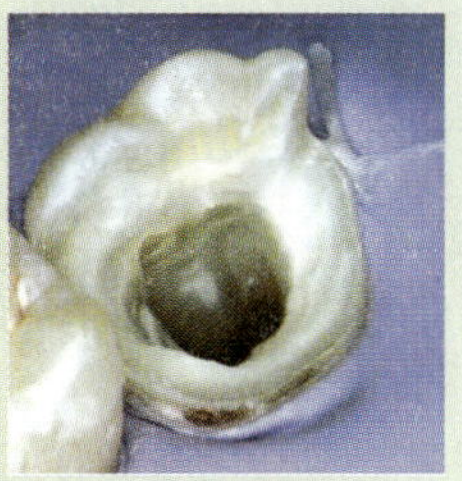	• Need of post • Select post followed by coronal coverage
Four walls missing	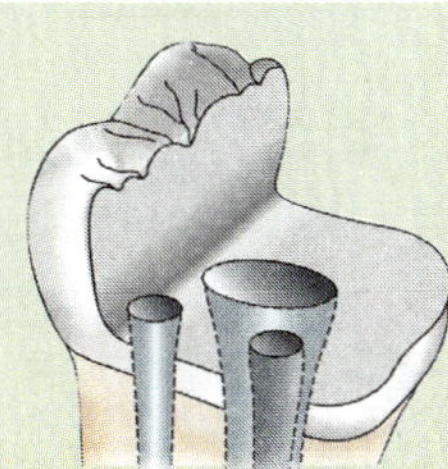	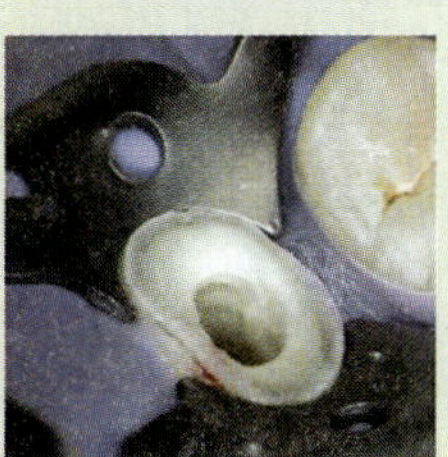	• Need of post • Crown lengthening/orthodontic extrusion may require • Final coronal coverage

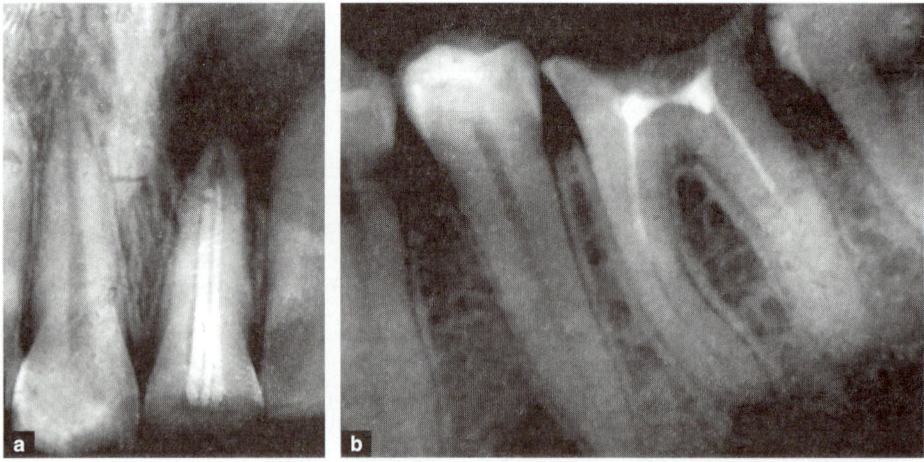

Fig. 22.6 Endodontic evaluation: (a) Faulty obturation; (b) Incomplete obturation

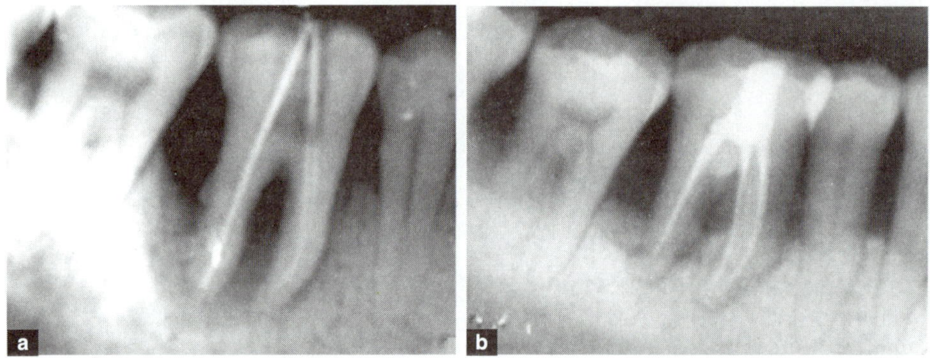

Fig. 22.7 Periodontal evaluation: (a) Insufficient bone support; (b) Insufficient crown-root ratio

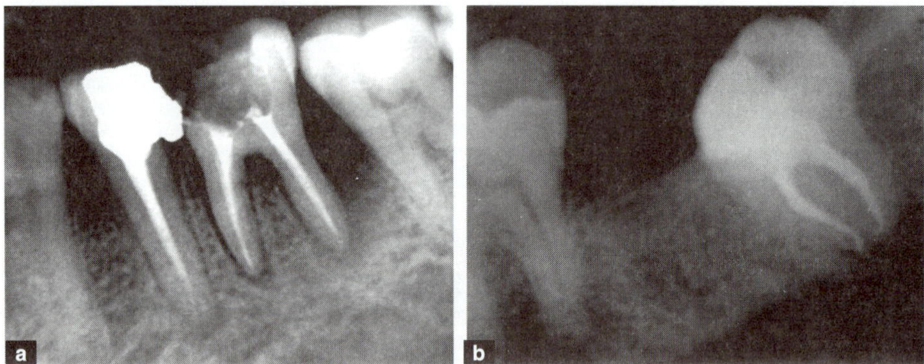

Fig. 22.8 Restorative evaluation: (a) Poor coronal restoration; (b) Position of tooth in the arch

POSTCORE RESTORATIONS

The substitution of the crown portion, with or without the help of pins, is referred to as 'core'. The root canal support of the core, may be metallic or of any other material, is referred to as 'post' or 'dowel'. Collectively the system is known as 'post and core' or 'postcore' system. The resistance and retention form is preferably achieved from the core only, without the root canal support. In case the post/dowel is mandatory, the root(s) should be thoroughly assessed before initiating the postpreparation.

The root/root canal should be assessed for following features:

- Remaining coronal/incisal tooth structure present along the root
- Quantum of occlusal load, which the restored tooth will be bearing
- Configuration of the root canal
- Thickness of dentin around the root canal

- Amount of dentin, which can be utilized in preparation of post
- Number of root canal(s) required for postplacement
- Caries/resorption inside the root, if any
- Periodontal (bony) support of the root
- Possibility of extra retentive devices, if any
- Sufficient length of the post, which can be achieved from the root canal.

Functions of Post

The post serves the following functions:

- It retains core, which helps in reinforcement of the lost tooth structure.
- It resists the tensile forces, which tend to pull the restoration away from the tooth.
- It distributes occlusal forces along the length of the roots to the periodontium (crowns of endodontically treated teeth are usually damaged to an extent that the remaining tooth structure cannot distribute the forces along the natural ways).
- It maintains the marginal integrity of the final restoration by providing sufficient rigidity at the margins; prevents breakdown of cement medium at the tooth-restoration interface.

Classification of Posts

The posts are classified as:

Class I: Self-retentive metal posts (post with self-cutting threads or different types of screws)

Class II: Metal posts with passive retention (no direct contact between the post and the root canal wall. The post needs luting cement for the space present between post and the root canal wall).

Class III: Non-metal posts with passive retention (fiber reinforced posts and ceramic posts along with adhesive cement).

Class IV: Biological posts (dentin posts along with adhesive cement).

The fiber posts have also been categorized as 'generation', based on radiopacity and their esthetic appearance. The categorized generations are:

1. Generation I (neither radiopaque nor esthetic) *(Mid 1980s)*
   - Composipost
   - C-post
2. Generation II (esthetic but not radiopaque) *(Mid 1990s)*
   - Esthetic-plus
   - Light-post
   - Fiber white
   - FiberKor
   - Lucent anchor
3. Generation III (Esthetics and radiopaque) *(2001 onwards)*
   - DT light post
   - DT light postillusion
   - Snow light (snow post)
   - Rely-X post
   - FRC postec plus.

Types of Posts

I. Metal posts
  A. Custom cast metal posts
  B. Prefabricated metal posts
    a. Passive posts
      i. Tapered
        - Smooth
        - Serrated
      ii. Parallel
        - Smooth
        - Serrated
    b. Active posts
      i. Tapered
        - Self-threaded
      ii. Parallel
        - Self-threaded

II. Fiber posts
  A. Custom fiber post
  B. Prefabricated fiber posts
    a. Carbon fibers
      i. Mirafit carbon
      ii. Endopost
      iii. Carbonite system
      iv. CF-post
    b. Silica fibers
      i. Quartz fibers
        - Aesthetic-post
        - Aesthetic-plus
        - Style-post
        - Light/light DT post
      ii. Glass fibers
        - Snow post
        - Mirafit white
        - Lucent anchor
        - FiberKor post
        - Fiber white parapost
    c. Polyethylene fibers
      - Ribbond/Ribbond THM
      - Construct
    d. Fiber post with gutta-percha
      - Fiberfill post system

III. All-ceramic posts

IV. Dentin posts (biological post)
V. Miscellaneous post systems
   a. Two piece custom post (split cast metal post and core)
   b. Post-inlay system
VI. Intraradicular rehabilitation with light transmitting plastic posts.

I. METAL POSTS

Metal posts can be custom cast and are also available as prefabricated metal posts.

A. Custom Cast Metal Posts

Custom cast metal posts are fabricated from a negative reproduction of the prepared root canal. The impression is made of the prepared postspace, using wax or cold cure resins; referred to as 'pattern'. The pattern is invested and the cast is prepared using an appropriate alloy. Type III and Type IV gold alloys are preferred alloys; however, the base metals and titanium alloys are also being used. The custom cast posts conform to the configuration of the prepared canal. The custom cast metal posts are preferred in single rooted teeth.

Indications

- Teeth with elliptical/flared canals
- Teeth where alignment of the proposed crown is significantly different from the inclination of the canal (mostly in anterior teeth)
- Availability of adequate space for bulk of the build-up material around the post
- When multiple teeth require posts, it is advisable to make an impression and fabricate the post in laboratory rather to build in clinic.

Advantages

- Conform to the root canal configuration (usually tapering)
- Strong
- Core is an inherent part of post (provide stability)
- Core can be fabricated at different angle, if need be
- More effective in single rooted teeth
- Do not induce any stress during installation.

Disadvantages

- May act as wedge during load transfer
- Venting is required during cementation
- Taper posts are less retentive than parallel posts
- Difficulty in retrieval during retreatment
- Rigidity may lead to fracture of root
- Certain metals may corrode (long-term failure).

22

B. Prefabricated Metal Posts

The different shapes and sizes of the post is prefabricated and designed to fit in a prepared canal space. This differs from the custom cast post; the canal is prepared according to the prefabricated post. The resulting fit may or may not be exact; however, clinically acceptable post can be selected.

The prefabricated posts are made of metal (usually steel and titanium) or plastic (plastic prefabricated posts are described in subsequent pages). The posts are available in tapered and parallel configuration. Further, the shapes can be smooth or serrated; the serrated ones offer better retention.

Advantages

- Easy manipulation
- Less time consuming
- Easy retrieval (passive post) as compared to custom metal posts
- Better retention; especially serrated, parallel posts
- Cost-effective.

Disadvantages

- Rigidity may lead to root fracture
- Active posts are difficult to remove
- Alloy may corrode (long-term failure)
- Not feasible in tortuous canals
- Extra removal of dentin may be required to adjust the size of post in the canal.

Prefabricated posts are mainly of two types:

a. Passive Posts

The passive posts drive retention from their close proximity to the dentin walls; mostly by adherence of the cementing medium. The types of passive posts are:

i. *Tapered posts*

The taper designs usually simulate the root canal configuration, thereby lessening the chance of a lateral perforation. Tapered posts exhibit least stresses during cementation; however, they may create a wedging effect inside the root.

The currently available tapered posts exhibit taper ranging from 1.1 to 6.2°. The tapered posts are selected according to the size of the reamer or file last used for the preparation of the canal.

The size at the apex is usually 1.0, 1.2, 1.3 and 1.6 mm and correspondingly the diameter is increased coronally. Two diameters (numbers) are indicated in one size; the diameters at the tip and second 10.0 mm from the tip.

The different tapers and sizes are available, suitable for different root canal configurations. The commonly available tapered passive (smooth sided) posts are Kerr endopost and Mooser post. These are the least retentive of all post designs.

ii. *Parallel posts*

The posts may have a serrated or smooth surface. Smaller diameter of such posts are also used as accessory retentive devices (as accessory pin into coronal dentin of root trunk). It is also necessary to evaluate the dentin available for placing the pin, if required. If there is insufficient available dentin, key-ways can be prepared around the post. The parapost (serrated parallel post) is manufactured with a groove running its entire length, which acts as a cement vent.

The post should be large enough to accommodate as far the coronal portion of the canal as possible, but must leave an adequate thickness of dentin at the apical end.

The parallel posts provide greater retention and create less stress than tapered posts, e.g. Whaledent parapost, the Boston post and the Parkell parallel post. A modified design of parallel-sided post with tapered apical end is also available (Schanker's design).

Parallel post	*Tapered post*
• More retentive	• Less retentive
• Create less stresses	• Creates more stresses
• No wedging effect	• Creates wedging effect
• Need of extraremoval of dentin	• No need of extraremoval of dentin
• Chances of perforation of dentinal apical end	• Wedging may lead to root fracture; no chance of dentin perforation

- *Whaledent parapost system*: This post system provides the most equitable distribution of masticatory forces. It has three designs; viz. parapost, parapost plus and unity post system. All are passive, parallel and vented (Fig. 22.9a to d).
  These are made of either stainless steel or titanium. The vertical channels on the parapost, spiral flutes and/or grooves on parapost plus and a raised diamond pattern on unity posts provide extra retention when used with luting cements.
- *Boston post system*: The Boston post resembles a parapost without the vertical venting channel. It is made of titanium with horizontal non-engaging serrations. These are also available with deeper grooves and rough surfaces.
- *Parkell parallel post system*: This is a passive, vented, serrated post with an antirotational lock that fits into the prepared root canal space.
- *Parallel post with tapered apical ends*: These posts were designed to provide better retention achieved by parallel posts (coronal half) along with tapered post conforming to the tapered apical half of the canal. It is of two types:
  - Degussa: The straight and tapered portions are generally of equal lengths and are smooth.
  - Unitek BCH system: Fine serrations are provided along parallel sides of the post and a smooth apical taper of 2.0 mm.
- *Integra-post system*: The integra-post system is made of the titanium alloy. It is biocompatible, corrosion resistant and stiff as well. The parallel passive design conserves tooth structure and minimizes stress. The mid-flange design of the post-effectively control stresses in the canal.

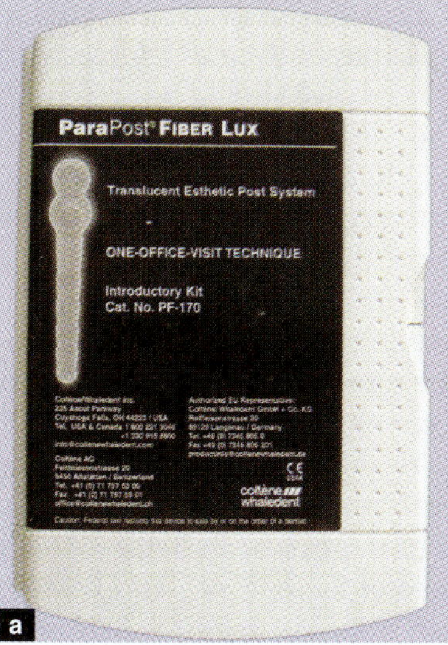

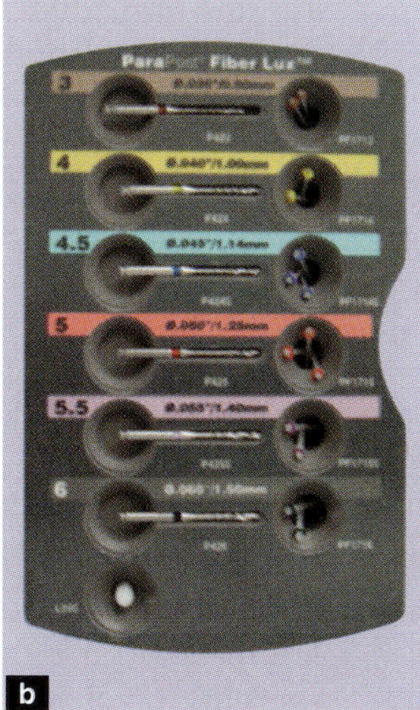

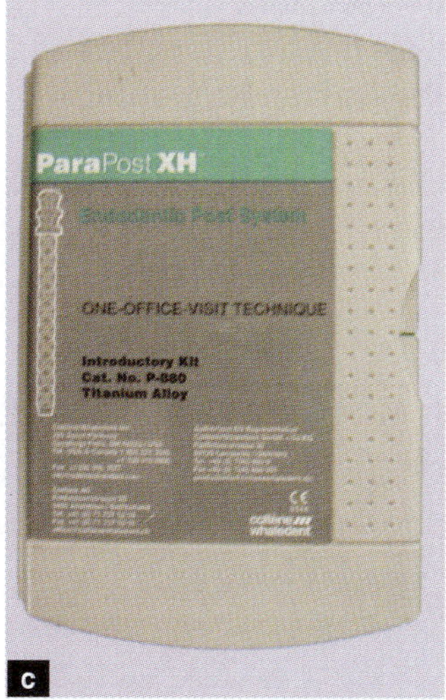

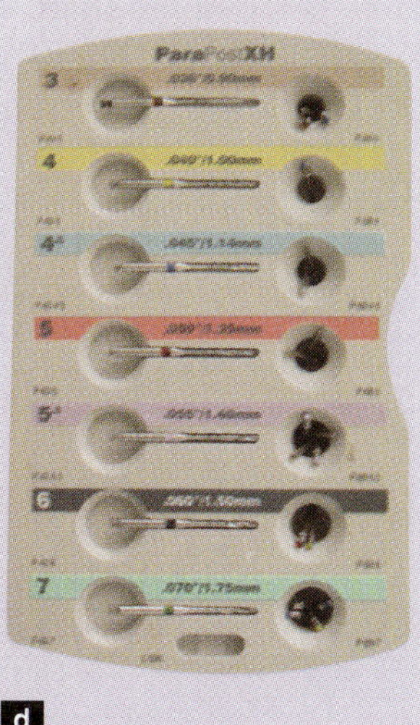

Fig. 22.9 (a) Parapost (outer); (b) Parapost (inner); (c) Parapost XH (outer); (d) Parapost XH (inner)

b. Active Posts

The active posts depend primarily on engaging the dentin directly. The threads on the post either screw into the dentin, or fit into threaded channels (prepared in the dentin) and 'tapped' like a bolt. These are more retentive than passive cemented posts. The self-threading posts produce the greatest stresses when installed in the root dentin. These posts act as a wedge and may induce fracture lines into the dentin. The types of active posts are:

i. *Tapered self-threaded*

The tapered self-threaded posts are available in different sizes, diameter and lengths. The overall taper varies from 3.0 to 30° (taper for the tip is 1.0 to 3.0°). It is frequently used on teeth having minimum of coronal tooth structure and multiple divergent canals (e.g. Dentatus screw posts) (Fig. 22.10).

The threads cut into dentin by 0.1–0.2 mm. The channel to receive the post is prepared by a drill sized 0.1 mm larger than the diameter of the shaft of the post. The blades (threads) extend beyond the shaft by 0.2 mm and engage into dentin. The retention is reinforced by cementing the post using any dual-cure resin cement.

ii. *Parallel self-threaded*

The parallel self-threaded posts are more retentive than tapered posts (offer maximum retention).

These posts produce stresses in the root, both at the apical end and coronal half of the root. It is recommended to 'back off' or reverse the post by half turn to minimize the stresses when slight resistance to threading is felt.

These posts are of three types. The first two have sharp threads and are vented to reduce hydraulic stress during cementation. They differ only in their length of threads along the shaft. The types are:

- *V-lock posts*: These posts have 'microthreads', extending 0.5 mm from the shaft and continue to the full length. V-lock posts are supplied with precise drills that prepare a parallel walled canal just slightly larger than the shaft. The post is inserted along with luting cement. V-lock posts are less retentive, comparable to passive paraposts.
- *Radix-anchor system*: It differs from V-lock posts by the quality of threads (sharp threads extend only partly down the shaft). It is vertically vented and fits along the root surface. Luting cements are utilized for the placement of post.
- *Post with pretapped channels*: These posts employ threads on their sides for retention and are inserted into the canal whose walls are prethreaded with a specially designed instrument. The luting cement is utilized for placement of posts in the root. These are two to three times more retentive than parallel-serrated posts. These posts are parallel in design with no vertical vent. They have rounded, high frequency threads that fit into counter threads 'tapped' into the dentin with a manual thread cutter. The *disadvantage* with this type of system is that there is a potential for root fracture because of inherent stresses.

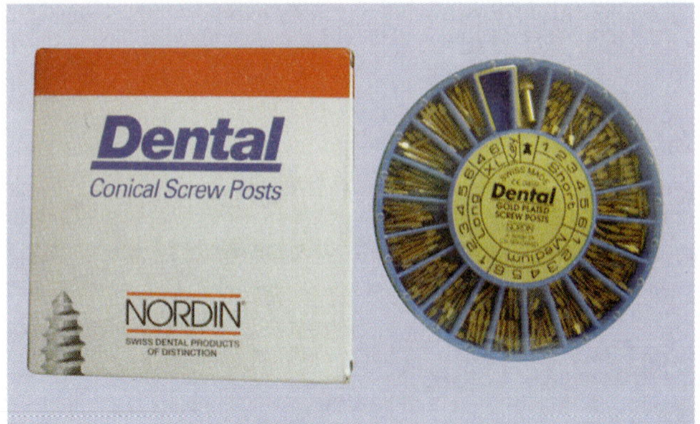

Fig. 22.10 Active screw post

Factors affecting Selection of Posts

The factors guiding selection of posts are:

a. *Root canal configuration*: Wider root canals are best suited for postpreparation, e.g. distal root canals of mandibular molars and palatal root canals of maxillary molars. However, additional retention (reinforcing post) can be achieved from adjacent smaller canals.
b. *Root canal morphology*: The shape of the prepared root canal affect post selection. The narrow root canals, especially in the apical third (mandibular incisors) are not indicative of parallel posts. The requisite dentin around the post may not be available with these root canals. A tapered post should be preferred. When the outline of the canal is oval, it is difficult to prepare a circular post channel to receive a parallel post. In such cases, a metal custom post is fabricated according to the shape of the canal.
c. *Remaining coronal tooth structure*: The 'thumb rule' says, when more than half the crown structure is lost, post and core should be considered. The use of a post should be considered for anterior teeth when one or both proximal walls are missing and for posterior teeth when two adjacent proximal walls are missing.
d. *Occlusal forces*: The occlusal forces on individual tooth are influenced by various factors, viz. tooth type, presence or absence of adjacent teeth, function of tooth in the arch and oral habits of the patient.

Factors affecting Post Retention

The factors affecting retention of post are:

1. Post Length

The accepted principle regarding the post length is '*more the length, more the retention*'. It is established that increase in length increases retention (3.0 mm increase in post length enhances 40% of the retention). The practical limitations, however, restrict the clinician to remain in the space properly surrounded by dentin. The length of the post can be increased as far as possible, provided the post all around its length, should be encircled by a minimum of 1.0 mm of dentin (Fig. 22.11).

The remaining gutta-percha length at the apical end should be 3.0–7.0 mm, depending upon the length of root. During removal of gutta-percha, as the apex is approached, the possibility of dislodging the root canal filling increases. The probability of uncovering the unfilled accessory/lateral canal increase, which may lead to reinfection. Above all, the requisite 1.0 mm of dentin may not be available at the apical end.

It is generally accepted that the length of post should be more than the crown, preferably one and a half-time the length of the crown. The post can be kept half-way between alveolar crest and root apex. Shorter posts besides being less retentive, may lead to fracture of root. If the end of the post is at or above the alveolar crest of bone, the part of the root investing the post uncovered by bone will not be able to transmit forces from post to tooth. The occlusal forces can produce stresses in the unsupported root, fracturing it diagonally from tip of the post down to the crest of bone.

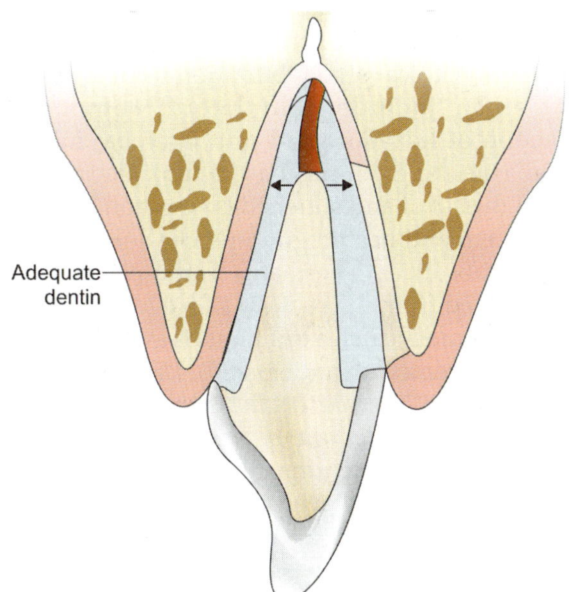

Fig. 22.11 Adequate post length

2. Post Taper

The parallel posts are approximately twice more retentive than tapered posts (Fig. 22.12). The tapered posts tend to produce greater stress in the shoulder area of the restoration, while the parallel post causes more stress in the apical area, especially during cementation. In an effort to minimize the splitting potential of a tapered post, a flat surface is created at the occlusal end of the preparation, which will resist apically directed forces and prevent wedging. The proximity of the apical end of a parallel post to the periphery of root canal may increase the danger of a lateral perforation, since the amount of dentin at the periphery of apical end of post would be much less. A combination of parallel and tapered posts (cervical half of the post parallel and the apical half-tapering) is designed to take advantage of the parallel post and to minimize the complications at the apical end (Fig. 22.13).

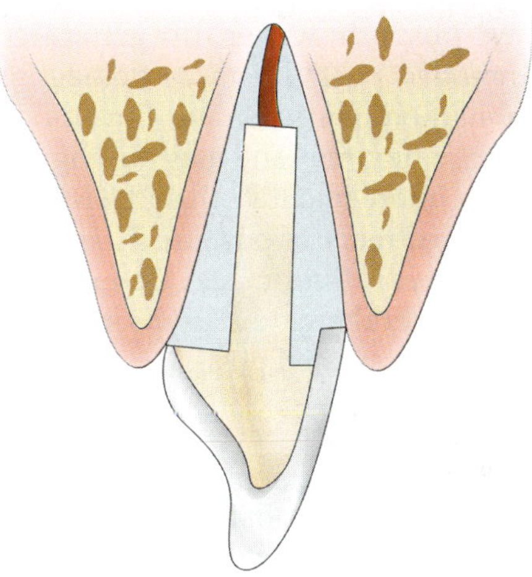

Fig. 22.12 Parallel post

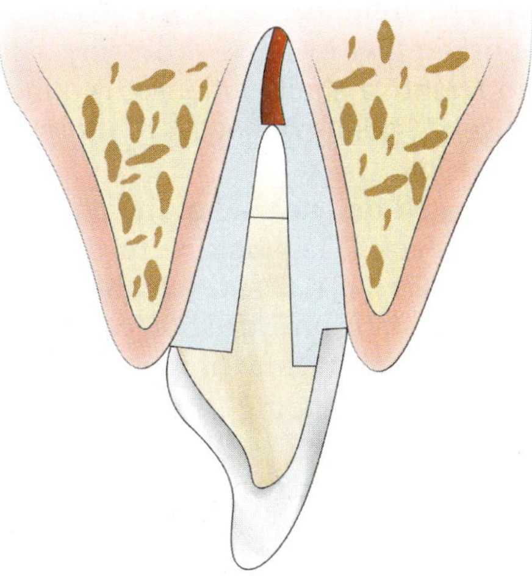

Fig. 22.13 Combination of parallel and taper post

3. Post Diameter

The diameter affects both resistance and retention of the restoration. The smaller diameter post may get displaced or fracture. Enlarging the diameter is not the safest way of improving retention because it does destroy dentin and weaken the root. The width of the post should not exceed one-third the diameter of root. 1.0 mm of dentin thickness around the post (the mesio-distal diameter of an average root is 3.0–4.0 mm at the apex) should always be preserved (Post should be one-third of the root diameter).

4. Surface Texture

The surface texture of the post (smooth, serrated or threaded) plays an important role in the retention. Threaded posts have been reported to be the most retentive. The pretapped, parallel-sided threaded posts are approximately twice as retentive as a parallel-sided serrated post and approximately six times as retentive as a smooth sided tapered post.

Threaded posts, however, do generate stresses. Tapered threaded posts are more damaging because of the combination of a taper and threads. Posts with serrated walls, which may and may not engage the sides of the canal are more retentive than the smooth surface post. Surface treatment of posts such as sandblasting, cleaning with hydrofluoric acid do aid in retention. Sandblasted prefabricated posts provide better retention than non-treated posts.

5. Cementing Medium

Several types of luting cements have been used for the placement of posts in the canal. Zinc phosphate cement, polycarboxylate cement and glass-ionomer cement are being used in routine. All cements are good in compressive strength, fairly good in shear strength but poor in tensile strength. Resin cements may provide improved tensile strength.

It is established that there is hardly any significant difference in retentive ability amongst routinely used cements; however, resins cements are more retentive than other cements.

A vent is created on one side of the post to relieve hydrostatic pressure. This may be in the form of a V-shaped groove or a flat side on the round post (Fig. 22.14). Hydrostatic pressure can lead to bouncing of post or even lead to fracture of root.

The new adhesive bonding agents are now being used for postretention. The 4-META product, C and B metabond have been found to be significantly superior in retention as compared to other bonding adhesives (Panavia, Gluma, Mirage Bond, Scotchbond, Tenure) as well as glass-ionomer and zinc phosphate cements.

22

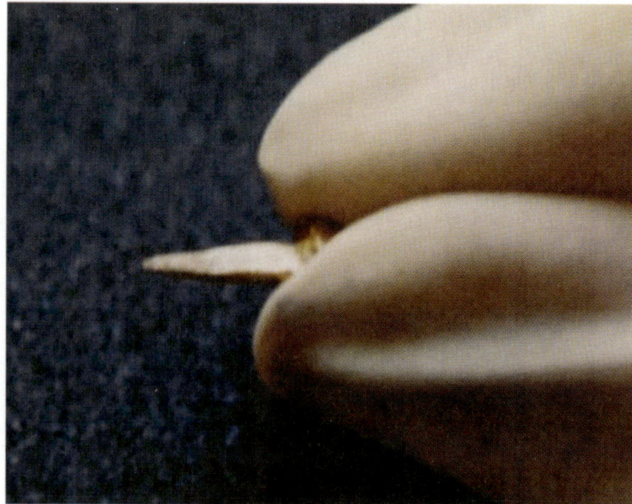

Fig. 22.14 Vent on one side of post

The 4-meta adhesives have the ability to adhere to tooth structure as well as metals, resins and porcelain.

The smear layer should be removed from the walls of the canal to open the dentinal tubules so that the cementing medium could flow into the tubules aiding mechanical lock. It is recommended to use 17% EDTA followed by irrigation with 5.25% sodium hypochlorite to flush away the decalcified dentin and the remaining organic material from the root canal before cementing the post.

Clinical Procedures

The clinical steps involved in preparation of postcore are as follows.

1. Removing the Gutta-percha

The first step in postpreparation is precisely removing the gutta-percha up to the predetermined length without disturbing the apical seal. Obturation techniques with gutta-percha include cold lateral compaction, compaction of heat-softened gutta-percha, injecting thermoplasticized gutta-percha (Obtura), placing gutta-percha in the canal and softened by mechanical means (Mc-Spadden) and heated gutta-percha surrounding a plastic/metal carrier (Thermafil). Gutta-percha can be safely removed from the root canal in every technique, except in Thermafil (such a technique is avoided in cases where postplacement in anticipated). *The pertinent question is whether gutta-percha should be removed immediately after the obturation or after a gap of some time.* A few authors observed no difference in immediate or delayed removal of the gutta-percha; however, it is advisable to remove the gutta-percha within 24 hours. The gutta-percha becomes brittle as the time passes and the removal would be difficult. More so, the apical seal is less disturbed if gutta-percha is removed within 24 hours.

The gutta-percha removal is facilitated by following methods:

i. ***Thermomechanical removal***: The gutta-percha removal is initiated using small round bur. The coronal/cervical 2.0–3.0 mm of gutta-percha should be removed rotating the round bur in slow motion (Fig. 22.15a to e). After the initial removal, bur should not be used in the root canal; otherwise the direction of the bur may lead to deviated track. A gently warm file is inserted in the gutta-percha and allowed to stay till it cool down (Fig. 22.16). The file is then rotated anticlockwise removing the entangled gutta-percha. The process is repeated till the gutta-percha is removed up to the desired length.

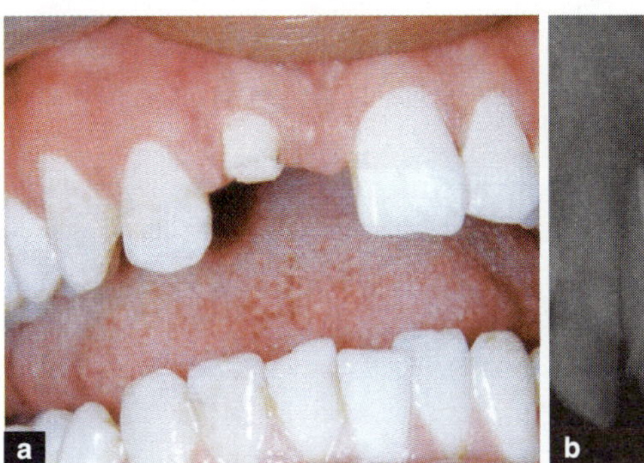

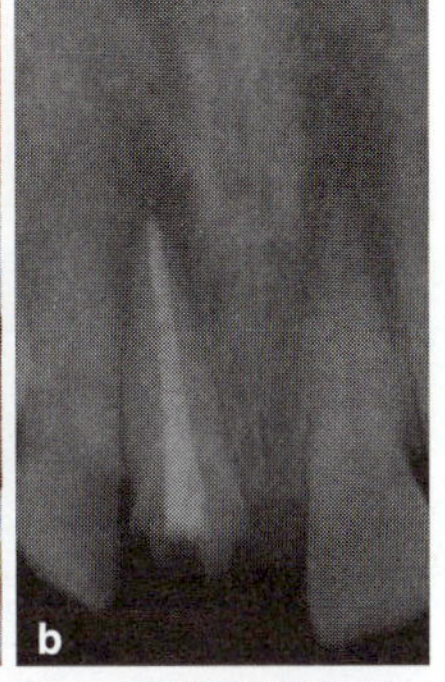

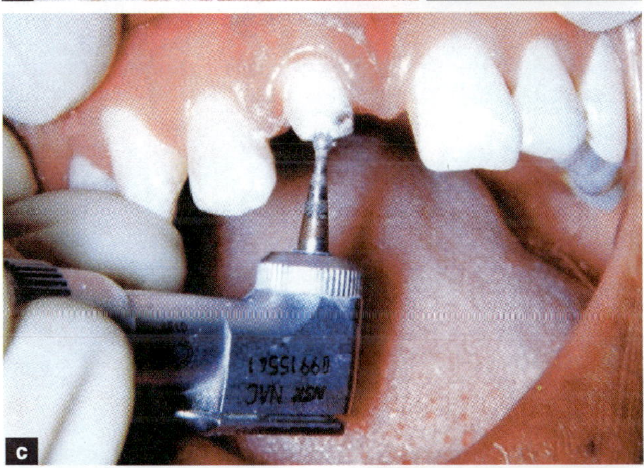

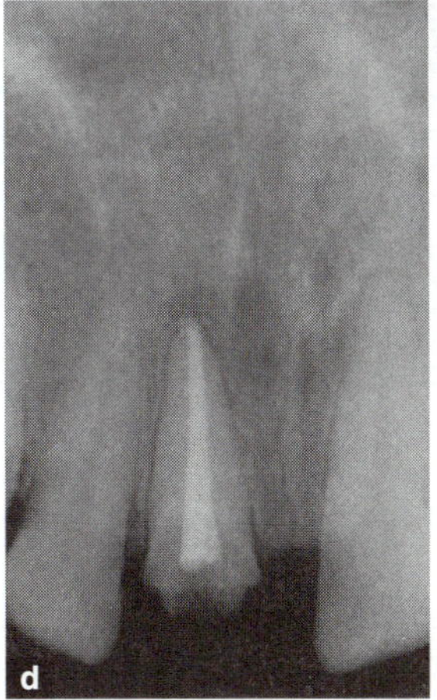

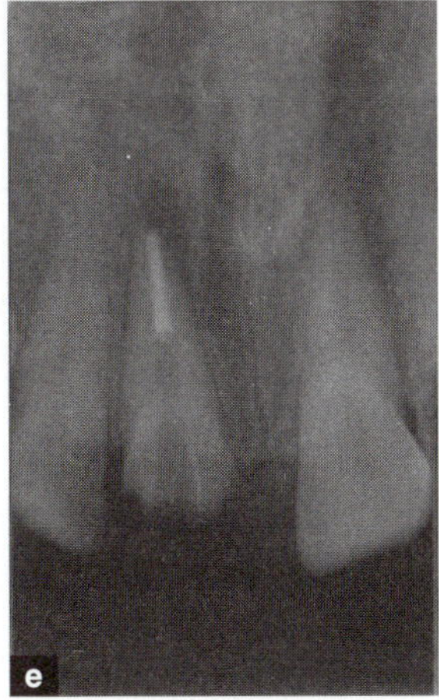

Fig. 22.15 (a) Fractured central incisor; (b) Preoperative radiograph; (c) Use of round bur (initial removal of gutta-percha); (d) Radiograph after removing coronal gutta-percha; (e) Radiograph after removing gutta-percha from the root canal

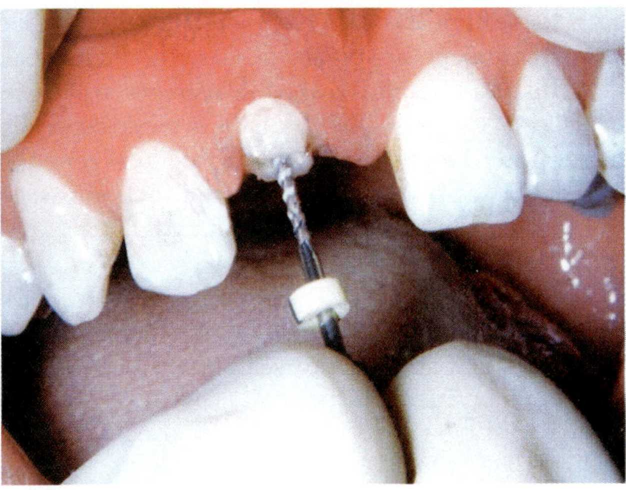

Fig. 22.16 Removing gutta-percha with warm file

ii. ***Chemical removal***: In case the gutta-percha is brittle, dissolving agents can be used to soften the gutta-percha. The commonly used solvents are euclyptol, halothane and turpentine oil. The chloroform being carcinogenic, is not used these days. Turpentine oil is less toxic but it may lead to dimensional changes in the gutta-percha, subsequently increasing the possibility of microleakage. *Commercial preparations as Endosolv-R is used for resin-based sealers and Endosolv-E is used for eugenol-based sealers around the gutta-percha.*

iii. ***Thermal removal***: A heated instrument (say plugger) is inserted into the root canal in a predetermined length; it softens and removes the gutta-percha. A system B spreader/plugger with a stopper is inserted into the root canal at pre-determined length, heated (up to 200°C) and kept for 3–5 seconds. The plugger is then twisted facilitating removal of gutta-percha. Another plugger (Buchanan plugger) can be used to compact the gutta-percha at the apical end. The thermal technique, though good for wider canal, pose difficulty for narrow canals.

2. Preparation of Postspace

Various instruments are being used for preparing the postspace. The initial preparation is carried out using long shank burs and reamers. Non-end cutting, slow speed instruments are preferred. Care should be taken not to disturb the apical seal while using rotary instruments (rotary instruments should be avoided especially in apical-third area). Iatrogenic perforations generally arise from use of end-cutting burs, failure to appreciate root anatomy and use of incorrect angulations.

The appropriate sized Gates glidden drill is used in straight and small canals. The final preparation should be completed with appropriate Peeso reamers.

In order to distribute stresses properly and also to avoid counter sinking of the post, a keyway is prepared in the root canal (Fig. 22.17a to c). In case of posterior teeth, two root canals should be taken to avoid rotation and to distribute the stresses properly (Fig. 22.18a to e).

The prepared postspace is washed thoroughly using 3.0% hydrogen peroxide followed by normal saline.

The prepared postspace should not be left empty for long. This may result in accumulation and reactivation of microorganisms in the postspace. In case the impression making procedure is to be delayed, the said space should be properly closed using paper points and temporary dressings.

In order to avoid perforation during preparation of root canals, it is recommended that the post diameter should not exceed one-third of the mesiodistal width

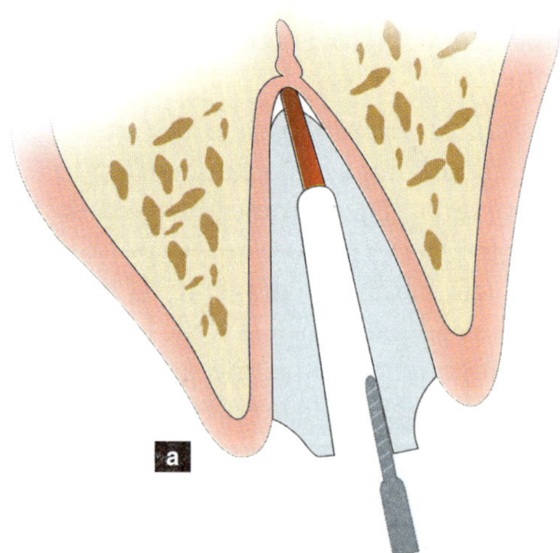

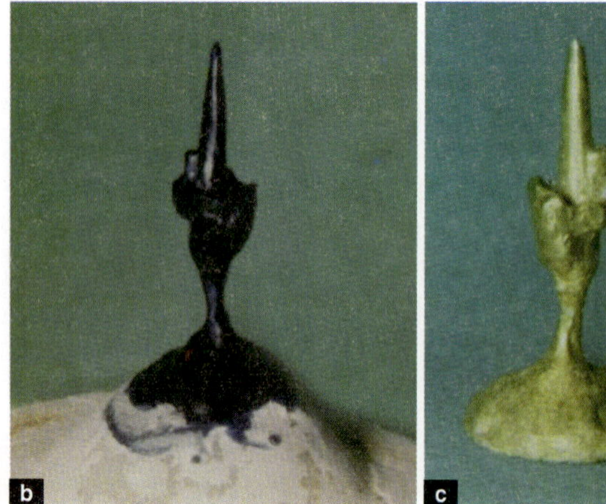

Fig. 22.17 (a) Preparation of keyway (diagrammatic); (b) Wax pattern showing keyway; (c) Casting showing keyway

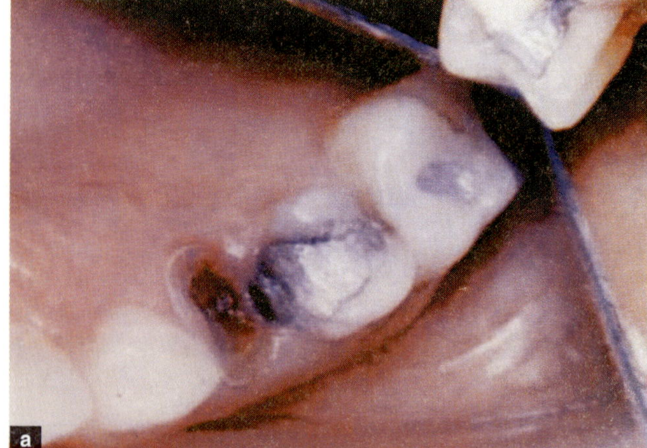

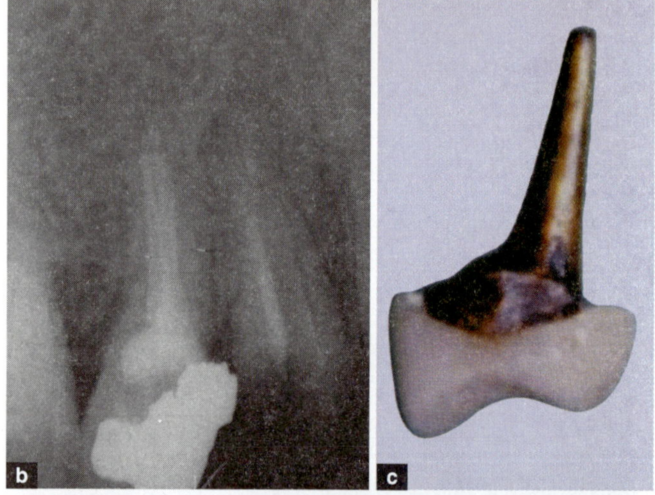

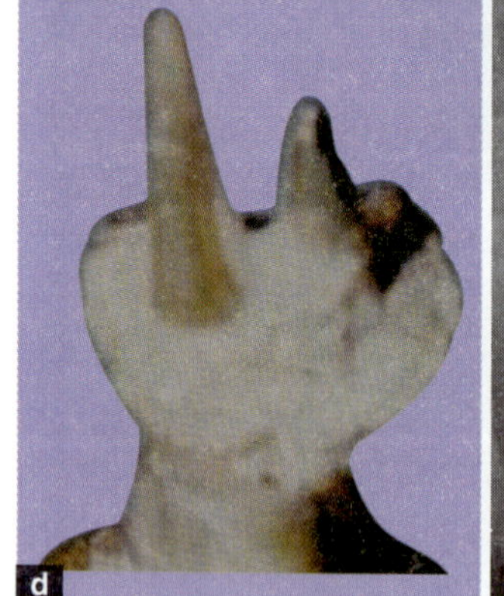

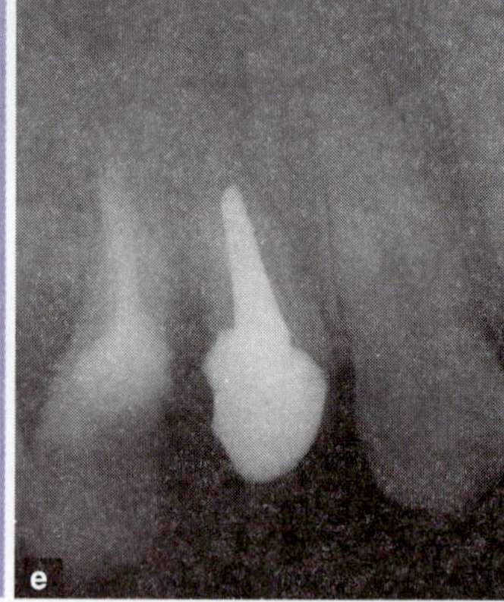

Fig. 22.18 (a) Maxillary first premolar (failed root canal treatment; one post for two root canals); (b) Preoperative radiograph; (c) Single post; (d) Two post; (e) Postoperative radiograph

of roots. It is hypothesized that post diameter of 0.7 mm for mandibular incisors and 1.7 mm for maxillary incisors is sufficient and adequate. It is important that the post diameter at the midpoint should be 2.0 mm less than the root and at least 1.5 mm less at the apical tip area.

Postspace preparation: Safety features

- Postplacement should be limited to a depth of 7.0 mm apical to the canal orifice
- Post diameter should be selected according to width of root/ root canal
- Only no. 2 peeso reamer should be used to prepare the canal (No. 3 and 4 may lead to perforation)
- Mesial roots of mandibular molars and buccal roots of maxillary molars should be avoided, because the root surface facing the furcation is the common site of perforation

Postspace preparation: Key features

- Use of non-end-cutting instruments, especially rotary
- Minimal canal enlargement
- Length to be decided on the basis of post material
- 4.0–5.0 mm gutta-percha should be retained at apical end
- Diameter should be one-third of the width of root
- Adequate space for ferrule
- Care should be taken not to lose the path

3. Impression Making of the Postspace

The impression making of the postspace is carried out in custom cast post system to fabricate metal post.

The techniques utilized in impression making are:

i. Direct method
ii. Indirect method

i. *Direct method*: The postimpression is fabricated directly from the prepared space using resin or wax pattern.

For making an impression, the selected pin (may be plastic or metal) is roughened with carborundum disc. Alternatively, an old file or reamer can be used. A thin layer of sticky wax is applied over the pin. The apical end should be properly covered by sticky wax. The pin with sticky wax is tried in the root canal. The instrument should be free in the root canal including the apical end. If not, the smaller diameter instrument is tried following the same protocol. Once tried, the instrument is coated with blue inlay wax, gently warm and inserted into the root canal. Keep it in the root canal for 60 seconds and then gently withdraw the instrument. The 'post' impression is ready. Check carefully for any voids, breakage and also the apical end. The process can be repeated, if need be. The 'post' is inserted back and the core is built in patient's oral cavity using blue inlay wax. While using blue inlay wax during core preparation of maxillary anterior teeth, care should be taken not to injure patient's tongue, as melted wax may fall over the tongue. Either a piece of cotton or operator's left thumb should be kept under the core during manipulation (Fig. 22.19a to f).

In case the impression is made in resin, the plastic pin is preferred. Ready-made plastic pins are available; alternatively, a blade of comb can be guided to make it round and can be used as a pin. Acrylic resin is coated over the plastic pin and inserted into the canal. Make the pin stable for a couple of minutes and then the pin along with the resin is taken out (Fig. 22.20a to f). It is checked for any voids or discrepancies and if found so, the process is repeated. The resin can be manipulated easily in the mouth without being distorted. The core is built over the post using the same resin.

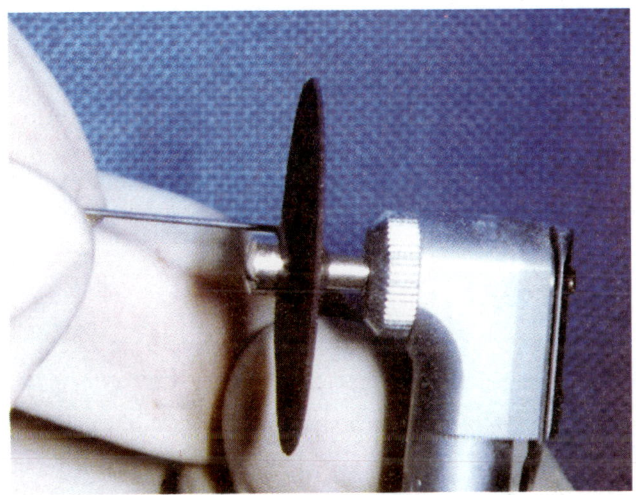

Fig. 22.19a Roughening the needle

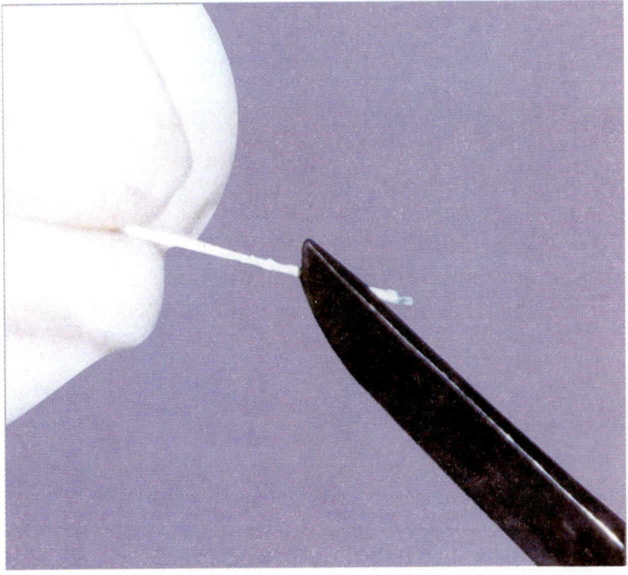

Fig. 22.19b Applying sticky wax

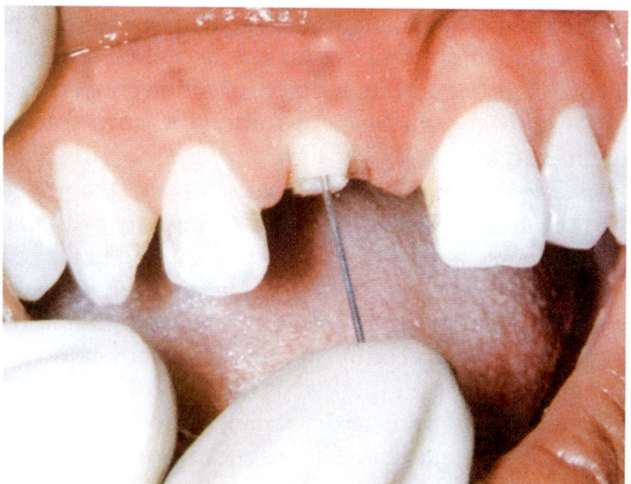
Fig. 22.19c Inserting into postspace

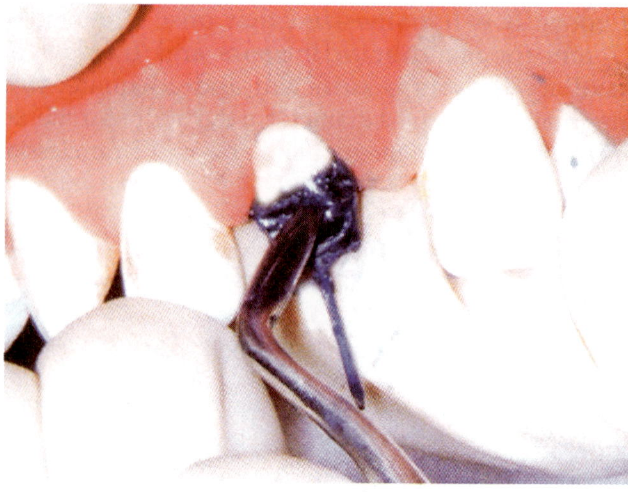
Fig. 22.19f Core fabrication

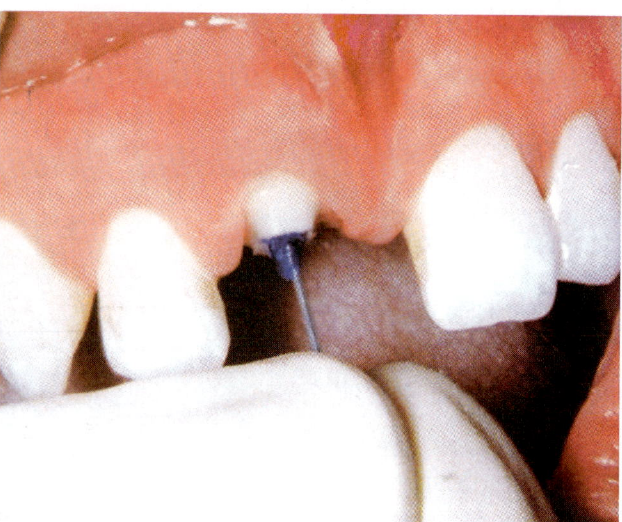
Fig. 22.19d Applying blue inlay wax and inserting again

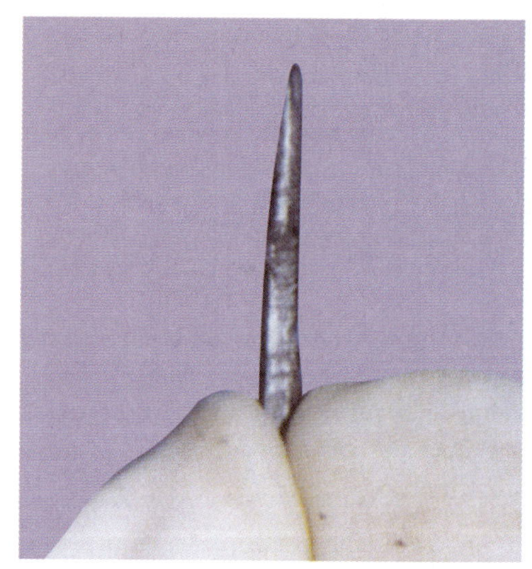
Fig. 22.20a Plastic pin

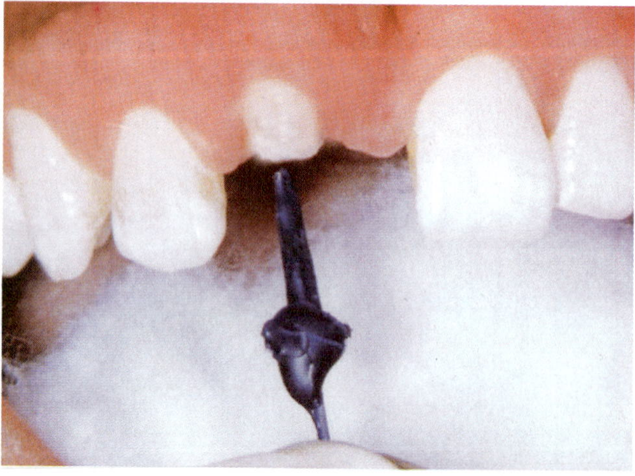
Fig. 22.19e Taking out the pattern

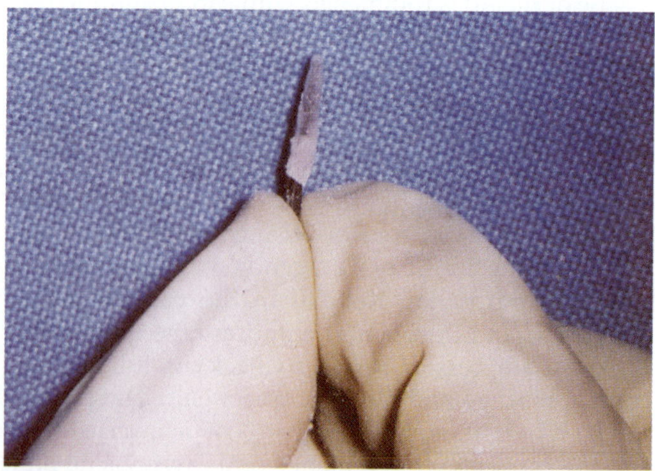
Fig. 22.20b Applying acrylic resin

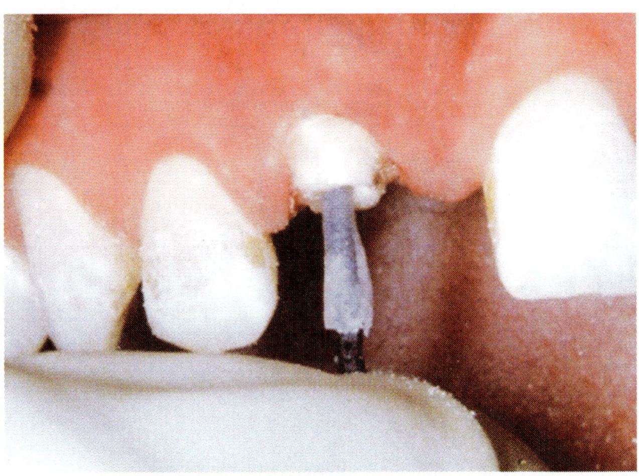

Fig. 22.20c Taking pattern

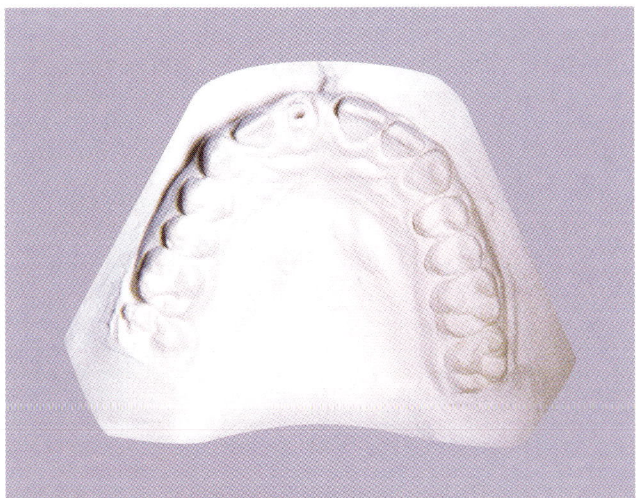

Fig. 22.20d Impression on the cast

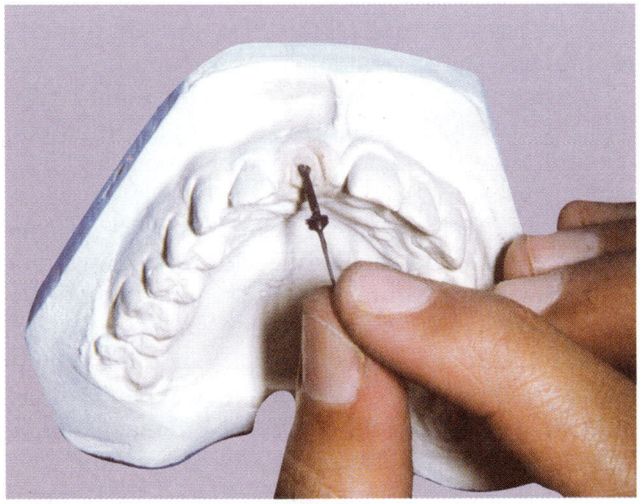

Fig. 22.20e Taking impression with blue inlay wax

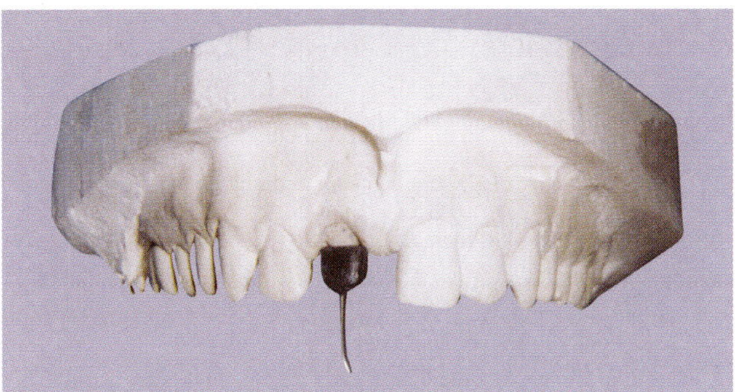

Fig. 22.20f Final impression

ii. *Indirect method*: The post is fabricated from the cast.

To prepare the cast, the impression material (preferably rubber base) is injected into the canal. The use of lentulo spiral ensures the elimination of entrapped air in the impression material inside the canal. The impression should be reinforced with some type of rigid material, viz. steel wire, plastic pin or a root canal instrument. The reinforcing devices not only strengthen the impression during fabrication, but also during pouring and separation.

The cast with prepared space for post is lubricated by applying machine oil or cocoa butter. The impression is made using blue inlay wax along with metal pin as described for direct methods. The indirect method saves time of the operator since, the impression can be made by some assistant in the clinic or laboratory.

Ferrule Effect

One major complication of the post-restored tooth is fracture of the root. The postcore should be so designed, that it should minimize the chances of root fracture.

A 'ferrule' is a metal ring or covering around the coronal part of the root intended for increasing the resistance form. The word originates from combination of two latin words 'ferrum' (iron) and 'viriola' (bracelet). A dental ferrule is an encircling band of cast metal round the coronal surface of the tooth. It can also be defined as '*the 360° metal collar covering/surrounding the parallel walls of the dentin extending coronal to the shoulder of the preparation*'. The ferrule resists all types of stresses, viz. functional forces, wedging effect of tapered posts and the lateral forces exerted during the post insertion.

During functional movements (the forward movement of mandibular anterior teeth Fig. 22.21), the forces exerted on the core portion of the post and core create pressure on the palatal surface of the root at the apical end of post. This process may lead to fracture of root (Fig. 22.22a and b). To increase resistance of the root to such fractures, the core portion is made to

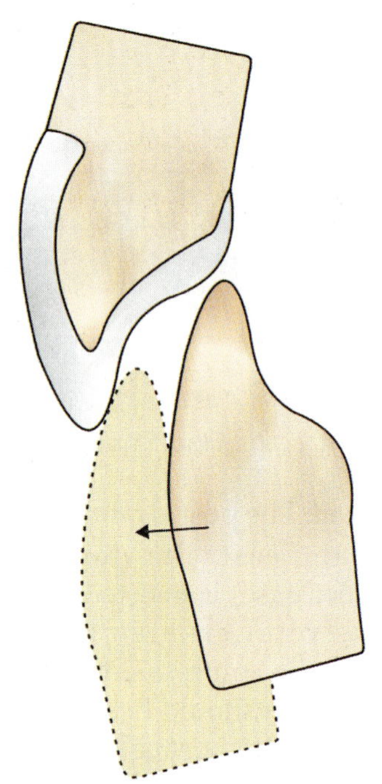

Fig. 22.21 Functional movement of mandibular anterior teeth

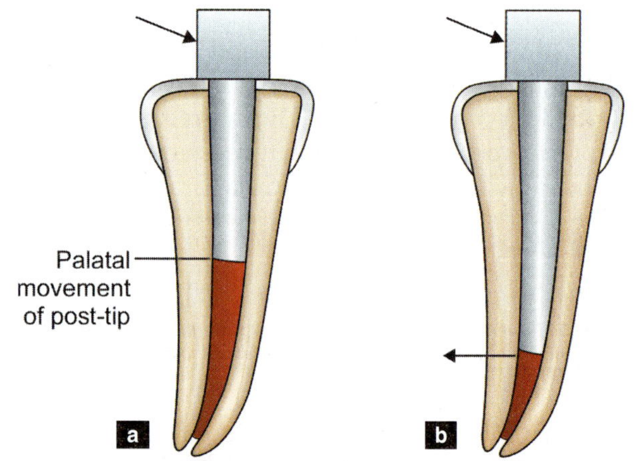

Fig. 22.22a and b Functional forces on core (arrow), pushing the post tip palatally (arrow)

encircle the root/remaining crown, so as the forces generated on core may dissipate within the total root. This covering of the core portion onto the root or crown portion is known as 'Core ferrule'. The full veneer crown over the core along with coronal tooth provides ferrule effect, known as 'Crown ferrule'. In case the length of the remaining crown is sufficient, there is no need to have additional core ferrule effect (the coronal portion of the remaining tooth would bear the forces generated by the functional movements as in normal tooth). The restored crown in such cases will be sufficient to provide ferrule effect (Fig. 22.23). In case the dislodging forces are severe in nature (traumatic deep bite, bruxism etc.), additional core ferrule may be

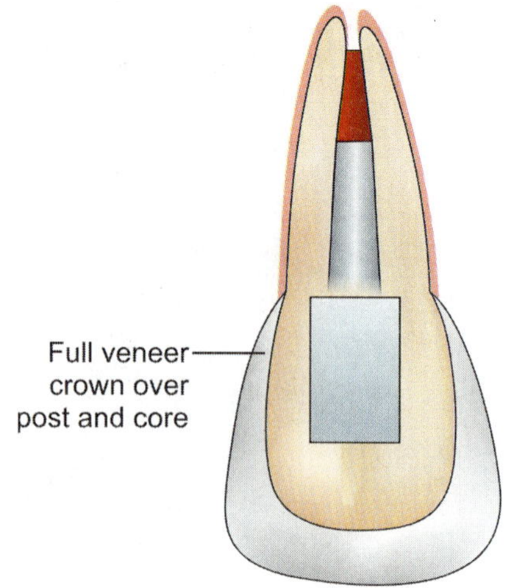

Fig. 22.23 Full veneer crown provides ferrule effect (crown ferrule)

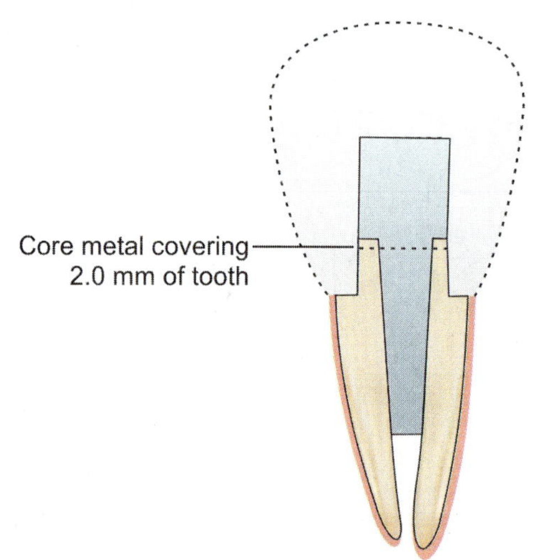

Fig. 22.24 Location of ferrule

required. The combined effect provides the requisite resistance to fracture of the root and/or postcore restorations. The cervical collar along the core increases the resistance of the post and core to torsional forces). The length/height of this covering is also important. The minimum ferrule length/height should be 1.5–2.0 mm while restoring maxillary anterior teeth (Fig. 22.24). The fracture resistance is increased with the increase in ferrule length/height. Ferrule width is also an important parameter; 1.5 mm width of the remaining dentin thickness is considered adequate and can provide requisite 1.5–2.0 mm width of ferrule (Fig. 22.25a and b).

Many a times, clinical conditions warrant thinning of dentin wall around the root canal and the remaining crown portion (the walls are considered 'too thin' when they are less than 1.0 mm in thickness). Covering of metal core over this thickness might not be practicable.

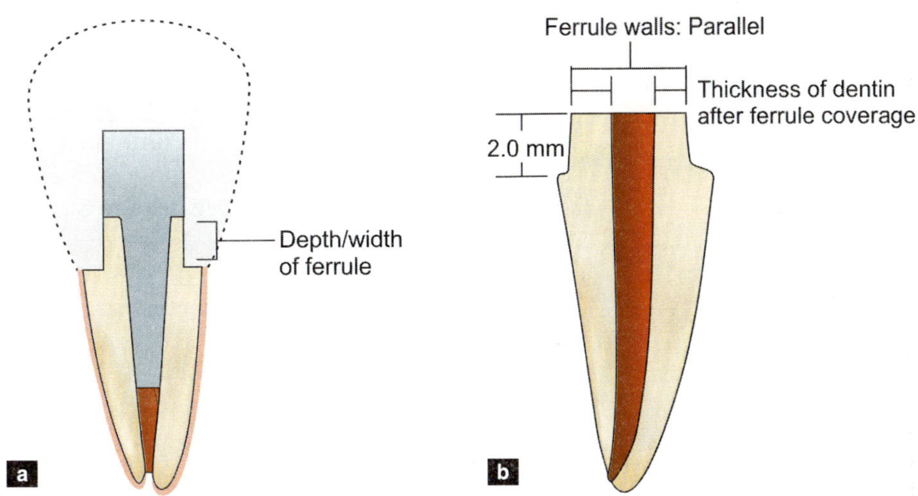

Fig. 22.25 Design of Ferrule (Diagrammatic representation) (a) Depth/width of Ferrule; (b) Ferrule width and remaining dentin thickness

In such cases, ferrule effect is achieved only by the full veneer crown.

The longevity of the restored endodontically treated tooth depends upon the presence of adequate height (1.5–2.0 mm) of sound tooth structure (ferrule), between the core and the crown margins. The ferrule provides the necessary bracing action to protect the integrity of the root. Inadequate ferrule may lead to root fracture, post fracture and/or loosening of post due to cement failure.

The ferrule effect is divided into two: 'complete ferrule effect' and 'partial ferrule effect'. In case it is practically feasible to encircle 1.5–2.0 mm of the coronal tooth structure with the core, it provides 'complete ferrule' effect (Fig. 22.26). Alternatively, covering only the side walls with core may provide 'partial ferrule' effect (Fig. 22.27).

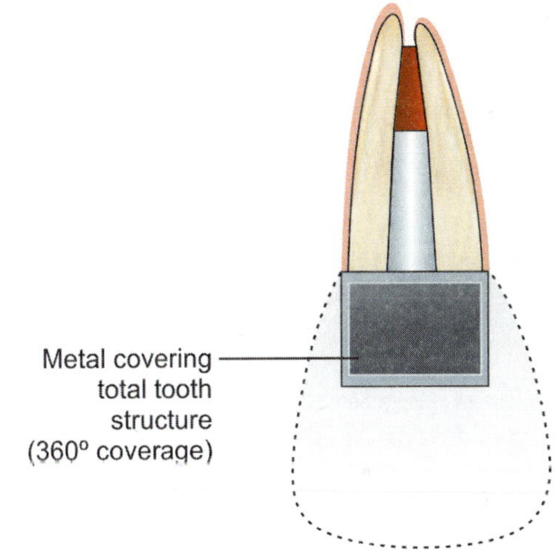

Fig. 22.26 Core ferrule—complete

Core ferrule: Key features

- The remaining dentin thickness should be at least 1.5 mm.
- The number of remaining dentin walls; preferably three or at least two wall must be present; if only one wall is left, alternative treatment planning, such as crown lengthening or orthodontic extrusion is planned.
- Excessive lateral forces need more of remaining tooth structure.
- 1.5–2.0 mm covering is adequate.
- Core metal encircling completely, i.e. 360° (complete ferrule); core metal encircling partially, i.e. 180° (partial ferrule)

In critical conditions where there is insufficient crown structure for achieving ferrule length, the clinician may consider crown lengthening procedures (Fig. 22.28a and b) or orthodontic extrusion (Fig. 22.29). This will allow the distance between crown margin and alveolar crest to be widened and increase the potential ferrule length. However, these methods may result in

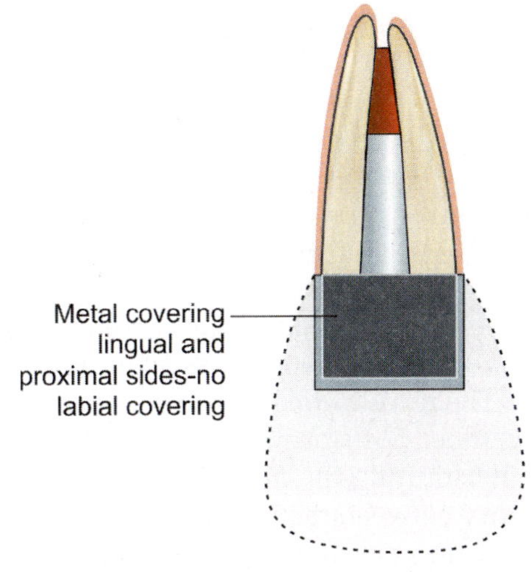

Fig. 22.27 Core ferrule—partial

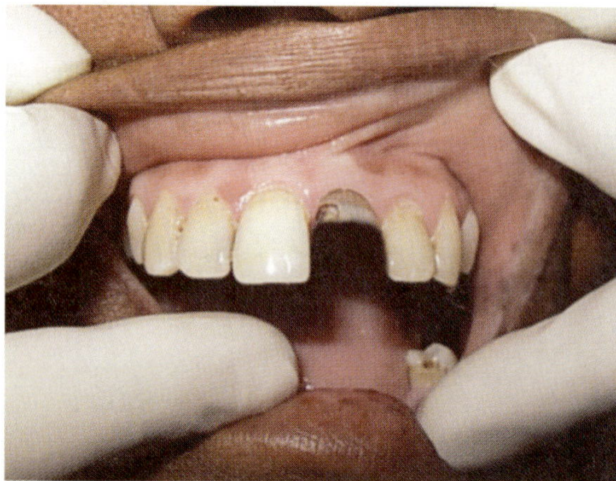

Fig. 22.28a Preoperative

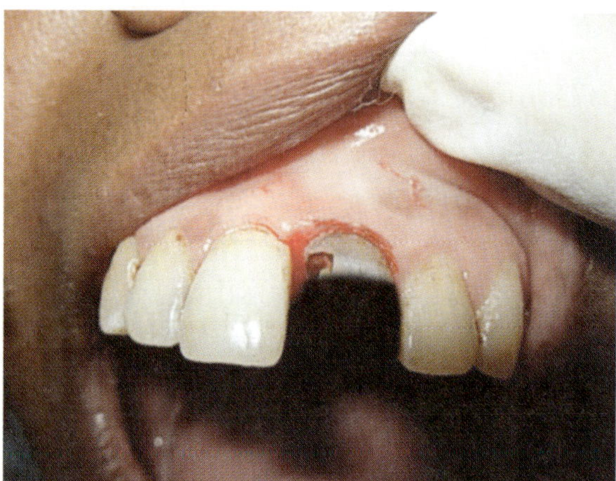

Fig. 22.28b Crown lengthening procedure

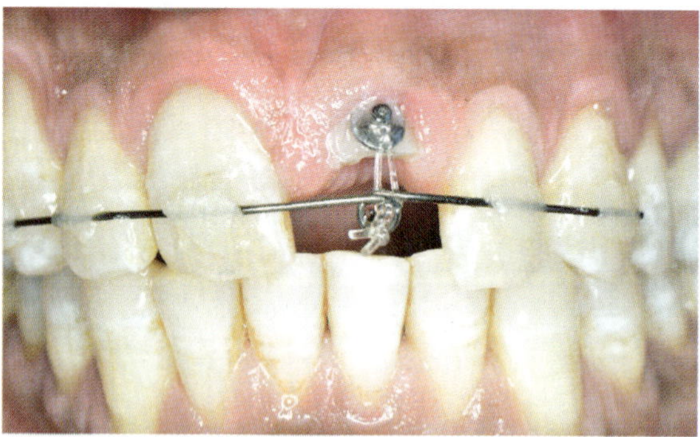

Fig. 22.29 Orthodontic extrusion

reducing the root length and making the crown-to-root ratio unfavorable. In such cases fiber postcores are preferred. The ferrule effect is not necessary in case of fiber posts (fiber posts provide monobloc effect within the root, substituting the ferrule effect). Thus balance is mandatory between the ferrule length achieved and the remaining root length. These considerations determine the choice of post and core material.

II. FIBER POSTS

The metal post and core provide optimum strength; however, need for color masking and discoloration of crown/gingiva with time, are the significant drawbacks. Furthermore, metal shines through all ceramic restorations and negates the transmission of light.

In an effort to overcome the disadvantages of metal posts, fiber reinforced posts have been developed and are widely being used as posts.

A. Custom Fiber Post

The fiber (plastic) post can be fabricated in clinics; however, prefabricated posts are preferred.

The steps employed in fabrication are (Fig. 22.30a to h):

- The root canal configuration is evaluated clinically and radiologically (Fig. 22.30a and b).
- Plastic pin of appropriate size is selected (plastic pins are available; alternatively, a blade of comb grinded to round shape can be used) (Fig. 22.30c).

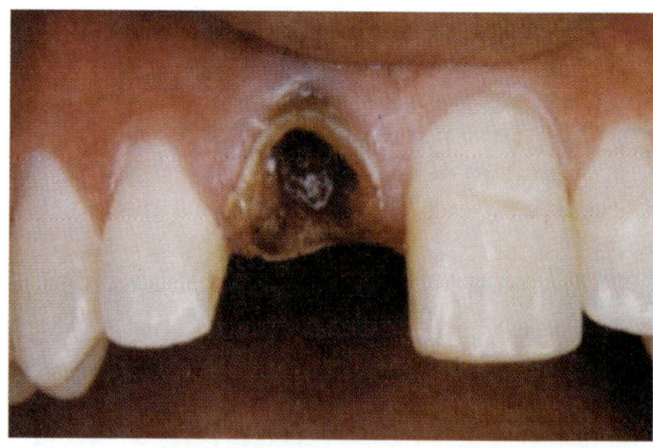

Fig. 22.30a Preoperative

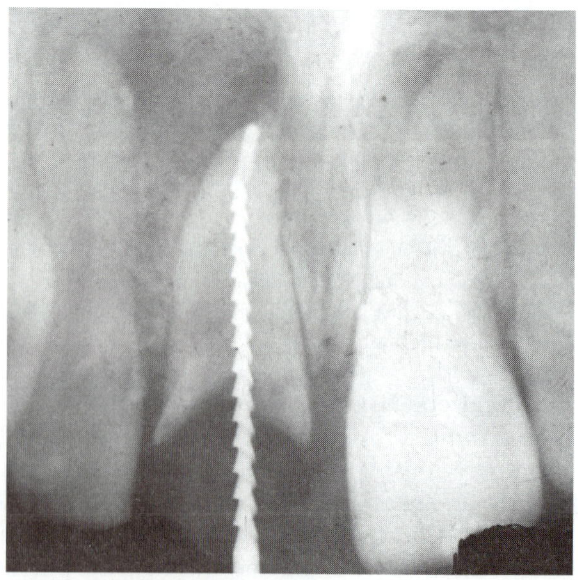

Fig. 22.30b Evaluating root canal

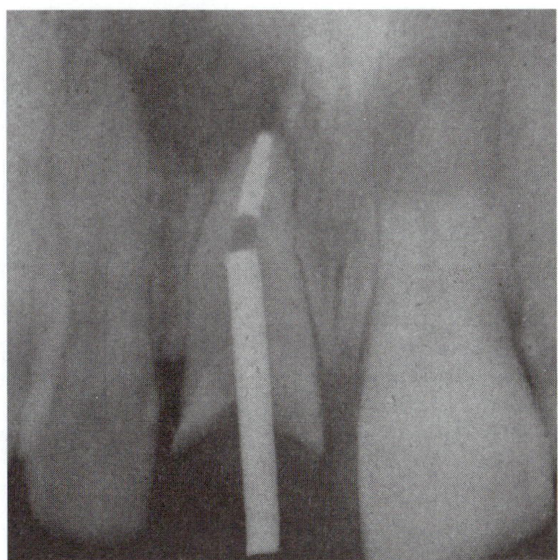

Fig. 22.30c Selection of plastic pin

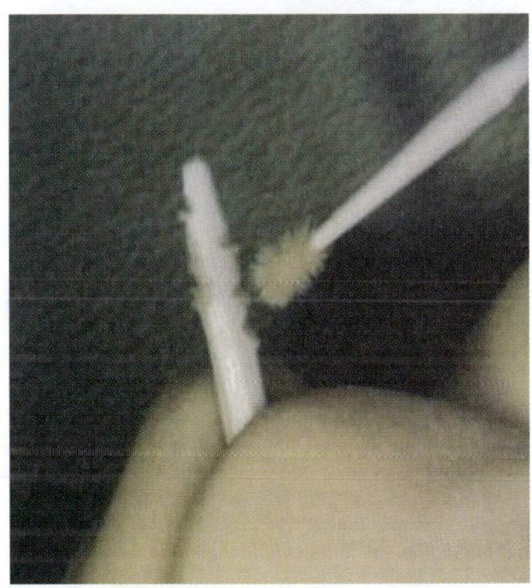

Fig. 22.30d Applying bonding agent

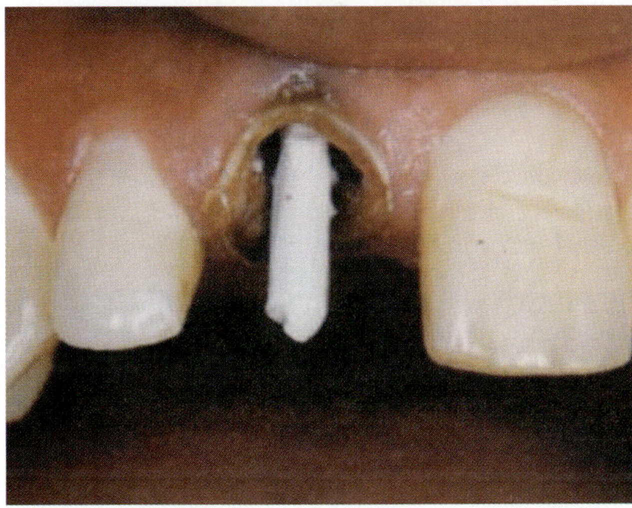

Fig. 22.30e Composite resin coated over the pin and inserted into the canal

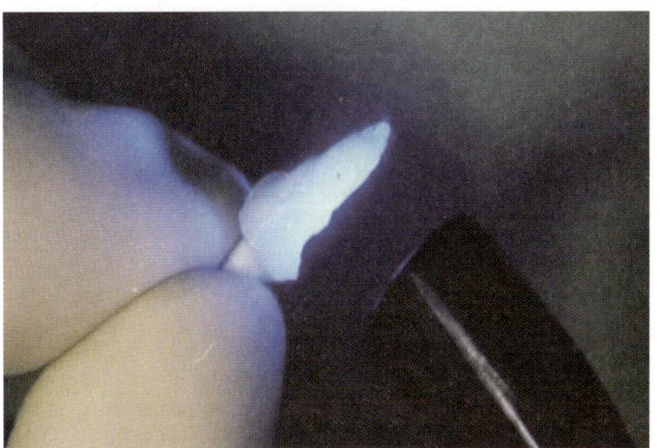

Fig. 22.30f Curing outside the canal

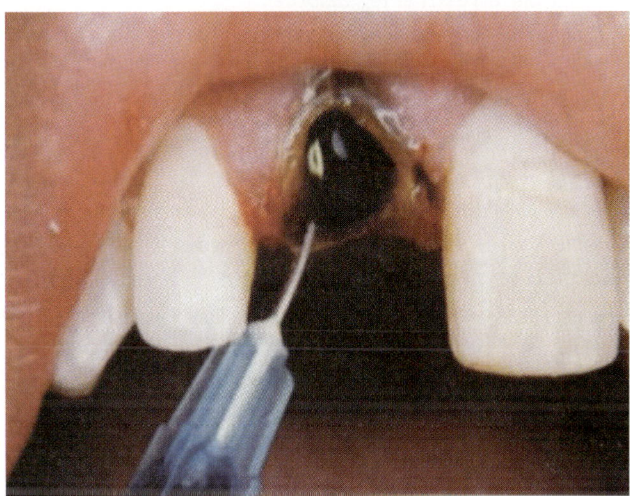

Fig. 22.30g Conditioning inside the canal

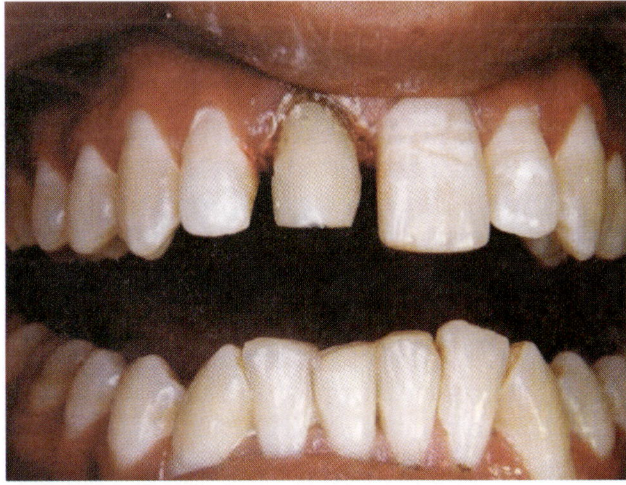

Fig. 22.30h Core build up

- The selected pin is roughened using old carbide burs or used carborundum discs.
- Bonding agent is applied over the prepared plastic pin (Fig. 22.30d).

- Composite resin is coated over the plastic pin and inserted into the root canal (lubricant is applied inside the canal) (Fig. 22.30e).
- The pin along with composite is removed when partly set and examined for any voids or irregularities; if so, the process is repeated (Fig. 22.30f).
- The partially set composite is cured outside the canal.
- The inside of the canal is 'conditioned' and the primer is applied (Fig. 20.30g).
- Flowable dual-cure composite is injected into the root canal and the pin coated with same resin is pushed into the canal. The material is cured from the coronal end.
- After curing and setting, the core is built with composite resin (Fig. 22.30h).
- The core is trimmed according to the anatomy of crown.
- Veneer crown of choice can be placed over the prepared core.

B. Prefabricated Fiber Post

A variety of fibers singly and in combination are being marketed as prefabricated fiber posts. Their classification is described earlier; the properties and technique of use is explained.

The commonly used posts, their properties and technique of use is described.

a. Carbon Fiber Posts

Carbon fiber posts (Mirafit carbon, Endopost, etc.) are considered viable alternatives to metals when properties like strength, stiffness, lightness and resistance to corrosion and fatigue are compared. The carbon fiber posts can bond to tooth structure and the modulus of elasticity (rigidity) is similar to dentin (significantly more flexible than metal posts). The carbon fiber posts are black in color and are radiolucent, which make it difficult to detect radiographically (Fig. 22.31a to c). Replacing carbon with quartz fibers result in a tooth colored posts.

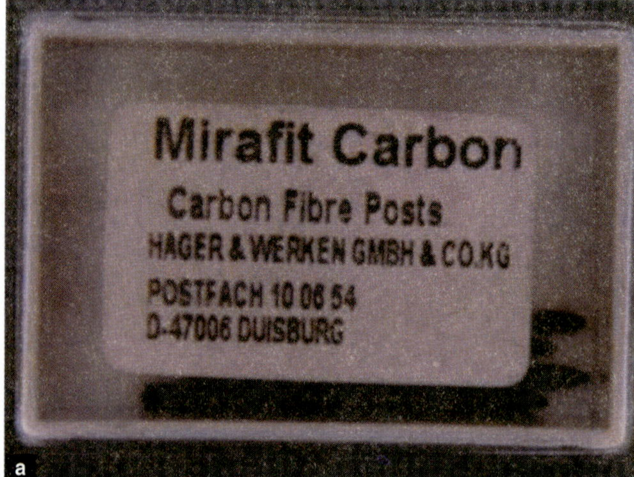

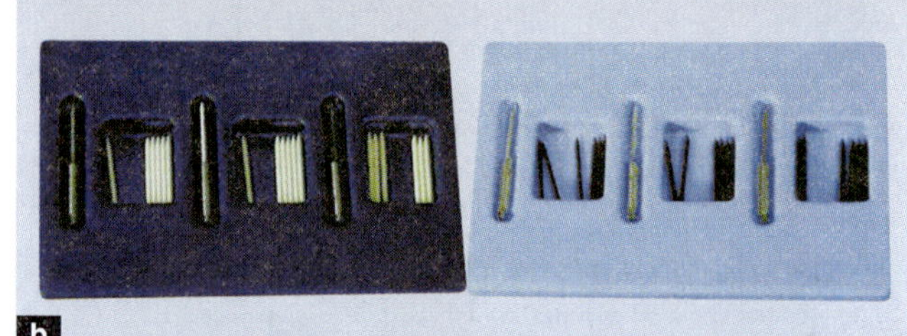

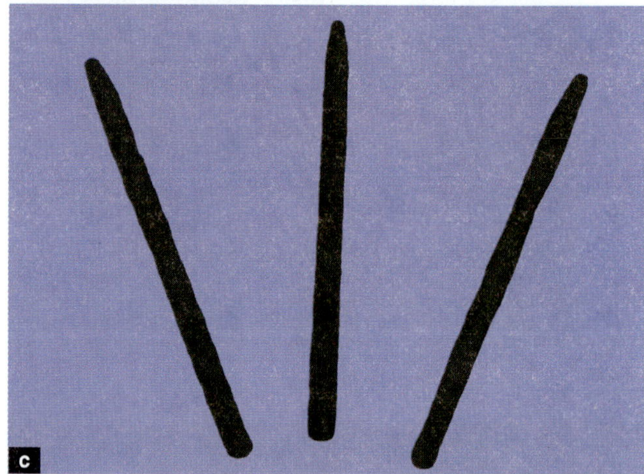

Fig. 22.31a to c Carbon fiber post

Technique

The suitable sized post is selected according to the configuration of the postspace prepared.

The inside of the canal is etched with 37% phosphoric acid for 10–15 seconds. The canals are washed thoroughly and dried with paper points. The primer is applied inside the canal and light cured. Similarly primer is applied to the post and light cured. The dual cure resin cement is applied inside the root canal and the post is inserted with gentle pressure. The exposed area of the post is coated with bonding agent and composite, creating initial shape of the core. The core portion is cured for 40 seconds. Finally trim and contour the core according to anatomy of the crown.

Advantages

- Superior mechanical properties
- Modulus of elasticity is similar to that of dentin
- Sufficient bonding to tooth structure and core composite.

Disadvantages

- Unesthetic (black color)
- Radiolucent.

b. Silica Fiber Posts

Silica fiber posts are either of quartz fibers or glass fibers.

i. ***Quartz fiber post***: The quartz fiber posts are the improved version of the carbon fiber posts. The types of quartz fiber posts are:

- *Light post/DT light post/DT light safety post*: These are available in different tapered designs for better adaptation to the prepared root canal. They are 20.0 mm long, available in three diameters (0.9, 1.0 and 1.2 mm at the apex) and three tapers, 0.06, 0.08 and 0.10. The matched set of reamers/drills is available to prepare the postspace (Fig. 22.32).
  Micromechanical tags are provided on the surface of the posts for better retention. The post has a modulus of elasticity similar to that of dentin; functional stresses get dissipated and not concentrated in the root, subsequently reducing the potential for root fracture. The translucent posts transmit light to the apical end and therefore may be used with light or dual cure cements.
  A retrieval kit for postremoval is available separately.
- *Aesthetic/Aesthetic plus post*: The posts utilizes white quartz fibers surrounding carbon fibers (aesthetic post) and all white quartz fibers (aesthetic plus). The posts have high flexure strength and low modulus of elasticity as good as carbon fiber posts.

  The technique for placement of quartz fiber post is similar to that of carbon fiber posts.
- *iLumi fiber optic post*: A post having ability to transmit light to the most apical part of root canal space improves postretention. When light is transmitted through root canal, its intensity is significantly reduced (less than 40%), subsequently decreasing the polymerization of resin cement. A new fiberoptic post, iLumi, was introduced, which can transmit light up to 12 mm into the postspace, thereby improving the retention of post.

Advantages

- Radiopaque (allow postoperative evaluation).
- Modulus of elasticity is similar to that of dentin; reduces the risks of tooth fracture.
- Complete and non-traumatic removal is possible.
- High tensile strength and superior fatigue resistance.
- Bond well to the tooth and core material.

ii. ***Glass fiber post***: The glass fiber posts are improved version of the quartz fiber posts. The glass fiber posts are esthetically pleasing along with maintaining the properties of fiber posts (glass fibers have lower modulus of elasticity than carbon/quartz fibers) (Fig. 22.33a and b).

The types of glass fiber posts are:

- *Lucent anchor post*: The Lucent anchor post is designed to transmit natural tooth colors for esthetic purposes. It is available in three diameters with 30° tapers. The lucent anchor post can be easily removed in case of retreatment.
- *FiberKor post*: The bundles of glass fibers are impregnated in resin matrix, which provide the requisite white color of the post. The post is available in four diameters and three degree taper along with matching drills (diameter 1, 1.2, 1.4 and 1.6 mm).
- *Fiber white parapost*: The post is parallel and has color coded ring around the head for identification. These are available in 4 sizes (diameter 1.14, 1.25, 1.4 and 1.5 mm).

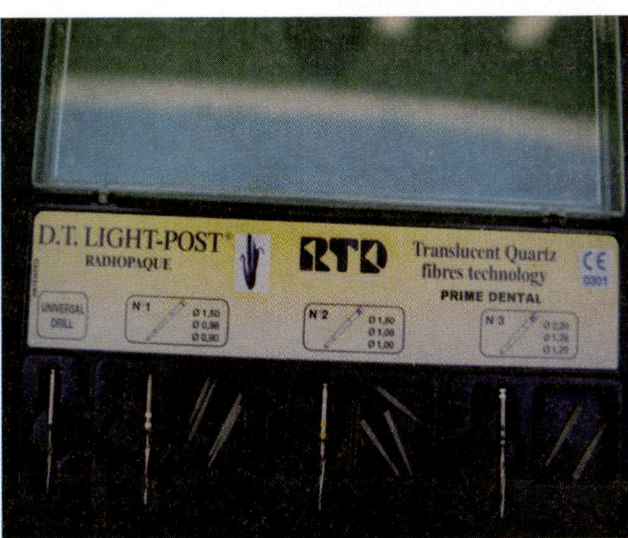

Fig. 22.32 DT light post

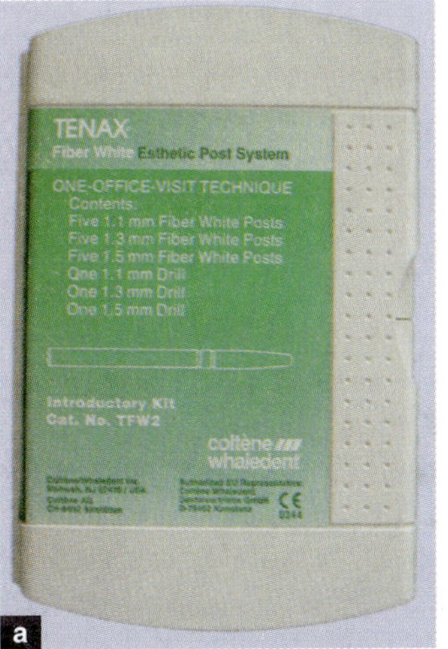

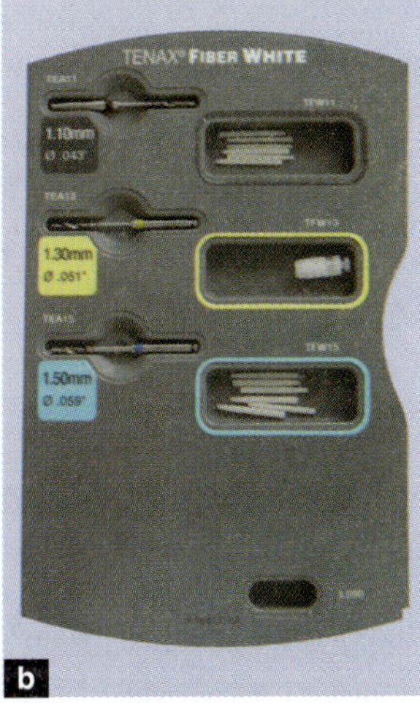

Fig. 22.33 Glass fiber posts: (a) Tenax fiber glass (outer); (b) Tenax fiber glass (inner)

The glass fiber posts are virtually radiolucent; a few contain silicone dioxide to impart radiopacity to the glass fiber posts. A new glass fiber post, AR glass fiber post, was introduced having radiopacity greater than enamel/dentin because of addition of zirconium oxide into the glass framework. A radiopaque post is preferred because it provides an easy evaluation at the interface with the root canal space.

The technique for placing glass fiber post is similar to that of carbon fiber posts.

Advantage of fiber posts

- Adequate bonding with the root dentin (bonding provides monobloc effect).
- Retentive; microretention achieved with fiber posts is far superior to other posts.
- Fiber posts are minimal invasive; one-half the length of root is sufficient as compared to metal posts where 'length' provides retention.
- Parallel posts or half-parallel-half-taper as envisaged in metal posts mandatory for retention and stress distribution is not required in fiber posts. Small taper posts provide good retention and good potential for distribution of stresses.
- Metal posts exhibit corrosion potential, which may contribute to decementation and even root fracture. Fiber posts overcome the problem of corrosion (titanium and ceramic also do not corrode).
- Removal of fiber post is easy, without disturbing the dentin substrate.
- Fiber posts are more fatigue resistant. Fiber posts may flex slightly, when necessary; some fiber posts have greater flexure strength than stainless steel and titanium.
- Most of the fiber posts are radiopaque.
- Fiber posts (except carbon fiber being black) are esthetically pleasing and overcome the need of applying masking over the post.

Disadvantages of fiber posts

- Fiber posts may undergo degradation because of repeated mechanical loading and under conditions of moisture.
- Degradation may lead to a reduction in the modulus of elasticity and flexural strength with an increased risk in debonding.

c. Polyethylene Fiber

Polyethylene fiber is available as Ribbond and Ribbond-THM (Thinner Higher Modulus). It is used both as post and core material. Ribbond—THM is made of thinner fibers with a higher thread count and is almost half as thick as original Ribbond. Fibers are composed of woven polyethylene (Fig. 22.34). The modulus of elasticity of these fibers is similar to that of radicular dentin; suitable for fabrication of post and core as one unit.

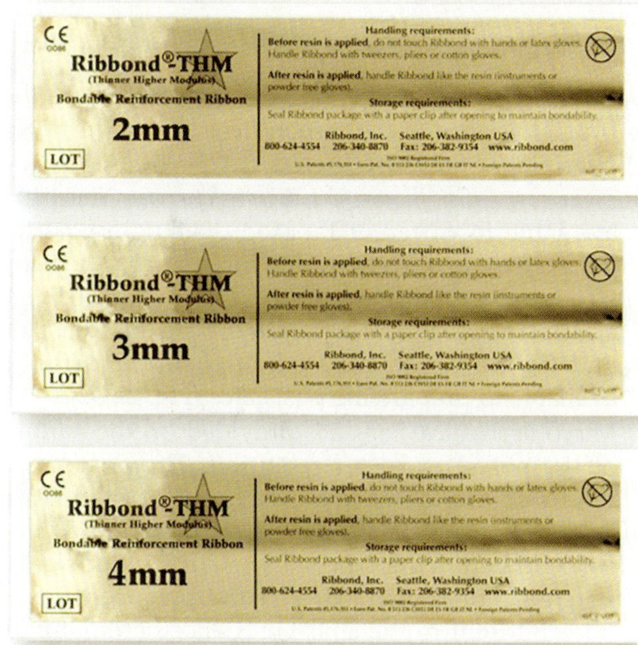

Fig. 22.34 Ribbond—polyethylene fiber

Technique

The steps involved are:

- The obturated material is removed up to pre-determined length (leaving gutta-percha at the apical end) as described earlier. The natural internal form of the pulp space is maintained. The final depth of the postdepends on the shape and diameter of the root canal. For single rooted teeth, the greater the irregularities and undercuts in the canal, the less depth of the post is required. For multirooted teeth, the greater the divergence of the canals, the less depth of the post is required.
- Verify the removal of gutta-percha/obturated material by evaluating radiograph of the prepared canal.
- The margins of the coronal opening of canal are rounded to eliminate sharp angles between the post and core; minimizes stress concentration and cracks at the post and core junction.
- Measures the depth of the prepared canal with a periodontal probe. Different thickness of Ribbond is available depending upon the need (for narrow canals, thin Ribbond is preferred). Cut a piece of Ribbond measuring twice the depth of the prepared canal and three to four times the height of the anticipated core. Use the widest Ribbond that will fit in the canal in a double thickness. The greater mass of Ribbond fibers is preferred.

- The canal is dried and etched for 10–15 seconds. Thoroughly rinse the canal and remove excess etchant. Apply primers and adhesive inside the root canal using a microapplicator.
- Wet the Ribbond with unfilled adhesive resin.
- Carry dual/self-cure luting composite in a small syringe, such as Endo-Eze or a Centrix syringe and place the syringe tip at the apical end of the canal before injecting the luting composite. Start injecting the composite slowly while withdrawing the syringe. Apply composite over the wet Ribbond also.
- Ribbond is pushed into the apical end of root canal. If space permits, insert an additional piece of wet Ribbond into the canal, even if second piece could be inserted half the depth of the canal preparation. The first piece is sufficient for retention of the post. The purpose of the second piece is to produce a greater density of Ribbond at the postcore junction. The free ends emerging from the canal will be used to form the core. Do not cure till now.
- After placement of the Ribbond in the canal, remove the excess flowing composite with a disposable brush. Complete the core build up using appropriate resin. Finish and shape the core using diamond rotary instruments. If the Ribbond becomes exposed and fuzz, place a layer of unfilled bonding adhesive over the exposed fibers and cure it.

Advantages

- A Ribbond post like a natural tooth is translucent and esthetically pleasing as compared to a metal post that is opaque.
- The Ribbond post along with resin adapts to the irregularities and undercuts within the root canals and becomes retentive and anti-rotational after curing.
- Since Ribbond post adapts to the irregularities and is bonded to the tooth, it acts to cross-splint the tooth. The wedging effect, subsequently leading to root fracture, is avoided.
- Ribbond post and core do not require additional preparation after root canal treatment, which eliminates possibility of root perforation.

d. Fiber Post with Gutta-percha

Fiberfill post system: The fiberfill system implies simultaneous obturation of the prepared root canal with the insertion of fiber reinforced post system. The system consists of an adhesive bonding agent, a light-curable calcium hydroxide based resin sealer and a fiber post with an apical terminus of gutta-percha. The primer in the system is a two-fold self-etching and priming liquid that allows the sealer to chemical bond to the root dentin. This system is time and cost-effective.

The main component and shape of some commercially available fiber posts are summarized in Table 22.1.

III. ALL CERAMIC POST

The major advantage of an all-ceramic post and core is its dentin like shade. The dentin like shade of ceramic postcore is related to the deeper diffusion and absorption of the transmitted light in the ceramic mass. All-ceramic restorations transmit a certain percentage of the incident light to the underlying core and post on

Table 22.1 Chemical composition and shape of routinely used fiber posts

Post (fiber)	*Main component*	*Shape*
Rely X Fiber Post (Glass fiber)	Resin matrix	Double tapered
FRC Post-Plus (Glass fiber)	UDMA, TEGDEMA, Ytterbium trifluoride, high dispersed silicon dioxide	Tapered
GC Fiber Post (Glass fiber)	Methacrylate	Double tapered
Light Post (Quartz fiber)	Epoxy resin	Double tapered
DT Light Post (Quartz fiber)	Epoxy resin	Double tapered
Macrolock Illusion Post (Quartz fiber)	Epoxy resin	Tapered, spiral head serrations
Radix Fiber Post (Zirconium enriched glass)	Epoxy resin	Double tapered
DT Light Safety Lock (Preconditioned quartz)	Epoxy resin	Double tapered
Dentin Post-X (Glass fiber)	Epoxy resin	Tapered
Snowpost (Zirconia-rich glass)	Epoxy resin	Cylindrical
Refor-post (Glass fiber)	BiS-GMA	Serrated
Fiber-Kleer-Serrated Post (Glass fiber)	BiS-GMA, UDMA, HDDMA	Serrated
Composi-post (Carbon fiber)	Epoxy resin	Two-stage parallel

which it has been placed. Thus, with all-ceramic posts and cores, the color of the final restoration will be derived from an internal shade of the ceramic post, similar to the optical behavior of the natural teeth. In addition, a ceramic post does not reflect intensively through thin gingival tissues, and provides translucency in the cervical root areas. All-ceramic posts and cores provide an excellent biocompatibility and do not exhibit galvanic corrosion.

The main obstacles for using ceramics, as post and core materials are their low flexural strength and toughness. High toughness ceramics, such as the glass infiltrated alumina ceramic, In-ceram, and the dense sintered alumina ceramic, show a three to six times higher flexural strength and toughness than do conventional feldspathic and glass ceramics (compost: available in two sizes; 1.4 and 1.7 mm). Contemporary zirconia powder technology contributes to the fabrication of new biocompatible ceramic materials with improved mechanical properties, i.e. further increase in flexural strength and toughness. The zirconium oxide ceramic have shown promising results for the fabrication of all-ceramic posts and cores.

Zirconium has several advantages over other ceramics owing to fundamental differences in their physical properties (ZiReal post is Zirconia ceramic with a small titanium insert at the apical part). Zirconia posts usually have smooth configuration without any serrations or threads. It is not possible to build a core of ceramic onto the zirconia ceramic post. Ceramic cores are fabricated indirectly and luted over the protruded end of the root.

The ceramic posts are inherently brittle. It is difficult to remove a fractured ceramic post. The modulus of elasticity of these posts is equal to metals, which make the post stiffer. The stiffer post produces more stresses.

Advantages

- Radiopaque
- Stiff and rigid
- Resistance to corrosion
- Biocompatible
- Esthetically pleasing (superior to metal posts).

Disadvantages

- Brittle
- Removal is difficult during retreatment
- Produce stresses, being stiff
- Not etchable (impossible to grind away the post)
- Core retention difficult; not possible to bond composite core material to post
- Weaker than metal posts
- Thicker posts (require additional removal of dentin)
- Bonding with root dentin may not be adequate.

22

IV. DENTIN POSTS (BIOLOGICAL POST)

The dentin post is a newer concept in which the post is fabricated from the root dentin of the stored extracted teeth. The extracted teeth, preferably incisors or single rooted, are stored in Hank's solution or other storage medium. The root canal of the tooth to be restored is prepared in routine. The cementum of the stored tooth is grinded by copy milling technique preferably to have two dentin posts; alternatively, the canal of the extracted tooth is filled with composite and the cementum is grinded to have single post (Fig. 22.35a and b). The shape of the post is fabricated according to the configuration of the prepared canal. The silicone impression of the prepared canal guides the fabrication of the dentin post. The post is finally luted into the root

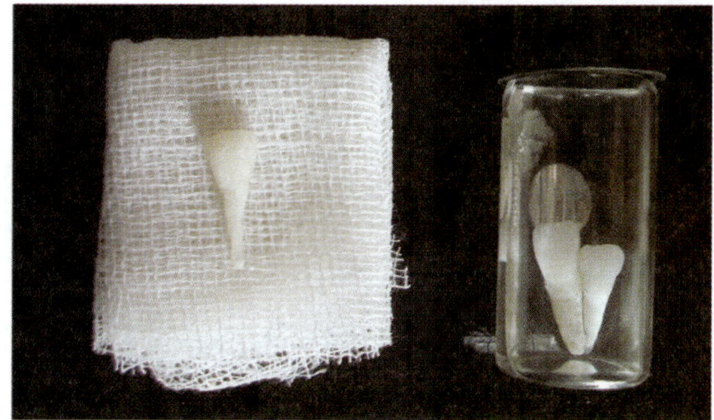

Fig. 22.35a Cementum removed and tooth stored

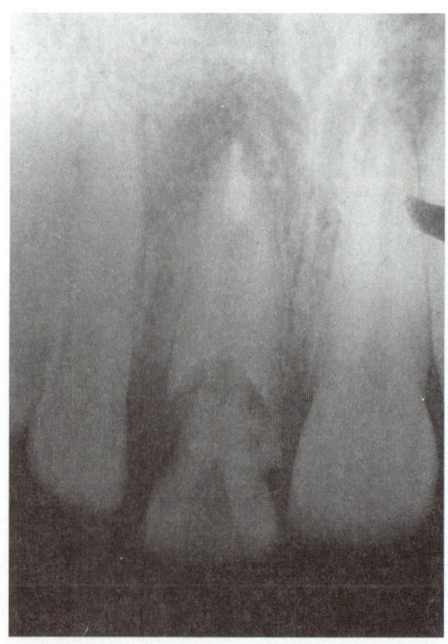

Fig. 22.35b Radiograph showing dentin post

canal using adhesive luting agents. The core portion can be fabricated with composites and finally restored with full veneer crowns.

The dentin posts have successfully been tried in deciduous teeth and are also showing promising results in permanent teeth.

V. INTRARADICULAR REHABILITATION WITH LIGHT TRANSMITTING PLASTIC POSTS

Occasionally, the post space presents a problem in routine postcore restorations, viz. flared canals, wider canal, internal resorption, and/or caries inside the root dentin. In such cases, the tooth is internally rebuilt with appropriate materials (composite, light cure glass-ionomer cement) to structurally reinforce the root to retain a post and core. A clear plastic light transmitting post is introduced, which can transmit light to polymerize composite resin placed deeply. The composite acts as a dentinal substitute and rehabilitate the weakened roots.

The light transmitting posts are also indicated in case of caries in the root dentin or trauma to the immature incisors. The internal resorption or any other mis-adventure leading to such type of canal configuration, warrant the use of light transmitting posts.

Technique

The light transmitting plastic post (Luminex light transmitting post) is selected according to the internal configuration of the root canal. The post is tried and adjusted in length. The internal root dentin is acid etched, rinsed and dried. A dual cured bonding agent is applied inside the root, air blown to make it uniform and cured. A microhybrid composite is injected into the canal and the light transmitted post is pushed into the uncured composite resin to its full depth. The light transmitting post allows the passage of light through its body but does not bond to the composite material. A hemostat is used to rotate and remove the light transmitting post, leaving an ideal shape for post-placement. Lucent anchor post of same matching size can then be inserted and cured in routine.

VI. MISCELLANEOUS SYSTEM

a. Two Piece Custom Post (Split Cast Metal Post and Core)

For the restoration of anterior teeth and premolars having straight canals, a single piece cast post is usually used along with core of same alloy or any core material. However, in case of molars or the key abutment teeth, which require more resistance and retention form, two-piece post is recommended. Because of the divergent roots in molars, fabrication of a single piece post and core is difficult. Therefore, a core with two or three posts should be employed. The postcore for a mandibular molar is usually divided into mesial and distal segments (Fig. 22.36a to j). The maxillary molar postcore is composed of labial and palatal components. The two piece system is also known as 'split cast metal post and core'.

The two-pieces must be bound together and remain stable after insertion. The core can be made in two halves held together by interlocking keys and key holes (interlocking is created by cutting a keyway/dovetail in one-half of core pattern).

b. Post-Inlay System

Many a times, teeth restored with crown may require endodontic treatment. Removing the crown may lead to fracture of the coronal portion of tooth or the crown or both. Long span bridges also pose difficulty in removal. In such cases, it becomes mandatory to initiate root canal treatment through the cast restoration.

An endodontic access through a crown is often larger because the crown obscures the morphology of the tooth and makes it difficult to locate the root canal.

After completion of the root canal treatment, the remaining unrestored part can be restored using prefabricated post along with appropriate cores or only the coronal part depending upon availability of the remaining dentin. The access cavity portion can also be restored as inlay along with custom post in one unit.

If a post with an attached inlay is fabricated, the combined restoration is retentive and also able to withstand laterally directed forces.

Because this restoration is a combination of a post and an inlay, it is designated as 'post-inlay' system.

Postretrievability (removal of post during retreatment)

The removal of post during retreatment of endodontically treated teeth always present great difficulties because of risk of fracture/perforation of the root, especially when the remaining root dentin is less. However, with the recent technical advances, these sequelae have been minimized.

The features which influence removal of posts are:

- It is easier to remove tapering post than parallel. Similarly, passive post is easier to remove than active post.
- The resins cement and glass-ionomer cement, being more retentive, pose difficulty in removal than zinc phosphate cement and zinc oxide eugenol cement.
- In case the coronal end of post lies above the orifice of the root canal, the removal is easy.

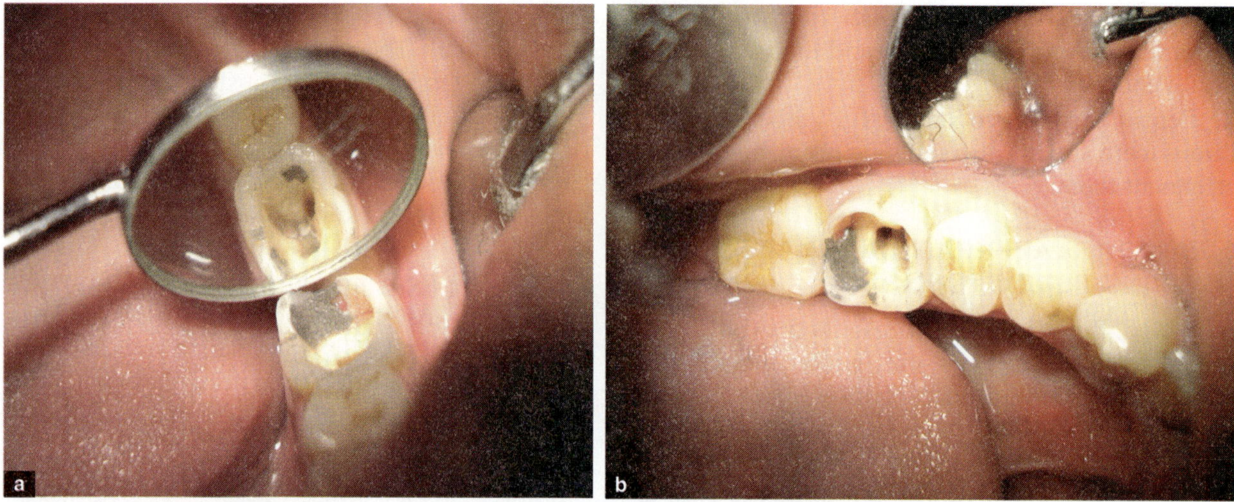

Fig. 22.36a and b Postspace preparation of the mesiobuccal and distal canals

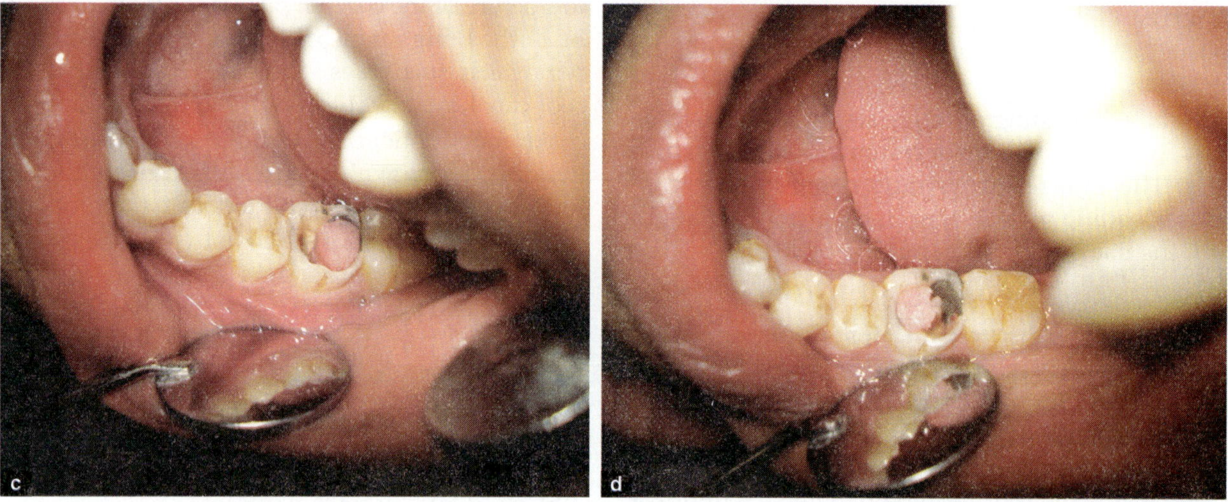

Fig. 22.36c and d Post patterns for mesiobuccal and distal inside the canals

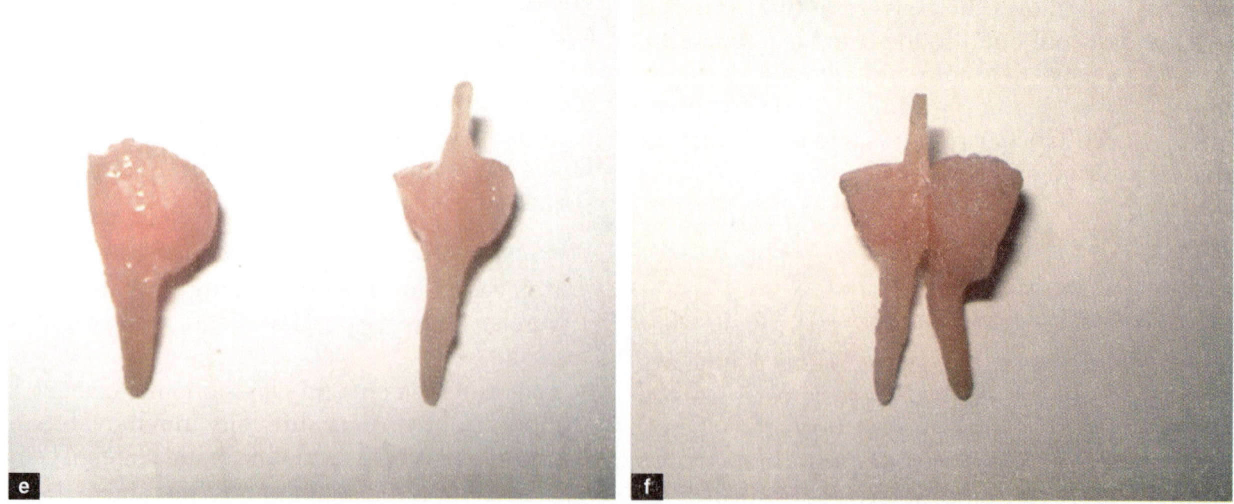

Fig. 22.36e and f Post patterns for mesiobuccal and distal

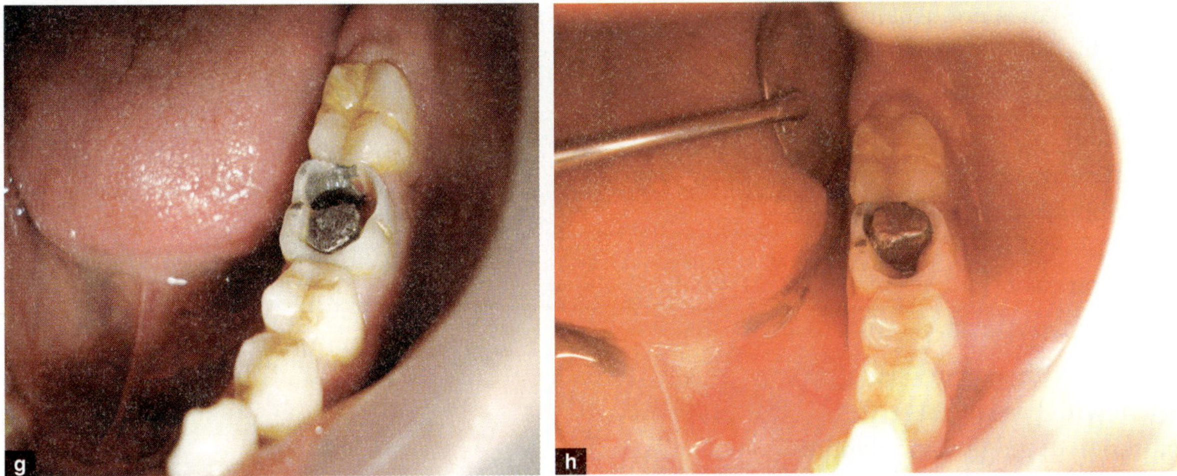

Fig. 22.36g and h Adjusted mesiobuccal and distal post

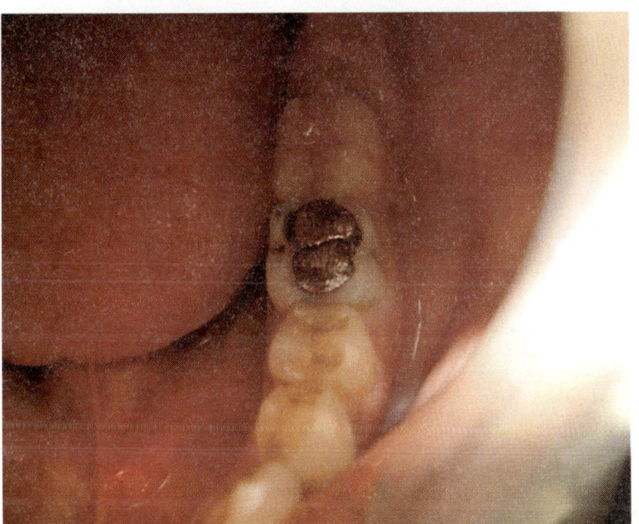

Fig. 22.36i Cementation of the post

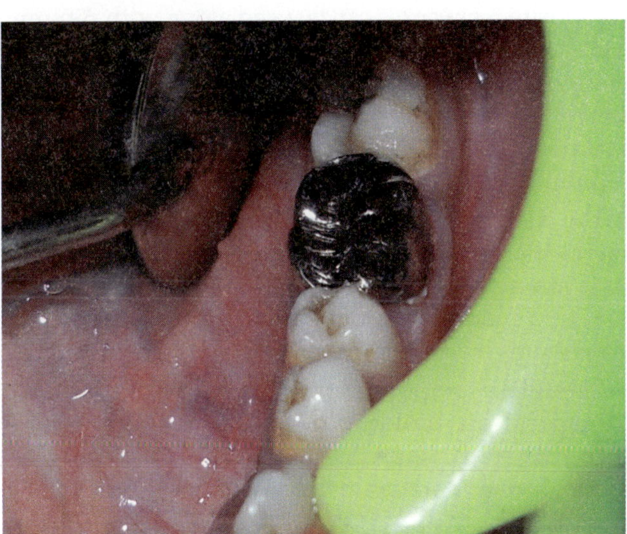

Fig. 22.36j Cast metal crown

- Fiber posts are easy to remove; metal posts and ceramic are difficult to remove.

The details of postremoval techniques are described in Chapter 36.

CORES

It is established that every endodontically treated tooth may not require a post. Most of the teeth, especially the molars can be successfully restored without a post. The remaining tooth structure usually supports the core, which is sufficient to withstand the occlusal forces.

The post is considered when the remaining tooth structure is not sufficient to support the core. Many a times, the cusps are destroyed and/or undermining of cusps warrants the use of posts along with core.

Various materials have been used and are being used as core without a post or along with the post. The commonly used materials are:

a. Amalgam

Amalgam was the most preferred core material; however, over the years, especially with the increasing popularity of all-ceramic crowns, it is no longer preferred. Pins are indicated for anchoring amalgam in teeth with extensive coronal damage. Amalgam pin cores are usually not employed for teeth where the appropriate dentin is not available.

A coronal radicular amalgam postcore has also been employed; the pulp chamber along with 2.0–4.0 mm of each canal is filled with amalgam (amalgapin used as secondary retentive devices). The bulk of amalgam is utilized for strength and retention.

The amalgam cores are usually given under metal crowns or metal ceramic crowns.

Advantages

- Reduced marginal leakage
- Better dimensional stability
- Good compressive strength
- Good modulus of elasticity
- Manipulation easy.

Disadvantages

- Safety issues with mercury use
- Corrosion with base metals
- Discoloration of gingiva and dentin.

b. Composite Resin

Composite resin cores can be used along with pins and posts as well. They are quite strong and easy to manipulate. The resin adapts well to retentive pins and possesses as much tensile strength as amalgam cores. Composites cores are recommended in teeth with minimum tooth structure loss (Fig. 22.37a and b).

The disadvantage with composite core is that the microleakage is greater than amalgam cores. Tensile bond strength for cast crowns is less during cementation; however, the retentive capacity is adequate. The crown margins should extend well past core margins.

Lumiglass composite has been tried as core material. Lumiglass core build-up composite is formulated to optimize with fiber posts. Light cure Lumiglass is translucent, and can be cured up to 8.0 mm thickness.

Lumiglass exhibits good handling characteristic for easy manipulation. It is radiopaque, and has better physical properties. The esthetic neutral shade is ideal for use with all-ceramic crowns.

Advantages

- Easy manipulation
- Good compressive strength
- Rapid/deep polymerization.

Disadvantages

- Poor dimensional stability
- Polymerization shrinkage.

c. Glass-ionomer Cement

Glass-ionomer cement has also been used as core material. It is preferred in cases where caries susceptibility is high and also in teeth with minimal tooth structure left. However, it is avoided in teeth under lateral load.

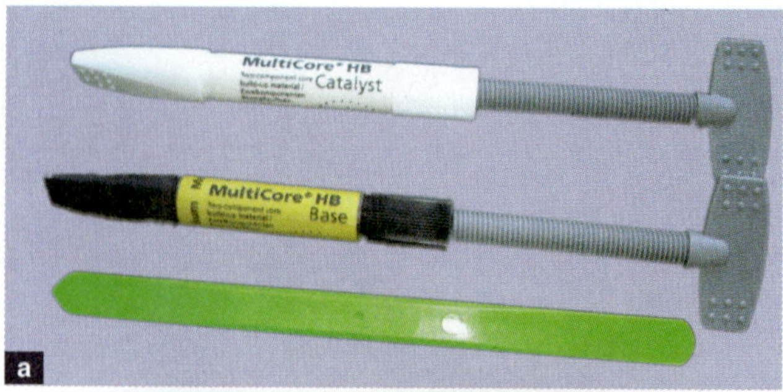

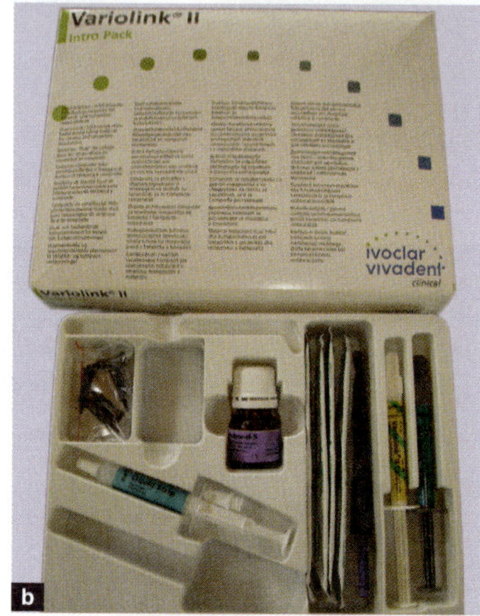

Fig. 22.37a and b Composite core material

Advantages

- Adhesive (chemical bonding with tooth)
- Anticariogenic
- Manipulation easy.

Disadvantages

- Low resistance to fracture
- Sensitive to moisture
- Solubility
- Low strength (fracture toughness).

d. Glass-cermet Cement

A combination of glass-ionomer cement and silver alloy in the ratio of 7 : 1 has been used as a core material. The glass-cermet cement possesses all the mechanical properties required for core and additionally helps in caries reduction by releasing fluorides. However, the black color of the glass-cermet limit its use only under metal crown or metal-ceramic crowns.

e. Resin modified Glass-ionomer Cement

Composite resin in combination of glass-ionomer cement has also been used as core material.

Advantages

- Anticariogenic
- Sufficient strength for smaller cores
- Good bonding
- Minimal microleakage.

Disadvantage

- Expansion of cement may displace crown.

ENDOCROWN

Use of high-strength ceramics coupled with adhesive technology has resulted in restorative treatment modality for posterior teeth without the use of post and core. The term 'endocrown' was coined to describe a ceramic crown extending into the pulp chamber/root canal orifices of the endodontically treated teeth in order to gain retention.

Endocrown is indicated for teeth with short clinical crowns or calcified/curved canals where postcore restoration is not feasible. These are also indicated in patients having limited interocclusal space, not providing adequate thickness for both the ceramic veneer and the metal/ceramic core framework.

It is established that endocrowns exhibit superior (higher) fracture strength than conventional postcore crowns.

Initially, endocrowns were fabricated using reinforced, acid etchable ceramics because they provide adequate mechanical strength to withstand occlusal load (ceramic reinforced with lithium disilicate provide high mechanical strength, excellent adhesion, and good esthetics).

Advantages of Endocrowns

- Short preparation time
- Less chair time
- Easy manipulation
- Esthetically pleasing
- Cost-effective.

A composite resin foundation along with indirect composite resin crown has also been tried. Recently, a high performance polymer, **polyetheretherketone (PEEK)** containing 20% ceramic filler has shown promising results. The material exhibits superior mechanical properties and is biocompatible.

Advantages of PEEK

- Better modulus of elasticity (4 GPa—as elastic as bone); act as stress breaker, dissipating occlusal load uniformly to tooth and the root.
- Good wear resistance
- Polishability is good (not in oral cavity after occlusal adjustments)
- Elimination of allergic reactions
- Good adhesive properties
- Radiolucent; facilitate caries detection.

Indirect composite resin over this material also act as stress breaker and reduce the occlusal load.

Endocrown using PEEK materials have shown good retention and without any microleakage. The esthetic appearance is equal to ceramics; however, intraoral occlusal adjustments may lead to unesthetic appearance.

RESTORATION OF TEETH AFTER ROOT AMPUTATION

In hemisection and radisectomy procedures, one root is extracted and the other root(s) along with the trunk (mostly) is utilized for restoration purposes (Fig. 22.38a to e).

Indications for root amputation are:

- Severe periodontal involvement of the single root
- Severe furcation involvement
- Severe root caries/resorption inside the root, which cannot be treated
- Endodontically unmanaged root (e.g. instrument fracture, perforation, etc.)

The restoration protocol differs in mandibular and maxillary molars.

Restoring Mandibular Molar

In mandibular molars, either mesial or distal root is retained.

a. *Retaining distal root*: In case the distal root is retained, it is advantageous being straight, has the widest canal and can accommodate the deepest post. Being posteriorly placed, it provides a greater arch length. It is wider in a buccolingual than mesiodistal direction and is handled like a bicuspid in its preparation for post and core. When the distal root has two canals, the distobuccal canal is usually the larger and should receive the post. The orifice is widened buccolingually to avoid perforation.
b. *Retaining mesial root*: In case the mesial root is retained, the straighter mesial canal (mesiolingual canal) is prepared to hold a single post. Additional retention may be gained by using a small preparation at the orifice of the unused canal. This also provides antirotational device for the post and core preparation. Because of the curved nature of these canals, care must be exercised not to make the posts so long that they deviate from the prepared canal space and lead to perforation. Both mesial canals can be used for twin posts. They must be parallel in the cervical third of canal, if a cast post is used but can deviate if fiber posts are used. Total retention is equal to the sum of post lengths. The root is treated as a bicuspid

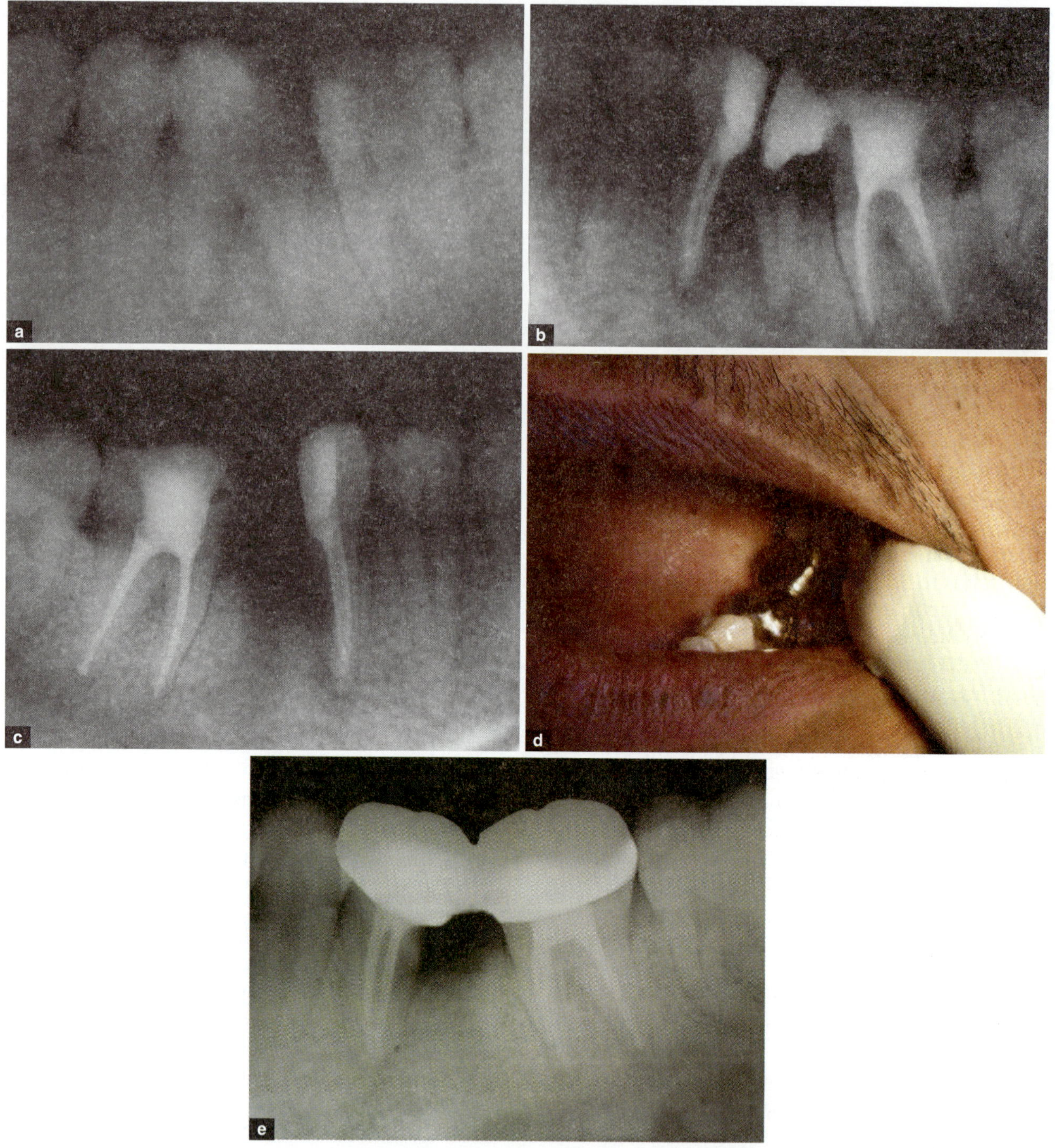

Fig. 22.38 Hemisection of mandibular first molar: (a) Preoperative: badly mutilated mandibular first molar; (b) Hemisection of molar; (c) Extraction of distal root; (d) Restoration with cast metal crown; (e) Radiograph showing final restoration (postoperative)

and is prepared along with the adjacent tooth to receive a restoration in a bridge form.

c. *Bisecting mesial and distal roots (retaining both)*: In case both the roots are retained, it is usually not possible to create a satisfactory environment for future cleaning around both the roots. The two roots are usually not divergent enough to gain a sizeable interproximal space where the furcation has been located. Minor orthodontic tooth movement can be helpful.

The recontouring is usually accomplished in two phases:

i. Initial contouring when the amputation is performed
ii. Final contouring during tooth preparation for crown fabrication.

The recontouring is mainly completed in first phase. The line angles are blended smoothly. Sharp projections or spurs are eliminated. The interproximal areas between the amputated root and adjacent tooth must be kept open to allow for optimal plaque control. The furcation area should be fluted to allow for proper tissue adaptation.

In the final phase of recontouring, the occlusal table should be narrowed and the excursive contacts should be eliminated.

Restoring Maxillary Molar

In maxillary molars, the root which most commonly needs extraction is the mesiobuccal root. The other roots are usually managed clinically. However, in certain cases distobuccal root is also extracted along with the mesiobuccal (palatal root is to be preserved for post and core restoration).

a. ***Retaining distobuccal and palatal roots***: The channel for post is prepared in the palatal root. The areas adjacent to the retained roots is critical because the trifurcation formed by the missing and remaining roots may pose clinical difficulties. This area is prepared to prevent the residual furcation from acting as a shelf for plaque accumulation.

The preparation at the gingival margin resembles a figure eight shape as the preparation is beveled in the furcation area between the remaining two roots. The shape of the final restoration at the gingival margin will depend on the horizontal depth of the concavity created between the two roots. Flat contours with mild concavities are preferred. The final coronal restoration should have an occlusal configuration similar to that of a molar but with the mesiobuccal or distobuccal portion reduced to lessen the occlusal stress where no root is present. At the gingival margin there is a large embrasure where the amputated root was formerly present.

b. ***Retaining palatal root only***: Sometimes, both the buccal roots are extracted and only palatal is retained. The palatal root is the widest of the maxillary roots and circumferential concavities on palatal roots are far more subtle than concavities on the other maxillary roots. The single remaining root must be used in conjunction with another tooth/teeth, since, it is not strong enough to function alone. The natural buccal curvature of the palatal root creates a severe undercut on its straight buccal surface. A beveled shoulder preparation of the buccal surface of the palatal root is required to parallel it with adjacent teeth and allow preparation of the undercut margin. The restoration must be narrow buccolingually, which may place the occlusal table in a cross-bite relation.

CEMENTATION OF POSTENDODONTIC RESTORATIONS

The postcore restorations and the indirect restorations (onlays, full veneer crowns) are to be cemented over the cores prepared for such restorations. A variety of luting agents are available with varied advantages and disadvantages. The commonly used luting agents are:

- Zinc phosphate cement
- Polycarboxylate cement
- Glass-ionomer cements
- Resin modified glass-ionomer cements
- Resin cements.

Requirements of a luting agent

The requirements of a luting agent are:

- *Wettability*: Seals the gap between restoration and the tooth surface.
- *Film thickness*: An ideal film thickness is considered as 25 μ; depends upon viscosity of the liquid.
- *Flow*: Ability to move into minor intricacies filling the gaps; lower powder: Liquid ratio enhances flow.
- *Dissolution in oral fluids*: Dissolution lead to marginal leakage; resin cements are less soluble followed by glass-ionomer cements.
- Should be biocompatible.
- Should be radiopaque.
- Sufficient strength to resist long-term fatigue stress at the margins.
- *Wear resistance*: May lead to caries and unesthetic appearance, if cement do not resist wear at the tooth-restoration interface.
- *Overhang control*: Extra cement is to be cleaned without disturbing the presence of luting agent at the margins.

Clinical Aspects

The clinical aspect of cementation is important as many factors play part in successful cementation of the restorations. The cementation procedure is divided into two:

a. Seating
b. Retention

a. *Seating*

The discrepancies in the prepared tooth and the castings coupled with cementing pressure lead to rebound of restoration. These discrepancies are to be compensated for proper seating of the restoration. The best method is to coat the die with multiple coats of die-spacer. Alternatively relieving the die or etching the casting can be helpful.

In seating the cemented restoration, the following features play important role.

i. Rheology of cement
ii. Working time
iii. Final film thickness
iv. Geometry of gap.

The failure usually occurs at cement-tooth interface. The flow of cement is the key factor for successfully cementing the restorations. To achieve sufficient cement flow, it is to be loaded rapidly and steadily maintained, until cement is set. The seating of restorations should be completed within a few seconds while the cement is sufficiently fluid.

The correct mix of zinc phosphate, polycarboxylate and ethoxy-benzoic acid cements has adequate flow with moderate pressure. The resin cements are less satisfactory in this respect.

The zinc oxide eugenol cement generates the lowest hydraulic pressures during seating, followed by polycarboxylate cement. Zinc phosphate cement exhibited the greatest hydraulic pressure. The tendency of rebound will not occur in case the seating force is maintained for sufficient time without any interruption while the cement is setting.

Mixing on a cool glass slab provide adequate working time.

The excess of cement is to be removed. In case of postcore preparation, a sort of path is created, known as *'venting'* which facilitates easy removal of cement and minimize the hydraulic pressure. Venting also provide minimal film thickness under cast restorations.

All cements have overhang after seating of the crowns or other indirect restorations (Fig. 22.39a and b). The criteria of time as regard removal of the overhang are very important. The 'cleaning' of set zinc phosphate and polycarboxylate cements is comparatively easier than glass-ionomers, composites and dual-cure cements. In such cases the 'cleaning' is carried out before the cement is set completely, i.e. partly set cements. Once the 'extra' cement is cleaned from all the sides, the patient is again asked to press the restoration. The pressing of restoration will fill the gaps between the tooth and restoration, if any. Once the cement is set, the probe should not be touched at the margins. Use of probe will remove the set cement, subsequently leaving the gap for caries and sensitivity (Fig. 22.40). The low viscosity luting agents should be used under easily accessible margins. Recently, the trend of using luting agents, which change color after setting is gaining importance. However, it is opined that such color may damage the overall esthetic nature of certain restorations.

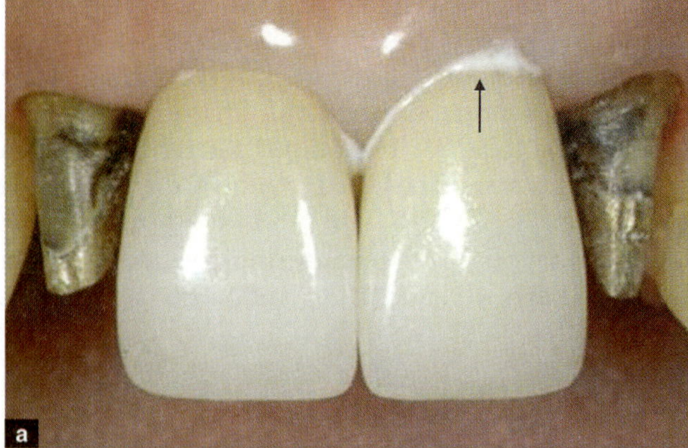

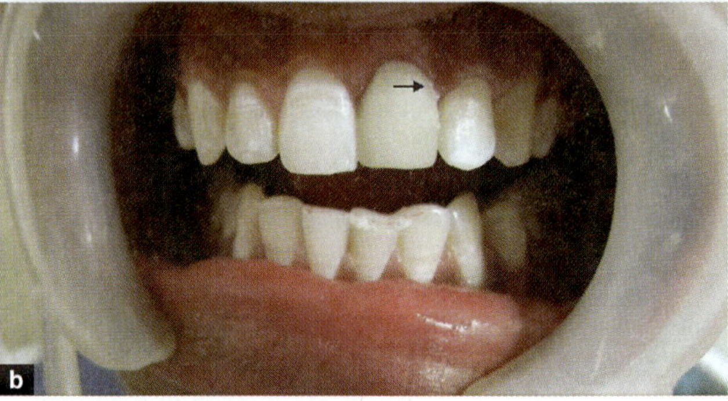

Fig. 22.39 (a) Extra cement at the cervical end; (b) Overhanging cement at the distal cervical area

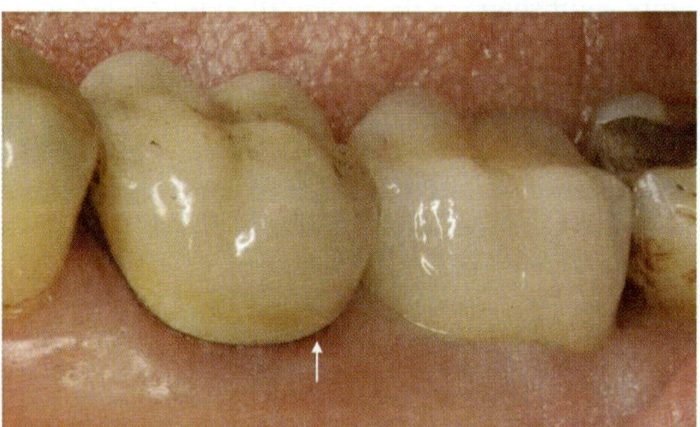

Fig. 22.40 Gap at the tooth-restoration interface

b. *Retention*

The luting agents do not help in retention directly; however, the tensile strength of the cement does aid in longevity of the restoration.

The retention of the restoration mainly depends upon the following:

i. The design of the tooth preparation, which in turn influences the stress distribution.
ii. Bonding efficiency of the luting cement to both the surfaces, i.e. tooth and the restoration.

iii. Durability of the cement, which includes its long-term resistance to mechanical breakdown and dissolution.

All cements are weak in tensile strength, thereby providing very little retention. It is recommended that the cement with a high tensile strength be used to cement crowns and long span bridges since shear stresses in marginal area can exceed the strength of cement.

Viscoelastic behavior and modulus of elasticity are also important features. Dentin exhibits viscoelastic behavior with a significant plastic deformation during fracture, which appears to be greater than that for the zinc phosphate and glass-ionomer cement. And also the modulus of elasticity of dentin in compression is slightly greater than that of zinc phosphate cements. The bonding of luting cements influence the stress transference between the cement, restoration and the tooth substrate.

BIBLIOGRAPHY

1. Abduljawad M, Samran A, Kadour J, Al-Afandi M, Ghazal M, Kern M and Habil MD. Effect of fiber posts on the fracture resistance of endodontically treated anterior teeth with cervical cavities: An *in vitro* study. J. Prosthet. Dent.: 2016; 116:80–84.
2. Abu Kasim NH, Madfa AA, Hamdi M and Rahbari GR. 3D-FE analysis of functionally graded structured dental posts. Dent. Mater.: 2011; 30:869–880.
3. Angerame D, De Biasi M, Cattaruzza M, Franco V, Turco G, Filingeri I, Zarone F and Sorrentino R. Resistance of endodontically treated roots restored with different fibre post systems with or without post space preparation: *in vitro* analysis and SEM investigation. Giornale Italiano di Endodonzia: 2016; 30:111–119.
4. Bandeca M, El-Mowafy O, Shebl A and Poro-Neto S. Non-metallic post endodontic restoration: a systematic review. Int. J. Dent.: 2010; 9:57–62.
5. Barcellos RR, Correia DP, Farina AP, Mesquita MF, Ferraz CC and Cecchin D. Fracture resistance of endodontically treated teeth restored with intra-radicular post: the effects of post system and dentine thickness. J. Biomech.: 2013; 46:2572–2577.
6. Bitter K and Kilebassa M. Post-endodontic restorations with adhesively luted fiber-reinforced composite post systems: A review. Am. J. Dent.: 2007; 20:353–360.
7. Brodbeck U. The Zi Real post: A new ceramic implant abutment. J. Esthet. Rest. Dent.: 2003; 15:10–23.
8. Brown PL and Hicks NL. Rehabilitation of endodontically treated teeth using the radiopaque fiber post. Compendium: 2003; 24:275–278.
9. Cagidiaco MC, Goracci C, Garcia-Godoy F and Ferrari M. Clinical studies of fiber posts: a literature review. Int. J. Prosthodont.: 2008; 21:328–336.
10. Cheron RA, Marshall SJ, Goodis HE and Peters OA. Nanomechanical properties of endodontically treated teeth. J. Endod.: 2011; 37:1562–1565.
11. Chieruzzi M, Pagano S, Cianetti S, Lombardo G, Kenny JM and Torre L. Effect of fibre posts, bone losses and fibre content on the biomechanical behaviour of endodontically treated teeth: 3D-finite element analysis. Mat. Sci. and Engg. C.: 2017; 74:334–346.
12. Chopra D, Singh NSK and Nehete P. Split cast metal post and core. J. Orofac. Res.: 2012; 2:95–98.
13. Daleprane B, Pereira CNB, Bueno AC, Ferreira RC, Moreira AN and Magalhaes CS. Bond strength of fiber posts to the root canal: Effects of anatomic root levels and resin cements. J. Prosthet. Dent.: 2016; 116:416–424.
14. Dietschi D, Duc O, Krejci I and Sadan A. Biomechanical considerations for the restoration of endodontically treated teeth: a systematic review of the literature – part 1: composition and micro- and macrostructure alterations. Quint. Int.: 2007; 38:733–743.
15. Eliyas S, Jalili J and Martin N. Restoration of the root canal treated teeth. Br. Dent. J.: 2015; 218:53–62.
16. Fishelberg G. Clinical response to a vacant post space. Int. Endod. J.: 2004; 37:199–204.
17. Furtos g, Baldea B and Dumitrescu LS. Development of new radiopaque glass fiber posts. Mat. Sci. and Engg. C: 2016; 59:855–862.
18. Gao H, Zhang ZT, Fan L, Wang DS, Zuo HJ and Sheng Y. Development of novel polyimide composite core materials reinforced with carbon fibres. Chinese J. Prosthodont.: 2007; 3:210–212.
19. Gegauff AG. Effect of crown lengthening and ferrule placement on static load failure of cemented cast post cores and crowns. J. Prosth. Dent.: 2000; 84:169–179.
20. Giachetti L, Scaminaci RD, Baldini M, Bertini F, Steier L and Ferrari M. Push-out strength of translucent fiber posts cemented using a dual-curing technique or a light-curing self-adhering material. Int. Endod. J.: 2012; 45:249–256.
21. Goracci C, Corciolani G, Vichi A and Ferrari M. Light-transmitting ability of marketed fiber posts. J. Dent. Res.: 2008; 87:1122–1126.
22. Goracci, C. and Ferrari, M. Current prospective on post systems: a literature review. Aust. Dent. J.: 2011; 56: 77–83.
23. Grande N, Butti A, Plotino G and Somma F. Adapting fiber-reinforced composite root canal post for use in non-circular shaped canals. Pract. Proced. Aesthet. Dent.: 2006; 18:593–599.
24. Grossmann Y and Sadan A. The prosthodontic concept of crown-to-root ratio: A review of literature. J. Prosth. Dent.: 2005; 93:559–562.
25. Guldener KA, Lanzrein CL, Guldener BE, Lang NP, Ramseier CA and Salvi GE. Long-term clinical outcomes of endodontically treated teeth restored with or without fiber post-retained single-unit restorations. J. Endod.: 2017; 43:188–193.
26. Hashim NS, Moaleem MM and Al-attas H. Tooth colored post system: review of literature. IJCD: 2013; 4:50–56.
27. Hayashi M and Ebisu S. Key factors in achieving firm adhesion in post-core restorations. Jap. Dent. Sci. Review: 2008; 44:22–28.
28. Jhavar N, Bhondwe S, Mahajan V and Dhoot R. Recent advances in post systems: a review. J. Appl. Dent. Med. Sci.: 2015; 1:128–136.
29. Juloski J, Gorraci C, Radovic I, Chieffi N, Vichi A and Vulicevic ZR. Post-retentive ability of new flowable resin composites. Am. J. Dent.: 2013; 26:324–328.

30. Juloski J, Radovic I, Gracci C, Vulicevic ZR and Ferrari M. Ferrule effect: a literature review. J. Endod.: 2012; 38:11–19.
31. King PA, Setchell DJ and Rees JS. Clinical evaluation of a carbon fiber reinforced endodontic post. J. Oral Rehab.: 2003; 30:785–789.
32. Koutayas S and Matthias K. All ceramic post and cores: The state of the art. Quint. Int.: 1999; 30:383–392.
33. Kumar M, Chauhan A, Olepu S and Sharma A. Advances in post systems—Pit and falls to avoid. Asian J. Sci. Tech.: 2014; 5:625–627.
34. Lamichhane A, Xu C and Zhang F. Dental fiber-post resin base material: a review. J. Adv. Prosthodont.: 2014; 6:60–65.
35. Lander E and Dietschi D. Endocrowns: a clinical report. Quint. Int.: 2008; 39:99–106.
36. Liaw DJ, Wang KL, Huang YC, Lee KR, Lai JY and Ha CS. Advanced polyimide materials: Syntheses, physical properties and applications. Prog. Polym. Sci.: 2012; 37:907–974.
37. Lindblad RM, Lassila LV, Salo V, Vallittu PK and Tjaderhane L. Effect of chlorhexidine on initial adhesion of fiber-reinforced post to root canal. J. Dent.: 2010; 38:796–801.
38. Lopes GC, Baratieri LN, Caldeira de Andrada MA and Maia HP. All-ceramic post, core, and crown: technique and case report. J. Esthet. Restor. Dent.: 2001; 13:285–295.
39. Mahasneh SA, Horner K, Cunliffe J, Al-Saehi S, Sengupta A and AlHadidi A.: Guidelines on radiographic imaging as part of root canal treatment: a systematic review with a focus on review imaging after treatment. Int. Endod. J.:2018; 51:e238-e249.
40. Mannocci F, Sherriff M, Watson TF and Vallittu PK. Penetration of bonding resins into fibre-reinforced posts: A confocal microscopic study. Int. J. Endodont.: 2005; 38:46–51.
41. Maroli A, Hoelcher KAL, Reginato VF, Spazzin AO, Caldas RA and Bacchi A. Biomechanical behavior of teeth without remaining coronal structure restored with different post designs and materials. Mat. Sci. and Engg. C.: 2017; 76:839–844.
42. Michalakis K, Hirayama H, Sfolkos J and Sfolkos K. Light transmission of posts and cores used for anterior esthetic region. Int. J. Periodontics and Rest. Dent.: 2004; 24:462–469.
43. Naumann M, Preuss A and Frankenberger R. Reinforcement effect of adhesively luted fiber reinforced composite versus titanium posts. Dent. Mater.: 2007; 23:138–144.
44. Northdurft FP and Pospiech PR. Clinical evaluation of pulpless teeth restored with conventionally cemented zirconia posts: a pilot study. J. Prosth. Dent.: 2006; 95:311–314.
45. Ozkurt Z and Kazazoglu IU. Zirconia ceramic post systems: a literature review and a case report. Dent. Mater.: 2010; 29:233–245.
46. Plotino G, Grande NM, Pameijer CH and Somma F. Influence of surface remodeling using burs on the macro and micro surface morphology of anatomically formed fiber posts. Int. Endod. J.: 2008; 41:345–355.
47. Poggio C, Chiesa M, Lombardini M and Dagna A. Influence of ethanol dying on the bond between fiber posts and root canals: SEM analysis. Quint. Int.: 2011; 42:e15–21.
48. Radovic I, Monticelli F, Goracci C, Vulicevic ZR and Ferrari M. Self-adhesive resin cements: a literature review. J. Adhes. Dent.: 2008; 10:251–258.
49. Rayyan MR, Aldossari RA, Alsadun SF and Hijazy FR. Accuracy of cast posts fabricated by the direct and indirect techniques. J. Prosthet. Dent.: 2016; 116:411–415.
50. Sadak FT, Monticelli F, Goracci C, Tay FR, Cardoso PE and Ferrari M. Bond strength performance of different resin composites used as core material around fiber posts. Dent. Mater.: 2007; 23, 95–99.
51. Sahafi A, Pentzfeldt A, Asmussen E and Gotfredson K. Effect of surface treatment of prefabricated posts on bonding of resin cement. Oper. Dent.: 2004; 29:60–68.
52. Sarkis-Onofre R, Fergusson D, Cenci MS, Moher D and Pereira-Cenci T. Performance of post-retained single crowns: A systematic review of related risk factors. J. Endod.: 2017; 43:175–183.
53. Sedgley CM and Messer HH. Are endodontically treated teeth more brittle? J. Endod.: 1992; 18:332–335.
54. Shamseddine L and Chaaban F. Impact of a core ferrule design on fracture resistance of teeth restored with cast post and core. Adv. In Medicine: 2016; Article ID5073459.
55. Slutzky-Goldberg I, Slutzky H, Gorfil C and Smidt A. Restoration of endodontically treated teeth: review and treatment recommendations. Int. J. Dent.: 2009; 1–9, Art.ID 150251.
56. Stankiewicz NR and Wilson PR. The ferrule effect: a literature review. Int. J. Endod.: 2002; 35:575–581.
57. Sterzenbach G, Franke A and Naumann M. Rigid versus flexible dentine like endodontic posts—clinical testing of a biomechanical concept: Seven-year results of a randomized controlled clinical pilot trial on endodontically treated abutment teeth with severe hard tissue loss. J. Endod.: 2012; 38:1557–1563.
58. Streacker AB and Geissberger M. The milled ceramic post and core: A functional and esthetic alternative. J. Prosth. Dent.: 2007; 98:486–487.
59. Stylianou A, Burgess JO, Liu P, Givan DA and Lawson NC. Light-transmitting fiber optic posts: An *in vitro* evaluation. J. Prosthet. Dent.: 2017; 117:116–123.
60. Tang W, Wu Y and Smales RJ. Identifying and reducing risks for potential fractures in endodontically treated teeth. J. Endod.: 2010; 36:609–617.
61. Theodosopoulou JN and Chochlidakis KM. A systematic review of dowel (post) and core materials and systems. J. Prothodont.: 2009; 18:464–472.
62. Valea MC and de la Pena VA. Titanium posts and bonded amalgam core longevity: a 22 year clinical survival retrospective study. JADA: 2017; 148:75–80.
63. Vlahova A, Kissovy C, Kazukova R and Popova E. Masking the metal color of cast post-and-core restorations by metal ceramic caps: a clinical report. JSM Dent.: 2014; 2:1024.
64. Yalcin E, Cehrili MC and Canay S. Fracture resistances of cast metal and ceramic post and core restorations: a pilot study. J. Prosthet. Dent.: 2005; 14:84–90.
65. Zhu Z, Dong XY, He S, Pan X and Tang L. Effect of post placement on the restoration of endodontically treated teeth: a systematic review. Int. J. Prosthodont.: 2015; 28:475–483.
66. Zoidis P, Bakiri E and Polyzois G. Using modified polyetheretherketone (PEEK) as an alternative material for endocrown restorations: a short-term clinical report. J. Prosthet. Dent.: 2017; 117:335–339.

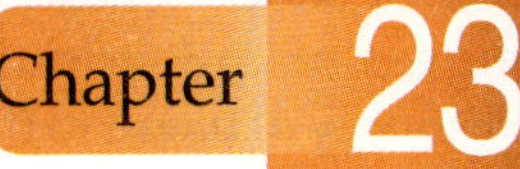

Endodontic Emergencies

The word 'emergency' literally means any condition which warrants immediate attention. Any biological condition usually of unforeseen and unscheduled occurrence, requiring immediate management is referred to as medical emergency. Endodontic emergency is defined as *'pathology (pain, swelling, fracture, avulsion, etc.) associated with pulp and periapical tissues, which need immediate attention (diagnosis and treatment) to provide relief to the patient.'* Pain in the oral cavity can have many causes although pulpal and periapical diseases are the most common. Due to confinement of the pulp tissue in dentin, nature of inflammatory response of pulp is more severe, leading to severe pain.

Prevalence of endodontic emergencies among all dental emergencies varied from 30 to 90%. The emergency is mainly the pain for which patient seeks immediate attention. The operator is to re-schedule the appointments to accommodate the emergency patient. The timely and quickly attention to such patients along with alleviating the pain builds confidence in the patient. The confidence so developed is useful in further planning and treating the problem.

CLASSIFICATION

The endodontic emergencies are classified as:

1. ***Pretreatment emergencies***
   a. Hyperreactive pulpalgia
      i. Dentinal hypersensitivity
      ii. Hyperemia
   b. Acute irreversible pulpitis
   c. Acute apical periodontitis
   d. Acute periradicular abscess
      i. Abscess without swelling
      ii. Abscess with localized fluctuant swelling
      iii. Abscess with localized non-fluctuant swelling
      iv. Abscess with diffuse swelling
   e. Crack tooth syndrome
   f. Tooth fracture
      i. Crown fracture
         - Enamel infraction
         - Uncomplicated crown fracture
         - Complicated crown fracture
      ii. Crown and root fracture
      iii. Root fracture
         - Transverse/horizontal root fracture
         - Vertical root fracture
   g. Luxation injuries
      i. Concussion
      ii. Subluxation
      iii. Extrusive luxation
      iv. Lateral luxation
      v. Intrusive luxation
   h. Avulsion.
2. ***Mid-treatment emergencies***
   a. Incomplete pulp tissue removal
   b. Apical periodontitis
      i. Due to over instrumentation
      ii. Due to chemical insult
   c. Phoenix abscess (mid-treatment flare up).
3. ***Post-treatment emergencies***
   a. Over instrumentation
   b. Over obturation/sealer extrusion
   c. High restoration
   d. Root fracture.

DIAGNOSIS

The initial and provisional diagnosis is achieved early since, the patient is in agony of pain and need immediate solution for the same. Pain must be considered in terms of quality (sharp, piercing, lancinating, dull, boring, gnawing and excruciating). The commencement, duration, provocation (hot, cold, chewing or biting, etc.), relief and localization of pain should also be noted. These characteristics of pain and any associated tenderness or swelling may be pathognomonic for specific conditions. The nature of the pain directs the operator to opt for either definitive treatment or palliative treatment.

The medical history facilitates identifying the risk patients (immunocompromised, hypertensive, allergic, diabetic, etc.) who may require a medical consultation, premedication or modification of the emergency treatment. Palpation and light percussion helps to identify periradicular inflammation. Periodontal probing and pulp vitality test helps in differentiating pain, which might be due to pulpal or periodontal origin. Response of patient on application of cold, heat, electricity and direct dentin stimulation usually indicate the status (vital or necrotic) of pulp. Additionally periapical and bitewing radiography may detect depth of caries, pulpal exposure, fracture, internal/external resorption, periradicular changes, etc.

1. Pretreatment Emergencies

a. Hyperreactive Pulpalgia

The sharp pain of short duration in the absence of pulpal inflammation is termed hyperreactive pulpalgia. This can be due to dentinal hypersensitivity or hyperemia.

i. *Dentinal hypersensitivity*: Patient complains of sharp and short duration pain, initiated due to contact of any thermal (usually cold), osmotic (sweet or sour), electrical (galvanic current on contact of two dissimilar metals) or physical (toothbrush, floss, interdental stimulator, fingernail or explorer) stimuli to the exposed dentin. Faulty brushing, curettage, usage of high abrasive toothpaste, cracks, etc. may lead to dentinal exposure. Clinically and radiographically, such abnormality is usually not detected.

Dentinal sensitivity is due to the movement of dentinal fluid leading to activation of nociceptors in the inner dentin or outer pulp.

Treatment

The treatment includes closure of open dentinal tubules and use of agents that inactivate pulpal nociceptors. The iontophoretic application of fluoride salts, complemented with fluoridated toothpastes and mouth washes, etc. help minimizing opening of dentinal tubules.

Excitability of pulpal axons can be reduced by potassium ions; use of toothpastes containing potassium facilitate early closure of dentinal tubules.

ii. *Hyperemia*: Patient complains of shock sensation which disappears on removal of the stimuli. Hyperemia implies increased supply of blood to the pulp; may be due to caries, leaky restorations, high restorations, finishing and polishing without coolant and also chemical cleaning of the cavity. Teeth are not tender to percussion except when occlusal trauma is a factor. Cold stimulates hyperemic pulp more readily than normal teeth. Radiographic examination reveals normal periodontal ligament space and lamina dura.

Treatment

- Causative factor is to be removed followed by palliative treatment.
- Occlusion should be checked; recontour the high points.
- Use pulp protection measures, such as, varnish, bonding agent, liner or bases under restorations.
- Placement of sedative dressing, such as, zinc oxide eugenol cement after removal of deep caries/any other irritant (usually from leakage).
- Microcracks, if detected and diagnosed, may be treated with bonding and flowable composites.

The pain gradually disappears once the causative factor is removed. However, if pain persists, pulpectomy should be performed.

b. Acute Irreversible Pulpitis

Irreversible pulpitis is defined as *'an inflammatory process in which the dental pulp has been damaged beyond repair.'* The classical symptoms of irreversible pulpitis are intermittent/spontaneous pain (not of short duration), which lingers on and does not resolve even after removal of the irritant. The pulpal pain may be sharp or dull, localized or referred, depending upon the type of nerve fibers involved. Pain is often worse during the night or on bending, because the recumbent position increases blood pressure in the pulp. Pulpal pain may be referred to adjacent teeth or even the teeth in opposing jaw. Occasionally, momentary relief may be provided by cold stimulus as vasoconstriction of the dilated vessels reduces pulpal tissue pressure. Since inflammation is mainly confined in the pulp, and periradicular changes might not be evident, the diagnosis of this condition becomes difficult. Pouring hot water on the isolated tooth may help in diagnosis. On electric pulp testing, less current may be required for response in early stages; whereas, more current is required when the tissue is necrosed. Differential diagnosis should be made between hyperemia and acute irreversible pulpitis, as the former is reversible but the latter is not.

Treatment

The preferred treatment modality is the root canal therapy. The emergency procedure may depend upon the stage of root formation (open or close apex) in both single and multirooted teeth.

- In case of close apex, root canal treatment is preferred (may be completed in single visit).
- In case of open apex, pulpotomy is preferred applying MTA or calcium hydroxide.
- In case of time constraints, emergency root canal opening (ERCO) is to be carried out followed by root canal treatment later.

c. Acute Apical Periodontitis

This is an acute inflammation of the periodontal ligament which may be associated with a vital or a non-vital tooth. Generally acute periodontitis is the extension of pulpal inflammation; however, traumatic occlusion, bruxism, sinusitis or orthodontic treatment may also lead to acute periodontitis. Rarely inflammatory reaction of the healing pulp may initiate periodontitis.

Signs and symptoms

Patient is presented with history of spontaneous, throbbing, sharp pain on exposure to thermal stimulus and persistence of pain following removal of stimulus. Classical manifestation is, heat causes intense pain, whereas cold relieves the pain. Tooth is tender on percussion (eating/biting on the affected side hurts).

Clinical examination reveals tenderness in the buccal sulcus on palpation. Presence of inflammatory exudates in the periodontal ligament causes elevation of tooth from within the socket; leading to pain, whenever tooth comes in contact with the opposing tooth.

Radiographical appearance may vary from small periapical radiolucency, thickening of periodontal ligament space to normal appearance. Occasionally all the three conditions can be seen around a multirooted tooth.

Treatment

- If the periodontitis is caused by extension of pulpal inflammation, the pulpotomy may not relieve the pain; root canal treatment is preferred (may be compiled in single visit, or in case of time constraint/ patient's long-sitting, multiple visit RCT is preferred). In case it is due to traumatic occlusion, selective grinding of the traumatic surface(s) will be sufficient.
- When acute periodontitis is associated with mandibular premolars and molars, achieving profound anesthesia is difficult. The so-called 'hot tooth syndrome' is mainly related to sensitization of nerve fibers. Supplementary anesthesia in the form of intraligamentary injection, intrapulpal injection, etc. can be effective (after access cavity preparation).
- Corticosteroid dressing as suggested by few authors, should be used sparingly; suppression of an inflammatory response by steroid allows bacteria to enter the bloodstream. This may be deleterious for certain patients having artificial valves, etc.
- Close dressing should be preferred to avoid bacterial contamination of clean canal. Occlusal adjustment to remove faulty contacts is often helpful. Relieving occlusion reduces pain, especially in teeth which are sensitive to touch.
- Antibiotics for this condition have no role. Only in the event of systemic signs or spread of the infection into facial planes, antibiotic can be prescribed. Routine analgesics can be effective.

d. Acute Periradicular Abscess (Acute Alveolar Abscess)

Acute periradicular abscess is also known as acute apical pericementitis. It may develop as a succession of acute apical periodontitis, which is caused due to extension of pulpal infection into periradicular areas. Acute abscess as an exacerbation of a chronic apical periodontitis is referred to as ***'Phoenix abscess'***.

The concerned tooth is tender to percussion. On palpation it may show minor mobility due to extrusion from the socket (mobility depends upon the amount of periapical exudates). Palpation may cause discomfort because of swelling, which may vary from undetected swelling to gross cellulitis. Swelling can be diffuse or localized and fluctuant or non-fluctuant. The tooth usually does not respond to pulp vitality tests. The patient feels pain due to pressure build-up in the periapical area because of toxic products. The pain continues until the purulent discharge crosses the cortical bone and enters the soft tissue.

The buccal vestibule is the most common site of swelling; however, orientation of root apex and muscular attachment, etc. may deviate the location of the swelling. Application of heat on that area may add to discomfort due to expansion of gases.

The acute lesions usually do not destroy sufficient periapical tissue for radiographic visualization. Radiographically, the lesion may remain undetected or show only widening of periodontal ligament.

Acute periradicular abscess and acute periodontal abscess is to be differentially diagnosed (tooth shows positive vitality if the cause is periodontal).

Treatment

The pulpal and periapical pressure is to be relieved immediately by establishing drainage and opening of root canals. The treatment protocol may be modified depending upon signs and symptoms of the case; the conditions described as follows:

i. *Abscess without swelling*: As the tooth is nonvital, there is no need of local anesthesia. However, if patient has discomfort or for psychological reasons, block anesthesia can be given. The access is achieved using high speed instruments, minimizing vibrations. In restored teeth, the restoration is removed completely; the access opening is evaluated and modified accordingly. Root canals should be thoroughly cleaned of the necrotic substrate. Access to the pulp chamber and root canals will relieve the gases present. The appropriate sized endodontic instrument can be extended beyond the apical foramen to establish drainage. Once complete drainage is established, the root canal should be irrigated and dried, followed by dressing and temporary closure of access opening. The occlusion should be relieved.

ii. *Abscess with localized fluctuant swelling*: In case of acute abscess with fluctuant swelling, immediate drainage is to be established, either through root canal or through soft tissues.

- *Drainage through root canal*: The drainage of abscess through the root canal is a preferred treatment modality. Block anesthesia is preferred, since local infiltration is not indicated (may cause pain due to the distended area). Access is gained with high speed instruments, minimizing vibrations. An appropriate sized endodontic instrument should be carefully extended beyond the apical foramen to establish drainage. A suction device can also be used. The root canals should not be left open to the oral environment as it may lead to severe contamination of microflora, including enteric bacteria and yeasts. Copious irrigation should be carried out while cleaning the canals and even after till the drainage is complete. The canals are dried, followed by dressing and sealing the access cavity. The tooth is disoccluded.
- *Drainage through soft tissues*: The drainage through soft tissues is established either using routine incision or trephination.

  The area is anesthetized using block anesthesia. Following routine protocol of incision and drainage, incise the swelling from inferior side with sharp scalpel blade. Hemostat can be used to open the incision adequately. Copious irrigation with saline and betadine should be carried out alternatively. Sometimes effective drainage is established using a 'drain' (a sterilized piece of gauge or a strip of rubber dam). Drains can be self- retentive (no need to suture to hold) or non-retentive (suture to edge of soft tissues to hold). Warm saline rinses are suggested for at least 48 hours after the drainage process.

  Artificial fistulation can also be established by incising the most dependent point of the swelling. The opening is enlarged with an excavator to facilitate the discharge.

  Trephination is carried out only if drainage through root canal and routine incision fails. Trephination implies cutting a hole through cortical bone into the cancellous space to relieve the build-up inflammation pressure. Block anesthesia is preferred. The location of the nerves and other anatomic structure are to be evaluated before incision. A horizontal incision should be made roughly in the middle to apical 1/3 of the root. An appropriate surgical bur is used to make a window in the cortical plate to locate the root. Proceed apically until the apex is reached. Once drainage is achieved, the apical area is curetted and irrigated. Drain is placed and resorbable suture should be placed to close the lateral extent of incision. The drain is removed after 24 to 48 hours. In case of multiple abscesses, drainage is established both through root canal and soft tissues.

iii. *Abscess with localized non-fluctuant swelling*: The conventional root canal treatment is initiated and drainage is established through the root canal. The incision through soft tissues should not be tried, as it may worsen the condition by spreading the infection. The patient is advised to rinse continually with warm saline.

iv. *Abscess with diffuse swelling*: In case of diffuse swelling, the patient also shows other systemic signs, such as, fever, malaise, nausea, lymphadenopathy, etc. These patients need immediate antibiotic coverage. Root canal treatment can be initiated in case the infection has not involved facial spaces; otherwise the patients should be referred to a hospital till the infection is under control to carry out further procedure.

In case sufficient drainage could be achieved, patient should be evaluated for next 24 hours and if symptoms persist, the antibiotics can be prescribed.

The effect of antibiotics, *vis-a-vis* patient's condition and the status of drainage is summarized in Table 23.1.

Table 23.1	Patient's condition, status of drainage and effect of antibiotics	
Patient's condition	*Status of drainage*	*Antibiotics effect*
No systemic involvement	Sufficient drainage achieved	Not required
No systemic involvement	Insufficient drainage	Partially effective
Systemic involvement	Sufficient drainage achieved	Partially effective
Systemic involvement	Insufficient drainage	Antibiotic required

e. Cracked Tooth Syndrome

The term 'Cracked Tooth Syndrome' refers to an incomplete fracture of a vital tooth that involves the dentin and occasionally extends into the pulp. The diagnosis of cracked tooth syndrome is usually difficult, since radiologically only normal features are visible. The early detection of cracks is important, because with passage of time the cracks progress and may lead to bacterial invasion.

Etiology

The etiologic factors are:

- Trauma
- Parafunctional habits, e.g. bruxism
- Holding objects like pencil, pipe, etc. in between teeth/opening bottle with teeth
- Chewing hard substances, e.g. sugarcane, nuts, bone, etc.
- Wedging effect of spreader/plugger during obturation
- Decreased remaining dentin inside the root (extensive postspace preparation)
- Stresses created due to placement of inlay, pins and posts, etc.
- Failure to place proper post endodontic restorations
- Long span bridges exerting excessive torque on the abutment teeth.

Incidence

Men and women are equally affected. Mandibular molars, especially second molars are the most frequently affected tooth; may be restored or unrestored. In a rough estimate, 3% molars and 1% premolars encounter fracture in males.

Signs and symptoms

Patient usually complains of momentary discomfort with cold stimulus or biting from that tooth. The pain is severe on release of biting force (Table 23.2). The reason may be that the pressure leads to separation along the crack line, resulting in movement of the dentinal fluid in the dentinal tubules. This movement stimulates odontoblasts in the pulp (crack line extending to the pulp directly stimulates the pulpal tissue). Patient's history occasionally reveals repeated restoration or repeated occlusal adjustment of same tooth without relief of symptoms.

Table 23.2	Signs and symptoms of tooth tissue involved in cracks
Involved tooth tissue	*Sign and symptoms*
Enamel crack	Asymptomatic
Crack involving dentin	Pain on biting, specially on release of biting force, sensitivity to cold, etc.
Crack involving pulp	Symptoms related to pulpitis (e.g. sensitivity to both hot and cold, referred pain, etc.)

The crown of tooth in doubt is painted with tincture iodine or methylene blue dye which is washed after two minutes. The crack will appear as dark line. Use of magnification can be a useful aid. Use of a fiber optic light often reveals the position of the crack. On periodontal probing, a narrow pocket may be located adjacent to the fracture site. Occasionally a sinus tract can be appreciated, which can be closer to the gingival margin than the apical area.

Pulp vitality tests remain normal until the cracks involve pulp. Tooth is normally not tender to percussion on an axial direction. Patient is asked to bite on an object, such as, applicator stick, Burlew rubber disk, folded rubber dam and wooden stick, etc. This results in separation of cracked fragments which elicits pain. The bite tests can confirm the diagnosis.

Since, the crack usually runs mesiodistally, radiographs do not reveal a fracture. The presence of a lateral diffuse widening of the periodontal ligament space is the characteristic radiographic appearance.

The pain due to cracked tooth syndrome is to be differentially diagnosed with pain due to periodontal causes, galvanic pain, orofacial and psychiatric disorders, etc.

Treatment

Site, extent and direction of fracture line are the three factors, which dictates whether the tooth can be restored or not.

The *direction of the fracture* can be:

- Horizontal, diagonal, vertical
- Mesiodistal or buccolingual.

The fracture may extend:

- Only in enamel
- Both enamel and dentin

- In enamel, dentin and pulp
  Further it may extend superficial to the alveolar crest or below the alveolar crest.
  The *site of the fracture* can be:
- Cervical third
- Apical third
- Peripherally located
- Centrally located.

Immediate treatment of crack tooth involves stabilization with orthodontic bands, followed by occlusal relief by selective grinding.

The crack line superficial to alveolar crest have better prognosis than the ones below the alveolar crest. Diagonal crack, if peripherally located separating a small fragment of tooth, the loose fragment can be extracted and the rest can be restored. Cracks extending subgingivally often require a gingivectomy to expose the margin. In case the crack is vertical and extends below the alveolar crest involving pulp, the tooth may be extracted. Full coverage restoration is preferred. Subsequently, if symptoms of irreversible pulpitis are evident treatment should be carried out accordingly.

f. Tooth Fracture

Tooth fractures in the anterior region are usually caused by direct trauma, while in posterior region, the causes can be other than trauma.

The fractures can be classified as follows:

i. Crown fracture
   - Enamel infraction
   - Uncomplicated crown fracture
   - Complicated crown fracture

ii. Crown and root fracture

iii. Root fracture
   - Transverse/horizontal root fracture
   - Vertical root fracture.

i. Crown fracture

- *Enamel infraction*: It is manifested as incomplete fracture of the enamel. The cracks can be easily seen in transillumination or by the use of dye. These teeth do not need any treatment but should be closely followed-up for further progress of the crack. Sealing the infarction line with unfilled resin may prevent further damage.
- *Uncomplicated crown fracture*: The fracture of enamel or enamel and dentin both without exposing the pulp is referred to as uncomplicated crown fracture. Most commonly the mesial or distal incisal edges in anterior teeth are fractured. When only enamel is fractured, the condition is asymptomatic; but depending upon the texture of tooth structure lost, it may cause injury to lips or/and tongue. The treatment varies from re-contouring the fracture edges to restoring with composites. Usually such injury pose no threat to the pulp; however, should be evaluated periodically.

  The fracture of dentin along with enamel exposes a large number of dentinal tubules to the oral environment, which may cause chemical and bacterial insult of the pulp. Depending upon the severity of irritants and host response, the outcome may be repair in the form of reparative dentin or lead to pulp inflammation. Patient may complain of thermal sensitivity or pain on mastication.

  In case where the fractured segment (may be enamel only or enamel and dentin) is not lost, then reattachment of the fragment can be tried. The primary aim is to protect the pulp from insult by sealing the open dentinal tubules with appropriate material (bonding agents, flowable composites, etc.). The missing tooth structure should be restored.
- *Complicated crown fracture*: The fractures of enamel and dentin involving pulp are referred to as complicated crown fracture. Patient may complain of sensitivity to hot and cold or/and pain on mastication. A small bleeding point or pinkish pulp can usually be seen.

Factors influencing the treatment options are, maturity of root apex, amount of tooth structure lost and associated injuries. If the root formation is incomplete, pulpotomy is preferred to preserve the pulp for a longer period facilitating normal root development. Mineral trioxide aggregate (MTA) and calcium hydroxide are the materials of choice for pulpotomy.

In tooth with mature root apex, root canal treatment followed by postendodontic restoration should be carried out. Depending upon the associated injuries, the tooth may need repositioning and splinting. Depending upon the amount of tooth structure loss, the restoration can be planned.

ii. Crown and root fracture

The fracture involves both crown and root. Mostly, the fracture line lies superior to the marginal gingiva on the facial aspect of the crown and runs in an oblique direction below the marginal gingiva on the lingual surface. The fractured fragment may or may not remain attached to the gingiva. Involvement of the pulp may complicate the treatment. When pulp is not involved and the fracture fragment is in one piece, reattachment can be tried. In case of multiple fractured fragments without pulp exposure, the fractured fragments are removed protecting the underlying pulp. If the fracture leads to pulp exposure, root canal treatment (orthodontic extrusion, if need be) followed by restoration is the treatment of choice.

iii. Root fracture

- *Transverse/horizontal root fracture*: The transverse/ horizontal root fractures involve cementum, pulp, dentin and periodontal ligament. Complete fracture line may not be visible in single routine radiographs. More than one radiograph with varying angulations are recommended.

Clinically, the tooth is slightly extruded with a lingually displaced crown. The coronal segment is laterally luxated. Mobility of the coronal segment depends upon the level of fracture line and the extent of associated injuries to supporting tissues. In undisturbed fractures the apical segment usually remains vital, whereas vitality of coronal segment depends upon the extent of injury. Pulp sensitivity test may not be helpful.

The healing of transverse/horizontal root fracture has been categorized into four types:

a. Union of the apical and coronal segment by hard tissue (the fragments remain undisplaced and non-mobile. Radiographically, the fracture line is seen as a thin radiolucent line).
b. Union of the apical and coronal segment by fibrous tissue (the fragments appear separated by a definite radiolucent line).
c. Union of the apical and coronal segment by bony in growth across the fracture line (the fragments are separated by a distinct bony ridge. This type usually occurs during growth spurts of the child).
d. Union of the apical and coronal segment by granulation tissue (the fragments usually do not join; fracture line communicates with the oral cavity. Granulation tissues in-between the fractured segments initiate healing. Response to pulp testing is negative).

Treatment

Treatment depends upon many factors, such as:

- Level of fracture line
- Vitality of pulp
- Mobility of fragment
- Degree of displacement of fragments.

Fracture line can be in apical, middle or coronal third of root. Mostly, the apical and middle third fracture do not lead to mobility of fragments; no need to stabilize. Fracture line in coronal third results in mobility of coronal fragment, which requires splinting for 2–4 weeks. In majority of cases the apical fragment retains its vitality, thus needs no treatment. Do not attempt any endodontic treatment and closely follow-up the case for any adverse reaction. If sign and symptoms indicate pulpal involvement, endodontic treatment is initiated. If the apical end of the coronal segment is wide open, apexification with calcium hydroxide/MTA is tried. If the pulp is nonvital and the coronal fragment is mobile, root canal treatment can be performed once the fragment is splinted in position (Table 23.3). In undisplaced fragments with nonvital pulp, root canal treatment of both the fragments can be carried out, followed by placement of rigid post to stabilize both segments. Unmanaged apical segment should be removed by surgical intervention.

If removal of coronal segments is necessary, the length of remaining root is evaluated. In case of sufficient length, orthodontic extrusion or surgical crown lengthening can be carried out, subsequently restoring with post and core.

If the length is not sufficient, then extraction becomes necessary. Maintenance of good oral hygiene is absolutely critical, especially when the fracture line is close to the alveolar bone margin. Gingival inflammation may result communicating the root fracture line with the oral environment.

Table 23.3 Treatment protocol for transverse/horizontal root fractures

Level of fracture	*Mobility*	*Vitality*	*Splinting*	*Endodontic treatment*
Apical 3rd	–	+	No	No
Apical 3rd	–	–	No	Yes
Middle 3rd	–	+	No	No
Middle 3rd	+	+	Yes	No
Middle 3rd	+	–	Yes	Yes
Coronal 3rd	–	+	No	No
Coronal 3rd	+	+	Yes	No
Coronal 3rd	+	–	Yes	Yes

- *Vertical root fracture*: This type of fracture extends vertically down the long-axis of the root and usually involves pulp and the periodontium. The etiological factors can be same as for cracked tooth syndrome. The operator related reasons are more prevalent for such a fracture. Most common orientation of vertical root fracture is mesiodistal involving both the marginal ridges.

Clinical features and diagnostic methods are same as for cracked tooth syndrome. CBCT images are considered better than conventional radiography in evaluating the vertical fractures.

Treatment

The vertical root fracture can be treated by extracting the fractured tooth atraumatically, bonding the fragments (adhesive resin/4-meta resin used as

Table 23.4 Treatment protocol for vertical root fracture

Symptoms	Segment mobility	Treatment
Absent	Absent	Bonded intracoronal restoration and full coverage crown
Present	Absent	Bonded intracoronal restoration and full coverage crown
Present	Present	Extraction

bonding agent) and then replanting the tooth with a 180° rotation. The rotation of the tooth facilitates connection of the healthy periodontal membrane to the fractured root. The application of bioresorbable membrane on root surfaces reinforces the periodontal healing. It allows regeneration of periodontal ligament cells, providing space for the in-growth of periodontal ligament tissues. The treatment protocol for vertical root fracture is summarized in Table 23.4 (for details *refer* to Chapter 26).

g. Luxation Injuries

Luxation injuries are classified into five distinct types:

i. ***Concussion***: Concussion is the injury to the supporting structure of the tooth. There is no loosening and the tooth is reactive to percussion. Splinting is not needed. Occlusion should be relieved. The tooth should be evaluated periodically for any adverse pulp reaction.

ii. ***Subluxation***: Loosening of the tooth with no clinical and radiological evidence of displacement. Usually splinting is not required, however if several teeth are subluxated, a splint may be effective. Splint should be removed in 7–10 days and follow- up is mandatory because of the greater chances of pulpal necrosis (6–47%) in such cases.

iii. ***Extrusive luxation***: The teeth are partially displaced from its alveolar socket. Radiographs at multiple angles may better depict severity of dislocation. The tooth is forcibly repositioned in the socket under local anesthesia. Formation of clot apical to the displaced tooth may pose difficulty in repositioning. A splint should be placed for one to two weeks. Follow-up is mandatory to evaluate any adverse pulpal sequelae.

iv. ***Lateral luxation***: The tooth is eccentrically displaced, may be due to fracture in the alveolar socket. Since, the laterally luxated tooth is part of the fractured alveolar socket, repositioning may be more difficult as compared to extrusive luxation injuries. Anesthesia should be given before repositioning. The thumb and index finger can be used to force the displaced tooth within the alveolar bone and then apply axial pressure in an apical direction and reposition the tooth into its natural position. Finally, the tooth is splinted. Follow-up is mandatory to evaluate any adverse pulpal changes.

v. ***Intrusive luxation***: Intrusive luxation is a type of injury that involves displacement of the tooth into the alveolar socket. This type of injury usually involves the maxillary anterior teeth and is more common in the primary than permanent dentition. Intrusion wound involves disruption of the marginal gingival seal, alveolar bone, periodontal ligament fibers, cementum and the neurovascular supply of the pulp. The injury may lead to complications such as, ankylosis, pulp necrosis, pulp obliteration, external root resorption and loss of marginal bone support. In teeth with incomplete root formation, slight movement of the apex may not lead to disruption of the blood vessels.

The **treatment modalities** include passive repositioning, active repositioning with orthodontic forces, and immediate surgical repositioning. Pulpal necrosis is a common sequel necessitating root canal treatment.

h. Avulsion

Avulsion implies total extrusion of tooth from the socket. Tooth avulsion is a physical and mental trauma for the patient.

Incidence of tooth avulsion ranges from 1–16% of all traumatic injuries to the permanent teeth. Maxillary teeth, particularly the central incisors are the most prone teeth for avulsion. Males are three times more prone than females.

The fate of avulsed tooth depends upon the biological reaction in periodontal ligament and pulp. Avulsion leads to the damage of the following tissues:

- Pulpal tissue due to detachment of blood and nerve supply
- Periodontal ligament due to separation of tooth from socket
- Cemental tissue due to physical trauma
- Fracture of alveolar socket wall
- Injuries to the lips and gingiva.

Management

The time factor plays a major role in the prognosis of treatment, therefore, emergency attention is important.

The following factors influence the treatment plan and the prognosis:

- Viability of periodontal ligament on the root surface
- Stage of root formation at the time of avulsion
- Duration for which the avulsed tooth remained outside the oral cavity
- Handling of avulsed tooth during procedure (root canal treatment)

- Transportation media
- Care of alveolar socket
- Care of associated dentoalveolar injury, if any
- Expiration of dental splint.

Replantation is the accepted treatment modality. Replantation is defined as *'replacement of tooth in its socket that has been removed from the alveolar socket either intentionally or by trauma.'* Periodontal ligament, pulp and alveolar socket are all important tissues to be handled with care.

a. ***Management outside dental office*****:** The extraoral time of the avulsed tooth should be kept as minimum as possible. The dehydration of periodontal ligament fibers should be avoided to retain normal metabolism of the periodontal ligament cells. Every effort should be made to replant the tooth within the first 15–20 minutes. The tooth is washed gently in the running water or saline and place it in the socket by the patient. Firm pressure should be applied to keep the tooth in socket till the patient reaches the dental clinic. If placement of tooth is not possible, the tooth should be transported to the dental clinic in suitable transportation medium (also *refer* to Chapter 26) such as:

- *Milk*: Milk is usually easily available at or near an accident site. It has a pH and osmolality compatible with vital cells and it is relatively free of bacteria. Patient's own saliva is preferred, as milk may contain many antigens that could act immunologically negative on the re-attachment process.
- *Vestibule of the mouth*: Vestibule of the mouth keeps the tooth moist but not ideal because of its pH, incompatible osmolality and presence of bacteria. Sometimes patient's condition due to accident does not allow placement of tooth in vestibule.
- *Saline/water*: Saline and water is the least desirable storage medium, because the hypotonic environment causes rapid cell lysis.
- *Cell culture media*: The cell culture media enhance the possibility of maintaining the viability of the periodontal ligament cell for an extended time after avulsion, e.g. Save-a-tooth that contain Hanks Balanced Salt Solution (HBSS).

An enamel matrix derivative, Emdogain, has been found to improve the periodontal regeneration after replantation.

b. ***Management in dental office*****:** After medical and dental history, carry out clinical examination of hard and soft tissue. Alveolar fracture is to be evaluated carefully. In case of serious injury, the patient is referred to physician/orthopedician as required.

During clinical examination, check for intactness of socket and the surrounding bone. Rinse the socket gently with normal saline to wash out the debris and clot. Do not curette the socket. If the alveolar bone is collapsed and prevents replantation, carefully insert a blunt instrument into the socket to reposition the bone to its original position. After replantation, manually compress facial and lingual bony plates. If the tooth was replanted at accident site, its position in the socket should be assessed by clinical and radiographic examination. If acceptable, then splinting, soft tissue management and adjunctive therapy are carried out. If unacceptable, then gently remove the tooth and replace it in correct position.

It is established that the success rate is higher when the avulsed tooth is immediately replanted at the accident site. The length of extraoral time and the stage of root formation determines the prognosis.

Preparation of root

i. If the root apex is closed and extraoral time is less than twenty minutes, revascularization might not be possible; however, as extraoral time is less, periodontal healing is expected to be excellent. The tooth and socket are gently rinsed with normal saline and the tooth is placed in the socket without causing further trauma.
ii. If root apex is open and the extraoral time is less than twenty minutes, the chances of revascularization are bright. Soak the tooth in 1.0 mg doxycycline and 20 ml of saline for five minutes before replantation. The doxycycline inhibits bacteria in the pulpal lumen which may otherwise prevent revascularization.
iii. If extraoral time varies between 20–60 minutes (apex may be closed or open), the tooth should not be replanted immediately, but placed in a solution of HBSS for 30 minutes before replantation. The necrotic cells and debris including bacteria float-off of the root during the soaking period, leaving less stimulus for inflammation.
iv. If extraoral time is more than 60 minutes (apex may be closed or open), the tooth loses almost all periodontal ligament cells thus soaking is ineffective. Now, all efforts will be focused to slow the inevitable resorption. The tooth should be soaked in citric acid for five minutes, in 2.0 mg stannous fluoride for five minutes and then doxycycline for another five minutes after which it can be replanted. Alendronate is equally effective as fluoride in slowing resorption; however, this material is costly. Emdogain is showing promising results in reducing resorption when put in the socket. The endodontic treatment can be completed prior to replantation.

Splinting

The requisite features of a splint are:

- Should be esthetically and hygienically acceptable
- Should not facilitate caries development
- Can be easily constructed in the dental clinic
- Should not hinder vitality tests and the endodontic treatment.

Semi-rigid splint is preferred, which allows slight vertical movement of the tooth during healing. The masticatory stimulus help reorienting necrotic periodontal ligament fibers with blood vessels and fibroblasts, minimizing the risk of ankylosis. A thin orthodontic wire (0.3 mm), fiber glass nylon splint and titanium trauma splint are routinely used to achieve functional immobilization. Prolonged and rigid immobilization increases the risks of external replacement root resorption. Occlusion should be checked as hyperocclusion impairs healing. For gaining proper periodontal support, splinting for one weak is sufficient; whereas, splinting for 4–8 weeks is mandatory for alveolar fractures.

Patient is advised to consume soft diet, use mouth rinses and maintain good oral hygiene. Biting on splinted teeth is to be avoided. Systemic antibiotics/ analgesics contribute to replantation success.

The replanted teeth with open apex (open apices have the potential to revascularize and continue root development) should be followed closely every two weeks for evidence of revascularization. If any sign of pathology is noted, root canal treatment is initiated. Vitality tests are usually not confirmative as open apex give false results; however, cold test with carbon dioxide snow (–78°C) or difluorodichloromethane (–50°C) can be effective. Laser Doppler flowmetry may also be useful.

Calcium hydroxide is preferred as dressing, as it favorably influences the local environment at the resorption site and promote healing. The alkaline pH of calcium hydroxide may slow the action of the resorptive cells and promote hard tissue formation. Other medicaments used to prevent resorption are antibiotic—corticosteroid paste (Ledermix) and hormone (Calcitonin). Periodic follow-up is necessary to evaluate any adverse changes.

2. Mid-treatment Emergencies

Mid-term emergencies can be because of the following factors:

a. Incomplete Pulp Tissue Removal

Incomplete removal of inflamed pulp tissue lead to survival of residual microorganisms, their by-products and toxins in the root canal; may cause pressure and subsequently pain to the patient. It is one of the principle factors contributing to the endodontic failures. Thorough débridement is mandatory for preventing such a problem.

b. Apical Periodontitis

i. ***Due to over instrumentation***: Instrumentation beyond the apical constriction causes trauma to the apical periodontal ligament. Over instrumentation may cause extrusion of significant amount of infected debris into the apical area. It also promotes the enlargement of apical foramen which may permit an increased flux of exudate and blood into the root canal, which further enhances the nutrient supply to the bacteria in the canal. Gross over-instrumentation can cause acute apical periodontitis leading to pain. It can be prevented by maintaining the working length and selection of an instrumentation technique that extrudes less amount of debris apically.

ii. ***Due to chemical insult***: Most irrigants and medications are cytotoxic, so their use should be restricted to the root canal. If such chemicals are extruded beyond the periapex, they may lead to inflammation and subsequently pain. Irrigants like sodium hypochlorite and hydrogen peroxide when accidentally injected beyond apex into the periradicular tissues may cause immediate pain and in a few hours, swelling, ecchymosis, neurological deficit and even necrotic ulcer. After few days, secondary infection and persistent pain may follow.

Management

The best management is prevention. Adequate control of the working length coupled with use of side-vent needles can prevent such accidents. However, in case of such an accident, carry-out immediate aspiration along with irrigation with saline. Patient is prescribed cold packs, analgesics and anti-inflammatory drugs. In severe cases, hospitalization is recommended for care of surgical wound.

c. Phoenix Abscess (Mid-Treatment Flare-Up)

The phoenix abscess is the synonym of mid-treatment flare-up. The flare-up is defined as '*an acute exacerbation of periradicular pathosis during root canal treatment*.' It is very annoying and upsetting both for the patient and the operator when the tooth under endodontic treatment suddenly becomes symptomatic (pain, swelling or both). The swelling in such cases is so profound that the patient avoids going to the same clinic.

The incidence of mid-treatment flare-ups vary between 1.0 and 25%. The root canal therapy in vital teeth exhibits minimum flare-ups. The problem mainly lies with chronic cases lying dormant for the last couple of years.

Patients with preoperative pain had a flare-up rate of 20%; whereas, patient with localized or defuse swelling show 15% incidence of flare-up.

The term Phoenix (rebirth) abscess relates to the sudden exacerbation of a previously symptom less periradicular lesion. The reasons for this phenomenon are not fully understood; however, it is hypothesized to be due to the alteration of the environment of bacterial flora in the root canal space during instrumentation. A few authors are of the view that facultative anaerobes multiply slowly in low oxygen environment of the periapical tissues. When root canal is opened, suddenly it receives oxygen, and in improved condition the bacteria fulminate violently and produce an acute reaction. Another opinion is that after initial canal instrumentation some strains are severely reduced, whereas other may be relatively unaffected. Since, there are fewer organisms with which to compete; a virulent strain may rapidly multiply.

Etiology

The probable causative factors are:

i. *Factors related to patient:*
   - Patient with preoperative pain or swelling.
   - Patient with dental phobias (prone because of their low psychophysiologic tolerance).

ii. *Factors related to periapical pathosis:*
   - Tooth with chronic necrotic pulp
   - Retreatment cases
   - Teeth with chronic periapical radiolucency.

iii. *Factors related to treatment procedure:*
   - Incomplete pulp tissue removal or undetected canals
   - Over instrumentation; trauma to the periapical tissues
   - Apical extrusion of debris during canal preparation
   - Extrusion of sealer/obturating material into the periapical area
   - Over medication of root canals
   - Improper sealing of access cavity
   - Traumatic occlusion.

Signs and symptoms

After an endodontic procedure or during inter appointment period, the patient had significant swelling, pain or both. Regional temporary paresthesia has also been reported. The problem is so severe, which warrants emergency attention.

Preventive measures

- Before initiating endodontic procedure, the patient should be mentally prepared and confident of the procedure. Fear and anxiety may exacerbate the patient perception, subsequently reducing the pain tolerance.
- Avoid half-hearted root canal therapy. All canals should preferably be prepared in one sitting. Missing canals should also be taken care of.
- Intracanal medicament should be used judiciously; too caustic materials or even excess amount of routinely used ones may leach in periapical area, resulting into painful reaction.
- Forced irrigation causes water-canon effect and trauma to periapical tissues resulting into violent tissue reaction; thus proper irrigation techniques should be followed.
- Debris extrusion is a problem with almost all the techniques of instrumentation. The technique which allows minimum debris extrusion should be selected followed by copious irrigation.
- Over instrumentation should be avoided. Occlusion should be relieved if apex is severely violated by over instrumentation.
- In retreatment cases, the patient should be informed about the chances of occurrence of flare-up.
- Proper coronal seal should be maintained to avoid recontamination of root canal system.
- Root canal should not be left open for drainage as that further contaminates the root canal.
- Calcium hydroxide is preferred in-between the appointments, as is effective during long inter-appointment delays.

Various hypotheses and preventive measures of mid treatment flare-up is summarized in Table 23.5.

Treatment

Reassurance is the most important aspect of treatment. Intravenous analgesic can be given. Triazolam (0.25 mg) given sublingually or orally has been found safe and effective. Antiallergic drugs should be prescribed since the allergy may be a causative factor. The root canal is opened. Sterilized paper point is inserted to evaluate any seepage. Incomplete canal preparation should be completed on the same sitting.

A corticosteroid-antibiotic intracanal medication is used to relieve the symptoms. The paste can be inserted with the help of paper point. Corticosteroids act as a anti-inflammatory agents, while the antibiotic prevents any possible over growth of microorganisms.

Table 23.5 Mid treatment Flare-up: Various hypotheses and preventive measures

Hypotheses	*Reasons*	*Preventive measures*
Extrusion of infected debris in the periapical area	Endodontic therapy may introduce medicaments, irrigating solutions or tissue proteins into the periapical lesion leading to violent reaction	• Prefer crown down instrumentation technique • Instruments should be used with rotation rather than pull and push action • Copious irrigation with mild irrigant
Changes in root canal/periapical environment	Endodontic therapy causes changes in the root canal environment that may favor the overgrowth of certain microorganisms. If these bacteria reach sufficient number, they can damage the periradicular tissues	• Completion of root canal preparation in single visit • Placement of a mild antimicrobial intra-canal medication with gentle pressure
Secondary infections	Microorganism that are not present in the primary infection may penetrate the root canal system during or after the treatment	• Prepare root canal under strict aseptic measures • Achieve coronal sealing • Do not leave the tooth open for drainage • Placement of an antimicrobial intra-canal medication
Increase of the oxidation-reduction potential	Entry of oxygen into the root canal during treatment may favor the overgrowth of facultative bacteria	• Completion of root canal preparation in single visit • Copious irrigation prior to intracanal medication

Access opening is closed with fast setting temporary cement and the occlusion is relieved.

3. Post-treatment Emergencies

a. ***Over instrumentation*:** Over instrumentation during root canal preparation, especially in case of single visit root canal treatment, lead to pain after obturation. The filling should be removed and the tooth is kept at rest; subsequently, re-filling after the symptomatic subside.

b. ***Over obturation/sealer extrusion*:** The over obturated teeth may create emergency; however, the mild symptom of pain and tenderness resolve within a day or so.

Over obturation will lead to higher incidence of discomfort, which may be related to the mechanical and chemical trauma exerted by the obturating material and/or sealer to the *periradicular tissues*. The pressure created by infected extrusion of sealer may also lead to severe pain.

c. ***High restoration*:** The high points in coronal restoration (may be interim or permanent) causes discomfort due to acute periodontitis. Relieving the occlusion immediately restore the inflammation and the pain.

d. ***Root fracture*:** The fracture occurs mainly due to unreasonable condensation of the obturating material. During postpreparation, similar fracture can occur if the proper direction is not followed.

The prognosis of root fracture, since mostly, the fractures are vertical, is very poor. Extraction may be the only solution. In multirooted teeth, however, hemisection can be planned.

Use of Antibiotics

It has been established that most of the endodontic emergencies do not require antibiotic coverage. Unnecessary use of antibiotics may lead to bacterial resistance. These are only indicated for febrile patients, lymphadenopathy, malaise, cellulitis, unexplained trismus, osteomyelitis and progressive and/or persistent swelling. Antibiotics are also indicated as prophylactic coverage in medically compromised patient. Pain is not an indication for continuity of antibiotics. High dose regimen for a short period is preferred to a low dose for a longer time. Most of the antibiotics may not demonstrate any significant clinical effects within the first 24 hours, which is not an indication of a failure of antibiotics or a need to change the antibiotic. Swelling may take a few days to one week for resolving. Reduction of pain is a good indication of effectiveness of treatment.

BIBLIOGRAPHY

1. Andreasen FM and Andreasen JO. Diagnosis of luxation injuries. The importance of standardized clinical, radiographic and photographic techniques in clinical investigations. Endod. Dent. Traumato.: 1985; 1:160–169.
2. Brain M, Hury and John F. Trephination for acute pain management. J. Endod.: 2003; 29:144–146.
3. Caglar E, Tanboga I and Susal S. Treatment of avulsed teeth with Emdogain–a case report. Dent. Traumatol: 2005; 21:51–53.

4. Christopher D, Lynch RJ and Mc Connell J. The crack tooth syndrome. J. Can. Dent. Assoc.: 2002; 68:470–475.
5. Cunha RF, Delbem ACB, Vietra AEN and Pugliesi DNC. Treatment of a severe dental lateral luxation association with extrusion in an 8-months old baby : A conservative approach. Dent. Traumatol.: 2005; 21:57–59.
6. Ernest H, Harold H. and Robert M. Flare ups in endodontics and their relationship to various medicaments. Aust. Endod. J.: 2007; 33:119–130.
7. Henry M, Reader A and Beck M. Effect of penicillin on post operative endodontic pain and swelling in symptomatic necrotic teeth. J. Endod.: 2001; 27:117–123.
8. Houck V, Reader A, Back M, Nis R. and Weaver J. Effect of trephination in post operative pain and swelling in symptomatic necrotic teeth. Oral Surg., Oral Med., Oral Path.: 2000; 90:507–513.
9. Iqbal M, Kurtz E and Kohli M. Incidence and factors related to flare-ups in a graduate endodontic programme. Int. Endod. J.: 2009; 42:99–104.
10. Keenan V, James GF, Allan F, Zbingniew NT and Jonothan A. A Cochrane systematic review finds no evidence to support the use of antibiotic for pain relief in irreversible pulpitis. J. Endod.: 2006; 32:87–92.
11. Levein L, Bryson EC, Caplan D and Trope M. Effect of topical alendronate on root resorption of dried replanted dog teeth. Dent. Traumatol.: 2001; 17:120–126.
12. Liesigner A, Marshall JF and Marshal GJ. Effect of variable doses of dexamethasone on post operative endodontic pain. J. Endod.:1993; 19:35–39.
13. McDougal RA, Olutayo, Delano E and Dan C. Success of an alternative for interim management of irreversible pulpitis. JADA.: 2004; 135:1707–1712.
14. Priyanka SR and Veronica. Flare-ups in endodontics – a review. IOSR J. Dent. Med. Sci.: 2013; 9:26–31.
15. Samuel S and Irving JF. Flare-ups in endodontics: I. Etiological factors. J. Endod.: 2004; 30:476–481.
16. Sathorn C, Parashos P and Messer H. The prevalence of post-operative pain and flare-up in single and multiple-visit endodontic treatment: A systematic review. Int. Endod. J.: 2008; 41:91–99.
17. Sathorn C, Parashos P and Messerj HH. Effectiveness of single versus multiple visit endodontic treatment of tooth with apical periodontitis: A systematic review and meta analysis. Inter Endod. J.: 2005; 38:347–355.
18. Segura-Egea JJ, Cisnero-Cabello R, Llamas-Carreras JM and Velasco-Ortega E. Pain associated with root canal treatment. Int. Endod. J.:2009; 42:614–620.
19. Strobl H, Haas M, Norea B, Gerhard S and Emshoff R. Evaluation of pulpal blood flow after tooth splinting of luxated permanent maxillary incisor. Dent. Traumatol.: 2004; 20:36–41.
20. Trope M. Clinical management of the avulsed tooth. Dent. Clin. North Am.: 1995; 39:93–112.
21. Turpo JC and Gobetti JP. The crack tooth syndrome: an elusive diagnosis. J. Am. Dent. Assoc.: 1996; 27:1502–1507.
22. Villanueva LE. Fustobacterium necleatum in endodontic flare-ups. Oral Surg., Oral Med., Oral Pathol., Oral Radiol. Endod.: 2002; 93:179–183.
23. Walker RT. Emergency treatment—a review. Int. Endod. J.: 2984; 17:29–35.

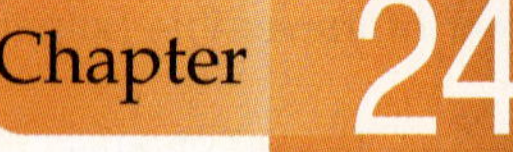

Chapter 24

Bleaching of Discolored Teeth

Esthetics is the science of beauty. Esthetic dentistry not only relates to disfigured teeth but also involves the needs of normal appearing people who wish to look younger, healthier and confident. The perception and description of color in a given object, coupled with the need and desire of an individual forms the basis of esthetics. One of the most frequent reasons warranting esthetic care is discoloration of anterior teeth. The improved technical ability of the dental surgeons along with better gadgets and also the increasing awareness of the public has paved the way for improving the esthetics of the discolored teeth and the surrounding tissues. The lightening of stained teeth without disturbing the biological tissues and the periodontal environment is the main goal of the practicing esthetic dental surgeon.

The lightening of the color of a tooth through application of chemical agent(s) to oxidize the organic pigmentation in the tooth, is referred to as 'Bleaching'. American Dental Association defined bleaching as, *'the treatment, involving an oxidative chemical that alters the light absorbing and/or light reflecting nature of the material structure, thereby increasing its value (whiteness)'*.

The term 'bleaching' and 'tooth whitening' are not exactly synonymous. Whitening restores teeth to their natural tooth color (removal of external stains on the tooth surface) and bleaching makes the teeth lighter than their natural color (modify colored substances within the tooth).

'Bleaching' or 'tooth whitening' dates back to 18th century when the chloride of lime was used as a bleaching agent. In early nineteenth century, hydrogen peroxide, alone and in combination with other materials, have been used as a bleaching agent. Over the years, various investigators have tried different materials and technique to aid in bleaching. Bleaching with lasers is also being familiarized.

TOOTH DISCOLORATION AND STAINING

The tooth discoloration and staining are multifactorial. A thorough knowledge of the etiology of tooth staining is essential in order to make a correct diagnosis. The factors and extent of discoloration influence the treatment options and also determine the prognosis. The vitality of the tooth also affects the treatment protocol and timings.

Etiology

The etiology of tooth discoloration is broadly divided into three categories, viz. intrinsic, extrinsic and internalized stains.

A. Intrinsic Discoloration

The factors causing intrinsic discoloration are classified as local and systemic factors. A few authors have categorized the causes of intrinsic discoloration as pre-eruptive and posteruptive causes.

a. Local factors

i. *Trauma*: Trauma leads to pulpal hemorrhage, causing grayish discoloration of the teeth. The obliteration of the pulp canal may add to dark yellow discoloration of the teeth.
ii. *Pulpal hemorrhagic products*: Pulp necrosis leads to the production of hemorrhagic products, which enter dentinal tubules and cause discoloration.
iii. *Aging*: Aging changes enamel and dentin structure, which eventually lead to discoloration.
iv. *Root resorption*: Root resorption, especially at a later stage, discolor the tooth.

b. Systemic factors

i. *Fluorosis*: It has been established that high concentration of fluorides (more than 4.0 ppm) causes moderate to severe discoloration; more prevalent in incisors followed by premolars and molars. Fluorosis is categorized as mild, moderate and severe. Mild fluorosis exhibits brown pigmentation on a smooth surface, moderate shows flecks on the enamel surface along with staining, and severe form shows pigmentation with pitted enamel surfaces. The severe form of fluorosis may not respond to bleaching.

ii. *Tetracycline staining*: Tetracycline is a widely used antibiotic. Discoloration due to tetracycline ingestion has been confirmed by various investigators. It was also established that the dose of tetracycline was more important than the duration. The different varieties of tetracycline produce yellow to yellowish brown stains; however, doxycycline does not produce any stain.

iii. *Amelogenesis imperfecta*: Amelogenesis imperfecta, the abnormal formation of the enamel, is of three types, viz. hypoplastic, hypomineralization and hypomaturation.

iv. *Dentinogenesis imperfecta*: Dentinogenesis imperfecta is an autosomal dominant developmental disturbance of the dentin. It leads to brownish violet to yellowish brown color of the dentin with a translucent hue.

v. *Dentin dysplasia*: Dentin dysplasia is a rare disturbance of dentin formation, may lead to slight amber translucency of teeth.

vi. *Congenital hyperbilirubinemia*: High level of bilirubin in the blood, may cause yellow green discoloration of teeth.

vii. *Congenital erythropoietic porphyria*: An inborn error of porphyrin-haem synthesis (inherited as an autosomal recessive trait); may lead to red brown/purplish red discoloration of the teeth.

viii. *Alkaptonuria*: An inherited genetic disorder of phenylalanine and tyrosine metabolism, may give brown discoloration to the teeth.

ix. *General diseases*: Diseases of genetic/idiopathic origin, such as epidermolysis bullosa, cleidocranial dysostosis, osteogenesis imperfecta, osteopetrosis, Morquio's disease, etc. Prenatal or congenital syphilis, trophic disturbances like infantile tetany, rickets, vitamin C deficiency, etc.

Causes of intrinsic stains have also been categorized as pre-eruptive and posteruptive

Pre-eruptive
- Tetracycline
- Fluorosis
- Trauma
- Genetic (amelogenesis imperfecta, hyperbilirubinemia)

Posteruptive
- Aging
- Root resorption
- Pulp necrosis
- Intrapulpal hemorrhage
- Pulp tissue remnants
- Materials (irrigants, sealers, etc.)

B. Extrinsic Discoloration

Extrinsic discoloration have been classified by various authors depending upon different criteria:

a. Classification according to the cause:
   - Staining, caused by chromogenic microorganisms derived from dietary sources; other factors may also be responsible
   - Indirect staining is associated with cationic antiseptics and metal salts.

b. Nathoo's classification:
   - *Type 1 (N1)*: Chromogens bind to tooth surface and cause discoloration. The color of the chromogen is similar to that of dental stains caused by tea, coffee, wine and various chromogenic bacteria.
   - *Type 2 (N2)*: Chromogen changes color after binding with teeth. The stain darkens with time
   - *Type 3 (N3)*: Prechromogen (colorless material) binds to tooth and undergoes chemical reaction to cause the staining.

c. Non-metallic stains:
   - Due to tea, coffee, blackcurrant juice, cola drinks etc.
   - Due to chemicals, like chlorhexidine.

d. Metallic stains:
   - Black staining seen in people using iron supplement and in iron foundry workers
   - Copper causes green stain after rinsing with copper salts
   - Potassium permanganate produces violet to black color
   - Silver nitrate salt causes gray discoloration
   - Stannous fluoride causes golden brown discoloration.

C. Internalized Discoloration

Internalized discoloration occurs due to incorporation of extrinsic stains within the tooth substance following some dental pathology. It occurs in enamel defects and in the porous surface of exposed dentin, e.g. in developmental defects like fluorosis, hypoplasia and enamel hypocalcification. These types of defects can also be seen in tooth wear, gingival recession and caries, etc.

The causes of discoloration are summarized in Flowchart 24.1.

Flowchart 24.1 Causes of discoloration

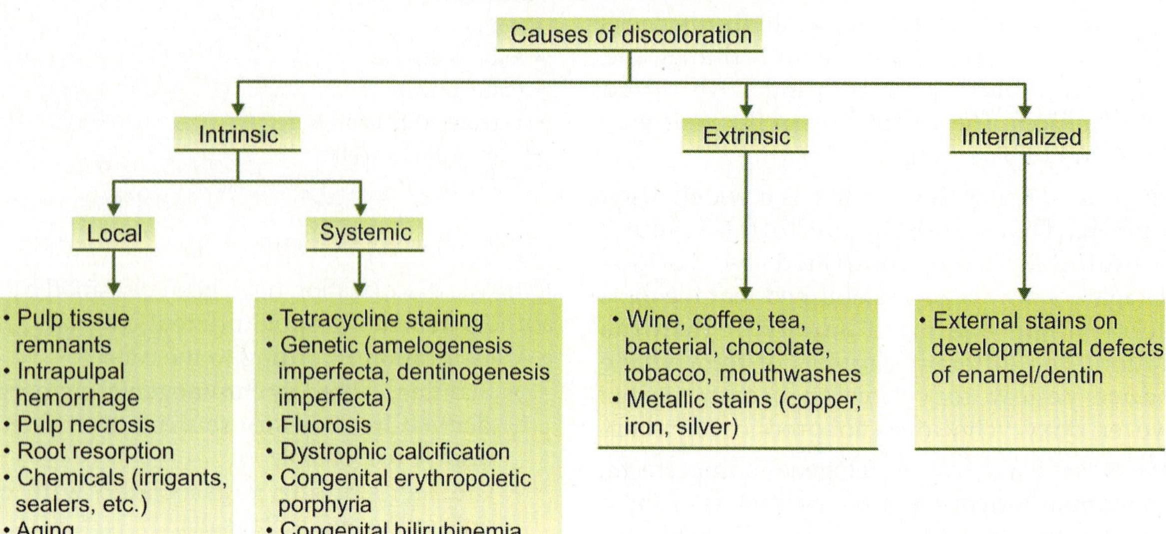

BLEACHING OF TEETH

Bleaching implies degradation of high molecular weight, complex organic molecules that reflect a specific wavelength of light, responsible for color of the stain. The degradation leads to lower molecular weight molecules, that reflect less light, resulting in reduction/elimination of discoloration.

Factors limiting the bleaching of teeth

- Dentin hypersensitivity
- Suspected or confirmed bulimia
- Generalized dental caries and leaking restorations
- Heavily restored teeth
- Teeth with opaque white spots
- Patient selection—patients with emotional or psychological problems do not make good candidates for bleaching
- Decreased bonding of adhesive materials to the tooth immediately after bleaching.

Indications

- Superficial color discrepancies
- Extrinsic/intrinsic stains of moderately dark and intense color
- General discoloration of teeth (yellow to brown).

Contraindications

- Severe discoloration from amalgam corrosion
- Extensive restorations
- Inherent sensitivity of the patient to bleaching agents.

Advantages

- Treatment is totally under control of the operator
- Potential for early results
- Soft tissue can be protected from the process.

Disadvantages

- Unknown duration of the treatment
- Discomfort of rubber dam application
- Temperature rise on the pulp
- Post-treatment sensitivity
- If etching is performed with bleaching (resulting in loss of small amount of enamel), polishing is required after each visit
- Cost factor.

The ***bleaching modalities*** are divided into vital and nonvital tooth bleaching.

I. Vital tooth bleaching
   A. In-office bleaching
      a. Thermocatalytic bleaching
      b. Nonthermocatalytic bleaching
      c. Power bleaching
      d. Microabrasion
   B. Home bleaching (nightguard vital bleaching).
II. Nonvital tooth bleaching
   a. Thermocatalytic technique
   b. Walking bleach technique
   c. Modified walking bleach technique
   d. Combination technique (inside/outside bleaching).
III. Laser assisted bleaching.
IV. Tooth bleaching with nonthermal atmospheric plasma.
V. Over the counter products.

I. VITAL TOOTH BLEACHING

Vital bleaching technique requires use of chemical agents that should not endanger the tooth structure and the adjoining soft tissues.

Bleaching Agents

The bleaching agents contain active and inactive ingredients.

The **active ingredients** include:

i. *Chlorine dioxide*: 0.5% chlorine dioxide when applied to enamel surface for 20 minutes, effectively bleach the tooth surfaces. However, its use may lead to roughness on enamel surface and decreased luster. Such teeth are more prone to restaining and usually develop sensitivity.

ii. *Hydrogen peroxide*: 30–35% hydrogen peroxide is a strong oxidizing agent that ionizes to produce different type of free radicals, such as hydroxyl ions (OH^-) and perhydroxyl ions (OOH^-).

iii. *Carbamide peroxide*: Carbamide peroxide is hydrogen peroxide combined with urea. 10–35% concentration of carbamide peroxide is being used for bleaching purpose (10% carbamide peroxide is equal to 3.0% hydrogen peroxide and 22% carbamide peroxide is equal to 7.5% hydrogen peroxide). Higher amount of peroxide is more effective; however, associated with increased risk of sensitivity. A few pH buffered products are available, which reduce likelihood of side effects.

iv. *Hydrochloric acid*: The hydrochloric acid(18–36%) causes decalcification of tooth substance along with removal of stain.

v. *Titanium dioxide nanoparticle doped with nitrogen* to bleaching agent having less concentration of hydrogen peroxide (3.0–10.0%) is recently tried as bleaching agent. The combination improves the biocompatibility of the solution reducing dental sensitivity during and after the procedure. Recent studies have confirmed the clinical efficacy of this newer bleaching agent with 3.0–6.0% hydrogen peroxide.

vi. *Other bleaching agents*: The whitening toothpastes and tooth whitening gels mainly contain calprox-baking soda-sodium bicarbonate (mild abrasive, dissolves protein pellicle layer and whiten teeth); Hydrated silica-silicone dioxide (mild abrasive, can be combined with calcium carbonate to increase effectiveness); sodium tripolyphosphate (detergent, removes stains) and polyvinylpyrrolidone (do not allow new stains adhering to tooth).

The **inactive ingredients** include:

i. *Preservatives*: Sodium benzoate is commonly used as preservative agent. It prevents bacterial growth and also accelerates the breakdown of hydrogen peroxide.

ii. *Thickening agents*: Carbopol (carboxypolymethylene), in a concentration of 0.5 to 1.5%, is commonly used thickening agent. It increases viscosity of the bleaching agent and also increases active oxygen releasing time of the bleaching material.

iii. *Surfactants* in bleaching agent act as surface wetting agent facilitating diffusion of hydrogen peroxide across the tooth surface.

iv. *Glycerine and propylene glycol added as carrier*, enhance viscosity and facilitate uniform distribution of bleaching agent.

v. *Certain flavoring agents*, such as peppermint, wintergreen, spearmint, etc. are added to improve taste and patient's acceptance.

vi. Potassium nitrate and fluorides are added to decrease post-treatment sensitivity.

vii. Certain remineralizing agents, such as calcium phosphate-casein phosphopeptide, are added to reduce sensitivity and also to get lustrous shine to the teeth.

Additional materials used during bleaching procedure

a. *Orabase paste*: Orabase paste is used to protect gingiva and oral mucosa during bleaching. It is composed of gelatin, pectin and sodium carboxymethylcellulose in plastibase (plasticized hydrocarbon gel).

Orabase paste adheres tenaciously and remains in intimate contact with mucous membranes, protecting the affected area in the oral cavity against irritation from chewing, swallowing, etc. It acts as an invisible bandage. A thin film of orabase paste is effective.

b. *Gingival dam*: The gingival dam is the polymerizable isolation barriers, which is used during bleaching process. The barrier material consists of:

- Monomers
- Curing agents (0.01–2%)
- Polymerization strength reducers (1–30%)
- Tissue adherence accentuators (0.01–9%)
- Reflective materials (1–50%).

The polymerizable isolation barrier consists of at least one monomer, one curing agent for curing the monomer and one of three preferred additives, i.e. the organic polymerization strength reducer, the tissue adherence accentuator, and the reflective material. The polymerizable isolation barrier material is preferably stored at or below room temperature. It is stable enough until activated by suitable light radiant energy.

The barrier material is made in a paste or gel form that can be expressed from a dental syringe. The barrier material is available in form of emulsion, dispersion/suspension solution depending upon selection of a preferred application.

c. *Diamond polishing paste*: The diamond polishing paste incorporates 3.0 μ diamond abrasive particles in a strand of fiber. These fibers form a three dimensional open weave design. This paste provides finishing and polishing in one step.

d. *First aid kit*: It contains antioxidants such as vitamin E in liquid or capsule form and aloe vera gel. A single spill of a droplet of hydrogen peroxide blanches and burns the gingival tissue. Vitamin E oil quickly relieves the symptoms within one minute.

The techniques involved in vital bleaching are:

A. In office bleaching
   a. Thermocatalytic bleaching
   b. Nonthermocatalytic bleaching
   c. Power bleaching
   d. Microabrasion.

B. Home bleaching (nightguard vital bleaching).

A. In-Office Bleaching

Preparation of the patient for bleaching

- Shade of the patient's existing dentition is recorded with a standardized shade guide tab; photograph of patient's teeth is taken for records
- Thorough prophylaxis is performed
- The patient is draped with a protective cap and is made to wear protective eyeglasses
- No local anesthesia is administered
- Teeth are isolated with heavy gauge rubber dam
- Before rubber dam application, oraseal (a light cured resin) or orabase paste is applied to protect the labial and lingual tissue
- Vaseline is applied to the patient's lips before mounting the rubber dam frame
- Wet gauze is placed over the patient's lips to prevent thermal trauma.

a. Thermocatalytic Bleaching

The thermocatalytic bleaching involves the use of heat alone or heat and light both. The units used for thermocatalytic bleaching are:

i. *Heat light unit*: The unit provides high intensity light and heat, required to activate bleaching agents. A narrow beam of light is concentrated at one specific site at a distance of approximately 13–15 inches. Calibrated rheostat controls the amount of light and heat.

24

ii. *Heat unit*: The unit with accurate temperature control provides the requisite heat to activate the bleaching agent. Two tips are available: one is directly applied (vital teeth) and the second is inserted through the coronal access opening (nonvital teeth). The recommended temperature for nonvital teeth is 60 to 70°C and 46 to 60°C for vital teeth.

After removing the heat source, tooth is allowed to cool to avoid sudden temperature change that can be deleterious to the pulp. After five minutes tooth is washed with warm water for one minute. Bleaching appointments are scheduled 2–4 weeks apart. Do not exceed 30 minutes of treatment in each appointment. A minimum of three treatments is required; ten are maximum. The color is checked one week after the third treatment.

The source of heat can be:

- Photoflood lamp
- Polymerization light
- Spirit lamp
- Commercial bleaching units
- Light-heat lamp
- Lasers.

The commercial preparation systems utilizing different activating light sources are:

- *Quartz tungsten halogen (QTH) curing light*: The standard curing light provides heat to activate the chemical reaction by stimulating light sensitive chemicals in the bleaching agent. Conventional light provide 17°C increase in temperature; whereas, with QTH light the temperature rises to 24.8°C above the baseline. The application time is approximately 40 seconds. Each application can be within 40–50 seconds.
- *Plasma arc*: Plasma arc provides slightly higher intensity of light/heat than halogen curing temperature. The four seconds application may lead to 2.2°C rise of intrapulpal temperature. The total increase in temperature varies from 37 to 39°C. The recommended time of application is 30 seconds per tooth.
- *Rembrandt tooth whitening system*: This system includes the use of a plasma arc light, named Rembrandt Sapphire. The unit can be fitted with a Rembrandt Whitening Crystal enabling the operator to treat both the arches simultaneously. The wavelength of light emitted from this source is in the range of 400–525 nm (blue green coloration).
- *Whitening accelerator*: This system utilizes high intensity blue light at a wavelength of 480–520 nm. The light is filtered to remove infrared and ultraviolet light. It is used with special whitening formula; the half-hour procedure can oxidize 16 or more teeth.
- *The Zoom! (Teeth whitening system)*: This system utilizes using mercury metal halide light with a wavelength of 300–450 nm (violet coloration). The

Zoom! Light unit has an infrared filter, which filters these radiations, thereby minimizing the amount of heat generated at the surface of tooth during the bleaching treatment.

Technique (Fig. 24.1a to c)

- Using a dropper, a small amount of bleaching solution (30–35% H_2O_2) is placed into a dappen dish.
- The teeth are properly isolated preferably with rubber dam.

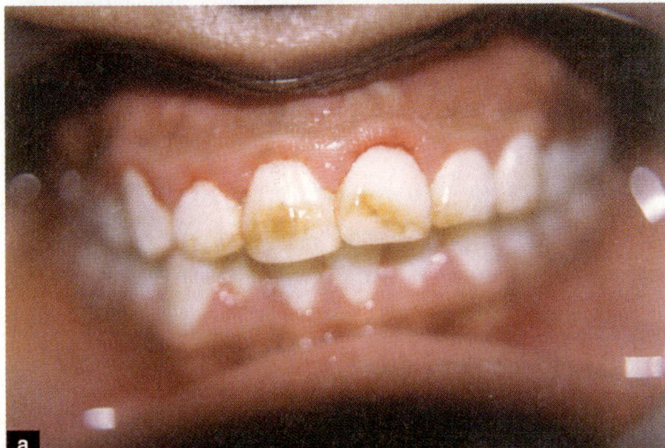

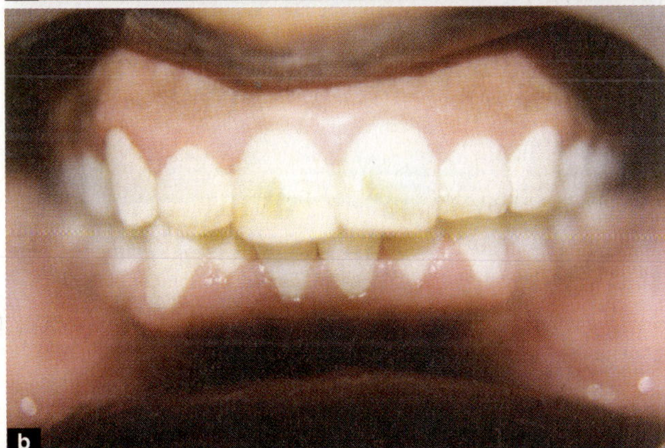

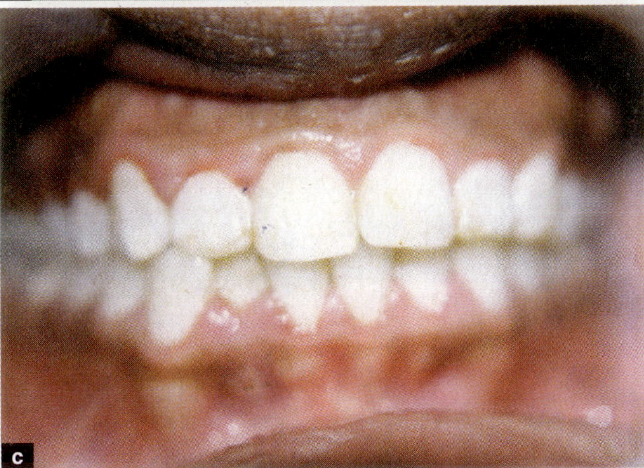

Fig. 24.1 Thermocatalytic bleaching: (a) Preoperative; (b) During bleaching process; (c) Postoperative

- A small piece of cotton/gauze piece, held in cotton pliers is dipped into the dappen dish and the saturated bleaching solution is applied onto the tooth surface.
- With a small plastic instrument, the gauze is shaped to cover the entire tooth surface.
- The selected heating unit is positioned.
- When the photo lamp is used, the bleaching solution is applied every 4 to 5 minutes.
- When the heat unit is used, the bleaching solution is applied after every heating cycle.
- After removing the gauze/cotton, the teeth and the entire rubber dam is washed with warm water and a high volume vacuum aspirator.
- The floss is removed by cutting with scalpel and removing slowly with cotton pliers.
- The rubber dam is stretched apically and labially to gain access to the interproximal areas. The clamps are removed and the rubber dam is gently teased off from the teeth.
- Wet, warm gauze pieces are used to remove the excess orabase/oraseal.
- The residues of bleaching agent on teeth are neutralized with a mild warm solution of ½ teaspoon salt, ½ cup warm water and ½ teaspoon sodium bicarbonate.
- Instruct the patient to avoid coffee, tea and cold drinks for two weeks.

b. Nonthermocatalytic Bleaching

The nonthermocatalytic technique does not utilize heat sources.

The bleaching solutions used are:

- Superoxol (5 parts of H_2O_2 + 1 part of ether) (Fig. 24.2).

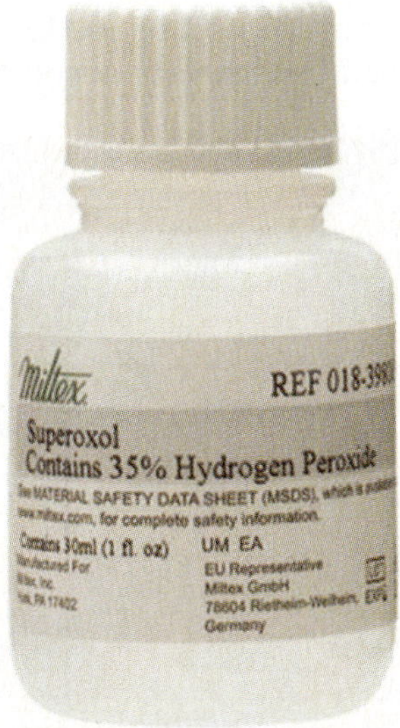

Fig. 24.2 Superoxol

- McInnes solution: 5 parts of 36% HCl (increases the penetration of solution) + 5 parts 30% H_2O_2 (bleaches the enamel by process of oxidation) + 1 part of 0.2% anesthetic ether (removes the surface debris).
- Modified McInnes bleaching solution consisting of 30% hydrogen peroxide and 20% sodium hydroxide in 1 : 1 ratio along with 0.2% ether has been introduced to overcome the deleterious effects of hydrochloric acid.
- Self-activating bleaching agent for vital teeth [(Composition: 35% hydrogen peroxide (0.4 ml), calcium oxide (0.12 gm) and aerosil (to alter/control the viscosity – 0.32/0.64 gm)].

Technique

After polishing the tooth surface and rubber dam application, paste is applied on the teeth and kept there for five minutes (Fig. 24.3a to f). The paste can be reapplied, if required, followed by copious irrigation with warm water.

c. Power Bleaching

Power bleaching utilizes higher concentration of hydrogen peroxide (35–45%).

The high intensity light used as a heat source in thermocatalytic bleaching is replaced with plasma arc lamps, Xe-halogen lights, lasers, etc. Power bleaching is mainly used on single tooth or even small area on the tooth surface that needs to be lightened. It is mainly indicated in deep tetracycline staining and dentin sclerosis, which take longer time with nightguard vital bleaching technique.

Advantage

- Produces immediate results.

Disadvantages

- The caustic nature of the 35–45% H_2O_2 makes isolation difficult; possibility of soft tissue injury

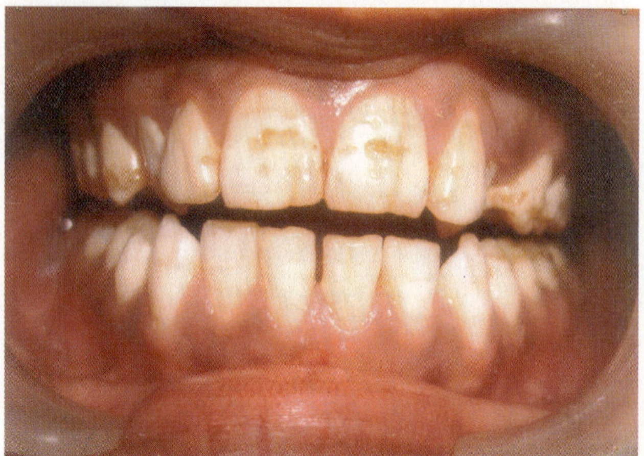

Fig. 24.3a Preoperative

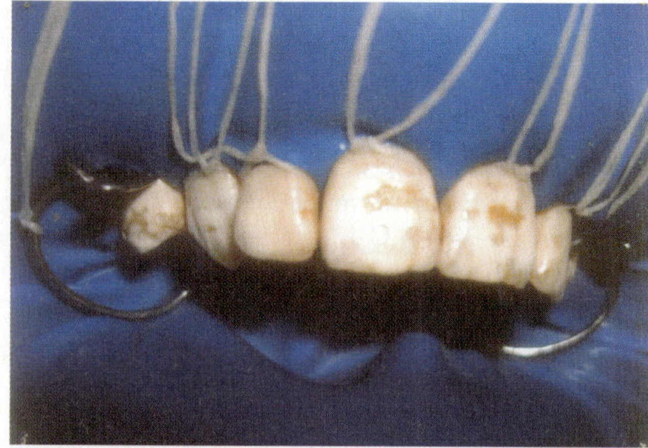

Fig. 24.3b Rubber dam isolation

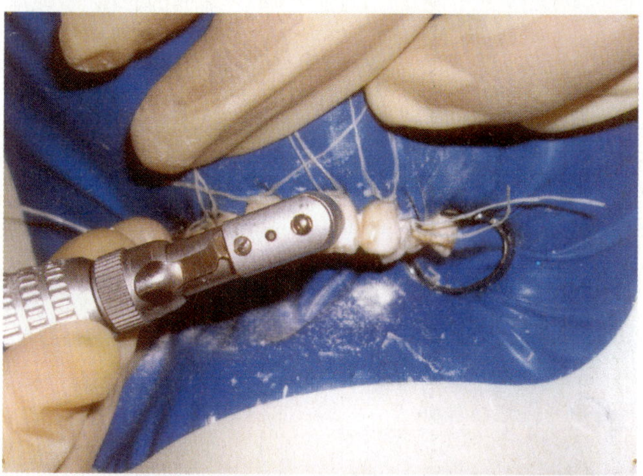

Fig. 24.3c Polishing with slurry of pumice and distilled water

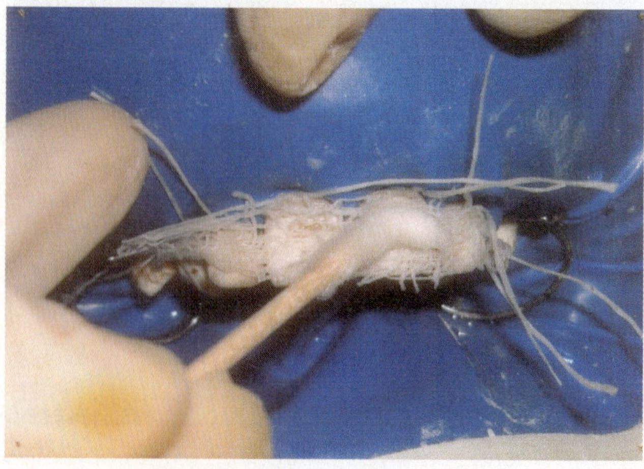

Fig. 24.3d Applying McInnes solution

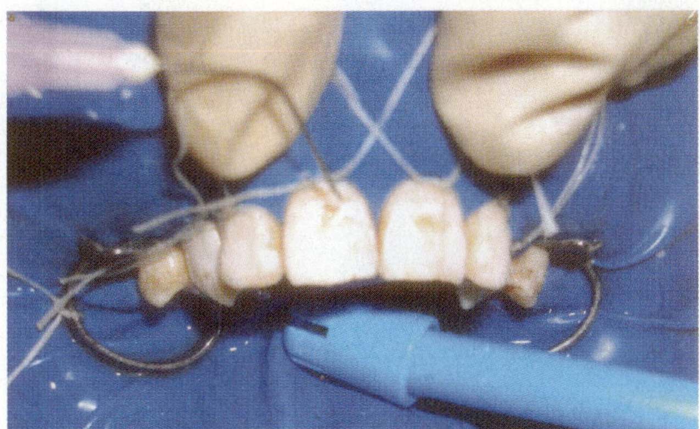

Fig. 24.3e Solution being neutralized by sodium bicarbonate

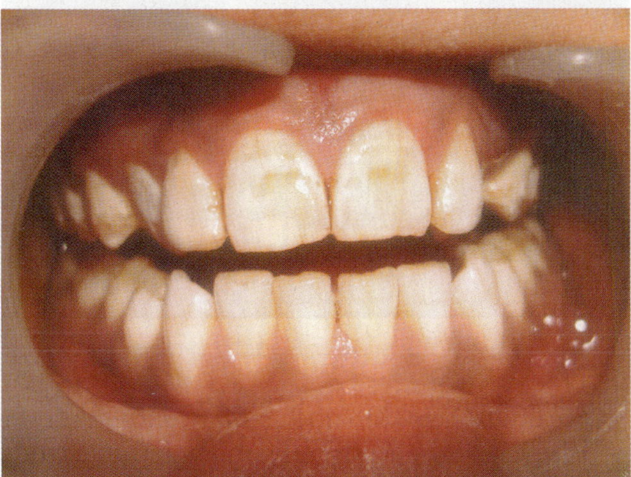

Fig. 24.3f Postoperative

- Lead to dehydration of teeth; may give false lighter shade
- Amount of lightening is not under control
- Greater risk of postoperative sensitivity.

d. Microabrasion

Microabrasion procedure involves surface dissolution of the stains of enamel by acids (preferably 18% hydrochloric acid) along with the abrasives (preferably pumice powder). Microabrasion is indicated for improvement of particular tooth color. This is also used in cases where routine bleaching is not effective.

Indications

- Stains limited to superficial enamel surface
- Enamel fluorosis (initial stages)
- Discoloration due to enamel hypo- or hyper-mineralisation
- Small decalcified lesions, may be due to orthodontic bands.

Contraindications

- Deep stains
- Stains of amelogenesis imperfecta, dentinogenesis imperfecta and tetracycline stains
- Hypoplastic lesion
- Decalcification areas leading to caries.

Technique (Fig. 24.4a to d)

- The selected tooth or teeth are cleaned with prophylaxis paste using rubber cups at slow speed
- The teeth are isolated using rubber dam
- Petroleum jelly is applied to adjacent soft tissue
- Microabrasive agent is applied to the tooth surface for 60 seconds, followed by rinsing
- The process is repeated till the requisite result is achieved
- Topical fluoride can be applied after the treatment
- Patient's consent is necessary for the final color achieved; if not satisfied, the process is repeated.

Advantages

- Helps to remove superficial stains and discoloration
- Minimal discomfort to patient
- Treated teeth display a smooth texture and shine
- Easy manipulation.

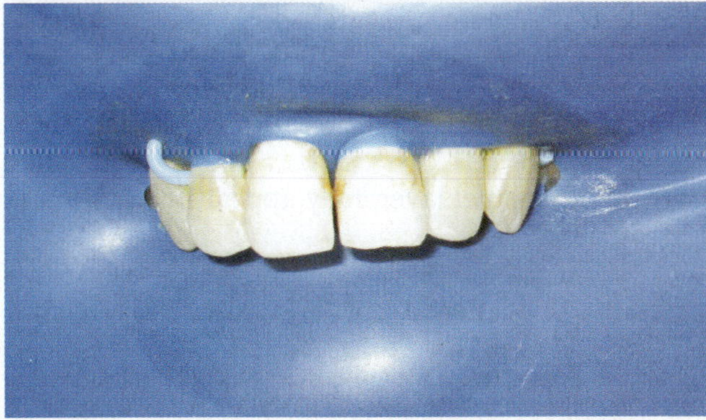

Fig. 24.4a Preoperative

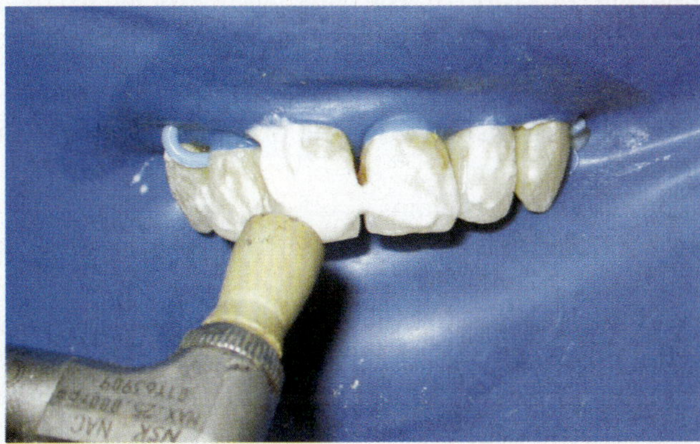

Fig. 24.4b Polishing the tooth surface

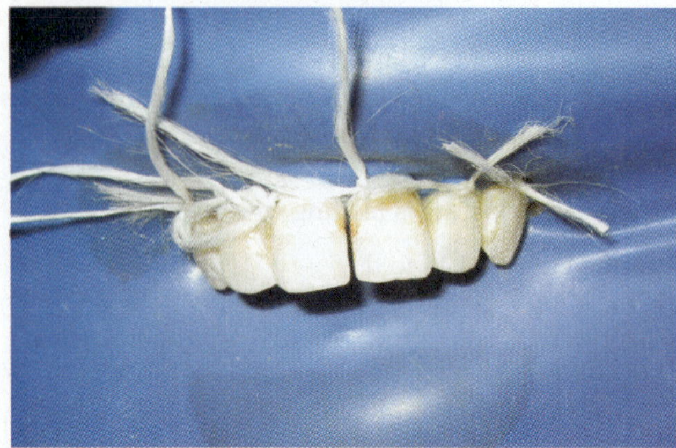

Fig. 24.4c Cleaned surface

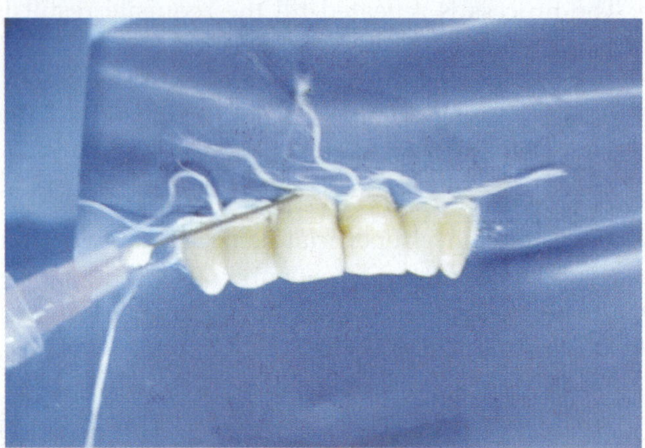

Fig. 24.4d Postoperative

Disadvantages

- Removes enamel layer; may appear yellowish after treatment
- Only effective on those stains, which are confined to outer layer of enamel (not effective for deeper stains)

B. Home Bleaching (Nightguard Vital Bleaching)

10% carbamide peroxide, in a custom fitting bleaching tray, is delivered to the patients for their use during night time (Fig. 24.5a and b). The patient is instructed to cover the teeth with the tray along with the medicament.

Indications

- People dissatisfied with the original color of their teeth
- Brown fluorosis stains
- Discolored teeth that have darkened from trauma but are still vital
- As retreatment of walking bleach after reversal of the treatment
- Lightening of discolored teeth prior to placement of porcelain veneers
- Lighten natural teeth to match ceramic crowns.

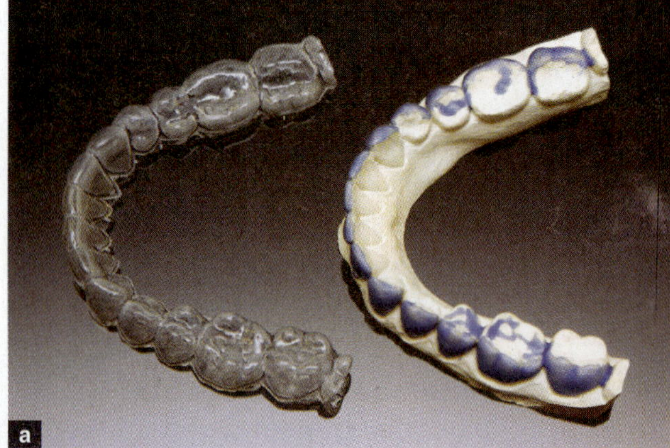

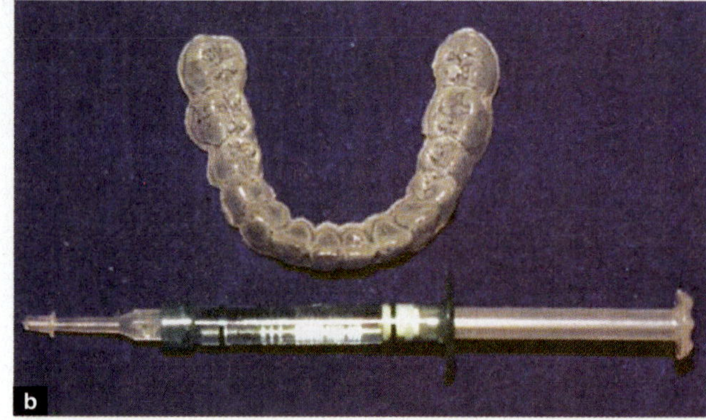

Fig. 24.5a and b Bleaching trays

Carbamide peroxide in different concentration is used as bleaching agent. As the solution is flown onto the tooth surface, carbamide peroxide being unstable dissociates into H_2O_2 and urea, in different concentrations depending upon the concentration of carbamide peroxide. The H_2O_2 further dissociates into water and oxygen. The oxygen radicals cause oxidation of pigmentation in the tooth. The urea degrades into ammonia and carbon dioxide. Carbopol is added to carbamide peroxide to prolong the release of oxygen and to counter carbon dioxide released by urea; subsequently, improving tissue adherence.

Commercial preparations

- 10% carbamide peroxide with carbopol (proxigel, ultralite, etc.) (Fig. 24.6)
- 10% carbamide peroxide without carbopol (fast oxygen releasing—glyoxide, dentalite, etc.)
- 15% carbamide peroxide (Nu smile)
- 1.0–10% hydrogen peroxide (peroxyl, brite smile, etc.)

Technique

There are three basic regimens for the application of the whitening solutions.

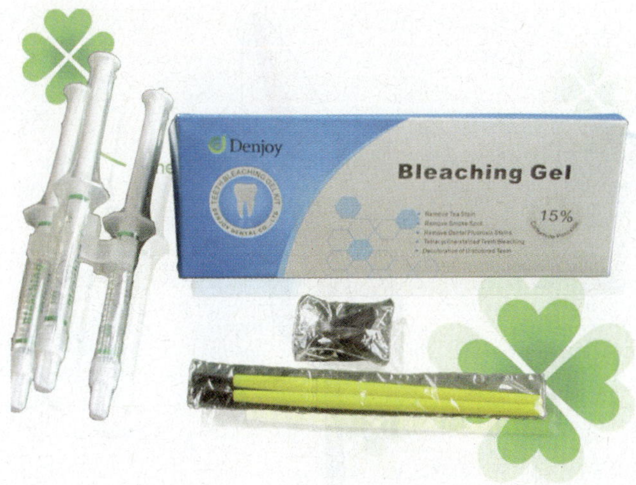

Fig. 24.6 Carbamide peroxide bleaching agent (web photo)

a. Sleeping with the nightguard tray filled with the bleaching solution (the solution is changed each night).
b. Wearing the loaded nightguard tray during the day time and changing the solution every 1.5–2 hours.
c. Polyethylene strips impregnated with 5.25% hydrogen peroxide are also used without tray.

The nightguard vital bleaching procedures usually require three appointments.

First Appointment

The shape and color of the teeth along with the gingiva is evaluated before initiating the bleaching procedure. The stone cast is formed after taking impressions with suitable materials. The tray material is selected (usually 0.040 inch or 0.035 inch ethyl vinyl acetate is used for fabricating the tray; 0.020 inch polypropylene has also been used).

The tray material is placed in the retainer frame on the vacuum forming unit. When the tray material (5″ × 5″ sheet) is sufficiently softened by heating, it is adapted slowly over the cast.

The tray material is allowed to cool on the casts. It is trimmed by scalloping the tray; the tray material should cover about 2.0 mm of tissue apical to gingival crest, both facially and lingually.

Variations in tray fabrication

i. Half round bur is used to cut groove along the gingival tooth margin on the cast.
ii. A trench is built into the tray by stretching a rectangular rubber band (2.0 × 2.0 mm) around the crest, centered on the clinical crowns of the teeth. This trench functions as a reservoir.
iii. Preparing tray with reservoir space (a reservoir is created between teeth and the tray using a viscous light cure composite gel).
    - The viscous composite spacer gel is applied to the selected teeth on the cast (about 0.5 mm)
    - The facial surface of the teeth is painted covering 1.0 mm from the gingival margin
    - The spacer gel is not allowed to flow onto the incisal edge or occlusal surface
    - A light curing unit can be used for curing the spacer
    - The oxygen inhibited resin layer is wiped away from the spacer
    - Tray material is selected and nightguard is constructed in a vacuum forming machine
    - The space of spacer gel in the bleaching trays forms the reservoir.

    Advantages of reservoir
    - Provides space for the bleaching agent
    - Facilitates seating of tray
    - Minimizes tooth sensitivity by avoiding the pinching effect of a light tray
    - Allows uniform transfer of bleaching gel.

    Disadvantages of reservoir
    - Increased cost of fabrication and time
    - Decreased tray retention
    - Gel may leak and irritate gingiva
    - Preparing tray with foam liner.
iv. Preparing tray using foam liner: The tray is also formed using foam liners, which are placed on the selected area of the cast. The trays are then fabricated, in routine, in a vacuum forming machine.

    Advantages of foam liner
    - Soft on patient's gingival tissues
    - 50% reduction in bleaching time.

    Disadvantages of foam liner
    - Esthetically less pleasing
    - Occlusal discrepancies are common
    - Does not help in retention.

Second Appointment

The second appointment involves inserting and fitting the tray. The bleaching material is applied into the tray as follows:

- Two to three drops of bleaching material are placed into the area of each tooth to be bleached
- After inserting the tray, the excess material is wiped out

- Patient is instructed not to drink or rinse during treatment
- The bleaching solution is replaced every one and a half to two hours during daytime regimen
- A single application of bleaching material is advised during night
- The daytime regimen requires one to three weeks; whereas, four to six weeks are required for night time bleaching.

Third Appointment

Third appointment includes postoperative photographs, patient's satisfaction and consent; a decision whether to continue bleaching or to opt for restorative treatment or to keep the patient under observation.

II. NONVITAL TOOTH BLEACHING

The nonvital teeth are discolored because of pulpal necrosis and related complications. Many a times, intentional root canal treatment is carried out in deeply stained (tetracycline stains) teeth so as to bleach the tooth both from inside and outside. Calcified root canals without any root canal treatment are also candidates for nonvital bleaching; however, this modality is contraindicated in teeth, which are discolored due to corrosion products and/or large restorations.

The commonly used solutions are:

- Hydrogen peroxide (H_2O_2)
  - Superoxol (30% H_2O_2)
  - Pyrozone (25% H_2O_2 and ether)
- Sodium perborate ($Na_2B_2O_4(OH)_4$)
- Sodium percarbonate ($2\ Na_2CO_3 \cdot 3\ H_2O_2$).

Preparation of the Tooth

- The restoration, if any, is removed from the coronal pulp chamber
- The access cavity is refined, exposing the surrounding dentin
- Approximately 2.0–3.0 mm of obturating material is also removed from coronal opening of root canals (Fig. 24.7)
- The tooth is washed with 3.0% H_2O_2 solution, rinsed with water and dried
- 1.5–2.0 mm thick glass-ionomer cement/zinc phosphate cement is sealed in direct contact with the obturation material (acts as a mechanical barrier) (Fig. 24.8)
- The color of the tooth is evaluated and noted.

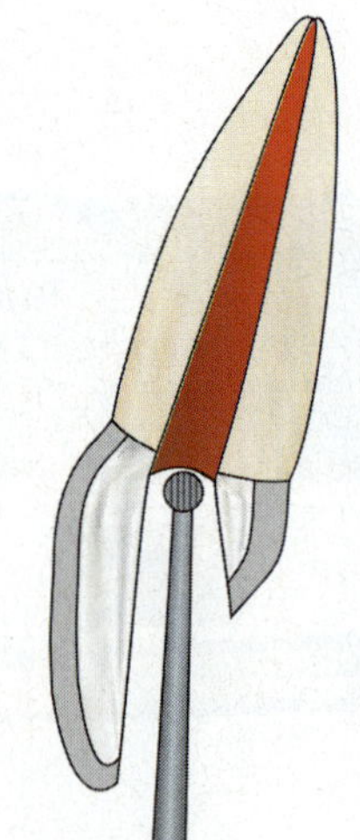

Fig. 24.7 Removal of gutta-percha and coronal filling

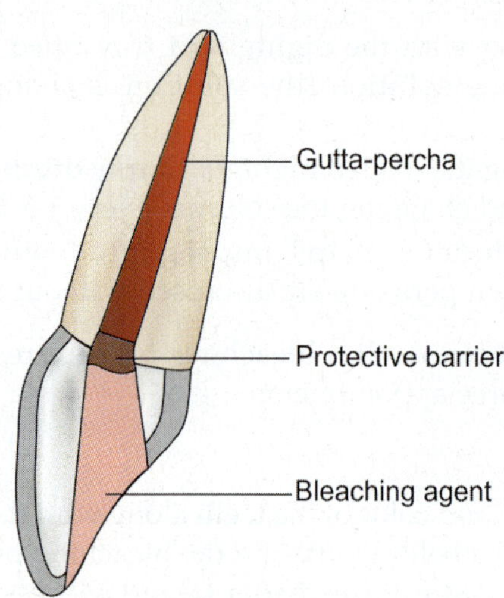

Fig. 24.8 Placement of barrier

The techniques involved in nonvital bleaching are as follows.

a. Thermocatalytic Technique

After preparation of the tooth as described, the technique followed in thermocatalytic nonvital bleaching is practically, the same as for vital tooth bleaching. The light and/or heat source is required to activate the bleaching solution.

Technique (Fig. 24.9a to g)

- The bleaching agent (superoxol and sodium perborate) separately or in combination soaked in cotton pellet is placed in the pulp chamber.
- The solution is activated using light or heat source (temperature 50–60°C).
- The solution is kept for 20–30 minutes in one appointment.

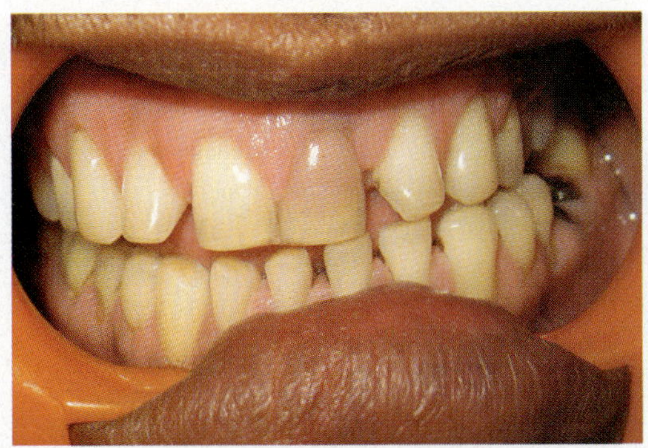

Fig. 24.9a Preoperative

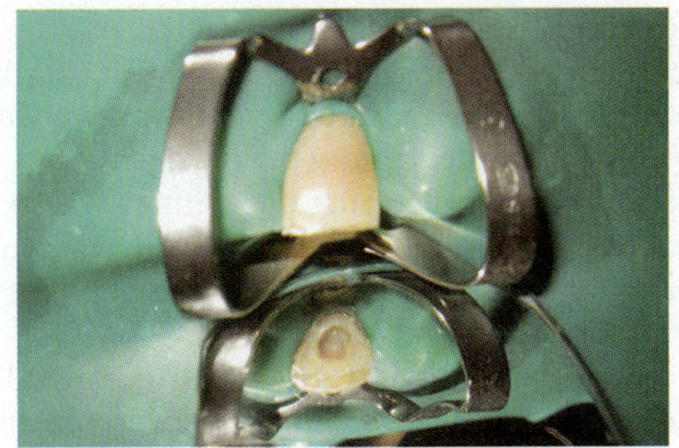

Fig. 24.9d Cleaning of pulp chamber

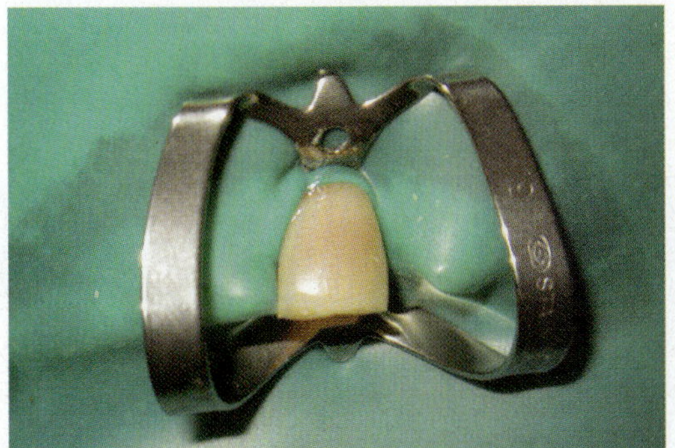

Fig. 24.9b Isolation

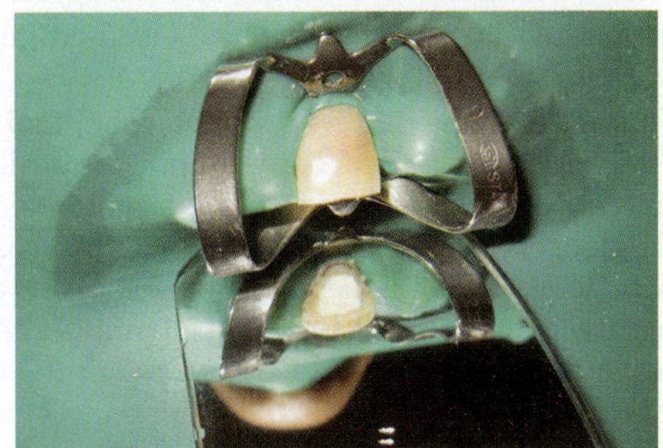

Fig. 24.9e Placing bleaching agent

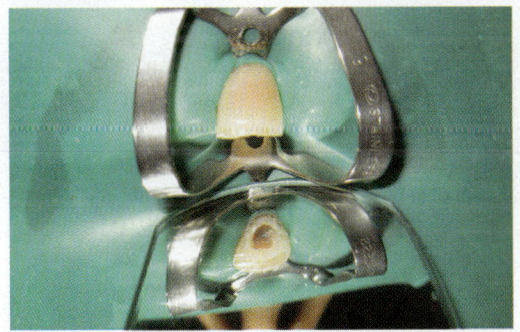

Fig. 24.9c Opening of pulp chamber

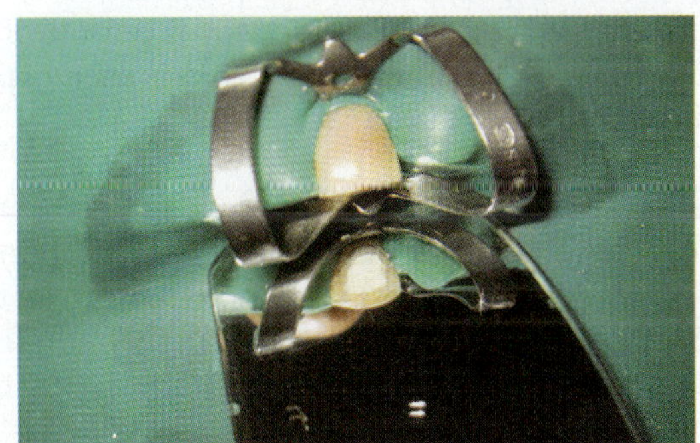

Fig. 24.9f Filling the chamber

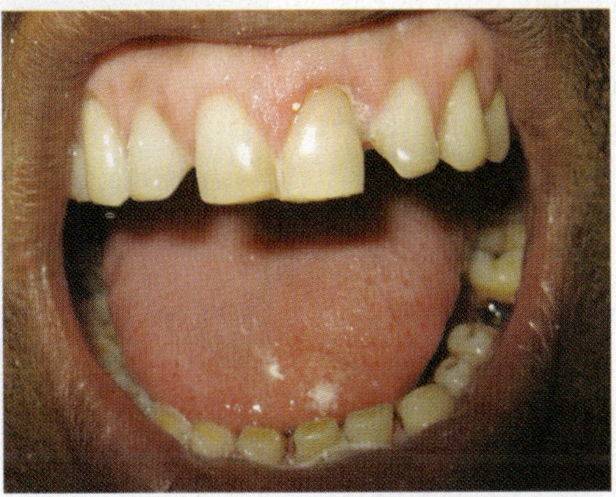

Fig. 24.9g Postoperative

- The process is repeated if required.
- The tooth is rinsed with water. A fresh, sterilized and dry cotton pellet is placed in the pulp chamber and sealed with temporary sealing agent.
- The patient is recalled after one to three weeks.
- The color is evaluated after removing the temporary seal and the cotton. If requisite color is not achieved, the process can be repeated.
- The final restoration of the cavity is carried out preferably with composite resin. It is recommended that acetone based adhesive systems should be used because these have been shown to reverse the adverse effects of bleaching on enamel bond strengths.

The thermocatalytic technique has been modified by various investigators. The modifications are:

i. A mixture of one part 95% ethyl alcohol and two parts chloroform is used for two minutes to desiccate the dentinoenamel surface. This is followed by placement of cotton pellet saturated with pyrozone in the access cavity. A thermocatalytic source is used to activate the solution for about 20 minutes. After this, a dressing of 30% H_2O_2 is placed in the pulp chamber and sealed with zinc phosphate cement.

ii. The dentinal tubules are dehydrated with 90% ethyl alcohol. The cotton saturated with superoxol/ pyrozone is placed into the pulp chamber and activated with a light source for a period of 30–40 minutes. A vulcanite rubber cone is used to press the cotton pallet during activation.

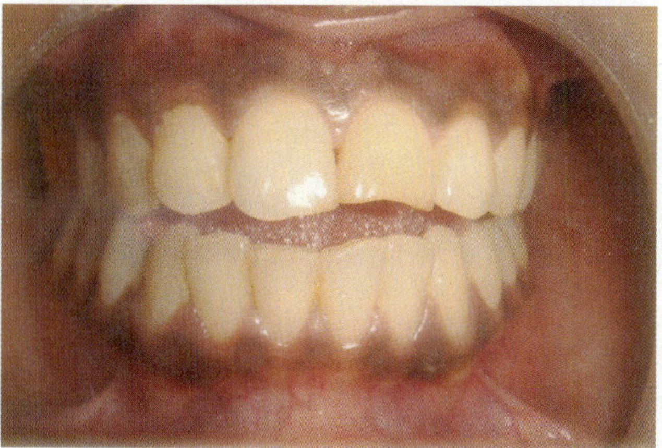

Fig. 24.10a Preoperative

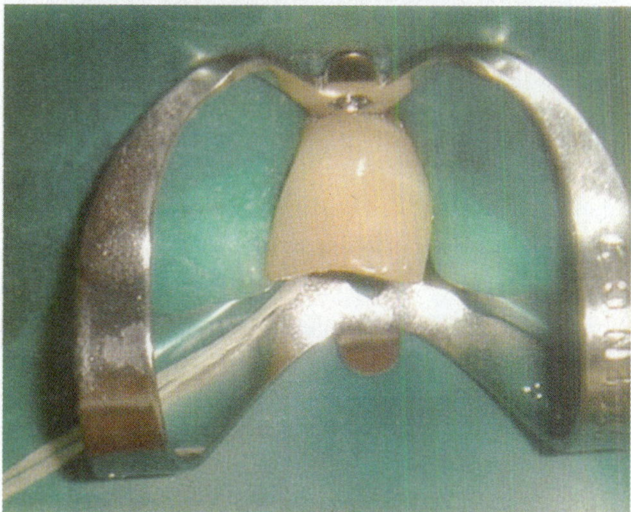

Fig. 24.10b Isolation and placing bleaching agent

b. Walking Bleaching Technique

The bleaching agent is placed in the pulp chamber (Fig. 24.10a to c) over an extended period of time (24–48 hours to 7–10 days). The commonly employed agents are superoxol, sodium perborate and their combinations.

Technique

- A thick paste of sodium perborate and 35% H_2O_2 is placed into the pulp chamber
- The access is sealed with a material capable of providing a good marginal seal (fast setting zinc oxide eugenol, zinc phosphate cement, glass-ionomer cement, etc.). The pressure created by these sealers facilitate bleaching.

c. Modified Walking Bleach Technique

The walking beach technique was modified by Aldecoa and Mayordomo (1992). After completion of walking bleach technique, a mixture of 10% carbamide peroxide and sodium perborate is placed in the pulp chamber for 4 to 6 weeks.

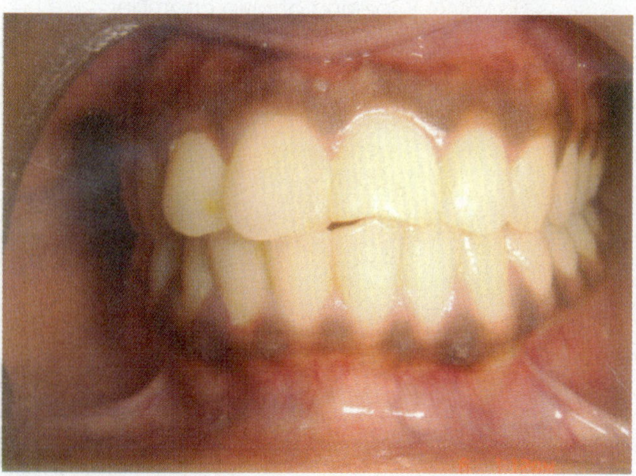

Fig. 24.10c Postoperative

Liebenberg (1997) placed 0.020″ poly-propylene splint soaked in 10% carbamide peroxide gel in the access cavity. The splint retained the bleaching agent and also prevented ingress of debris into the access cavity.

d. Combination Technique (Inside/Outside Bleaching)

This technique involves the combined use of thermo-catalytic in-office nonvital bleaching technique along with nightguard bleaching as in vital tooth bleaching (Fig. 24.11). The synergistic effect significantly improves bleaching. It is indicated where an endodontically treated tooth is present within an arch and the whole arch is to be bleached. As the nonvital tooth gets bleached, the access cavity is restored with suitable composite resin, followed by continuation of night-guard bleaching, if required.

III. LASER ASSISTED BLEACHING

Laser tooth whitening is not a new phenomenon. The procedure utilizes 30–35% hydrogen peroxide, which is applicable in routine bleaching. Laser whitening gel is highly processed fumed silica crystals impregnated in 35% H_2O_2.

Bleaching gel is applied and is activated by high intensity light source/plasma arc light. Crystals in gel absorb thermal energy from light, allow dissociation and penetration of oxygen into the enamel matrix, thus increasing the lightening effect on teeth.

In general, lasers enhance the bleaching effect through photo-oxidation of colored molecules of teeth, which interact with ingredients of bleaching gel via photochemical reactions.

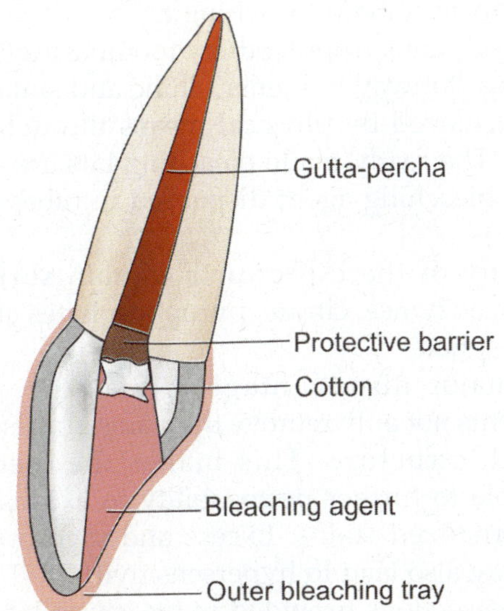

Fig. 24.11 Inside/outside bleaching (diagrammatic)

A few factors, which can enhance hydrogen based bleaching are:

- *Alkaline pH*: Hydrogen peroxide is more reactive at alkaline pH (pH above 7). An alkalinizing agent is mixed with hydrogen peroxide prior to its application to achieve the enhanced effect.
- *Thermal enhancement*: Heating of bleaching agent enhances efficiency of bleaching. The reaction becomes faster and also the penetration of H_2O_2 into dental tissues improves (care is exercised, since heat may lead to irreversible damage of the pulp).
- *Photobleaching*: Green light is considered optimal for photobleaching, since it is not absorbed by hydroxy-apatite water. It can penetrate deeper, removing chromophores (oxidised color particles) that absorb green light. Laser light is more efficient in photo-bleaching.
- *Photolysis*: The light is absorbed by a molecule, effectively breaking down the chemical binding. Hydrogen peroxide, when absorb ultraviolet light, releases hydroxyl ions, which are more potent bleaching agent; enhance the bleaching efficiency.

Following dental laser wavelengths have been cleared by the Food and Drug Administration (FDA) for tooth whitening.

a. Argon laser (488 nm)
b. Carbon dioxide (CO_2) laser (10,600 nm)
c. Diode laser (980 nm)
d. Photochemical laser whitening (smart bleach) (532 nm).

a. Argon Laser

Argon lasers are in the form of a blue light with the wavelength of 480 nm in the visible part of the spectrum. Such a spectrum having affinity to dark color ensures easy removal of stains.

The argon laser excites the unstable and reactive hydrogen peroxide molecule; the energy is absorbed into intramolecular bonds. The H_2O_2 molecules disintegrate into extremely reactive ionic fragments that combine with the chromophilic structure of the organic molecules of the tooth tissue, producing simple chemical chains. The process leads to white tooth surface.

Argon lasers emit photons with short wavelength (480 nm) and higher energy; fairly effective in bleaching (higher wavelength laser may create unfavorable pulp response).

b. Carbon Dioxide (CO_2) Laser

The carbon dioxide (CO_2) lasers (wavelength of 10,600 nm) have been used for enhancing the effect of argon lasers. The effect of initial bleaching with argon laser is enhanced using CO_2 laser.

The argon laser (emits visible blue light) is used first to activate the bleaching gel. The emitted blue light will be absorbed by the dark stains and becomes less effective as the tooth whitens (the blue light will be reflected rather than absorbed by the whiter tooth surface). Then, the CO_2 laser (emits invisible infrared energy) is used to achieve deeper penetration resulting in more efficient tooth whitening.

CO_2 laser, however, has been discontinued because of its thermal effects on the pulp.

c. Diode Laser

These are semiconductor lasers with varying wavelengths; 980 nm wavelength is usually used for bleaching procedure. 38% H_2O_2 is used as bleaching agent.

d. Photochemical Laser Whitening (Smart Bleach)

Lasers effectively bleach teeth; however, use of 30% hydrogen peroxide may transiently reduce the microhardness of enamel and dentin. It may also result in post-treatment sensitivity.

With the smart bleach technique (KTP laser) these problems do not occur as the pH of the bleaching gel is alkaline (approximately 9.5). The primary action of smart bleaching is photochemical and not photothermal. The perhydroxyl ion produced, is more reactive than the superoxide and other radicals. Also, under alkaline conditions, etching of the tooth surface does not occur.

Smart bleach is particularly useful in bleaching tetracycline stained teeth. The chelate formed between tetracycline and hydroxyapatite is a red quinine product, dimethylamino tetracycline. This colored product is relatively resistant to oxidation from peroxide, but can be broken down (photo-oxidised) by green light in a particular narrow spectral range (512 to 540 nm). Because this energy aligns particularly well with the wavelength of KTP laser (532 nm), energy from this laser can cause terminal photo-oxidation of the quinone molecule, which renders it colorless. The use of the KTP laser in combination with a hydrogen peroxide based gel ensures that complete and irreversible bleaching of red quinone occurs.

In addition to driving photo-oxidation reactions within the tooth, some of the visible green laser energy applied to the site is absorbed in Rhodamine B red dye, which is present in the bleaching gel. The photochemical process results in the production of free oxygen radicals. A portion of the KTP laser energy absorbed into the Rhodamine B dye is also transferred from the excited molecule into the bleaching gel in the form of thermal energy. This transfer results in controlled heating of the gel and not the tooth, thus minimizing the possibility of thermal insult to the dental pulp. This superficial heating of the gel accelerates the breakdown of H_2O_2, which boosts the free oxygen radicals over a given time.

The currently marketed laser whitening systems are laser smile whitening system (Biolase) and PearlinBrite laser whitening system.

IV. TOOTH BLEACHING WITH NONTHERMAL ATMOSPHERIC PLASMA

Plasma is considered as the fourth state of matter and it is the most abundant state in the universe. Plasma can be divided into two main categories: hot plasma (near-equilibrium plasma) and cold plasma (non-equilibrium plasma). Hot plasma consists of very high temperature particles and they are close to the maximal degree of ionization. Cold plasma is composed of low temperature particles and relatively high temperature electrons and they have low degree of ionization. Various investigators (Lee et al 2009) have demonstrated that room temperature plasma could be used for tooth bleaching. The authors opined that the tooth bleaching method with plasma can be complementary to conventional method because it provides effective bleaching without thermal damage.

V. OVER THE COUNTER PRODUCTS

A considerable number of home tooth whitening products, viz. tooth polish, toothpastes and bleaching kits are available in the market. Mostly, the tooth polish and toothpastes contain ingredients that remove extrinsic stains on teeth rather than bleaching them (a few products contain bleaching agents). The removal of extrinsic stains from teeth by toothpastes (Close up whitening, Amway whitener, Shine and smile, etc.) is mainly achieved by physical means through organic solvents. The ready-made bleaching kits are available with the bleaching agent dispensed in tubes (Colgate Platinum).

Majority of these products contain surfactants, peroxide, enzymes, citrate, pyrophosphates and hexametaphosphate.

The major disadvantage is that the abrasive constituents not only remove the stains but also abrade the tooth structure. This makes the teeth more susceptible to further permeability to extrinsic stains and internalized stains. Excess and vigorous use of pastes may also lead to hypersensitivity.

The instructions provided in bleaching kits are not sufficient. The prefabricated trays may not fit accurately in the patient's oral cavity causing occlusal discrepancies, temporomandibular joint dysfunction and leaching of the bleaching agent; subsequently, leading to soft tissue injury.

ADVERSE EFFECTS OF BLEACHING

The bleaching process, both vital and nonvital, has side effects, adversely influencing the tooth and the surrounding tissues. The adverse effects reported in animal and human studies include:

a. Hydrogen peroxide toxicity
b. Cervical root resorption associated with nonvital bleaching
c. Increased sensitivity associated with vital bleaching
d. Effect on gingiva and mucous membrane
e. Alteration in the structure of enamel
f. Effect on dentin
g. Effect on pulp
h. Effect on resin-based restorative materials
i. Effect on marginal seal
j. Vital tooth bleaching may activate caries progression.

Adverse effects of bleaching	
Vital tooth bleaching	• Sensitivity • Alteration in enamel structure • Effect on dentin and pulp • Minor ulceration of gingiva • Caries progression
Nonvital tooth bleaching	• Cervical root resorption • Effect on marginal seal
General	• Hydrogen peroxide toxicity and toxicity of other bleaching agents • Effect on restorative materials

a. Hydrogen Peroxide Toxicity

Hydrogen peroxide is a toxic product, especially at higher concentrations. The adverse effects of hydrogen peroxide are:

i. Hydrogen peroxide can cause burns on contact with skin or eyes. When 30% H_2O_2 was applied to the tip of rat tongue at 15 minute intervals (four applications), it lead to edema. However, prior application of catalase may prevent such edema.
ii. The inadvertent flow of H_2O_2 into the periodontal ligament and periapical tissues during root canal treatment, produce effervescence and liberate oxygen; may lead to tissue emphysema.
iii. The adverse effects of hydrogen peroxide mouth rinses (6% H_2O_2) include mouth irritation and discomfort, dryness, loss of taste, elongation of filiform papillae and diffuse mucosal whitening of tongue.
iv. Use of hydrogen peroxide may lead to change in epithelial morphology and its proliferation rate. The proliferating cell nuclear antigen (PCNA) index, an indication of cell proliferation, increases in basal and parabasal layers of epithelium. Usually smokers had a significantly higher PCNA index than nonsmokers, this difference disappeared following bleaching, indicating simulation of cell division activity by peroxide similar to that produced by smoke. It has been established that 10% carbamide peroxide would act as a tumour promoter in the presence of mutated cells.
v. Dental pulp is reported to have a low peroxidase enzyme activity due to a sparse population of fibroblasts. Studies have reported the inhibition as well as inactivation of pulpal enzymes by H_2O_2. The quantity of peroxides penetrating the pulp chamber, even in small amounts, are sufficient to produce toxic effects on cultured fibroblasts.

b. Cervical Root Resorption associated with Nonvital Bleaching

The most commonly seen complication of nonvital bleaching is cervical root resorption (an inflammatory mediated external resorption of the root). The incidence of cervical root resorption after nonvital bleaching ranges from 0 to 7%. This is more commonly seen in teeth, which become pulpless at a young age and when no barrier is placed between endodontic filling material and pulp chamber during bleaching. In such cases, the dentinal tubules remain patent and communicate with periodontal space through the defects of cementoenamel junction. This allows the bleach solution to reach the periodontal ligament from root canal system and an inflammatory reaction can be initiated, resulting in external cervical root resorption.

The features affecting the root resorption are:

- 10% of anterior teeth have cervical areas in which enamel and cementum do not meet
- Cervical resorption occurs coronal to the endodontic seal.

The critical region for the root resorption is the proximal area, where the cementoenamel junction dips and cervical root resorption begins. Location, shape and the barrier between endodontic filling material and the pulp chamber can effectively curtail this problem.

The barrier placement involves periodontal probing from three sides, viz. labial, mesial and distal. The probing is carried out from the epithelial attachment to the labial contour of the tooth followed by mesial and distal. The internal level of barrier should be one millimeter incisal to the corresponding external probing of the epithelial attachment.

The intention of barrier placement is to cover dentinal tubules apical to the epithelial attachment so that the bleaching agents are contained within the pulp chamber.

Cavit and light cure glass-ionomer cements are the most commonly used barrier materials.

c. Increased Sensitivity associated with Vital Bleaching

Vital tooth bleaching uses high concentration of hydrogen peroxide (35–50%) or carbamide peroxide (35–40%), often supplemented with a heat source; or in a bleaching tray to be used at home.

The exact mechanism of tooth sensitivity is not clear; however, on the basis of *in vitro* studies, it is assumed that H_2O_2 in the bleaching gel is capable of penetrating through enamel and dentin and reaching the pulp chamber.

It has been established that the bleaching procedure increases intrapulpal temperature, which is detrimental to pulp. The heat when applied to hydrogen peroxide may lead to diffusion of H_2O_2 into dentin and pulp. However, inflammatory changes get recovered within one month.

In-office bleaching procedures with high concentrations of hydrogen peroxide were associated with high post-treatment sensitivity; however, nightguard bleaching with lower concentration of hydrogen peroxide (3.0%) or carbamide peroxide (10%) has resulted in decreased sensitivity.

The pH of the bleaching agent and desiccation of the tooth surface are causative agents for sensitivity. Potassium nitrate and sodium fluoride when added to 10% carbamide peroxide, considerably reduce sensitivity without any significant change in bleaching results. Use of anti-inflammatory drugs prior to bleaching may also be effective.

Tooth sensitivity is a common adverse effect of external tooth bleaching. Various studies have confirmed that use of 10% carbamide peroxide had led to increased tooth sensitivity in at least 50% of the patients. Higher incidences of tooth sensitivity (65–78%) have been reported after bleaching with H_2O_2 in combination with heat.

Tooth bleaching in younger individuals (less than 18 years) should be avoided; and also on teeth with caries, exposed dentin and/or defective restorations.

24

d. Effect on Gingiva and Mucous Membrane

Bleaching trays which are ill-fitting, overextended, or not properly trimmed, can irritate soft tissue directly or through bleaching agents leaking onto gingival soft tissues. Higher concentration of H_2O_2 produce soft tissue burns; the color changes to white. It is hypothesized that rehydration and application of antiseptic ointment return the color to its original. Effective protection of gingiva and mucosa, with good isolation will minimize the risk of irritation.

The barrier must be checked for any sign of leakage. The barrier should cover all buccal gingival surface. In case of ulceration, the site is extensively washed with water and/or the anesthetic solution. In severe cases, vitamin E can be applied over the ulceration, which will help healing the wound. The position of light should also be adjusted; should not be too near to mucous membrane.

e. Alteration in the Structure of Enamel

Vital tooth bleaching using carbamide peroxide or hydrogen peroxide significantly alters enamel topography. High concentrations of carbamide peroxide damage enamel surface integrity; however, lesser than phosphoric acid etch. As a result of this increased surface roughness, the teeth may be more susceptible to extrinsic discoloration after bleaching. A few studies have reported that after bleaching, enamel gets weakened by oxidation of organic/inorganic elements, which may appear as porous or pitted surface. The oxygen radicals released from peroxide bleaching material may affect chemical structure of enamel, reducing calcium/phosphate ratio, enamel microhardness and surface morphology; subsequently, lead to increased caries risk. Various studies have also confirmed that use of 10% carbamide peroxide daily for six months did not adversely affect the surface texture of human enamel.

f. Effect on Dentin

Bleaching agents effect tooth color (primarily of dentin). McCaslin et al (1999) placed 10% carbamide peroxide directly on enamel and observed a uniform color change throughout the dentin surface.

The majority of studies investigating surface morphology of dentin found no significant changes. However, Zalkind et al (1996) found that Ca and PO_4 ions ratio of dentin was modified following 7 days of continuous treatment with 30% H_2O_2 or 10% carbamide peroxide solutions.

A transient decrease in surface micro hardness has been observed; however, it is recovered following treatment with 0.05 fluoride solution.

It is established that oxygen radicals damage the dentin substrate (hybrid layer), which is mainly responsible for adhesion of composite resin to dentin surface. Recent studies have also confirmed that the durability of adhesive restorations are detrimentally influenced by carbamide peroxide bleaching. It is concluded that the damage caused to restoration-dental tissue bond strength by the bleaching agent is proportional to the increase in carbamide peroxide concentration; the dentin-composite bond was less sensitive as compared to enamel-composite bond.

g. Effect on Pulp

A 3.0% solution of hydrogen peroxide is capable of causing transient reduction in pulpal blood circulation and occlusion of pulpal blood vessels. The most common side effect experienced by patients using home bleaching technique is mild, transient temperature sensitivity. This sensitivity appears to be dose-related rather than pH related.

h. Effects on Resin-based Restorative Materials

Bleaching may increase the solubility of glass-ionomer and other cements and reduce the bond strength between enamel and resin-based fillings, especially in the first 24 hours, but not later. Following bleaching, hydrogen peroxide residues in the enamel may inhibit the polymerization of resin-based materials and reduce bond strength. Therefore, tooth-bleaching agents should not be used at least 24 hours prior to treatment with resin-based materials.

To improve the bond strength of previously bleached teeth, 10% sodium ascorbate has been found to be effective in reversing the compromised bonding of composite with enamel previously bleached with 10% carbamide peroxide.

It has been established that sodium ascorbate gel when applied following bleaching increased the resin-enamel bond strength (the increase was proportional to the duration of application).

A few authors opined that use of catalase or catalase like substances can effectively neutralize the residual hydrogen peroxide on the bleached teeth. α-tocopherol and grape seed extract have also been found to be effective. It is recommended to postpone the bonding procedure for a sufficient time after the bleaching; 24 hours to four weeks have been quoted in various studies.

i. Effect on Marginal Seal

The nonvital bleaching procedures adversely affect the marginal seal leading to marginal leakage. Various studies have concluded that use of mouthrinses (Oral-B, Listerine, etc.) after bleaching can increase post-restoration microleakage of composite restorations.

j. Vital Tooth Bleaching may activate Caries Progression

It is established that vital bleaching alters surface enamel structure (pitting, etc.). Such altered enamel surface becomes the potential sites for caries progression.

BIBLIOGRAPHY

1. Abouassi T, Wolkewitz M and Hahn P. Effect of carbamide peroxide and hydrogen peroxide on enamel surface: an *in vitro* study. Clin. Oral Investig.: 2011; 15:673–680.
2. Almas K and Al-Harbi M. The effect of 10% carbamide peroxide home bleaching system on the gingival health. J. Contemp. Dent. Pract.: 2003; 1:32.
3. Alonsodela V and Balboa CO. Comparison of the clinical efficacy and safety of carbamide peroxide and Hydrogen peroxide in at-home bleaching gels. Quint. Int.: 2006; 37:551.
4. Alqahtani MQ. Tooth-bleaching procedures and their controversial effects: A literature review. Saudi Dent. J.: 2014; 26:33–46.
5. Arora V, Nikhil V, Suri NK and Arora P. Cold atmospheric plasma (CAP) in dentistry. Dentistry: 2014; 4:1–5.
6. Auschill TM, Hellwig E, Schmidale S, Sculean A and Arweiler NB. Efficacy, side effects and patients acceptance of different bleaching techniques (OTC, in office, at home). Oper. Dent.: 2005; 30:156.
7. Bartlett JD, Dwyer SE, Beniash E, Skobe Z and Ferreira TL. Fluorosis: A new model and new insights. J. Dent. Res.: 2005; 84:832.
8. Bastings RT, Rodrigues AL and Serra MC. The effect of 10% carbamide peroxide, carbopol and/or glycerine on enamel and dentin microhardness. Oper. Dent.: 2005; 30:608.
9. Bortolatto JF, Pretel H and Floros MC. Low concentration H_2O_2/TiO-N in-office bleaching: a randomized clinical trial. J. Dent. Res.: 2014; 93:66S–71S.
10. Briso A, Forseca M, de Almeida L, Mauro S and Dos SP. Color alteration in teeth subjected to different bleaching techniques. Laser Physics: 2010; 20:2066–2069.
11. Browning WD, Chan DC, Frazier KB and Callan RS. Safety and efficacy of a nightguard bleaching agent containing sodium fluoride and potassium nitrate. Quint. Int.: 2004; 4:26.
12. Buchalla W and Attin T. External bleaching therapy with activation by heat, light or laser - a systematic review. Dent. Mater.: 2007; 23:586–596.
13. Burrows S. A review of the safety of tooth bleaching. Dent. Update: 2009; 36:604.
14. Dahl JE and Pallesen U. Tooth bleaching—a critical review of the biological aspects. Crit. Rev. Oral Biol. Med.: 2003; 14:292–304.
15. D'Arce M, Lima D, Aguiar F, Ambrosano G, Munin E and Lovadino J. Evaluation of ultrasound and light sources as bleaching catalysts—an *in vitro* study. Eur. J. Esthet. Dent.: 2012; 7:176.

16. De Moor RJG, Verheyen J, Diachuk A, Verheyen P, Meire MA, De Coster PJ, Keulemans F, De Bruyne M and Walsh LJ. Insight in the chemistry of laser-activated dental bleaching. The Scientific World J.: 2015; Article ID650492:1–6.
17. Deliperi S, Bardwell DN and Papathanasiou A. Clinical evaluation of a combined in-office and take home bleaching system. JADA: 2004; 135:628.
18. Dias HB, Carrera ET, Bortolatto JF, de Andrade MF and de Souza RAN. LED and low level laser therapy association in tooth bleaching using a novel low concentration H_2O_2/N-doped TiO_2 bleaching agent. Laser Physics: 2015; 26:015602.
19. Dietschi D, Rossier S and Krejci I. *In vitro* calorimetric evaluation of the efficacy of various bleaching methods and products. Quint. Int.: 2006; 37:515.
20. Felman D and Parashos P. Coronal tooth discoloration and white mineral trioxide aggregate. J. Endod.: 2013; 39:484–487.
21. Fernandez E and Bortolatto J. New trends on in-office tooth bleaching. J. Dent. Sci. and Ther.: 2016; 1:26–28.
22. Gianluca G, Luca T and Giovanni D. Clinical evaluation of a novel liquid tooth whitening gel. Am. J. Dent.: 2003; 16:147.
23. Goldberg M, Grootveld M and Lynch E. Undesirable and adverse effects of tooth-whitening products: a review. Clic. Oral Invest.: 2010; 14:1.
24. Heymann HO. Tooth whitening: facts and fallacies. Br. Dent. J.: 2005; 198:5–14.
25. Joiner A. Review of the effects of peroxide on enamel and dentin properties. J. Dent.: 2007; 35:889.
26. Joiner A. The bleaching of teeth: a review of the literature. J. Dent.: 2006; 34:412–419.
27. Joiner A. Tooth color: a review of the literature. J. Dent.: 2004; 32:3–12.
28. Joshi SB. An overview of vital teeth bleaching. J. Inderdiscip. Dent.: 2016; 6:3–13.
29. Kielbasa AM, Maire M, Gieren AK and Eliav E. Tooth sensitivity during and after vital tooth bleaching: A systematic review on an unsolved problem. Quint. Int.: 2015; 46:881–97.
30. Kihn PW. Vital tooth bleaching. Dent. Clinic. North Am.: 2007; 51:319–331.
31. Kwon SR and Wertz PW. Review of the mechanism of tooth whitening. J. Esthet. Restor. Dent.: 2015; 27:240–257.
32. Kwon SR. Whitening the single discolored tooth. Dent. Clinic. North Am.: 2011; 55:229.
33. Lee HW, Kim GJ, Kim JM, Park JK, Lee JK and Kim GC. Tooth bleaching with non-thermal atmospheric pressure plasma. J. Endod.: 2009; 351:587–591.
34. Lee HW, Nam SH, Mohamed AAH, Kim GC and Lee JK. Atmospheric pressure plasma jet composed of three electrodes: application to tooth bleaching. Plasma Processes and Polymers: 2010; 7:274–280.
35. Lenherr P, Allgayer N, Weiger R, Filippi A, Attin T and Krastl G. Tooth discoloration induced by endodontic materials: a laboratory study. Int. Endod. J.: 2012; 45:942–949.
36. Leonardo NGS, Almeida LHS, Kodama A, Jacobovitz M, Msotti AS, Ferrari JCL and Pappen FG. Influence of different pulp capping materials to induce coronal tooth discoloration. Giornale Italiano di Endodonzia: 2016; 30:22–26.
37. Li Y and Greenwall L. Safety issues of tooth whitening using peroxide-based materials. Br. Dent. J.: 2013; 215:29–34.
38. Markowitz K. Pretty painful: why does tooth bleaching hurt? Med. Hypotheses.: 2010; 74:835–840.
39. Meincke DK, Prado M, Gomes BP, Bona AD and Sousa EL. Effect of endodontic sealers on tooth color. J. Dent.: 2013; 41:93–96.
40. Mokhlio GR, Matis BA, Cochrm MA and Eckert GJ. A clinical evaluation of carbamide peroxide and hydrogen peroxide whitening agents during daytime. JADA: 2000; 131:1269.
41. Naik S, Tredwin CJ and Scully C. H_2O_2 tooth-whitening (bleaching): Review of study in relation to possible carcinogenesis. Oral Oncology: 2006; 42:668.
42. Nam SH, Lee HJ, Hong JW and Kim GC. Efficacy of non-thermal atmospheric pressure plasma for tooth bleaching. The Sci. World J.: 2015; Article ID 581731.
43. Pan J, Yang X and Sun K. Tooth bleaching using low concentrations of hydrogen peroxide in the presence of a non-thermal plasma jet. IEEE Transactions on Plasma Science: 2013; 41:325–329.
44. Presoto CD, Bortolatto JF, de Carvalho PPF, Trevisan TC, Floros MC and de Oliveira OB. New parameter for in-office dental bleaching. Case Report in Dent.: 2016; Article ID 6034757, 1–4.
45. Pretty IA, Ellwood RP, Brunton PA and Aminian A. Vital tooth bleaching in dental practice: 1. Professional bleaching. Dent. Update: 2006; 33:293.
46. Soares DG, Marcomini N, Basso FG, Pansani TN, Hebling J and de Sourza CA. Indirect cyto-compatibility of a low-concentration hydrogen peroxide bleaching gel to odontoblast-like cells. Int. Endod. J.: 2016; 49:26–36.
47. Souza GDM, Santos LM, Fernandes CA, Dantas EDV, Galvao MR, de Assuncao IV and Borges BCD. Sensitivity in dental bleaching and the use of anti-inflammatory agents. JSM Dent.: 2014; 2:1023.
48. Sulieman M. An overview of tooth discoloration: Extrinsic, intrinsic and internalized stains. Dent. Update: 2005; 32:463.
49. Sulieman M. An overview of two bleaching techniques: Nightguard vital bleaching and non-vital bleaching. Dent. Update: 2005; 32:37.
50. Toh CG. Clinical evaluation of a dual activated bleaching system. Asia J. Aesthet. Dent.: 1993; 1:65–70.
51. Tredwin CJ, Naik S, Lewis NJ and Scully C. Hydrogen peroxide tooth whitening (bleaching) products: review of adverse effects and safety issues. Br. Dent. J.: 2006; 200:371.
52. Tsubura S and Yamaguchi R. Clinical evaluation of a new bleaching product 'Polanight' in a Japanese population. Odontology: 2005; 93:52.
53. Walsh LJ, Liu JY and Verhejen P. Tooth discoloration and its treatment using KTP Laser assisted tooth whitening. J. Oral Laser Appl.: 2004; 4:7.
54. Watts A and Addy M. Tooth discoloration and staining: A review of the literature. Br. Dent. J.: 2001; 12:191.
55. Wetter NU, Barroso MC and Pelino JEP. Dental bleaching efficacy with diode laser and LED irradiation: an *in vitro* study. Lasers in Surgery and Medicine: 2004; 35:254–258.
56. Zimmerli B, Jeger F and Lussi A. Bleaching of non-vital teeth: A clinically relevant literature review. Schweiz Monatsschr Zahnmed: 2010; 120:306–313.

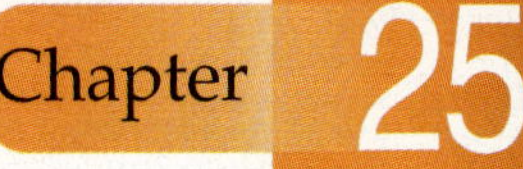

Chapter 25 Vital Pulp Therapy

Importance of dental pulp in a healthy tooth is unquestionable. It provides inductive, formative, nutritive, protective and reparative function. Throughout the life of the tooth, it forms secondary, reparative and sclerotic dentin. Vital pulp is essential for routine functioning. Endodontic treatment carried out in nonvital teeth is not free of side effects. Therefore, every precaution should be taken to preserve the vitality of tooth. The defense cells in the dental pulp and potential new odontoblasts can form reparative dentin maintaining the pulp vitality.

It has been observed that when local inflammation is induced in the pulp, the tissue pressure increases only in inflamed area. This fluid is absorbed into capillaries in adjacent uninflamed tissues resulting in increased lymphatic drainage. The healing process usually prevails when injurious agents are removed and therapeutic measures are instituted.

Etiology of Pulpal Diseases

A. *Mechanical*

a. Trauma
  i. Accidental
  ii. Parafunctional habits
    - Bruxism
    - Bruxomania
    - Clenching
  iii. Iatrogenic dental procedures
    - Tooth preparation
    - Pins
    - Malleting gold foil
  iv. Chronic trauma from occlusion

b. Pathologic wear
  i. Attrition
  ii. Abrasion
  iii. Abfraction

c. Deep tooth preparation where remaining dentin thickness is less than 2.0 mm

d. Crack through body of tooth

e. Barometric changes leading to aerodontalgia

f. Orthodontic movement of heavily restored abutment teeth.

B. *Thermal*

Slight rise in intrapulpal temperature (100°F) affects pulp. The following factors raise the intrapulpal temperature.

- Heat from cavity preparation (with coolant)
- Setting of cements leading to an exothermic reaction
- Inadequate pulp protection beneath metallic restorations
- Polishing of restorations
- Impression materials.

C. *Chemical*

- Dental materials with high acidity
- Irritants like resin monomers
- Erosion with acids
  - Soft drinks
  - Gastrooesophageal reflux.

D. *Bacterial*

- Caries
- Trauma leading to direct invasion of bacteria in pulp
- Systemic (anachoresis)
- Chronic periodontal diseases.

Healthy Pulp and Primary Trauma

The sequelae of trauma to the healthy pulp is described in Flowchart 25.1.

Clinical Status of Pulp

The healthy pulp, under the influence of abovementioned factors, may get stressed, inflamed or necrosed. The stressed pulp is a clinical concept and

Flowchart 25.1: Sequelae of trauma to the healthy pulp

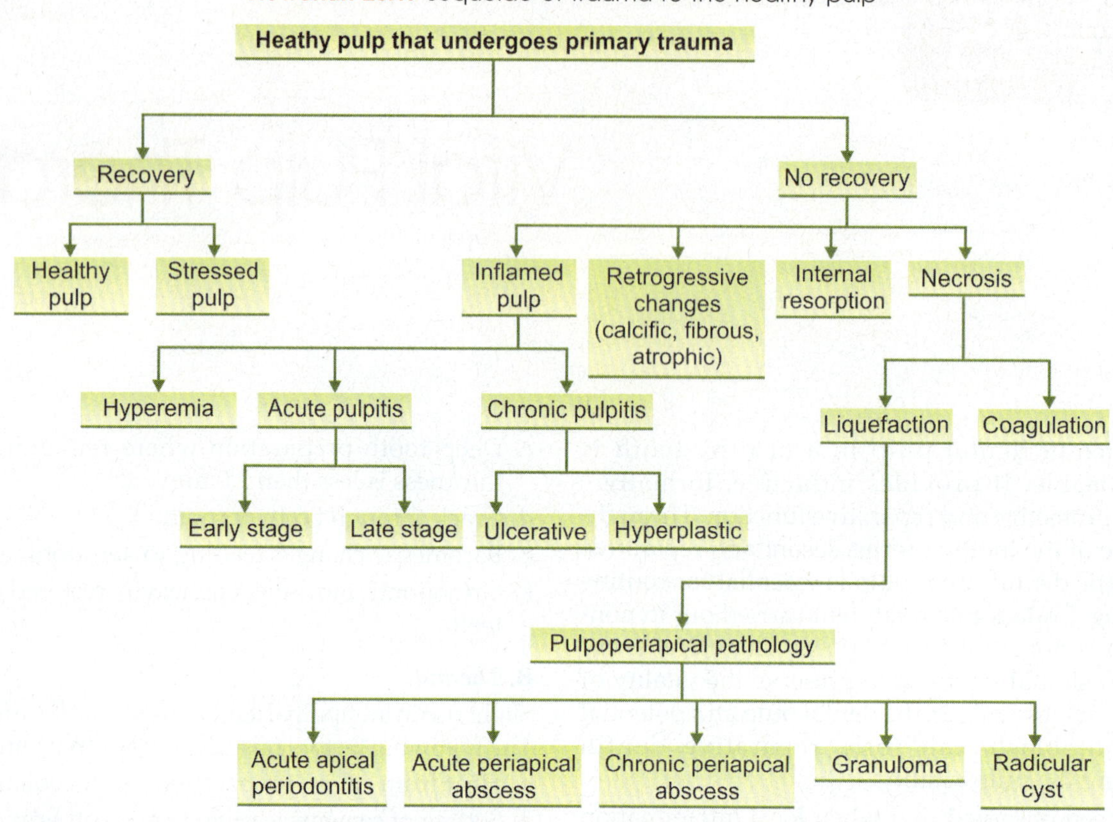

not a histologic entity. Although stressed pulp is usually asymptomatic clinically, it may deteriorate rapidly to a diseased condition. Crown preparations, pin buildups, restorative failures and tooth structure cracks can transform the pulp from a state of asymptomatic stress to a state of pulpal disease.

The clinical evaluation of healthy, stressed, inflamed and necrotic pulp is tabulated in Table 25.1.

VITAL PULP THERAPY

It is the treatment of an exposed or nearly exposed pulp by a medicament to repair and maintain its vitality.

Table 25.1 Clinical evaluation of healthy, stressed, inflamed and necrotic pulp

Clinical evaluation	*Healthy pulp*	*Stressed pulp*	*Inflamed pulp*	*Necrotic pulp*
Patient's history	• No significant dental history • Effective mastication after dental procedures	• Asymptomatic (no pain) • History of long dental procedures, caries or trauma	• Symptomatic (pain) • Previous complex dental history	• Usually no pain or pain on mastication only • Pain with hot stimulus
Radiographic features	• Well-defined pulp chamber and root canals • Acceptable remaining dentin • No calcification	• Deep restorations or caries • Pulp spaces altered by calcification or internal resorption	• Pulp chamber recession • Narrow pulp chamber (partial calcification) • Deep restorations	• May show any of the findings of healthy, inflamed or stressed pulp
Examination of teeth and surrounding tissues	• Minimal caries or restorations • Normal color of tooth and surrounding tissues	• Normal surrounding tissues • Teeth normal	• Defective restorations/ multiple restorations • Surrounding tissues may be normal	• May show any of the findings of healthy, inflamed or stressed pulp
Pulp response to external stimuli	• Nil	• Very rapid or very late response, provoked on stimulus and may linger on	• Late, weak, inconsistent response requiring high degree of stimulation and longer time	• No response to stimuli • Sometimes pain with hot stimulus

Vital pulp therapy has a high success rate under following conditions:

- Pulp is not inflamed.
- Hemorrhage is properly controlled.
- Application of nontoxic capping material.
- Capping material and restoration able to seal out bacteria.

Vital pulp therapy includes following treatment modalities:

1. Indirect pulp capping/indirect pulp treatment
2. Direct pulp capping
3. Pulp curettage
4. Partial pulpotomy
5. Pulpotomy
6. Apexogenesis (physiological root formation).

Apexification, a procedure, wherein root closure/apical barrier is achieved in nonvital teeth with incompletely formed root apex, is also described.

1. Indirect Pulp Capping/Indirect Pulp Treatment

Indirect pulp capping implies treating pulps, which are not exposed and may be near exposure; whereas, indirect pulp treatment is a technique in which an effort is made to avoid pulp exposure during the treatment of teeth with deep carious lesions without any evidence of pulp degeneration or periapical pathology.

Indirect pulp capping is two appointment procedure, whereas indirect pulp treatment is a single appointment procedure.

Indication

- Deep carious lesion with minimal pulpal inflammation (complete removal of caries may lead to pulp exposure).

Contraindications

- A tooth with existing pulp inflammation
- A tooth with periapical pathology.

Objectives

- Minimize pulp injury
- Promote dentin sclerosis
- Minimize postoperative sensitivity
- Arrest progression of carious lesion
- Stimulation of reparative dentin formation
- Remineralize affected dentin.

Rationale

In a carious lesion, dentin decalcification precedes bacterial invasion within dentin. In an active carious lesion, two distinct layers are seen:

i. ***Infected dentin***: It is necrotic, soft dentin, not painful to stimulation and grossly infected with bacteria. Collagen is irreversibly denatured.

ii. ***Affected dentin***: It is demineralized, discolored but hard dentin, painful to stimulation containing very few bacteria. It is reversibly denatured and capable of being remineralized.

When outer layer is removed, most of the bacteria are removed and the substrate on which they thrive is also removed. When cavity is sealed with a suitable material, any remaining bacteria are either killed or lie in a stage of dormancy. However, affected dentin can be left on pulpal and axial walls and never on dentinoenamel junction and cavity margins. The two layers can be differentiated with either 0.5% basic fuchsin or 1.0% acid red dyes. Acid red is preferred since basic fuchsin has carcinogenic potential.

The remaining dentin thickness also plays an important role. If remaining dentin thickness is more than 1.0 mm, no significant disturbance in the pulp is seen. 0.25 to 0.5 mm remaining dentin leads to maximal reparative dentin formation and remineralization of demineralized dentin; whereas, 0.25 mm or less remaining dentin provoke bacterial growth in pulp. Reparative dentin formation and remineralization is greatly decreased.

Technique

The technique involves the following steps:

A. Removal of caries

a. *Mechanical method*

- Soft caries can be removed with a spoon excavator by removing flakes of carious dentin in layers.
- The discolored dentin can be removed with large round steel burs revolving at slow speed. Pulp damage may result from reaction of frictional heat with the use of bur while excessive pressure with a spoon excavator may force the microorganism into the dentinal tubules or expose the pulp. Removal of infected dentin should continue until the remaining dentin feels as hard as normal dentin.

b. *Chemomechanical methods*

The conventional caries excavation methods usually induce pain and fear in patients, especially the children. To make the caries removal painless, selectively softening the carious lesion will facilitate removal by excavation without any pressure.

The chemical agents used to soften dentin are:

i. *Sodium hypochlorite-based agents*: Earlier 5.0% sodium hypochlorite has been used to soften carious lesions.

Later, the use of 5.0% sodium hypochlorite was observed to be toxic to adjacent healthy tissues. A new solution, *GK-101* was developed, which consisted of sodium hydroxide, sodium chloride and glycine in addition to 5.0% sodium hypochlorite. GK-101 was more effective than the hypochlorite alone; however, the carious softening effect was very slow.

Caridex, a commercial preparation, is consisted of sodium hypochlorite solution buffered with mixture of aminobutyric acid, sodium chloride and sodium hydroxide. The ability of sodium hypochlorite to selectively soften carious lesion is attributed to the buffering effect of the amino acids, which enhances disrupting effect on the degenerated collagen of the carious dentin. The resultant friable collagen fibrils can be easily removed with excavators.

Caridex was not fully successful in clinical practice because of the need for a specific apparatus to deliver the solution into the cavity, short shelf-life, longer treatment time, and higher treatment cost.

Another caries removing chemical agent based on sodium hypochlorite was introduced in the name of *Carisolv*. It is available in the form of a gel. It consists of two components, one is transparent liquid containing 0.5% sodium hypochlorite and the other component contain an amino acid mixture (glutamic acid, leucine and lysine), sodium carboxymethyl cellulose to enhance the viscosity; sodium hydroxide provide pH of 11 and water acts as vehicle.

The chemical composition and microstructure of dentin after excavation with Carisolv remained unchanged. The calcium and phosphorus content remain similar after excavation; however, the hardness values of residual dentin were same as for sound dentin. The etch pattern of dentin in Carisolv-excavated lesions is deeper than caries removed with a conventional bur. Carisolv excavated dentin shows better bonding characteristics, viz. patent dentinal tubules, not covered by smear layer, irregular surface and the improved wetting potential. Carisolv has superior property in reducing the counts of viable bacteria in residual dentin, as compared to conventional bur excavation. Carisolv has bactericidal activity due to formation of chloramines compounds. The *disadvantages* include its high cost and need of special instruments. Children usually dislike the chlorine taste and odor (Table 25.2).

ii. *Pepsin-based agents*: An enzyme pepsin in a phosphoric acid/sodium bisphosphate buffer has also been tried as a chemical agent to soften caries. *SFC-VIII* (3M ESPE, Germany) is the commercially available pepsin based agent. The *advantage* of this pepsin-based agent is that it acts on more specific denatured collagen than the sodium hypochlorite-based agents. The phosphoric acid dissolves the inorganic component of carious dentin, while at the same time pepsin gets access to the organic part of the carious mass, selectively dissolving the denatured collagen. For effective caries removal, SFC-VIII gel should be used along with an excavator having hardness between that of sound and infected dentin. The *limitation* of SFC-VIII excavation is that the heavily pigmented and arrested dentin caries pose problem in pepsin digestion.

iii. *Papacarie*: Papacarie (Sao Paulo-Brazil) is another chemomechanical caries removing agent, which contains papain, chloramines, toluidine blue and certain salts. Papain is a proteolytic enzyme similar to pepsin. Papain comes from latex of leaves and fruits of green

Table 25.2 Comparison of Caridex and Carisolv

Characteristics	*Caridex*	*Carisolv*
Composition	Solution I: 1.0% sodium hypochlorite Solution II: i. 0.1M glycine aminobutyric acid ii. 0.1M sodium chloride iii. 0.1M sodium hydroxide	Solution I: 0.5% sodium hypochlorite Solution II: i. 0.1M glutamic acid/leucine/lysine ii. Sodium carboxymethyl cellulose iii. Sodium hydroxide
Dye	Nil	Erythrocin pink
pH	11	11
Physical form	Liquid	Gel
Volume needed	100–500 ml	0.2–1.0 ml
Time required	5 to 15 minutes	5 to 15 minutes
Activity after mixing	Remains active up to one hour	Remains active up to 20 minutes
Biocompatibility	No adverse effects	No adverse effects
Bactericidal activity	Satisfactory	Much better
Bonding characteristics	Satisfactory bonding	Better bonding characteristics

adult papaya, (carica papaya). Papacarie is available in syringes having 3.0 ml gel. The papacarie gel is allowed to act in a cavity for 60 seconds. As the collagen fibrils gel dissolved, the clear gel becomes dark in color. The papain digests dead cells and breaks the partially degraded collagen molecules, contributing to the degradation of the collagen fibrils formed by the carious process.

iv. *Carie-care*: It is an enzyme derived from papaya plant, "the Carica Papaya". It is composed of papaya extract, therapeutic essential oil, coloring gel, sterile water, chloramines and sodium chloride.

Carie-care (papain) acts on the carious tissue, which lacks alpha-antitrypsin (a plasmatic antiprotease system, which inhibits proteolysis). The absence of anti-protease allows papain to act on the partially degraded collagen by breaking the peptide bonds. In addition to papain, the chloramine dissolves carious dentin by means of chlorination of the partially degraded collagen. The gel also contains therapeutic oils (clove oil), which induce analgesic and antiseptic action. It minimizes pain sensation and has a pleasant taste, acceptable by children and the adults as well.

The procedure is explained in detail in Chapter 15, Dental Caries book by the author—Vimal Sikri.

Two-Appointment Technique (Indirect Pulp Capping)

1st Sitting

Local anesthesia is administered and the tooth is isolated with a rubber dam. Cavity outline is established with a high-speed handpiece. Peripheral carious dentin/infected dentin should be removed with sharp spoon excavators (Cohen recommends the use of a large round bur for better results) (Fig. 25.1a). Cavity should be irrigated and dried with cotton, followed by placement of hard setting calcium hydroxide over the remaining affected dentin (Fig. 25.1b). The remainder of the cavity is filled with reinforced zinc oxide eugenol cement or a glass-ionomer cement to achieve a good seal (Fig. 25.1c). This seal should not be disturbed for 6–8 weeks, as the carious process in the deeper layer gets arrested.

2nd Sitting (6–8 Weeks Later)

In the second sitting, all temporary filling material, especially calcium hydroxide dressing over deep portions of the cavity floor is removed. The color changes from deep red rose to light gray/light brown; the texture would change from spongy-wet to hard and caries appears to be dehydrated. Thus, the remaining affected carious dentin appearing dehydrated and "flaky" can be easily removed. Do not disturb pre-dentin, which is the area around the potential exposure appearing whitish and may be soft. The cavity preparation should be restored in the similar way as 1st sitting.

Re-enter or not?

The re-entry restorative procedure is still questionable. It is recommended only if the tooth is asymptomatic, surrounding soft tissues are free from swelling, temporary filling is intact, bitewing radiographs of the treated tooth shows the presence of reparative dentin. Research has shown that carious dentin will re-mineralize within the restoration. So, if "all system go" on recall, the restoration should not be redone.

With re-entry there could be a risk of creating pulp exposure and further insult to the pulp. If a pulp exposure occurs during re-entry, a more invasive vital pulp therapy techniques, such as direct pulp capping or pulpotomy would be indicated.

One Appointment Technique (Indirect Pulp Treatment)

One appointment indirect pulp capping is termed indirect pulp treatment. The selection for one appointment indirect pulp treatment must be based on

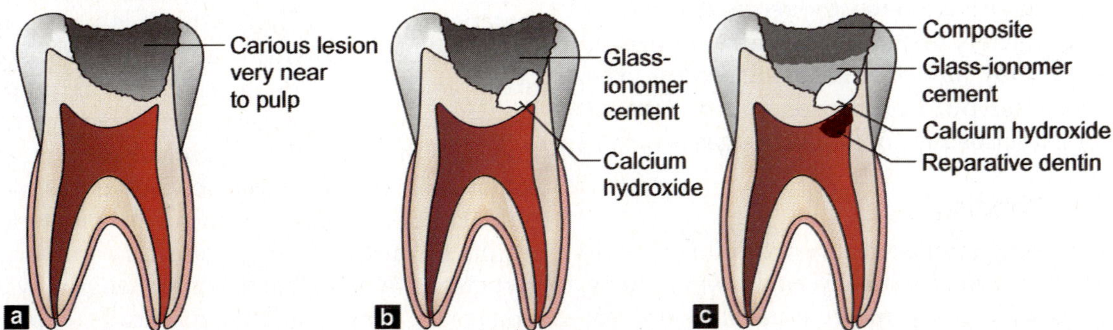

Fig. 25.1 Indirect pulp capping: (a) Carious lesion near pulp (pulp not exposed); (b) Placement of calcium hydroxide on affected dentin; (c) Tooth restored after formation of reparative dentin

clinical judgment and experience with many cases. In recent years, rather than complete caries removal in two appointments, the focus has been to excavate caries as close as possible to the pulp, i.e. some caries be left in the tooth to avoid an exposure, placement of a protective liner, and restoring the tooth without a subsequent re-entry to remove any remaining affected dentin.

Stepwise Excavation

The stepwise excavation of deep caries has shown promising results in managing reversible pulpitis without pulpal perforation and/or endodontic therapy. This approach involves a 2-step process.

i. The first step is the removal of carious dentin along the dentinoenamel junction (DEJ) and excavation of only the outermost infected dentin, leaving a carious mass over the pulp. The objective is to change the cariogenic environment in order to decrease the number of bacteria, close the remaining caries from the biofilm of the oral cavity, and slow arrest the caries development.
ii. The second step is the removal of the remaining caries and placement of a final restoration. The most common recommendation for the interval between steps is 3–6 months, allowing sufficient time for the formation of tertiary dentin and a definitive pulpal diagnosis. Critical to both steps of excavation is the placement of a well-sealed restoration.

The research is inconclusive as regard the decision to use one-appointment caries excavation or stepwise technique. The decision should be based on the individual patient circumstances.

Atraumatic restorative technique (ART) is considered as one form of indirect pulp treatment. The procedure is based on excavating and removing caries using hand instruments only and then restoring the tooth with an adhesive filling material.

B. *Pulp protection*

The open dentinal tubules after the removal of caries need to be completely sealed to minimize ingress of bacteria, which may hinder pulp repair process. The materials used for pulp protection (pulp capping materials) are described in subsequent pages.

2. Direct Pulp Capping

Direct pulp capping implies treating exposed pulps. It is defined as *'treatment of an exposed vital pulp by sealing the pulp wound with an appropriate material to facilitate formation of reparative dentin and maintenance of vital pulp'*. Exposure caused by trauma or by operator's fault during tooth preparation can be successfully treated; whereas, exposure caused by caries usually need root canal treatment. The younger the patient, the better are the chances of healing and repair.

Indications

- Size of exposure should be less than 0.5 mm.
- No profuse hemorrhage or serous/purulent exudate.
- In case of trauma, exposure should not be more than a few hours old.
- Nontender to percussion (a recently traumatized tooth may be reversibly tender to percussion).

Contraindications

- Instrument has penetrated the pulp; infected dentin chips may settle in the pulp.
- Periodontally involved tooth.
- Symptoms of irreversible pulpitis.

Requirements

Ideal requirements for pulp capping material are:

- Stimulate reparative dentin formation
- Maintain pulp vitality
- Bactericidal/bacteriostatic
- Release fluoride to prevent secondary caries
- Adhere to dentin/restorative material
- Resist forces during restoration placement and thereafter functional forces
- Provide appropriate seal
- Radiopaque.

Technique

Tooth is isolated with rubber dam. Caries, if present, are removed from side walls using spoon excavators (Fig. 25.2a). The exposed pulp is not allowed to dry. The exposed site is washed with weak disinfectant and covered with a moist cotton pellet dipped in disinfectant solution. Bleeding is controlled with 5.0% sodium hypochlorite. After controlling bleeding, pulp capping material is placed (Fig. 25.2b). It is placed with little pressure, because with heavy pressure displacement of capping material/dentin chips into the pulp may lead to further pulpal damage. It is followed by a restoration that seals the tooth from microleakage (Fig. 25.2c). It is established that bacterial leakage is responsible for pulpal response rather than toxicity of materials, which results in only mild and transitory pulpal response. Hypersensitivity to temperature change may persist for a day or so. Tooth is tested periodically for pulp vitality. Symptoms usually subside in 4–6 weeks. If tooth remains vital, a permanent restoration may be placed.

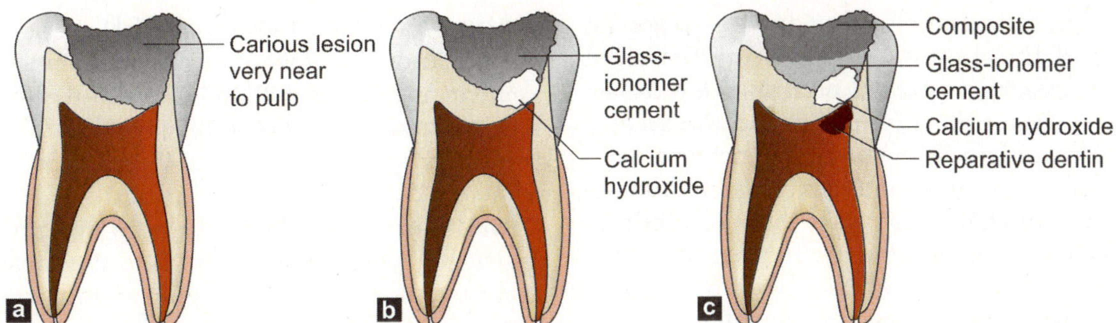

Fig. 25.2 Direct pulp capping: (a) Carious lesion leading to pin-point exposure of pulp; (b) Placement of calcium hydroxide on exposed pulp; (c) Tooth restored after formation of reparative dentin

If tooth becomes painful, or exhibits decreased reading on vitality testing or becomes nonvital, root canal treatment becomes mandatory.

Pulp Capping: Key points

- *Avoid exposing the pulp*
- *Even if residual caries present, cover carious dentin and seal properly*
- *Follow-up for at least six weeks for any symptoms*
- *If pulp gets exposed, control hemorrhage with appropriate astringent agents (sodium hypochlorite is effective hemostatic agent and is also antibacterial)*
- *Calcium hydroxide and mineral trioxide aggregate (MTA) are suitable pulp capping agents*
- *Newer agents, such as morphogenic proteins, enzymes, plant extracts, resorcinol, etc. are also effective*
- *Zinc oxide eugenol, glass-ionomer cement and bonding agents are not successful (should be avoided)*
- *The cavity should be sealed immediately after pulp capping; protect underlying tissues from leakage and bacterial contamination*
- *The tooth should be assessed clinically and radiologically at periodic intervals; restore with suitable restorative material*

The materials used as pulp capping are:

a. Zinc oxide eugenol
b. Calcium hydroxide
c. Mineral trioxide aggregate (MTA)
d. Bonding agents
e. Resin-resorcinol
f. Polycarboxylate cement
g. Cyanoacrylates
h. Antibiotics and corticosteroids
i. Growth factors
j. Enzymes
k. Stem cells
l. Propolis
m. Emdogain
n. TheraCal LC
o. Biodentine
p. Dentin shavings
q. Tricalcium phosphate
r. Laser
s. Miscellaneous

Other techniques for pulp tissue excision and disinfection are:

- Laser
- Electrosurgery

a. *Zinc oxide eugenol*

The use of zinc oxide eugenol as pulp capping agent is controversial. It does provide anodyne effect to the pulp. Because of better marginal adaptability, it provides environment for pulp healing; may not induce calcific bridge formation.

b. *Calcium hydroxide*

Hermann (1930) demonstrated that when vital pulps were covered with calcium hydroxide, it led to the formation of secondary dentin. Calcium hydroxide, applied directly to pulp tissue lead to coagulation necrosis of the adjacent tissues. Beneath the region of coagulation necrosis, cells of underlying pulp differentiate into odontoblast and other cells, which help to form dentin matrix. However, a blood clot should not be left between calcium hydroxide and pulp. Such cases, (hydroxyl ions trapped in the clot) do not allow differentiation of odontoblasts.

Calcium hydroxide maintains a local state of alkalinity necessary for bone/dentin formation. Earlier, it was postulated that calcium (Ca) from calcium hydroxide would diffuse into pulp and participate in the formation of reparative dentin. Later, it was established that calcium ions from calcium hydroxide do not help formation of new dentin; however, it may come from blood. Commercially available pastes of calcium hydroxide are less alkaline and less caustic; a bridge is formed in contact with capping material and some of the tissue underlying the bridge may get degenerated/resorbed, leaving a void between capping material and the dentin bridge. Under calcium hydroxide dressings, an area of necrosis is formed on the surface of the pulp stump. Beyond the area of induced necrosis, undifferentiated mesenchymal cells in the cell rich zone proliferate and differentiate into odontoblasts. Another theory says that new odontoblasts develop from fibroblasts. In case of severe inflammation, reparative dentin devoid of dentinal tubules is formed. In case of mild inflammation, varying number of dentinal tubules are present. Calcium hydroxide induced dentinal bridge contains multiple tunnel defects facilitating bacterial microleakage. Calcium hydroxide in due course of time (one to two years) also becomes soft and allows leakage resulting in pulpal inflammation and necrosis. The concerned tooth may show evidence of calcification or internal resorption; subsequently, root canal treatment is to be initiated.

Calcium hydroxide has been used in various forms, viz. powder alone, paste form or commercially available calcium hydroxide.

Powder alone is found to be highly irritating. Also prolonged exposure to atmosphere leads to the formation of calcium carbonate, which forms an ineffective capping material (upper portion of the powder in a jar should be discarded before use).

Calcium hydroxide paste is applied in a thickness of 1.0 mm. Antibiotics should not be incorporated since high degree of alkalinity of calcium hydroxide destroys/severely decreases the efficiency of antibiotics.

Disadvantages

- No curative effect on inflammation.
- No anodyne effect.
- Chronic inflammation may lead to necrosis, abscess.
- Internal resorption may occur.
- Sclerosis of root canals; subsequent root canal treatment would be difficult.
- High alkalinity may lead to surface tissue necrosis.

c. *Mineral trioxide aggregate (MTA)*

Mineral trioxide aggregate (MTA), a modified Portland cement, is an accepted and successful alternative to calcium hydroxide. It is of three types, gray, white and modified. The composition of three types is tabulated in Table 25.3.

MTA is mixed according to manufacturer's instructions (MTA: H_2O is 3 : 1) to the consistency of wet sand. It is carried to the pulp surface with a spoon excavator or MTA carrier gun. It is patted down with a moist cotton pellet. 1.5 mm thick layer of MTA is considered effective pulp capping agent. The chamber is filled with flowable composite/any other interim restorative materials. MTA should be covered in wet conditions; dry MTA loses its cohesiveness and becomes hard to handle. Patient is recalled after one week. Patient is questioned about sensitivity and any other discomfort. If comfortable, final restoration is planned. In case discomfort persists, keep the patient under observation for 4–6 weeks. If still not comfortable, root canal treatment is initiated.

Bridge formed under MTA is tubular, thicker and continuous than that formed under calcium hydroxide. Pulp exhibits very less inflammation. MTA resists microleakage, even in presence of blood.

Properties

- Setting time: sets within 24 hours
- Compressive strength: 70 MPa after one day
- pH of the set MTA: 11–13 after setting
- Biocompatible and nonmutagenic
- Antibacterial effect is similar to calcium hydroxide.

d. *Bonding agents*

It is established that healing is directly related to capacity of pulp capping agent to provide a biological seal against immediate and long-term microleakage. Adhesive bonding agents have been tried as pulp capping agent. They do provide immediate seal; however, when adhesive agents were compared with calcium hydroxide, they showed more pulp necrosis.

Table 25.3 Composition of three types of mineral trioxide aggregate (MTA)

Gray	*White*	*Modified*
• Tricalcium silicate • Dicalcium silicate • Tricalcium oxide • Tricalcium aluminate • Bismuth oxide (radiopacifier) • Traces of free crystalline silica, calcium oxide, magnesium oxide, potassium, iron and sodium sulfate	All others except iron	Three versions: i. Free of aluminium oxide ii. Percentage of calcium oxide was increased to have more alkalinity iii. Addition of 1% methylcellulose increases compressive strength

Histological studies have shown persistent inflammatory reactions and hyaline alteration of extracellular matrix inhibiting complete pulpal repair or bridge formation when bonding agents were used. Direct bonding agents are not preferred as it can lead to inflammatory reaction, delay in pulpal healing and failure of dentin bridge formation.

e. *Resin-resorcinol*

Resin-resorcinol has also been successfully tried as pulp capping material (details in Chapter 37).

f. *Polycarboxylate cement*

Polycarboxylate cement is well-tolerated by the pulp. Its adhesive character provides the requisite marginal seal. Initially polyacrylic acid in polycarboxylate cement irritates the pulp tissue, which may subside over the time. However, induction of calcific bridge has not been reported.

g. *Cyanoacrylates*

Isobutyl cyanoacrylates have been used with varying success.

h. *Combination of antibiotic and corticosteroids*

Combination of antibiotics and corticosteroids have also been used. These effectively provide bactericidal effect, which may lead to partial bridge formation. The narrowing of root canals has also been reported with their use. The material is clinically not preferred.

i. *Growth factors*

Growth factors regulate growth and development and also induce wound healing and tissue regeneration.

Various forms of growth factors have been used as pulp capping agents to induce repair of pulp.

Bone Morphogenic Protein (BMP), belonging to β-transforming growth factor (TGF-β), is a potent modulator of tissue repair. Bone morphogenic proteins plays a vital role in the differentiation of adult pulp cells into odontoblasts during pulpal healing.

The differentiated odontoblasts lead to deposition of osteodentin and tubular dentin.

Other growth factors, such as insulin like growth factor-I, epidermal growth factor, insulin-like growth factor II, platelet-derived growth factor have also been tried. Insulin like growth factor-I has shown dentin bridge formation.

j. *Enzymes*

Enzymes, such as heme-oxygenase-I and simvastatin are being tried as pulp capping agent because of their potential to induce functional odontoblasts and improved dentin formation. Earlier, alkaline phosphatase when applied to exposed pulp stimulated the differentiation of other pulp cells into odontoblast, subsequently stimulating dentin matrix formation. It has been reported that heme oxygenase-1 (HO-1) might play a cytoprotective role against proinflammatory cytokines and nitric oxide in human pulp cells.

Simvastatin improves the osteoblast function and suppresses osteoclast function, resulting in enhanced bone dentin formation. It stimulates the function of odontoblasts, thus leading to improved dentin formation.

The enzymes induce angiogenesis and increases neuronal cells, indicating the possible effectiveness in pulp regeneration along with dentin regeneration. It has an anti-inflammatory effect; considered as an active pulp capping material to accelerate reparative dentin formation.

k. *Stem cells*

Stem cells are a group of undifferentiated biological cells, which are capable of self-renewal and multilineage differentiation. Their potential to stimulate tertiary dentin formation is effectively explored as pulp capping material.

Dental pulp stem cells and Stem cells from Human Exfoliated Deciduous Teeth (SHED) have been identified having the capacity of self-renewal and multi lineage differentiation.

The disadvantage of stem cells might be their rejection because of immunological reasons (stem cells are derived from embryos that are not patients own and the patient body may reject these cells).

l. *Propolis*

Propolis is a natural biological derivative containing flavonoids, phenolics, iron, zinc and other aromatic compounds. It is traditionally used as anti-inflammatory and antibacterial agent.

Propolis has great potential as pulp capping agent. It has been effectively used as an antioxidant, reducing hypersensitivity. Propolis has shown comparable results with MTA and Dycal, as regard dentin bridge formation. It may exhibit mild to moderate inflammation, which stimulates dentin bridge formation.

m. *Emdogain*

Emdogain is enamel matrix derivative secreted from Hertwig's epithelial root sheath during porcine tooth development. It is rich in amelogenin and amelin protein, capable of inducing reparative process. It stimulates the regeneration of acellular cementum, periodontal ligaments, and alveolar bone.

Emdogain contains biomolecular proteins, which promote odontoblast differentiation and reparative dentin formation. It has been established that emdogain suppresses the inflammatory cytokine production and contains β-TGF growth factor; create a favorable environment for promoting wound healing in the pulp.

Emdogain is used as an adjunct along with other pulp capping agents to achieve desired results.

Various investigators have reported that MTA produced a better quality reparative hard tissue with the adjunctive use of emdogain as compared with calcium hydroxide.

Emdogenic gel when applied directly to exposed pulp without the use of other pulp capping agent could not produce the requisite hard tissue barrier (Emdogain possess poor sealing ability).

n. *TheraCal LC*

TheraCal LC is a light cured, resin modified calcium silicate liner, mainly used in direct/indirect pulp capping, as a protective base/liner under restorative materials. Being radiopaque, the material can be easily identified during routine radiographic examination.

TheraCal LC contains tricalcium silicate particles in a hydrophilic monomer, providing significant calcium release. Calcium release stimulates dentin bridge formation. The alkaline pH promotes apatite formation. The barrier provides insulation and is moisture resistant.

It is established that TheraCal LC displayed higher calcium releasing ability and low solubility than MTA or Dycal. TheraCal LC can be cured to a depth of 1.7 mm, which stabilizes the material at the site of placement.

o. *Biodentine*

Biodentine is bioactive cement, simulating dentin in its physical properties. A modified form of calcium silicate cement, it is mainly used as dentin substitute reinforcing lost coronal and radicular dentin. Biodentine has shown promising results as an alternative to calcium hydroxide. It is biocompatible with high strength; also exhibit excellent marginal adaptability. Its strong antibacterial activity provides effective results when placed over deep carious lesions. It has also been used as retrograde filling materials, pulp capping agent, in internal/external resorption and also in apexification procedures.

It has been established that biodentine induces secondary dentin formation by stimulating odontoblastic cell differentiation. Biocompatibility and capability of providing bacteria-free seal make Biodentine a material of choice in pulp capping/pulpotomy procedures.

p. *Dentin shavings*

The sterilized dentin shavings when placed on exposed pulp stimulate the formation of reparative dentin. Both analogous and homologous dentin chips have been successfully tried as pulp capping agent; however, creating and placing dentin shavings over the pulpal site is clinically difficult.

q. *Tricalcium phosphate*

Tricalcium phosphate, when implanted in bone stimulate new bone formation. It does induce dentin bridge formation; however, severe initial inflammation may lead to necrosis of pulp. Practically, it has been replaced by MTA.

r. *Laser*

Lasers have shown promising results, especially in pulpotomy. Lasers effectively excise the surface pulp tissue, create bacteria-free environment, stimulating collagen production and fibroblast proliferation. CO_2 laser and ND-YAG laser have been extensively used in direct/indirect pulp capping.

Lasers induce secondary dentin formation. The targeted tissues are sterilized, providing sustained bactericidal effect. However, the use of Laser is technique sensitive; high doses may damage the underlying pulp tissue.

s. *Miscellaneous*

A few materials like endosequence, castor oil bean cement, calcium enriched mixture (endodontic cement), Freeze dried bone matrix, etc. have also been tried as pulp capping materials, with varying success.

Table 25.4 summarizes the advantages and disadvantages of various pulp capping agents.

3. Pulp Curettage

It is well-documented that pulp exposure due to caries usually lead to pulp necrosis with passage of time. During caries removal, carious dentin chips may be inadvertently pushed into pulp tissue resulting in inflammation, resorption and encapsulation of dentin chips which after capping may show foreign body reaction. It is suggested to remove superficial layer of pulp tissue by enlargement of the exposure site. This procedure is known as 'Pulp curettage'. It is followed by control of hemorrhage, placement of pulp capping material and sealing the cavity as in direct pulp capping.

Advantages

- Preserves cell rich zone due to minimal excision; chances of better healing.
- Physiologic apposition of dentin is maintained.
- Natural color/translucency of tooth is maintained.
- Less chances of root canal obliteration.

Table 25.4 Pulp capping agents: Advantages and disadvantages

Pulp capping agent	*Advantages*	*Disadvantages*
Zinc oxide eugenol	• Reduces inflammation • Act as obtundant	• Lack of calcific bridge formation • Eugenol released might be cytotoxic
Calcium hydroxide	• Accepted pulp capping material • Antibacterial (high alkalinity) • Induction of mineralization (calcific bridge formation) • Low cytotoxicity	• Highly soluble in oral fluids (potential of dissolution over time) • Extensive dentin bridge formation • Lack of adhesion • Acid etching may degrade layer of calcium hydroxide
Mineral Trioxide Aggregate (MTA)	• Less pulpal inflammation • Hard tissue barrier formation is better than calcium hydroxide • Antibacterial • Radiopaque • Releases bioactive dentin matrix proteins • Biocompatible	• Poor handling characteristics • Long setting time • Grey MTA may cause tooth discoloration • High solubility
Bonding agents	• Provide adhesion to hard tissues • Provide effective seal against microleakage	• Absence of calcific bridge formation • May lead to chronic inflammatory pulpal response • Potential of toxicity
Resin-resorcinol	• Excellent sealing ability	• Calcific bridge formation is natural, may be due to bacteria-free seal
Polycarboxylate cement	• Chemically bond to tooth structure	• Do not stimulate calcific bridge formation
Isobutyl cyanoacrylate	• Reduces pulp inflammation	• Dentin bridge formation is not satisfactory
Corticosteroids and antibiotics	• Reduces pulp inflammation • Combination may lead to reparative dentin bridge	• Should not be used in patients at risk from bacteremia
Growth factors [Insulin like growth factor 1, Bone Morphogenic Protein (BMP)]	• Formation of osteodentin and tubular dentin • Superior to calcium hydroxide as regard mineralization inducing properties (formation of more homogeneous reparative dentin)	• Fail to stimulate reparative dentin in inflamed pulp • Technique sensitive (appropriate dose required for positive results) • Possibility of immunological problems • All growth factors may not induce reparative dentin formation
Enzymes (alkaline phosphatase, heme-oxygenase 1, simvastatin)	• Anti-inflammatory action • Promote angiogenesis • Improve the function of odontoblasts; lead to superior dentin formation	• May lead to pulp tissue damage • Sensitive to appropriate concentration when applied directly to pulp tissue
Stem cells (pulp and other dental origins)	• Regeneration of dentin-pulp complex	• Technique sensitive • Still under investigations
Propolis	• Superior bridge formation (stimulate reparative dentin formation) • Reduces pulp inflammation and degeneration • Antioxidant, antibacterial, antifungal, antiviral and anti-inflammatory properties	• May exhibit mild/ moderate inflammation after two to four weeks
Emdogain	• Induce odontoblast differentiation and reparative dentin formation • Suppresses the inflammatory cytokine production • Create a favorable environment for promoting pulp healing • Amount of hard tissue formed with Emdogain was twice as compared to calcium hydroxide	• Emdogain gel when applied on exposed pulps without the adjunctive use of a pulp-capping material was ineffective in producing a hard tissue barrier (effective only as an adjunct)

(Contd...)

Table 25.4 Pulp capping agents: Advantages and disadvantages (*Contd.*)

Pulp capping agent	*Advantages*	*Disadvantages*
TheraCal LC	• Stimulate regeneration of dentin-pulp complex • Bond to deep moist dentin • Minimum solubility (solubility lower than MTA and Dycal) • Radiopaque • Display higher calcium releasing ability	• Opaque and 'whitish' color may show through composite/ceramic materials affecting esthetics
Biodentine	• Biocompatible • Good antimicrobial activity • Stimulate tertiary dentin formation • Less soluble • Produces bacteria-free seal comparable to calcium hydroxide • Less setting time and good handling characteristics	• Initially successful; long-term evaluation is not documented
Dentin shavings	• Induce secondary dentin deposition	• Placing and creating dentin shavings is difficult
Tricalcium phosphate	• Significant absence of pulp inflammation • Good physical properties • Induce calcific bridge formation	• Not much documented • Clinically difficult
Lasers	• Stimulate secondary dentin formation • Effective sterilization of targeted tissue • Bactericidal	• May cause thermal damage to pulp • Technique sensitive • Secondary dentin formation is natural under sterile environment
Miscellaneous (castor oil bean cement)	• Antibacterial • Less cytotoxic • Promote tissue healing • Induce calcific barrier	• Bioinert rather than bioactive • Not much documented

4. Partial Pulpotomy

Partial pulpotomy is the removal of only outer layer of damaged and hyperemic tissues in exposed pulps. (If 2.0–3.0 mm of pulp is removed, it is called 'partial pulpotomy').

Rationale

The rationale of partial pulpotomy is that following surgical amputation of the affected or infected pulp tissue at the exposure site, the remaining tissue is capable of healing.

Indications

- A small and recent pulpal exposure in a noncarious primary teeth.
- A very young tooth with a wide-open apex and very thin root dentin walls.
- Only if sufficient tooth structure is present to allow adequate restoration.

Contraindication

- If the exposure is very large (oral contaminants may cause extensive infection or inflammation beyond 2.0 to 3.0 mm of the exposure)
- When more than two weeks have passed between injury and treatment time.

25

Partial pulpotomy for carious exposures (Fig. 25.3a to d)

Procedure

- The inflamed pulp tissue beneath an exposure is removed to a depth of 1.0 to 3.0 mm or deeper to reach healthy pulp tissue.
- Pulpal bleeding is controlled by a bactericidal agent, such as sodium hypochlorite.
- Site is covered with calcium hydroxide or MTA.
- Calcium hydroxide has been demonstrated to have long-term success; MTA has shown more predictable dentin bridging and pulp health.

Partial pulpotomy for traumatic exposures (Cvek pulpotomy) (Fig. 25.4a to e)

Procedure

- The procedure is similar to partial pulpotomy for carious exposures. In case of MTA, white, rather than gray, is recommended, especially in anterior teeth to decrease the chance of discoloration (although both the versions have shown similar properties).
- Tooth is sealed with an appropriate restorative material to prevent microleakage.
- If hemostasis is not achieved, cervical pulpotomy should be performed.

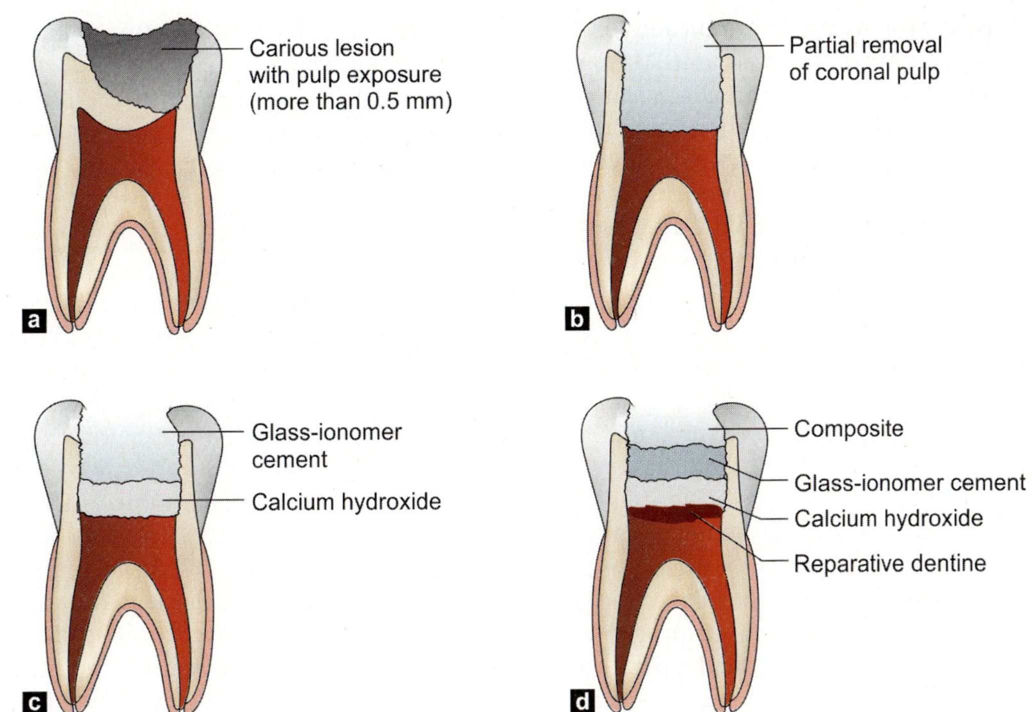

Fig. 25.3 Partial pulpotomy for caries exposure: (a) Pulp exposure (more than 0.5 mm); (b) Partial removal of coronal pulp; (c) Placement of calcium hydroxide; (d) Tooth restored

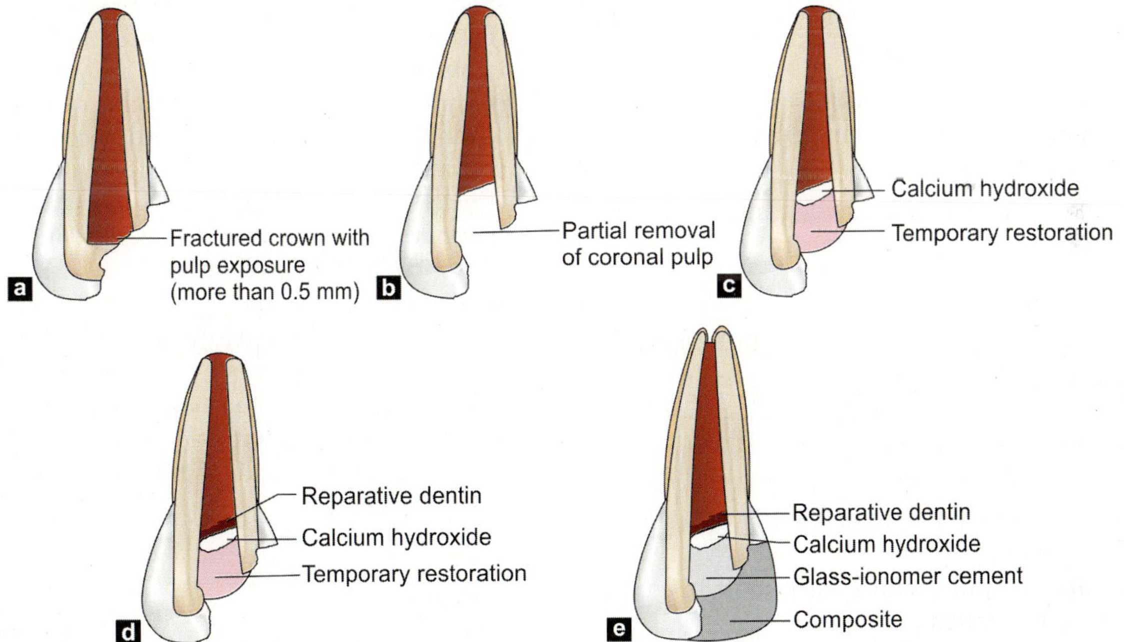

Fig. 25.4 Partial pulpotomy for traumatic exposure: (a) Fractured crown with pulp exposure (more than 0.5 mm); (b) Partial removal of coronal pulp; (c) Placement of calcium hydroxide over remaining pulp; (d) Formation of reparative dentin; (e) Tooth restored

Advantages of partial pulpotomy

- Procedure is quick and easy to perform.
- Maintains the natural tooth color and preserves the tooth structure for better retention of restoration.
- It is advantageous over complete pulpotomy in the preservation of cell-rich coronal pulp tissue.
- Allow continuation of normal development of the tooth, including further root development and maturation.

The patient should be evaluated periodically for 2–4 years to determine outcome of the treatment. Although histologic success cannot be determined, clinical success is judged by the absence of clinical/radiographic signs of pathology and evidence of continued root development in teeth with incompletely formed roots. The remaining pulp should continue to be vital after partial pulpotomy.

5. Pulpotomy

Pulpotomy procedure implies surgical removal of partly/completely inflamed coronal pulp and protecting the radicular pulp with a suitable material to retain its vitality. It is followed by filling the coronal chamber with a suitable base and restoring the tooth with a material that seals the tooth from microleakage.

Pulp inflammation results in local tissue necrosis and microabscess formation. The local destruction releases more chemical mediators and results in progress of inflammation. Healing depends on radicular pulp only. There is no physiological apposition of dentin in cervical area. So, the tooth is prone to fracture, and may discolor over time. Lack of coronal pulp does not provide reliable results with vitality tests. Root canal obliteration may occur.

Objectives

- Infected/inflamed area of pulp is removed leaving vital, uninfected pulp tissue in root canal.
- Apexogenesis in immature teeth.
- Pain relief in teeth with irreversible pulpitis. (Carried out as an emergency procedure).

Indications

- Teeth with incomplete apical development: Pulpotomy keeps apical portion of the pulp vital to allow normal root development and closure when routine endodontic therapy can be instituted.
- As an emergency procedure before pulpectomy.
- Attempted in selected cases of chronic hyperplastic pulpitis in young patients.
- Mildly inflamed pulp with a very short history of pain in a young patient.
- Crown fracture exposing pulp.
- Teeth posing difficulty in root canal treatment, e.g. sharp apical dilacerations or inaccessible molars.

Contraindications

25

- Traumatized teeth with little clinical crown.
- Teeth to be used as bridge/partial denture abutment.
- Teeth involved in complex periodontal therapy.
- Marked constriction of pulp chamber as evident radiographically.
- Teeth with symptoms of irreversible pulpitis.
- Pulp bleeds excessively after caries removal, which could not be controlled early.

Technique

- Anesthetize the tooth.
- Isolate the tooth. If part of the tooth is fractured, a metal band is applied, which facilitates isolation.
- Carious tooth structure is removed with an appropriate, sterilized bur in a high speed handpiece and air water coolant so that a straight line access is gained to the pulp chamber. In posterior teeth, approach is gained through occlusal surface and in anterior teeth, it is gained from the site of trauma or palatal/lingual surface in intact teeth. Overheating should be avoided because it can lead to damage to radicular pulp due to decreased circulation because of anesthesia.
- Roof of the pulp chamber is removed with an appropriate sized round bur. Shelf of dentin around the periphery of roof of coronal chamber is removed to create funnel-shaped access.
- Pulp is removed from coronal pulp chamber with a sharp endodontic excavator or periodontal curette (Fig. 25.5a and b). Twisting of pulp tissue is avoided. In anterior teeth, since floor of the pulp chamber is continuous, the incisal pulp is severed with an end-cutting bur in a high speed handpiece with air-water coolant. Any strands of pulp tissue extending coronally from the pulp periphery are removed, otherwise they may become necrotic and jeopardize the outcome of the treatment.
- Achieving hemostasis:
  Hemostasis is achieved by one of the following way/material:
  - Direct pressure at the exposure site with a cotton pellet moistened with sterile saline
  - Iron sulfate (not used if adhesive restorations are to be given)
  - Epinephrine
  - Sodium hypochlorite
  - MTAD
  - Aluminium chloride.

  (2.5–5.0% of sodium hypochlorite is used in routine. In addition to hemostasis, sodium hypochlorite allows for removal of dentin chips, chemical amputation of blood clot, fibrin and disinfection of cavity interface. It has been observed that hemostasis with sodium hypochlorite does not impair the biological repair. If pulpal hemostasis cannot be obtained in 5–10 minutes, the diagnosis is irreversible pulpitis and pulpectomy should be considered).

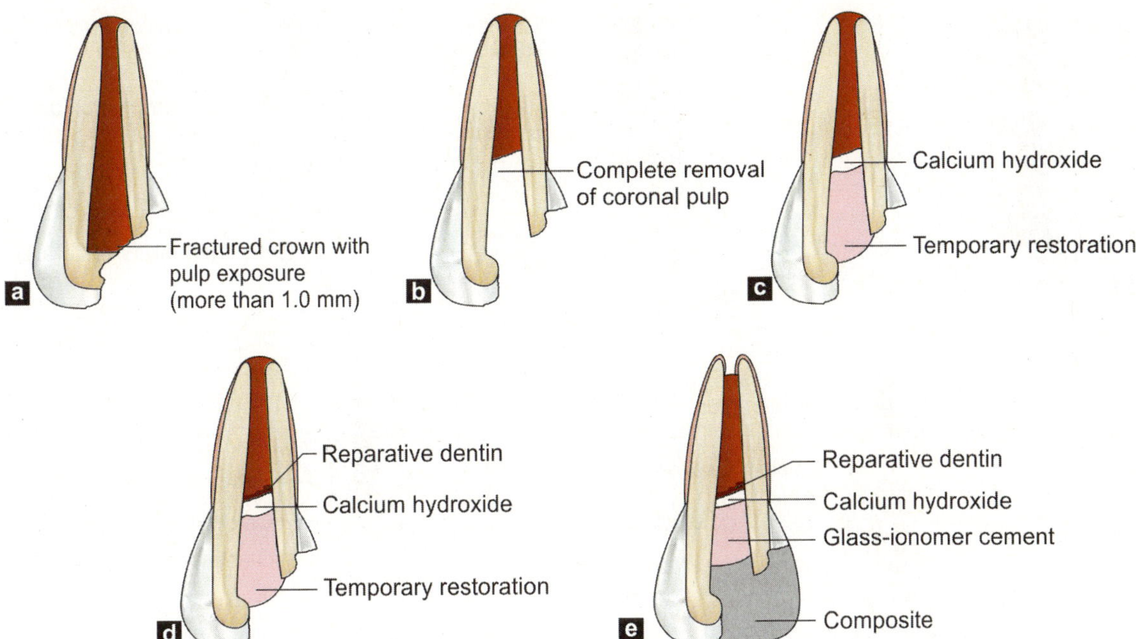

Fig. 25.5 Pulpotomy: (a) Pulp exposure (more than 1.0 mm); (b) Complete removal of coronal pulp; (c) Placement of calcium hydroxide over remaining pulp; (d) Reparative dentin formation; (e) Tooth restored

- The materials used for pulpotomy are the same as for pulp capping. Formocresol/glutaraldehyde is usually preferred for pulpotomy in primary teeth and avoided in permanent teeth. However, it may be used as an emergency measure to relieve pain in permanent teeth. It sanitizes and fixes pulp tissue. No calcific bridge is formed. Apical third of the pulp may retain its vitality for an extended period of time.
- Calcium hydroxide/any suitable material is placed over the remaining pulp (Fig. 25.5c).
- The tooth is restored after the signs of reparative dentin are evident (Fig. 25.5d and e).

Disadvantages

- Causticity
- Carcinogenicity/mutagenicity
- Fixes even healthy radicular pulp tissue
- Internal resorption
- Calcific metamorphosis.

6. Apexogenesis (Root Formation)

Apexogenesis is a histological term used to describe the continued physiologic development and formation of the root's apex. It can be regarded as a very deep pulpotomy. Harrison and Raskun (1985) termed apical closure with continued root development as apexogenesis with vital pulp.

Apexogenesis is defined as *'a vital pulp therapy procedure performed to encourage continued physiological development and formation of the root end'*.

Various materials have been used for pulpal wound dressing; however, the use of calcium hydroxide has been shown to be the most predictable with regard to long-term clinical success. Mineral Trioxide Aggregate has also shown favorable clinical and histological results in pulp capping, apexogenesis and apexification cases.

Indications

- In immature teeth when part of the pulp tissue remains vital and uninflamed, as in carious exposures.
- In some trauma cases in which pulp exposure occurred.

Goals

- Sustaining a viable Hertwig's sheath, thus allowing continued development of root length for a more favorable crown-to-root ratio.
- Maintaining pulpal vitality, thus allowing the remaining odontoblasts to lay down dentin, producing a thicker root and decreasing the chance of root fracture.
- Promoting root-end closure, thus creating a natural apical constriction for root canal filling.
- Generating a dentinal bridge at the site of the pulpotomy.

Procedure

It involves removal of the inflamed coronal pulp and the placement of calcium hydroxide on the remaining

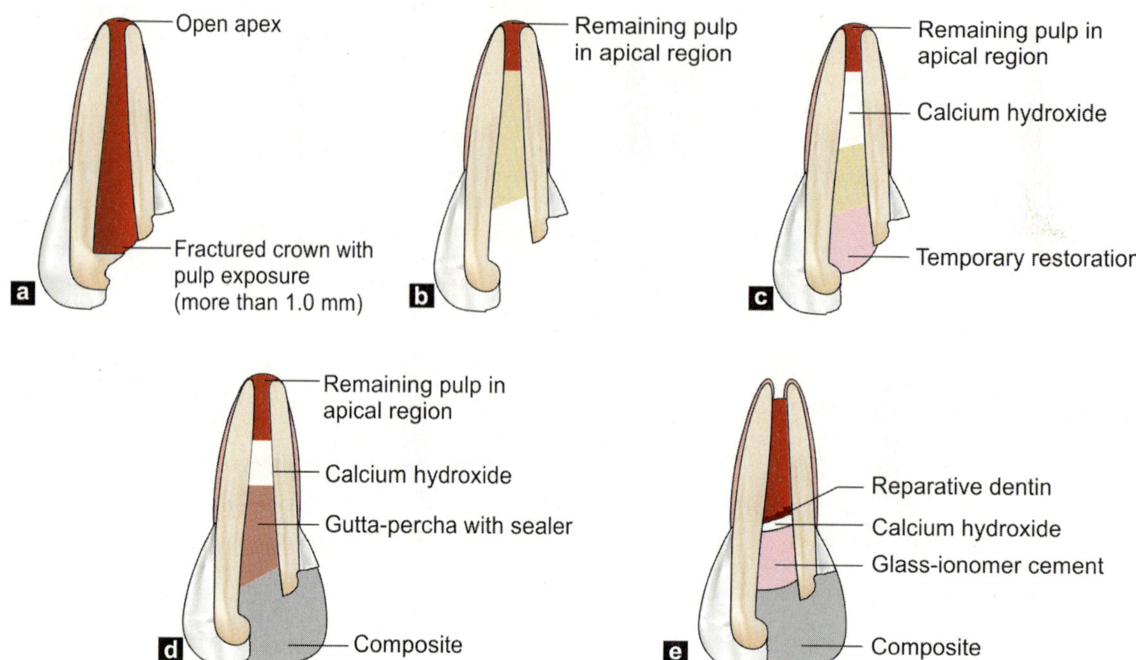

Fig. 25.6 Apexogenesis with calcium hydroxide: (a) Pulp exposure (more than 1.0 mm); (b) Removal of pulp, except in apical third area, (c) Placement of calcium hydroxide over remaining pulp; (d) Obturation with gutta-percha over calcium hydroxide; (e) Tooth restored after closure of apex

healthy pulp tissue. However, the depth to which the tissue is removed should be determined by clinical judgment. Calcium hydroxide is placed over vital pulp stump after hemostasis. For deeper amputation calcium hydroxide powder packed in an amalgam carrier is carried at the site (Fig. 25.6a to e). Radiographic and clinical follow-up is mandatory.

The total time for achievement of positive result of the apexogenesis ranges between one and two years depending on the degree of tooth development at the time of the procedure. The patient should be recalled at 3-monthly intervals in order to determine the vitality of the pulp and the extent of apical maturation. If it is determined that the pulp has become irreversibly inflamed or necrotic, or if internal resorption is evident, the pulp should be extirpated and apexification therapy initiated.

Controversy exists as to whether further endodontic intervention should be carried out following the completion of root development. Since, it is not possible to determine the pulp vitality or the health of the remaining pulp tissue, it has been advocated that once root development appears to be completed, the tooth should be re-entered and root canal therapy performed. However, it is emphasized that initiation of endodontic treatment prior to development of root resorption, canal obliteration and the development of apical periodontitis will lead to long-term success.

APEXIFICATION (ROOT END CLOSURE)

Endodontic management of the pulpless permanent teeth with a wide open blunderbuss apex has always been challenging. Endodontic treatment of young permanent teeth may also present difficulties due to the incomplete root development and associated open apices. Such teeth usually have thin, fragile walls, making it difficult to clean and subsequently attain the required apical seal. To achieve the apical barrier for effective endodontic treatment, apexification procedure is undertaken, facilitating formation of calcific barrier in a root with open apex or continued apical development of an incomplete root with necrotic pulp.

Apexification is defined as *'a procedure of inducing apical closure through the formation of mineralized tissue in the apical pulp region of a nonvital tooth with an incompletely formed root and an open apex'*.

(Apexification is indicated in nonvital permanent teeth with incomplete formed roots; whereas, Apexogenesis is carried out in vital teeth).

Aims

- Induce the formation of hard tissue barrier across the open apex, allowing proper condensation of obturating material in the root canal spaces.
- The hard tissue barrier, so formed, will not allow the irrigant/filling material to extrude out of the apical foramen.
- The procedure should not lead to periapical pathology.

Procedure

Many techniques have been advocated to manage open apex in nonvital teeth. The techniques managing the open apex in nonvital teeth are mostly confined to fill conventional paste (calcium hydroxide and combination) periodically, till calcific barrier is formed at the apex. This type of procedure is carried out in multivisits (may take 9 to 18 months for calcific bridge formation) (Fig. 25.7a to e).

The procedure was modified over the years and carried out in one visit. The rationale is to establish an apical stop that would enable the root canal to be filled immediately. A number of materials have been proposed, including tricalcium phosphate, calcium hydroxide, freeze dried bone and mineral trioxide aggregate in one-visit apexification. The materials provide scaffolding for the formation of hard tissue and the potential of a better biological seal.

Various materials have been tried for apexification; the important ones are:

a. Calcium hydroxide
b. Triple antibiotic paste
c. Mineral trioxide aggregate (MTA).

a. Calcium Hydroxide

Calcium hydroxide is used with different medium such as, camphorated paramonochlorophenol (CPMC), distilled water, metacresol acetate, cresanol (CPMC + metacresol acetate), methylcellulose base, normal saline solution, Ringer's solution and Anesthetic solution. The addition of barium sulfate enhances its radiopacity.

The concerned tooth is prepared and disinfected in routine. Sodium hypochlorite and chlorhexidine solutions are preferred as irrigants. The clean canal is filled apically with calcium hydroxide paste, followed by sealing the coronal end with interim filling materials. Various combinations of calcium hydroxide, as described above, have been used as apical seal material; calcium hydroxide and methylcellulose (pulpdent), because of better consistency and less solubility, is preferred over other materials.

The calcium hydroxide 'dressing' is to be repeated every six to eight weeks for better results (controversy exist as regard re-filling of calcium hydroxide and after how long a time; a few authors prefer no re-filling, whereas others prefer changing calcium hydroxide every month, after 3 and 6 months).

It is hypothesized that the high pH of calcium hydroxide is an important factor in its ability to induce hard tissue formation. The antimicrobial activity is related to the release of hydroxyl ions, which are highly oxidant and show extreme reactivity. These ions damage the bacterial cytoplasmic membrane, protein denaturation and the bacterial DNA.

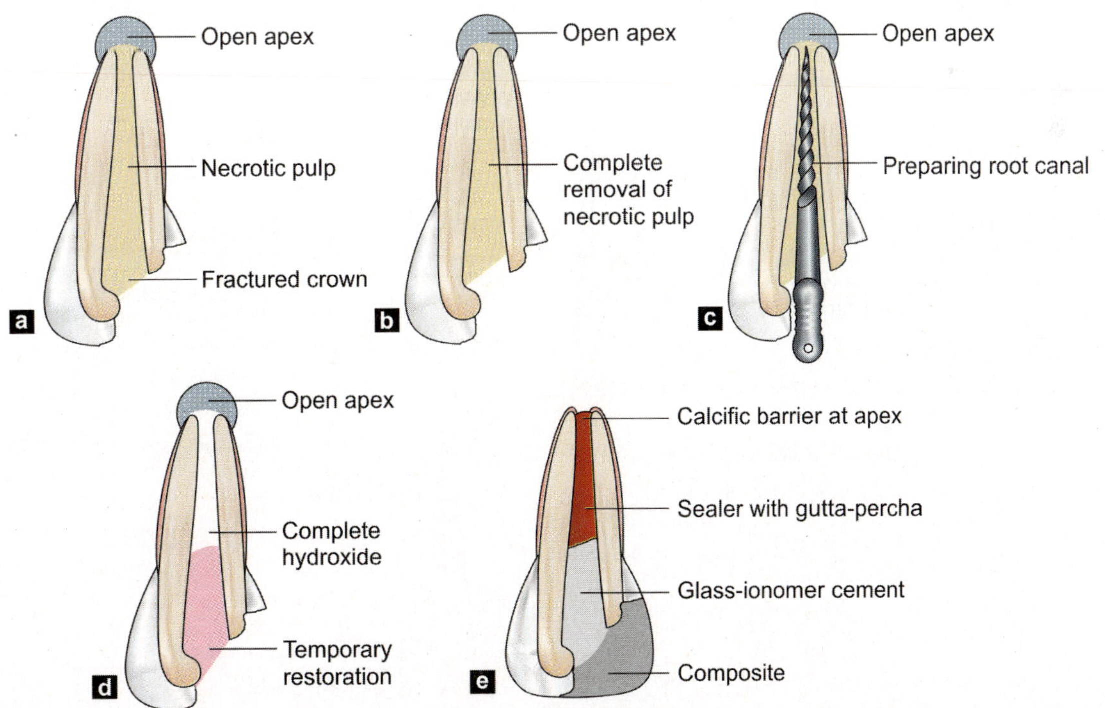

Fig. 25.7 Apexification with calcium hydroxide: (a) Open apex with periapical rarefaction; (b) Removal of necrotic pulp; (c) Preparation of root canal; (d) Placement of calcium hydroxide dressing; (e) Tooth restored after formation of calcific barrier

However, if there is remaining vital pulp tissue in the canal, the direct contact of calcium hydroxide paste with the tissue will induce the formation of a layer of calcific tissue, which may occupy the pulp space; thereby preventing the pulp tissue to regenerate into that space. Another concern is that calcium hydroxide may damage the Hertwig's epithelial root sheath and thereby losing its ability to induce the nearby undifferentiated cells to become odontoblasts.

Limitations

- Long span of the treatment
- Procedure requires multivisits; clinical protocol to be followed in each visit
- Risk of re-infection; periapical exudate may dissolve calcium hydroxide.

b. Triple Antibiotic Paste

The bactericidal efficacy of triple antibiotic paste (metronidazole, ciprofloxacin, minocycline) has been successfully tested against microbes from carious dentin and infected pulp. It is established that triple antibiotic paste is sufficiently potent to eradicate the bacteria from the root canal systems. Intracanal medication with triple antibiotic paste for four weeks is an effective approach to manage nonvital open-apex teeth promoting continuing root development.

The main concern of using the antibiotic paste is that it may lead to bacterial resistance [The paste contains both bactericidal (metronidazole and ciprofloxacin) and bacteriostatic (minocycline) antibiotics]. Additionally, minocycline causes tooth discoloration (minocycline can be replaced with cephalexin to avoid discoloration). Triple antibiotic and double antibiotic pastes have been successfully used in apexification procedures.

c. Mineral Trioxide Aggregate (MTA)

Mineral trioxide aggregate (MTA) has shown promising results when used to create apical barrier in open apex teeth. In nonvital open-apex teeth with short root lengths, the root can completely be filled with MTA (Fig. 25.8a to e).

The root canal system should be thoroughly cleaned and disinfected using sodium hypochlorite irrigation. A calcium hydroxide paste is placed in the root canal for at least one week to effectively eradicate the residual microorganisms. Thereafter, calcium hydroxide paste is rinsed out and the root canal is irrigated with 5.0% sodium hypochlorite and 17% EDTA and dried with sterile paper points. A thick mix of MTA is prepared by mixing MTA powder with sterile water and is carried to the canal with a specific carrier. MTA is condensed to the apical end of the canal with an appropriate plugger. A 3.0–4.0 mm apical plug is created and its density, position and extension are checked radiographically. If an ideal plug is not created in the first attempt, MTA should be rinsed out with sterile water and the procedure should be repeated. The

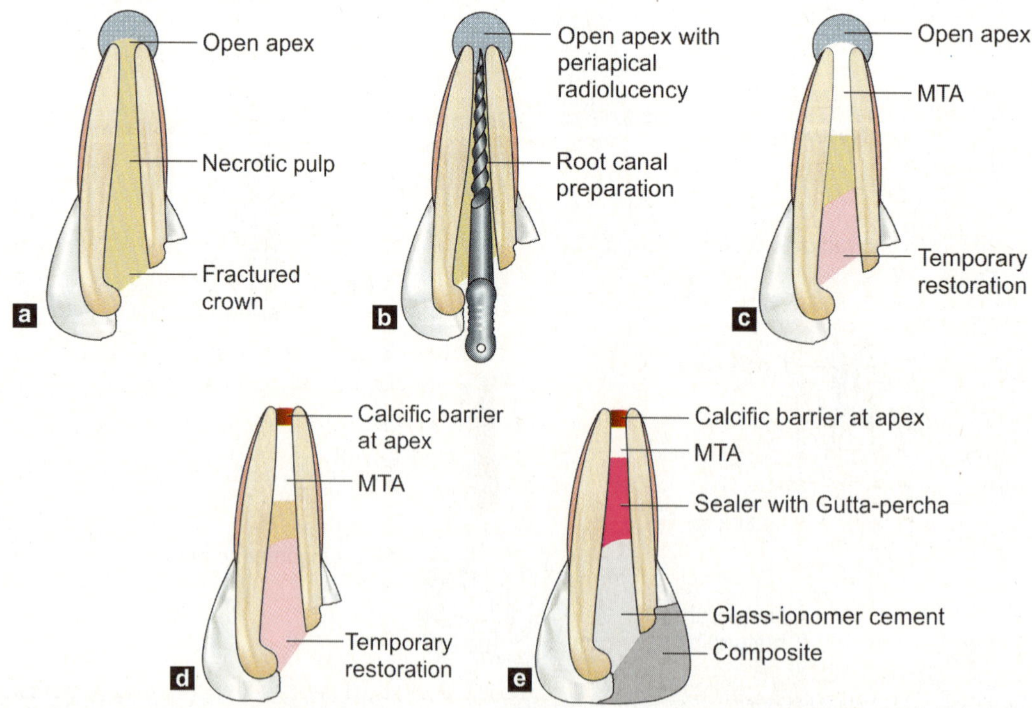

Fig. 25.8 Apexification with MTA: (a) Open apex with periapical rarefaction; (b) Preparation of root canal; (c) Placement of MTA at the apical end; (d) Formation of calcific barrier at apex; (e) Tooth restored

25

coronal end is sealed with appropriate interim material, such as Cavit. After two weeks, if the tooth is asymptomatic, the canal is evaluated for any pathological exudates. If no pathological feature, the coronal cavity is filled with glass-ionomer cement. The tooth should be followed up periodically to observe the formation of calcific barrier at the root apex. Gutta-percha is used to fill the remaining canal space. If the canal walls are thin, the canal space can be completely filled with MTA to strengthen the tooth against fracture. Adverse post-treatment signs or symptoms, such as sensitivity, pain, or swelling should not be evident. There should be no radiographic evidence of external root resorption, root fracture, or breakdown of periradicular supporting tissues during or following therapy. The tooth should continue to erupt, and the alveolus should continue to grow in conjunction with the adjacent teeth. Apexification with MTA in maxillary central incisor is depicted in Fig. 25.9a and b.

MTA is biocompatible and has good sealing ability. Coronal sealing with glass-ionomer further provide the requisite bacteria-free seal. An internal matrix created by platelet rich fibrin (PRF) along with MTA as apical barrier has also been successfully tried (PRF is an immune platelet rich concentrate, when placed as matrix, promote healing and repair; also control adequate filling of MTA).

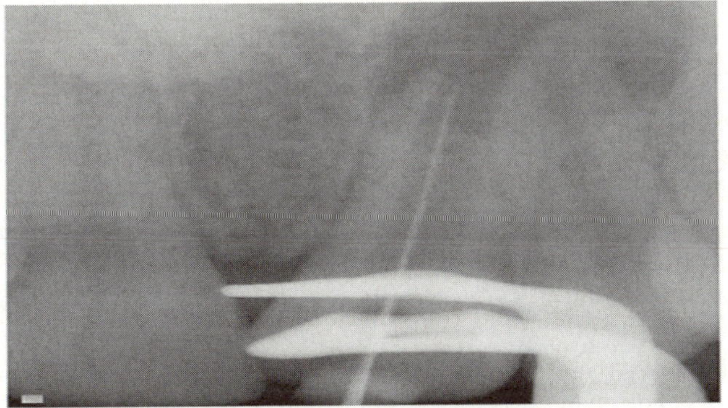

Fig. 25.9a Working length determination (open apex)

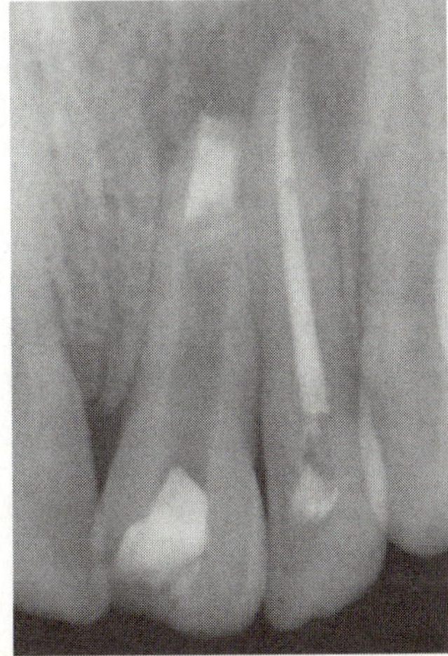

Fig. 25.9b Apexification with MTA

The necessity of the use of medicament for induction of apical barrier formation is questioned. Nygaard-Ostby hypothesized that laceration of the periapical tissues until bleeding occurred might produce new vital vascularized tissue in the canal. He suggested that this treatment may result in further development of the apex. Infected necrotic pulp tissue induces strong inflammatory reactions in the periapical tissues. Therefore, its removal should create an environment conducive to apical closure without use of a medication. It was believed that instrumentation may in fact hamper root development.

Hemorrhage was induced by an endodontic explorer penetrating slightly into the periapical tissue allowing the blood clot to form in the canal and stopped at a level 3.0 mm apical to cementoenamel junction. Mineral trioxide aggregate was then placed over the blood clot. Calcium hydroxide is not preferred as intracanal dressing after blood clot. The calcific tissue initiated by calcium hydroxide may prevent pulpal tissue from regeneration. Secondly, presence of calcium hydroxide can damage Hertwig's epithelial root sheath; also do not facilitate undifferentiated viable cells to differentiate into odontoblasts. It was considered that the blood clot acts as a scaffold and source of growth factors to facilitate the repair and regeneration of tissues into the canal; however, there is lack of histological evidence confirming blood clot for the formation of repaired tissues. This is the basis of regenerative endodontics, described in detail in Chapter 38.

Because of the thin dentinal walls, the incidence of root fractures in teeth after apexification is high. Restorative efforts should be directed towards strengthening the immature root. Newer dentin bonding techniques have found to significantly increase the resistance to fracture of these teeth, as good as of intact teeth.

A technique is tried, in which the access is restored with a composite restoration and a clear curing post is inserted into the soft composite and cured. The post is then removed leaving a patent channel for calcium hydroxide replacement and subsequent obturation.

Mechanism of Continued Root Formation

Vitality of Hertwig's epithelial root sheath (HERS) is important for continued formation of the apical portion of the root. Mesenchymal cells in the periapical region and the organizing influence of HERS may differentiate into formative cells which form the apex.

There are four clinical possibilities in apexification:

- Definite apical closure with minimal recession of the root canal.
- No reduction in the space of the root canal; canal may be shaped like a blunderbuss.
- Radiographically, a calcified barrier located coronally to the root apex.
- Evidence of pathology in the periapex or in the root canal (sign of failure of apexification).

The calcified apical barrier mainly consists of cementum along walls of root canal along with dentinal/bony tissue.

Hertwig's epithelial root sheath may and may not be present. The calcified tissue is not exactly dentin or cementum; however, it simulates characteristics of dentin, cementum and bone.

BIBLIOGRAPHY

1. Abu-Tahun I and Torabinejad M. Management of teeth with vital pulps and open apices. Endod. Topics: 2012; 23:79–104.
2. Aguilar P and Linsuwanont P. Vital pulp therapy in vital permanent teeth with cariously exposed pulp: A systematic review. J. Endod.: 2011; 37:581–587.
3. Albuquerque MTP, Nagata JY, de Jesus SA and Zaia AA. Pulp revascularization: an alternative treatment to the apexification of immature teeth. Rev Gauch Odontol.: 2014; 62:401–410.
4. Asgray S and Ehsani S. Permanent molar pulpotomy with a new endodontic cement: a case series. J. Conserv. Dent.: 2009; 12:31–36.
5. Bergenholtz, G. Factors in pulpal repair after oral exposure. Adv. Dent. Res. 2001, 15, 84. Waterhouse, P.J. "New age" pulp therapy: Personal thoughts on a hot debate. Pediat. Dent. 2008; 30, 247–252.
6. Bergenholtz G, Axelsson S, Davidson T, Frisk F, Hakeberg M, Kvist T, Norlund A, Petersson A, and Portenier I. Treatment of pulps in teeth affected by deep caries—a systematic review of the literature. Singapore Dent. J.: 2013; 34:1–12.
7. Beeley JA, Yip HK and Stevenson AG. Chemochemical caries removal: a review of the techniques and latest developments. Br. Dent. J.: 2000; 188:427–430.
8. Bindsley PH and Lvschall H. Treatment outcome of vital pulp treatment. Endod. Topics: 2002; 2:24–34.
9. Camilleri J, Montesin FE, Brady K, Curtis RU, Sweeney R and Pittford TR. The constitution of mineral trioxide aggregate. Dent. Mater.: 2005; 21:297–303.
10. Desouza CA, Hebling J and Hanks CT. Current status of pulp capping with dentin adhesive systems: a review. Dent. Mater.: 2000; 16:188–197.
11. Dominguez MS, Witherspoon BE, Gutman JL and Operman LA. Histological and scanning electron microscopy assessment of various vital pulp-therapy materials. J. Endod.: 2003; 29:324–333.
12. Duncan HF, Nair PNR and Pittford TR. Vital pulp treatment: a review. Endod. Practice: 2008; 2:247–258.
13. European Society of Endodontology. Quality guidelines for endodontic treatment: Consensus report of the European Society of Endodontology. Int. Endod. J.: 2006; 39:921–930.
14. Kumar A, Yadav A and Shetty N. One-step apexification using platelet rich fibrin matrix and mineral trioxide aggregate apical barrier. Ind. J. Dent. Resch.: 2014; 25:809–812.
15. Lim KC and Kirk EEJ. Direct pulp capping: a review. Endod Dental Traumatol.: 1987, 3; 213–219.
16. Mjor IA, Dahl E and Cox CF. Healing of pulp exposure: an ultrastructural study. J. Oral Pathol. Med.: 1991; 20:496–501.
17. Modina KC, Casas-Apayco LC Atta MT, Costa CA, Hebling J, Sipert CR, Navarro MF and Santos CF. Cytotoxicity and biocompatibility of direct and indirect pulp capping materials. J Appl Oral Sci.: 2009, 17; 544–554.
18. Nosrat A and Asgray S. Apexogenesis of a symptomatic molar with calcium enriched mixture. Int. Endod. J.: 2010; 43: 940–944.
19. Olivi G, Genovese MD, Maturo P and Docimo R. Pulp capping: Advantages of using laser technology. Eur. Arch. Pediat. Dent.: 2007; 8:89–95.
20. Olsson H, Petersson K and Rohlin M. Formation of a hard tissue barrier after pulp capping in humans—a systematic review. Int. Endod. J.: 2006; 39:429–442.
21. Paulindraraj S, Venkatesan R, Suprakasam S and Christopher A. Apexification – Then and Now: A review. Int. J. Dent. Med. Res.: 2015; 1:193–196.
22. Roberts HW, Toth JM, Berzins DW and Charlton DG. Mineral trioxide aggregate material use in endodontic treatment: A review of literature. Dent. Mater.: 2008; 24:149–164.
23. Shabahang S. Treatment options: Apexogenesis and Apexification. J Endod.: 2013, 39; 526–529.
24. Sikri V and Sikri P. Direct pulp capping with resorcinol: a clinical and histological evaluation. JCD: 1998; 1:90.
25. Siqueira Jr JF and Lopes HP. Mechanisms of antimicrobial activity of calcium hydraulic: a critical review. Int. Endod. J.: 1999; 32:361–369.
26. Stabholz A, Sahar-Helft S and Moshonov J. Lasers in Endodontics. Dent. Cl. North Am.: 2004; 48:809–832.
27. Swift EJ, Trope M and Ritter AV. Vital pulp therapy for the mature teeth – can it work? Endod. Topics: 2003; 5:49–56.
28. Tziafas D, Smith A and Lesot H. Designing new treatment strategies in vital pulp therapy. J. Dent.: 2000; 28:77–92.
29. Quershi A, Soujanya E and Nandkumar. Recent advances in pulp capping materials: An overview, J Clinical Diag. Res.: 2014, 8:316–321.
30. Zhang W and Yelick PC. Vital pulp therapy: current progress of dental pulp regeneration and Re-vascularization. Int. J. Dent.: 2010; 1 (Online).

Chapter 26

Traumatic Dental Injuries and Management

Traumatic injury refers to physical injuries of sudden onset and severity which require immediate attention. The injury may lead to systemic shock called 'shock trauma' and may require medical interventions.

Traumatic dental injuries are often unanticipated events mainly affecting children and adolescents. Traumatic injury is one of the common cause of damage to tooth and the supporting structures. Such injuries involve perioral soft tissues, teeth and the supporting tissues. The management involves overall treatment of all the affected tissues. These injuries are to be attended immediately to avoid serious consequences. The careful examination of the clinical findings and immediately planned treatment modality can favor a successful outcome. Dr Anderson, a pioneer in dental traumatology, has contributed a lot as regards diagnosis, etiology and incidence of dental injuries.

Incidence

Maxillary incisors are more frequently involved in traumatic injuries as compared to mandibular incisors. Males sustain injuries two or three times more as compared to females. It is documented that children in the age of 8–12 years are more prone to dental injuries. The protrusion of the maxillary incisors is one of the predisposing factor in these traumatic injuries. Children with Angle's class II Div. I malocclusion are three times more prone to traumatic injuries.

Traumatic injuries may involve only crown or only root or both crown and the root. Injuries to the tooth structure depend on the severity of the blow; i.e. mild, moderate or severe. Mild impact usually leads to concussion or luxation without fracture of the tooth. Moderate impact lead to crown fracture with or without pulpal involvement or only intrusive luxation; however, crown-root fracture or displacement of the tooth is the common finding with severe impact.

Root fractures in permanent teeth are less frequent, comprising 0.5 to 5% of all traumatic injuries. Horizontal root fracture occurs mainly in the anterior region of maxilla, usually owing to the frontal impact. It is usually observed in fully erupted teeth with complete root formation. It occurs more frequently in the middle third of the root and rarely in the apical third. The prognosis is poor if the fracture level is at the coronal third.

Etiology

i. Accidental fall; may be at home/school or road traffic accidents.
ii. Domestic violence due to child abuse or physical trauma.
iii. Collision during sports activities.
iv. Bruxism and age related attrition.
v. Bacteriological (extensive caries lesion).
vi. Iatrogenic
   - Extensive tooth preparation for restorations
   - Tooth structure loss due to endodontic procedures

Traumatic Dental Injuries: Types and Nomenclature

The luxation injuries are:

- *Avulsion*: The complete displacement of the tooth out of its socket.
- *Concussion*: An injury to the tooth-supporting structures without any displacement; but with pain to percussion.
- *Intrusion*: Displacement of the tooth into the alveolar bone, characterized by crushing of alveolar socket.
- *Extrusion*: Partial displacement of the tooth out of its alveolar socket, characterized by separation of the periodontal ligament. Apart from axial displacement, the tooth will usually have an element of protrusion. The alveolar socket bone remains intact.
- *Subluxation*: An injury to the tooth-supporting structures, but without displacement of the tooth. Bleeding from the gingival sulcus in early case.

- *Lateral luxation*: Displacement of the tooth out of its socket other than axially, characterized by separation of the periodontal ligament. Fracture of either the labial or the palatal/lingual alveolar bone (one side). If both sides of the alveolar socket have been fractured, the injury should be classified as an alveolar fracture.

The injuries affecting tooth and/or bone are:

- *Enamel fracture*: A fracture confined to the enamel with loss of tooth structure.
- *Enamel infraction*: An incomplete fracture or crack in the enamel without a loss of tooth structure.
- *Incomplete tooth fracture*: A demonstrable fracture with no visible separation of the segment along the plane of fracture.
- *Fissured fracture*: A crack in the crown of the tooth.
- *Root fracture*: A fracture of root, may be horizontal or vertical
- *Alveolar fracture*: A fracture of the alveolar process, involving the alveolar socket. Teeth with alveolar fractures are characterized by mobility of the alveolar process; several teeth move as a unit.
- *Uncomplicated crown and root fracture*: A fracture through the enamel, dentin, and cementum which caused a loss of tooth structure; without pulp involvement.
- *Uncomplicated crown fracture*: A fracture through the enamel and dentin which caused a loss of tooth structure; without pulp involvement.
- *Complicated crown fracture*: A fracture through enamel and dentin which caused a loss of tooth structure; involving pulp.
- *Complicated crown and root fracture*: A fracture through the enamel, dentin, and cementum which caused a loss of tooth structure; involving pulp.
- *Cracked tooth syndrome*: It refers to the incomplete fracture of the vital tooth that involves the dentin and occasionally extends into the pulp.

The injuries affecting soft tissues/oral mucosa are:

- *Abrasion*: A superficial bleeding wound caused by the rubbing or scraping of tissues with an object or surface.
- *Contusion*: A bruise of the gingiva/oral mucosa caused by a blunt object often associated with an adjacent bone fracture.
- *Laceration*: A wound in the gingiva or oral mucosa caused by a penetrating sharp object.

CLASSIFICATION

26

Many attempts have been made over the years to classify dental injuries. The currently accepted system is based on the World Health Organization's application of international classification of diseases to dentistry and stomatology. The classification is applicable to injuries to the teeth and supporting structure and can be applied to both primary and permanent dentition. The classifications suggested by different authors are as follows:

Author (Year)	Classification
Sweet (1955)	Classified fractures of anterior teeth into eight classes
Rabinowitch (1956)	Classified injuries of the primary teeth into six types
Ellis (1961)	Classified anterior teeth fracture into six groups
Garcia-Godoy (1968)	Classified traumatic injuries of primary and permanent teeth into nine classes
Ellis and Davey (1970)	Modified Ellis classification and classified anterior teeth fracture
Silvestri and Singh (1970)	Classified posterior teeth fractures into four types
WHO (1978)	Classified oral structures injuries using code numbers for both primary and permanent teeth
Andreasen (1978)	Modified WHO classification by including terms, uncomplicated/complicated crown-root fracture and concussion/ subluxation/ lateral luxation
Heithersay and Morile (1982)	Classified root fractures into five classes
Pulver (1982)	Combined the classifications of Ellis and Davey, Andreasen, Hargreaves and Craig, McDonald and Avery: classified traumatized teeth into five classes
McDonald, Avery and Lynah (1983)	Modified Ellis and Davey classification into four classes
Ulfohn (1985)	Classified crown fractures into three classes
International classification of diseases in dentistry and stomatology (1992)	Accepted WHO Classification of traumatic dental injuries with codes
Feiglin (1995)	Classified transverse root fractures into three zones
Filippi, Tschan Pohl, Berthold and Ebeleseder (2000)	Classified tooth injuries using a new scoring system
Spinas and Altana (2002)	Classified crown fractures of teeth into four classes
Berman, Branco and Cohen (2007)	Classified dental injuries into hard injuries and soft injuries
Loomba et al (2010)	Classified tooth fractures based on treatment needs into four types

Classification by Ellis

Class 1: Simple fracture of crown involving little or no dentin

Class 2: Extensive fracture of the crown involving considerable dentin but not the pulp

Class 3: Extensive fracture of the crown involving considerable dentin and exposing the pulp

Class 4: Traumatized teeth that become non-vital with or without loss of the crown structure

Class 5: Teeth lost as a result of trauma

Class 6: Fracture of the root with or without the loss of crown structure

Ellis and Davey modified the Ellis classification and added two more classes:

Class 7: Displacement of a tooth without fracture of the crown or root

Class 8: Fracture of crown en-masse and its replacement

Hargreaves and Craig further modified Ellis and Davey classification and added one more class:

Class 9: Traumatic injuries to primary teeth

Classification by Andreasen

A. Injuries to Hard Dental Tissues and Pulp

1. *Crown infraction (N873.60)*: An incomplete fracture of the enamel without loss of the tooth substance.
2. *Uncomplicated crown fracture (N873.61)*: A fracture contained to the enamel or involving enamel and dentin but not exposing the pulp.
3. *Complicated crown fracture (N873.62)*: A fracture involving enamel and dentin and exposing the pulp.
4. *Root fracture (N873.63)*: A fracture involving dentin, cementum and the pulp.
5. *Uncomplicated crown root fracture (N873.64)*: A fracture involving enamel, dentin and cementum but not involving the pulp.
6. *Complicated crown root fracture (N873.65)*: A fracture involving enamel, dentin and cementum and exposing pulp.

B. Injuries to the Periodontal Tissue

1. *Concussion (N873.66)*: An injury to the tooth supporting structures without abnormal loosening or displacement of the tooth, but with marked reaction to percussion.
2. *Subluxation (N873.66)*: An injury to the tooth supporting structures with abnormal loosening but without displacement of the tooth.
3. *Intrusive luxation (N873.67)*: Displacement of the tooth into the alveolar bone. This injury is accompanied by comminution or fracture of the alveolar socket.
4. *Extrusive luxation (N873.66)*: Partial displacement of the tooth out of its socket.
5. *Lateral luxation (N873.66)*: Displacement of the tooth in a direction other than axially. This is accompanied by comminution or fracture of the alveolar socket.
6. *Ex-articulation complete avulsion (N873.68)*: Complete displacement of the tooth out of its socket.

C. Injuries to the Supporting Bone

1. *Comminution of the alveolar socket (Mandible N802.20, Maxilla N802.40)*: Crushing and compression of the alveolar socket.
2. *Fracture of the alveolar socket wall (Mandible N802.20, Maxilla N802.40)*: A fracture contained to the facial or lingual socket wall.
3. *Fracture of the alveolar process (Mandible N802.20, Maxilla N802.40)*: A fracture of the alveolar process which may or may not involve the alveolar socket.
4. *Fracture of the mandible and maxilla (Mandible N802.21, Maxilla N802.42)*: Fracture involving the base of the mandible or maxilla. It may and may not involve alveolar socket.

D. Injuries to Gingiva or Oral Mucosa

1. Laceration of gingival or oral mucosa (N873.69)
2. Contusion of gingiva or oral mucosa (N902.00)
3. Abrasion of gingiva or oral mucosa (N910.00)

Classification by Garcia Godoy (Fractures of Primary Teeth)

Class I: Enamel fracture

Class II: Enamel and dentin fracture without pulp exposure

Class III: Enamel and dentin fracture with pulp exposure

Class IV: Enamel, dentin and cementum fracture

Class V: Root fracture

Class VI: Concussion

Class VII: Luxation

Class VIII: Extrusion

Class IX: Avulsion

Classification by Filippi et al

Filippi et al (2000) used a new scoring system to classify tooth injuries.

The new scoring system designates the tissues involved in trauma to anterior teeth, i.e. dental tissues (enamel, dentin), endodontium (pulp), periodontium, alveolar bone and gingiva. Depending upon the severity of injury, each of five tissues is given a number between 0 and 5 (Table 26.1). Assessment of the complete tooth which also takes the form of number; the so called 'score' is made after diagnosing the individual tissues and allocating the corresponding numbers. The lowest value is then multiplied by the sum of the other four values. For example, a healthy uninjured tooth, allotted five tissues the value five, is thus given the maximum score of 100 and if one of the tissues cannot be treated anymore, is given the value zero, then the tooth also may be considered as not worth saving and scores zero.

A score of 80 signifies that the tissues are healthy; only pulp vitality could not be diagnosed with certainty. A score of 60 means that the tissues are healthy but endodontic treatment was required. All scores under 60 signify failure or complication in any one of the tissues examined.

Spinas and Altana's Classification

Spinas and Altana classified traumatic injuries into four classes:

Class A: Simple enamel lesion involving one proximal angle or only incisal edge.

Class B: Enamel dentin lesions involving one proximal angle or only the incisal edge; subclass B1: with pulp exposure.

Class C: Enamel dentin lesion involving the incisal edge and at least one-third of the crown; subclass C1: with pulp exposure.

Class D: Enamel dentin lesions involving the mesial or distal angle/incisal or palatal surface and root involvement.

When necrotic pulp is present, the letter 'h' is placed after the main class.

Berman, Blanco and Cohen's Classification

Berman, Blanco and Cohen classified injuries to the dentition into two main types:

A. *Hard tissue injuries*: Involving the teeth, alveolar bone and other facial bones.

B. *Soft tissue injuries*: Involving facial skin, lips, mucosa (cheeks and periodontium), soft tissues of the hard/soft palate and tongue.

A. Hard Tissue Injuries

a. *Crown fracture*: Crown fracture includes:
   i. Enamel infraction
   ii. Uncomplicated crown fracture
   iii. Complicated crown fracture

b. *Root fracture*: There may be an injury of the tooth that does not directly affect the crown of the tooth, but rather causes a fracture through the root. This fracture may be vertical, horizontal or oblique in relationship to the long axis of root.
   i. Crown—root fracture
   ii. Intra-alveolar root fracture—the injury involves fracture of the root that is completely encased within bone. The fracture may be horizontal or more diagonal and typically divides the root into two fragments—a coronal fragment and the apical fragment.

Table 26.1 Numerical allocation after diagnosis of individual tissues (Filippi et al 2000)

Score	*Hard (enamel dentin) tissues*	*Endodontium (pulp)*	*Periodontium*	*Alveolar bone*	*Gingiva*
5	Intact crown	Intact endodontium (pulp not involved)	Intact periodontium	Intact alveolar bone	Intact gingiva
4	Enamel infraction, fracture of root apex	Exposure of dentin	Concussion	Contusion of marginal bone	Contusion
3	Enamel-dentin fracture, intraalveolar root fracture	Large pulp exposure internal contusion (root fracture)	• Subluxation • Extrusion • Lateral luxation	Fracture of alveolar socket	Rupture of papilla
2	Crown root fracture (directly restorable)	Infection of pulp	• Intrusion • Reimplantation with vital periodontium	Fracture of alveolar process	Vertical laceration
1	Crown root fracture (indirectly restorable)	Endodontic complication (e.g. internal root resorption)	• Luxation and periodontal infection	Fracture and infection	Infected laceration
0	Vertical fracture or lost tooth	Endodontic periodontal lesion	Reimplantation with necrotic periodontium	Loss of alveolar socket	Loss of gingiva

c. *Luxation injuries*: When a traumatic injury to a tooth causes its displacement from the socket, it is termed as luxation injury; such as:
   i. Concussion
   ii. Subluxation
   iii. Lateral luxation
   iv. Intrusion (intrusive luxation)
   v. Extrusive luxation
   vi. Avulsion

d. *Alveolar injuries*: There are several types of fractures of bone tissues secondary to dental injuries.
   i. Comminuted fracture
   ii. Lateral, facial or lingual fracture of alveolar socket
   iii. Fracture of the alveolar bone with or without involvement of any tooth socket

B. Soft Tissue Injuries

Concomitant with most dental injuries is trauma to the surrounding soft tissues including the facial skin, lips, oral mucosa, gingiva, frenum, soft tissues of hard/soft palate and the tongue.

Loomba's Classification

Loomba et al (2010) classified tooth fracture based on treatment need.

***Type I*:** Fractures of the anterior teeth in horizontal or transverse plane

Division I: Fractures of tooth crown

A. Fracture in incisal one-third up to the junction of the incisal and middle third of the crown either partial or complete
B. Fracture in the middle one-third up to the junction of the middle and cervical third of the crown, either partial or complete
C. Fracture in the cervical one-third up to the cervical line of the crown, either partial or complete

Division 2: Fractures of the tooth root

A. Fracture in the cervical one-third up to the junction of the cervical and middle third of the root
B. Fracture in the middle one-third up to the junction of the middle and apical third of the root
C. Fracture in the apical one-third of the root

Division 3: Fractures involving both the crown and root or at multiple sites

***Type II*:** Fractures of the posterior teeth in horizontal or transverse plane

Division 1: Fractures involving the cusp/cusps

A. Fractures involving one cusp
B. Fractures involving two cusps
C. Fractures involving three cusps
D. Fractures involving four or more cusps

Division 2: Fracture of crown en masse

Division 3: Fracture involving root or roots

***Type III*:** Fractures of teeth in the vertical or longitudinal plane

Division 1: Incomplete tooth fracture or cracked tooth syndrome

Division 2: Vertical fractures involving tooth crown

A. Fracture in an anterior or posterior tooth where the fracture line passes buccolingually in the crown
B. Fracture in an anterior or posterior tooth where the fracture line passes mesiodistally through the crown

Division 3: Vertical fractures involving tooth roots

A. Fracture in an anterior or posterior tooth where the fracture line passes buccolingually in both the crown and root or in the root only
B. Fracture in an anterior or posterior tooth where the fracture line passes mesiodistally through both the crown and root or the root only.

***Type IV*:** Oblique fractures involving crown, root or both in the anterior or posterior teeth.

ROOT FRACTURE

Root fracture is defined as '*the fracture involving dentin, cementum and pulp*'. Root fracture is mainly categorized as (i) horizontal/transverse fracture and (ii) vertical fracture. Horizontal fracture is more prevalent; occur mainly in anterior region of maxilla (maxillary incisors). The middle region of the root is mostly involved followed by apical and coronal. The vertical root fracture (extends through long axis of root towards the apex) is comparatively rare.

Vertical root fracture is characterized by an incomplete or complete fracture line that extends through the long axis of the root towards the apex (Fig. 26.1a to c). In anterior teeth, the fracture occurs most commonly in a buccolingual direction. In molar teeth, the fracture is buccolingual in orientation to individual roots. Mesiodistal fractures are less common in both anterior as well as posterior teeth.

The diagrammatic representation of types of root fracture is summarized in Table 26.2.

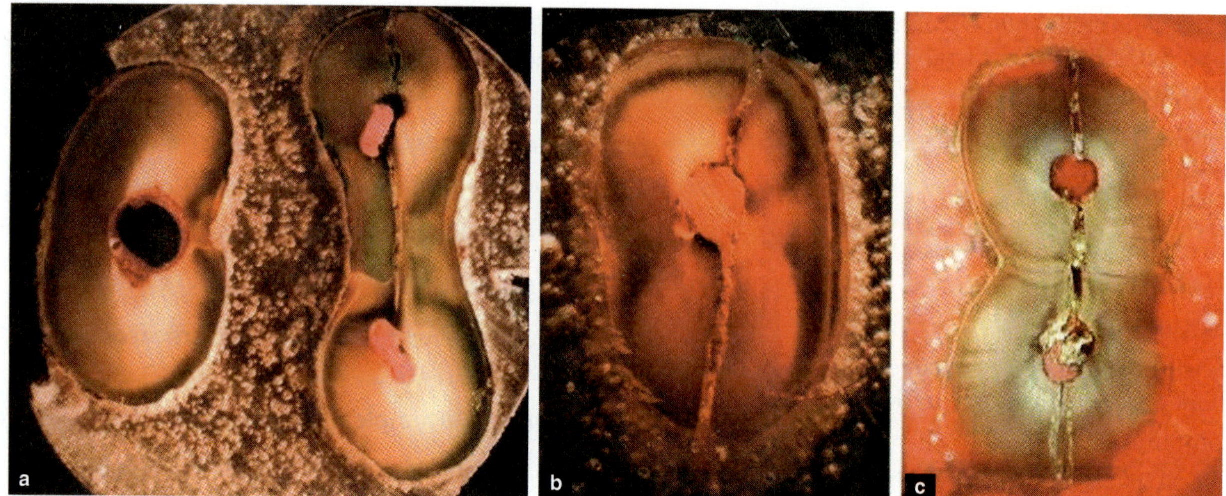

Fig. 26.1 Vertical root fracture: (a) Incomplete fracture at the buccal aspect of mesial root of a mandibular molar; (b) Cross-section of a vertically fractured maxillary premolar showing complete fracture from the buccal to the lingual aspect: One root canal; (c) Complete fracture from the buccal to the lingual aspects of maxillary premolar: Two root canals

Table 26.2 Types of root fractures (diagrammatic representation)

	Horizontal/transverse		*Vertical*
Location	Cervical	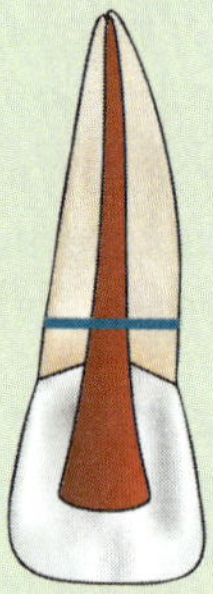 Separation of fragments	Complete (fragments move independently) 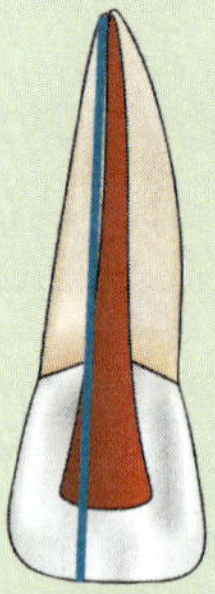
	Middle	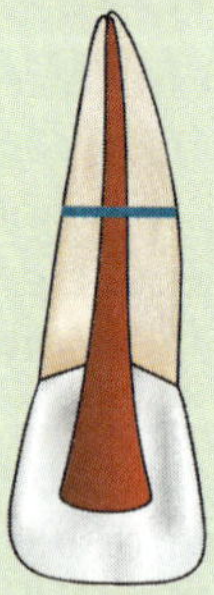	Incomplete (fragments string together) 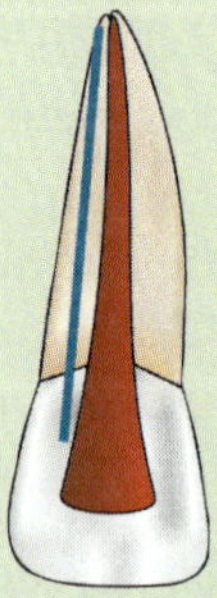
	Apical 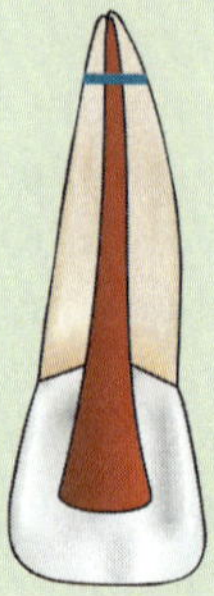		

(Contd...)

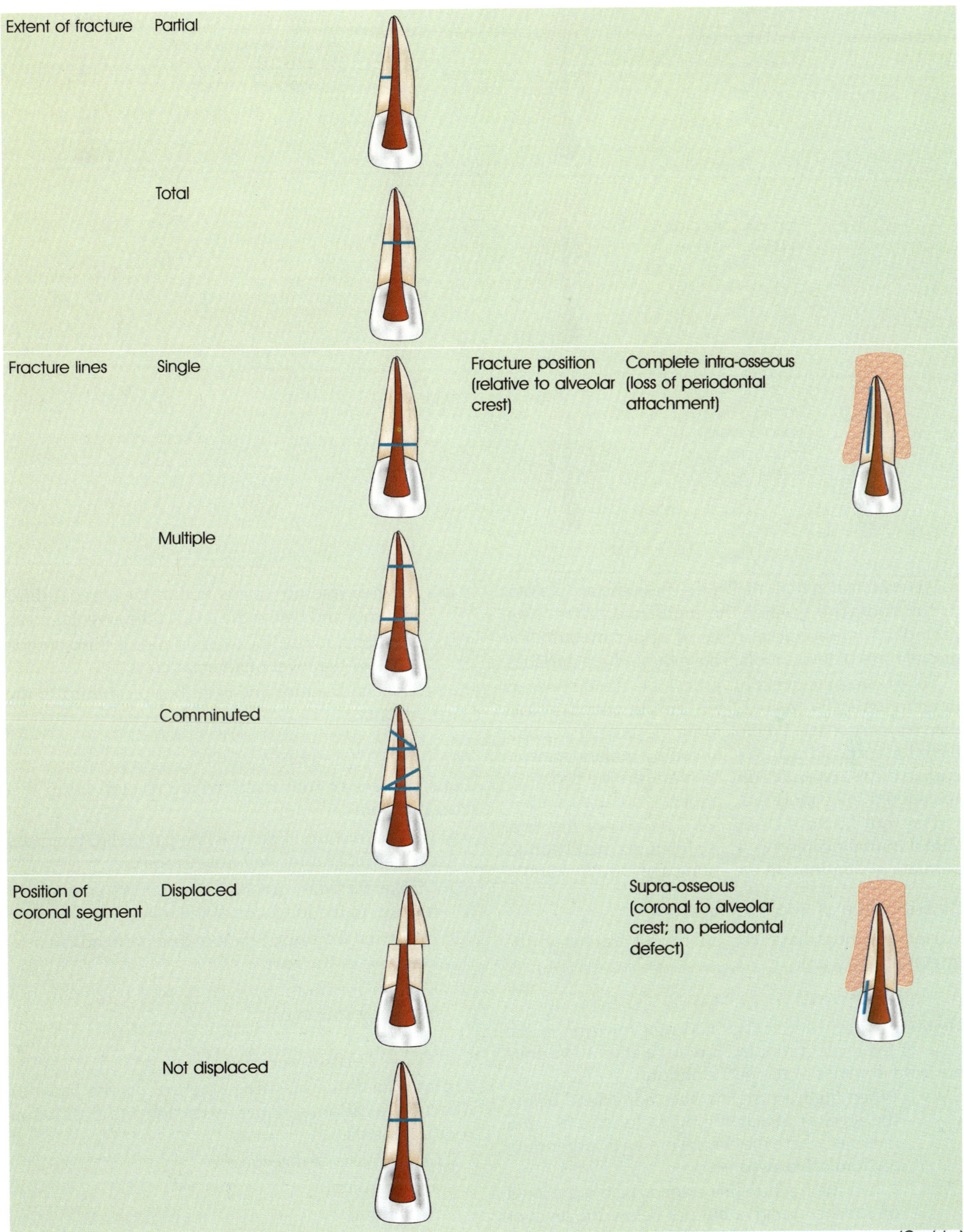
Extent of fracture
Partial
Total
Fracture lines
Single
Multiple
Comminuted
Fracture position (relative to alveolar crest)
Complete intra-osseous (loss of periodontal attachment)
Position of coronal segment
Displaced
Not displaced
Supra-osseous (coronal to alveolar crest; no periodontal defect)

(Contd...)

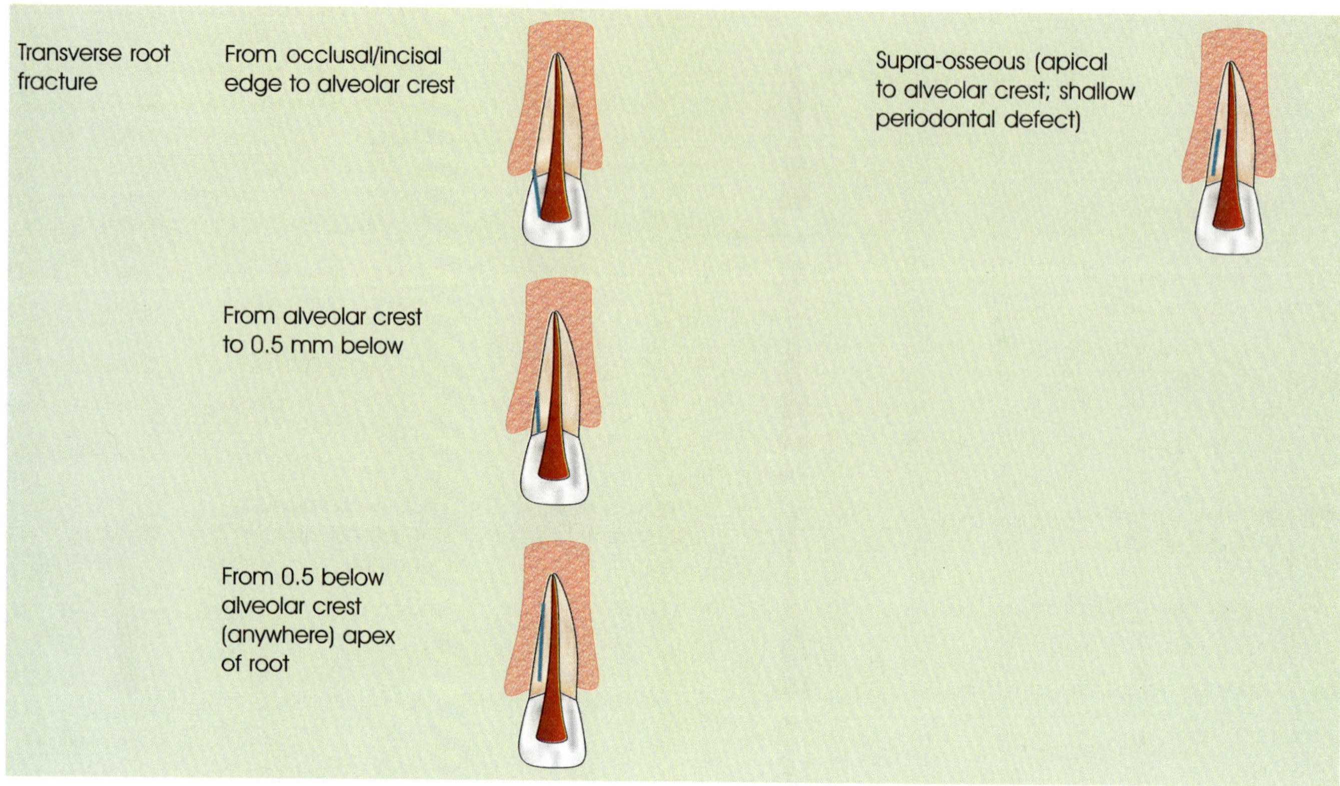

It is established that smaller the mesiodistal diameter of the root, the greater the incidence of fracture. Premolars, mesiobuccal roots of upper molars, and mesial roots of lower molars have these characteristics.

The greatest incidence of vertical root fracture occurs in endodontically treated teeth, and in patients older than 40 years of age. Premolars are the most susceptible teeth for vertical fracture followed by molars, incisors and canines. Mesial root of mandibular molar is considered to be more susceptible.

The root fracture comprises 1.0–7.0% of the total dental traumatic injuries. These fractures mainly affect permanent dentition in the young age (10–20 years).

Classification of Root Fractures

Various authors have classified root fractures; the important ones are:

a. Heithersay and Morile Classification

Heithersay and Morile classified root fracture on the basis of the level of root fracture in relation to various horizontal planes of the periodontium.

Class 1: When the fracture line does not extend below the level of attached gingiva (occurs in aged patients where the clinical crown is larger than anatomical crown).

26

Class 2: When the fracture line extends below the level of attached gingiva but not below the level of alveolar crest.

Class 3: When fracture line is within the coronal third of root and below the level of the alveolar crest.

Class 4: When fracture line extends middle third of root, below the level of alveolar crest.

Class 5: When fracture line is in the apical third of the root.

b. Chin-Jyh Yeh Classification

Four patterns of root fractures are recognized in this classification:

i. *Vertical fractures*: Fracture line parallel to long axis of the root and located only in root.
ii. *Oblique fractures*: Fracture line follows an angle in relation to the long axis of the root.
iii. *Horizontal fractures*: Fracture line perpendicular to long axis of the root.
iv. *Laminar fractures*: A piece of root fragment, not involving root canal.

c. Enrique Basrani Classification

Enrique Basrani classified fracture on the basis of direction, location, number, extension and position of root fragments.

i. On the basis of direction
   - Horizontal
   - Oblique
   - Vertical

ii. On the basis of location
- Cervical third
- Middle third
- Apical third

iii. On the basis of number of root fragments
- Simple
- Multiple
- Comminuted

iv. On the basis of extension of fracture line
- Partial
- Total

v. On the basis of position of root fragments
- Without displacement
- With displacement

The accepted ***classification for horizontal/transverse root fracture*** is based on the following features:

1. Location of fracture line
   - Cervical
   - Middle
   - Apical
2. Extent of fracture
   - Partial
   - Total
3. Fracture lines
   - Single
   - Multiple
   - Comminuted
4. Position of coronal segment
   - Displaced
   - Not displaced
5. Transverse root fracture
   - From occlusal/incisal edge to alveolar crest
   - From alveolar crest to 0.5 mm below
   - From 0.5 below alveolar crest towards (anywhere) apex of root

The accepted ***classification for vertical root fracture*** is based on the following features:

1. Position of fracture in relation to alveolar crest
   - Incomplete supraosseous fracture, terminating coronal to the alveolar crest (no periodontal defect)
   - Incomplete supraosseous fracture, terminating slightly apical to the alveolar crest (creating shallow lesion)
   - Complete/incomplete intraosseous fracture resulting in loss of periodontal attachment.
2. Based on separation of fragments
   - Total separation; fragments move independently (complete fracture)
   - No separation; fragments string together (incomplete fracture)

Etiology

The etiology of vertical root fracture may not be definite; however, following factors play an important role.

- Excessive canal shaping during endodontic treatment contributing to weakening of the root; subsequently, the vertical root fracture.
- Excessive pressure during lateral or vertical compaction.
- Wedging effect of endodontic posts (diameter and shape of the post).
- Corrosion of posts, leading to expansion.
- Inappropriate choice of abutment; unfavorable forces on abutment.

Clinical Features

The clinical signs and symptoms vary according to the type of fracture, position of fracture, periodontal and bony architecture around the fractured tooth. The clinical features are:

- Swelling of soft tissue over the root
- Presence of sinus tract around the affected root
- Tenderness
- Repeated dislodgement of post and post-core restoration
- No resistance during compaction of gutta-percha
- Cracking sound during compaction or cementation of post

Diagnosis

The patient's dental history along with clinical and radiographic findings are important to diagnose vertical root fracture. The following features are helpful:

- Age of patient
- Root canal treated teeth
- Degree of mobility
- Type of post and core restoration
- Pain/tenderness
- Presence/absence of swelling
- Presence of sinus
- Periodontal defect adjoining one tooth/root

The following tests can be significant in diagnosing vertical root fracture:

i. Bite test

The bite test is carried out to simulate masticatory forces. Rubber wheels or cottonwood sticks are placed on mesial/distal/palatal areas of tooth to replicate masticatory stresses.

ii. Periodontal probing test

A periodontal probe can be used to evaluate periodontal defect in the gingival attachment. In the absence of any other associated periodontal disease, this defect may be consistent with an underlying bony dehiscence that is secondary to a vertical root fracture (Fig. 26.2a).

A common feature of vertically root fractured teeth is the development of deep and narrow periodontal pockets adjacent to the fracture site.

The probing pattern for a tooth with a vertical root fracture is different as compared to teeth with periodontal disease. Deep probing in one position around the circumference of the tooth usually indicates that the tooth is fractured (Fig. 26.2b). Deep probing in two positions on opposite sides is also indicative of fracture.

iii. Pulp vitality tests

The pulp vitality tests may not be reliable, especially during early stages. The injured pulp may not response to such tests for at least 6 to 8 weeks after the injury.

The pulps usually retain vitality following an intra-alveolar root fracture. The collateral circulation established by a fracture line often allows for maintenance of pulp vitality. In vertical root fracture, the tooth may become hypersensitive to electric pulp testing.

iv. Radiographic examination

The following features should be evaluated:

- Separation of root fragments
- Fracture lines along the root or root fillings: A fracture line that deviates from the long axis of the canal may be radiographically more obvious; whereas, a fracture line running parallel and adjacent to a root filling may be less prominent.
- Vertical root fracture is suspected if the root filling appears well condensed but is in close contact with only one wall of the root canal.
- Appearance of a space between the post and the edge of a root canal.
- Overlapping of the fragments may result in double images of the external root surface.
- Certain specific patterns of bone loss evident with vertical root fracture are:
  - 'Halo like' bone loss: In case of a vertical root fracture the bone loss has a tendency to give a 'halo like' appearance, traversing circumferentially around the root. The radiolucent area may also superimpose upon one side of the root. The bone loss is dependent on the extent of destruction, the plane of fracture and the architecture of the bone adjacent to the fracture. Bone destruction associated with anterior teeth will be easier to detect than those associated with molars.
  - The widening of periodontal ligament space around the whole length of the root is an indicative of vertical fracture.
  - Step-like bone defects appear when the fracture runs obliquely across the root or where the fracture does not extend into the apical portion. Additional radiographic examination with the X-ray beam angled 15° to the mesial/distal may provide a better view of the defect.
  - Isolated horizontal bone loss in molars
  - Resorption along the fracture line
  - Dislodgement of retrograde filling material

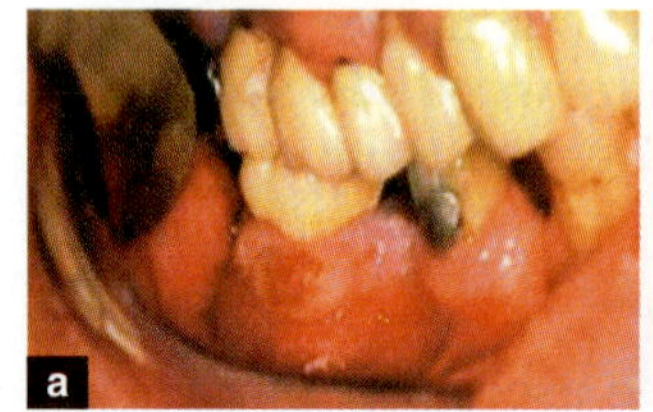

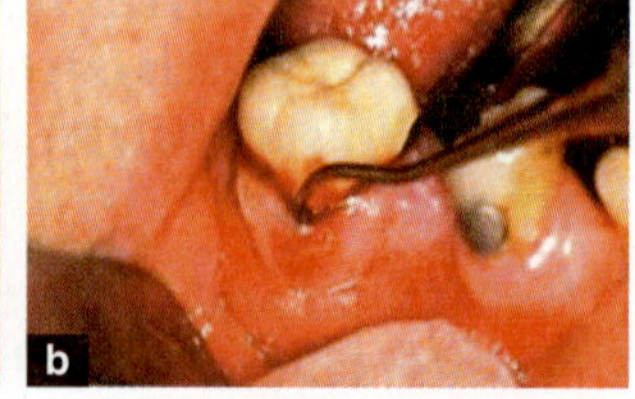

Fig. 26.2 Periodontal probing: (a) Soft tissue swelling over fractured site; (b) Periodontal pocket at the fracture site

The clinical features and diagnosis of traumatic dental injuries are summarized in Table 26.3.

CRACKED TOOTH SYNDROME

It is reported that 80% of patients over 40 years of age may exhibit cracked teeth. The incidence and prevalence of cracked teeth were commonly associated with intracoronal restorations; most prevalent in mandibular molars. The wedging effect of the prominent mesiopalatal cusp of the maxillary first molar may account for this fracture. Non-functional cusp may be more susceptible to fracture than functional cusp because they are subjected to lateral excursive occlusal forces. Cracks may initiate from the coronal structure or from within the pulpal side.

Cracked tooth syndrome has been defined as *'an incomplete fracture of a vital posterior tooth involving the dentin and possibly the dental pulp.'* Cameron coined the term *'cracked tooth syndrome'*.

Incomplete tooth fracture is defined as *'a fracture plane of unknown depth and direction passing through tooth structure that if not already involving, may progress to communicate with the pulp and/or periodontal ligament'*.

Diagnosis and management of cracked tooth is always a challenge in clinical practice. It is important to differentiate between dentinal, pulpal and periodontal pain before planning any treatment. Early diagnosis is important in the treatment of cracked teeth to limit the propagation of the cracks.

Table 26.3 Clinical features and diagnosis of traumatic dental injuries

Injury	*Clinical signs*	*Percussion test*	*Mobility test*	*Pulp test*	*Radiological findings*
Avulsion	Teeth are completely displaced out of their socket	Not indicated	Positive	Not indicated	Tooth seems elongated in socket
Intrusion	Tooth intruded axially in socket	Not indicated	Negative	May respond abnormal	Periodontal space reduced
Extrusion	Tooth partially displaced out of socket	Tender to percussion	Mobile	May respond abnormal	Periodontal space increased
Subluxation	Tooth not displaced in socket	Tender to percussion	Slight mobility	May respond abnormal	No change
Luxation	Tooth slightly displaced in socket	Not indicated	Slight mobility	May respond abnormal	Periodontal space increased
Concussion	Injured tooth is not displaced	Tender to percussion	Negative	Normal response	No radiological abnormality
Enamel infraction	Fracture of enamel without affecting tooth	Not indicated	Negative	Not indicated	No change
Alveolar fracture	Several teeth move as a unit when mobility is checked	Tender to percussion	Several teeth move as one unit	May respond as hyper-active pulp	A visible fracture at alveolar bone
Root fracture	Tooth may be displaced slightly	Tender to percussion	Upper portion mobile	May respond as hyper-active pulp	A visible fracture in root
Crown fracture (no pulp involvement)	Fractured crown without involving pulp	Non-responsive	Only crown mobility	Normal response	Fracture visible in crown
Crown fracture (pulp involved)	Fractured crown with an exposed pulp	Tender to percussion	Only crown mobility	Abnormal response, depends upon pulp involvement	Fracture visible in crown
Crown-root fracture	Fractured crown-root structure	Not indicated	Positive	Abnormal response, depends upon pulp involvement	Fracture may and may not be visible

Classification of Cracks

Over the years, various authors have classified cracks; the routinely mentioned are:

A. ***American Association of Endodontists Classification*** identifies five types of cracks that are located in the crown and root as well as vertical root fractures that originate from the root (Table 26.4).

B. ***Luebke's classification*:** Luebke classified cracks into three classes:

Class 1: Incomplete, supraosseous with no periodontal defect

Class 2: Incomplete, intraosseous with a minor periodontal defect

Class 3: Complete or incomplete, intraosseous with a major periodontal defect

Table 26.4 American Association of Endodontists classification for cracked teeth

Nomenclature	*Diagrammatic*	*Origin*	*Direction*	*Symptoms*	*Pulp status*	*Prognosis*
Craze lines		Crown	Variable	None	Vital	Excellent
Fractured cusp		Crown	Mesiodistal and faciolingual	Mild pain generally, only to biting and cold	Usually vital	Good
Cracked tooth		Crown ± root	Mesiodistal often central	Acute pain on biting, occasionally sharp pain to cold	Variable	Questionable; depends on depth and extent of the crack
Split tooth		Crown ± root	Mesiodistal	Marked pain on chewing	Often root filled	Poor; unless crack terminates just subgingivally
Vertical root fracture		Roots	Faciolingual	Vague pain, mimics periodontal disease	Mainly root filled	Poor; root resection in multi-rooted teeth

C. *William's classification*: William divided cracks into four categories:

Category 1: Incomplete vertical fracture through the enamel into the dentin but not into the pulp.

Category 2: Incomplete crown fracture involving the pulp.

Category 3: Incomplete vertical fracture crossing the attachments.

Category 4: Fracture divides the tooth completely.

D. *Talim and Gohil's classification*: Talim and Gohil classified cracks into four classes:

Class 1: Fracture involving the enamel

a. Horizontal or oblique.
b. Vertical
  i. Complete
  ii. Incomplete

Class 2: Fracture involving enamel and dentin without involving the pulp

a. Horizontal or oblique.
b. Vertical
  i. Complete
  ii. Incomplete

Class 3: Fracture involving enamel, dentin and the pulp

a. Horizontal.
b. Vertical
  i. Complete
  ii. Incomplete

Class 4: Fracture of roots (based on direction of the fracture line)

a. Vertical or oblique
  i. Involving the pulp
  ii. Not involving the pulp
b. Horizontal
  i. Cervical third
  ii. Middle third
  iii. Apical third.

E. *Pruden's classification*: Pruden classified cracks as:

a. Crack line
  i. No separation of parts, no pain symptoms.
  ii. No apparent separation, but tooth is sensitive to percussion or patient has a persistent/vague pain, not definitely related to the tooth.
b. Fractured cusp
  i. No pain or pulpal involvement
  ii. Possible pulpal involvement
c. Fractured crown
  i. No pulpal involvement
  ii. Pulp involved
d. Fractured root tip

F. *Clark's classification*: Clark classified cracks into three types:

Type 1: Little or no risk of underlying pathology.

Type 2: Moderate risk of underlying pathology.

Type 3: High risk of underlying pathology.

G. *William Kahler's classification*: William Kahler classified cracks into following five types:

i. Craze line
ii. Fractured cusp
iii. Cracked tooth
iv. Split tooth,
v. Vertical root fracture

MANAGEMENT OF PATIENT WITH DENTAL TRAUMA

Traumatic dental injuries, as a part of emergency, need immediate attention. The urgency is both for the patients and the operator. The planned and organized approach to diagnosis and treatment help overcome psychological problems of the patient and get better outcome of the results. The long term prognosis of traumatized teeth is dependent on the quickly provided emergency management.

The traumatic injury may involve intraoral and/or extraoral sites, which is usually contaminated with blood and debris. The injury sites must be cleaned with mild detergents prior to examination.

The following steps provide necessary information to establish the correct diagnosis and plan the treatment.

A. *Medical and dental history*: It is essential to establish any possibility of drug or any other allergies, blood disorders or other systemic conditions that may influence the treatment. The dental history should include the following questions:

a. ***Whether the patient is conscious or unconscious?***
   If unconscious, provide immediate medical attention.
b. ***When did the injury occur?***
   The time elapsed since the injury occurred is important, especially in avulsion and displacement cases.
c. ***Where did the injury occur?***
   The site of injury is important in evaluating the extent of trauma; for example, blow to the chin may transmit to the condyles.
d. ***Is there a change in bite?***
   Changes in occlusion following an injury would indicate a possible tooth luxation, alveolar bone fracture, or condylar fracture.

e. ***Is there increased sensitivity to temperature changes?*** Observe and note in teeth with crown fractures exposing the dentin and/or pulp.

B. *Clinical examination*: Clinical examination includes evaluation of any soft tissue wounds, including examination for the presence of impacted foreign bodies in the wounds. Almost all lip wounds have impacted foreign bodies. The teeth are examined for any fracture or craze lines. The former is easily observed visually while the latter requires directing the light parallel to the tooth's labial surface. If the crown fracture has occurred, note whether the pulp is exposed and also the extent of pulp exposure. Any displacement of teeth must be noted and recorded as lateral or axial luxation.

C. *Diagnostic tests*: The following tests are helpful in arriving at the diagnosis:

a. *Mobility test*: The degree of mobility of individual tooth or group of teeth is determined and noted.
b. *Percussion test*: The percussion test is carried out to analyze damage to periodontal ligament. It should be performed gently. Tap first with the finger tip, followed by mirror handle. Adjacent tooth should be percussed first. Percussion can provide information about the relationship of the tooth and the adjacent bone; a high, metallic tone indicates lateral or intrusive displacement. Such a percussion tone would indicate ankylosis of the tooth in follow-up examination.
c. *Pulp sensitivity test*: The pulp sensitivity of a traumatized tooth can be evaluated by the use of a heat, cold and/or electrical pulp tester. The placement of the electrode should be at the junction of middle and cervical third of the crown of anterior teeth. Pulp sensitivity tests are usually helpful in anterior teeth.

The lack of response to electric pulp tester should not be taken as pulp necrosis. The response immediately after injury may not provide accurate information.

D. *Radiographic examination*: A couple of radiographs from different angulations provide the most reliable information about the changes in the dentoalveolar complex. This is important in case of root fractures since the single exposure may fail to demonstrate the diagonal root fractures. CBCT is also helpful in diagnosing vertical/oblique fractures. Another application of radiography is to analyze the presence of impacted foreign bodies in the lips and adjoining soft tissues.

26

E. *Follow-up evaluation*: Follow-up evaluation is important to confirm the diagnosis, determine need for change in treatment and also evaluate the treatment outcome or complications, if any. The splint applied to the luxated teeth can usually be removed after three to four weeks. Radiographic examination should be performed to analyze the possible initiation of root resorption or periradicular lesion. After 6 weeks, clinical and radiographic examination may reveal evidence of pulp necrosis and infection. At 3–6 months, it is necessary to establish definitive diagnosis of pulpal/periodontal healing. One year is a minimum observation period to assess the final outcome of traumatic dental injuries.

Management

The traumatized teeth should be repositioned to achieve acceptable function and appearance. The repair of fractures and proper positioning of periodontal soft tissues provide the requisite function and appearance.

The treatment protocol can be:

- *Early treatment*: Injuries like tooth avulsions, alveolar fractures, extrusive and lateral luxations and possibly root fractures require early treatment. The passage of time affects the treatment outcome. Early repositioning and stabilizing promote the healing.
- *Partially delayed treatment*: Injuries like subluxation and crown fracture with pulpal exposure can be delayed up to 24 hours without much affecting the results.
- *Delayed treatment*: The treatment of crown fractures without pulpal exposure can be delayed as per desire of the patient or the operator.

The management involves treatment of both soft and hard tissues.

Management of Soft Tissue Injuries

Following the initial evaluation of any life threatening condition and resuscitation, injuries to the soft tissues should be evaluated.

Facial injuries can be superficial or may involve adjacent structures including bones, muscles, glands, and/or dentoalveolar structures. Lacerations involving the scalp can occasionally be difficult to control with pressure and may require clamping and/or electrocautery.

The length of time from initial injury to treatment is important in any injury, so is in soft tissue injury. The risk of secondary infection increases as time lapses. Healing of facial wounds is usually unaffected by interval between injury and repair. The tetanus prophylaxis is recommended as:

- If the patient has not received a booster injection within the last 10 years, a booster injection is given for any wound.

- Patients who are immunized and have received a booster injection within the last 10 years do not require tetanus prophylaxis if the wound is not tetanus prone (Tetanus-prone wounds are those which are heavily contaminated, devitalized tissue, or deep puncture wounds). If the wound is tetanus prone and the patient has not received a booster injection within 5 years prior to the injury, a 0.5 ml tetanus toxoid booster injection should be given.

Sequence of Treatment

Treatment of soft tissue injuries involves early reconstructive procedures addressing both the soft tissue and the underlying bony injury, if any. The common soft tissue injuries are categorized as follows:

i. ***Lacerations*:** Lacerations, caused by sharp injuries, contributes approximately 50% of such wounds. Lacerations usually have sharp and ragged margins. Laceration wound should be sutured in the center to avoid creating excessive tissue on the end of the laceration. Ragged margins should be excised to provide perpendicular skin edges to prevent scar formation.

ii. ***Abrasions*:** Abrasion wound implies removal of superficial layer of skin. The wound should be gently cleaned with a mild soap solution and irrigated with normal saline. Foreign bodies, if embedded in the wound, should be properly removed. After the wound is cleaned, abraded skin is covered with a layer of topical antibiotic ointment to minimize desiccation and secondary infection.

iii. ***Contusions*:** Contusions, caused by blunt trauma usually lead to edema and haematoma formation in the subcutaneous tissues. Extensive swelling, ecchymosis are associated features. Small sized haematomas heal without any treatment, however, large haematomas should be drained preferably to prevent secondary subcutaneous atrophy.

iv. ***Avulsion*:** A loss of segment of soft tissue is referred to as avulsion injury. Small defects are closed by primary closure; whereas, large wound areas are allowed to heal by secondary intention or surgically grafting soft tissue grafts.

Local anesthesia is used effectively to clean the soft tissue wounds. Local anesthetics containing epinephrine have been used in routine in all areas of the face; however, epinephrine is avoided where extensive undermining of the soft tissue is necessary. One should avoid injecting directly into the wound. Regional nerve blocks are considered beneficial since the blocks prevent distortion of the tissues.

The wound is thoroughly debrided excising non-vital tissue in an attempt to salvage most of the tissue. Soft tissue wounds are often contaminated with bacteria and foreign material. Foreign bodies, if present, are removed properly (continuous irrigation is mandatory).

Thumb rule is to avoid irrigating the wound with any solution that is not considered suitable for irrigating the eye. A scrub brush and detergent soap may be necessary to remove deeply embedded foreign material. However, soaps may cause cellular damage and necrosis. Polymyxin B sulfate can be used to remove the greasy portion in the wounds. Infections are rare when the wound is properly closed removing devitalized tissue and/or foreign bodies from beneath the sutured skin.

Suturing is preferred for facial lacerations maintaining the esthetic considerations. A layered closure is necessary to eliminate dead space beneath the wound. If the dead space is not obliterated, it may lead to accumulation of inflammatory exudates, subsequently tension and necrosis of the skin edges due to impairment of the vascular supply.

Deep layers should be re-approximated with suitable resorbable sutures. Margins should be undermined to allow slight eversion of the wound margin. Skin sutures should be removed 6–7 days after placement. As the wound heals, the collagen contract along its length and width and become inverted. Initial management is aimed at producing a slightly everted wound edge. Tissue adhesives, such as cyanoacrylates, have been used where esthetics was a priority; however, its use should be avoided in complex lacerations.

Management of Hard Tissue Injuries

A. *Enamel infraction*

Enamel infraction does not require any specific treatment. However, in case of multiple infraction lines, the enamel surface is sealed with an unfilled resin. The surface, if not sealed, may take stains from food, drinks or even chromogenic bacteria.

B. *Uncomplicated crown fracture*

The fractured portion of crown should preferably be restored. Bonding of original fragments can also be tried if the separation is minimal. The tooth may not respond initially to pulp test (vitality should be checked periodically).

C. *Complicated crown fracture*

Complicated crown fracture generally lead to pulp exposure. Root canal treatment is preferred; rarely pulpotomy can also be effective. Mineral Trioxide Aggregate is the material of choice; however, calcium hydroxide can be also used. Fiber post reinforcement is effective along with splinting (Fig. 26.3 a to e).

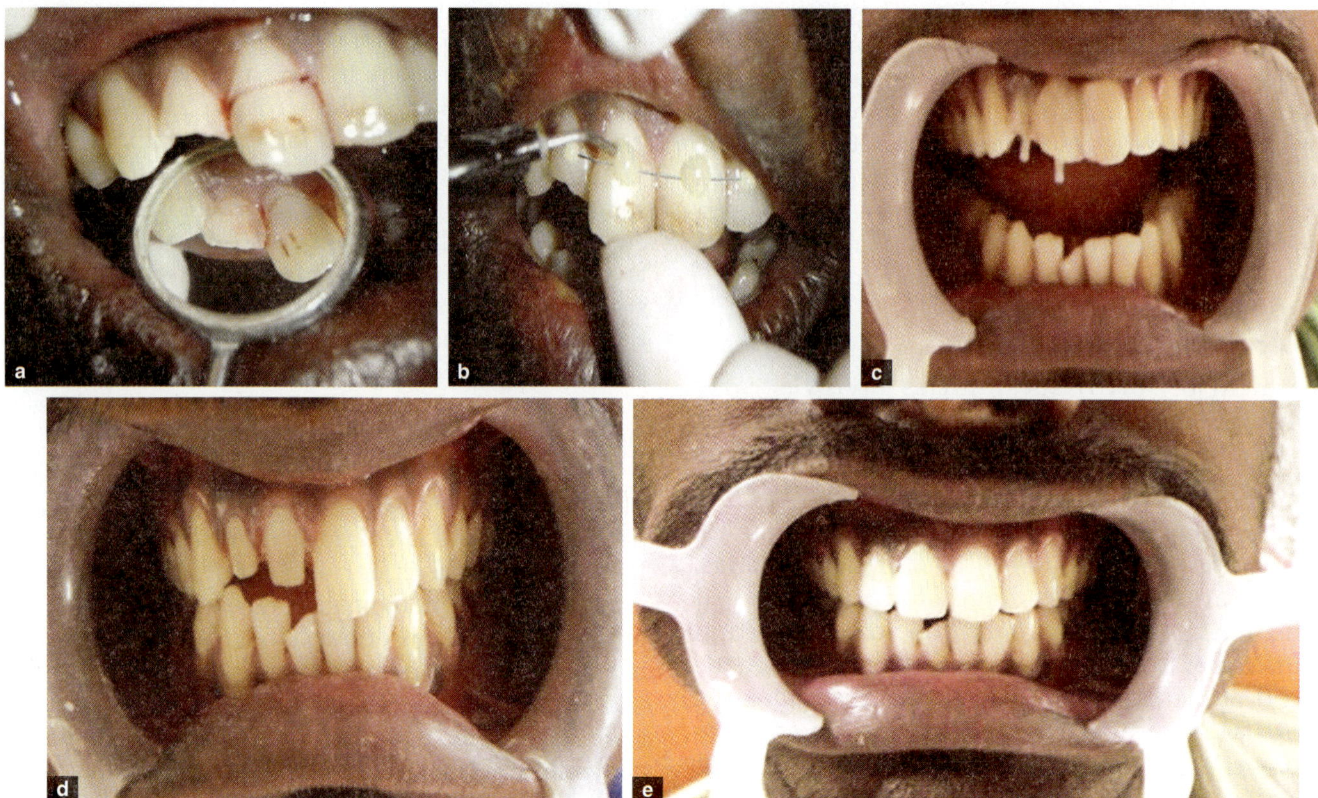

Fig. 26.3 Management of complicated crown fracture with fiber post reinforcement and resin splinting. (a) Crown fracture; (b) Resin splinting; (c) Fiber post reinforcement; (d) Tooth preparation; (e) Restored tooth

D. *Cracked tooth syndrome*

The treatment protocol for cracked teeth is explained in Flowchart 26.1.

E. *Crown-root fracture*

The management of crown-root fracture may have the following options depending upon the clinical condition:

- Removal of mobile fragment when approximation is difficult.
- Reattachment of fractured fragment with bonding procedure.
- When fracture extends subgingivally, bonding is difficult; hence, gingivectomy is performed to convert the subgingival fracture into a supragingival fracture. The fiber reinforced esthetic post may also be used to aid in the retention of fractured segment.
- Orthodontic extrusion of the apical fragment may help bring the subgingival margin to supragingival position.
- Surgical extrusion of the apical fragment can be carried out in teeth with long roots.

F. *Root fracture*

Root fracture can be either horizontal or vertical. The common factors which lead to root fracture are related to root morphology, deviant masticatory habits and excessive occlusal forces.

a. *Horizontal root fracture*

Horizontal root fracture is usually located at the apical and middle half of the root. Such fractures are characterized by rupture of hard structures of the root; subsequently separating the tooth into two fragments; the apical segment is not usually displaced and the coronal segment is often displaced.

The following factors should be considered before planning the treatment (treatment mainly depends upon status of pulp and mobility of coronal segment):

i. Position of the coronal segment after fracture
ii. Mobility of coronal segment
iii. Site of fracture
iv. Status of the pulp
v. Access to oral environment
vi. Age and sex

***i. Position of tooth following fracture*:** The teeth following fracture are usually lingually placed and slightly extruded. The treatment protocol involves reduction of displaced coronal fragment and immobilization. It is established that if treatment is initiated immediately, repositioning of the fragment is easily achieved. If resistance is felt during repositioning, it is most likely due to fracture of the labial socket wall. In this case repositioning of the fractured bone is

Flowchart 26.1 Treatment protocol of cracked teeth

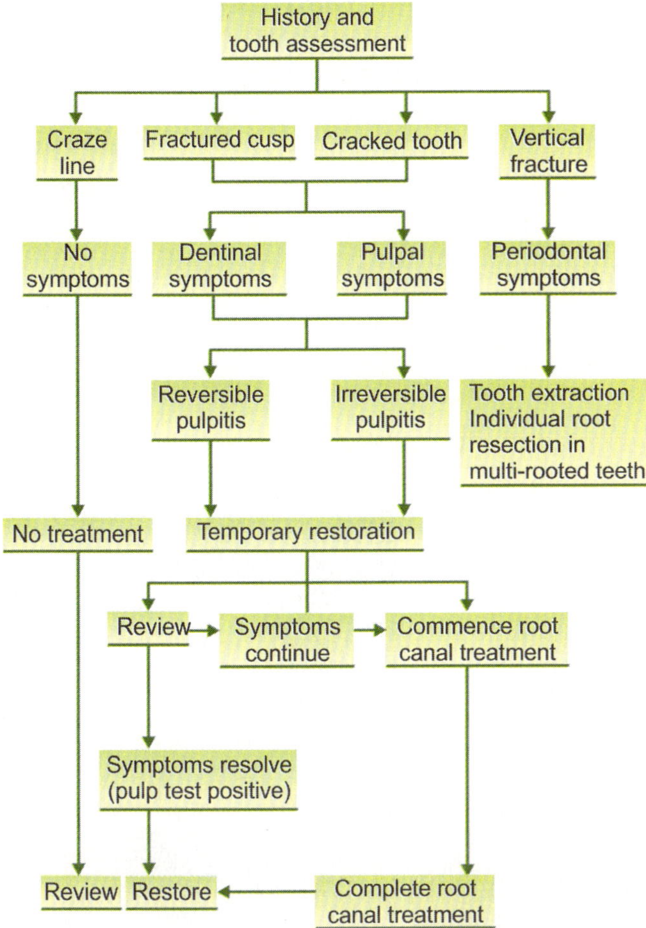

necessary before reducing the root fracture. After reduction, the position should be verified radiographically. Splinting for 6 to 8 weeks effectively reduces the fractured segments.

***ii. Mobility of coronal segment*:** Root fractures in the apical third of the root without displacing the coronal fragment do not require any splint. It has been shown that there is no difference in the outcome of treatment between splinted and non-splinted teeth in such cases. However, splinting is necessary in mid root or cervical root fractures.

***iii. Site of fracture*:** A root fractured in apical third area has an excellent prognosis because the pulp in the apical fragment usually remains vital, and the tooth may remain firm in its socket. If the pulp in the coronal fragment remains vital and the tooth is stable (with or without ligation), then no additional treatment is required. If the pulp in the coronal fragment gets necrosed, then endodontic treatment limited to the coronal fragment can be performed. If the tooth fails to recover, the apical root fragment can be removed surgically.

Generally the prognosis is good for apical and mid-root fracture, while it is questionable in case of cervical root fracture.

Horizontal root fractures at the level of the periodontal attachment have generally a poor prognosis. The treatment involves a combination of endodontic, orthodontic, periodontic and restorative therapy.

In case of cervical-third fractures, the treatment depends upon length of the remaining root and the availability of coronal segment. The treatment options can be:

- Fractures below the alveolar crest can be treated by conventional means by stabilizing the fractured segments. The splinting should be kept for a longer period (say 4–6 months), maintaining proper oral hygiene. The occlusal/functional load should be kept to a minimum.
- In case the coronal fragment is available and the fracture is coronal to the alveolar crest, reattachment of the fractured segment should be attempted. Both the fractured surface areas are etched and bonded with flowable adhesive restoration (slight undercut can be created on both the fragments or a plastic pin can be inserted on both the sides to achieve better retention).
- In case the coronal fragment is not available; fracture line extends below the alveolar crest, the remaining root is endodontically treated and restored with appropriate post-core restorations.
- The remaining root can be extracted carefully and adjusted at the requisite position; the fractured segment is stabilized by interdental suturing and dressing (Intra-alveolar transplantation of fractured root segment).
- In case the above mentioned modalities fail or not feasible, extraction followed by implantation can be carried out.

***iv. Status of the pulp*:** Horizontal root fracture, especially in a tooth with an open apex warrants maintenance of radicular pulp vitality to allow continued root formation.

Immature teeth with incomplete root fractures may heal by hard tissue union. However, these teeth may be splinted for better results. The tooth should be observed radiographically and with vitality tests in order to detect changes in pulp status, if any.

***v. Access to oral environment*:** In case the fracture line develops communication with oral environment (through gingival sulcus), the prognosis of union is poor (usually the site of fracture gets contaminated with oral micro-organisms, which hinder with the repair process).

***vi. Age and sex*:** Younger age is favorable for healing (mostly traumatic injuries occur in young age); better blood supply coupled with immunity facilitate hard tissues formation at the fractured site.

Healing of fractured segments is not related to sex; however, girls have shown early healing as compared to boys.

The treatment protocol of root fracture depending upon condition of pulp and the mobility of coronal segment is explained in Table 26.5.

The various options are:

- Root canal therapy of both the segments.
- Root canal therapy of coronal segment and removal of separated apical segment (Fig. 26.4a to i)
- Root canal therapy of coronal segment and no treatment for intact vital apical segment (Fig. 26.5a to d)

Table 26.5 Condition of pulp and mobility of coronal segment; recommended treatment of root fracture

Vitality (condition of pulp)	*Mobility of coronal segment*	*Root canal treatment required*	*Splinting required*
+	–	No	No
+	+	No	Yes
–	–	Yes	No
–	+	Yes	Yes

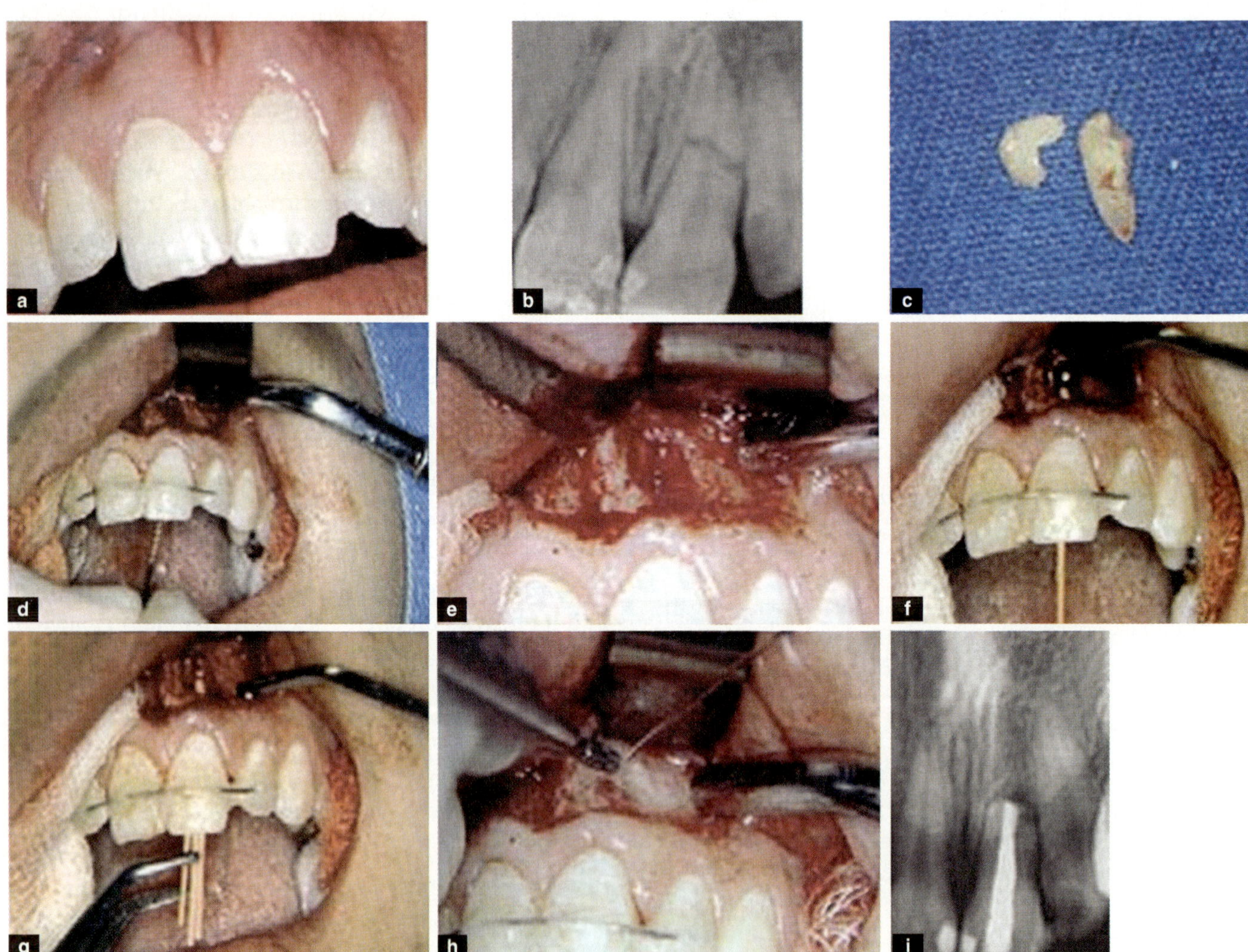

Fig. 26.4 Root canal treatment of coronal segment and removal of fractured apical segment: (a) Fracture of left maxillary central incisor (central incisor bonded to the lateral incisor); (b) Preoperative radiograph revealing root fracture; (c) Removed apical fragments; (d) Root canal preparation of coronal fragment; (e) Evaluating root canal with endodontic file; (f) Filling of the coronal fragment; (g) Completing obturation of coronal fragment; (h) Apical segment removed surgically (four anterior teeth splinted); (i) Postoperative radiograph showing healing

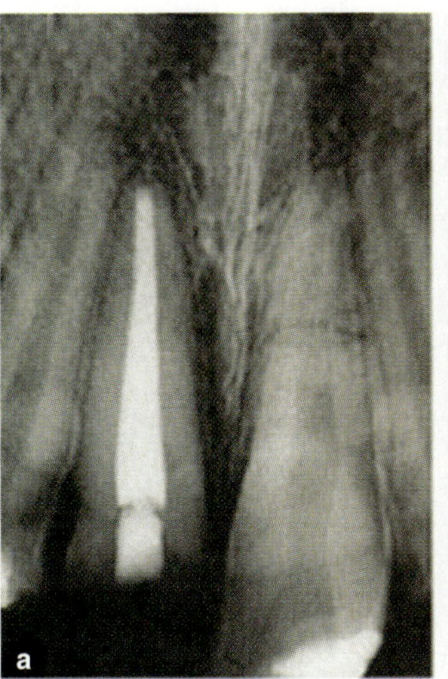
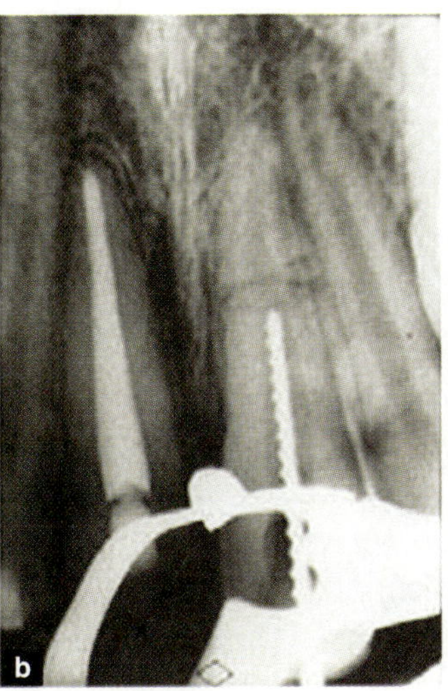
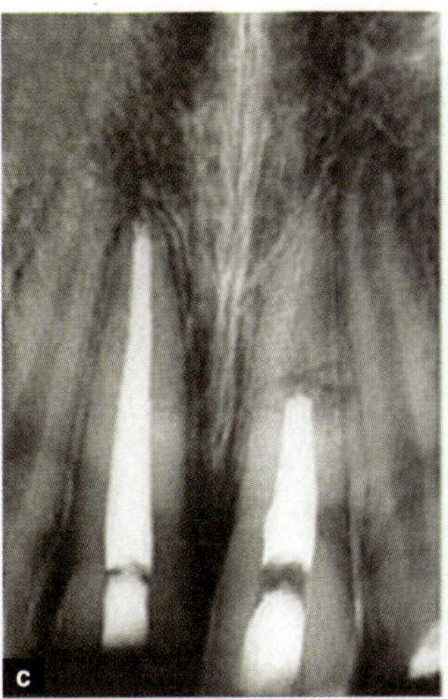
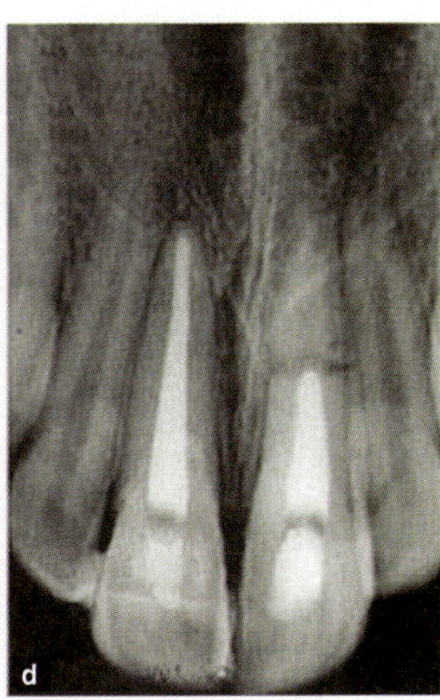

Fig. 26.5 The coronal portion is root canal treated up to the fracture line; the apical portion is left untreated (healing with interposition of hard and soft tissue): (a) Preoperative radiograph showing horizontal root fracture of the left upper central incisor; (b) Assessing the fracture segments; (c) Coronal fragment obturated with gutta-percha; (d) Postoperative radiograph

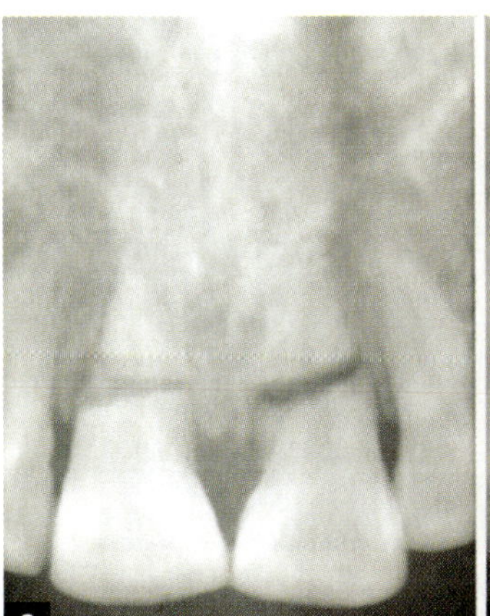
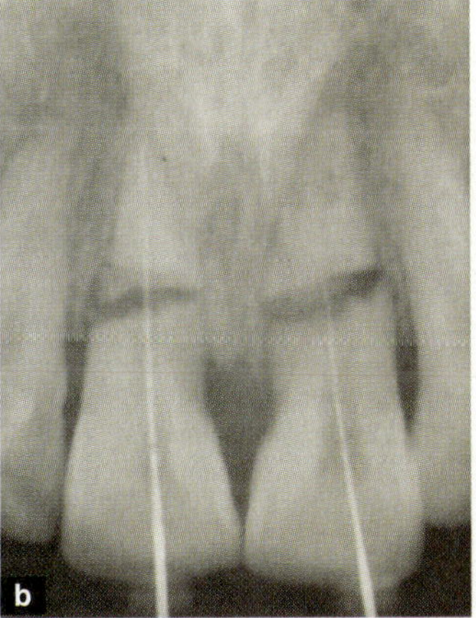
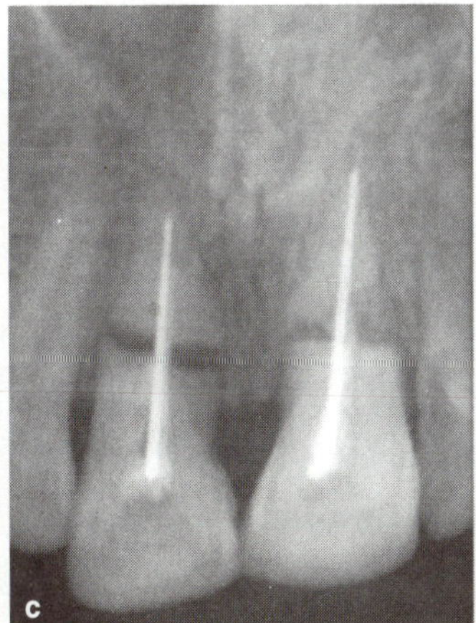
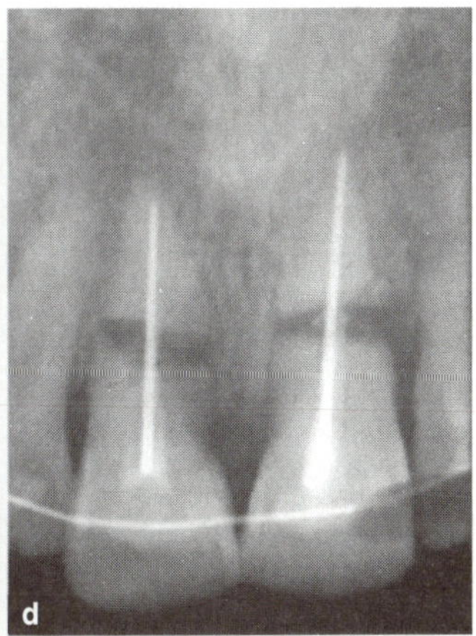

Fig. 26.6 Use of intraradicular splint connecting fractured segments: (a) Horizontal root fracture in the middle third of root; (b) By-passing the fracture segment; (c) Interradicular splint inserted; (d) Splinting of the fractured teeth with healthy teeth

- Root canal therapy of coronal segment with mineral trioxide aggregate (MTA) as apical barrier
- The use of intraradicular splint connecting both the segments (Fig. 26.6a to d)
- Root extrusion—removal of coronal segment and subsequent orthodontic or surgical extrusion of the remaining apical fragment

The horizontal mid root fracture with clinical signs of pulpal necrosis can be treated by performing root canal treatment on both the segments. The fragments should be stabilized by inserting stainless steel endodontic file inside the root canal. Anderson recommended that detection of a sinus tract emanating from the coronal fragment requires root canal treatment of that portion only.

Mineral trioxide aggregate has also been used in managing mid root fractures. There is not sufficient documentation to evaluate clinical outcomes of root canal treatment using mineral trioxide aggregate in teeth with horizontal root fractures; however, individual case reports (Fig. 26.7a to i) are positive.

The management of root fracture is summarized in Table 26.6.

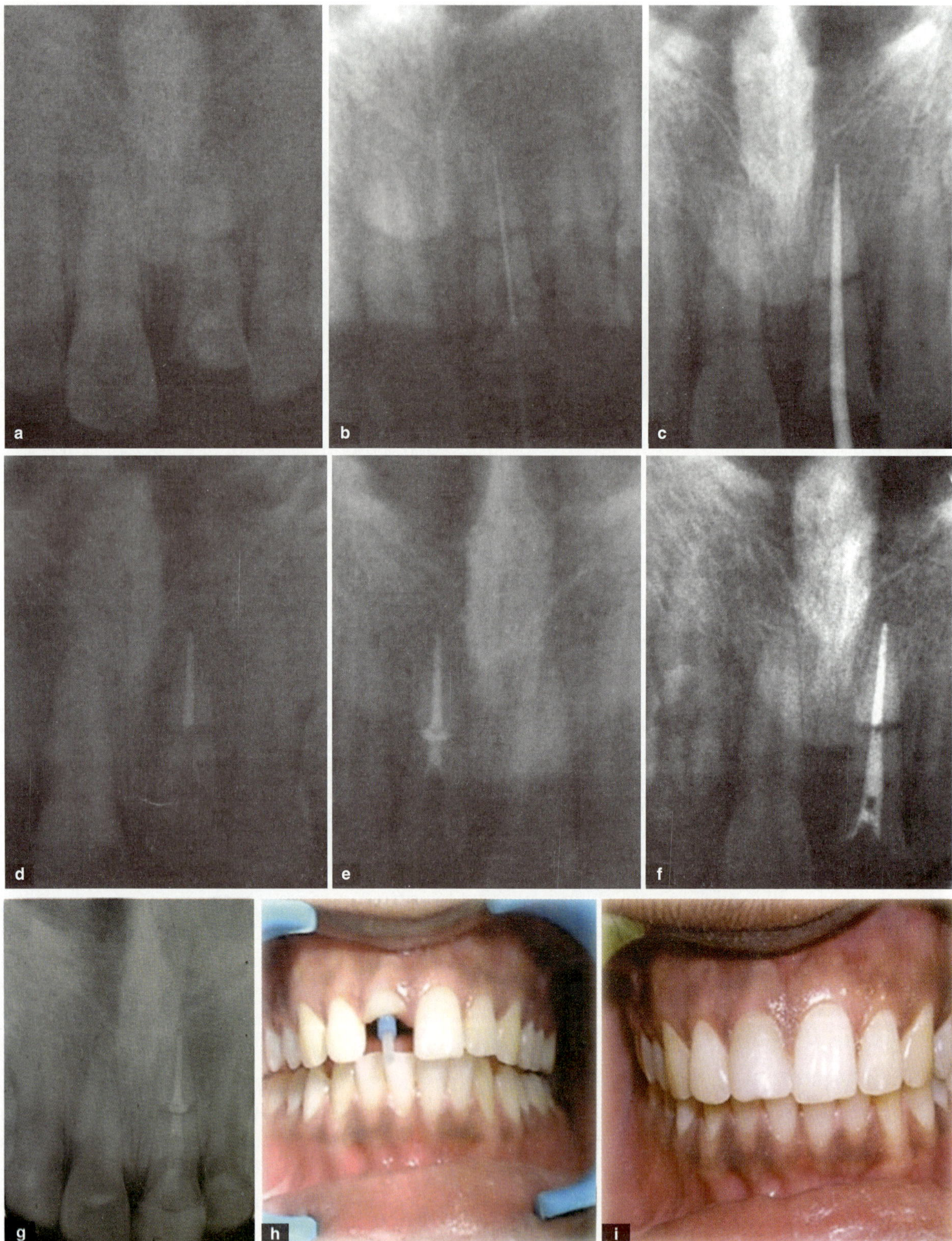

Fig. 26.7 Mid-root fracture managed by mineral trioxide aggregate (MTA): (a) Preoperative radiograph showing mid-root fracture; (b) By-passing the fracture segment; (c) Assessing the fracture segments with gutta-percha cone; (d) Obturation of apical segment with gutta-percha; (e) Apical barrier between coronal and apical segments with mineral trioxide aggregate; (f) Obturation of coronal segment with gutta-percha; (g) Postoperative radiograph; (h) Coronal segment reinforced with fiber post and core; (i) Final restoration with a crown.

Table 26.6 Management of root fracture

Horizontal	
Fracture at apical third	• Retain the fragments (wait for natural healing) • Root canal treatment of both the fragments (minimum or no mobility of fragments) • Root canal treatment of both the fragments followed by stabilizing the fractured segments (mobility of fractured segments)
Fracture at middle third	• Reduction and stabilization • Root canal treatment of both the fragments followed by stabilizing the fractured segments (mobility of fractured segments)
Cervical third area	• Reattachment if coronal segment available and fracture is above the alveolar crest • Stabilization, if fracture site below the alveolar crest • Crown lengthening if fracture site is within 3.0 mm of the gingival crevice area, followed by conventional root canal treatment and post-core restorations • Surgical extrusion/orthodontic extrusion, followed by conventional root canal treatment and post-core restorations • Extraction, if other treatments fail/not feasible
Vertical	
Partial/complete	• Extracting the fractured root; bonding the fractured segments with adhesive and reimplanting in 180° rotation (rotation facilitates periodontal ligament attachment) • Application of bioresorbable membrane followed by stabilization and reduction

Prognosis

Successful treatment of horizontal root fractures have been reported in literature. Additional findings, such as pulp canal obliteration, external and internal surface resorption have been observed along with healing modalities.

b. Vertical root fracture

Generally, prognosis is poor with vertical root fracture, especially in single rooted teeth. In multirooted tooth, radisectomy can be helpful.

The vertical root fracture can be treated by extracting the fractured tooth atraumatically, bonding the fragments (adhesive resin/4-meta resin used as bonding agent. Lasers have also been tried) and then replanting the tooth with a 180° rotation. The rotation of the tooth facilitates connection of the healthy periodontal membrane to the fractured root. The application of bio-resorbable membrane on root surfaces reinforces the periodontal healing. It allows regeneration of periodontal ligament cells, providing space for the in-growth of periodontal ligament tissues.

Fractured roots that radiographically reveal less space between the fragments after repositioning usually heal with hard tissue repair than those with more space between the fragments. Reduction is also important for eliminating the blood coagulum between the fragments, which is the substrate for bacterial growth.

Ankylosis is a common complication of replanted teeth leading to a gradual resorption of the dental hard tissues and their replacement by bone. The vitality of the periodontal membrane was reported to be of critical importance in preventing ankylosis.

Healing of Root Fracture

The healing of root fracture depends upon the site of fracture and the status of pulp. The wound healing is initiated both from pulpal and periodontal ligament side.

If the pulp is intact after fracture, the odontoblastic progenitor cells create a hard tissue bridge uniting the fractured fragments, followed by cementum deposition derived from the periodontal ligament cells obliterating the fracture site.

The fate of the injured pulp depends upon revascularization from the periodontal ligament sites. In case the pulp is severely stretched at the level of fracture, the revascularization process is initiated from the coronal pulp. If bacteria gain access during the process, it may lead to necrosis of coronal pulp.

Clinical and radiographic follow-ups are necessary to evaluate pulp necrosis. Extrusion of the coronal fragment, tenderness to percussion, and the radiographic signs of pulp necrosis can usually be detected within the first two months after injury.

A negative sensibility response immediately after injury does not necessarily indicate pulp necrosis. However, it has been observed that teeth which did not respond to pulp testing immediately following root fracture demonstrated significantly greater risk of pulp necrosis.

The periodontally derived cells help in root fracture healing by interposition of connective tissue. During the initial stage of wound healing, the inflammatory response trigger series of osteoclastic activities, subsequently obliterating the fracture site. The pattern of healing may eventually lead to resorption. The types of resorption can be:

- External surface resorption surrounding the proximal fracture edges at the periodontal side of the fracture.
- Internal surface resorption surrounding the fracture edges centrally at the pulpal side of the fracture.
- Internal tunneling resorption burrows behind the predentin layer and along the root canal walls of the coronal fragment.

The resorption processes are usually self-limiting and resolve within first one to two years after injury.

The pattern of healing of root fracture may vary. The possible patterns can be:

i. Healing with calcified tissue

The calcified tissue, simulating dentin, osteodentin and/or cementum is formed at the fracture site. The innermost layer of repaired tissue simulate dentin; whereas, the peripheral portion is repaired with cementum. The connective tissue may not completely bridge the gap between the fracture surfaces, but is interspersed all along the fractured area. A slight widening of the root canal close to the fracture site may be seen after the hard tissue formation.

This type of healing depends upon the intact pulp and is seen primarily in cases with little or no dislocation of the coronal segment. Clinically, the tooth appears normal in these conditions.

ii. Healing with interproximal calcified tissue

The healing is characterized by the presence of connective tissue between the fragments. The fracture surfaces are covered with connective tissue fibers running parallel to the fracture surface or from one fragment to the other.

A common finding is peripheral rounding of the fracture site. In-growth of bony tissues into the fracture area may also be seen. Radiographically, peripheral rounding of the fracture edges and a radiolucent line separating the fragments can be visible.

Initially, external and internal surface resorptions are often seen, as well as pulp canal obliteration of both apical and coronal aspect of the root canal. Clinically, the teeth are firm or may be slightly mobile. Long term follow-up is mandatory, because the resorptive process may lead to ankylosis.

This type of healing is related to extrusion or lateral luxation with moderate pulp injury.

iii. Healing with interposition of bone and connective tissue

26

This mode of healing is a sequelae of trauma prior to complete growth of the alveolar process (the coronal fragment continues to erupt while the apical fragment remains stationary). Interposition of bone and connective tissues is seen along the fracture site.

Radiographically, a bony bridge is seen separating the fragments with a periodontal ligament space around both the fragments. Pulp canal obliteration of the root canals in both fragments is a common finding. Clinically, the teeth are firm and react normally to pulp tests.

iv. Interposition of granulation tissue

The fractured site is obliterated with granulation tissue. The coronal portion is usually necrotic, while the apical portion remains vital. The necrotic pulp tissue is responsible for inflammatory changes along the fracture line. Radiographically, widening of the fracture line, loss of lamina dura and rarefaction of the alveolar bone corresponding to the fracture line are common findings.

Follow-up

A standard follow-up protocol should be followed based on clinical information and sensitivity tests. Laser Doppler evaluation can be helpful in demonstrating early revascularization of the coronal pulp. The radiographic examination should be carried out periodically to evaluate the healing pattern.

G. Luxation injuries

Luxation injuries account for 15.0 to 60.0% of traumas in primary and permanent teeth. Accidents and fights are the main reasons for such injuries. Six types of luxation lesions are recognized (Fig. 26.8):

i. Concussion
ii. Subluxation
iii. Extrusive luxation
iv. Lateral luxation
v. Intrusive luxation
vi. Tooth avulsion

i. ***Concussion***: It is a mild form of luxation injury, characterized by sensitivity to percussion only. No displacement and no mobility is seen as a result of the injury (Fig. 26.8a). Treatment for concussion is symptomatic. Tooth is allowed to rest to promote recovery of trauma to periodontal ligament and apical vessels. Pulp status should be monitored by pulp tester and the tooth should be periodontically clinically examined for any evidence of color changes (Table 26.7).

ii. ***Subluxation***: Subluxated tooth is mobile and sensitive to percussion (Fig. 26.8b). The pulp tests may result in 'no response' or may be 'positive'. Treatment may not be required; alternatively, the tooth may be stabilized for a short period of time (Table 26.7). Subluxated teeth need to be evaluated and monitored regularly to evaluate the pulp status.

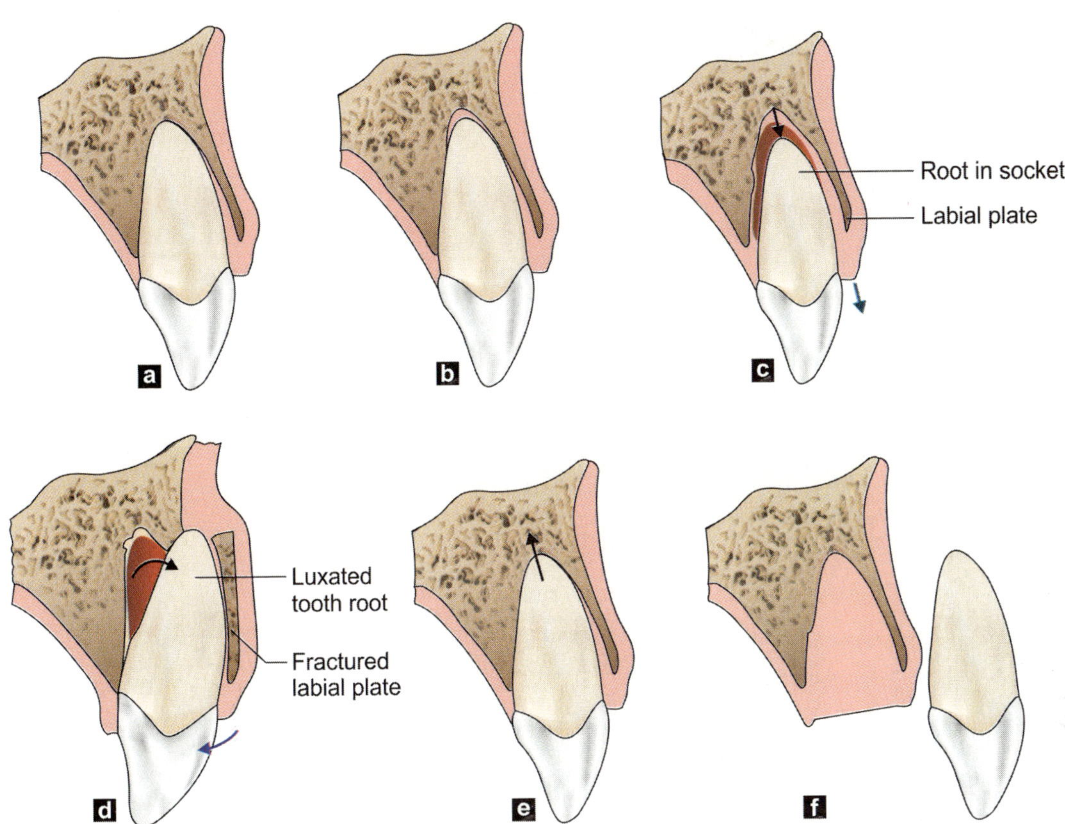

Fig. 26.8 Luxation injuries: (a) Concussion; (b) Subluxation; (c) Extrusive luxation; (d) Lateral luxation; (e) Intrusive luxation; (f) Tooth avulsion

iii. ***Extrusive luxation***: The tooth is axially displaced in a coronal direction (Fig. 26.8c). The luxated tooth is mobile and likely to have a premature contact with opposing teeth. The tooth is immediately stabilized by functional splint for 4 to 8 weeks (Table 26.6).

    Long stabilization period is preferred to realign the periodontal ligament fibers. Generally, the extrusive luxated teeth require root canal therapy except in young, developing teeth in which the pulps are more prone to recover.

iv. ***Lateral luxation***: Traumatic injuries may result in displacement of a tooth labially, lingually, distally or mesially. Such displacement is called lateral luxation (Fig. 26.8d).

    The lateral luxation cases are managed by repositioning and stabilization the tooth. Repositioning a laterally luxated tooth may require pressure application at the apical end of the root in the direction of the original root apex. Definitive treatment may include root canal therapy (Table 26.6).

v. ***Intrusive luxation***: A tooth, during trauma, is pushed apically; mostly firm in the socket (Fig. 26.8e). Treatment depends upon the stage of tooth development (Table 26.6). No treatment is advised for immature teeth (it is expected that tooth with wide open apex has the potential to re-erupt and establish a normal occlusal alignment within few weeks/months).

    Monitor the progress of re-eruption of teeth; if tooth erupts in a natural position, no other treatment is needed. Pulp status of tooth is also evaluated periodically. Root canal therapy is usually not required.

    Recent guidelines advise no treatment if intrusion is within 3.0 mm; however, intrusion up to 7.0–8.0 mm need repositioning using surgical/orthodontic/combination of two means. Tooth is likely to get ankylosed if not treated on time.

vi. ***Tooth avulsion***: An avulsed tooth is completely displaced out of its socket (Fig. 26.8f). Avulsion is considered as a dental emergency, since timely attention could save such teeth. It has been established that immediate reimplantation of avulsed teeth leads to clinical success (Table 26.8).

    The most important factor from the moment the tooth is avulsed from the alveolar socket is 'time'. The increase of time between avulsion to reimplantation increases the danger of replacement resorption and decreases revascularization; subsequently compromising success.

    Long term success depends on the storage medium and also management of the root surface.

Table 26.7 Luxation injuries: Signs, symptoms and management

Tooth status	*Concussion*	*Subluxation*	*Lateral luxation*	*Intrusion*	*Extrusion*
Clinical findings	• No change in tooth position • No mobility • Sensitive to percussion	• Sensitive to percussion may increase • May be slightly mobile • No change in tooth position	Tooth laterally repositioned	• No mobility • Metallic sound upon percussion	• Tooth sensitive to percussion • Extruded tooth may be mobile • Visible gingival damage
Radiological findings	No radiolucency	No radiolucency	Widened periodontal ligament	Absence of periodontal ligament	Widened periodontal ligament
Treatment/ Management	No treatment indicated	Non-rigid splint for one to two weeks	• Anesthetize area and push the tooth to original position • Non-rigid splint for four weeks • The tooth is selectively grinded to minimize occlusal forces	• Closed apex: Immediately return tooth to original position by orthodontic eruption or surgical • In case of open apex, wait for natural eruption • Periodic evaluation of pulp status	Anesthetize area and push the tooth to its original position
Periodical follow-up	Follow-up at 4 weeks, 8 weeks; up to one year	Evaluate pup status	• Evaluate pulp status • Root canal treatment may be required • Radiographic confirmation	• Evaluate pulp status • Root canal treatment may be required • Radiographic confirmation	• Evaluate pulp status • Root canal treatment may be required • Radiographic confirmation
Patient instructions	• Soft diet initially • Brush/rinse with 0.2% chlorhexidine twice daily • Antibiotics/analgesics according to the need				

Table 26.8 Management of avulsed teeth

On-site treatment	• Hold the tooth by the crown • Wash and keep the tooth in oral cavity (saliva) • Can be kept in milk/other storage medium, as available • Refer patient to dental clinic immediately		
Treatment in clinic	**Condition A** • Tooth replanted in the socket	**Condition B** • Tooth stored in medium, such as saline solution or saliva (up to 2 hours after injury) or milk (up to 3 hours after injury) or dry (less than 60 minutes)	**Condition C** • Tooth remained dry for more than 60 minutes or longer than recommended time in other media
	• The tooth is stabilized and splinted	• Remove tooth from medium and gently apply antibiotic solution to the root surface	• Remove periodontal ligament fibers with gentle brushing and place tooth in a topical fluoride (APF 1.23% F^-) solution for 15 minutes. • Remove blood clot from socket with normal saline. Perform root canal extraorally, reimplant the tooth and splint
Follow-up of the case	• Ensure correct tooth position within the socket • Selective grinding to relieve tooth from occlusal forces • Periodic examination to evaluate status of pulp and surrounding tissues		
Postoperative instructions	• Soft diet for two weeks • Rinse mouth with 0.2% chlorhexidine twice daily for a week • Put patient on antibiotics, etc.		

Storage medium

Tooth should be immediately placed in a storage medium to diminish injury to the periodontal ligaments cells.

The storage media are:

i. Water
ii. Normal saline
iii. Saliva
iv. Coconut water
v. Egg white
vi. Green tea/propolis
vii. Milk
viii. Viaspan
ix. Hanks balanced salt solution (HBSS)
x. Dulbecco's storage medium
xi. Soymilk

i. *Water*: Water is not a good medium for storage. Its non-physiological pH/osmolality, hypotonicity and bacterial contamination favor cell lysis of attached periodontal ligament.

ii. *Normal saline*: Normal saline has physiological pH/osmolality; however, it does not contain any essential nutrient (mainly glucose and proteins) for the survival of cells. Saline is not considered as an effective storage medium.

iii. *Saliva*: Buccal vestibule is considered as a safe storage medium for avulsed teeth. However, saliva has unfavorable characteristics, such as non-physiologic pH/osmolality, hypotonicity and bacterial contamination.

Artificial saliva is also not effective. Both artificial and human saliva is considered only if other adequate media are not available.

iv. *Coconut water*: Coconut water is pure, sterile natural product, rich in nutrients (amino acids, vitamins and minerals). It is an effective storage medium; comparable to milk and HBSS.

v. *Egg white*: Egg white is an excellent storage medium because of its nutrients (proteins, vitamins, water) along with absence of microbial contamination. It provides cell viability for a long period of time.

vi. *Green tea/propolis*: Both green tea and propolis are anti-inflammatory, antibacterial and anti-oxidants. These have the potential to inhibit prostaglandin synthesis facilitating phagocytic activities and promoting healing effects. Both are very good storage medium.

vii. ***Milk***: Milk has physiological pH/osmolality, is isotonic and contains growth factors/nutrients. Milk contains epithelial growth factor, which proliferates epithelial growth factor, which proliferates epithelial cell rests of Malassez. It is very good storage medium.

viii. ***Viaspan***: Viaspan has physiological pH/osmolality and sufficient nutrients favoring cell growth. It is an excellent storage medium; however, it is not easily available. The high cost of the medium makes it unviable for routine use.

ix. ***Hank's balanced salt solution (HBSS)***: Hank's balanced salt solution has physiological pH/ osmolality, considered an excellent storage medium. It contains nutrients for preserving the vitality of cells.

x. ***Dulbecco's solution***: Dulbecco's solution has physiological pH. It maintains intracellular/ extracellular osmotic balance. It provides nutrients (mainly glucose) for survival of cells. It is considered as an excellent storage medium.

xi. ***Soymilk***: Soy milk has physiological pH (as compared to cow's milk, it contains no cholesterol and is fat free). It has the potential for cell proliferation. Soymilk, as a storage medium, is comparable to HBSS solution and is superior to Egg white and coconut water.

The characteristic features and efficacy of storage media are summarized in Table 26.9.

Table 26.9 Characteristics and efficacy of storage medium

Storage medium	*Characteristics*	*Efficacy*
Water	• Non-physiological pH • Contaminated with bacteria and other aerosols	Nil (Poor)
Normal saline	• Physiological pH • Osmolality • Easy availability	Poor
Saliva	• Non-physiological pH • Hypotonic • Contaminated with micro-organisms • Accessibility to patient's own saliva	Poor
Coconut water	• Sterile and natural • Contain nutrients • Availability varies	Good
Egg white	• Contains nutrients (protein)/ water • Minimum bacterial contamination	Good
Green tea/propolis	• Antibacterial • Antioxidant • Anti-inflammatory	Very good
Milk	• Physiological pH/osmolality • Contains growth factors and nutrients • Minimum bacterial contamination • Isotonic	Very good
Viaspan	• Physiological pH/osmolality • Favors cell growth	Excellent
Hank's balanced salt solution	• Physiological pH/osmolality • Contains nutrients	Excellent
Dulbecco's solution	• Physiological pH • Maintain intracellular/ extracellular osmotic balance • Provide nutrients	Excellent
Soymilk	• Physiological pH • Facilitate proliferation of cells	Very good

Management of root surface

The management of root surface depends on the amount of time elapsed from the time of injury, coupled with type of storage medium, if used.

A tooth that remains out of oral cavity and remained in dry condition for less than 60 minutes or stored in one of the recommended mediums, the root surface is soaked in 1.0 mg/10 ml doxycycline for five minutes before reimplantation. The use of antibiotics enhances the potential for revascularization and even lower the frequency of inflammatory root resorption. In the event that 60 minutes have passed in dry condition or the tooth remained in recommended medium for longer period, then the tooth should be soaked in a fluoride solution before reimplantation. In such cases, replacement resorption is inevitable. Therefore the goal is to make root more resistant to resorption. Soaking the root in topical fluoride (APF 1.23% F^-) for 15 minutes slows down the process of resorption. It is advisable to perform root canal therapy outside the oral cavity (Fig. 26.9a to g).

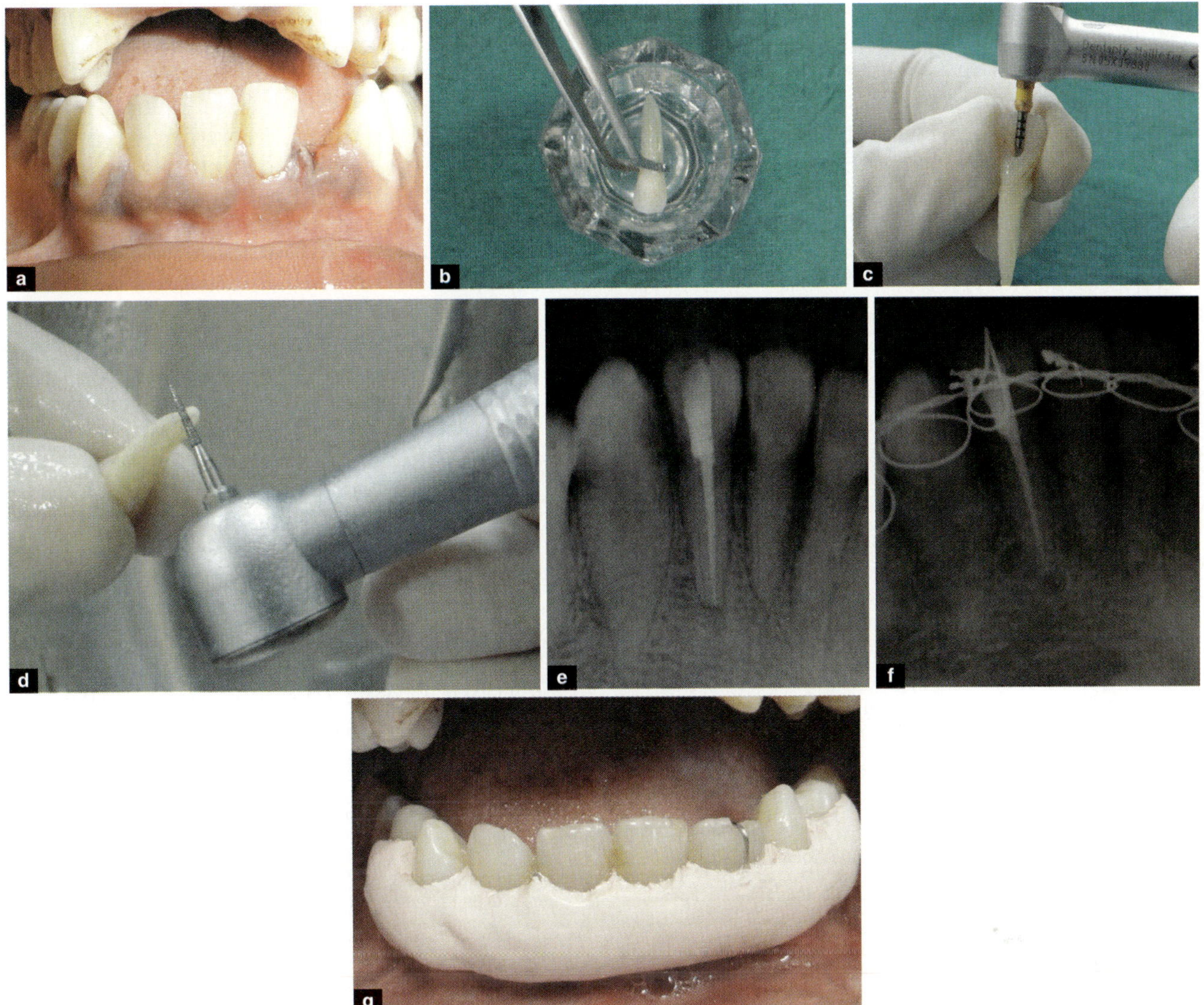

Fig. 26.9: Reimplantation of mandibular incisor: (a) Preoperative; (b) Avulsed tooth dipped in APF solution; (c) Preparing root canal; (d) Apex resected; (e) Avulsed tooth placed back in the socket after root canal treatment; (f) Radiograph showing splinting; (g) Periodontal pack placed

Fracture of Alveolar Process

The fracture involves socket wall and the alveolar process. A transitory negative response is common during pulp testing.

Initial treatment consists of reduction of the fracture and stabilization by splinting for three to four weeks. Follow-up evaluation should be carried out periodically after initial treatment.

BIBLIOGRAPHY

1. Abbott PV and Salgado JC. Strategies to minimize the consequences of trauma to the teeth. OHDM: 2014; 13:229–232.
2. Aggarwal VS, Kapoor S and Shah NC. An innovative approach for treating vertical root fracture of mandibular molar-hemisection with socket preparation. J. Interdiscip. Dent.: 2012; 22:141–143.
3. Andrade ES and de Campos AL. Root healing after horizontal fracture: a case report with a 13-year follow up. Dental Traumatology: 2008; 24:1–3.
4. Arakawa S, Gobb CM, Rapley JW, Killoy WJ and Spencer P. Treatment of root fracture by CO2 and Nd:YAG lasers: An in-vitro study. J. Endod.: 1996; 22:662–665.
5. Bastone EB, Freer TJ and McNamara, JR. Epidemiology of dental trauma: a review of the literature. Aust. Dent. J.: 2000; 45:2–9.
6. Bhattacharya V. Management of soft tissue wounds of the face. Indian J. Plast. Surg.: 2012; 45:436–439.
7. Cvek M, Meja`re I and Andreasen JO. Healing and prognosis of teeth with intra alveolar fractures involving the cervical part of the root. Dental Traumatology: 2002; 18:57–65.
8. da Costa KM and Caldas AF. A systemic review of the diagnostic classifications of traumatic dental injuries. Dental Traumatology: 2006; 22:71–76.

9. Deshpande A and Deshpande N. Flexible wire composite splinting of root fracture of immature permanent incisors: A case report. Pediat. Dent.: 2011; 33:63–66.
10. Duggan D, Quinn FO and Sullivan M. A long-term follow up of spontaneously healed root fractures later subjected to orthodontic forces—two case reports. Dental Traumatology: 2008; 24:231–234.
11. Filippi A, Tschan J, Pohl Y, Berkhold, H. and Ebeleseder K. A retrospective classification of tooth injuries using a new scoring system. Clin. Oral Invest.: 2000; 4:173–175.
12. Floratos SG and Kratchman SI. Surgical management of vertical root fractures for posterior teeth: Report of four cases. J. Endod.: 2012; 38:550–555.
13. Hassan B, Metska ME, Ozok AR, Stelt PV and Wesselink PR. Comparison of five cone beam computed tomography systems for detection of vertical root fractures. J. Endod.: 2010; 36:126–129.
14. Kahler W. The cracked tooth conundrum: Terminology, classification, diagnosis and management. Am. J. Dent.: 2008; 21:275–282.
15. Katz A, Wasenstein-Kohn, Tamse A and Zuckerman O. Residual dentin thickness in bifurcated maxillary premoalrs after root canal and dowel space preparation. J. Endod.: 2006; 32:202–205.
16. Kawai K and Masaka N. Vertical root fracture treated by bonding fragments and rotational replantation. Dental traumatology: 2002; 18:42–45.
17. Khasnin SA, Kidiyoor KH, Patil AB and Kenganal SB. Vertical root fractures and their management. J. Cons. Dent.:2014; 17:103–107.
18. Kishen A. Biomechanics of fractures in endodontically treated teeth. Endod. Topics: 2015; 33:3–13.
19. Kocak S, Cinar S, Kocak MM and Kayaoglu G. Intraradicular splinting with endodontic instrument of horizontal root fracture-Case report. Dental Traumatology: 2008; 24:578–580.
20. Lin S, Zuckerman O, Fuss Z and Ashkenazi M. New emphasis in the treatment of dental trauma: avulsion and luxation. Dental Traumatology: 2007; 23:297–303.
21. Loomba K, Loomba A, Bains R and Bains VK. A proposal for classification of tooth fractures based on treatment need. J. Oral Science: 2010; 52:517.
22. Main BG and Adair SR. The changing face of informed consent. Br. Dent. J.: 2015; 219:325.
23. Majorana A, Pasini S, Bardellini E and Keller E. Clinical and epidemiological study of Traumatic root fractures. Dental Traumatology: 2002; 18:77–80.
24. Metska ME, Aartman IH, Wesselink PR and Ozok AR. Detection of vertical root fracture in vivo in endodontically treated teeth by cone beam computed tomography scans. J. Endod.: 2012; 38:1344–1347.
25. Molina1 JR, VannJr WF, McIntyre JD, Trope M and Lee JY. Root fractures in children and adolescents: Diagnostic considerations. Dental Traumatology: 2008; 24:503–509.
26. Mozami F, Mirhadi H, Geramizadeh B and Sahebi S. Comparison of soymilk, powdered milk, Hank's balanced salt solution, and tap water on periodontal ligament cell survival. Dent. Traumatol.: 2012; 28:132–135.
27. Ozer SY. Detection of vertical root fractures of different thickness in endodontically enlarged teeth by Cone Beam Computed Tomography versus digital radiography. J. Endod.: 2010; 36:1245–1249.
28. Pagadala S, Tadikonda DC. An overview of classification of dental trauma. IAIM: 2015; 2:157–161.
29. Panzarini SR, Gulinelli JL, Poi WR, Sonoda CK, Pedrini D and Brandini DA. Treatment of root surface in delayed tooth replantation: a review of literature. Dent. Traumatol.: 2008; 24:277–282.
30. Poi WR, Sonoda CK, Martins CM, Melo ME, Pellizzer EP, de Mendonca MR and Panzarini SR. Storage media for avulsed teeth: a literature review. Braz. Dent. J.:2013; 24:437–445.
31. Qin M., Ge LH and Bai RH. Use of a removable splint in the treatment of subluxated, luxated and root fractured anterior permanent teeth in children. Dental Traumatology: 2002; 18:81–85.
32. Rosen E, Tsesis I, Tamse A, Bjorndal L, Taschieri S and Givos N. Medicolegal aspects of vertical root fracture in root filled teeth. Int. Endod. J.:2012; 45:597–613.
33. Sikri V and Sikri P. Management of fractured posterior teeth: A new technique. JIDA: 1996; 67:198–202.
34. Silva EJ, Rollemberg CB, Coutinho-Filho TS, Krebs RL and Zaia AA. Use of soymilk as a storage medium for avulsed teeth. Acta. Odontol. Scand.: 2013; 71:1101–1104.
35. Souza BDM, Luckemeyer DD, Reyes-Carmona JF, Felippe WT, Simoes CMO and Felippe MCS. Viability of human periodontal ligament fibroblasts in milk, Hank's balanced salt solution and coconut water as storage media. Int. Endod. J.:2011; 44:111–115.
36. Spinas E and Altana M. A new classification for crown fractures of teeth. J. Clin. Pediat. Dent.: 2002; 26:225–231.
37. Terata R, Minami K and Kubota M. Conservative treatment for root fracture located very close to gingiva. Dental Traumatolgy: 2005; 21:111–114.
38. Toure B, Faye B, Kane AW, Lo CM, Niang B and Boucher Y. Analysis of reasons for extraction of endodontically treated teeth: A prospective study. J. Endod.: 2011; 37:1512–1515.
39. Tsesis I, Rosen E, Tamse A, Taschieri S and Kfir A. Diagnosis of vertical root fractures in endodontically treated teeth based on clinical and radiographic indices: A systematic review. J. Endod.: 2010; 36:1455–1458.
40. Versiani1 MA, De Sousa CJ, Cruz-Filho AM, Da Cruz Perez DE and Sousa-Neto MD. Clinical management and subsequent healing of teeth with horizontal root fractures. Dental Traumatology: 2008; 24:136–139.
41. Walton RE, Michelich RJ and Smith GN. The histopathogenesis of vertical root fractures. J. Endod.: 1984; 10:48–56.
42. Wang J and Li M. Multidisciplinary treatment of a complicated crown-root fracture. Pediatric Dentistry: 2010; 32:250–254.
43. Westphalen VP, De Sousa MH, Da Silva Neto UX, Fariniuk LF and Carneiro E. Management of horizontal root-fractured teeth. Report of three cases. Dental Traumatology: 2008; 24:e11–e15.
44. Zadik Y, Sandler V, Bechor R and Salehrabi R. Analysis of factors related to extraction of endodontically treated teeth. O.Surg, O. Med, O. Path.: 2008; 106:e31–e35.

Chapter 27

Root Resorption

Root resorption, a multidisciplinary problem, is of concern to the clinicians, especially the endodontists. Root resorption is defined as '*the progressive loss of dentin and cementum through the continuous action of osteoclastic cells (odontoclasts, cementoclasts and all clast cells, derived from monocytes, which form macrophages)*'. In bone, continuous apposition and resorption occur as a part of remodeling process. Early diagnosis, removal of the cause, proper treatment and reinforcement of the resorbed root is mandatory for achieving success. Efforts should be directed towards maintaining integrity and vitality of the periodontal ligament of luxated and the displaced teeth.

The resorption can be physiological and pathological. The resorption in primary dentition is physiological (Fig. 27.1); whereas, in permanent dentition, it is pathological (Fig. 27.2). Roots of permanent teeth do not undergo resorption normally. The cellular surface layer of odontoblasts and cementoblasts usually provide immunity to the permanent dentition (root cementum from the side of periodontal ligament is coated with precementum and cementoblasts; odontoblasts and predentin protect dentin from resorption). Physical/chemical injuries to this cellular layer may lead to resorption. Atypical resorption of external root surface has been reported in primary dentition. This is not associated with pulp necrosis and the tooth is generally asymptomatic. Radiologically, dome-shaped or cone-shaped area can be seen on the root surface involving periodontal ligament. It is co-related with the habit of thumb sucking, which may induce low intensity constant trauma. The resorption is self-limiting and gets repaired as the cause is removed. Rarely, abnormal positioning of permanent tooth germ may lead to its resorption along with deciduous tooth.

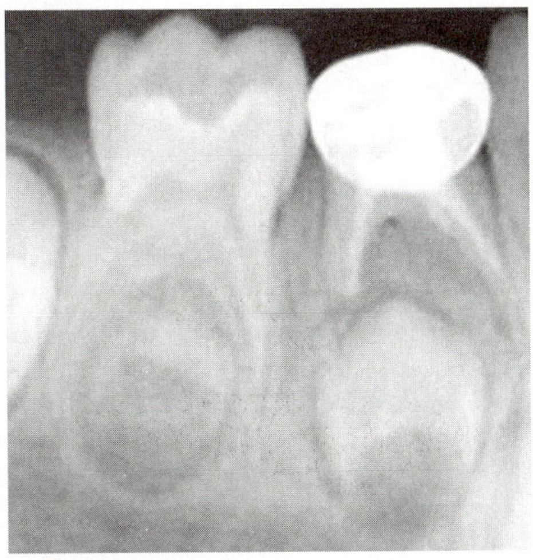

Fig. 27.1 Physiological root resorption

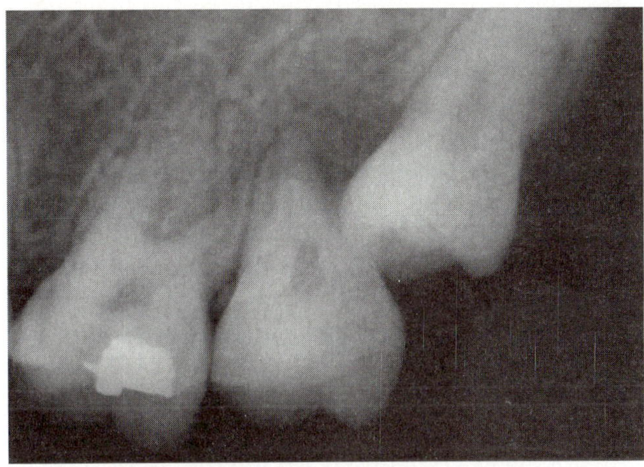

Fig. 27.2 Pathological root resorption

Etiology

The phenomenon of root resorption has multiple causes with varying hypothesis. The causes are broadly divided into three; local, systemic and iatrogenic. High temperature during cavity preparation/tooth preparation and calcium hydroxide in vital pulp therapy has also been the source of stimulation of resorption.

The causes of root resorption are summarized in Table 27.1.

Table 27.1 Causes of root resorption

Local causes	*Systemic causes*	*Iatrogenic*
• Tooth reimplantation (damage to periodontium) • Injuries/trauma • Improper habits • Orthodontic force • Bleaching procedures • Pressure of tumor or cyst • Invaginated teeth/dental abnormalities • Aggressive periodontal treatment • Malocclusion • Impacted teeth putting pressure on adjacent teeth • Materials like silver nitrate may stimulate resorption	• Genetic disorders • Radiotherapy • Hormonal disorders (hyperthyroidism/hyperparathyroidism) • Kidney/hepatic impairment • Paget's disease • Turner's syndrome • Papillon-Lefèvre syndrome • Vitamin deficiencies, especially vitamin A • Hypertension • Bone dysplasia	• High temperature during tooth preparation • Vital pulp therapy with calcium hydroxide • Irregular eruption of permanent teeth • Acute mechanical injury

Pathogenesis

It is established that cementum and periodontal ligament protect external root surface and predentin protect the internal root surface. Damage to these surfaces allow osteoclasts to bind to the surface of root; and an inflammatory response may stimulate resorption. Persistent stimulation may lead to clinical resorption. It is hypothesized that cementum lacks those proteins found in bone that stimulate osteoclastic activity. It also has inhibiting factors for osteoclastic activity. It is also hypothesized that non-collagenous components in predentin resist internal resorption.

The resorptive process is linked to osteoclasts (large multinucleate cells found within crypts on hard tissue surfaces). Mechanism of hard tissue destruction by osteoclasts involves:

- Dissolution of inorganic hydroxyapatite by acids produced by ruffled border of osteoclasts and enzyme carbonic anhydrase II and acid phosphatase.
- Dissolution of organic matrix containing type 1 collagen by enzymes, such as collagenase and cysteine proteinase.

A significant stimulation is also associated with bacteria. In the presence of bacterial lipopolysaccharides, leukocytes differentiate into osteoclasts. Certain gram-positive species have been demonstrated to stimulate osteoclastic activity through osteoclast differentiation factors.

Odontoclasts, morphologically similar to osteoclasts, (odontoclasts are smaller in size and have fewer nuclei as compared to osteoclasts), resorb the largest tissue in a similar manner. Both cells possess similar enzymatic activity and create resorptive lacunae on the surface of mineralized tissue. Damage to the odontoblastic layer and predentin is a prerequisite for the initiation of internal root resorption. The advancement of internal root resorption depends upon bacterial stimulation of the clastic cells involved in hard tissue response. There might be no resorption without this stimulation. The pulp tissue apical to the resorptive lesion should have viable blood supply to provide clastic cells and their nutrients; whereas, the infected necrotic pulp tissue provide stimulation for these clastic cells.

Classification

Root resorption may be categorized as internal and external, depending upon the location of the resorption. It may also be categorized as inflammatory and replacement, depending upon the initiating factors. Few authors have also categorized root resorption as systemic, inflammatory and idiopathic (Table 27.2).

Table 27.2 Classification of root resorption

Based on process	• Physiological resorption • Pathological resorption
Based on location	• Internal • External/cervical
Based on initiating factor	• Inflammatory • Transient • Progressive • Replacement • Idiopathic

The modified Andreasen classification is given in Table 27.3.

Table 27.3 Andreasen's classification

Internal resorption	*External resorption*
• Internal inflammatory resorption • Internal surface resorption • Internal replacement resorption • Internal transient apical breakdown	• External inflammatory resorption (infection related) • External cervical resorption • External replacement resorption (ankylosis) • External surface resorption • External transient apical breakdown

The classification and terminology as proposed by Andreasen is widely acknowledged; however, many analogous terminologies are also prevalent.

Andreasen terminology	*Analogous terminology*
• Internal inflammatory resorption • Internal surface resorption	• Internal root resorption • Transient surface resorption • Transient inflammatory resorption
• External surface resorption	• Surface resorption
• External inflammatory resorption	• Peripheral inflammatory resorption • Periapical replacement resorption • External root resorption
• External replacement resorption	• Progressive inflammatory resorption • Replacement resorption • Ankyloses • Osseous replacement
• External cervical resorption	• Invasive cervical resorption • Hyperplastic tooth resorption • Odontoclastoma • Sub-epithelial external root resorption

A. EXTERNAL RESORPTION

External resorption involves the lateral/external surface of root, normally covered with cementum and periodontal ligament. The pathological stimulation which disturbs the balance between activities of cementoblasts and osteoclasts, lead to resorption. Minor irritants can cause transient resorption, usually reversible after eliminating the cause; whereas, chronic stimulus lead to external resorption.

Clinically, external root resorption is categorized as:

a. External inflammatory resorption (infection related)
b. External cervical resorption
c. External replacement resorption (ankylosis)
d. External surface resorption
e. External transient apical breakdown

a. External Inflammatory Resorption (Infection Related)

This type of resorption is mainly related to endodontic infection. Bacteria present in root canals and dentinal tubules trigger osteoclastic activity on the root surface. Bacterial toxins, when diffused to periodontal ligament via exposed dentinal tubules stimulate osteoclastic activity, leading to resorption of bone and cementum. Practically all teeth with apical periodontitis will exhibit apical resorption (Fig. 27.3a and b). Clinically, this condition is rarely of concern, since after the root canal treatment the resorption gets resolved or do not progress.

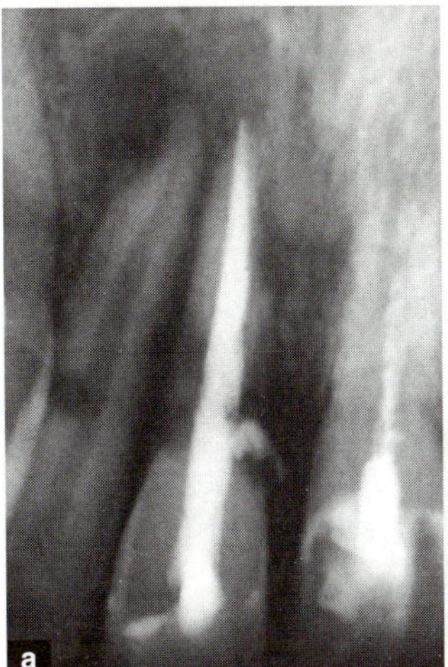

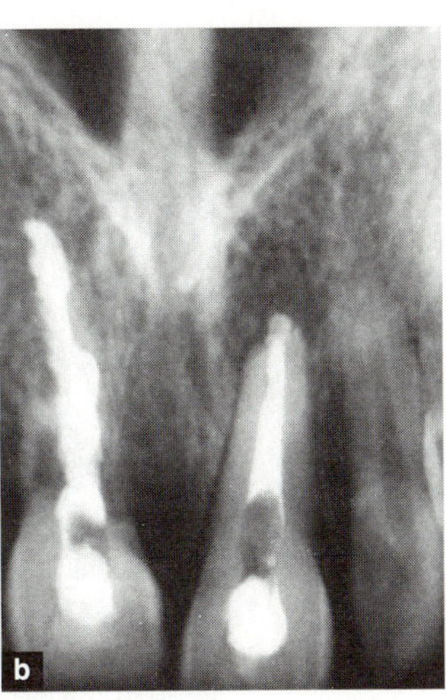

Fig. 27.3a and b External inflammatory resorption

However, in teeth that have suffered displacement injuries, external root resorption may become extensive. Extrusion or intrusion of teeth, as well as the subsequent repositioning procedures, inevitably lead to denuded areas on the root surface, which acts as chemotactic to hard tissue-resorbing cells. Root resorption will then ensue (Fig. 27.4).

Apical root resorption is common in purulent inflammation and cysts and less common in granulomas; whereas, lateral resorption is observed due to infected pulp.

Clinically, such resorption is rapidly progressing and may involve the total surface of roots (Fig. 27.5). The tooth show mobility and may be slightly extruded because of inflamed periodontal ligament. Radiographically, a small radiolucency with ragged, irregular margins is evident.

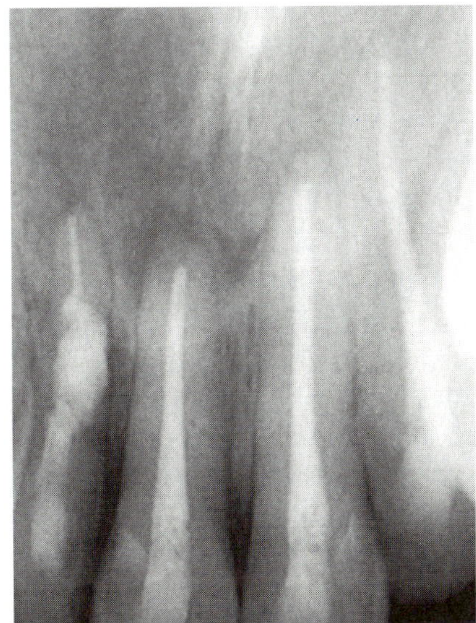

Fig. 27.4 External resorption due to displacement

27

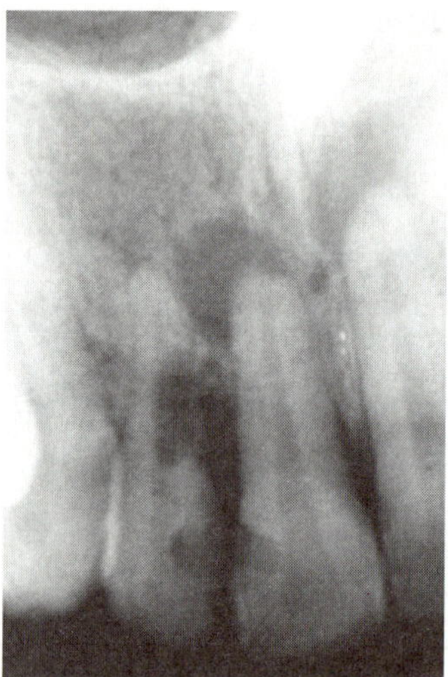

Fig. 27.5 External resorption involving almost total surface

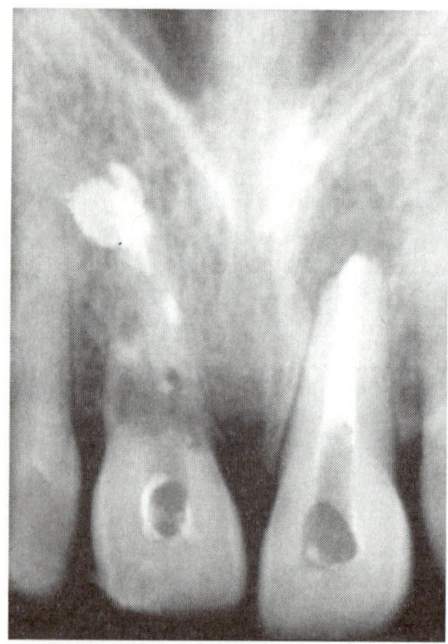

Fig. 27.6 Cervical resorption

The displacement of the teeth may lead to a disruption of the blood vessels at the apical foramina, subsequently ischemic pulp necrosis. Micro-organisms will ingress into the root canal through enamel-dentin cracks and exposed dentinal tubules. At this point in time the root resorption induced by the denuded areas of the root surface may have exposed tubular root dentin. Bacterial products from the infected root canal will then reach the resorptive lacunae on the root surface through the dentinal tubules and sustain the resorption of the root.

Management

Root canal treatment is effective; calcium hydroxide can be used along with obturating materials [combination of calcium hydroxide and calcitonin (hormone) inhibits clastic activities when placed in the root canal].

Acetazolamide, a carbonic anhydrase inhibitor, is also used as intracanal medicament to manage root resorption (both inflammatory and surface resorption). Ledermix paste (combination of antibiotic and steroids) have been effective in controlling external inflammatory root resorption.

b. External Cervical Resorption

Cervical resorption (Fig. 27.6) is a kind of external inflammatory resorption. It is localized resorptive lesion of the cervical area of the root below the epithelial attachment (may not always be in cervical region). Cervical resorption can be associated with vital teeth, a feature which distinguishes it from external inflammatory resorption (infection is prerequisite). It is seen clinically and radiographically as a single resorption lacuna in the cervical area of the tooth. It appears to follow injury to the cervical attachment apparatus, most importantly to an area of the cervical root surface (precementum) below the epithelial attachment. The damaged area of the root surface is then colonized by hard tissue-resorbing cells. Predisposing factors may include trauma, periodontal treatment, intracoronal bleaching and associated factors as bruxism, developmental defects, etc.

Classifying external cervical resorption defects into four classes, Heithersay (1999) opined that careful case selection is mandatory for achieving successful outcome. The classification (Fig. 27.7) is as follows:

Class 1: A small invasive resorptive lesion near the cervical area with shallow penetration into dentin.

Class 2: A well-defined invasive resorptive lesion that has penetrated close to the coronal pulp chamber, but shows little or no extension into the radicular dentin.

Class 3: A deeper invasion of dentin by resorbing tissue, not only involving the coronal dentin, but also extending into the coronal third of the root.

Class 4: A large invasive resorptive process that has extended beyond the coronal third of the root.

The classification is useful for assessing the extent of cervical resorptive defects; however, classification detects lesions on proximal sides only. The lesions on labial/lingual sides are challenging. CBCT can be effective in evaluating these lesions.

Management

Mostly the cervical resorption defects are transient, which means, the cementum repair may occur within two to three weeks without any treatment. Treatment, if necessary, will depend upon severity, location and whether the defect has perforated the root canal system. Mainly, the treatment involves removal of resorptive

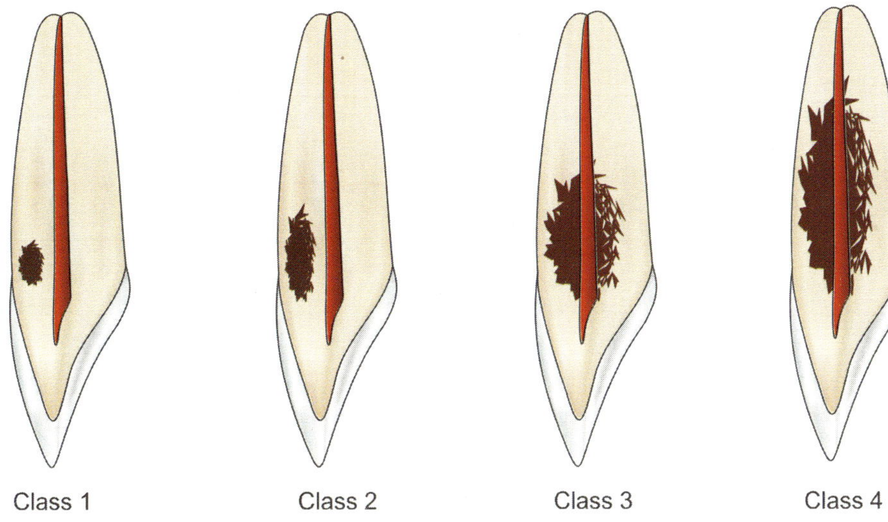

Fig. 27.7 Heithersay classification

lesion and restoring the resultant defect with appropriate filling materials. The objective of the treatment is to arrest resorptive process, restore damaged root surface and improve esthetics of the tooth.

The treatment protocol involves:

- Smaller lesions (classes 1 and 2) where pulp is not involved, can be treated by raising the flap and excavating the defect with appropriate instruments. The defect can be filled with glass-ionomer cement and composite resin.

  Heithersay recommended use of topical application of 90% trichloroacetic acid after curettage of chronic resorptive defect, which contains fibro-osseous tissue (trichloroacetic acid results in coagulation necrosis of the defect without damaging the adjacent periodontal tissues). Other solutions, such as 3.0% sodium hypochlorite and 17% EDTA have also been used.
- Orthodontic extrusion is required in some cases where defect is undermined.
- Root canal treatment may be required in case of class 3 and class 4 defects or any lesion approaching pulp tissue.
- Biodentine can be filled up to occlusal plane, as three-dimensional obturation (MTA has also been tried).
- A few authors have suggested dressing of root canals with calcitonin to prevent further progression of resorption [calcitonin, a hormone synthesized by the thyroid gland (potent inhibitor of clastic cells), inhibits osteoclastic activity and also suppress inflammation].
- Combination of calcitonin and calcium hydroxide as intracanal medicament effectively controls inflammatory root resorption.
- Surgical approach may be necessary in some cases to access resorption area and removal of granulomatous tissue.

The clinical and radiological signs of external cervical resorption are summarized in Table 27.4.

It is important to differentiate external cervical resorption and subgingival caries (Table 27.5).

Table 27.4 Clinical and radiological signs of external cervical resorption

Clinical signs	*Radiological signs*
• Cervical area of the tooth is involved • Tooth is generally vital (pulp involvement in advanced cases) • Clinically pink tooth or pink spot is recognized • Cavity margins are thin and sharp • May bleed on probing	• Irregular radiolucency with irregular cervical/proximal margins • Advanced lesions may show mottled appearance because of fiber-osseous deposition • Intact root canal(s) visible • Detected accidentally by radiographs

Table 27.5 Differences between external cervical resorption and subgingival caries

External cervical resorption	*Subgingival caries*
• Present with pink spot	• No such spot
• The base will feel hard; scraping sound on probing	• Sticky on probing
• Probing will lead to profuse bleeding (underlying highly vascular tissue)	• No such bleeding
• Positive to pulp testing	• May not be positive (depend upon extent of lesion)
• Cavity has sharp edges	• Irregular edges

External cervical resorption should also be differentiated from cervical burnout, which usually appears as a radiolucent band across the entire neck of the tooth. Three-dimensional imaging with CBCT help assessing the nature of the lesion.

c. External Replacement Resorption (Ankylosis)

External replacement resorption is the process of replacement of root surface with bone, termed as 'ankylosis'. It is not a result of a disease process, but occurs as a 'mistake' because the cells involved in the remodeling of bone are not able to distinguish between the dental tissues and bone (common occurrence is young people, 8–16 years).

The damage to the innermost layer of the periodontal ligament initiates competitive healing. Healing from the socket wall (bone marrow-derived cells) and healing from adjacent periodontal ligament (cementum and Sharpey's fibers) occur simultaneously. If less than 20% of the root surface is involved, a transient ankylosis may occur, which can be resorbed due to functional stimuli, provided the tooth in that period is stabilized with a splint (transient replacement resorption) (Fig. 27.8). In larger injuries, where 40% or more root is involved, a permanent ankylosis is created (progressive replacement resorption) (Fig. 27.9). The tooth thus becomes an integral part of the bone remodeling system; the resorbing cells remain the osteoclasts. Subsequently, osteoblasts replace the resorbed areas of the root with bone.

Bony trabeculae develop within the periodontal ligament space and fuse to the root surface.

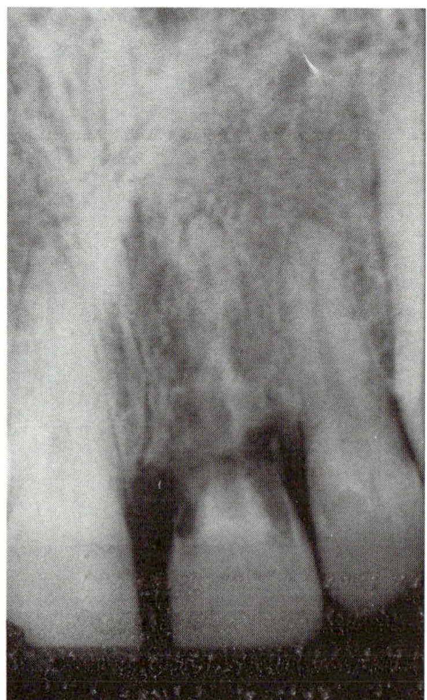

Fig. 27.8 Transient replacement resorption

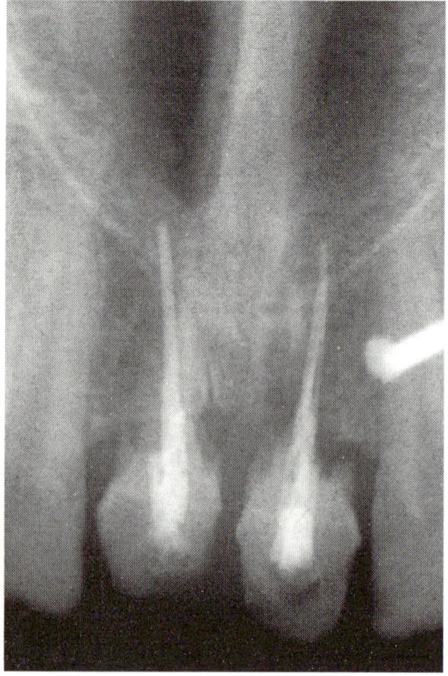

Fig. 27.9 Progressive replacement resorption

Clinically, the tooth is immobile, and exhibits a high percussive tone. Radiographically, the periodontal ligament space is absent, and a direct union is seen between alveolar bone and the root. Total loss of cementum and dentin has been seen in few cases, especially after replantation (Fig. 27.10). Infraocclusion relative to adjacent teeth can be evident both clinically and radiographically (ankylosis prevents physiological mesial movement of teeth inhibiting the local growth of alveolar bone, which is sinking into the surrounding alveolar ridge).

Concurrent internal and external root resorption has also been reported (Fig. 27.11a and b).

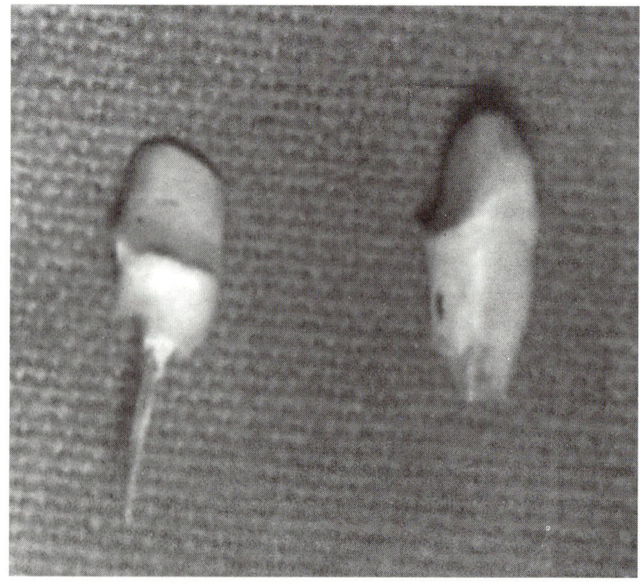

Fig. 27.10 Total loss of cementum

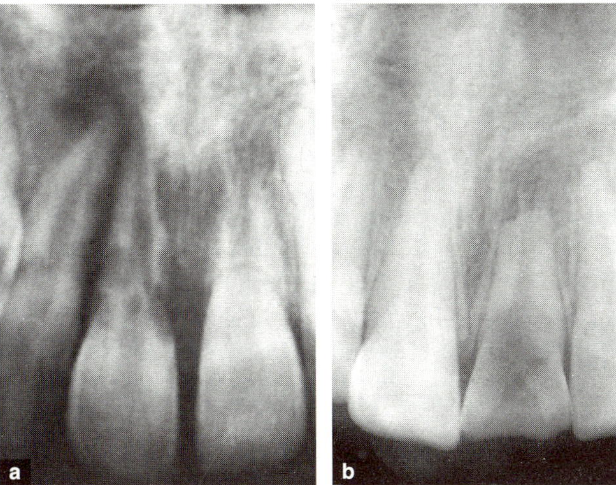

Fig. 27.11a and b Concurrent external and internal resorption

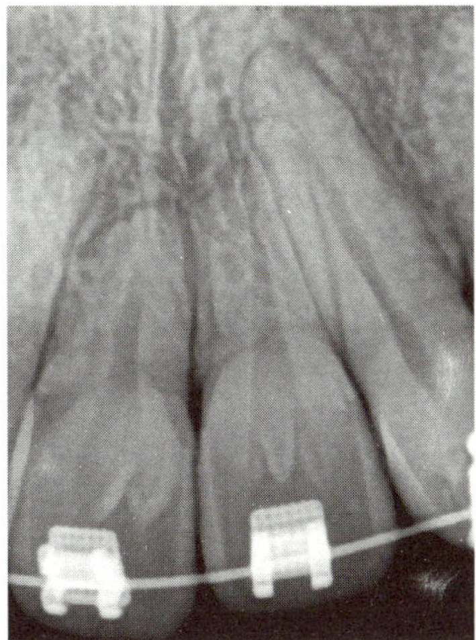

Fig. 27.12 External resorption due to orthodontic pressure

Management

While appropriate endodontic therapy is effective in the treatment of external inflammatory resorption, replacement resorption cannot be arrested or repaired. Fluoride solution (1.0% stannous fluoride and 2.0% sodium fluoride) effectively decrease replacement resorption and ankylosis.

Ascorbic acid (vitamin C) is effective when applied in replanted teeth (stimulate osteogenesis by the activation of alkaline phosphatase, increasing functional activity of osteoblasts). Citric acid and phosphoric acid, used earlier, were not effective in controlling resorption.

It is hypothesized that in young patient decrowning is carried out, stimulating the growth of alveolar bone for future implant prosthesis. Even in replanted teeth, a layer of fluoride over the roots delays the process of ankylosis.

Emdogain, an enamel matrix derivation, has been successfully employed to restore periodontal ligament, cementum and alveolar bone in patients with severe attachment loss (usual phenomenon in replanted teeth). Conditioning of roots with amelogenin (the enamel protein) in replanted/avulsed teeth stimulates regeneration of tooth attachment apparatus. It is recommended to take anti-inflammatory drugs to suppress ankylosis.

d. External Surface Resorption

External surface resorption is mainly because of chronic mechanical injuries or as a result of continuous pressure of the impacted teeth, expanding cysts/tumors and abnormal occlusal contacts. Orthodontic forces also affect such resorption (Fig. 27.12).

The location and extent of the defect depends upon the direction, time of action and the amplitude of the force applied. Radiographically, the periodontal ligament space may be missing; a cavity like depression can be seen at the site of pressure.

Treatment involves eliminating the cause of the treatment and rehabilitating the defect with appropriate filling material. Rarely, root canal treatment is warranted.

e. External Transient Apical Breakdown

Orthodontic application of force over a period of time may lead to biological changes in periodontal ligament. Root resorption associated with orthodontic movement pressure frequently occur in maxillary anterior teeth (Fig. 27.12).

Transient apical breakdown, a type of root resorption, is considered as a temporary process in which apex of a tooth exhibit evidence of resorption radiographically because of orthodontic forces. The teeth respond normally to pulp tests; radiographically blunting of root apices and widening of periodontal ligament may be seen. The affected tooth may also display color changes (Fig. 27.13a and b).

Genetic factors have also been related to such resorption; with many genes such as IL-1B and TNFRSF 11A contributing to the problem.

No treatment is recommended for transient apical breakdown; the root apex and the surrounding tissues returns to normal within one year after the removal of the forces applied. This type of resorption is to be distinguished from periapical replacement resorption without ankylosis (apex of the tooth is involved and do not heal after removal of the cause).

External Root Resorption of Non-dental Origin

Various types of cysts and tumors of the jaws, not of dental origin, may present signs of external root resorption. The cysts/tumors causing external root 27

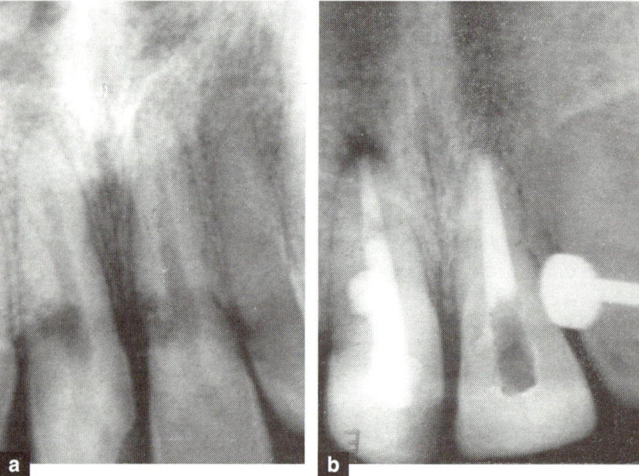

Fig. 27.13a and b Transient apical breakdown

resorption includes chondrosarcoma, ossifying fibroma, giant cell reparative granuloma, etc. Such lesions should be diagnosed prior to initiating any treatment for root resorption. Unnecessary dental treatment should be avoided and the appropriate surgical/medical treatment be provided to the patient.

Systemic disorders may also lead to root resorption, though the frequency is less. Many systemic abnormalities have been associated with root resorption, such as hormonal imbalances, hyperparathyroidism, liver and renal diseases, Papillon-Lefèvre syndrome, osteogenesis imperfecta, etc. These diseases may be diagnosed using blood chemistry tests, Weise analysis, etc. and should be treated accordingly.

Alendronate is being used to inhibit pathologic osteoclastic-mediated root resorption in systemic diseases (Paget's disease, osteoporosis and osteoclastic malignancies of bone). A few authors observed that Alendronate limited the root resorption, but could not impair its occurrence.

B. INTERNAL RESORPTION

Internal resorption involves root dentin and cementum from within the root canal. It can be apical or intraradicular. Radiologically, a small radiolucent area is seen around the pulp spaces. Internal resorption mainly affects incisors and mandibular molars. Radiographs are mandatory for diagnosing internal resorption. However, sometimes it may manifest clinically as *'pink spot'* when resorption progresses to an extent that the vascular pulpal tissue is seen through the overlying thinned dental hard tissues. Also, during pulp extirpation if excessive bleeding occurs clinically, internal resorption should be suspected.

The vascular changes in the pulp subsequent to trauma, orthodontic tooth movement, chronic pulpitis, direct and indirect pulp capping and pulpotomy may lead to internal resorption. Circulatory changes produce active hyperemia which increase local oxygen tension, thereby lowering the pH. These collectively alter the metabolism of the pulp. Vascular changes attract numerous macrophages which eventually differentiate into osteoclasts. Multinucleated giant cells are also described in lacunae next to polymorphonuclear neutrophils. Finally, the connective tissue may undergo metaplasia and be changed to granulation tissue.

Clinically, internal resorption is categorized as:

a. Internal inflammatory resorption
b. Internal surface resorption
c. Internal replacement resorption
d. Internal transient apical breakdown

a. Internal Inflammatory Resorption

Internal inflammatory resorption, also known as 'Radial pulp enlargement resorption', is characterized by ovoid or fusiform enlargement of root canal; expansion mainly on lateral side. The pulp is chronically inflamed (bacteria may enter pulp tissue via dentinal tubules or cracks in the cervical root) (Fig. 27.14a and b). Internal inflammatory resorption is usually asymptomatic and discovered through routine radiographic examination. In rare cases, the resorption may perforate lateral root surface and appear similar to external resorption. The process is analogous to external inflammatory resorption.

b. Internal Surface Resorption

Internal surface resorption, also referred to as 'Transient root resorption' (Fig. 27.15), occurs frequently in traumatized teeth and in teeth that have undergone orthodontic and periodontal treatment, but is also seen in other teeth, apparently as a result of wear and tear.

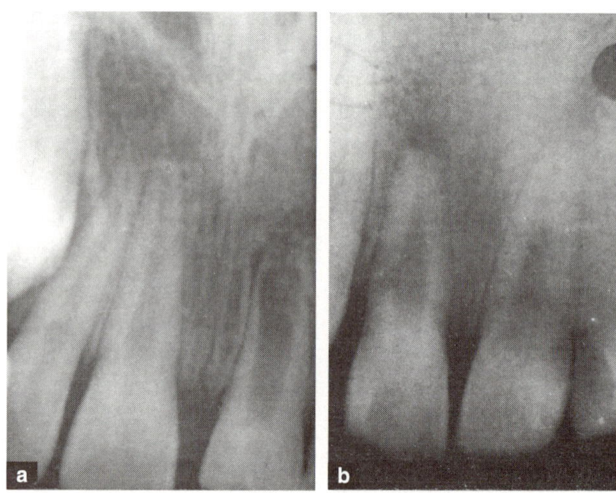

Fig. 27.14a and b Internal resorption

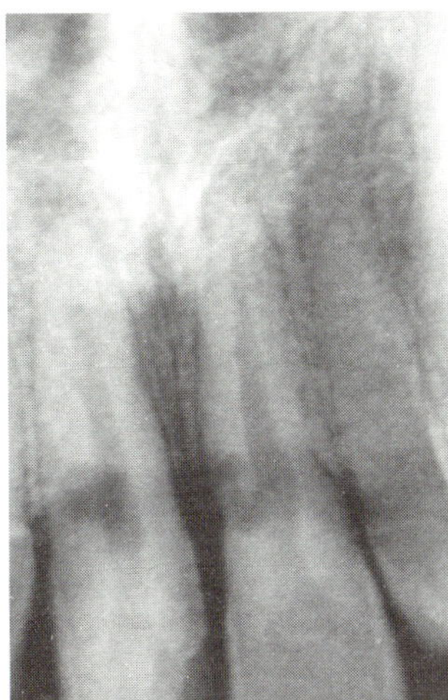

Fig. 27.15 Transient root resorption

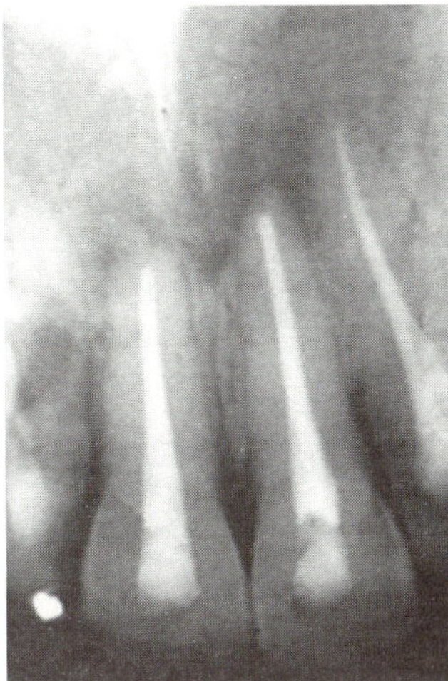

Fig. 27.16 Transient apical breakdown

Mineralized or denuded areas of the root surface will attract hard tissue-resorbing cells that will colonize the damaged areas of the root. However, resorbing cells require continuous stimulation during phagocytosis and stimulation by a denuded dentin or cementum surface appears to be insufficient to sustain the resorptive process for more than 2–3 weeks. A phagocytic colonization of denuded areas of the root, therefore, will be transient without additional stimulation of the cells, and repair with formation of a cementum-like tissue will occur both in the root canal and on the root surface.

Transient root resorption as such is without clinical importance and the resorption defects are usually too small to even be detected radiographically.

c. Internal Replacement Resorption

Internal replacement resorption is very rare; may occur along with external replacement resorption. The canal spaces may be obliterated with cancellous-like bony tissue. It is hypothesized that dental pulp cells produce osteoid material as a result of reparative mechanism. A few authors have proposed that cells are non-pulpal in origin and have migrated into pulp from periapical tissues.

d. Internal Transient Apical Breakdown

The process of internal transient breakdown is analogous to external transient breakdown. The apical resorption is caused by orthodontic forces; no treatment is recommended, because the resorption gets healed once the orthodontic force is removed (Fig. 27.16).

Management

In case where the root canal is perforated, mineral trioxide aggregate (MTA) should be considered the material of choice to seal the perforation. Biodentine has also been tried along with thermoplasticized gutta-percha in case of perforation in internal resorption. A few authors advocate hybrid obturation, whereby apical area is filled with gutta-percha and the resorbed area and below is filled with MTA or Biodentine.

Prompt endodontic treatment is imperative in all diagnosed cases of internal root resorption. Calcium hydroxide is preferred as sealer along with gutta-percha. Calcium hydroxide reduces the inflammatory response and initiates prompt healing (because of its higher pH, it neutralizes the lactic acid produced from macrophages and osteoclasts). It arrests the osteoclastic activity and stimulates repair. Success depends upon filling the canal as well as the resorptive defects. As long as no communication exists with oral fluids (no perforation of root canal wall) and the site is covered with epithelial attachment, calcium hydroxide treatment is quite successful. However, in case of perforation, the treatment of choice is surgery, and filling the defect with appropriate filling material.

The distinguishing features of external and internal resorption are summarized in Table 27.6.

The management (treatment) protocol of resorption is summarized in Table 27.7.

Internal Root Resorption of Non-dental Origin

Root resorption of non-dental origin is important, since these type of resorption need medical therapy; whereas, conventional endodontic treatment is effective in resorption of dental origin.

Internal resorption caused by herpes zoster infection is a common occurrence. Herpes zoster (varicella-zoster virus) may impact the trigeminal nerve and subsequently dental tissues are involved. Oral complications involve devitalization of teeth along with

Table 27.6 Distinguishing features of external resorption and internal resorption

External resorption	*Internal resorption*
• May occur at any surface of root; distribution is not symmetrical	• Mainly within the root surface; distribution is symmetrical
• Ragged/rough margins on the side of defect	• Well-demarcated margins; ballooning of root canals
• Radiodensity varies	• Radiodensity uniform
• Resorption of bone along with root surface	• Resorption confined to root
• Normal root canal shape	• Shape of root canal distorted
• No pink spot	• Pink spot is a usual sign
• The defect moves away from the canal as the angulation of radiograph changes	• The defect remain close to canal, even if angulation of radiograph changes

Table 27.7 Management protocol of resorption

Type of resorption	*Surface(s) involved*	*Management*
Inflammatory resorption (infection related)	Internal	Root canal treatment with calcium hydroxide dressing before placement of root filling. MTA can be filled into the resorption site.
	External	Root canal treatment with intracanal medication with Ledermix paste or calcium hydroxide. Once resorption is controlled, root canal can be filled.
	Concurrent	Root canal treatment with intracanal medication as above.
Surface resorption (trauma/pressure)	Internal	Monitor radiographically, endodontic treatment only if signs of infection or discolouration.
	External	Remove cause (unerupted cuspid, impacted tooth, orthodontic force, cysts etc.). In severe cases (e.g. immature tooth in infraocclusion), surgically reposition and treat root surface with Emdogain, or decoronate and submerge for future implant therapy.
Replacement (hyperplastic) resorption	Internal	If pulp involvement, pulpectomy and root filling after intracanal dressing with Ledermix paste. Orthodontic extrusion if necessary.
	External (cervical)	Classes 1, 2: Topical application of 90% trichloracetic acid, curettage and glass ionomer cement restoration. Class 3: Topical application of 90% trichloracetic acid to resorptive tissue, curettage, intracanal dressings with Ledermix. Class 4: Resorptive area filled with MTA/Biodentine and monitor; extraction and implant placement, if not responding. Surgical intervention may be required in some cases.
Idiopathic	Internal/external	Conventional root canal treatment with calcium hydroxide as intracanal medication.

external/internal resorption. Herpes zoster infection is suspected when unexplained dental pain and root resorption occur in multiple adjacent teeth on one side of the dental arch.

Conventional root canal therapy is effective along with antiviral medication to control further progress of neuralgia.

C. IDIOPATHIC ROOT RESORPTION

27 Idiopathic root resorption of a single or multiple teeth is common in literature. The causative factors may not be same as for inflammatory or other types of resorptions. It is assumed that the excessive occlusal loading may result in dystrophic changes in the periodontium.

External cervical resorption may affect multiple teeth, described as *'multiple idiopathic cervical resorption'* (MICR). MICR affects number of teeth (minimum three). Such lesions are usually asymptomatic. A few authors have linked this resorption to feline herpes virus 1, though not documented.

Osteosclerotic areas that do not seem to be associated with infection and/or inflammation are frequently observed on radiographs. These might be part of the reparative process or a compensatory response of unknown cause. There may not be any family history or any medical/dental ailment which can be considered as a possible cause for this type of resorption.

Kjaer et al (2012) have reported couple of cases of idiopathic root resorption occurring regionally. The authors linked this type of resorption to virus spreading along nerve path (the resorption process stopped at the area, which might be innervated differently and not infected with virus). They emphasized that neural pattern is important for diagnosis and also for predicting the course of such root resorption.

Management

There may not be any definite treatment for such teeth; however, endodontic treatment is beneficial. The teeth treated with calcium hydroxide and conventional root canal treatment exhibited evidence of healing.

BIBLIOGRAPHY

1. Bergmans L, Cleynenbreugel J, Van Meerbeek, B and Lambrechts P. Cervical external root resorption in vital teeth. X-ray microfocus-tomographical and histopathological case study. J. Clin. Periodontol.: 2002; 29:580–585.
2. Consolaro A. The concept of root resorptions or root resorptions are not multifactorial, complex, controversial or polemical. Dent. Press J. Orthodont.: 2011; 16:1–5.
3. Darcey J and Qualtrough A. Resorption: Part 1. Pathology, classification and etiology. Br. Dent. J.: 2013; 214:439–451.
4. Finucane D and Kinirons MJ. External inflammatory and replacement resorption of luxated and avulsed replanted permanent incisors: a review and case presentation. Dent. Traumatol.: 2003; 19:170–174.
5. Fishcher WG and Guggenheine J. Concurrent internal and external resorption. Oral Surg Oral Med Oral Pathol.: 1977; 43:161.
6. Fuss, Tsesis I and Lin S. Root resorption—diagnosis, classification and treatment choices based on stimulation factors. Dent. Traumatol.: 2003; 19:175–182.
7. Gonzalez OL, Vera J, Orozco MS, Mancera JT, Gonzalez KV and Malagon GV. Transient apical breakdown and its relationship with orthodontic forces: a case report. J. Endod.: 2014; 40:1265–1267.
8. Goultschn J, Nitzan D and Azaz B. Root resorption: review and discussion. Oral Surg. Oral Med. Oral Pathol.: 1982; 54:586–591.
9. Gunraj MN. Dental root resorption. Oral Surg. Oral Med. Oral Pathol. Oral Radiol.: 1999; 88:647–653.
10. Haapasalo M and Endal U. Internal inflammatory root resorption: the unknown resorption of the tooth. Endod. Topics: 2006; 14:60–79.
11. Harokopakis-Hajishengallis E. Physiologic root resorption in primary teeth: molecular and histological events. J. Oral Sci.: 2007; 49:1–12.
12. Heithersay GS. Invasive cervical resorption. Endodontic Topics: 2004; 7:73–92.
13. Heithersay GS. Management of tooth resorption. Aust. Dent. J.: 2007; 52:S105–S121.
14. Herrera H. Treatment of external inflammatory root resorption after autogenous tooth transplantation: a case report. O. Surg. O. Med. O. Pathol.: 2006; 102:e51–e54.
15. Jacobovitz M and Lima RKP. Treatment of inflammatory internal root resorption with mineral trioxide aggregate: a case report. Int. Endod. J.: 2008; 41:905–912.
16. Kaiwar A, Ranjini, MA, Pasha, MF and Meena, N. Internal resorption managed by root canal treatment: Incorporation of CT with 3D reconstruction in diagnosis and monitoring of the disease. J. Int. Oral Health: 2010; 2:86.
17. Kjaer I, Strom C and Worsaae N. Regional aggressive root resorption caused by neuronal virus infection. Case Report in Dent.: 2012; Art. ID 693240.
18. Krishna R, Ali SN, Pannu D, Peacock ME and Bercowski DL. An orderly review of dental root resorption. Int. J. Med. Dent. Sci.: 2005; 4:669–673.
19. Lad N, Hosey, MT and Hunter KD. Localized idiopathic internal resorption in primary dentition. J. Clin. Pediatr. Dent.: 2010; 34:339–341.
20. Maini A, Durning P and Drage N. Resorption: within or without? The benefit of cone-beam computed tomography when diagnosing a case of an internal/external resorption defect. Br. Dent. J.: 2008; 204:135–137.
21. Mohammadi Z, Cehreli ZC, Shalavi S, Giardino L, Palazzi F and Asgary S. Management of root resorption using chemical agents : a review. Iran Endod. J.: 2016; 11:1–7.
22. Ne RF, Witherspoon DE and Gutmann JL. Tooth resorption. Quint. Int.: 1999; 30:9–25.
23. Nilsson E, Bonte E, Bayet F and Lasfargues JJ. Management of internal root resorption on permanent teeth. Int. J. Dent.: 2013; Art. ID 929486.
24. Panzarini SR, Gulinelli JL, Poi WR, Sonoda CK, Pedrini D and Brandini DA. Treatment of root surface in delayed tooth replantation: a review of literature. Dent. Traumatol.: 2008; 24:277–282.
25. Patel S and Pitt Ford TR. Is the resorption external or internal? Dent. Update: 2010; 34:218–229.
26. Patel S, Kanagasingham S and Pitt Ford T. External cervical resorption: a review. J. Endod.: 2009; 35:616–625.
27. Patel S, Ricucci D and Tay F. Internal Root Resorption: A Review. J. Endod.: 2010; 36:1107–1121.
28. Rajasekharan S, Martens LC, Cauwels RG and Verbeeck RM. Biodentine material characteristics and clinical applications: a review of the literature. Eur. Arch. Paediatr. Dent.: 2014; 15:147–158.
29. Re D, Ceci C, Cerutti F, Del Fabbro M, Corbella S and Taschieri S. Natural tooth preservation versus extraction and implant placement: patient preferences and analysis of the willingness to pay. Br. Dent. J.: 2017; 222:467–471.

30. Sak M, Radecka M, Karpinski TM, Wedrychowicz-Welman A and Szkaradkiewicz AK. Tooth root resorption: etiopathogenis and classification. MicroMedicine: 2016; 4:21–31.
31. Samir PV, Dhull KS, Dutta B, Bachi A and Verma T. Invasive cervical resorption: An insidious form of external root resorption. IOSR J. Dent. Med. Sci.:2017; 16:24–32.
32. Santos BO, Mendonca DS, de Sousa DL, Neto JJ and Araujo RB. Root resorption after dental traumas: classification and clinical, radiographic and histologic aspects. RSBO: 2011; 8:439–445.
33. Sikri VK. Root resorption—An enigma. IJCDC: 2011; 1:11–15.
34. Sogur E, Sogur HK, Baksi BG and Sen BH. Idiopathic root resorption of the entire permanent dentition: systemic review and report of a case. Dent. Traumatol.: 2008; 24:490–495.
35. Solzano S and Tirone F. Mini-invasive non-surgical treatment of class 4 invasive cervical resorption: a case series. Giornale Italiano di Endodonzia: 2016; 30:52–63.
36. Stamos DE and Stamos DG. A new treatment modality for internal resorption. J. Endod.: 1986; 12:315–319.
37. Thomas P, Pillai RK, Ramakrishnan BP and Palani J. An insight into internal resorption. ISRN Dent.: 2014; Art. ID 759326.
38. Tronstad L. Root resorption—etiology, terminology and clinical manifestations. Endod. Dent. Traumatol.: 1988; 4: 241–252.
39. Umashetty G, Hoshing U, Patil S and Ajgaonkar N. Management of inflammatory internal root resorption with biodentine and thermoplasticised gutta-percha. Case Report in Dent.: 2015; Art. ID 452609.
40. Vatanpour M, Javidi M, Zarel M and Shirazian S. External root resorption: Arrested or progressing?. Int. Endod. J.: 2008; 41:997–1004.
41. Vier FV and Figueiredo JA. Internal apical resorption and its correlation with the type of apical lesion. Int. Endod. J.: 2004; 37:730–737.

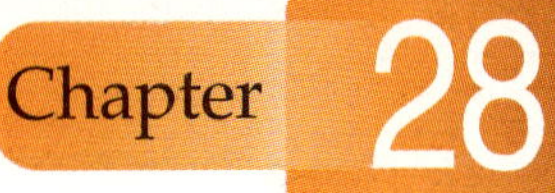

Chapter 28 Pediatric Endodontics

The importance of retaining deciduous teeth in the long-term prognosis of maintaining the arch is gaining significance over the years. The root canal treatment in primary teeth is to be planned keeping in mind the remaining teeth, age of the child and also the probable effects of early extraction.

Extensive dental decay in the primary dentition, that easily progresses to the dental pulp (dentin thinner than permanent teeth), remains a serious problem in pediatric dental practice. The first treatment decision for the young patient with one or more grossly carious primary teeth is whether to retain or to extract. Root canal treatment is the treatment of choice to retain them; however, it should be carried out after evaluating patient's existing dentition (age and strategic importance of developing teeth) and also the associated clinical implications. The basic aims and treatment protocol of endodontic therapy in children are the same as those in adults; however, certain areas need special consideration in deciduous and young permanent teeth.

DIFFERENCES IN PRIMARY AND PERMANENT TEETH

a. Difference in Morphology

- The primary teeth are smaller in dimensions than their permanent counterparts. Their crowns are wider mesiodistally than cervico-occlusal length (key feature during access opening).
- The enamel in primary teeth is thinner with consistent depth. The thickness of dentin between the pulp chambers and enamel in primary teeth is less. Primary molars have larger pulp chambers with higher pulp horns, especially the mesial. The advancing carious lesions may involve pulp of primary teeth far earlier than permanent teeth.
- The primary teeth have thin pulpal floor as compared to permanent teeth (periradicular lesions associated with infected primary molars are usually inter-radicular rather than periapical as in permanent teeth, due to the presence of accessory canals in the thin floor of the pulp chamber).
- The crowns of anterior primary teeth have prominent facial and lingual cervical thirds of crown.
- The primary teeth exhibit marked constriction at cementum-enamel junction (cervical portion of crown); the area susceptible to perforate.

b. Differences in Root Formation

- Primary teeth have characteristic ribbon-like radicular pulp, i.e. narrower and longer roots as compared to permanent teeth. In addition, their root-to-crown length is greater than permanent.
- Molar roots flare out from cervix to the apex to accommodate permanent tooth crowns (care to be taken while cleaning and shaping).
- In permanent teeth, root length is not completed until 1–4 years after a tooth erupts into oral cavity; whereas, in primary teeth it is completed in a short period of time because of shorter length of the primary roots.
- Root resorption and deposition of additional dentin within the root canal system may change number, size and shape of the root canals within the primary tooth.
- The primary tooth root will begin to resorb as soon as the root length is completed. The resorption continually changes the position of the apical foramen; no such phenomena in permanent teeth (care to be taken while cleaning, shaping and obturation).

c. Differences in Root Canals

- The root canals of anterior primary teeth are relatively simple, have few irregularities, and can be easily managed; whereas, the posterior primary teeth may have ramifications and deltas between canals, making debridement difficult and subsequently success of the treatment.

- The maxillary primary molars may have two to five canals, with the palatal root usually rounder and longer than the two buccal roots. The primary mandibular first and second molars usually have three canals which generally correspond to the external root canal anatomy.

  The general features of deciduous tooth are depicted in Fig. 28.1.

Variations in Root and Root Canal Morphology of Deciduous Teeth

The root and root canal morphology of deciduous teeth, especially molars show wide anatomical variations (aberrant internal anatomy might be attributed to secondary dentin formation and physiologic root resorption, which are able to reconfigure the root canal system).

- Two rooted maxillary first molars have been reported in approximately 50% cases.
- Two rooted second maxillary molars have been observed to be 10%.
- Mandibular first molars are mostly two rooted.
- Mandibular second molars may be three-rooted in 30% cases.
- Maxillary first molar usually exhibit one canal in one root; 10% cases may have two root canals in mesiobuccal root (five and six root canals in three roots have also been reported).
- Number of root canals in maxillary second molar are usually similar to first molar.
- Mostly mandibular first and second molars exhibit canals in two roots (four and five canals have also been reported).
- Radix entomolaris is also seen in deciduous first molar (Fig. 28.2a).

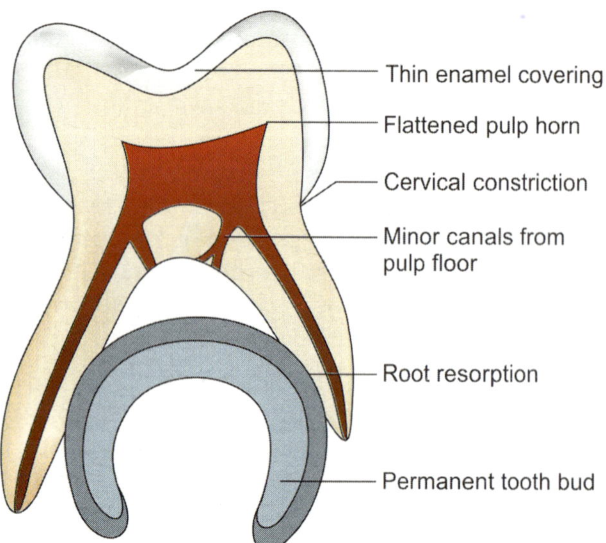

Fig. 28.1 Features of deciduous tooth

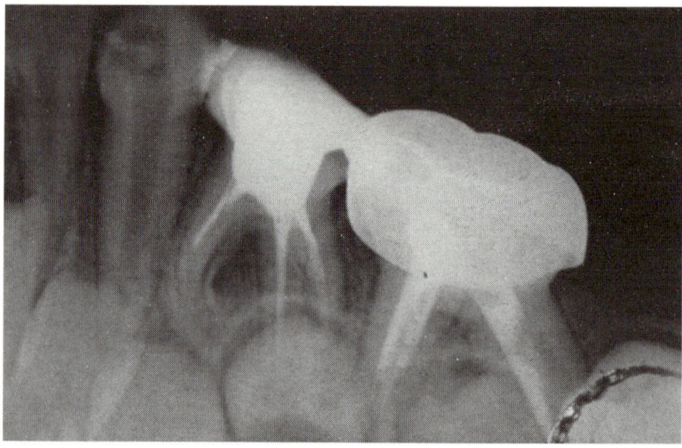

Fig. 28.2a Radix entomolaris

- Usually maxillary molars present ovoid-shaped canal; whereas, mandibular molars may present with ovoid-shaped and ribbon-shaped canal outlines (75% molars have consistent cross-sectional root canal outline from cervical to apical area).
- Three canals in maxillary canine (Fig. 28.2b to e); a less documented case.
- The complex pulp and periodontal tissues interrelationship in primary molars may result in appearance of radiolucency anywhere along the root or in the furcation area.

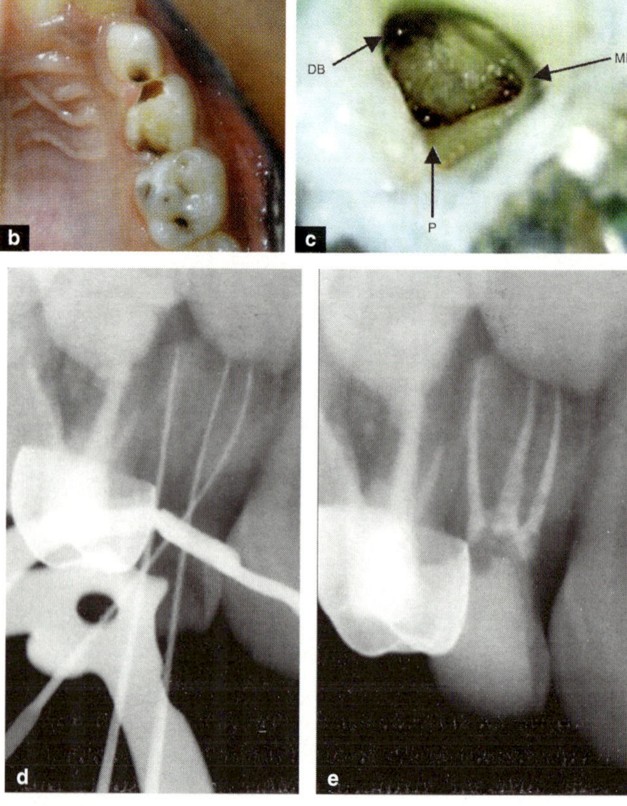

Fig. 28.2b to e Primary maxillary canine (three root canals)

- Radicular resorption of the deciduous tooth may create pulpal-periodontal communications in areas other than the apical foramen.

Rimondini and Baroni (1995) studied 80 primary molars in children 4 to 12 years old, 75 of which were extracted because of pulpal involvement. The teeth were measured and the apices and areas of resorption were located.

They observed as follows:

- Roots that were longer than 10 mm were related to a curved root shape with no external resorption.
- Roots with length between 4.0 mm and 7.0 mm were associated with advanced root resorption.
- Roots that were shorter than 4.0 mm were associated with resorption and perforation at the furcation.

The authors were of the view that resorption up to 4.0 mm length of a root can be successfully treated.

DIAGNOSIS

Diagnosis of pulp involvement in deciduous teeth as well as in young permanent teeth present difficulties due to rapid spread of inflammation in the coronal and radicular pulp. Early stages may not indicate the extent of tissue damage; even pain is felt when periradicular tissues are involved.

The clinical diagnosis may be derived from the following.

a. *Medical and dental history*

Children usually do not give accurate details of their symptoms; parents should be involved in noting the history. Systemic illness is not usually a contra-indication for root canal therapy in primary teeth, except in severe cases like congenital heart disease. Root canal therapy is the treatment of choice in hemophiliacs. Pre-treatment and post-treatment antibiotic coverage is indicated for most of the systemic conditions. The past dental treatment, including current symptoms coupled with chief complaints should be noted and evaluated before proceeding to endodontic treatment.

b. *Clinical examination*

A careful extraoral and intraoral examination will present an overview of the general conditions of teeth and the surrounding tissues. Palpation and percussion are considered helpful diagnostic tools; however, they are not reliable in children due to the psychologic aspects.

c. *Radiographs*

Radiographs are essential prior to the commencement of treatment, though it may not provide adequate information of early pathological changes. Radiographs help us evaluate the condition of the pulp chamber and the root canals, the status of the furcal area, periapical area and the surrounding bone. Intraoral radiographs are usually not possible due to poor cooperation of the children; alternative methods can be preferred.

Interpretation of radiographs is usually complicated in children. The superimposition of the furcation of the maxillary molars on the palatal root makes accurate reading difficult in maxillary molars. In addition, young permanent teeth with incompletely formed roots also pose a problem. The factors which complicate the interpretation of radiographs are, large bone narrow spaces, superimposition of developing tooth buds and normal resorption of deciduous roots.

d. *Pulp vitality tests*

Pulp testing in children is usually unreliable because children usually do not cooperate. The incomplete innervations of newly erupted teeth may also affect the results. In addition, each test is subjective that depends on patient's perceived response to a stimulus as well as the operator's interpretation. The validity of children's response in pulp vitality testing has always been questioned (may elicit false positive or false negative results).

i. *Traditional methods*: The traditional methods of pulp vitality testing like electric pulp test, thermal pulp test, anesthetic test, preparing a test cavity, etc. are based on stimulation of nerve fibers and may not be accurate. The use of traditional tests help establish an empirical diagnosis; may not be accurate and reliable.
ii. *Newer tests*: The blood circulation is considered as the accurate way of assessing pulp vitality. The blood supply of the pulp is evaluated through light absorption and reflection (photoplethysmography, pulse oximetry and dual wavelength spectrophotometry) or the shift in light frequency as it is reflected back from a tooth (laser Doppler flowmetry). They offer the advantages of being objective, non-invasive and atraumatic and are accurate and reliable.

e. *Color and amount of blood at the exposure site*

The color and amount of blood at the exposure site may be a reliable guide as regards pulpal inflammation in primary teeth. Light-red blood and hemorrhage that can be arrested easily is limited to the coronal pulp. Profuse hemorrhage from the exposure site, with deep-red blood, is associated with inflammation extending into the root canals. The former is indicated for pulpotomy while the latter would require pulpectomy.

The diagnostic features for pulp status in deciduous teeth is tabulated in Table 28.1.

Table 28.1 Diagnostic features for pulp status in deciduous teeth

Diagnostic features	*Pulp condition*		
	Reversible pulpitis	*Irreversible pulpitis*	*Pulp necrosis*
Mobility	No	May be mobile	May be mobile
Tender on percussion	No	Yes	Mostly
Widening of periodontal ligament	No	Often	Yes
Excessive bleeding at the pulp stumps	No	Often	No
Swelling	No	Rare	May be present

PULP THERAPY

Pulp therapy in primary teeth is aimed at retaining the tooth in a symptom-free state until it is lost naturally during the transition from primary to permanent dentition.

Goals

- To retain the tooth in the oral cavity in a non-pathological state
- Maintenance of the arch length and tooth space
- To restore the tooth to its function and form
- To prevent possible deviation of speech
- Preventing psychological trauma to the child

Indications

i. *General*

- Cooperative child
- Child with blood dyscrasias or bleeding abnormality (e.g. hemophilia) for whom extraction is not advisable

ii. *Dental*

- The patient exhibiting sign and symptoms of pulpitis
- Loss of interproximal marginal ridge, due to progress of caries.
- Radiographic evidence of caries extending more than half way from the dentinoenamel junction to the pulp.
- Primary tooth need to be retained due to absence of its permanent successor.

Contraindications

i. *General*

- Uncooperative child
- A child with congenital heart disease or a history of rheumatic fever.

ii. *Dental*

- Tooth, which cannot be restored
- Caries penetrating sub-pulpal floor of the pulp chamber
- A tooth close to natural exfoliation (i.e. less than two-thirds of root length remaining)
- Extensive pathological root resorption in a tooth

The treatment modalities of pulp therapy are:

I. Indirect pulp capping/treatment
II. Direct pulp capping
III. Pulp curettage
IV. Pulpotomy/cervical pulpotomy/complete pulpotomy
V. Non-vital pulpotomy
VI. Partial pulpectomy
VII. Pulpectomy
VIII. Apexification/Apexogenesis

I. Indirect Pulp Treatment/Capping

The procedure involves removal of gross caries followed by sealing rest of the cavity with an appropriate bactericidal/obtundant agent.

Indirect pulp treatment is a technique in which an effort is made to avoid pulp exposure during the treatment of teeth with deep carious lesions, without any evidence of pulp involvement. All the carious dentin is removed, leaving a thin non-carious dentin, which is then covered with calcium hydroxide or any other suitable materials.

Indirect pulp capping involves excavating deep caries and the deeper layers of softened dentin is covered with a pulp capping agent. After a period of 6–8 weeks, the tooth is reopened, and the remaining soft caries, if any, is removed (technique is no longer recommended). It has been established that all caries is to be removed, even in case of exposure; direct pulp capping or pulpotomy procedure is recommended in case of pulp exposure.

Objectives

- To arrest the carious process and provide conditions conducive to the formation of reactionary dentin and remineralization of remaining carious dentin.
- To preserve the vitality of pulp tissues
- To promote pulpal healing and dentinal sclerosis

Indications

Indirect pulp capping treatment is indicated when:

- History of mild discomfort from chemical and thermal stimuli with the absence of spontaneous pain.

28

- Clinically, the tooth should reveal a large carious lesion in close proximity to the pulp without any signs or symptoms of pulp involvement. Radiographic examination should exhibit normal lamina dura and periodontal ligament space with no inter-radicular or periapical radiolucency.
- In case of minimal pulpal inflammation (for example, reversible pulpitis), complete removal of caries may lead to a pulp exposure.

Contraindications

- Any signs of pulpal/periapical pathology
- Soft dentin covering large area of the cavity
- Swelling/fistula
- Tenderness to percussion
- External/internal root resorption
- Periapical/inter-radicular radiolucency

It is established that carious dentin consists of two distinct layers having different ultramicroscopic and chemical structures.

- *Infected dentin*: The outer carious layer, which is irreversibly denatured and incapable of being re-mineralized should be removed (contains significant number of bacteria).
- *Affected dentin*: The inner carious layer, which is reversibly denatured, not infected (with no demonstrable bacteria) and capable of being re-mineralized should be preserved.

The clinical challenge in indirect pulp treatment is the assessment of how much caries should be kept at pulpal/axial floor. Whether an area is an infected carious lesion or a bacteria-free demineralized zone is the quality of the dentin; soft, mushy infected dentin should be removed without exposing pulp, and hard discolored affected dentin can be indirectly capped. These two layers can be differentiated clinically by caries detector dyes. It can help in determining the extent of outer infected layers of caries.

Step-wise caries removal, also known as interim restorative treatment, implies removal of caries with hand instruments in steps. Various authors have concluded that in deep lesions, partial caries removal is preferable to complete caries removal to minimize the risk of carious exposure.

Various materials, calcium hydroxide, mineral trioxide aggregate (MTA) and glass-ionomer cement have been used in indirect pulp capping.

The indirect pulp treatment is considered as the most appropriate treatment for symptom-free primary teeth with deep caries provided the cavity is filled with leakage-resistant restoration. The indirect pulp treatment has been quite successful in primary teeth. Healing of the pulp can be confirmed by the formation of reparative dentin under the affected tubules. Follow-up of teeth receiving vital pulp therapy is very important. The follow-up radiographs should be compared with the preoperative radiographs to observe any change. No change between the pre-operative and follow-up radiograph is the standard for success.

Should Calcium Hydroxide be used in Deciduous Teeth?

It is established that calcium hydroxide, when placed in permanent teeth, results in calcific (dentin) bridge formation. It is hypothesized that certain properties of calcium hydroxide that produces healing in permanent teeth, may provoke untoward reactions in the pulps of primary teeth. These intense inflammatory responses to calcium hydroxide in deciduous teeth may trigger macrophages to fuse and transform into odontoclasts; subsequently leading to root resorption. Though the exact mechanism of such odontoblastic activity is not clear, various hypothesis have been proposed, such as:

- Calcium hydroxide-induced resorption in deciduous teeth may be attributed to inflammatory cytokines, which contribute to transformation of preodontoclasts to odontoclasts.
- The high pH of calcium hydroxide has beneficial effects, viz. neutralization of acid products, antimicrobial property, and the activation of alkaline phosphatase. When calcium hydroxide is placed in deciduous teeth, it is hypothesized that the high alkaline pH could trigger existing preodontoclasts (undifferentiated mesenchymal cells) to transform into odontoclasts.
- It has been established that resorption can occur when the protective un-mineralized tissues such as pre-cementum and pre-dentin are mechanically damaged, allowing osteoclasts/odontoclasts to gain access to calcified dental tissues. It is known that the placement of calcium hydroxide produces a superficial zone of necrosis because of its high alkalinity. This could also cause damage to the pre-dentin, which may lead to exposure of the underlying dentin to resting odontoclasts. These odontoclasts, after being activated, result in tooth resorption.

II. Direct Pulp Capping

Direct pulp capping is defined as *'the placement of a medicated/non-medicated material on the pulp that has been exposed while excavating the last portions of caries or as a result of trauma'*. The objective of direct pulp capping is to encourage the formation of a dentin bridge at the point of pulp exposure with preservation of pulpal health and vitality, and to seal the pulp against bacterial leakage. Pulp capping procedures in primary teeth should be reserved for teeth with small mechanical or traumatic exposures or in cases in which the teeth will exfoliate within 1 or 2 years. It is hypothesized that the high cellular content of primary pulp tissue may be responsible for the failure of direct pulp capping in primary teeth. Undifferentiated mesenchymal cells may differentiate into osteoclastic cells in response to either the caries or direct pulp capping which could lead to internal resorption. Direct pulp capping has limited application and is not recommended for deciduous teeth.

Pulp capping: Key features
- Avoid exposing the pulp; tooth can survive even if residual caries remain.
- Calcium hydroxide is the material of choice; MTA is equally effective.
- Zinc oxide eugenol, glass ionomers and adhesives are poor pulp capping agents.
- The rest of the cavity is to be filled with leakage-resistant restoration.
- In case pulp is exposed, control haemorrhage with sodium hypochlorite (possess antibacterial properties).

III. Pulp Curettage

It is a modification of the direct capping technique, wherein the exposure site is enlarged prior to the placement of capping material. Exposure site enlargement serves three purposes:
- Removes inflamed and/or infected tissue in the exposed area.
- Facilitates removal of carious and non-carious debris particularly dentin chips.
- Ensures intimate contact of the capping material with healthy pulp tissue.

The location of exposure is important as there should be no pulp tissue coronal to the exposure. Exposure in a cervical cavity would lead to reactionary dentin formation, which would restrict the blood supply to the tissue more coronal to it, leading to necrosis and failure. These teeth should preferably be root canal treated.

IV. Pulpotomy/Cervical Pulpotomy/ Complete Pulpotomy

28

Pulpotomy procedure in primary teeth is defined as *'amputation of the affected or infected coronal portion of the dental pulp, preserving the vitality and function of the remaining radicular pulp'*. The main approaches to this technique are:
- Preserving the radicular pulp in a healthy state
- Rendering the radicular pulp inert
- Encouraging tissue regeneration and healing at the site of radicular pulp amputation

Indications
- A carious or mechanical exposure of vital coronal pulp
- Aggressive progress of carious lesion
- Tooth free of radicular pulpitis (elicited by hemorrhage from amputation site)
- At least two-thirds of the primary tooth root is still present
- Asymptomatic tooth or only transient pain
- Where extraction of the primary tooth is contraindicated

Contraindications
- Tooth which cannot be restored
- History of spontaneous pain/pain on percussion
- Presence of an abscess
- Permanent successor close to eruption
- Presence of necrotic pulpal tissue/suppuration from the root canal
- If hemorrhage from pulpal tissue is uncontrollable

Pulpotomy procedure is categorized as single-visit or two-visit pulpotomy

A. Single-visit pulpotomy
B. Two-visit pulpotomy
   a. Desensitizing pulpotomy
   b. Devitalization pulpotomy
      i. Devitalization using paraformaldehyde
      ii. Devitalization using formocresol (formocresol pulpotomy)
   c. Preservative pulpotomy
   d. Regenerative (inductive/reparative) pulpotomy

A. Single-visit Pulpotomy

The concerned tooth is anesthetized and isolated. The pulp chamber is opened using appropriate armamentarium and the roof of the pulp chamber is removed carefully. The inflamed pulp from the coronal chamber is removed using sterilized excavators. The exposed site is disinfected with formocresol and covered with calcium hydroxide, followed by restoring the tooth with appropriate restorative material.

B. Two-visit Pulpotomy

a. *Desensitizing pulpotomy*

Desensitizing pulpotomy is carried out to reduce pulpal inflammation, in order to facilitate subsequent pulpotomy or pulpectomy procedure.

Indications

- Hyperalgesic pulp (adequate analgesia not achieved)
- Carious pulp exposure with no signs/symptoms of loss of vitality
- Non-compliant child

Procedure

Tooth is anesthetized and isolated. Caries is removed and a small pledget of cotton wool loaded with steroid-antibiotic paste (Ledermix, Septomix) is placed directly over exposure site (tooth is usually too sensitive to remove entire roof of pulp chamber). A temporary dressing is placed over the cotton pledget. After 6–8 weeks recall, the operator may proceed with a pulpotomy or pulpectomy technique, depending on clinical findings.

b. *Devitalization pulpotomy*

Devitalization implies 'mummifying' the pulp tissue. The term 'mummified' has been described to chemically treat pulp tissue that is inert, sterilized, metabolically suppressed, and incapable of autolysis. This two-stage procedure mummifies and fixes the coronal pulp tissue, while the major part of the radicular pulp may remain vital.

Indications

- Inability to arrest hemorrhage from the amputated pulp stumps during a single-visit pulpotomy.
- Hyperalgesic pulp (adequate analgesia not achieved).

i. *Devitalization using paraformaldehyde* [Paraformaldehyde paste, camphorated paramonochlorophenol (CMCP) and Cresol etc. are used to devitalize the coronal part of the pulp]. The constituents of Paraformaldehyde pastes are: paraformaldehyde (1.0 g), lignocaine (0.06 g), carmine (10 mg), carbowax 1500 (1.3 g), and propylene glycol (0.5 ml).

Procedure

First visit: After gaining access to the pulpal exposure area, a pledget of cotton wool soaked with small amount of paraformaldehyde devitalizing paste is applied to the exposed pulp tissue. Formaldehyde vapor liberated from the dressing permeates through the pulpal space causing fixation of the tissues. A layer of zinc oxide-eugenol is placed passively without applying pressure. The patient must be informed of possibility of mild discomfort.

Second visit: After a couple of weeks, the devitalized coronal pulp may be removed, without the need for local anesthesia. Zinc oxide-eugenol mixed with formocresol is then placed over the radicular stumps and the tooth is restored with appropriate material (Fig. 28.3a to d). If vital tissues remain in the coronal pulp chamber, a further dressing of paraformaldehyde paste can be applied.

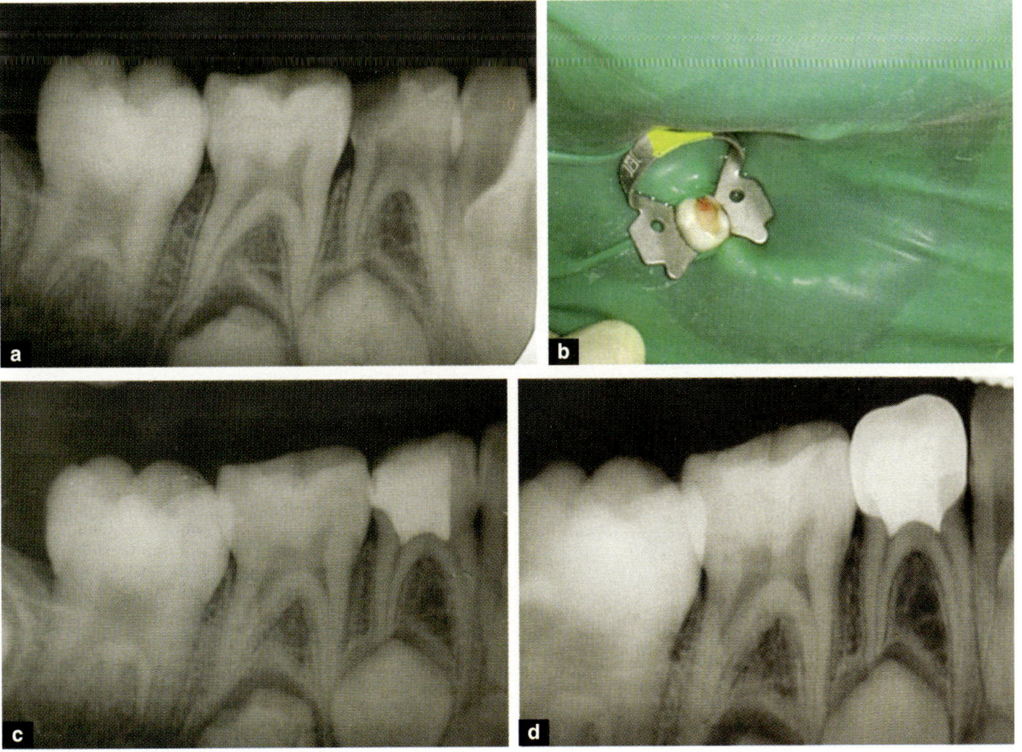

Fig. 28.3a to d Pulpotomy (first deciduous molar)

ii. *Devitalization using formocresol (formocresol pulpotomy)*: Formocresol is the standard medicament in both vital and non-vital pulp therapy techniques in the primary dentition. Despite its potential risks it continues to be one of the treatment choices for primary teeth.

Buckley's formocresol solution consists of 35% tricresol, 19% aqueous formaldehyde, glycerine, and water. A 1:5 dilution of Buckley's formocresol is recommended as the pulp medicament, as it is less damaging.

The histologic studies on formocresol pulpotomy have shown distinct zones in the pulp as follows:

- Superficial debris along with dentinal chips at the amputation site
- Eosinophil-stained and compressed tissue
- A pale stained zone with loss of cellularity
- An area of fibrotic and inflammatory activity
- An area of normal-appearing pulp tissue considered to be vital.

Earlier investigators have used 5.0% sodium hypochlorite as a pulpotomy agent in primary molars. The success rate of sodium hypochlorite is comparable to formocresol and ferric sulphate pulpotomies.

Toxicity

Formocresol has demonstrated high clinical and radiographic success; however, this medicament may exhibit certain potential risks. The concerns over use of formocresol are tabulated in Table 28.2. The International Agency for Research on Cancer (IARC) has documented that there was sufficient evidence that formaldehyde might cause nasopharyngeal cancer in humans. Studies linking formocresol with nasopharyngeal cancer are based on chronic exposure to formaldehyde (both humans and animals) at very high doses. There is also evidence of a causal relationship between formaldehyde exposure and leukemia.

Table 28.2 Concerns over use of formocresol
• It is caustic and toxic at high doses
• Histologically, pulp responds with inflammation and necrosis
• Potential systemic absorption and distribution throughout the body; may lead to liver and kidney changes
• May effect the enamel of succedaneous teeth
• Possibility of reversible fixation leading to autoantibody formation
• Mutagenicity and carcinogenicity
• Destruction of cellular integrity due to cresol
• May lead to nasopharyngeal cancer and leukemia

c. *Preservative pulpotomy*

Preservative pulpotomy involves medicaments and techniques that provide minimal insult, maintain the vitality and normal histologic appearance of the entire radicular pulp.

The medicaments commonly used in preservative pulpotomy are:

i. Glutaraldehyde: Application of 2.0–4.0% glutaraldehyde produces rapid surface fixation of the underlying pulp tissue; however, its depth of penetration is limited.

Advantages of glutaraldehyde over formocresol

- It has mild effects on pulp tissue and does not perfuse into the pulp tissue to the apex; demonstrate less systemic distribution immediately after its application.
- Large dose caused little toxic effects.
- Provides superior fixation with relatively little immunogenicity.
- Exhibits very low tissue binding and is readily metabolized mostly in the kidneys, lungs, liver, heart and muscle tissues and is eliminated in urine.

Histologic features

- Less damage/necrosis of apical tissue.
- Clearly demarcated zones within radicular tissue are minimum.
- Absence of multizones in the root pulp (a homogenous, eosinophilic stained zone may be present below amputated surface).
- No evidence of ingrowth of granulation tissue.
- Less dystrophic calcification and limited to coronal portion of canal.
- Fibroblastic proliferation is observed immediately below glutaraldehyde fixed tissue in coronal 3rd indicating repair/replacement.

Limitations

- Neither the optimum concentration of glutaraldehyde nor the amount of time of application has been established.
- It has lower clinical success rate than with formocresol. (*It is no longer preferred concerning about the handling of glutaraldehyde and its hypersensitivity.*)

ii. Hemostatic agents: The commonly used hemostatic agents are:

- 20% ferric sulphate (Monsel solution)
- 1.0% feracrylum solution (Repalum)

Procedure

Hemostatic agents are available in solution form along with an applicator tip. Following hemorrhage control, ferric sulphate (commonly used hemostatic agent) is gently applied to the pulp stumps for 10–15 seconds (it requires only 15 second for manipulation as compared to 5 minutes for formocresol.) The pulp chamber should then be gently rinsed with water and dried with cotton pellets. A thick mix of zinc oxide eugenol is placed in the chamber and tightly packed against the pulp stumps. A few authors have cautioned, fearing that the eugenol may promote internal resorption following the ferric sulphate pulpotomy.

Ferric sulphate prevents problems arising from clot formation after the removal of the coronal pulp. It also minimizes the chances of inflammation and internal resorption, an important factor for the failure of pulpotomy with calcium hydroxide.

Ferric sulphate is preferred instead of formocresol for pulpotomy of primary teeth. It has shown significant clinical and radiological success over a period of three years.

iii. Electrosurgery: Electrosurgery is a non-pharmacological hemostatic pulpotomy for primary molars; a non-chemical devitalization approach.

It carbonizes and denatures superficial pulp tissue producing a layer of coagulation necrosis. It provides a barrier between healthy radicular tissue and any base material placed in the pulp chamber. The odontoblasts are stimulated to form a dentin bridge and the tooth is maintained in the arch with vital radicular tissue until it exfoliates.

Procedure

The procedure is basically the same as for the formocresol technique. Following removal of coronal pulp tissue, a sterile cotton pellet is placed in contact with the pulp, and pressure is applied to obtain hemostasis. A dental electrode is used to deliver the electrical arc. The cotton pellet is quickly removed, and the electrode is placed 1.0–2.0 mm above the pulp stump. The electrical arc is allowed to bridge the gap at the pulp stump for one second, followed by cooling for five seconds. The pulp stumps appear dry and completely blackened after the procedure. Zinc oxide eugenol is placed directly over the pulp stumps filling the pulp chamber.

iv. Lasers: Lasers are an effective alternative for treating pulps, as no chemical is being introduced into the young canals.

Lasers used in pulpotomy are:

- *Carbon dioxide laser*: The advantage of carbon dioxide laser over other lasers is that the bloodless tissue incisions can be attained at a practical cutting speed and also the edges of the irradiated tissue are covered by only a thin layer of necrotic material.
- *Nd:YAG laser*: The successful effects of Nd:YAG laser on the wound healing of amputated pulps has been established.
- *Er:YAG laser*: Er:YAG laser has been successfully used in treating both vital and non-vital primary teeth.
- *Argon laser*: Argon laser pulpotomy for primary teeth has shown formation of reparative dentin.

d. *Regenerative pulpotomy*

Regenerative pulpotomy implies use of agents that have cell-inductive capacity to replace lost cells or induce existent cells to differentiate into hard tissue-forming elements.

Calcium hydroxide was the first medicament to be used in a 'regenerative capacity' because of its ability to stimulate hard tissue barrier formation. Calcium hydroxide stimulates dentin bridge formation, leading to healing of pulp tissue. Its regenerative capacity has been questioned owing to the fact that its response is more reactive than inductive.

A high failure rate using calcium hydroxide for pulpotomy in primary teeth has been demonstrated, which is explained by the presence of an extrapulpal clot separating the calcium hydroxide from the pulpal tissue and thus impairing healing.

It is established that use of calcium hydroxide lead to internal root resorption, which might result from overstimulation of the primary pulp by its highly alkaline nature. This alkaline-induced overstimulation could cause metaplasia within the pulp tissue, leading to the formation of odontoclasts.

In addition, undetected microleakage could allow large numbers of bacteria to cover the pulp and nullify the beneficial effects of calcium hydroxide.

Mineral trioxide aggregate (MTA) allows for bone regeneration and overgrowth of cementum when used as a root-end filling material. It is biocompatible material, with sealing ability superior to amalgam and zinc oxide eugenol. It has many positive properties such as alkaline pH, radiopacity, high sealing capacity and ability to induce the formation of dentin, cementum and bone.

The true cell-inductive agents include transforming growth factor-β (TGF-β) in the form of bone morphogenetic proteins, and Freeze-dried bone. These materials are also being tried in pulpotomy of primary teeth.

Failures of pulpotomy

- The first sign of failure is often internal resorption; subsequently, external resorption may occur
- Pulp canal obliteration can be seen
- Radiolucency might develop at the bifurcation and trifurcation area

- Presence of fistula/excessive mobility of operated tooth
- Inflammatory follicular cysts may develop

V. Non-vital Pulpotomy

Non-vital pulpotomy is technically a misnomer. It is followed when root canal treatment is to be delayed for some reasons.

Indications

- When the inflammatory process affecting the coronal pulp has extended to the radicular pulp leading to irreversible changes in the pulp tissue
- When the pulp is non-vital, along with periradicular involvement
- Where pulpectomy is to be delayed for some reasons

Procedure

At the first visit, the necrotic contents of the pulp are removed and the infected radicular pulp is treated with beechwood creosote solution [composition: D-methoxyphenol (47%), p-methoxyphenol (26%), cresol (13%), m-methoxyphenol (7%) and incipients (7%)]. In the next visit, the tooth is checked for any adverse signs and symptoms. If there is evidence of infection (sinus, pain, swelling, etc.), beechwood creosote dressing should be placed. If symptoms have resolved, the tooth may be restored with suitable restorative material.

VI. Partial Pulpectomy

Partial pulpectomy is considered as an extension of the pulpotomy procedure, whereby the radicular pulp is amputated, short of total length of canal leaving vital tissue in the apical half. Technically, it is a vital pulp therapy technique. Pulpotomy refers only to coronal extirpation of vital pulp tissue, while any amount of pulp removal short of total extirpation may be referred to as partial pulpectomy.

Indication

To control hemorrhage from the radicular orifice; when even after removing the coronal pulp, the hemorrhage remains uncontrolled.

Procedure

The coronal pulp is removed from the chamber. After controlling the hemorrhage, approximately one half of the coronal portion of the radicular pulp is also removed (Fig. 28.4a and b).

The canals and chamber are irrigated. If hemorrhage is still not controlled, the pulpectomy procedure is initiated.

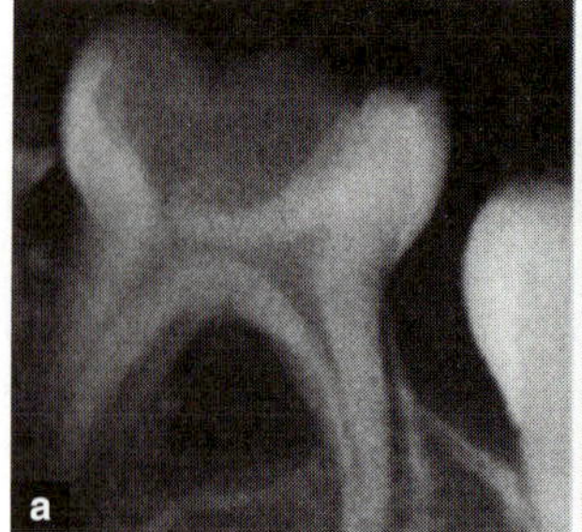

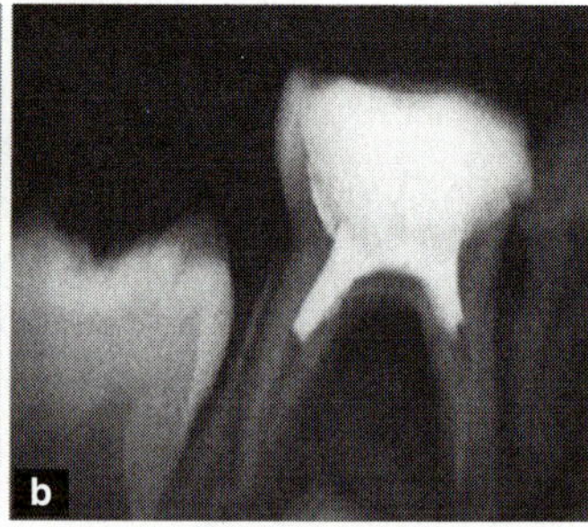

Fig. 28.4a and b Partial pulpectomy

After successful hemorrhage control, a formocresol dampened cotton pellet, squeezed dry, is placed in the pulp chamber for a day or so.

The pellet is removed, and zinc oxide eugenol cement is packed with gentle pressure.

The tooth is restored in routine after 6–8 weeks follow-up of the procedure (permanent restoration is usually delayed, since partial pulpectomy is for short duration; subsequently, pulpectomy is to be carried out).

VII. Pulpectomy

Pulpectomy can be defined as *'removal of the inflamed/necrotic pulp, cleaning and shaping the root canals, and obturation of the tooth with a resorbable filling material'*.

Earlier authors treated endodontically involved deciduous teeth with beechwood creosote and iodine. Various materials and techniques have been tried to treat pulp involved deciduous teeth, with varying success.

Indications

- Signs of irreversible pulpitis
- Non-vital radicular pulp with/without associated infection
- Minimal periapical changes with sufficient bone support
- Two-thirds of the root length should be available
- Internal resorption without any obvious perforation
- Strategically important tooth (for example, in case of the deciduous second molar where the permanent first molar has not erupted)
- Good patient compliance

Contraindications

- Systemic conditions like infective endocarditis
- Lack of patient cooperation
- Excessive mobility
- Non-restorable tooth
- Perforations of the floor of pulp chamber

- Pathologic root resorption involving more than one-third of the root
- Excessive loss of bone support (pathological)
- Presence of dentigerous cyst
- Periapical or interradicular lesion involving the crypt of the developing permanent successor.

Implications of Pulpectomy (Root Canal Treatment) in Deciduous Teeth

Root canal treatment in children may present difficulties due to the following reasons:

- The root canal system in primary teeth usually have numerous lateral and accessory canals, areas of internal resorption, communication with the furcation and deviated canal shape, especially at the apical area.
- Mobility of the tooth, even if minor, pose difficulty in instrumentation.
- The root canals must be obturated with resorbable materials, which should not interfere with the eruption of the succedaneous tooth.
- The problem is further complicated by the reluctance among general practitioners to treat such teeth due to the difficulty of managing young, apprehensive children and also the lack of experience of treating the deciduous teeth.

Procedure

The pulpectomy procedure can be completed in one visit or in two multiple visits.

A single/two-multiple visit pulpectomy may be undertaken depending on whether the radicular pulp is irreversibly inflamed or non-vital, with/without an associated periradicular pathosis.

A. Single-visit pulpectomy

Single-visit pulpectomy (Fig. 28.5a to c) is preferred in following cases:

- Presence of inflamed but remnants of vital radicular pulp
- An asymptomatic primary tooth with necrotic pulp tissue, without any acute symptoms such as cellulitis
- Presence of a chronic buccal lesion without any active discharge or acute symptoms.

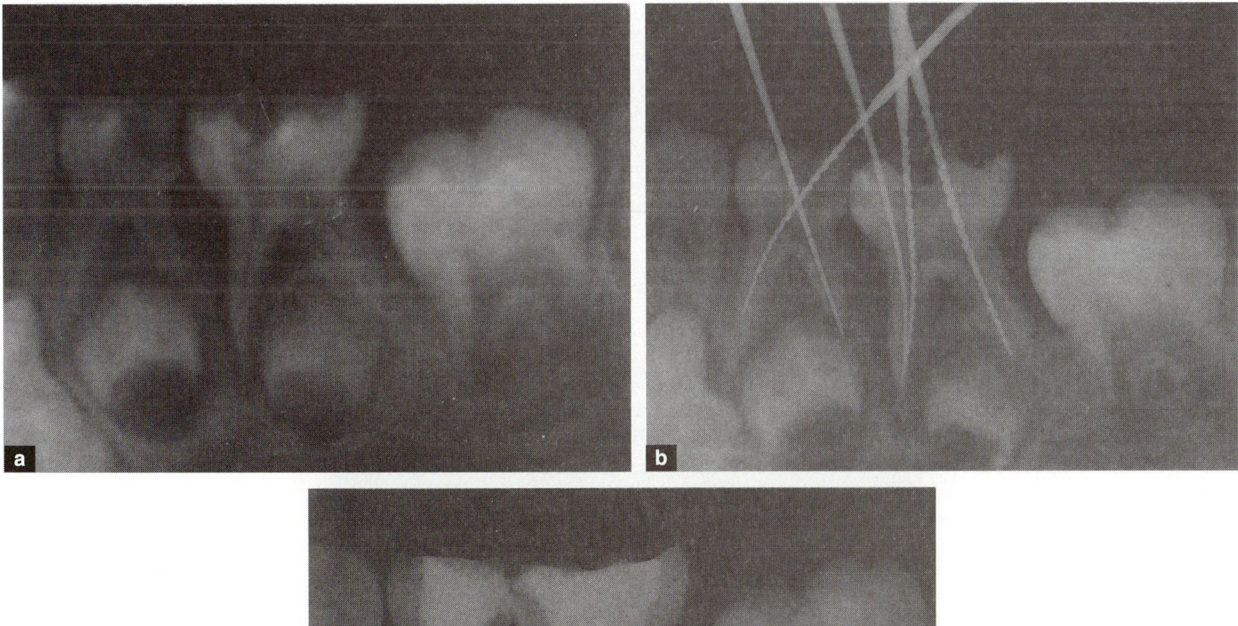

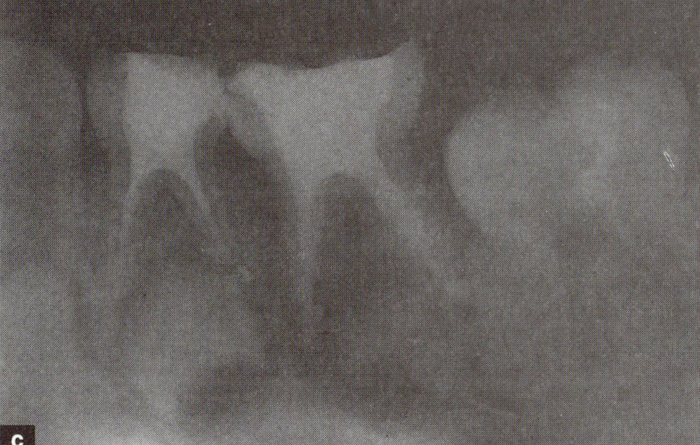

Fig. 28.5 Single-visit pulpectomy (a) Preoperative; (b) Diagnostic radiograph; (c) Postoperative

B. Two-visit/multi-visit pulpectomy

Two-visit technique is preferred where acute/chronic infection/exudate is present with or without associated cellulitis (Fig. 28.6 a to c).

Procedure

The steps involved are:

a. Access cavity preparation: The access cavity preparation is the most important phase of root canal treatment in deciduous teeth just like permanent teeth. The basic objectives of access preparation, viz. gaining straight line access and conserving the tooth structure are followed in primary teeth also.

i. *Anterior teeth*: Access cavity preparation for primary anterior teeth have traditionally been through the lingual surface, except for the maxillary primary incisors. Since endodontically treated primary incisors would be discolored, it has been recommended to use a facial approach. The access cavity is filled with composite restoration immediately after the obturation to maintain esthetics.

The anatomy of maxillary primary incisors also facilitate access from the facial surface. The only variation would be the more extension to the incisal edge than with the normal lingual access in order to provide straight line approach into the root canal.

ii. *Posterior teeth*: Access cavity preparation for the primary posterior teeth are essentially the same as for the permanent teeth; however, following differences between the primary and permanent teeth are to be kept in mind during access cavity preparation.

- Configuration (bulbous shape) of the crowns.
- Thin dentinal wall at the pulpal floor and in the root.
- The depth necessary to penetrate into the pulp chamber is quite less than that in the permanent teeth.
- The distance from the occlusal surface to the pulp floor of the pulp chamber is much less than in permanent teeth (in primary molars, perforation of pulpal floor is common).

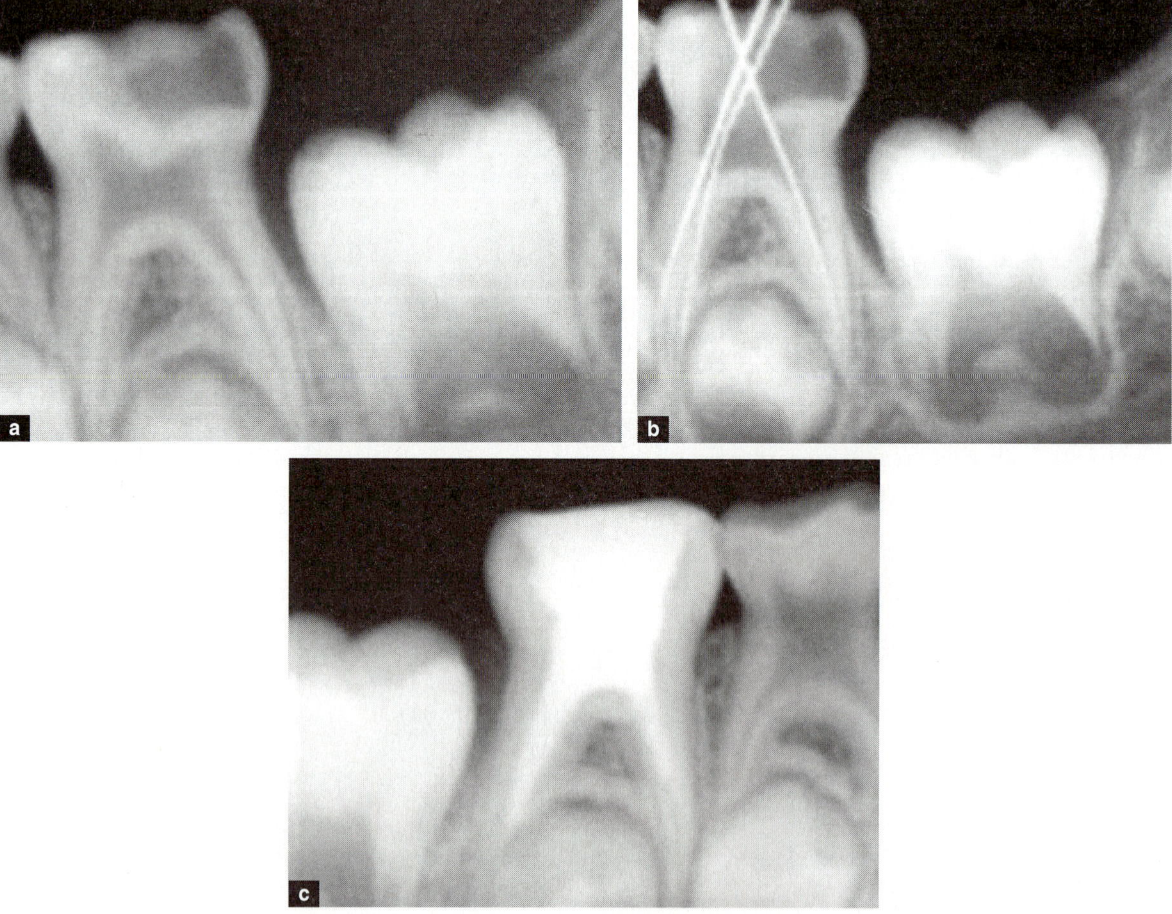

Fig. 28.6 Two-visit pulpectomy: (a) Preoperative; (b) Diagnostic radiograph; (c) Postoperative

- When the roof of the pulp chamber is identified and perforated, the entire roof should be removed. Since the crown of the primary teeth are bulbous, less extension towards the exterior of the tooth is necessary to uncover the openings of the root canals than in the permanent teeth.

b. Working length: Accurate determination of the working length is a crucial step prior to pulpectomy in primary molars. Due to limitations of radiographic interpretation and high possibility of over-instrumentation of the unevenly resorbed roots and subsequent overfilling, the application of electronic apex locators is recommended regardless of the stage of root resorption.

Garcia-Godoy's method of determining working length

The root resorption in primary teeth is initiated at the site of the root which is closest to the permanent successor. As the growth proceeds, the developing tooth moves under the divergent roots of primary molar. The position and size of the follicle affects the pattern of resorption showing uneven root resorption in one or more roots at any given time. This poses a great difficulty in determining the exact working length in primary teeth. To overcome this problem, Garcia-Godoy (1987) suggested a new method of working length determination in primary molars.

- If permanent tooth bud is within the furcation area, use of instruments should be limited to a plane just occlusal to the occlusal plane of permanent tooth bud (Fig. 28.7).

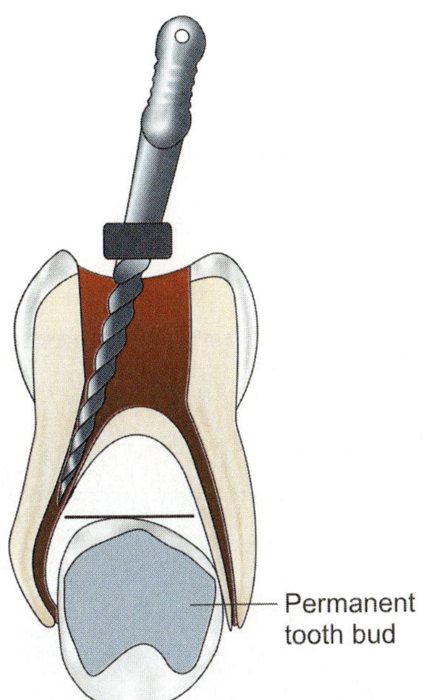

Fig. 28.7 Working length measurement in deciduous teeth (permanent tooth bud within the furcation area)

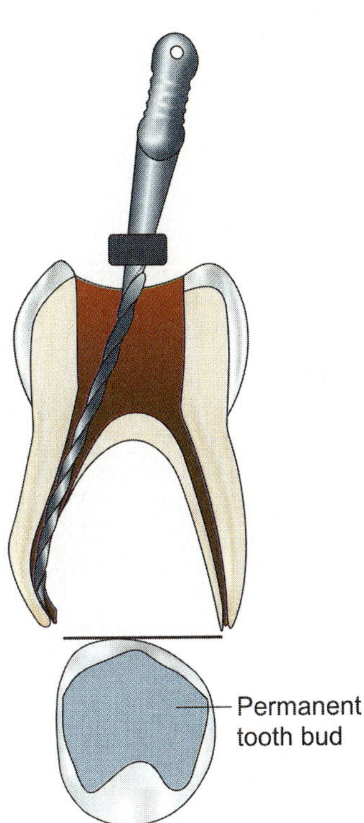

Fig. 28.8 Working length measurement in deciduous teeth (permanent tooth bud below the apices of molar)

- If permanent tooth bud is below the apices of the deciduous molar, instruments can be used for the entire length of canals (Fig. 28.8).

Figure 28.9a and b exhibits lateral resorption of mesial root; subsequently obturated.

c. Cleaning, shaping and irrigation: Cleaning and shaping of root canals in deciduous teeth is carried out using stainless steel hand files (usually not larger than size 30) in routine cases. Flexible files are recommended in curved/S-shaped canals. Operator should carefully choose irrigating solutions due to possible chemical interactions among different irrigants. Use of intermediate solutions, such as saline or sterile distilled water can prevent such toxic interactions.

d. Obturation: Various materials have been tried for obturating primary root canals; no single material could meet the requirements as described. Gutta-percha is not a resorbable material, therefore, its use in primary teeth is contraindicated.

Ideal root canal—filling material for primary teeth should have the following characteristics:

- Should resorb at a similar rate as the primary root
- Should be harmless to the periapical tissues and to the permanent tooth germ
- Resorb readily if extruded beyond the apex
- Should be antiseptic

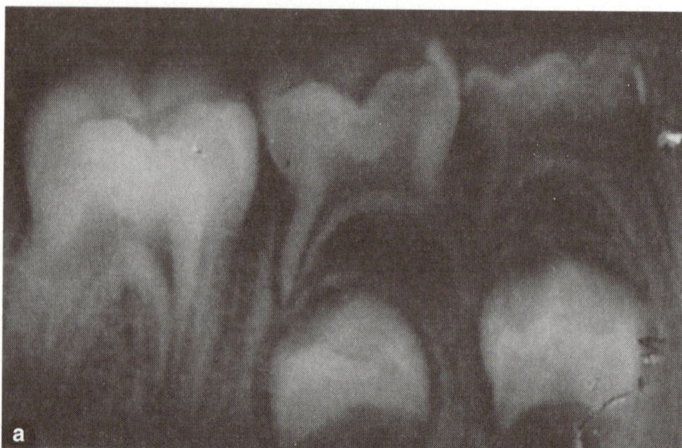

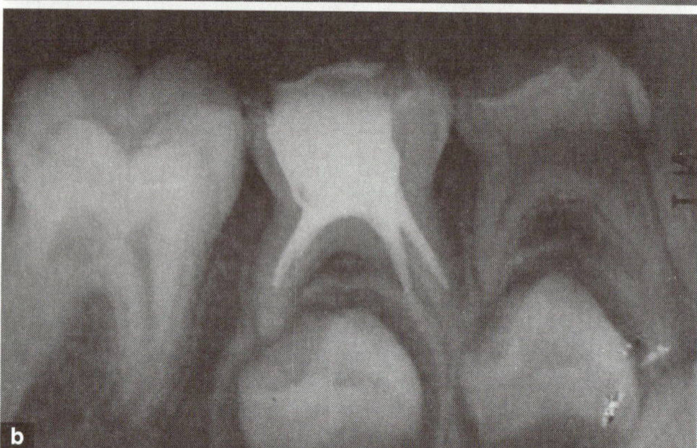

Fig. 28.9a and b (a) Lateral resorption of mesial root; (b) Obturated root

- Should fill the root canals easily and adhere to root dentin
- Should not shrink and discolor the tooth
- Should be easily removed, if necessary
- Should be radiopaque

The commonly used **obturating materials** for deciduous teeth are:

i. *Zinc oxide eugenol*

Zinc oxide eugenol alone and in combination with formocresol/formaldehyde, paraformaldehyde and cresol has been widely used as obturating material in deciduous teeth. A combination of zinc oxide eugenol with iodoform has also been effective as obturating material.

Limitations

- Limited antimicrobial action (tends to resorb at a slower rate than the roots of the deciduous teeth).
- Causes irritation to periapical tissues; may lead to necrosis of bone and cementum.
- May alter path of eruption of succedaneous tooth (chances of retention of the overfilled material in periapical region).
- Not bactericidal (combination materials do have bactericidal properties).

ii. *Calcium hydroxide*

Calcium hydroxide has been used as obturating material due to its antimicrobial properties. It is easily resorbed when inadvertently extruded beyond the apical foramen. Calcium hydroxide, in combination with iodoform has shown favorable results in deciduous teeth.

Advantages

- Biocompatible
- Antibacterial
- Resorbable

Disadvantages

- Depletion of material from root canal prior to physiologic resorption of root.
- May lead to internal resorption (early resorption in root canal may become a hollow tube for bacteria to induce re-infection).

iii. *Vitapex*

Vitapex is a pre-mixed paste of 30.3% calcium hydroxide and 40.4% iodoform (Fig. 28.10). It is packed in a sterile syringe; the paste is injected into the canal with disposable plastic needles.

When extruded into furcal or apical areas, it can either be diffused away or resorbed in part by macrophages within a week or two and causes no foreign body reaction.

This technique is easy to use for primary incisors; however, pushing paste in narrow canals is difficult, especially in primary molars.

Advantages

- Resorbable
- Harmless to successors
- Easy to remove
- Suppresses residual bacteria in root canal/periapical region

Disadvantage

Low anti-bacterial effect

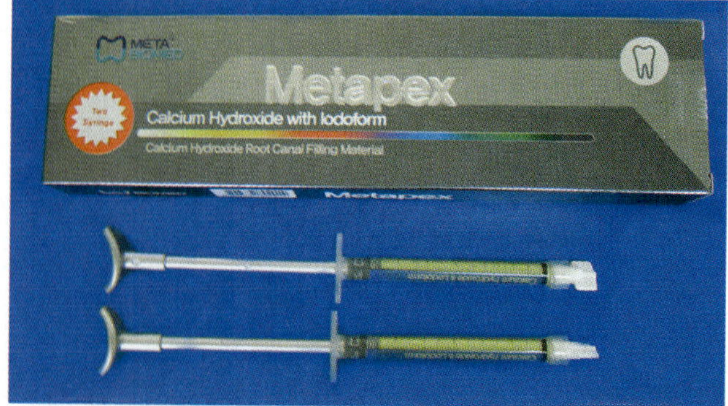

Fig. 28.10 Calcium hydroxide and iodoform paste

iv. *Iodoform paste*

Iodoform pastes have better resorbability and disinfectant properties than zinc oxide eugenol. It has excellent healing properties and is bactericidal. Different formulations of root canal filling materials containing iodoform are available:

- *Walkoff paste* (parachlorphenol, camphor, menthol).
- *KRI paste* (parachlorphenol, camphor, menthol and iodoform).
- *Maisto paste* (parachlorphenol, camphor, menthol, iodoform, zinc oxide, thymol and lanolin).
- *Guedes-Pinto paste* (iodoform, camphorated parachlorophenol).

Advantages

- Bactericidal
- Easy to remove
- Biocompatibility

Disadvantage

- May produce a yellowish-brown discoloration of the tooth crowns compromising esthetics.

v. *Endoflas*

Endoflas is available in powder: liquid form. The powder contains zinc oxide eugenol (56.5%), triiodomethane/iodine (40.6%), calcium hydroxide (1.07%) and barium sulphate (1.63%). Liquid contains eugenol and pentachlorophenol (Fig. 28.11).

Advantages

- Hydrophilic material; can be used in mild humid root canal
- Firmly adheres to root dentin provide a good seal
- Ability to disinfect dentinal tubules and accessory canals that cannot be disinfected/cleaned mechanically
- Broad spectrum antibacterial effect
- Biocompatible
- Easily removed by phagocytosis; making the material resorbable.

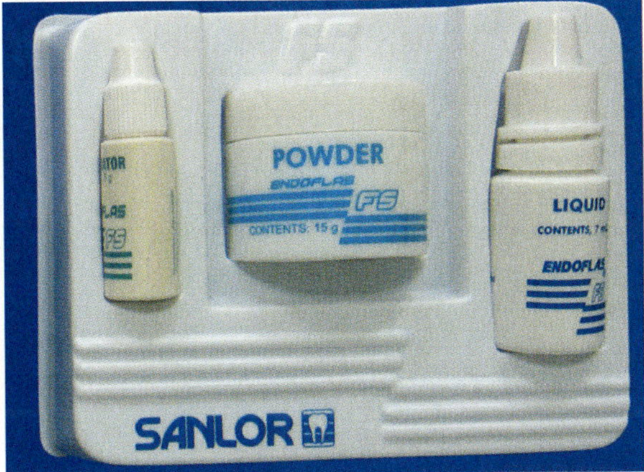

Fig. 28.11 Endoflas

Disadvantages

- May lead to periapical irritation
- Yellowish brown tooth discoloration
- May lead to cemental necrosis
- Cannot be removed completely from the root canals

Obturation Techniques

The ultimate goal of obturation is to create hermetic seal in the root canals, so as to prevent re-infection of the pulp spaces. The selected filling technique should fill the root canals without any over-fill and voids. Various techniques are being used to obturate the primary root canals.

The commonly employed techniques are as follows.

i. Endodontic Pressure Syringe

The apparatus consists of a syringe barrel, threaded plugger, wrench and threaded needle (different sizes are available). The needle is inserted into the root canal until resistance is felt. The obturating material is injected into the root canal with mild pressure. The needle is withdrawn of 3.0 mm intervals, pushing the material, till the canal can be visibly filled at the orifice. Small gauge needles are flexible and can easily be maneuvered in the tortuous canals of primary molars. The disadvantage of this method is, the needle is to be repeatedly withdrawn and inserted, which may disrupt placement of obturating material in the canal. Air gets entrapped and the voids can be created using this technique. More so, the technique is time consuming.

Mechanical syringe with plunger system has also been used, but with little success. The screw mechanism of endodontic pressure syringe could generate sufficient pressure for placement of the obturating material.

ii. Lentulo Spiral

Lentulo spiral is one of the commonly used instrument for applying paste into primary root canals (also effectively used in permanent teeth). The flexibility of the instrument facilitate carrying paste even to narrow and curved root canals. Various authors in their respective studies have concluded that calcium hydroxide when inserted using a Lentulo spiral technique showed better radiodensity, especially in curved canals. The disadvantages of using this technique are, frequent fracture of instrument and also the probability of extrusion of obturating material beyond the apex.

A reamer (Fig. 28.12) is also used as a paste carrier (reamer coated with obturating paste is inserted into canal with clockwise rotation along with up and down

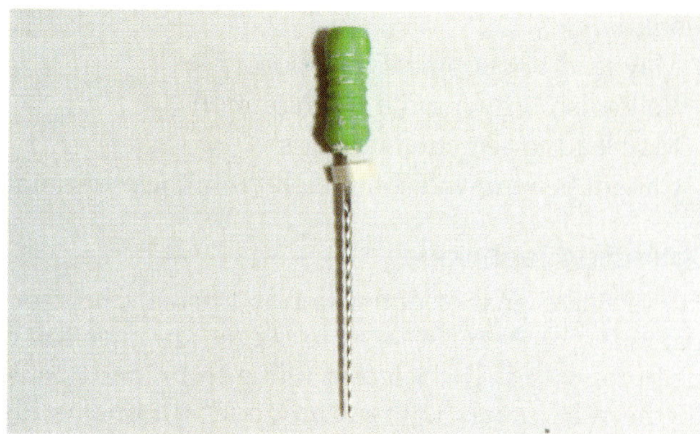

Fig. 28.12 Reamer

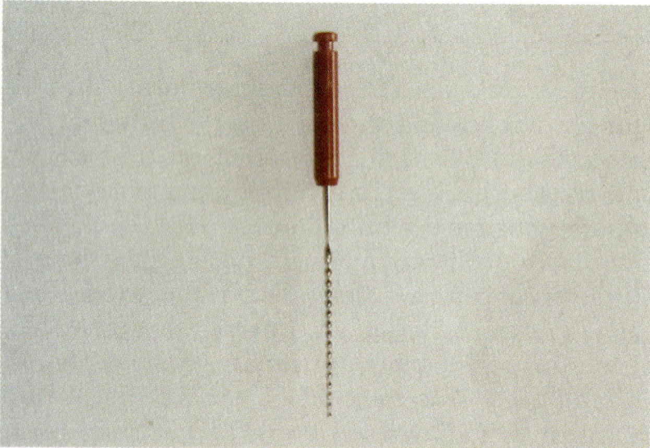

Fig. 28.13 Past inject

motion. A rubber stop can be used to keep the reamer in a predetermined length. Past inject (micromega), a paste carrier, with improved blade design (flat blades) has also been introduced (Fig. 28.13). Manufacturer claims better placement of obturating material with this carrier. Another carrier, Bi-directional spiral (EZ-fill), effectively control the obturating paste placement in the root canal. The spirals at the coronal end spin the material down to apex and the spiral at apical end spin the material coronally. The chances of apical extrusion is minimum with bi-directional spiral obturating paste carrier.

iii. Incremental Filling Technique

An endodontic plugger corresponding to the size of the canal is selected. A rubber stop is fixed 2.0 mm short of the root canal length. Pre-mixed zinc oxide eugenol or any other obturating paste is inserted into the root canal in small increments. The process is repeated until the canal is filled to the cervical area. A few authors prefer placing the material in bulk and pushing it into the canals with endodontic pluggers. The disadvantage of this technique is, since the flexibility of endodontic pluggers is limited, the paste cannot be placed in narrow/curved canals (effective only in wider canals).

iv. Jiffy Tube

The premix slurry of zinc oxide eugenol is coated in the root canal walls with the help of paper points. The zinc oxide eugenol mixture is loaded in the tube (Jiffy tube). The tube is gently squeezed, placing tip of tube at the canal orifice and pushing the material into the root canal. Since no apical pressure is applied, chances of apical extrusion are minimum.

v. Conventional/Insulin/Tuberculin Syringe

The pre-mixed zinc oxide eugenol is loaded into the syringe with a standard 3/8-inch needle and 26–30 gauge. The material is expressed into the canal by slow finger pressure on the plunger until the canal is filled. The disadvantage of syringe technique is the choice of needle gauge; if small sized, may pose difficulty in pushing the material, and if large sized, may not fit into many canals. Placement of obturating material may also create voids in the canal.

Insulin syringe (Fig. 28.14) is also available with smaller gauge size. A thin and flexible metal tip (viz. NaviTip) has been introduced to deliver root canal sealer. The NaviTip is available in different sizes with the provision to adjust rubber stop.

It has been pointed out that pulpally treated primary teeth may occasionally present a problem of over-retention. It is hypothesized that the large amount of zinc oxide in the canals may impair the physiological resorption and lead to prolonged retention of the crown. The teeth should be periodically evaluated for any signs of failure or over-retention and managed accordingly. The success rate of pulpectomy in deciduous teeth is quite satisfactory.

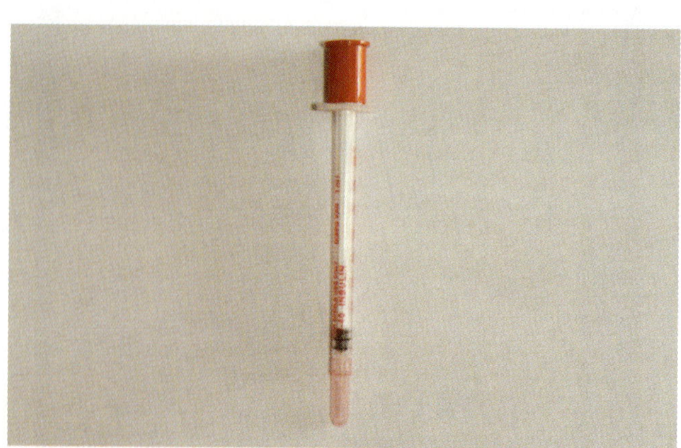

Fig. 28.14 Insulin syringe

VIII. Apexification/Apexogenesis

The diseased anterior primary teeth are usually extracted because they have shown to create developmental defects in permanent successors. In rare conditions (aggressive rampant caries), apexification using calcium hydroxide/tricalcium phosphate has been tried.

In permanent teeth the closure of apex may take three years after eruption. Certain factors may interfere with the normal development of the root. Because of the important role of Hertwig's epithelial root sheath in continued root development after pulp injury, effort should be made to maintain its vitality.

The clinical situation may vary:

- In case of immature tooth with vital pulp, apexogenesis is undertaken to preserve the vitality and allowing completion of root development (Fig. 28.15a and b).
- In case the immature tooth with necrotic pulp, apexification is performed to induce a calcific barrier at the open apex (Fig. 28.16a and b).

The details of the procedure being followed is described in Chapter 25.

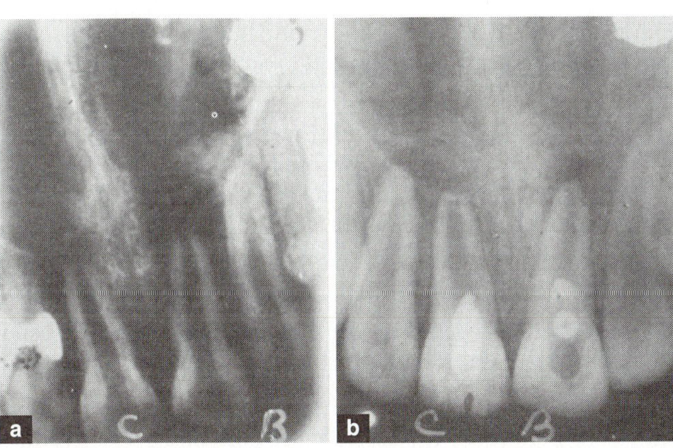

Fig. 28.15 (a) Immature tooth with vital pulp; (b) Normal development of root

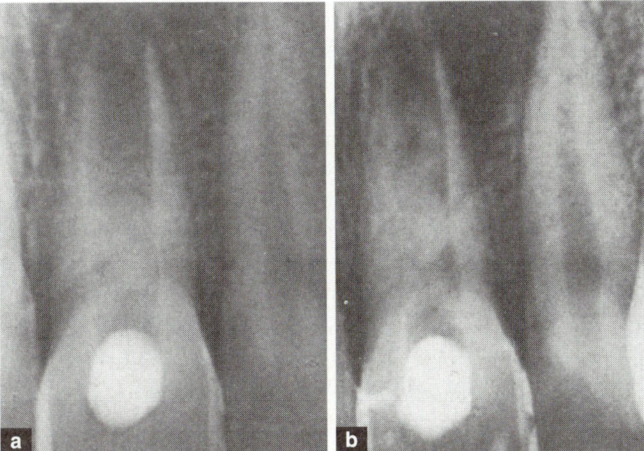

Fig. 28.16 (a) Immature tooth with non-vital pulp; (b) Apexification undertaken

USE OF ANTIBIOTICS IN PEDIATRIC ENDODONTICS

Antibiotics play an important role in pediatric endodontics. Systemic antibiotics have been extensively used for the management of odontogenic infections. The antibiotics should be selected based on age, overall state of the patient's health and up to date microbiological knowledge. The ideal duration of antibiotic therapy should be capable of preventing both clinical and microbiological relapse.

The majority of infections of endodontic origin can be effectively managed without the use of antibiotics. Chemo-mechanical debridement with drainage through the root canal system or by incision and drainage of soft tissue, help in healing process.

Topical antibiotics have been widely used as intracanal medicaments. Bacteria within the root canals are inaccessible to irrigation and the mechanical cleaning process. It is opined that antibiotics induced within the canal may be able to diffuse into inaccessible areas to reduce the number of viable bacteria and improve periapical healing.

Prophylactic antibiotics should be given to prevent infective endocarditis as recommended by American Heart Association. These can also be prescribed before long duration procedures.

BIBLIOGRAPHY

1. AAPD. Guidelines on pulp therapy for primary and immature permanent teeth. Pediatric Dent.: 2012; 34:222–229.
2. Ahmed HM. Anatomical challenges, electronic working length determination and current developments in root canal preparation of primary molar teeth. Int. Endod. J.: 2013; 46:1011–1022.
3. Ahmed HM. Pulpectomy procedures in primary molar teeth. Eur. J. Gen. Dent.: 2014; 3:3–10.
4. Aminabadi NA, Farahani RMZ and Gajan EB. Study of root canal accessibility in human primary molars. Journal of Oral Sci.: 2008; 50:69–74.
5. Andreasen JO, Farik B and Munksgaard EC. Long-term calcium hydroxide as a root canal dressing may increase risk of root fracture. Dent. Traumatol.: 2002; 18:134–137.
6. Ansari G. and Ranjpour M. Mineral trioxide aggregate and formocresol pulpotomy of primary teeth: a 2-year follow-up. Int. Endod. J.: 2010; 43:413–418.
7. Barcelos R, Santos MP, Primo LG, Luiz RR and Maia LC. ZOE cement paste pulpectomies outcome in primary teeth: A systematic review. J. Clin. Pediatr. Dent.: 2011; 35:241–248.
8. Barja-Fidalgo F, Moutinho-Ribeiro M, Oliveira MAA and de Oliveira BH. A systematic review of root canal filling materials for deciduous teeth: Is there an alternative for Zinc oxide eugenol? ISRN Dent.: 2011; ID367318, 1–7.
9. Bawazir OA, Salama FS. Clinical Evaluation of Root Canal Obturation Methods in Primary Teeth. Pediatr Dent.: 2006; 28:39–47.

10. Caicedo R, Abbott PV, Alongi DJ and Alarcon MY. Clinical, radiographic and histological analysis of the effect of mineral trioxide aggregate used in direct pulp capping and pulpotomies of primary teeth. Aust. Dent J.: 2006; 51:297–305.
11. Carrotte P. Endodontic treatment for children. Br. Dent. J.: 2005; 198:9–15.
12. Cerqueira DF, Mello-Moura AC, Santos EM and Guedes-Pinto AC. Cytotoxicity, histophathological, microbiological and clinical aspects of an endodontic iodoform-based paste used in pediatric dentistry: A review. J. Clin. Pediatr. Dent.: 2008; 32:105–110.
13. Chandrashekhar S and Shashidhar J. Formocresol, still a controversial material for pulpotomy: A critical literature review. J. Rest. Dent.: 2014; 2:114–124.
14. Chen J and Jorden M. Materials for primary tooth pulp treatment: The present and the future. Endod. Topics: 2012; 23:41–49.
15. Cleghorn BM, Boorberg NB and Christie WH. Primary human teeth and their root canal systems. Endod. Topics: 2010; 23:6–33.
16. Coll JA, Josell S and Casper JS. Evaluation of a one-appointment formocresolpulpectomy technique for primary molars. Pediatr. Dent.: 1985; 7:123–129.
17. Coll JA. Indirect Pulp Capping and Primary Teeth: Is the primary tooth pulpotomy out of date? Pediat. Dent.: 2008; 30:230–236.
18. Dean JA, Mack RB, Fulkerson BT and Sanders BJ. Comparison of electrosurgical and formocresolpulpotomy procedures in children. Int. J. Pediat. Dent.: 2002; 12:177–182.
19. Fidalgo FB, Ribeiro MM, Oliveira MAA andde Oliveira BH. A systematic review of root canal filling materials for deciduous teeth: Is there an alternative for zinc oxide eugenol? ISRN Dent.: 2011; 1–7.
20. Fuks AB, Guelmann M and Kupietzky A. Current developments in pulp therapy for primary teeth. Endod. Topics: 2012; 23:50–72.
21. Fuks AB. Vital pulp therapy with new materials for primary teeth: New directions and treatment perspectives. J. Endod.: 2008; 34:S18–24.
22. Gangwar A. Antimicrobial effectiveness of different preparations of calcium hydroxide. Ind. J. Dent. Res.: 2011; 22:66–70.
23. Garcia-Godoy F. Evaluation of an Iodoform paste in root canal therapy for infected primary teeth. J. Dent. Child: 1987; 54:30–34.
24. Georgi AC and Camp JH. Root canal treatment in primary teeth: a review. Pediatric Dent.: 1983; 5:33–37.
25. Gould JM. Root canal therapy for infected primary molar teeth—Preliminary report. J. Dent. Child.: 1972; 39:269–273.
26. Hegde V. Pediatric Endodontics- Endodontist's view. People's J. Sci. Resch.: 2001; 4:71.
27. Hibbard ED and Ireland RL. Morphology of the root canals of primary molar teeth. J. Dent. Child: 1957; 24:250–257.
28. Hill MW. The survival of vital and non-vital deciduous molar teeth following pulpotomy. Aust. Dent. J.: 2007; 52:181–186.
29. Hori A, Poureslami HR, Parirokh M, Mirzazadeh A and Abbott P. The ability of pulp sensibility tests to evaluate the pulp status in primary teeth. Int. J. Pediat. Dent.: 2011; 21:441–445.
30. Karayilmaz H and Kirzioglu Z. Evaluation of pulpal blood flow changes in primary molars with physiological root resorption by laser Doppler flowmetry and pulse oximetry. J. Clin. Pediatr. Dent.: 2011; 36:139–144.
31. Liu H, Zhou Q and Qin M. Mineral trioxide aggregate versus calcium hydroxide for pulpotomy in primary molars. Chin. J. Dent. Res.: 2011; 14:121–125.
32. Liu JF, Chen LR and Chau SY. Laser pulpotomy of primary teeth. Pediat. Dent.: 1999; 21:128–129.
33. Lucas Leite AC, Rosenblatt A, da Silva Calixto M, da Silva CM and Santos N. Genotoxic effect of formocresol pulp therapy of deciduous teeth. Mutat. Res.: 2012; 747:93–97.
34. Markovic D, Zivojinovic V and Vucetic M. Evaluation of three pulpotomy medicaments in primary teeth. Eur. J. Pediat. Dent.: 2005; 6:133–138.
35. Mesbahi M, Talei Z, Mollaverdi F and Kadkhodazadeh M. Comparison of root canal system configuration in primary teeth. Res. J. Biol. Sci.: 2010; 5:488–491.
36. Milnes AR. Is formocresolobsolete? A fresh look at the evidence concerning safety issues. J. Endod.: 2008; 34:S40–46.
37. Moghaddam KZ, Mehran M and Zadeh HF. Root canal cleaning efficacy of rotary and hand files instrumentation in primary molars. Iran. Endod. J.: 2009; 4:53–57.
38. Moretti ABS, Sakai VT, Oliveira TM, Fornetti APC, Santos CF, Machado MAand Abdo RCC. The effectiveness of mineral trioxide aggregate calcium hydroxide and formocresol for pulpotomies in primary teeth. Int. Endod. J.:2008; 41:547–555.
39. Moskovitz M, Sammara E and Holan G. Success rate of root canal treatment in primary molars. J. Dent.: 2005; 33:41–47.
40. Moskovitz M, Yadav D, Tickotsky N and Holan G. Long-term follow up of root canal treated primary molars. Int. J. Pediatr. Dent.: 2010; 20:207–213.
41. O'Sullivan SM and Hartwell GR. Obturation of a retained primary mandibular second molar using mineral trioxide aggregate: A case report. J. Endod.: 2001; 27:703–705.
42. Odabas ME, Bodur H, Barus E and Demir C. Clinical, Radiographic, and Histopathologic Evaluation of Nd:YAG Laser Pulpotomy on Human Primary Teeth. J.Endod.: 2007; 33:415–421.
43. Oncag, O, Gogulu D and Uzel A. Efficacy of various intracanal medicaments against enterococcus faecalis in primary teeth: an in vivo study. J. Clin. Pediat. Dent.: 2006; 30:233–237.
44. Ounsi HF, Debaybo D, Salameh Z , Chebaro A and Bassam H. Endodontic considerations in pediatric dentistry: A clinical perspective. Int. Dent. South Afr.: 2009; 11:40–50.
45. Ozalp N, Saroglu I and Sonmez H. Evaluation of various root canal filling materials in primary molar pulpectomies: An in vivo study. Am. J. Dent.: 2005; 18:347–350.
46. Peng L, Ye L, Guo X, Tan H, Zhou X, Wang C and Li, R. Evaluation of formocresol versus ferric sulfate primary molar pulpotomy: a systematic review and meta-analysis. Int. Endod. J.: 2007; 40:751–757.

47. Praveen P, Anantharaj A, Venkataragahavan K, Rani P, Sudhir R and Jaya AR. A review of obturating materials for primary teeth. SRM Univ. J. Dent. Sci.: 2011; 20:1–3.

48. Ranly DM and Garcia-Goday F. Current and potential pulp therapies for primary and young permanent teeth. J. Dent.: 2000; 28:153–161.

49. Robinson S and Chan MF. New teeth from old: Treatment options for retained primary teeth. Br. Dent. J.: 2009; 207:315–320.

50. Rocha CT, Rossi MA, Leonardo MR, Rocha LB, Nelson-Filho P and Silva LA. Biofilm on the apical region of roots in primary teeth with vital and necrotic pulps with or without radiographically evident apical pathosis. Int. Endod. J.: 2008; 41:664–669.

51. Rodd HD, Waterhouse PJ, Fuks AB, Fayle SA and Moffat MA. Pulp therapy for primary molars. Int. J. Pediat. Dent.: 2006; 16:15–23.

52. Ruby JD, Cox CF, Mitchell SC, Makhija S, Chompu-Inwai P and Jackson J. A randomized study of sodium hypochlorite versus formocresol pulptotomy in primary molar teeth. Int. J. Pediatr. Dent.: 2003; 23:145–152.

53. Sari S and Okte Z. Success rate of Sealapex in root canal treatment for primary teeth: 3-year follow up. Oral Surg. Oral Med. Oral Path. Oral Radiol. Endod.: 2008; 105:e93–96.

54. Sarkar S and Rao AP. Number of root canals, their shape, configuration, accessory root canals in radicular pulp morphology. A preliminary study. J. Ind. Soc. Pedo. Prev. Dent.: 2002; 20:93–97.

55. Sheller B and Morton TH. Electrosurgical pulpotomy: A pilot study in humans. J. Endod.: 1987; 13:69–76.

56. Somnez A, Oba A and Almaz ME. Revascularization/ regeneration performed in immature molars: case reports. J. Clin. Pediat. Dent.: 2013; 37:231–234.

57. Takushige T, Cruz E, Asgor MA and Hoshino E. Endodontic treatment of primary teeth using a combination of antibacterial drugs. Int. Endod. J.: 2004; 37:132–138.

58. Tan JME, Parolia A and Pau AKH. Intracanal placement of calcium hydroxide: A comparison of specially designed paste carrier technique with other techniques. BMC Oral Health: 2013; 13:1–7.

59. Torres CP, Apicella MJ, Yancich PP and Parker MH. Intracanal placement of calcium hydroxide: A comparison of techniques, revisited. J. Endod.: 2004; 30:225–227.

60. Trairatvoraku C and Chunlasikaiwan S. Success of pulpectomy with zinc oxide-eugenol vs calcium hydroxide/ iodoform paste in primary molars: a clinical study. Pediat. Dent.: 2008, 30:303–308.

61. Tunc ES and Bayrak S. Usage of white mineral trioxide aggregate in a non-vital primary molar with no permanent successor. Aust. Dent. J.: 2010; 55:92–95.

62. Vostatek SF, Kanellis MJ, Weber-Gasparoni K and Gregorsok R. Sodium hypochlorite pulpotomies in primary teeth: a retrospective assessment. Pediat. Dent.: 2011; 33:327–332.

63. Wang YL, Chang HH, Kuo CI, Chen SK, Guo MK, Huang GF and Lin CP. A study on the root canal morphology of primary molars by high-resolution computed tomography. J. Dent. Sci.: 2013; 8:321–327.

64. Waterhosue PJ, Nunn JH and Whitworth JM. An investigation of the relative efficacy of Buckley's formocresol and calcium hydroxide in primary molar vital pulp therapy. Br. Dent. J.: 2000; 188:32–36.

65. Waterhouse PJ. Formocresol and alternative primary molar pulptotomy medicaments: a review. Endod. Dent. Traumatol.: 1991; 11:157–162.

66. Witherspoon DE, Small JC, Regan JD and Nunn M. Retrospective analysis of open apex teeth obturated with mineral trioxide aggregate. J. Endod.: 2008; 34:1171–1176.

67. Zarzar PA, Rosenblatt A, Takahashi CS, Takeuchi PL and Costa Junior LA. Formocresol multagenicity following primary teeth pulp therapy: An in vivo study. J. Dent.: 2003; 31:479–485.

68. Zoremchhingi JT, Varma B and Mungara J. A study of root canal morphology of human primary molars using computerized tomography: An in-vitro study. J. Ind. Soc. Pedod. Prev. Dent.: 2005; 23:7–12.

Chapter 29

Geriatric Endodontics

Geriatric dentistry is defined as the delivery of dental care to 'old population' involving treatment of problems associated with normal aging and age-related diseases. Presently, population over the age of 65 is considered as older adults, whereas 'old' individual is over the age of 75 (the chronological age may vary in different parts of the world). In order to provide better oral health care, it is mandatory to focus on the knowledge and education in the field of geriatric dentistry.

Clinical management in elderly patients is becoming increasingly challenging as older people are aware of their health and related ailments. The challenges include biological and psychological differences from the younger patients as well as treatment complications in older population. Older adults now prefer saving their teeth at any cost. Over the years, the preservation of the natural dentition has been so successful that tooth loss is no longer accepted as inevitable. Endodontic treatment is less traumatic than extraction/implantation, etc. especially in older patients; systemic problems may also necessitate opting for less traumatic procedure in older adults.

The quality of life for older patients can be improved by saving teeth through endodontic treatment, which can have a significant impact on oral, physical and mental health. The National Institute on Aging has suggested that all oral health professionals should receive education concerning treatment of older adults as part of their basic professional learning.

As the body ages, retrogressive changes take place in body tissues. Similarly age changes do affect oral-dental tissues.

CHANGES DUE TO AGING IN ORAL DENTAL TISSUES

i. *Changes in enamel*

- Loss of enamel (tooth substance loss) due to attrition, abrasion and erosion
- Decrease in permeability
- May become brittle

ii. *Changes in pulp-dentin complex*

- The number and size of odontoblasts and fibroblasts in pulp decrease; odontoblastic processes degenerate with age (fewer odontoblastic processes extend to dentinoenamel junction).
- Remaining cells of pulp become less active.
- Number of collagen fibers of pulp increase (increased fibrosis with age may not be due to formation of collagen; persistence of connective tissue sheath in an increasingly narrow pulp space may be the reason).
- Number of blood vessels and nerve fibers decrease.
- Prevalence of occurrence of denticles (pulp stones) increases both in coronal and radicular pulp.
- Pulpal arteries may demonstrate arteriosclerotic changes; decrease of the lumen size, resulting in thickening and hyperplasia of elastic fibers.
- Calcification of pre-capillaries and arterioles may be seen (Fig. 29.1).
- Pulp tissues recede due to secondary and tertiary dentin formation (Fig. 29.2a and b).

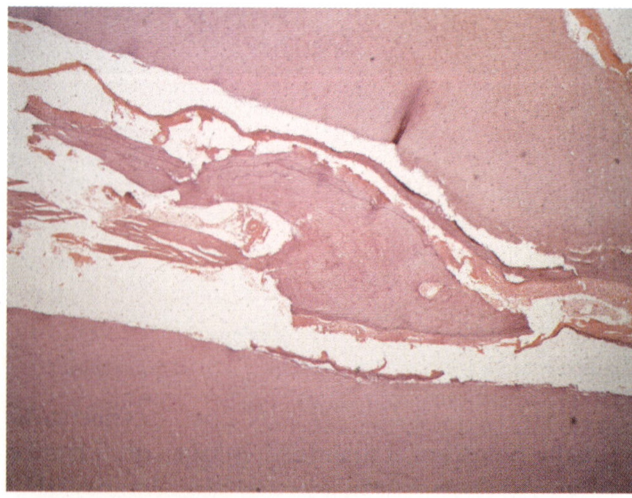

Fig. 29.1 Diffuse calcification in an aged pulp

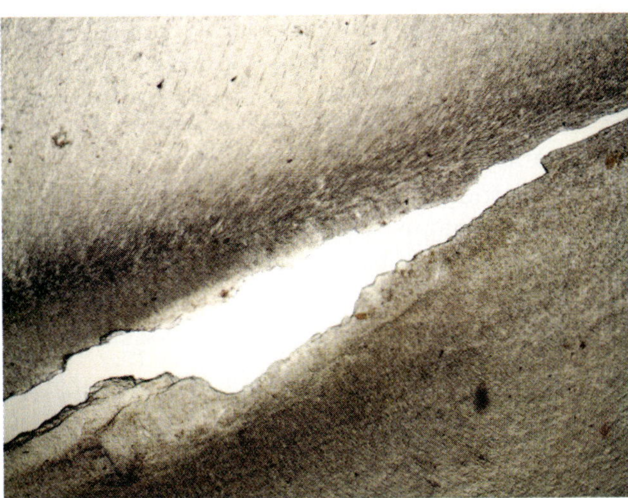

Fig. 29.2a Decreased pulp volume by continuous deposition of dentin

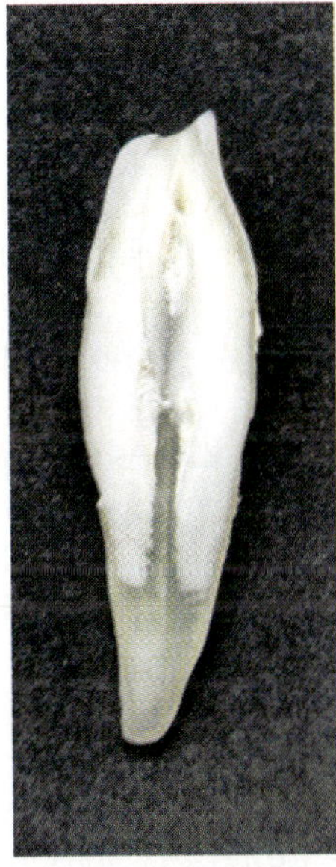

Fig. 29.2b Cut section of an old tooth showing attrition, reduced pulpal space and sclerotic dentin

- Primary dentin is formed before tooth eruption; whereas, secondary and tertiary dentin is formed as the age advances. The deposition of secondary and tertiary dentin varies in different teeth, such as:
  - In anterior teeth, secondary dentin deposition is in incisal area and in lingual wall of pulp chamber
  - In posterior teeth, secondary dentin deposition is in the floor of pulp chamber.
  - Tertiary dentin is also formed due to irritation by caries, trauma, etc. The tertiary dentin can fill the entire pulp chamber.
  - In general, pulp volume is inversely proportional to age; as age increases, pulp size decreases. The overall canal size decreases as the cementodentinal junction moves farther from the radiographic apex with continued cementum deposition.
  - The calcification process associated with aging appears to be of a linear type. Dentinal tubules become more occluded with advancing age; decreasing tubular permeability. Lateral and accessory canals can calcify; thus decreasing their clinical significance.

iii. *Changes in cementum/root*

- Continuous deposition of cementum (hypercementation)
- Apical root resorption
- Cementodentinal junction recedes

iv. *Miscellaneous changes*

- It is hypothesized that the older adults may exhibit adverse reaction to injury or they might be more resistant because of decreased permeability of dentin (no proven documentation).
- No change in periradicular tissues as regard cellularity and vascularity with age.
- Similar pattern of healing in young and old (critical to healing is vascularity).
- Systemic conditions may affect endodontic treatment prognosis at any age.

ENDODONTIC TREATMENT IN ELDERLY PATIENTS

Endodontic procedures in the elderly have always been challenging due to various psychological and technical perspective. The long-term planning for the older adults has become more critical. Every phase of the treatment is important from geriatric point of view. The endodontic treatment protocol in elderly is described as follows.

a. History and Clinical Examination

It is important to focus on factors that indicate the probable risks involved in treating the older patient. Clinician must recognize that the biological age of an individual is far more important than chronologic age.

In general, aging may lead to changes in the cardiovascular, respiratory and central nervous systems that warrant intake of drugs. The decline in renal and liver function in older patient should also be considered when predicting interaction of drugs that may be used in dental treatment. The elderly usually takes more drugs than the general adult population and so the adverse drug reactions are more common in these patients. It is important that the clinician take a careful history and regularly update the same in consultation with the patient's physician.

The intraoral and extraoral examination provides valuable information about the previous treatment. The factors that contribute to oral cancers accumulate with age; many systemic diseases may manifest such signs and symptoms.

Missing teeth contribute to reduced functional ability. The resultant loss of chewing efficiency leads to intake of softer and more cariogenic foods. Saliva plays a significant role in the maintenance of oral and general health. Aging may not have direct role on salivary secretion; however, salivary hypofunction can be due to excessive use of medications. Xerostomia affects more than 30% of population above the age of 65. Xerostomia leads to increased susceptibility of dysphagia and caries.

The compensating bite produced by missing and tilted teeth can cause temporomandibular joint dysfunction or loss of vertical dimension. Diminished eruptive forces with age, however, reduce the amount of mesial drift and supraeruption.

Gingival recession exposes cementum and dentin, which creates sensitivity. The excavation of root caries may irritate the pulp; may lead to pulp exposures. Exposures of pulp on one root surface of a multi-rooted tooth can result in uncommon clinical situation of the presence of both vital and non-vital pulp tissue in the same tooth.

Attrition, abrasion and erosion also expose dentin through a slower process that allows the pulp to respond with dentinal sclerosis and reparative dentin. The reduced organic component of the dentin may increase susceptibility to cracks and cuspal fractures. Pulpal exposures caused by cracks may not present acute problems in older patients.

Periodontal disease may be the principal problem for older adults. The relationship between pulpal and periodontal disease can be expected to be more significant with age. Patients with diabetes have increased periodontal disease and may have a reduced likelihood of success of endodontic treatment, especially in case with preoperative periradicular lesion.

The dental pain usually has a pulpal or periapical origin that may require root canal treatment or extraction. The status of pulpal or periapical disease is to be ascertained to finalize treatment modality. It is emphasized that pulpal symptoms are usually chronic in older patients; the sources of pain should be ruled out before some diagnosis is arrived at. Older patients may have had the experience of both the treatments and know the practical implications.

29

Orofacial pain is more common in elderly and significantly more prevalent in females. This might be due to hormonal changes that occur in females with age. The possibility of non-odontogenic pain should be kept in mind when treating elderly. Pain associated with vital pulps usually reduces with age. The severity also diminishes over time. The healing capacity may and may not be reduced; however, necrosis may occur quickly after microbial invasion.

The geriatric patients usually do not complain about signs and symptoms of pulpal and periapical disease, considering these to be of minor nature as compared to other ailments.

b. Diagnosis

Initial examination, such as palpation, percussion, etc. is carried out in routine. Transillumination can be effective to detect cracks, a common occurrence in elderly patients. The presence of micro cracks might not be significant in older teeth; however, vertical cracks can be the cause of pulpal or periapical diseases. The diagnostic features are:

i. *Pulp testing*

The response to stimuli may be weaker in elderly patients because of the fewer nerve branches present in older pulps. This may also be due to retrogressive changes resulting from mineralization of the nerve and nerve sheath.

- Slow and gentle testing should be carried out to determine status of pulp and periapical tissues (electric stimulus in patients with pacemakers is not recommended. The same caution holds true for electrosurgical units).
- Pulps with a high degree of pulpal calcification may give false negative result to thermal tests; electrical pulp testing can be effective as there is no difference of electric stimulation threshold between young and old pulps.
- A test cavity is generally less useful because of reduced dentin innervations.
- Discoloration of single teeth usually indicate pulp necrosis; however, in geriatric individual the reason may be different. Dentin gets thicker in older adults and the tubules become less permeable to breakdown products from the pulp. A yellow opaque color produced with age indicate progressive calcification.

ii. *Radiographs*

Radiographs are adjunct to diagnostic aids even in older adults. However, several physiologic, anatomic changes can significantly affect their interpretation. Film placement may be a problem in older patients; therefore, film holders are preferred. Sometimes, exposure time need to be increased to accommodate dense bone (bony changes can be effectively detected by digital radiography as compared to conventional radiography).

In older patients, pulp recession is accelerated by reparative dentin and complicated by pulp stones and dystrophic calcification. Minute pulp calcifications may not be visible on radiographs; however, receding pulp horns are apparent. Radiographs do detect a number of roots, root canals, size and configuration of pulp spaces and also the proximal caries.

c. Treatment Planning

The limited life expectancy coupled with psychological constraint in older adults should not alter the requisite treatment plan; do not plan compromised treatment in any case. It is important that all older patients be well informed of the probable risks and also the alternatives. Such patients deserve thorough explanation for their disease and treatment planning. Geriatric individuals are mostly cooperative and appreciative patients.

One-appointment procedures are usually preferred in older patients. The time span of one appointment should also be taken care of, as the elderly people may not be able to sit on the chair for long. The waiting period should also be managed.

The older patient should be evaluated psychologically to determine the ideal time of the day and length of time necessary to schedule treatment. Morning appointments are usually preferred for older patients. Some patients prefer afternoon visits to avoid early morning stiffness.

The retention of roots of excessively worn teeth is a desirable objective in older adults, as it maintains the alveolar bone. The loss of tooth roots is a known cause of alveolar bone resorption. The absence of tooth roots leads to resorption of alveolar bone. Moreover, loss of teeth alters the physical properties of the cortical mandibular bone, such as thickness, elastic/shear moduli and stiffness, subsequently weakening the mandible.

The procedures, such as, pulp capping, etc. are not as successful in older teeth as in younger ones; because of reduced blood supply.

d. Preparation before Endodontic Treatment

Before initiating endodontic procedures, the patient should be mentally prepared for the minor implications during and after the treatment. Patient's consent is important; patient's physicians consent and instructions, if any, should also be recorded. Patients should be made comfortable adjusting the chair position, light, etc. as per need of the patient. The use of pillow to support the neck improves patient comfort. A few patients prefer keeping pillow under the legs as well.

e. Endodontic Procedure

The endodontic procedure involves:

i. *Anesthesia*

The cutting of dentin does not produce the same level of response in an older patient as in young patients. The number of nerve endings in dentin is reduced, and they do not extend as far into the dentin as required. In addition, the dentinal tubules are more calcified. A painful response may not be encountered until very near to pulp or actual pulp exposure has occurred.

Older patients may accept treatment without anesthesia; preferably should be persuaded that anesthesia is necessary for their routine operative procedures.

Anatomic landmarks that are used as guides to needle placement during block and infiltration injections are usually more distinguishable in older patients; however, during supplementary intraligamentary injections, reduced width of periodontal ligament makes needle placement difficult.

The reduced volume of the pulp chamber makes intrapulpal anesthesia difficult in single-rooted tooth and almost impossible in multi-rooted teeth.

ii. *Isolation*

Reduction in salivary flow and gag reflex reduces the need for a saliva ejector and other isolation procedures. There might be a need to use artificial saliva. Elderly patients usually do not accept rubber dam placement.

iii. *Access cavity preparation*

The identification of canal orifices are usually difficult for older patients. The access cavity need to be deepened to visualize and negotiate the canal orifices. Aging may reduce the volume and coronal extent of the pulp chamber; however, the position of canals remain the same and can be negotiated during conventional, but deep access cavity preparation.

Location and penetration of the canal orifice are often difficult and time consuming in older adults because of narrow/calcified canals. Very few canals of older teeth, even maxillary anterior teeth, have adequate diameter to allow the effective use of broaches. Small files along with lubricants are preferred for negotiation.

Magnification aids are mandatory in identification and instrumentation of geriatric root canals.

iv. *Preparation (cleaning and shaping)*

The physiological narrowing of root canals resulting from the aging process presents a different clinical situation as compared to calcification/obliteration resulting in younger individuals. The physiological narrowing of root canals (calcification) is more concentric and linear. This allows easier preparation of canals once they are negotiated.

The canal in the elderly should be flared to facilitate irrigation procedure; it reduces stress on root canal.

Calcified canals may reduce the clinician's tactile sense in identifying the constriction clinically. Increased incidence of hypercementosis makes it difficult to assess the accurate positioning of the terminus. Reduced periapical sensitivity in older adults may lead to inadvertent penetration of apical foramen. Instrumentation with crown-down technique reduces instrument stress and also chances of instrument separation.

v. *Obturation*

The obturation procedures in geriatric patients should not generate pressure in the mid-root area, which may lead to root fracture. Passive placement of the obturating material is preferred. Resilon/thermoplasticized gutta-percha provides an effective seal in older adults. Permanent restoration should also be placed as soon as possible to maintain stomatognathic system.

vi. *Repair after endodontic treatment*

Repair of elderly patients is normally delayed due to increase in atherosclerotic changes in blood vessels and also decrease in stimulation of bone formation (porosity of bone increases and mineralization decreases with age).

Managing elderly endodontic patient: Key features

- Detailed history of systemic problems; intake of medication
- Short appointments, preferably during noon time
- Psychological motivation required
- Pillow for neck comfort in dental chair (may also be for legs)
- Mouth props for limited jaw opening
- Magnification to negotiate narrow/calcified canals
- Isolation should be managed without rubber dam
- Modification in access preparation (deep access cavity)
- Rotary crown-down instrumentation to reduce treatment time
- Gentle pressure during instrumentation and obturation
- Vital pulp therapy may have lower success rate (not preferred in elderly)
- Judicious approach in case of retreatment
- Repair is delayed

Challenges in Treating Elderly Patients

Treating elderly patients are always challenging for the clinicians. The operator must exercise patience and satisfy these patients according to their needs. The features, which can be challenging during endodontic procedures are:

- Heavy restorations (already restored teeth) may interfere with endodontic diagnosis and treatment
- Pulp calcification may create problems in negotiating the canals
- Periodontal problems in geriatric patients affect prognosis of the treatment.
- Isolation procedures pose difficulties as these patients may suffer from breathlessness, gagging, etc.
- Since healing may take longer period, the geriatric individual should be kept informed and assessed periodically.
- Geriatric patients should be given utmost respect to keep them psychologically motivated.

Management of Root Exposure

Root exposure is universally prevalent in older individuals. The root exposure may lead to root caries and/or loss of cementum leading to exposure of dentin. It may involve pulp. Gingival recession is the apical shift of marginal gingiva from its normal position on the crown of the tooth to the level on the root beyond the cementum-enamel junction. The esthetics is also compromised in case of recession and/or root caries (Fig. 29.3a and b).

The exposed root(s) should be covered to overcome the problem of sensitivity and to improve upon the esthetics. The following conditions are mandatory for successful root coverage.

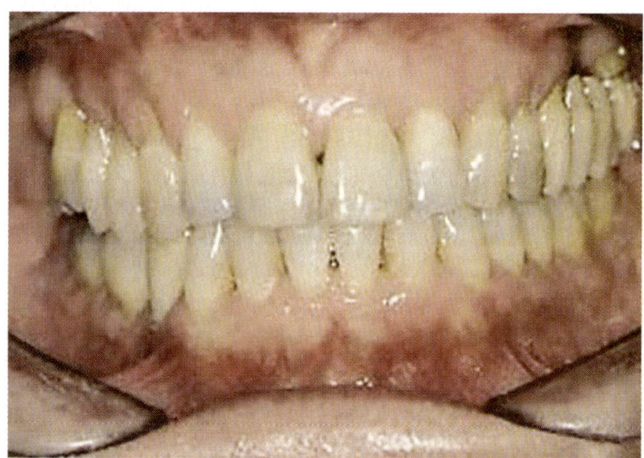

Fig. 29.3a Recession in multiple teeth

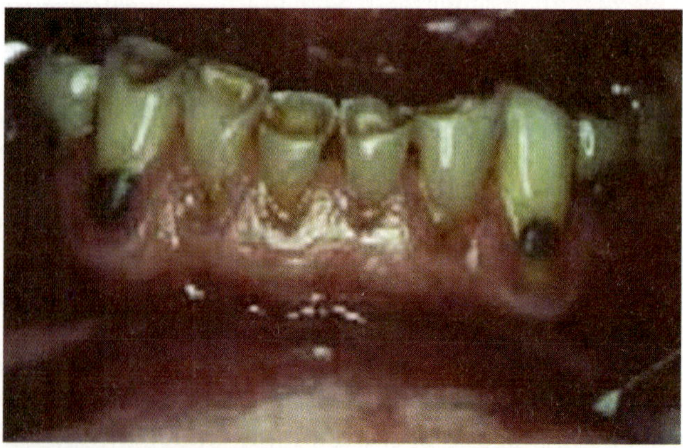

Fig. 29.3b Caries in multiple teeth

- Sufficient interdental papilla adjacent to gingival recession area
- Sufficient blood supply ensured to the donor tissue
- The decay/abrasion of root surface be managed prior to covering.

Minimum of 1.0–2.0 mm attached gingiva is adequate for covering; inflammation be kept under control.

The root coverage can be managed either by surgical or non-surgical methods.

a. Surgical Methods

- Pedicle soft tissue graft
- Free soft tissue graft
- Double papillary flaps
- Coronally advanced flaps
- Connective tissue grafts
- Guided tissue regeneration procedures

b. Non-surgical Methods

- Pink glass-ionomer cement (Fig. 29.4a and b)
- Gum veneers (Fig. 29.5a and b)

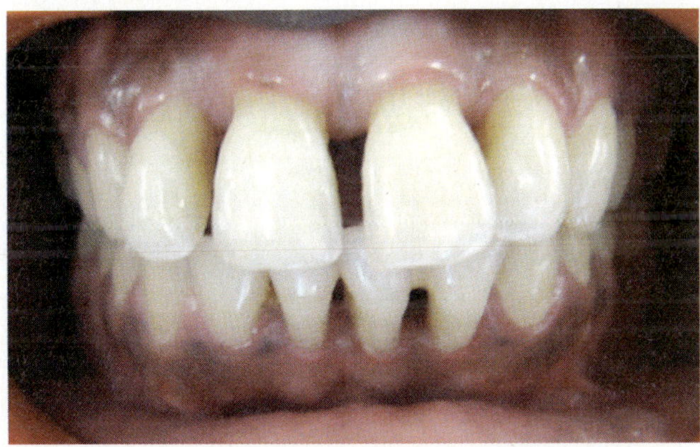

Fig. 29.4a Recession in aged patient (preoperative)

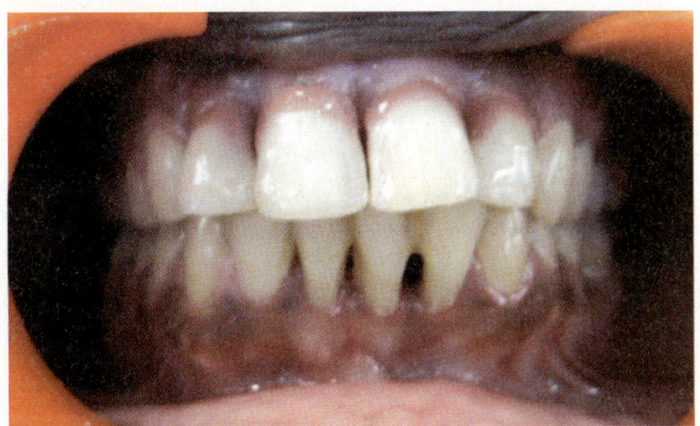

Fig. 29.4b Recession restored with pink glass-ionomer cement (postoperative)

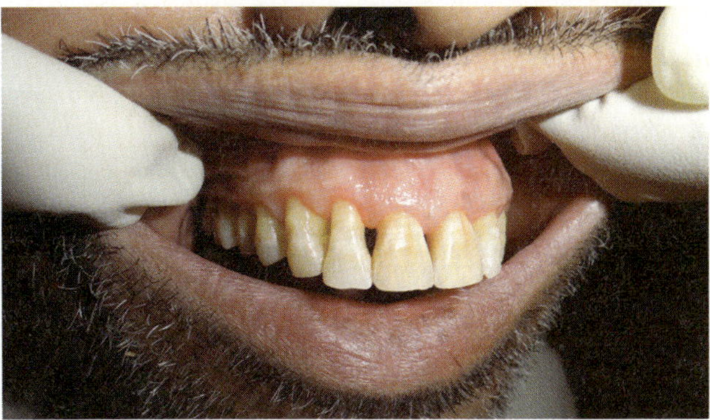

Fig. 29.5a Recession of anterior teeth in an old patient (preoperative)

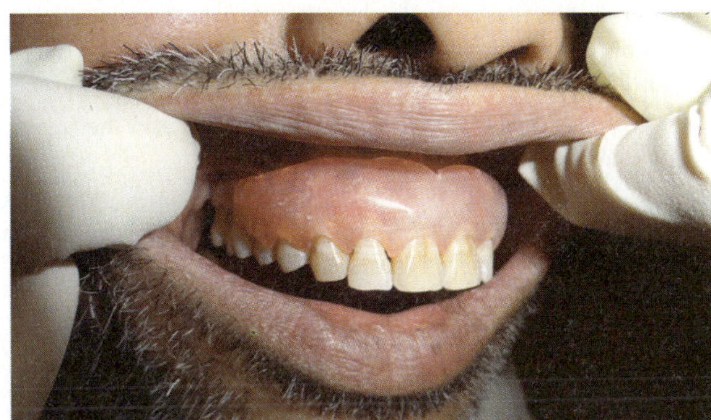

Fig. 29.5b Gum veneers to mask the recession (postoperative)

The non-surgical procedures are preferred in older adults as surgical procedures might not be very successful. The non-surgical methods improve esthetics, relatively inexpensive, painless and easily maintained by the older patients. They can also be used as interim measures till final treatment is being planned.

BIBLIOGRAPHY

1. Allen PF and Whitworth JM. Endodontic considerations in the elderly. Gerodontology: 2004; 21:185–194.
2. Arola D and Reprogen RK. Effects of aging on the mechanical behavior of human dentin. Biomaterials: 2005; 26:4051–4061.
3. Atkinson JC, Grisius M and Massey W. Salivary hypofunction and xerostomia: diagnosis and treatment. Dent. Clin. North Am.: 2005; 49:309–326.
4. Barjilay I and Tamblyn I. Gingival prosthesis—A review. J. Can. Dent. Assoc.: 2003; 69:74–78.
5. Bennett CG, Keelln EE and Biddington WR. Age changes of the vascular pattern of the human dental pulp. Arch. Oral Biol.: 1956; 10:995–998.
6. Berkey D, Berg RG, Ettinger RL, Mersel A and Mann J. The old-old patient: the challenge of clinical decision making. JADA: 1996; 127:321–332.

7. Bernick S and Nedalman C. Effect of aging on the human pulp. J. Endod.: 1975; 3:88–94.
8. Ciancio SG. Medications' impact on oral health. J. Am. Dent. Assoc.: 2004; 135:1440–1448.
9. De Rossi SS and Slaughter YA. Oral changes in older patients: a clinician's guide. Quint. Int.: 2007; 38:773–780.
10. Fridman M J.: Gingival masks: a simple prosthesis to improve the appearance of teeth. Compend. Contin. Educ. Dent.: 2000; 21:1008–1010.
11. George C. Evidence-based approach for treatment planning options for the extensively damaged dentition. CDA.: 2004; 32:983–990.
12. Gorduysus MO. Geriatric endodontics, clinical changes and challenges. EC Dent. Sci.: 2016; 7:38–40.
13. Gunay H, Guertsen W and Luhars A. Conservative treatment of periodontal recession with Class V defects using gingiva shade composite—a systematic treatment concept. Dent. Update: 2011; 38:124.
14. Johnstone M and Parashos P. Endodontics and the ageing patient. Aust. Dent. J.: 2015; 60:20–27.
15. Joshi N, Parolia A, Kundbala M and Manuel ST. A conservative method to reproduce lost gingival tissue—an innovative approach. Nepal Med. Coll. J.: 2009; 11:214.
16. Liu P, McGrath C and Cheugn G. What are the key endodontic factors associated with oral-health related quality of life? Int. Endod. J.: 2014; 47:238–245.
17. Mekayarajjananoth T, Kiat-annuary S, Sooksuntisakoonchal N and Salinen T. The functional and esthetic deficit replaced with an acrylic resin gingival veneer. Quint. Int.: 2002; 33:91.
18. Mysore AR and Aras MA. Understanding the psychology of geriatric edentulous patients. Gerodontology: 2012; 29: e23–27.
19. Perlea P, Nistor CC, Iliescu MG, Iliescu A, Aminov L, Vataman M and Iliescu AA. High risk in root canal neogiation in elderly patients: clinical case series. Endodontics: 2015; 5:52–58.
20. Qualtrough AJ and Mannocci F. Endodontics and the older patient. Dent. Update: 2011; 38:559–566.
21. Ranjitkar S, Taylor JA and Townsend GC. A radiographic assessment of the prevalence of pulp stone in Australians. Aust. Dent. J.: 2002; 47:36–40.
22. Ship JA, Pillemer SR and Baum BJ. Xerostomia and geriatric patient. J. Am. Geraiatr. Soc.: 2002; 50:535–543.
23. Singh SK, Kanaparthy A, Kanaparthy R, Pillai A and Sandhu G. Geriatric Endodontic. J. Orofac. Res.: 2013; 3:191–196.
24. Sperber GH and Yu DC. Patient age is no contradiction to endodontic treatment. J. Can. Dent. Assoc.: 2003; 69:494–496.
25. Toto PD, Kastelic EF, Duyvejonck KJ and Rapp GW. Effect of age on water content in human teeth. J Dent Res 1971; 50:1284–1285.
26. Walton RE. Endodontic considerations in the geriatric patient. Dent. Cl. North Am.: 1997; 41:795–816.
27. Zander HA and Hurzeler B. Continuous cementum apposition. J. Dent. Res.: 1958; 37:1035–1044.

Chapter 30

Magnification in Endodontics

The art of dentistry is based on precision. The human eye may not be able to achieve the requisite precision on all occasions. Visualizing the oral cavity, more so the morphology of pulp spaces, always pose a challenge to the clinician. The unaided human eye can visualize only up to 0.2 mm (200 microns). This means that when two lines are drawn parallel to each other with a distance of 0.2 mm between them, the human eye can visualize it as two separate lines. If the separation is less than 0.2 mm, the eye will detect it as a single line.

Since long, higher magnifications have been used to study cell growth, division and mutation, etc. When working without magnification, head is to be forwarded at an angle which may cause muscle fatigue leading to a disease entity called *Tension Neck syndrome (TNS)*. Such patients complain of headache and pain in inter-scapular muscles leading to cervical disc degeneration or spondylosis. The magnifying devices can enhance working posture by maintaining set focal range (loupes) or by location of fixed binoculars (microscope) or on LCD screen (procedure scope). It is also emphasized that improper adjustments of these devices may worsen the existing pain and injury to neck muscles.

MAGNIFICATION TYPES

In earlier days magnifying lenses have been tried but with little success. The lenses had to be hand held by the operator. The magnification provided was not sufficient and also they suffered from spherical and chromatic aberrations.

There are three basic types of magnification; the loupes, procedure scope and the operating microscopes. Endoscope and orascope are also magnification gadgets.

i. Loupes

Loupes, also referred to as telescope, are usually used magnification device in dentistry. The loupes allow working with less than 25° forward movement of head leading to less muscle fatigue (Fig. 30.1).

There are three types of loupes:

- *Flat plane (single-lens) loupe*: It consists of a single lens, which is fairly inexpensive. However, plastic lens used might not be always correct. This type of loupe creates stresses compromising with posture [TTL-through the lens (fixed loupe)].
- *Galileian lens (two-lens) loupe*: Two lens system is a compact system providing up to 4.5X (magnification) [TTL—through the lens (fixed loupe)].
- *Prism loupe (prism roof design) folding the path of light*: Prism loupes are advanced type of loupes providing up to 6.0X. The lens can be flipped-up during a procedure. They provide a larger field of view from longer distance minimizing stress factor (flip up loupe).

Loupes, despite of providing the required magnification, have their own limitations. It limits to only one magnification. The loupe becomes heavier as the magnification increases. Loupes have a fixed focal

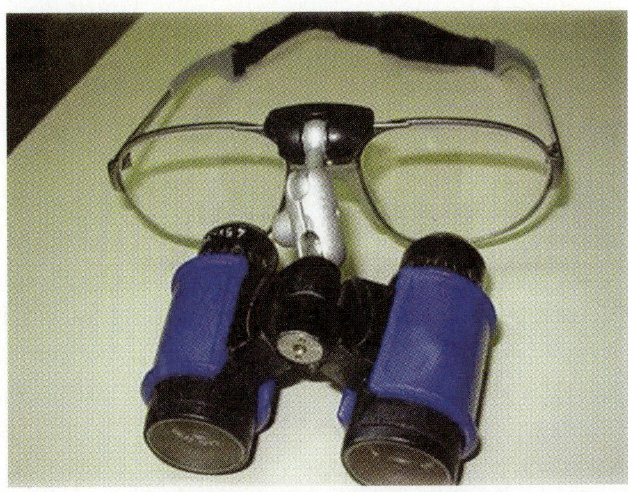

Fig. 30.1 Magnifying loupe

length; hence, do not contribute to ergonomics. Since the focal length of the loupes is fixed and cannot be changed, the distance from the lens to the object being narrow; the operator has to bend forward towards the patient in order to see the operative field clearly. The occupational stresses cannot be prevented. Illumination is achieved with a head gear, which casts shadow over the operating field.

Advantages

- Easy manipulation; no training required
- Inexpensive

Disadvantages

- Maximum magnification is 6X
- Accessories like beam—splitter and video camera cannot be attached to a loupe for better field magnification
- Higher magnification loupes are heavy (flip-up loupes)
- Image is not stable due to head movement

ii. Procedure Scope

The procedure scope offers optimal ergonomic benefits by facilitating neutral head posture. A camera is placed above the patient's oral cavity projecting up to 20X image onto a large flat LCD screen. The operator moves the camera freely over the patient's oral cavity while visualizing at the screen.

iii. Operating Microscope

The first microscope used in clinical procedures was introduced by Apotheker in 1981. In early eighties, Noah Chivian, an endodontist, introduced 8X microscope in the field of endodontics. Dr Carr introduced the first ergonomically configured operating microscope for routine endodontic procedures. The use of the dental operating microscope in endodontics has progressed over the years. Dr Carr's statement, *'You cannot treat what you cannot see'*, has inspired a great number of endodontists to add microscope to their normal armamentarium. He is aptly known as the *'Father of Microscopic Endodontics'*. According to Dr Carr, the microscope is simply an avenue for greater competence and that there are some procedures that can only be performed with a microscope and almost all procedures are performed more competently using a microscope. Microscopes provide us the ability to observe and evaluate at low power; subsequently, a higher power can be used for working and inspection. A well-illuminated field visualizing any area of the oral cavity is required to perform any procedure under the microscope.

The visual information provided by the operating microscope is, in fact, not indicative of the magnification that is being employed. The actual amount of visual information is the area under the scope (the number of horizontal pixels multiplied by the number of vertical pixels). A microscope at 10X (magnification) provides 100 times the amount of visual information compared to the naked-eye view (Table 30.1).

The comparison of different magnification aids is tabulated in Table 30.2. The comparative clinical implications are summarized in Table 30.3.

Table 30.1 Magnification and resolution of various magnification systems

Magnification device	*Magnification*	*Resolution (mm)*	*Resolution (microns)*
Unaided human eye	Nil	0.2	200
Low magnification loupes	2.5X	0.08	80
High magnification loupes	6X	0.05	50
Microscope (low)	6.4X	0.031	31
Microscope (med)	10X	0.02	20
Microscope (high)	20X	0.01	10

Table 30.2 Magnification and resolution of various magnification systems

Loupes	*Procedure scope*	*Microscope*
Usually fixed magnification (2 to 6X)	Variable magnification (2 to 20X)	Variable magnification (2 to 20X)
Focusing by neck	Focusing by camera	Focusing by microscope
No light	Standard light	Standard light
20°–40° forward head posture	Head posture near neutral	Head posture near neutral
Ordinary/standard equipment	Standard equipment	Micro equipment
3-D image convergence angle	2-D image on screen	3-D image binocular vision
Less expensive	Less expensive	Expensive

Table 30.3 Comparative clinical implications of magnification aids

Magnification type	*Head position*	*Vision*	*Operator movement*	*Direction of light*
TTL (fixed) loupes	20° to 40° forward	Three-dimensional (convergence angle)	Moderate movement, depends on working range of loupes	At an angle (less than 15°)
Flip-up loupes	20° to 30° forward	Three-dimensional (convergence angle)	Moderate movement, depends on working range of loupes	At an angle (less than 15°)
Procedure scope	Neutral	Two-dimensional (on screen)	Free movement	Parallel to operator's sight
Microscope	Neutral	Three-dimensional (binocular vision)	Restricted movement	Parallel to operator's sight

iv. Endoscope

The traditional endoscope consists of rigid glass rods with flexible and non-flexible variants. An optical lens with a diameter of 0.9 mm provides the clinician a magnification up to 20X.

An improved version of endoscope (2.7 mm lens diameter and 3.0 cm long rod-lens) is recommended for non-surgical procedures. The rod-lens endoscope provides greater magnification and a clear view of the field as compared to the loupes.

The Endoscope should not be used to retract gingival tissue while viewing a surgical field (assistant should preferably retract the gingival tissues). Hemostasis of the surgical site, is also important before using endoscope.

v. Orascope

An orascope is a fiberoptic endoscope. Fiberoptics are made of plastics; they are light weight and are flexible. The fiberoptic endoscope (orascope) is designed for intracanal visualization.

The focus and depth of field of orascope is from 0.0 mm to infinity (∞). This allows the orascope to provide imaging of apical end of the canal without actually inserting up to that level. Orascope facilitates visualization of the treatment field at various angles and distances without losing focus and depth of field.

A 0.8 mm fiberoptic size enables the orascope to go down into canal (canal is prepared up to size 80 or 90 at the coronal half before inserting orascope). Orascope visualization may be difficult in curved canals, because of limited flexibility of the instrument. The canal should be dried before viewing with orascope.

ERGONOMICS

Ergonomics is derived from Greek words, *'ergon'* meaning work and *'nomoi'* means natural laws; science of refining the design of products to optimize them for human use (literally known as engineering of human factors). One of the major advantages of the use of the dental operating microscope is the ergonomics associated with its use. The operating microscope allows the operator to sit in an upright, neutral and balanced posture with minimum neck, shoulder and lower back muscle fatigue. The increased comfort allows the operator to work more efficiently for longer periods of time. Since the eyes are focused at infinity, the eye strain is minimum. The operators working with the aid of a microscope use micro movements and light pressure.

Researchers studying human biometrics have measured the load on the neck and shoulder muscles and have found that the load doubles with every 2.0–3.0 centimeters the head shifts forwards from the ideal upward posture.

The ideal operator zones are in the 7 to 12 o'clock positions for right-handed operators, and 5 to 12 o'clock for left-handed operators. The key to proper ergonomics is to seat yourself first in the most comfortable and neutral position. The operator sits with his/her thighs parallel to the floor with the hips slightly elevated, feet planted firmly on the ground, shoulders erect, straight and perpendicular to the floor and arms stretched forwards with the elbows close to the body. The microscope is then adjusted to the eyes in this position without bending forward. The patient is adjusted between the hands to maintain this neutral position of the operator.

It has been reported that the most common reason for not using a microscope is the difficulty in positioning and adjusting the eyes of the operator. Mirrors are essential to examine the beveled root-end preparation in surgical endodontics, although direct vision is preferred over indirect, if convenient. An optimal operating position with a good front surface mirror is a critical factor in the successful use of operating microscope.

The most comfortable position of the operator is the 12 o'clock position for visualization of almost all teeth (Fig. 30.2). Right quadrant of the lower arch can also be visualized in the 9 to 11 o'clock positions. Advantage of the 9 to 11 o'clock positions is that they allow direct visualization of the occlusal surfaces of the teeth in the 3rd and 4th quadrant.

Common Terms used in Magnification

i. *Usable power*: Usable power is the maximum object magnification that can be used in a given clinical situation relative to the depth and size of the operative field. Increasing the magnification decreases the depth of field and narrows its size.
ii. *Viewing angle*: Angular position of optics allowing comfortable position of the operator.
iii. *Field of view*: Area visible under magnification.
iv. *Depth of field*: The distance between the nearest and the farthest objects.
v. *Working distance*: The distance from operator's eye to the treatment field.
vi. *Convergence angle*: Aligning of two oculars pointing at the identical distance and angle to the object or the field.
vii. *Declination angle*: The angle of operator's eyes that is inclined downward toward the work area is the declination angle.

Advantages of Microscope

- Detailed view of root canal intricacies enabling the operator to be more precise.
- Multiple choices of magnification with the twist of a knob, from 2X to 20X.
- Solve many traditional ergonomic problems associated with posture.

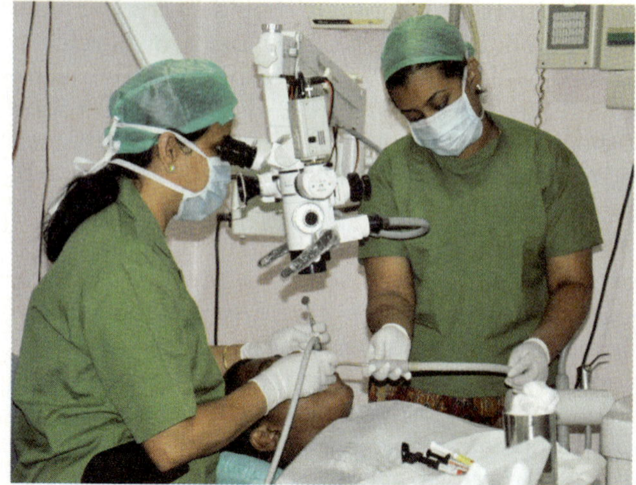

Fig. 30.2 Position of the operator

- A more relaxed eye position, as the optical properties of viewing through a microscope eliminate the need to converge the eyes for focus
- Illumination without shadows due to coaxial lighting from the microscope
- An apparent increase in fine motor skills due to increased visual acuity and visibility
- Documentation benefits from attachments in the form of digital photography and video productions.
- "Work satisfaction" in practice. Clinicians who utilize a dental microscope enjoy more during clinical procedures due to ideal working conditions and predictable treatment outcomes.

Disadvantages of Microscope

- Indirect vision with mirrors is inevitable in non-surgical endodontics. Left to right and right to left coordination is difficult initially.
- As magnification increases, the size and depth of field decreases and also the illumination.
- Four or six handed dentistry is mandatory. The assistant should be well trained to be able to anticipate and pass on the relevant instruments without the operator removing his/her eyes from the eyepiece.
- It slows down the operator; each procedure takes more time to perform under the operating microscope.
- The normal instruments are too bulky; hence smaller sized instruments are required.
- Cost of the microscope and accessories.
- Learning takes time.

Parts of the Microscope

The basic components of operating microscope include:

1. Magnification
   a. Eyepiece
   b. Binocular
   c. Magnification changers
   d. Objective lens
2. Illumination
3. Accessories

1. Magnification

Microscopes can provide magnification in the range of 2X to 20X and even more. Low magnifications are excellent for routine work having a wide field of view and a good depth of focus. Midrange magnifications are used for operative procedures. In endodontics, these are known as the "working magnification". Higher magnifications are used for specific tasks such as inspection of finer details, check resected root surfaces, locating extra canals, retrieving separated instruments, etc. The field of view and the depth of focus is reduced. Overall magnification is determined by the power of the eyepiece, focal length of the binoculars, the magnification change factor and the focal length of the objective lens.

The total magnification of a microscope is represented by the following formula:

$$\text{Total magnification} = \frac{\textbf{Focal length of tube}}{\textbf{Focal length of object length}} \times \text{Eyepiece power} \times \text{Magnification value}$$

Magnification: Point to remember

- If the focal length of the objective lens is increased, the magnification and the illumination is decreased, while the field of view is increased.
- If the focal length of the binoculars is increased, the magnification is increased and the field of view is decreased.
- If the magnification factor is increased, the magnification is increased and the field of view is decreased.
- As the magnification increases (may be the power of eyepiece), the field of view and the depth of field decreases.

a. *Eyepiece*: The eyepiece is available in powers of 6.3X, 10X, 12.5X ... and so on. They provide the desired magnification of an object along with the focal length and magnification change factors. The viewing side of each eyepiece has a rubber cup, which is turned down if the operator wears eyeglasses (Fig. 30.3).

It has adjustable diopter settings, which range from –5 to +5 and are used to adjust for accommodation (the ability to focus the lens of the eyes). The ability to accommodate decreases with age. They also adjust for refractive error (the degree to which a person needs to wear corrective eye glasses).

b. *Binoculars*: The function of the binoculars is to hold the eyepieces. It allows the adjustment of interpupillary distance. They are aligned manually or with a small knob until the two divergent circles of light combine to affect a single focus. It projects an intermediate image into focal plane of the eyepieces. As in a typical pair of field binoculars, the interpupillary distance is set by adjusting the distance between the two binocular tubes.

Binoculars are of different focal lengths. Longer the focal length of the binocular, the greater is the magnification. They are available as straight, inclined or inclinable forms.

i. *Straight Binocular*: Straight binocular is oriented parallel to the optical axis of the microscope. They have the advantage of allowing the use of direct vision in both the arches.

ii. *Inclined Binocular*: Inclined binocular is off set at an angle of 45°.

iii. *Inclinable Binocular*: Inclinable binocular (Fig. 30.4) is adjustable for positions up to and sometimes beyond 180°. This type of binocular is most useful for endodontic procedures including surgeries. It allows the operator to look directly at the maxillary and mandibular arches. It also provides postural comfort and flexibility.

c. *Magnification changers*: The dental microscopes have magnification changers (Fig. 30.5) to increase or decrease

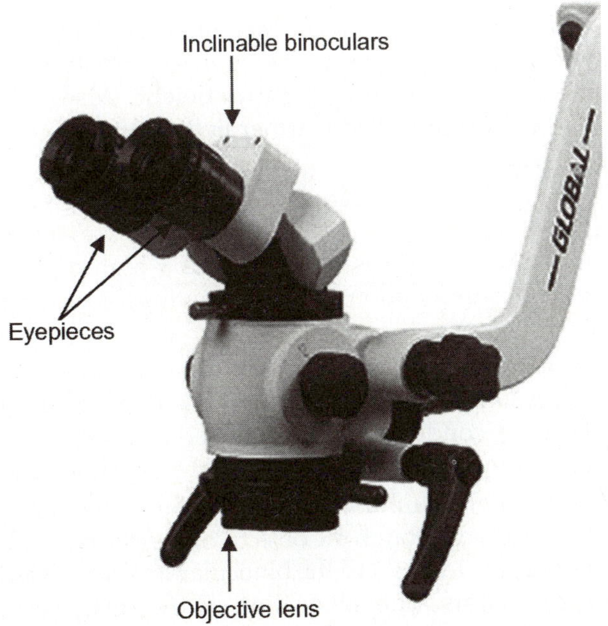

Fig. 30.3 Eyepieces and objective lens

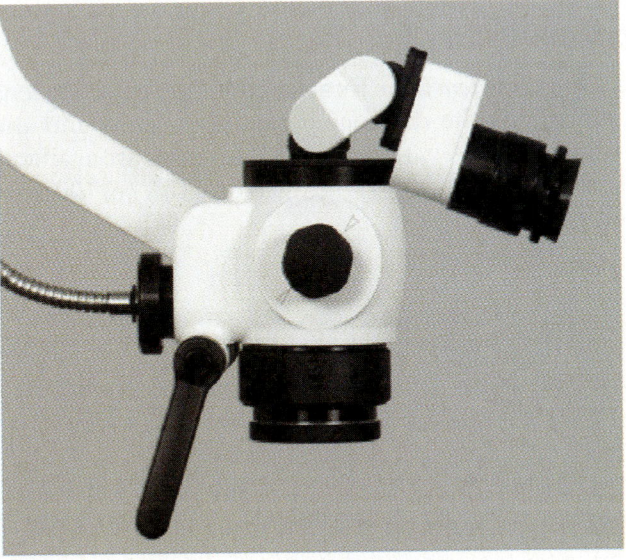

Fig. 30.4 Inclinable binocular

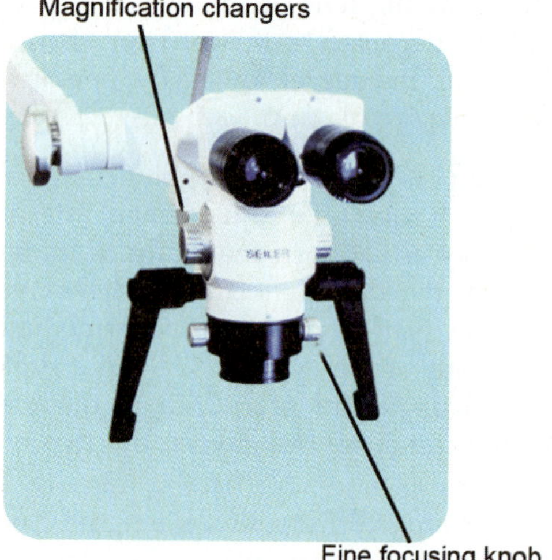

Fig. 30.5 Magnification changers

the magnification during operative procedures. These are available as 3 or 5 steps manual changers or power zoom changers. Located in the head of the microscope, it consists of lenses that are mounted on a turret. This turret is connected to a dial that is located on the side of the microscope housing. The dial positions (one lens in front of the other within the changer) produce a fixed magnification factor. Five-step changer has a second set of lenses mounted on the turret and produce five fixed powers of magnification. Rotating the dial reverses the lens position and produces a second magnification factor.

Power zoom changer is a series of lenses that move back and forth on a focusing ring to give a wide range of magnification factors. Advantage of power zoom changers is that it avoids momentary visual disruption, which is common using a 3 or 5 steps manual changer.

d. *Objective lens*: The focal length of the objective lens determines the distance between the lens and the surgical field. A variety of objective lenses are available with focal lengths ranging from 100 to 400 mm (Table 30.4).

Table 30.4 Distance between lens and operative field vs focal length of objective lens

Focal length of objective lens	*Distance between lens and operative field*
100 mm	4 inches
175 mm	7 inches
200 mm	8 inches
400 mm	16 inches

A 200 mm focal length and 8 inches distance is recommended so as to have adequate room to place surgical instruments and will be close to patients.

The dental operating microscope is focused much like a laboratory microscope. The manual focusing knob, which is usually located on the side of the microscope housing, changes the distance between the microscope and the surgical field.

Before the microscope is used, it is made parfocal (the process of setting the focus for the entire range of magnification for the operator). Parfocaling is operator specific. To parfocal a microscope, a flat object is placed under the scope and focused at the highest magnification. The right eye/left eye diopter settings are unique to each person and must be set individually. Once the microscope is parfocused, accessories such as cameras and auxiliary binoculars are also adjusted accordingly.

A microscope set up should have the following features for use in endodontic applications:

- 12.5x eyepiece power
- 125 mm inclined binocular
- 200 mm objective lens
- 5-step changer, ranging from 4X to 28X.

2. Illumination

The illumination in a microscope is from the light source. Three light source systems are available; 100W xenon halogen light bulb, metal halide light source and a quartz halogen bulb. The xenon light is brighter and produces light almost comparable to daylight; whereas, the halogen light produces a yellow picture.

The xenon light is better than quartz halogen, since the fiberoptic cables of halogen absorb light and have a tendency to be light deficient. Also, xenon projects a brighter and warmer light against bone and soft tissues.

The metal halide light is a compact, powerful, and efficient light source. It works under high pressure and temperature. Light is delivered via a high efficiency fiberoptic illumination, thus maintaining a cool surgical site.

The intensity of the light is controlled by a rheostat and the lamp is cooled by a fan. The light is reflected through a condensing lens to a series of prisms and then through the objective lens to the surgical field.

As the light illuminates the field, the reflected image is transmitted through the objective lens (the magnification changer lenses and the binoculars) as two separate optical beams. The separation of the image beams produces the stereoscopic effect necessary to assess the depth of field.

The illumination with the operating microscope is coaxial, i.e. the light is focused between the eyepieces in such a fashion that the clinician can look into the surgical site without any shadow. The microscope uses Galilean optics, which forms at infinity and send parallel beam of light to each eye. The eye fatigue is minimum. Loupes, on the other hand, rely on convergent vision that essentially requires an overlap of two images. This form of magnification leads to eye fatigue soon (Fig. 30.6).

In order to document the surgical proceedings, the reflected light after splitting made available to camera or auxiliary observation tube. This is known as *'beam splitter'* (Fig. 30.7). The beam splitter when inserted in the optical pathway of the microscope splits the light reflected from the surgical field and direct the image to a camera and/or an auxiliary observation tube. Depending on the split ratio, most of the light is available for the operator. A traditional 50/50 beam splitter contains two cube prisms. These prisms reflect 50% of the available light across the area of each prism through partially reflective coatings. The reflected portion of the light then goes through an iris diaphragm to a video camera. The other 50% is transmitted across the area of the cube prism to the primary user (Fig. 30.8).

3. Accessories

Many accessories are provided to facilitate movement during operative procedures.

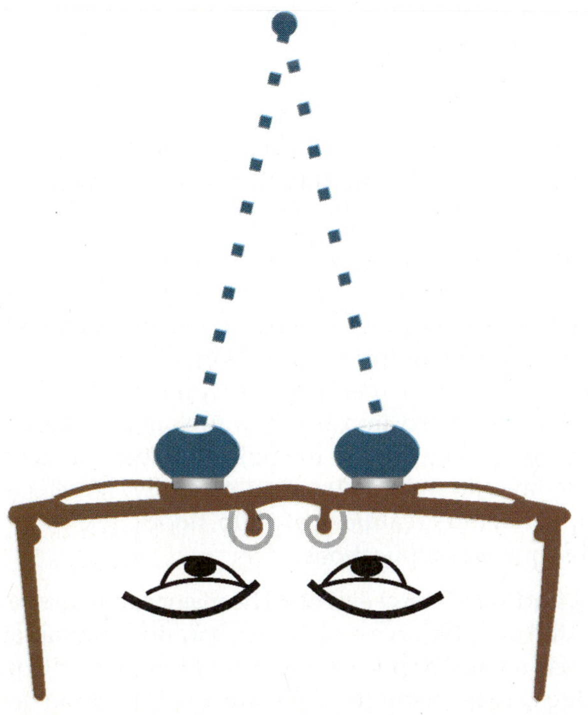

Fig. 30.6 Convergent vision leading to eye fatigue in loupes

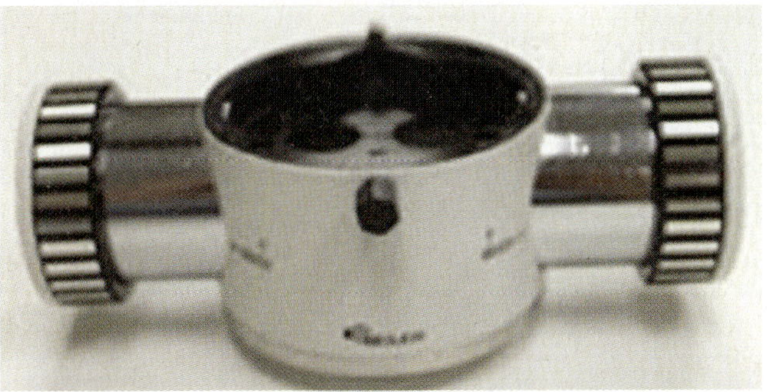

Fig. 30.7 Beam splitter

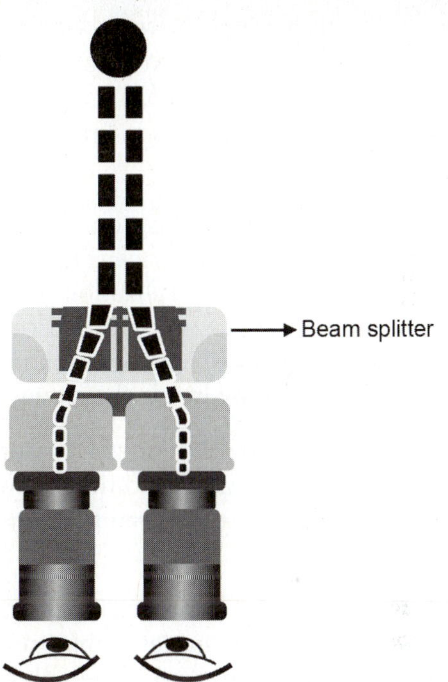

Fig. 30.8 Parallel vision created by beam splitter minimizing eye fatigue

- Pistol grip or bicycle style handles can be attached to bottom of the microscope to facilitate movement of the microscope during operative procedures. Either of these two types is essential for maneuverability.
- Observer tubes (auxiliary monocular or binocular) for assistants to see what the operator performs so that they can assist at the same magnification. LCD screen can also be provided for assistants.
- Camera and video adapters (Fig. 30.9) are used to attach video and digital cameras to the beam splitters for documentation of photographs and videos. These adapters should have the same focal length as the eyepiece so that the camera can record an image with the same magnification and field of view as that seen by the operator.

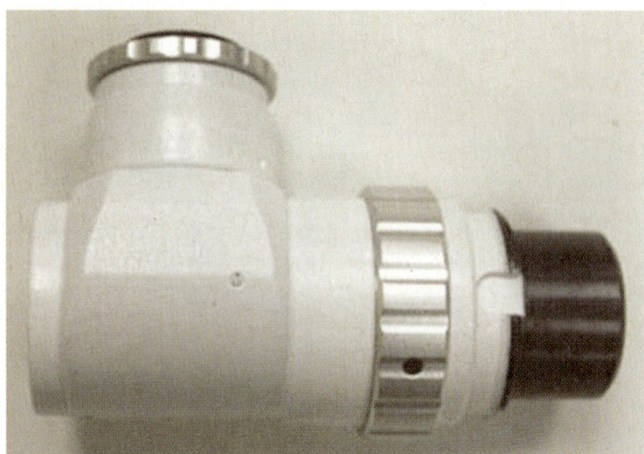

Fig. 30.9 Camera and video adapter

Uses of Operating Microscope in Endodontics

1. Diagnosis

a. *Diagnosis of caries*: Magnification is essential for diagnosing incipient dental caries (Fig. 30.10). The initial color alteration/demineralization on the tooth surface can only be diagnosed by microscope. High magnification makes it possible to detect hidden caries (microscopic signs of decay inside the crown).

b. *Soft tissue evaluation*: Soft tissue evaluation, in routine, may not require magnification. However, at times, inconspicuous sinus tract can be located using higher magnification.

c. *Identification of cracks*: The superficial fracture lines in the enamel are relatively undetectable with normal vision; however, when viewed under high power, definite cracks can be diagnosed (Fig. 30.11a and b).

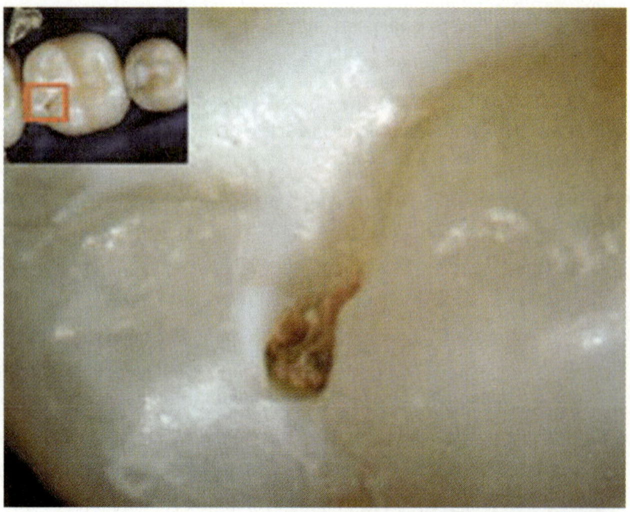

Fig. 30.10 Incipient caries

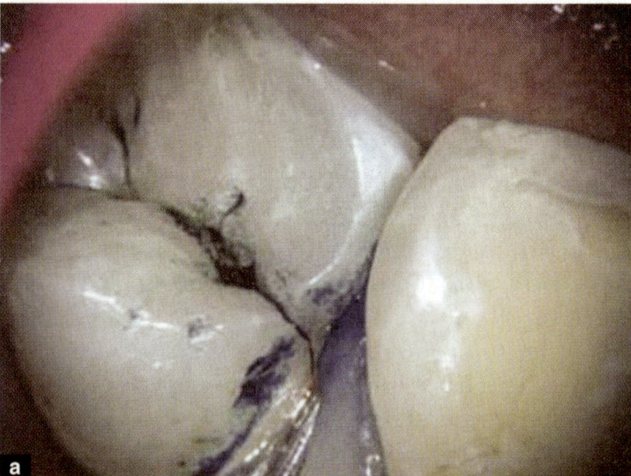

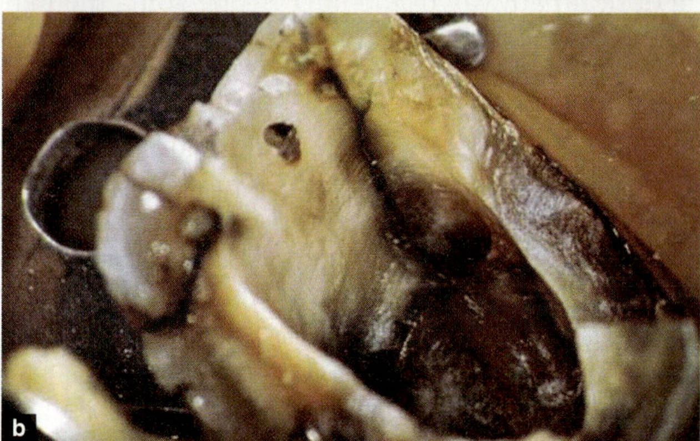

Fig. 30.11a and b Identification of cracks

2. Non-surgical Endodontic Procedures

The use of microscope has revolutionized non-surgical endodontics. The ability to visualize the root canal system in fine details help the operator to clean and shape it more efficiently. The dryness of root canal before obturation and distribution of sealer on the wall of the root canal during obturation can be better assessed. The microscope is helpful in following situations:

a. *Identification of anatomical landmarks*: The anatomy of pulp chamber and the anatomical landmarks in the pulp chamber, viz. overhanging walls of the roof of pulp chamber (Fig. 30.12), are better viewed using microscopes. The pulp stones, if any, are also removed in a better way using microscopes (Fig. 30.13). The floor of the pulp chamber is a delicate structure and is to be handled carefully. Microscopes help in better treatment of pulp floors, which avoid subsequent complications.

b. *Location of canal orifices*: The major canals are easily located once the access cavity preparation is completed. In case where the pulp chamber is obliterated with pulp stones, it is difficult to locate the canals orifices. Magnified views make it easier to recognize the dentin

30

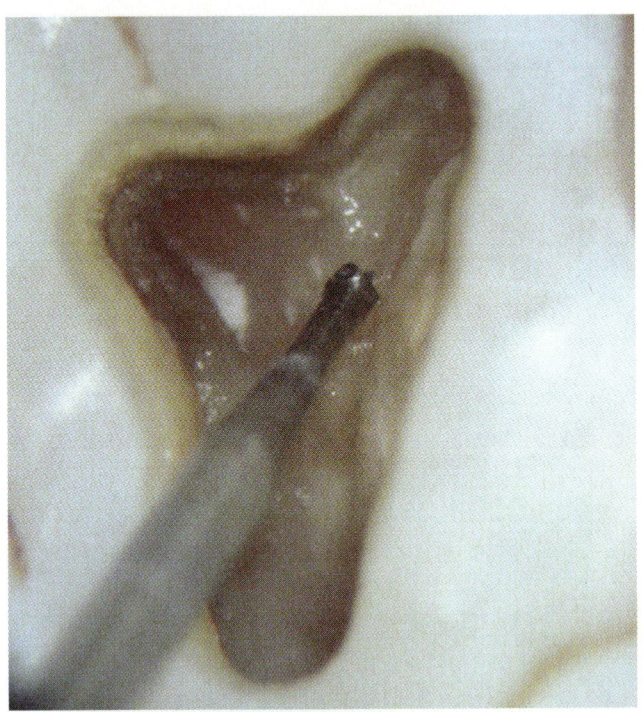

Fig. 30.12 Overhanging wall of roof of pulp chamber

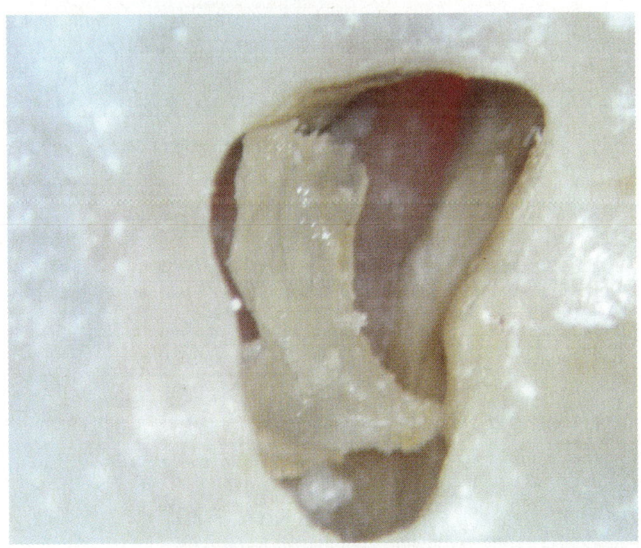

Fig. 30.13 Pulp stones

coverage over the orifice, which can be removed precisely with an ultrasonic instrument (Fig. 30.14).

c. ***Negotiating calcified canals***: Use of magnification along with ultrasonic troughing of the pulp chamber helps to identify and remove the calcifications including denticles. The operator can identify, which aspects of the pulp chamber walls prevent endodontic files from making straight line access. This ability allows for more conservative removal of tooth structure to improve endodontic access (Fig. 30.15).

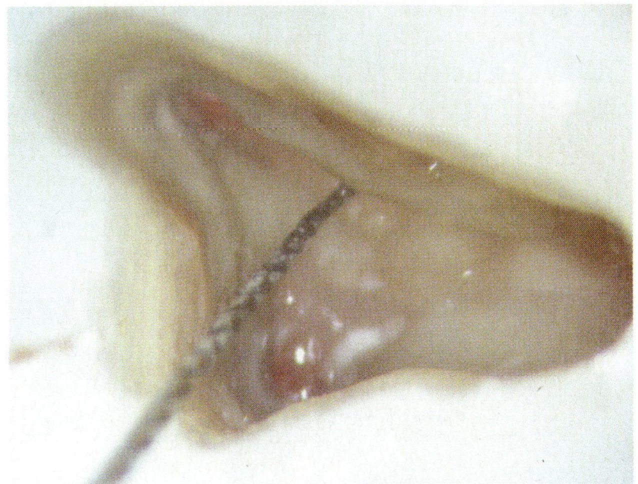

Fig. 30.14 Location of MB2 (removing dentin cover from the orifice)

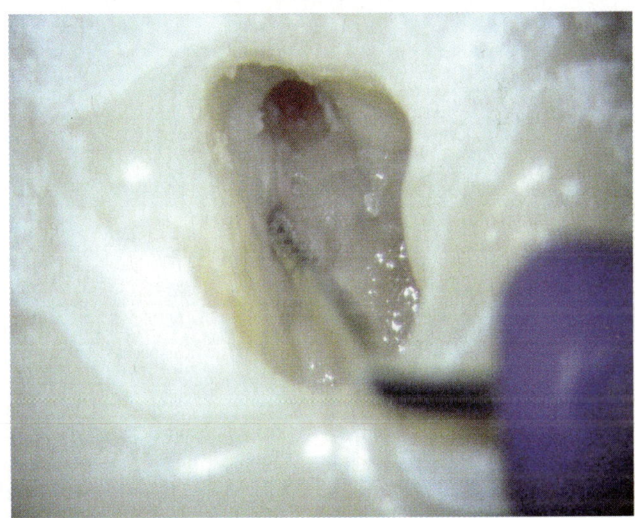

Fig. 30.15 Negotiating calcified canals

d. ***Identification of extra canals***: The variation in morphology of the pulp spaces is not an unusual phenomenon. The use of magnification and fiberoptic illumination has the better chances of locating extra root canals. The prevalence of second mesiobuccal canal in maxillary first molars has increased from 73% from the premagnification era to 93% in the microscope era (Fig. 30.16a). The identification of a middle mesial and middle distal canal in the mandibular first molars has also improved with microscope (Fig. 30.16b and c).

e. ***Identification of cracks and fractures***: After the access preparation, cracks can be detected on the floor of the pulp chamber. Radicular cracks, which may and may not extend vertically can also be identified (Fig. 30.10).

f. ***Removal of pulp tissue completely***: Magnification helps in identifying pulp tissue remnants from crevices

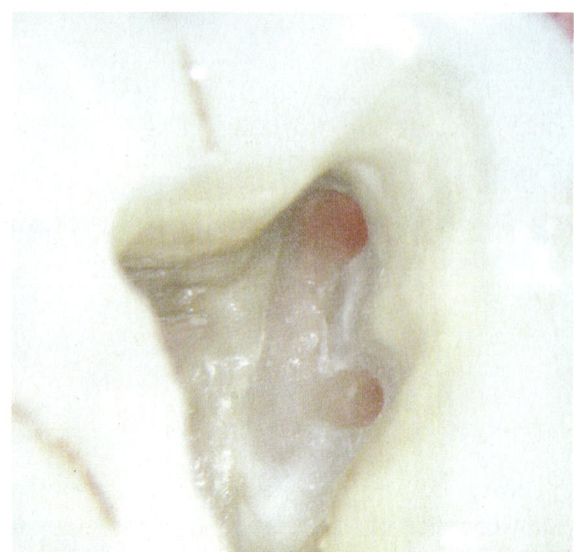

Fig. 30.16a Location of extra root canal

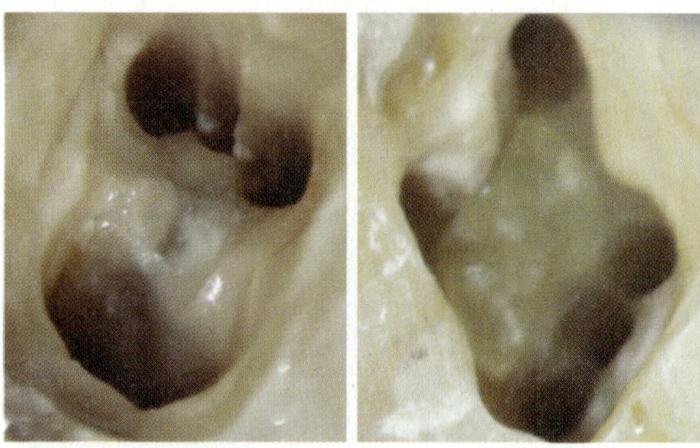

Fig. 30.16b Middle-mesial Fig. 30.16c Middle-distal

within the pulp chamber. Magnification can help removing pulp remnants from root canals, ensuing a cleaner canal (Fig. 30.17a and b).

g. *Retreatment*: The operating microscope has brought significant advantages of being able to perform successful non-surgical retreatment without the need for surgery. Procedures such as bypassing a ledge, removing a separated instrument or repairing a perforation have become more predictable (Fig. 30.18a and b). During post removal, identification of residual cement and the remaining dentin can be better carried out using microscope.

3. Surgical Endodontics

The operating microscope has improved the visualization of surgical field. The operator can visualize root and tooth anatomy in a better way and understand the reasons of errors during surgical procedures. The magnification, illumination and micro instruments constitute a microsurgical trial.

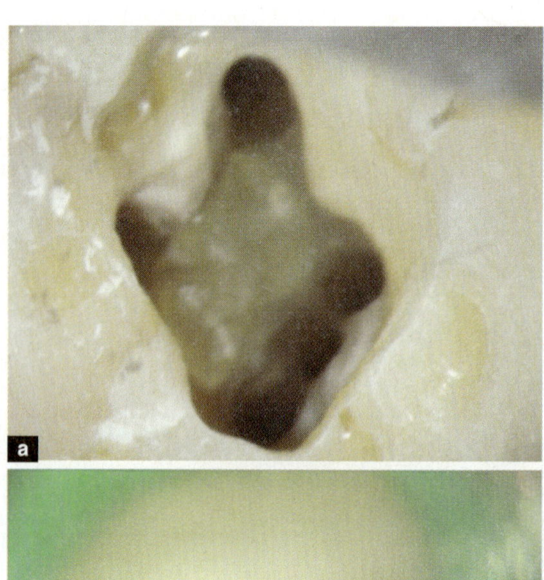

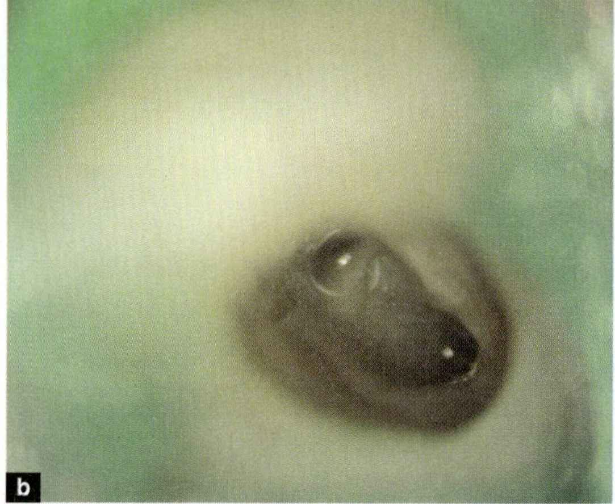

Fig. 30.17a and b Removal of pulp tissue

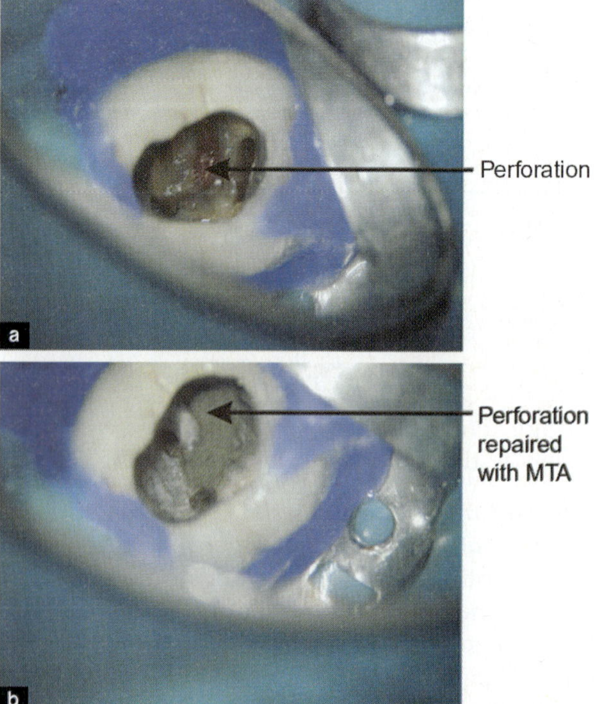

Fig. 30.18a and b Perforation repaired with MTA

A resected root under higher magnification easily reveals anatomical details, such as isthmus, canal fins and lateral canals. The ultrasonic instruments help in preparing the root-end in a precise manner (Fig. 30.19a and b). The differences between conventional and microsurgery are tabulated in Table 30.5.

Use of mini (micro) instruments

Magnification in endodontics facilitated miniaturization of routine and surgical endodontic instruments. The most important instrument required for micro endodontics is the micro-mirror (Fig. 30.20). These mirrors differ from the traditional mirrors in their size and shape. Smaller micro-mirrors are required since the operating field under the microscope has a limited area. A front surface mirror is preferred to eliminate the double image distortion seen with the normal mirrors. Micro mirrors are available as round (2.0 mm, 3.0 mm, 4.0 mm and 5.0 mm diameter), oval or rectangular mirrors. The size and shape can be selected depending upon the area available at the surgical site. Mini head handpieces are also available for inaccessible areas (Fig. 30.21)

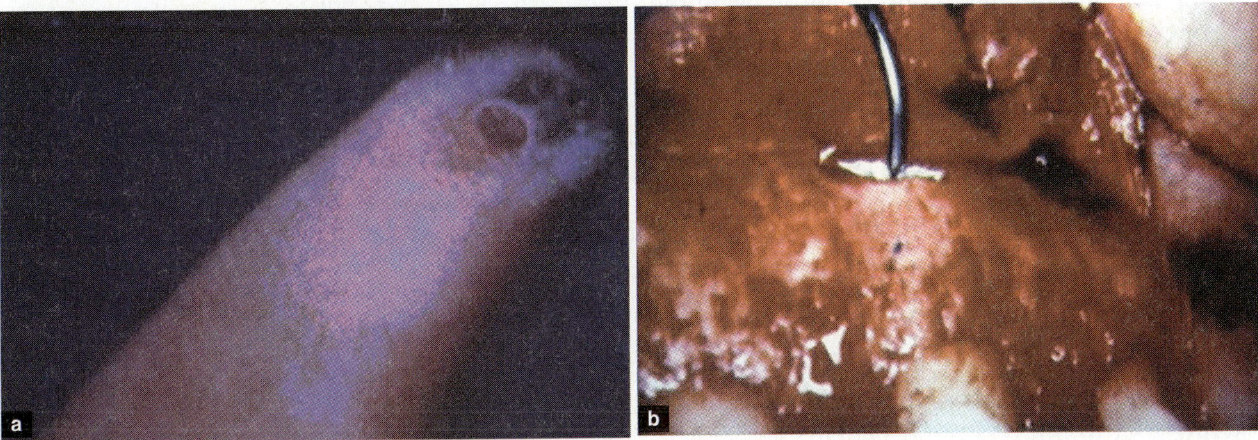

Fig. 30.19a and b Root-end prepared and retrograde filling

Table 30.5 Differences of conventional surgery and microsurgery

Procedure	*Conventional surgery*	*Microsurgery*
Identification of root apex	Difficult	Comparative easy
Size of osteotomy	Large (more than 1.0 cm)	Small (0.5 cm is sufficient)
Bevel angle	Acute (45°)	Shallow (10°)
Isthmus identification	Very difficult	Easy
Inspection of preparation	Difficult	Easy
Retrofilling	Approximate	Precise

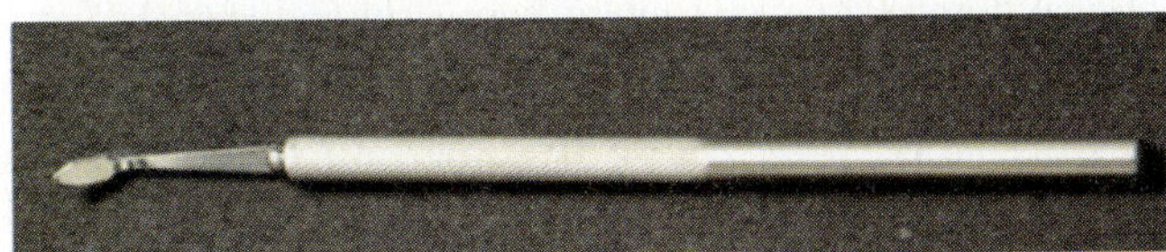

Fig. 30.20 Micro mirrors

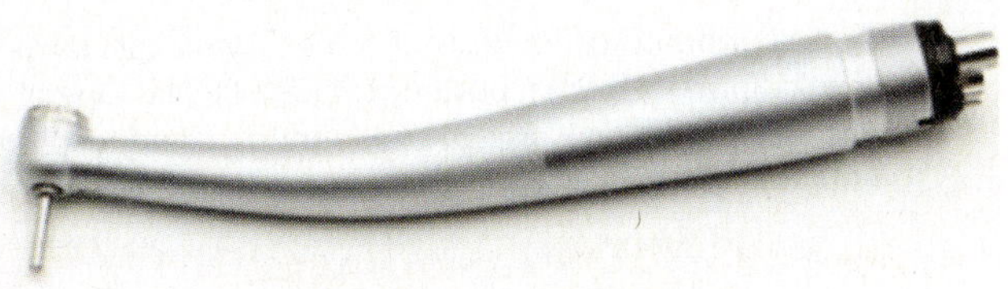

Fig. 30.21 Mini head handpiece

Use of ultrasonics in combination with microscopes

The advantages of operating microscope-ultrasonic combination are:

- Ultrasonic tips can be more effective to "move" the coronal shaping away from furcations, flutings, and other high-risk anatomical sites.
- Microscopic visualization is improved because the bulky head of a traditional handpiece is not a factor.
- Ultrasonics can be more effective and conservative at "sweeping" the access to de-roof the chamber
- The MB2 or calcified chambers in posterior teeth rely on a lateral, not apical, motion that benefits from the micro-ultrasonic combination.
- The cleaning and shaping of the canals can be better visualized rather than just relying on the "feel".

Various ultrasonic tips are available for different procedures, viz. tips for removal of calcifications, tips for root-end preparations, etc.

4. Documentation and Patient Education

The endodontic procedures can be videotaped using camera provided with microscope. The photographic evidence of the procedure, not only help in legal implications, but also in patient education. The clinical and radiographic features can be shown to the patient, in case some controversy arises, or for motivating the patient and family members.

Documentation is an important benefit of using the dental operating microscope. In this era of evidence based dentistry, cameras attached to the microscope help in recording and documenting the treatment procedures. It serves three purposes:

- Helps to educate the patients as well as the students.
- It is a mode of communication with the referral dental surgeon.
- Helps maintain legal documentation of the diagnosis and the subsequent treatment.

5. Marketing and Practice Management

The photography with microscope can be utilized as a marketing tool to impress upon patients and others regarding dental procedures being carried out in the clinic. These features definitely effect growth of the practice.

BIBLIOGRAPHY

1. Bachall JK and Barss JT. Orascopy: A vision for the new millennium, part 2. Dent. Today: 1999; 18:82–85.
2. Bahcall JK. Visualization in endodontics. Eur. J. Gen. Dent.: 2013; 2:96–101.
3. Bowers DJ, Glickman GN, Solomon ES and Jianing H. Magnification's effect on Endodontic fine motor skills. J. Endod.: 2010; 36:1135–1138.
4. Carr G. Microscopes in Endodontics: J Calif. Dent. Assoc.: 1992; 11:55–61.
5. Cunha RS, Davini F, Fontana CE, Miguita KB and Bueno CES. The micosonics concept: Maxillary first molar with five root canals: case report. South Braz. Dent. J.: 2011; 8:231–235.
6. De Carvalho MC and Zuolo ML. Orifice locating with a microscope. J. Endod.: 2000; 26:532–534.
7. Del Fabbro M and Tascheiri S. Endodontic therapy using magnification devices: a systematic review. J. Dent.: 2010; 38:269–275.
8. Dhingra A and Nagar N. Recent advances in endodontic visualization: a review. IOSR J. Dent. Med. Sci.: 2014; 13:15–20.
9. Donald EA. Introduction to Magnification. J Esthet. Restor. Dent.: 2003; 15:426–439.
10. Engelke W, Leiva C, Wagner G and Beltran V. In vitro visualization of human endodontic structures using different endoscope systems. Int. J. Clin. Exp. Med.: 2015; 8:3234–3240.
11. Fabbro MD. Endodontic therapy using magnification devices: a systematic review. J. Dent.: 2010; 38:269–275.
12. Feix LM, Boijink D, Ferreira R, Wagner MH and Barletta FB. Operating microscope in endodontics: Visual magnification and luminosity. South Brazilian Dent. J.: 2010; 7, 340–348.
13. Garcia A. Dental magnification: a clear view of the present and a close-up view of the future. Compend. Contin. Educ. Dent.: 2005; 26:459–463.
14. Girsch WJ and McClammy TV. Microscopic removal of dens invaginatus. J. Endod.: 2002; 28:336–339.
15. Lins CC, Silva EM, Lima GA, Menezes SE and Travassos RM. Operating microscope in endodontics: A systematic review. Open J. Stomatology: 2013; 3:1–5.
16. Louis JB, Michael JB, Ellen AB and Christopher SW. Effect of magnification on locating the MB2 canal in maxillary molars. J. Endod.: 2002; 28:324–327.
17. Mamoun JS. A rationale for the use of high powered magnification or microscopes in general dentistry. Gen. Dent.: 2009; 57:18–26.
18. Moshonov J and Nahlieli O. Endoscopy in endodontics. Alpha Omegan: 2011; 104:26–34.
19. Perrin P, Neuhaus KW and Lussi A. The impact of loupes and microscopes on vision in endodontics. Int. Endod. J.: 2014; 47:425–429.
20. Robinstein R. Magnification and illumination in apical surgery. Endodontic Topics: 2005; 11:56–77.
21. Rubinstein R. The anatomy of the surgical operating microscope and operating positions. Dent. Clinic. North Am.: 1997; 41:391–413.
22. Schwarze C, Baethge T, Stecher and Geurtsen W. Identification of second canals in the mesiobuccal root of maxillary first and second molars using magnifying loupes or an Operating Microscope. Aust. Endod. J.: 2002; 28, 57–60
23. Takatomo Yoshioka, Chihiro Kobayashi and Hideaki Suda. Detection rate of root canal orifices with a microscope. J. Endod.: 2002; 28:452–453.
24. Valachi B. Magnification in Dentistry: How ergonomic features impact your health. Dent. Today: 2009; 28, 132–134.
25. Von AT, Steiner RG and Tay FR. Apical surgery: endoscopic findings at the resection level of 168 consecutively treated roots. Int. Endod. J.: 2011; 44:290–302.
26. Yoshifumi Kinomoto, Fumio Takeshige, Mikako Hayashi, Shigeyuki Ebisu J. Optimal positioning for a Dental Operating Microscope during nonsurgical endodontics. J. Endod.: 2004; 30:860–862.

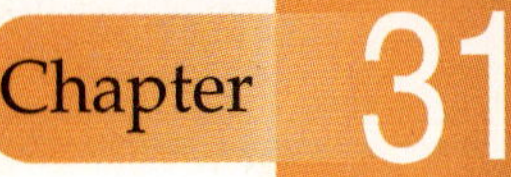

Chapter 31

Lasers in Endodontics

The development of Lasers has revolutionized every field of medical science, including endodontics. The investigators have been studying the effects of Lasers on oral hard and soft tissues. The areas of interest have been the reduction of dental caries through increased resistance of enamel due to alteration of enamel's structure, caries detection and removal, sterilization of dental instruments, disinfection and preparation of root canals, welding of orthodontic appliance and fixed prosthesis, therapy for soft tissue lesions and laser acupuncture.

Laser is a device that transforms light of various frequencies into a chromatic radiation in the visible, infrared and ultraviolet regions with all the waves in a phase capable of mobilizing immense heat and power when focused at a close range.

Laser is acronym for *'Light amplification by stimulated emission of radiation'*. The concepts of stimulated emission of radiant energy, the foundational basis for modern laser physics, were initially discussed in the literature by Einstein in 1917. The first laser was constructed by Theodore Harold Maiman in 1960 using synthetic Ruby (aluminium oxide doped with chromium oxide). The first lasers to be marketed for intraoral use were carbon dioxide lasers. The application of lasers for endodontics was first carried out by Weichman and Johnson.

PRINCIPLE OF LASER

If a microwave beam containing photons passes through a cloud of ammonia gas, the gas molecules will be raised to a higher energy state as energy is absorbed. Earlier, Einstein predicted that if a photon of correct size struck a molecule already in an excited state, that molecule would fall back to lower energy level and would emit a photon of exactly the same size and moving in the same direction as the entering photon. Thus, in case of ammonia gas, the molecules can undergo two possible changes, i.e. either moving to a higher state or being pushed back to a lower one. Normally, the first process would predominate but if the majority of molecules are already in a higher energy state (termed as population inversion) then the released photon will move in speed with the original photon. These two photons will strike two further molecules causing production of another two photons and the vicious reaction starts. This effect is known as MASER (Microwave amplification by stimulated emission of radiation). This principle was applied to the electromagnetic waves of light and the process was called LASER.

COMPONENTS OF LASER DEVICE

The laser device consists of:

1. ***Laser medium***: Laser medium determines the wavelength of the light emitted from laser. The names of dental lasers are based on the active medium that is to be stimulated. The active medium can be a gas (argon, carbon dioxide), a liquid (dyes) or a solid state crystal rod [neodymium: yttrium-aluminium-garnet (Nd:YAG), erbium-doped yttrium aluminium garnet (Er: YAG) or a semiconductor (diode lasers)].
2. ***Optical cavity/Laser tube/Optical screen***: It consists of two mirrors, one fully reflective and other partially transmissive; located on either end of the optical cavity.
3. ***Power source***: The power source excites or pumps the atoms of laser medium to their higher energy levels (Fig. 31.1).

Laser is a beam of very high intensity light. It differs from ordinary sun light and light of other sources, as lamps, etc. The striking features of laser light are:

- *Monochromatic*: Radiation in which the waves have single wavelength (color). Lasers are often designated by visible color, i.e. red light/green light laser.

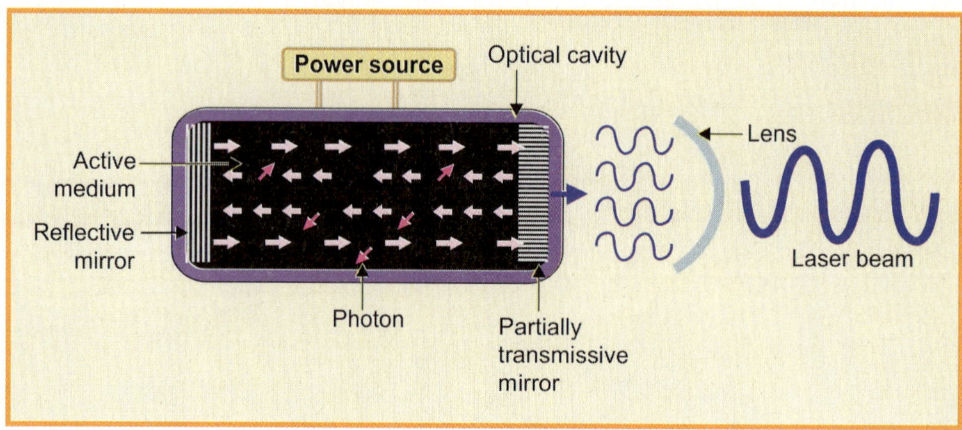

Fig. 31.1 The laser device

- *Coherent*: The waves are in a certain phase relationship to each other, both in space and time.
- *Collimated (directional)*: The emitted waves are nearly parallel and collimated; do not diverge (source even at a distance can be focused).
- Produce *intense and powerful* beam of light (power and beam quality affects this property).

Laser Delivery System

There are three delivery systems:

- *Articulated arms (with mirror at joints)*: For ultraviolet, visible and infrared lasers.
- *Flexible hollow waveguide*: A flexible hollow waveguide or tube has an interior mirror finish. The laser energy is reflected along this tube and it exits through the handpiece at the surgical end with the beam striking the tissue in a non-contact fashion.
- *Glass fiberoptic cable*: The third delivery system is a glass fiberoptic cable. This cable can be more pliant than the waveguide as it has a corresponding decrease in weight and resistance to movement, and is usually smaller in diameter (the delivery system of choice).

Laser Emission Modes

The dental laser device can emit the light energy mainly in two modalities as a function of time (third is the running mode):

- *Continuous (constant on) emission*: It is the continuous wave in which the beam is emitted at only one power level for as long as the operator depresses the foot switch.
- *Pulsed (pushed on and off) emission*: It is termed as a gated pulse mode having periodic alterations of the laser energy, much like a blinking light. This mode is achieved by the opening and closing of a mechanical shutter in front of the beam pathway of a continuous wave emission. It can be super-pulsed or ultra-pulsed depending upon the timings.
- *Running pulse mode*: Another mode is the running pulse mode, wherein large laser energy is emitted for an extremely short span, followed by no laser beam for a relatively long time.

The types of lasers and their mode of emission are tabulated in Table 31.1.

Table 31.1 Types of lasers and their mode of emission

Type of laser	*Active medium (wavelength in nm)*	*Mode of emission*
Gas laser	• Argon (488, 515) • Helium-Neon (633) • Carbon dioxide (10600, 10300, 9600)	• Continuous • Continuous • Continuous
Solid-state laser	• Nd:YAG (1064) • Er:YAG (2940) • Er:Cr:YAG (2780) • Ho:YAG (2100)	• Continuous/pulsed • Continuous/pulsed • Continuous/pulsed
Semiconductor laser (Diode)	• Gallium-Arsenide (GaAs) (904) • Gallium-Aluminium-Arsenide (GaAlAs) (780,890) • Indium-Gallium-Aluminium Phosphide (GaAlP) (630, 700)	• Continuous/pulsed • Continuous/pulsed • Continuous/pulsed

Mechanism of Laser Action

The possible mechanisms of laser action can be:

- *Photothermal ablation*: Photothermal ablation is used to vaporize or coagulate tissue through absorption in a major tissue component (occurs in high powered lasers).
- *Photomechanical ablation*: It causes the disruption of tissues due to a range of phenomena, such as shock wave formation, cavitations, etc.
- *Photochemical effects*: Light sensitive substances are used to treat specific tissues, such as cancer.

LASER TISSUE INTERACTION

Laser tissue interaction implies interaction of photons with the atoms or molecules of the target tissue. Lasers differently interact with the target tissue, depending on the optical properties of the tissue. The different ways of interaction are:

a. *Photobiological interactions*: The photobiological interactions are of four types:

i. *Absorption*: The desired interaction is the absorption of laser energy by the intended target tissue. This amount of energy that is absorbed by the tissue depends on the tissue characteristics, such as pigmentation (melanin of skin, hair and hemoglobin in blood), proteins and water content; and also on the laser wavelength and emission mode. Argon has a high affinity for melanin and hemoglobin in soft tissue.

ii. *Transmission*: This interaction is inverse of absorption; transmission of laser energy directly through the tissue without effecting it.

iii. *Reflection*: The incident laser beam redirects itself without affecting the target tissues.

iv. *Scattering*: Scattering of the reflected light weakens the intended energy and possibly produces no useful biologic effect; may transfer heat to the adjacent tissues.

b. *Photochemical interactions*: The basic principle of photochemical process is that specific wavelength of laser light is absorbed by naturally occurring chromophores (tissue compounds), which are able to induce certain biochemical reactions. Photosensitive compounds, when exposed to laser energy, can produce a single oxygen radical for disinfection of the root canals.

c. *Photothermal interactions*: The radiant energy absorbed by tissue substances are transformed into heat energy, which then produces the requisite effects (Table 31.2).

Table 31.2 Tissue effects with rise in temperature

Tissue temperature (°C)	*Observed effect*
50–60°C	Hyperemia
60°C to 100°C	Protein denaturation, welding, hemolysis, coagulation, shrinkage
100°C–150°C	Water in soft and hard tissue boils (vaporization or ablation)
200°C–400°C	Carbonization of organic material may occur
400–1400°C	Inorganic constituents melt and/or recrystallize and may vaporize

d. *Photomechanical and photoelectrical interactions*: These include photodisruption, photoplasmolysis and photoacoustic interactions. The pulse of laser energy on the dental tissues can produce a shock wave (photo acoustic effect of laser light), which may explode or pulverize the tissues with mechanical energy. Photoplasmolysis describes the removal of tissues through the formation of electrically charged ions.

Classification

Lasers have been classified depending upon the following features:

1. According to wavelength
   a. Excimer laser (wavelength 150–350 nm)
   b. Visible light laser (wavelength 350–750 nm)
      - Ruby laser
      - Argon laser
      - Helium-neon laser
   c. Infrared laser (wavelength 750–12000 nm)
      - Neodymium: Yttrium-aluminium-garnet (Nd:YAG)
      - Holmium: Yttrium aluminium garnet (Ho:YAG)
      - Erbium-doped yttrium aluminium garnet (Er:YAG)
      - Carbon dioxide laser
2. According to the type of laser medium
   a. Gas laser (argon, helium-neon, carbon dioxide)
   b. Solid-state laser (Nd:YAG, Er:YAG, Er:Cr:YAG, Ho:YAG)
   c. Semiconductor laser (Gallium-Arsenide, Gallium-Aluminium-Arsenide, Indium-Gallium-Aluminium-Phosphide)
3. According to tissues to be lased
   a. Soft tissue laser
   b. Hard tissue laser

4. According to potential hazards, lasers are classified according to American National Standard Institute's safety norms.
   - *Class I*: Do not pose a health hazard; inherently safe for eyes and skin (e.g. laser printers).
   - *Class II*: Emit only visible light with low power output (1.0 mW) and do not normally pose a hazard because of the normal blinking (aversion reactions) of eye, e.g. surgical laser [continuous staring should be avoided; staring more than 10000 seconds produce burning in retina; e.g. commercial laser scanner (referred to as class IIa)].
   - *Class III*:
     - Class IIIa: Any wavelength and output power less than 5 mW of visible light. It will not harm the unprotected eye within the blinking reflex (one-fourth of a second) period (e.g. laser printers).
     - Class IIIb: Can produce a hazard to the unprotected eye if viewed directly/from reflective light. Power output 500 mW (e.g. diode laser cutter).
   - *Class IV*: Extremely hazardous from direct viewing where the laser power is above 500 mW (e.g. lasers used in surgery).

This classification was accepted till 2002 and is designated as 'old classification'. The classification is modified now including concepts of 'maximum permissible exposure' (MPE) (The highest power or energy density, i.e. W/cm^2 of a laser source that is considered safe) and the 'accessible emission limit' (AEL) (the maximum power or energy, which can be emitted in a specified wavelength range and exposure time that passes at a specific distance).

The modified classification

Class 1: Safe under all conditions; maximum permissible exposure (MPE) cannot be exceeded when viewing a laser with naked eye or with microscope.

Class 1M: Safe under all conditions, except when passed through microscopes and telescopes.

Class 2: Safe because of blink reflex; applies to visible-light lasers (400–700 nm). Laser pointers and measuring instruments are in class 2.

Class 2M: Safe because of blink reflex, if not viewed through optical instruments.

Class 3R: Visible continuous lasers are limited to 5 mW (for pulsed lasers, this limit varies). 3R is considered safe with restricted beam viewing.

Class 3B: 3B laser is hazardous if exposed directly (direct viewing need protective eyewear). The accessible permissible emission limit (AEL) for continuum laser is 0.5W and wavelength 400–700 nm.

Class 4: Lasers exceeding 3B level of AEL; mostly unsafe for eyes and skin.

TYPES OF LASERS

a. Soft Tissue Lasers

The soft tissue lasers are athermic, low energy lasers that generally utilize the semiconductor laser diodes. Their wavelength stimulates cellular activity. They aid in tissue regeneration and wound healing by increasing collagen production by fibroblast stimulation (Figs 31.2 and 31.3). Soft tissue lasers are used to relieve pain, inflammation, edema and also accelerate healing.

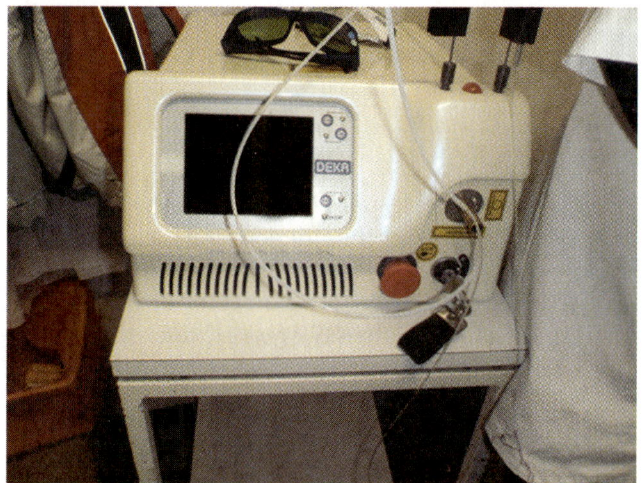

Fig. 31.2 Soft tissue laser by DEKA

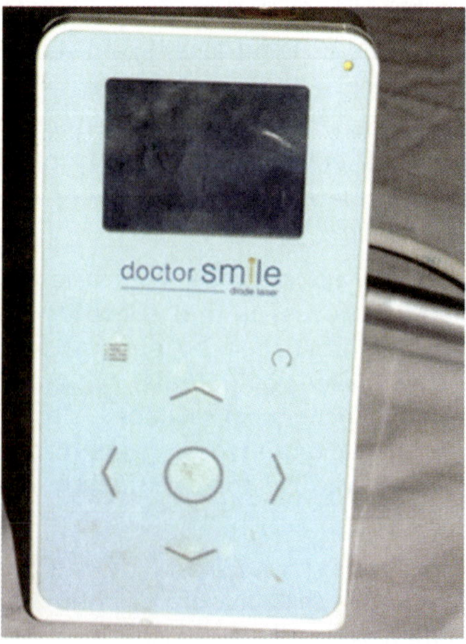

Fig. 31.3 Diode soft laser

In dentistry, soft tissue lasers are used for:

- Desensitization of hypersensitive dentin
- Healing of dry socket
- Reducing pain and promoting healing of ulcers, etc.

The examples of soft tissue Lasers are:

- Helium – Neon (He-Ne)
- Gallium – Arsenide (Ga-Ar)
- Gallium – Aluminium–Arsenide (Ga-Al-Ar)

b. Hard Tissue Lasers

The hard tissue lasers are thermic and of high energy, that are utilized in surgery as precise energy source, i.e. cut, coagulate and vaporize (Fig. 31.4a and b). These are mostly used for caries removal, cavity preparation and etching of enamel and cementum surfaces.

The examples of hard tissue lasers are:

- Argon
- Carbon dioxide

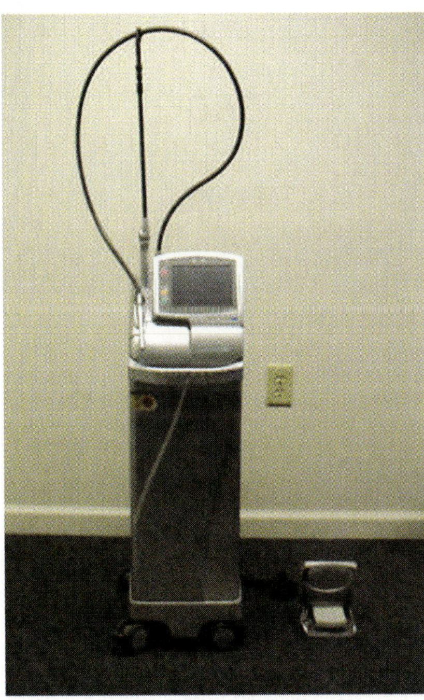

Fig. 31.4a Hard tissue laser (BIOLASE)

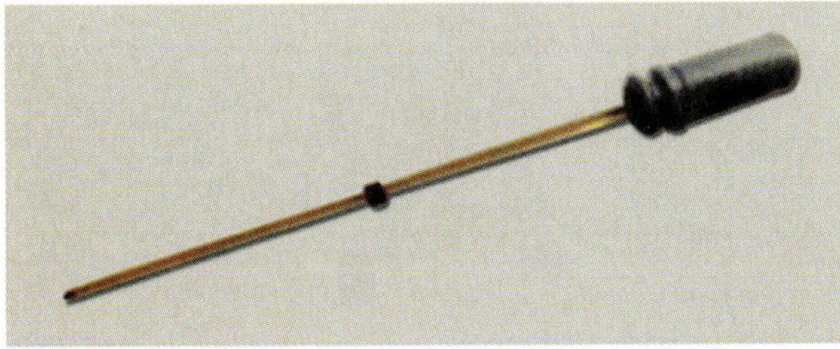

Fig. 31.4b Radial firing tip used with BIOLASE

- Neodymium: Yttrium aluminium garnet (Nd:YAG laser)

The *routinely used Lasers* are described:

a. Carbon Dioxide (CO_2) Laser

Carbon dioxide laser (active medium CO_2 and nitrogen) produces a beam of infrared light centering in 9.4 µm to 10.6 µm (Fig. 31.5). CO_2 laser was thought to be suitable for selected surface applications on teeth, such as sealing of pit and fissures, welding of ceramic materials to enamel and prevention of dental caries. However, generating extremely high surface temperatures and inability of the beam to be transmitted via a fiberoptic cable to a handpiece limited its use for above applications. As principally absorbed by water molecules, it can cut many hard and soft tissues (used both for hard tissues ablation and soft tissue surgeries). The wavelength has the highest absorption in hydroxyapatite out of any dental laser. Therefore, structures adjacent to surgical site must be shielded from laser beam.

Advantages

- Excellent hemostasis, reduce bacteremia
- Minimum postoperative pain/discomfort
- Remove tissue quickly and efficiently
- Minimize mechanical trauma

Disadvantages

- Lack of feed back (CO_2 laser used in a non-contact mode)
- Black-brown pigmentation of the treated tissues
- Costly

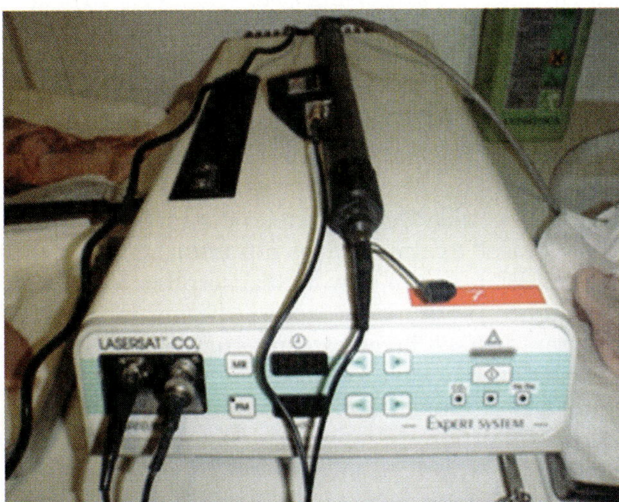

Fig. 31.5 Carbon dioxide laser

b. Argon Laser

The argon laser uses argon gas as the active medium, which generate coherent visible light with primary wavelengths of 488 and 514 nm. The 488 nm (blue color) wavelength emission is for activating camphoroquine during polymerization of composites. The 514 nm (blue green color) light wavelengths have peak absorption in red pigment such as hemoglobin; thus, laser light is well absorbed in pigmented tissues with abundance of hemoglobin, hemosiderin and melanin. Argon laser light is not well absorbed by enamel and dentin or other non-pigmented tissues. These characteristics make argon laser very useful for cutting, vaporizing, coagulating and providing hemostasis on gingival and oral mucosa. The argon laser is primarily used for root planing and curettage, gingival retraction, gingivectomy/gingivoplasty, frenectomy, treatment of oral lesions, tissue welding and for caries detection.

c. Neodymium: Yttrium Aluminium Garnet (Nd:YAG) Laser

Nd:YAG laser systems are usually large and bulky. This system emits its pulsed energy at 1064 nm (near infrared) and this energy is directed through a 320 µ silica fiber, using the high peak powers and free running pulse emission. When this beam is used in non-contact, defocused mode, this can penetrate deep and is used for hemostasis, treatment of aphthous ulcers or pulpal analgesia. The main disadvantage is the direct exposure of pulp by laser light through crown or root, leading to denaturation of pulp tissues. The common clinical applications are for cutting and coagulation of the dental soft tissues. It has an affinity for pigmented tissues (more for melanin and less for hemoglobin). It minimizes the heat build-up in tissues.

d. Erbium Laser

Erbium laser is a promising laser system because of its emission wavelength (Er:YAG—2940 nm and Er:Cr:YAG—2780 nm), which coincides with main absorption peak of water, resulting in good absorption in all biologic tissues including enamel and dentin. Infrared laser systems like carbon dioxide or Nd:YAG laser have reported the presence of zones of carbonization and necrosis due to high temperatures. In contrast, Er:YAG laser treatment does not induce any thermal changes. Water has a very high absorption for Er:YAG laser light. The incident laser radiation is absorbed in a thin surface layer causing sudden heating and vaporization of water. A high steam pressure then leads to micro-explosions with erupting particles. Because the tissue is not vaporized completely but only disintegrated into fragments, radiant energy is converted into ablation that alters the morphological structure of tissue. Er:YAG laser can be used for the removal of healthy hard tissue as well as carious decay without causing any thermal injury to adjacent tissues. Restorative materials like composites and cements can be ablated without using mechanical bur. Gold crowns and cast fillings cannot be removed because the laser beam is reflected by metals. No ablation effect is observed on ceramics. This laser is recommended for osteotomy, cyst removal and apicoectomy because of bone healing properties.

The thermal side effects are greatly reduced with Er:YAG laser. However, this laser beam is not easily transmitted through optical fibers and therefore is usually applied via mirror and arm delivery systems. A root canal preparation is not possible due to lack of suitable delivery system (Fig. 31.6 a and b).

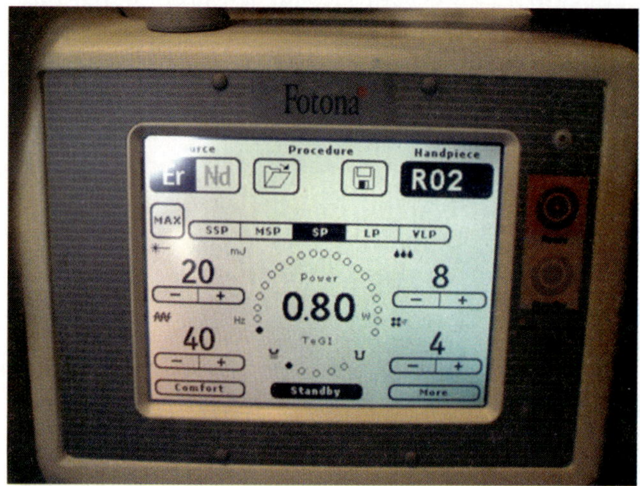

Fig. 31.6a Fotona Fidelis (screen projection)

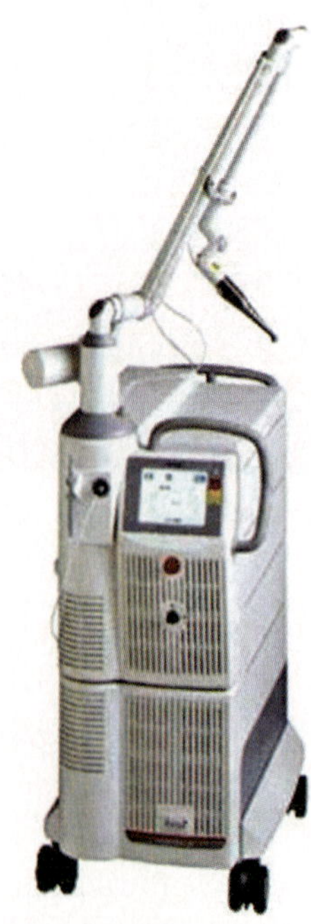

Fig. 31.6b Fotona Fidelis—dual wavelength dental laser Er:YAG and Nd:YAG

e. Semiconductor/Diode Laser

Gallium-Arsenide (GaAs) 904 nm, Gallium-Aluminium-Arsenide (GaAlAs) 780–890 nm and Indium-Gallium-Aluminium Phosphide (InGaAlP) 630–700 nm are the common diode lasers (Fig. 31.7). In diode lasers, the active medium is sandwiched between silicon wafers. The discharge of current from one silicone wafer to another releases photons from the active medium. Diode lasers are used for the treatment of dentin hypersensitivity, wound healing and for relieving post-surgical pain.

Laser type, wavelength and their clinical potential are summarized in Table 31.3.

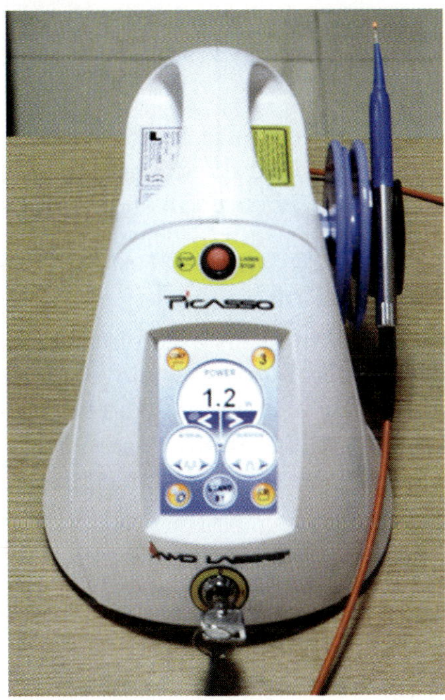

Fig. 31.7 Different wavelength diode laser

Advantages of laser

- Interaction with diseased tissue is selective and precise
- Damage to surrounding tissues is minimum
- Easy osseous tissue removal and contouring
- Provide good hemostasis
- Help reduction in pain
- Minimal need for anesthesia
- No whining sound or vibration of dental drill
- Less chair time
- Fast healing
- Less antibiotics and analgesics required

Disadvantages of laser

- High cost
- Delivery systems are bulky
- Difficult access to the surgical area
- Air embolisms may be produced by air and water
- Precise selection of wavelength is mandatory for different procedures

APPLICATION OF LASER TECHNOLOGY IN ENDODONTICS

The rapid development of laser technology coupled with better understanding of interactions with biological tissues, has widened the scope of applying this technology in endodontics.

In endodontics, laser energy is being tried in the following procedures:

i. Analgesia
ii. Reducing permeability of dentin and fusing dentin plug at apical end
iii. Sterilization of endodontic instruments
iv. Pulp testing (assessment of flow of pulpal blood by laser Doppler flowmetry)

Table 31.3 Laser type, wavelength and their clinical potential

Medium	*Wavelength (nm)*	*Enamel surface characteristics*	*Clinical use*
Carbon dioxide	10,600	• Surface fusion • Charring/cracking • Roughness • Partially fused crystallization	• Resin bonding • Enamel etching • Caries reduction
Argon	514	• Reflection of beam produces minimal effect on surface	• Resin polymerization
Er:YAG	2940	• Etched and flaky, rough surface	• Cavity preparation • Enamel etching
Nd:YAG	1,064	• Reflection of beam is seen, until photo-absorptive is placed	• Removal of debris • Enamel etching
Diode/semiconductor	630–890	• Slight etching, smooth, lacking in charring, planed enamel prisms	• Cavity preparation • Enamel etching

v. Pulp capping and pulpotomy
vi. Preparation of access cavities and root canal walls
vii. Disinfection of root canals
viii. Obturation of root canals
ix. Removing gutta-percha and separated instruments
x. Endodontic surgery
xi. Endodontic mishaps
xii. Laser bleaching
xiii. Stimulate healing and relieving postoperative pain
xiv. Retrograde cavity preparation

i. Analgesia

Certain wavelengths of laser energy interfere with the sodium pump mechanism, change cell membrane permeability, alter temporarily the endings of sensory neurons and block depolarization of C and Aδ fibers of the nerves. The pulsed Nd:YAG laser has been successfully used for achieving analgesia.

ii. Reducing Permeability of Dentin and Fusing Dentin at Apical End

It is established that the laser irradiation of 10 pulses/second for two minutes on dentin melts normal dentinal surface and closes the exposed dentinal tubule orifices without creating any surface cracks (Fig. 31.8a and b). The dentin surface after Nd:YAG laser treatment showed no protrusive rods (protrusive rods are a measure of open dentinal tubules). Lasers can effectively treat dentin hypersensitivity. The laser treatment is also effective in fusing the dentin at the apical end.

iii. Sterilization of Endodontic Instruments

A significant reduction in the microbial loads due to raised temperatures has been reported after the sterilization of endodontic instruments by lasers. Carbon dioxide, argon and Nd:YAG lasers effectively sterilize the instruments used in endodontics.

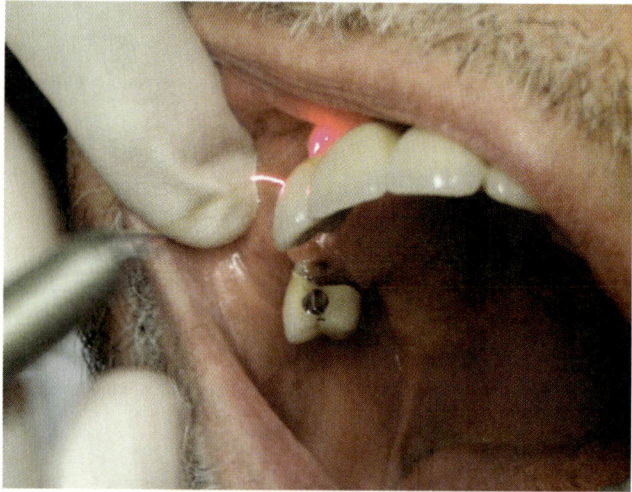

Fig. 31.8b Laser irradiation for treating dentin hypersensitivity in cervical abrasions

iv. Pulp Testing (Assessment of Flow of Pulpal Blood by Laser Doppler Flowmetry)

Laser Doppler flowmetry is a non-invasive technique that detects net red blood cell movement in small volumes of a tissue and monitor the total blood flow through that tissue (Fig. 31.9).

It utilizes light beam from a He-Ne laser (632.8 nm), which is carried to and from the tissues by a fiberoptic probe that carries light by one fiber and receives back the scattered light (by moving red cells which undergo frequency shift according to the Doppler principle) by another fiber to the instrument (Fig. 31.10).

Details of the technique are described in Chapter 9.

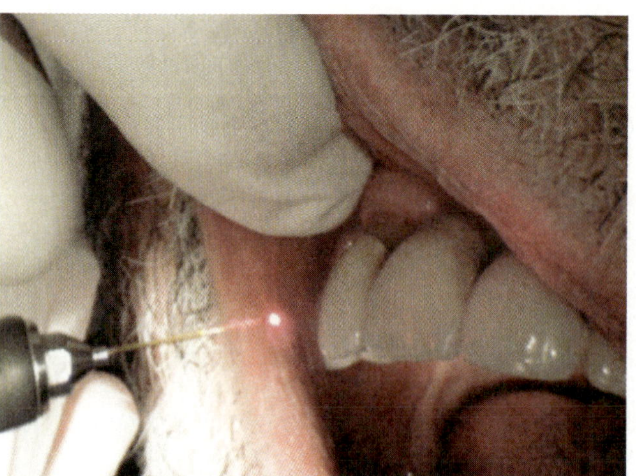

Fig. 31.8a Laser irradiation for treating dentin hypersensitivity in cervical abrasions

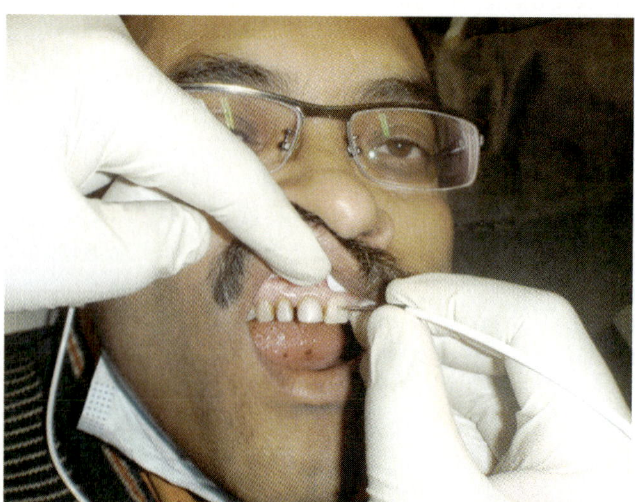

Fig. 31.9 He-Ne laser used for pulp testing

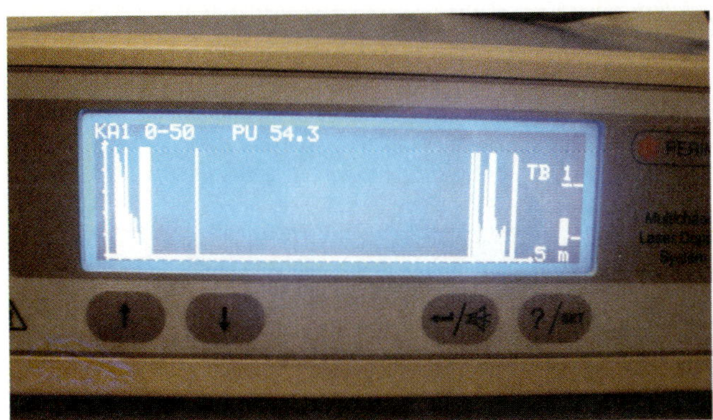

Fig. 31.10 Frequency shift (laser Doppler flowmetry)

Lasers (Nd:YAG) has also been used to differentially diagnose types of pulpitis from normal pulp.

v. Pulp Capping and Pulpotomy

Practically, all types of lasers have been used in pulp treatment procedures, especially in deciduous and young permanent teeth. For direct pulp capping, an energy level of 1 W at 0.1 second exposure time with one second pulse intervals is applied until the exposed pulps are completely sealed.

For indirect pulp capping, reduction in the permeability of dentin is achieved by sealing the dentinal tubules using Nd:YAG and carbon dioxide lasers. The energy is well absorbed by the hydroxyapatite of enamel and dentin, causing tissue ablation, melting and re-solidification.

It is established that laser therapy stimulates odontoblast activity (calcium and collagen production), leading to secondary dentin formation. Carbon dioxide laser has been very effective in pulp treatment procedures. It sterilizes and heals the irradiated area, reduce inflammation and the size of blood clot, ensuring close contact of the pulp with the capping materials (fast mode for hemostasis, disinfection and sealing of exposed pulp tissue).

Nd:YAG, Er:YAG and Er:Cr:YAG have also been tried successfully in pulp capping and pulpotomies. These are equally effective in hemostasis and coagulation of exposed pulp.

The factors rationalizing the effect of lasers on pulp are:

- The bactericidal effect of laser creates a sterile area over exposed pulp.
- Facilitates sealing of exposed pulp.
- The coagulating effect provides dry area with no bleeding.
- Controlled thermal effects of laser allow formation of barrier against contamination.

The Nd:YAG laser and formocresol tooth pulpotomies, when compared at 6th and 12th week of postoperative period, depicted no significant differences in radiological findings. Histologically, the frequency of dentin bridge formation was higher for laser group than formocresol group.

vi. Preparation of Access Cavities and Root Canal walls

Various Lasers in different forms have been tried for preparation of access cavities and root canal walls (Er:Cr:YSGG—2780 nm, Er:YAG—2940 nm). The root canals prepared with Lasers are cleaner as compared to conventional techniques.

Technique

The apical region of canal is initially hand instrumented with a No. 15 K-file. The laser energy set at 150 mJ through fiberoptic was inserted into root canal up to working length. The canal is prepared circumferentially in apical third, middle third and the coronal third, sequentially increasing the size, as required.

The laser preparation shows remarkable cleanliness of all canals. The dentin reveals a crusty, wavy aspect with open tubules and no apparent smear layer; however, carbonization has been observed in irradiated root canals.

The Er:YAG laser is equally effective for debris removal, producing a cleaner surface with a higher number of open tubules compared to other lasers.

Nd:YAG laser may present melted and recrystallized dentin and smear layer removal. Argon laser irradiation of root canal system also efficiently removes intracanal debris. Recently, Xe-Cl (308 nm) Excimer laser effectively lead to melting and lasing dentinal tubules.

Photon Induced Photoacoustic Streaming (PIPS) Technology

It is a revolutionary method for cleaning and debriding the root canal system using Er:YAG laser energy at subablative power levels.

Photon induced photoacoustic streaming (PIPS) harness the power of the Er:YAG laser to create photoacoustic shock waves within the cleaning/debriding solutions (sodium hypochlorite, distilled water, EDTA, etc.) introduced in the root canal. The shock waves effectively stream the solutions through the entire canal system. The canals are left clean and the dentinal tubules are free of smear layer. Photon induced photoacoustic streaming (PIPS) is equally effective for final rinsing prior to obturation (Fig. 31.11a to d).

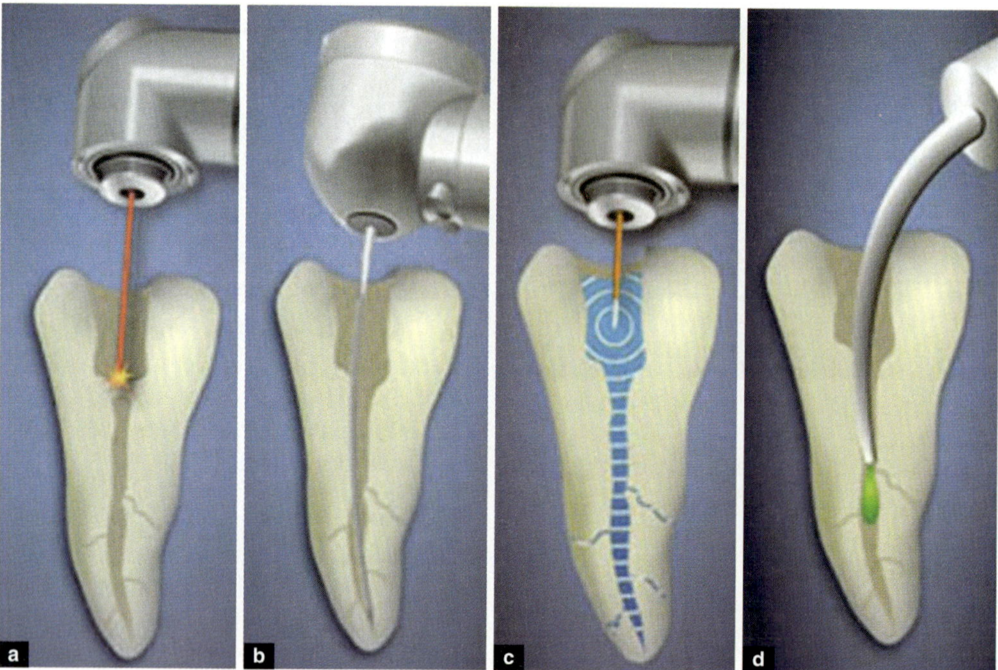
Fig. 31.11a to d PIPS technology (Web-photo)

PIPS technology eliminates the need to introduce the tip into the root canals. Unlike traditional laser techniques (placement of tip at 1.0–5.0 mm from apical constriction), PIPS tip is placed at the coronal chamber, allowing acoustic waves to spread into the root canals.

A combination of laser wavelength is being used in twinlight endodontic treatment (TET). The authors used deep penetrating Nd:YAG laser wavelength for deep thermal disinfection and better absorbed wavelength for non-thermal acoustic cleaning of root canal system. The procedure facilitates clean canals with open dentinal tubules free of smear layer.

vii. Disinfection of Root Canals

The efficacy of Nd:YAG laser in sterilizing contaminated root canals has been established. Various studies have confirmed the efficacy of diode and Nd:YAG lasers in eradicating bacterial load from the root canals; however, a few authors have cautioned the undesirable thermal effects of root dentin. An average of 34% decrease in colony forming units (CFU) for *Actinomyces* and 15.7% for *Pseudomonas aeruginosa* with 5 Hz laser treatment and a decrease of 77.4% for Actinomyces and 85.8% for Pseudomonas with 10 Hz laser have been reported. It is further documented that Nd:YAG laser is significantly more bactericidal than other lasers (Fig. 31.12a to c).

Photoactivation disinfection (PAD)/light activated disinfection (LAD)/photodynamic antimicrobial chemotherapy (PACT) work on the principle that photosensitive molecules get attached to the membrane of the bacteria. The specific wavelength of laser

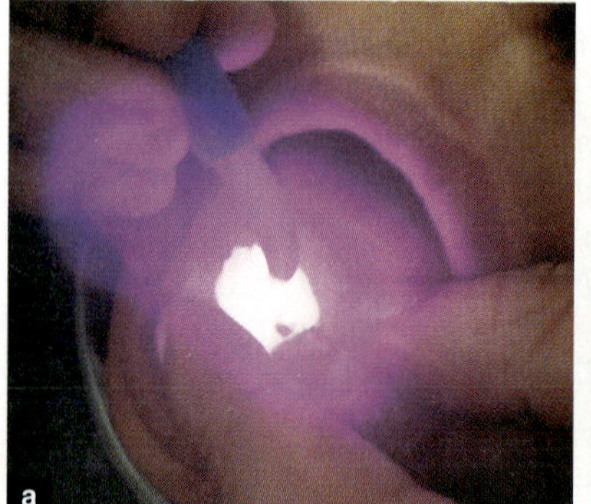
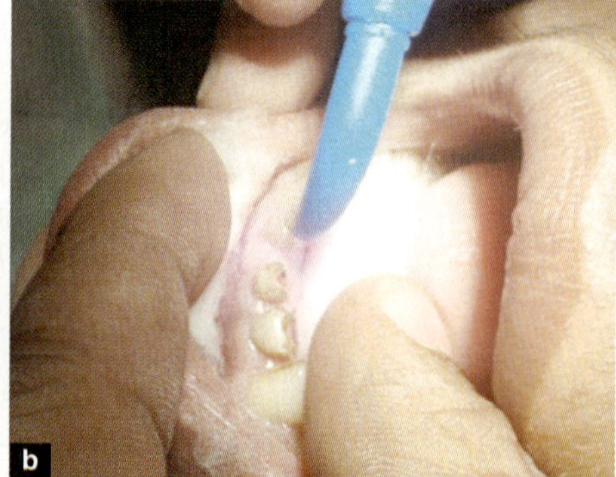
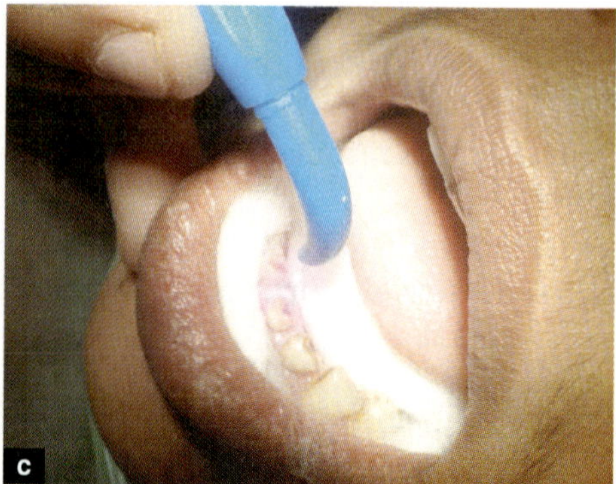
Fig. 31.12a to c Disinfection of root canals using Nd:YAG laser

irradiation leads to the production of singlet oxygen, which may cause bacterial cell wall to rupture, killing the bacteria. Virtually, all kinds of micro-organisms can be inactivated by this technology (specifically gram-positive pathogens are more sensitive than gram-negative pathogens). It is established that this technique effectively destroys bacteria remaining in the canal spaces after using conventional irrigants in root canal treatment.

viii. Obturation of Root Canal Spaces

Argon laser has been used as a heat source to compact the gutta-percha during root canal obturation. The quality of apical seal achieved has not been established yet.

ix. Removing Gutta-percha and Separated Instruments

Nd:YAG laser has successfully used to remove gutta-percha and broken files from the root canals. Nd:YAG and Er:YAG lasers are effective in removing zinc oxide sealers and other filling materials. Biolase laser is used to remove gutta-percha and other filling materials following the hydrokinetic process. It involves removal of tissues with laser-energized water droplets. Hydrokinetic energy is produced by combining a spray of atomized water with laser energy. The resulting energy gently and precisely removes a wide range of materials and human tissue.

x. Endodontic Surgery

Lasers have been tried in endodontic surgery to irradiate the surgical site during apicoectomy. It effectively achieves hemostasis and visualization of the operating field. Laser has also been used for biostimulation of abscess (Fig. 31.13a and b). Er:YAG laser in a low-output power, when used in apical surgery (Fig. 31.14a and b), lead to smooth and clean surface devoid of charring. Diode lasers have been tried to improve healing at the surgical sites.

The *advantages* of using lasers in endodontic surgery are:

- Effective hemostasis by sealing the blood vessels.
- Minimal postoperative pain due to minimum tissue damage and sealing off nerve endings.

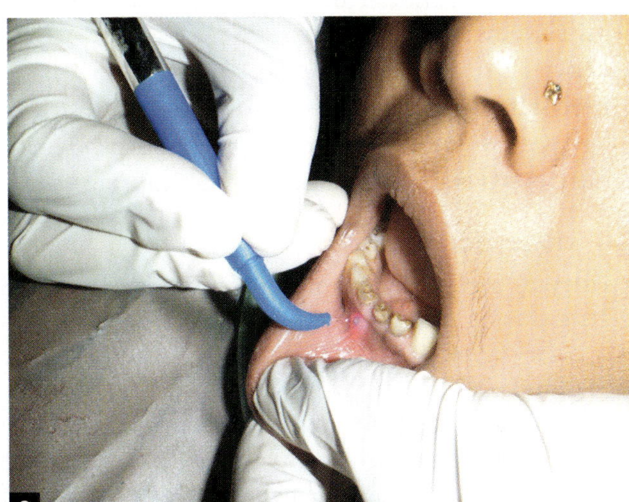

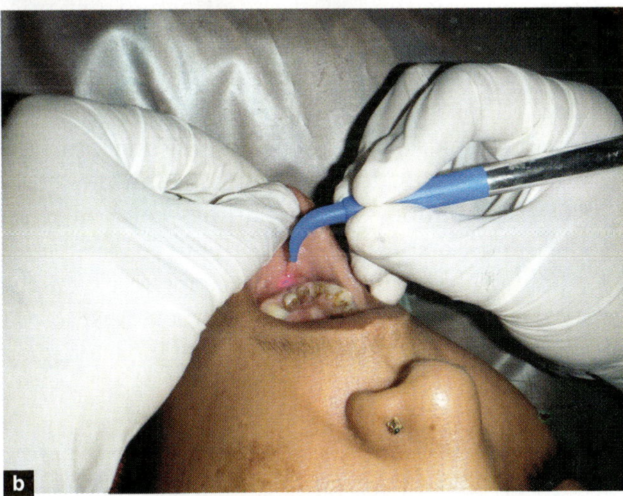

Fig. 31.13a and b Biostimulation of abscess

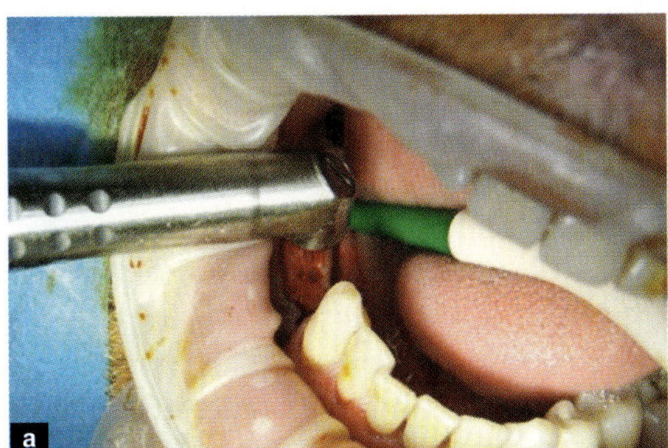

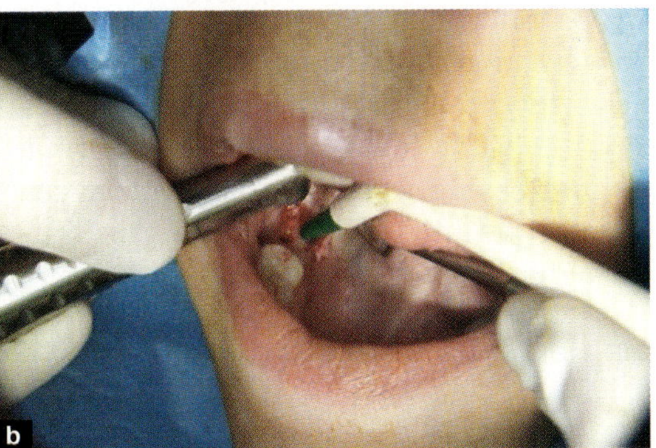

Fig. 31.14a and b Laser (Er:YAG) used in endodontic surgery

- Clean incision resulting in minimal edema and scarring.
- During surgery for malignancies, no danger of splattering blood and lymph.
- Many surgical procedures can be carried out without local anesthesia. The procedure is not painful because laser pulse is shorter than time required for transmission by nerves.
- Leave a dry and sterile field.
- Precisely interact with diseased tissues
- Reduce the amount of bacteria in the surgical field
- Easy osseous tissue removal and contouring

xi. Endodontic Mishaps

Accidental perforation of pulp chamber is a common feature during tooth preparations. Such perforations may occur anywhere along the root during endodontic procedures.

Lasers have been tried to sterilize the affected area and seal the perforation effectively. Nd:YAG laser has been observed to be effective in disinfecting the area of perforation and removing the attached organic/ inorganic smear layer followed by sealing the area with laser irradiated composites.

Nd:YAG laser was tried to seal the vertical root fracture fragments and other cracks. The crack surfaces were filled with tricalcium phosphate and melted by the laser irradiation (various studies confirmed the presence of tricalcium phosphate along the crack lines). A few authors have successfully tried melting bioactive glass paste over the crack site using carbon dioxide laser (higher temperature of laser could melt bioactive glass paste in a very short span of time).

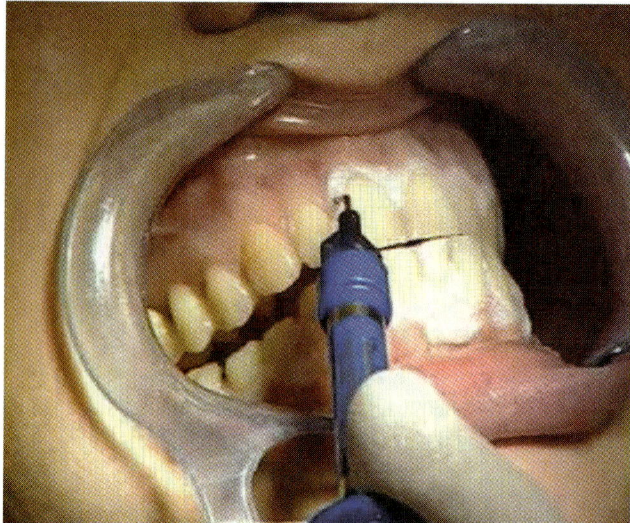

Fig. 31.15 Laser bleaching

xii. Laser Bleaching

The procedure utilizes 30–35% hydrogen peroxide, which is usually applicable in routine bleaching. Laser whitening gel has a unique mix of thermal absorption crystals integrated into gel of highly processed fumed silica and 35% hydrogen peroxide. Bleaching gel is applied and is activated by high intensity light source or plasma arc light. Crystals in gel absorb thermal energy from light allowing better dissociation of oxygen and easy penetration into the enamel matrix thus increasing the lightening effect on teeth (Fig. 31.15).

xiii. Stimulate Healing and relieving Postoperative Pain

Laser causes an anti-inflammatory effect in the irradiated area, which accelerates healing and decreases pain. It has got a stimulating action on bone morphogenic proteins, which further stimulates undifferentiated mesenchymal cells into osteoblasts, resulting in increased osteogenesis. Laser also stimulate fibroblasts for more collagen production, accelerate cell reproduction and also cause increased prostaglandin levels, which help in healing and regeneration of tissues (Fig. 31.16).

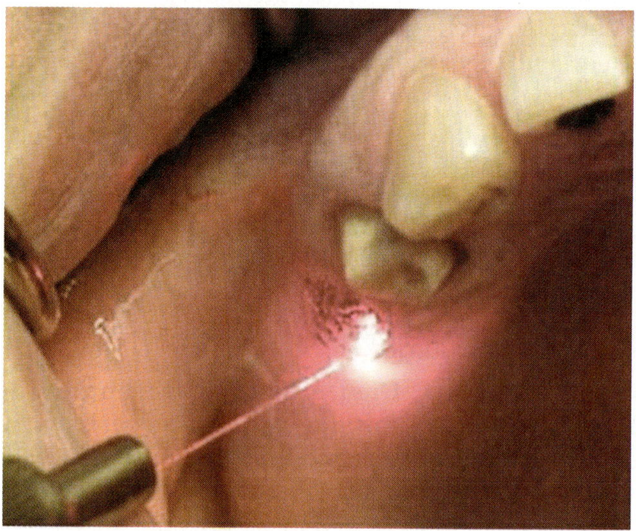

Fig. 31.16 Laser on surgical site for healing

xiv. Retrograde Cavity Preparation

Er:YSGG and Cr:YSGG laser have been used for root-end cavity preparation. The root-surface cracking that produced by ultrasonic retropreparation tips/ conventional preparation using a bur have been overcome by lasers (Fig. 31.17).

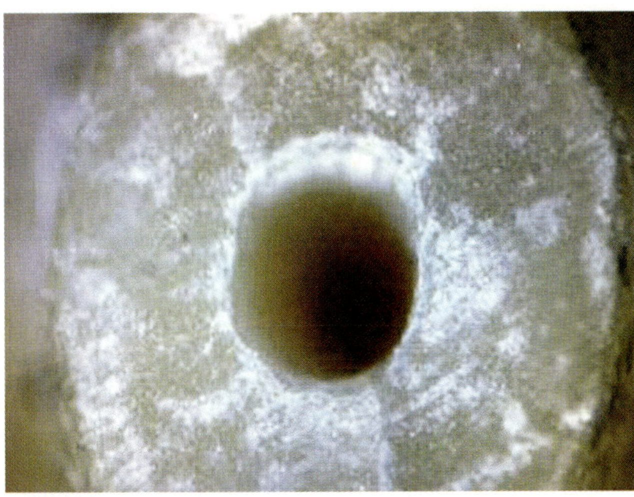

Fig. 31.17 Retrograde cavity prepared by laser

LASER HAZARDS

Lasers, although beneficial in endodontics, may have certain hazards in clinics. The hazards can be:

a. Ocular injuries
b. Tissue damage
c. Environmental hazards
d. Electrical hazards

a. Ocular Injuries

Potential injury to the eye can occur either by direct emission from laser or by reflection from a specular surface. The primary ocular injury that may result from a laser accident is a retinal or corneal damage. Retinal injury is possible with emissions in the visible (400–780 nm) and near infrared (780–1400 nm) wavelengths.

The effects of different wavelength of Lasers on eyes are summarized in Table 31.4.

b. Tissue Damage

Laser induces damage to skin and other tissues as a result from thermal interaction of radiant energy with tissue proteins. Temperature elevation of 21°C above normal body temperature can produce cell destruction by denaturation of cellular enzyme and structural proteins, which interrupts basic metabolic processes.

Factors affecting laser-tissue interaction are:

- Relative absorption and transmission of particular wavelength.
- Pulse duration and pulse repetition rate.
- Level of radiation exposure.
- Relative degree of vascularity of tissue.

The deleterious effects of lasers on enamel and dentin are as follows:

- Enamel exhibits gross cratering from 0.1 to 1.1 mm deep depending on amount of energy delivered to target area. In deeper penetration, dark speckling of exposed dentin can be seen. Examination under polarized light may show crystallographic changes.
- Dentin shows shallow, irregular craters 0.1 mm deep. Three distinct zones of dentinal destruction are: Central zone of complete dentinal destruction; an immediate surrounding area of partial dentinal destruction and a scattered zone of dark specks beyond first two zones.

Table 31.4 Laser wavelength and pathological effect on eyes

Wavelength (nm)	*Effect on eyes*
180–315 (ultraviolet)	Inflammation of the cornea (like sunburn)
315–400 (ultraviolet)	Clouding of eye lens
400–780 (visible)	Retinal burn (photochemical damage to retina)
780–1400 (near infrared)	Retinal burn; cataract
1400–3000 (infrared)	Cataract, corneal burn
3000 and above	Corneal burn

c. Environmental Hazards

Airborne contaminants can be emitted in the form of smoke or plume generated through thermal interaction of laser with tissue or through accidental escape of toxic chemical and gases from laser itself. These airborne contaminants may damage the functioning of respiratory system.

d. Electrical Hazards

Because laser use high currents and high voltage power supplies, these are potentially hazardous. Electrical hazards of lasers can be grouped as electrical shock hazards, electrical fire hazards or explosion hazards.

LASER SAFETY

It is established that even small amount of laser light can lead to eye injuries. Laser safety designs utilize implementation of laser to minimize the risk of laser accidents, especially involving skin and eyes. American National Standard Institute (ANSI) provides control measures for laser hazards. The maximum permissible exposure (MPE) limit should strictly be looked into prior to use of lasers.

ANSI has provided guidance for the use of lasers in a series, ANSI 136. The standard protocol is:

136.1: Safe use of lasers

136.2: Safe use of optical fibers and LED sources

136.3: Safe use of lasers in health care

136.4: Laser safety measurements for hazard evaluation
136.5: Safe use of lasers in educational institutions
136.6: Safe use of lasers outdoors
136.7: Labelling laser protective equipment
136.8: Lasers in research and development
136.9: Lasers in manufacturing environment

Safety Measures

- A laser warning signal outside the clinic (aware of the risks).
- Use of barriers within the operatory.
- Use of eyewear to protect against reflected laser light or accidental direct exposure (high intensity beams should be guided through opaque tubes).
- The residue left after tissue ablation should be evacuated using high volume suction.
- Equipment should be serviced and checked regularly (high temperature and fire hazards may result from operation of high powered lasers).
- The operator should take adequate precautions to prevent injury/damage to adjacent soft and hard tissue (alignment of beams and optical components should be performed at a reduced beam power).

Everyone uses laser should be aware of the risks involved. The routine complacency dealing with invisible risks can lead to health hazards, which should be avoided following safety measures.

BIBLIOGRAPHY

1. Andrew LS. DiagnoDent laser fluorescence assessment of endodontic infection. J. Endod.: 2009; 35:1404–1407.
2. Attrill DC, Davies RM and King TA. Thermal effects of Er:YAG laser on simulated dental pulp: a quantitative evaluation of effects of water spray. J. Dent.: 2004; 32:35–40.
3. Benedicenti S, Cassanelli C, Signore A, Ravera G and Angiero F. Decontamination of root canals with the gallium-aluminium-arsenide laser: An in vitro study. Photomed. Laser Surg.: 2008; 26:367–70.
4. Cankat K and Recep O. Comparative evaluation of Nd:YAG laser and fluoride varnish for treatment of dentin hypersensitivity. J. Endod.: 2009; 35:971–974.
5. Chaudhary S, Yadav S, Oberoi G, Talwar S and Verma M. Evaluation of root-end cavity preparation using erbium, chromium:yttrium, scandium, gallium, and garnet laser, ultrasonic retrotips, and conventional burs. J. Dent. Lasers: 2016; 10:43–46.
6. Claudio HV. Obturation of root canal system treated by Cr, Er:YSGG laser irradiation. J. Endod.: 2007; 33:1091–1093.
7. Daniel HP. CO2, Er:YAG and Nd:YAG lasers in endodontic surgery. J. Appl. Oral Sci.: 2009; 17:596–599.
8. Enwemeka CS, Parker JC, Dowdy DS, Harkness EE, Sanford LE and Woodruff LD. The efficacy of low-power lasers in tissue repair and pain control: A meta-analysis study. Photomed. Laser Surg.: 2004; 22:323–329.
9. Gutknecht N. Lasres in Endodontics. J. Laser and Health Acad.: 2008; 4:1–5.
10. Kimura Y, Yonaga K, Yokoyama K, Kinoshita J, Ogata Y and Matsumoto K. Root surface temperature increase during Er:YAG laser irradiation of root canals. J. Endod.: 2002; 28:76-78.
11. Linc CH, Chou TM and Chen JH. Evaluation of effect of laser tooth whitening. Int. J. Prosthodont.: 2008; 21:415–418.
12. Marcelo TS, Bocangel JS and Nogueria GEC. SEM evaluation of interaction pattern between dentin and resin after cavity preparation using Er:YAG laser. J. Dent.: 2003; 31:127.
13. Marchesan MA. Effects of 980-nanometer diode laser on root canal permeability after dentin treatment with different chemical solutions. J. Endod.: 2008; 34:721–724.
14. Mathew A, Lajevardi M, Al Juboori HA. An in vivo study on comparison of disinfection of root canal with chemical disinfectants and disinfectant-diode laser-photodynamic treatment combined system. J. Dent. Lasers: 2015; 9:2–10.
15. Meire M and De Moor R. Laser disinfection, an added value? Endod. Pract. Today: 2007; 1:159–172.
16. Nishad SG, Thyath MN, Sharma M and Zaidi I. Laser in Endodontics. J. Adv. Med. Dent. Sci. Res.: 2015; 3:137–141.
17. Norberto Batista de Faria-Junior. Evaluation of ultrasonic and ErCr:YSGG laser retrograde cavity preparation. J. Endod.: 2009; 35:741–744.
18. Pawar SS, Pujar MA, Makandar SD and Khaiser MI. Post-endodontic treatment pain management with low-level laser therapy. J. Dent. Lasers: 2014; 2:60–63.
19. Qian-qian W. Evaluation of bactericidal effect of Er, Cr:YSGG and Nd:YAG lasers in experimentally infected root canals. J. Endod.: 2007; 33:830–832.
20. Roy G and Ian AM. Laser activation of endodontic irrigants with improved conical laser fiber tips for removing smear layer in apical third of root canal. J. Endod.: 2008; 34: 1524–1527.
21. Roy G. Lasers in dentistry—Review. Int. J. Dent. Clinics.: 2009; 1:13–19.
22. Shoj S and Nakamana M. Histopathological changes in dental pulp irradiated by CO2 laser; a preliminary report on laser pulpotomy. J. Endod.: 1985; 11:379–384.
23. Viducic D. Removal of gutta-percha from root canals using Nd:YAG laser. Int. Endod. J.: 2003; 36:670–673.
24. Wang HL, Bor SL and Hsin CL. Morphological study of Nd:YAG laser usage in treatment of dentinal hypersensitivity. J. Endod. 2004; 30:131–134.
25. Wong WS and Rosenberg PA. A comparison of apical seals achieved using retrograde amalgam and Nd:YAG laser. J. Endod.: 1994; 20:595–597.
26. Yuichir N. Effect of Er:YAG laser irradiation on biofilm-forming bacteria associated with endodontic pathogens in-vitro. J. Endod.: 2008; 34:826–829.

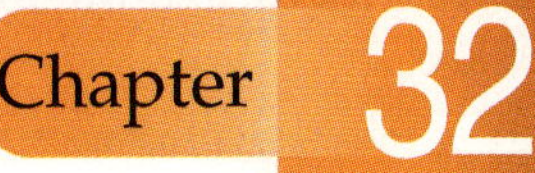

Chapter 32 Surgical Endodontics

Endodontic surgery refers to the removal of tissues other than the contents of root canal space, before or after root canal treatment. Surgical intervention using advanced technologies coupled with availability of better diagnostic aids has led to greater success in retaining a tooth with pulpal and/or periapical involvement.

The most common endodontic surgical procedures are periradicular curettage and apicoectomy (root end resection). Other procedures include crown lengthening, replantation/intentional replantation, hemisection/radisectomy, incision/drainage and perforation repair.

The surgical intervention should be selective in the best interest of the patients.

Indications

- Need for surgical drainage
- Failed nonsurgical endodontic treatment
  - Irretrievable root canal filling material
  - Irretrievable intraradicular post
- Calcific metamorphosis of the pulp space
- Procedural errors
  - Instrument separation
  - Non-negotiable ledges
  - Root perforation(s)
  - Symptomatic overfilling
- Anatomic variations
  - Root dilacerations
  - Apical root fenestration
- Corrective surgery
  - Hemisection/bicuspidization/radisectomy
- Replacement surgery
  - Replantation/intentional replantation
  - Autotransplants

Contraindications

The contraindications for surgery are mostly relative and not absolute.

The *absolute contraindication* is:

- Where the tooth cannot be restored or saved to serve the functions.

The *relative contraindications* are:

Medical conditions

- Patients with uncontrolled diabetes mellitus, tuberculosis, nephritis, etc.
- Active leukemia with neutropenia
- Recent cardiac/tumor surgery
- Immunocompromised patients
- Uncontrolled hypertension
- Bleeding disorders
- Radiation therapy of face (within six months)
- First trimester and third trimester of pregnancy
- Psychologically distressed patients

Anatomic considerations

- Proximity of roots to nasal floor, maxillary sinus, mandibular canal or mental foramen
- Inadequate visual and mechanical access such as thick buccal plate and lingually inclined roots in mandibular second molars

Skill and experience

- The skill and experience of the operator is mandatory to carry out surgical procedures

Classification of Surgical Endodontic Procedures

I. Periradicular surgery
- Curettage
- Apicoectomy (root end resection)

II. Fistulative surgery
- Incision and drainage
- Trephination
- Decompression

III. Corrective surgery
- Perforation repair
- Replantation/intentional replantation

IV. Biopsy

PREOPERATIVE ASSESSMENT

Preoperative assessment involves following features.

Patient Considerations

The type of procedures planned for the patient and health status of patient must be noted. Healthy patients tolerate a surgical procedure better than medically compromised patients. A thorough medical history and assessment of vital signs is mandatory.

The American Society of Anesthesiologists (ASA) has categorized risk for surgical patients as follows:

ASA 1: Healthy patients (require no modification of surgical treatment plan).

ASA 2 and 3: Patients having mild to moderate systemic disease (require medical consultation and modification of surgical treatment plan).

ASA 4, 5 and 6: Patients having significant systemic problems (preferably not treated in dental clinic).

Patients with sub-acute bacterial endocarditis and prosthetic joints should be administered with prophylactic antibiotics. Patients on anticoagulant therapy (such as warfarin) are required to stop medication two days before treatment. Patients on aspirin therapy should stop medication 4–5 days before surgery. International normalized ratio (INR) and prothrombin test should be carried out at least a day before surgery.

Anatomic Considerations

A thorough clinical and radiographic examination should be carried out to evaluate access to surgical site. The anatomical problems can be:

- Restricted access
- Root tips inclined lingually
- Small oral opening
- Active facial muscles
- Shallow vestibule
- Thick buccal alveolar bone
- Proximity to mandibular canal, mental foramen, maxillary sinus or nasal floor

Informed Consent

Any postoperative complication specific to a particular situation/medical condition should be informed; written consent may also be obtained from the patient.

PRESURGICAL EVALUATION

Presurgical evaluation includes the following.

32

Case History

Case history comprises data recording with regard to chief complaint, history of present illness, family history and general health of the patient. The medical ailments influencing surgical procedures are:

- Cardiovascular diseases
- Metabolic/hepatic disorders
- Bleeding disorders
- Drug allergies
- Respiratory problems
- Renal problems
- Neurological problems
- Miscellaneous conditions, like pregnancy, nutritional deficiency, addiction, etc.

Physical Examination

It includes inspection, palpation, percussion and auscultation.

The general physical examination is followed by local examination of the maxillofacial region.

Laboratory Investigations

a. Hematological investigations like Hb, BT, CT, TLC, DLC, platelet count (complete blood count), diabetic screening (fasting blood sugar, glucose tolerance test, etc.).
b. Urine investigations
    - *Gross examination*: Like color, odor, etc.
    - *Chemical examination*: For presence of glucose, ketones, etc.
    - *Microscopic examination*: For presence of RBC, epithelial cell, etc.
c. Biochemical investigations: For uric acid, serum cholesterol, blood urea, serum bilirubin, etc.
d. Radiological examination
    - Extraoral radiographs
    - Intraoral radiographs
    - Special radiographic examinations
e. Histopathological investigations
    - Biopsy
f. Microbiological investigation: For bacterial, viral and protozoal infections, etc.

Special Investigations

Special investigations includes ELISA, tuberculin test, Widal test, VDRL test, etc.

Presurgical Preparation

The tolerance of the surgical procedure, the incidence of complications, and the quality and rate of healing are all affected by the health of the patient. Therefore, it becomes goal of the surgeon to maximize physical condition of the patient prior to surgery.

The most important decisions concerning surgical procedures are made long before any anesthetic agent is administered. The decision to perform surgery should be the culmination of several diagnostic steps.

The important steps prior to surgery are as follows.

A. Premedication

Premedication can be defined as *'the preliminary drugs with specific pharmacological actions, given prior to surgery to achieve the requisite goals'*.

The *requisite goals* are:

- Relief of apprehension/anxiety
- Sedation
- Analgesia
- Amnesia of preoperative events
- Antisialagogue effect
- Reduction of stomach acidity and volume
- Prevention of nausea and vomiting

The *premedication agents* are:

- Sedative and hypnotic agents
  - Benzodiazepines (diazepam, midazolam, etc.)
  - Barbiturates (phenobarbitone)
- Analgesic agents: Opioids (morphine, pethidine)
- Anticholinergic agents (atropine, glycopyrrolate, etc.)

B. Preparation of the Surgeon and the Patient

a. Hand Scrub

Clean hands beneath gloves are necessary. The purpose of hand scrub is to remove the superficial contaminants and loose epithelium and to reduce bacterial count on the skin. 20% chlorhexidine and 7.5% povidone iodine are the routinely used agents for hand scrubbing.

It is recommended that the scrubbing procedure (using soap) should take approximately 10 minutes.

The steps followed are:

- Before beginning of hand scrub, the nails should be checked for cleanliness.
- The scrub begins at the tip of one finger of one hand. The long axis of the finger is divided into four surfaces and 30 scrub strokes are applied to each surface. After this, the inter webbing is given 30 strokes and the next finger is begun. Then the ventral, dorsal and lateral surfaces of the hands are cleaned along with forearms.
- Then scrubbing is progressed towards the elbow, extending two inches above it.
- When one area is scrubbed, it should not be touched again because of the possibility of contamination from unscrubbed area.
- The arms are rinsed of excess soap after scrubbing. The rinse should be carried out with the elevated arms so that the water will drain from the finger tips, progressing down the hands, arms and finally elbow. The hands and arms are not rubbed during rinse and only superficial soap is removed in the process; the residual soap provides about three hours of anti-bacterial action for the surgeon's hands.
- The drying with sterile towel begins at the fingertips of one hand and progress down the hand and arm in a similar manner.

b. Gloving

There are two types of gloves. The most common type is clean latex. For those who are allergic to latex, milled rubber gloves are available. These are thinner than the latex gloves and may provide better tactile sensation, but are more fragile.

C. Preparation of the Surgical Site

The operative site may not be sterilized thoroughly; however, the gross cleaning action can significantly reduce the incidence of postoperative infection.

The scrub should begin in the center of the area of preparation and then moved concentrically. This will minimize contamination of already cleaned region from unscrubbed one. The area may be scrubbed a second time with a new sterile gauze in the same manner as the first. The area near eyes and ears should be taken care of.

Draping the Patient

The purpose of draping the patient is to isolate the surgical areas from other parts of the body. A double layered drape is necessary for effective isolation.

A sterile head drape is used around patient's head and is secured with towel clips.

The anesthetist and the equipment are isolated from the operating team by a drape covered screen.

LOCAL ANESTHESIA

Local anesthesia is defined as *'the loss of sensation in a circumscribed area of the body caused by inhibiting the excitation of nerve endings or blocking the conduction process in peripheral nerves, without inducing loss of consciousness'*.

Common Terms used in Local Anesthesia

Analgesia: It is loss of pain sensation without loss of consciousness.

Regional analgesia: It is loss of pain sensation over a given region without loss of consciousness.

***Regional anesthesia*:** It is loss of all sensations, i.e. pain as well as temperature, pressure and motor function without the loss of consciousness.

***Topical analgesia*:** It renders the free nerve endings in accessible structure (intact mucous membrane, abraded skin, etc.) incapable of stimulation by the application of a suitable solution directly to the surface area.

***Local infiltration*:** The small terminal nerve branches in the area of surgery are flooded with local anesthetic solution rendering them insensible to pain or preventing them from becoming stimulated and creating an impulse.

***Field block*:** It consists of depositing local anesthetic solution in close proximity to a large terminal nerve branch so that a circumscribed area is walled off to prevent central passage of afferent impulses.

***Nerve block*:** It consists of depositing local anesthetic solution within close proximity to the main trunk and thus preventing afferent impulses traveling beyond that point.

Ideal Requirements of Local Anesthetic

An ideal local anesthetic should possess the following properties:

- Action must be reversible.
- Remain stable in solution and undergo biotransformation readily within the body.
- Should be either sterile or capable of being sterilized without deterioration.
- Must be non-irritating to the tissues and produce no secondary reaction.
- Should have a low degree of systemic toxicity.
- Should not produce any allergic reactions.
- Should have a rapid onset and be of sufficient duration.
- Should have sufficient penetration to be effective for topical use.
- Should have sufficient potency to provide proper anesthesia.

Although the present local anesthetics do not fulfill all these requirements, but still possess sufficient properties for safe and effective use.

Selection of Method of Local Anesthesia

The selection of the method of local anesthesia depends upon the following factors:

32

- Age of the patient
- Area to be anesthetized
- Profoundness of anesthesia required
- Duration of anesthesia as required for specific procedures
- Presence and extent of infection
- When anesthesia of a single tooth or a small area is required, extraoral block is not used. Where profound anesthesia is required, an intraosseous method or a nerve block should be preferred.
- When longer duration of anesthesia is required, a nerve block is the method of choice. The nerve block may be preferred even if a small area is to be anesthetized. Also, if infection in the region precludes the use of local infiltration, nerve bock becomes a preferred choice even if a small area is to be anesthetized.

Indications

In endodontics, local anesthesia is used for:

- During radiography, especially in sensitive patient who are prone to gagging during placement of film
- For access cavity preparation
- For pulpotomy and pulpectomy
- Incision and drainage of abscess
- In surgical endodontic procedures like apicoectomy, hemisection, etc.
- For diagnostic purposes; when the patient is not able to pinpoint the offending tooth.
- During surgical procedures as an adjunct with a vasoconstrictor for bloodless field.

Contraindications

The contraindications can be 'absolute' or 'relative'.

Absolute

- Allergy to anesthetic solution(s).

Relative

- Local infections may render the drug ineffective.
- Un-cooperative patients.
- Patient refuses regional anesthesia because of fear or apprehension.
- Surgical procedures, which need prolonged anesthesia.
- Anomalies make regional analgesia difficult or impossible.
- Systemic conditions, like renal and liver diseases affect the metabolism and excretion of the drug.

Advantages

- Patient remains awake, co-operative and well oriented.
- Very low incidence of morbidity.
- Minimal distortion of normal physiology.
- Techniques are simple.

- No additional trained person is necessary.
- Failure rate is less.
- Patient need not omit the previous meal.

Mode of Action

The anesthetic salts are formed by a reaction of a weak base and a strong acid. Water solubility is necessary for their diffusion through the interstitial fluids to the nerve fiber. The salts exist both as uncharged molecules (free base) and the positively charged molecules (cation) in equilibrium with each other in an anesthetic solution. The relative proportion between the uncharged base and the charged cation depends on the pH of the solution and the pKa of the specific chemical cation form. The uncharged form (Free base) is responsible for optimal diffusion through the nerve sheath. After penetration, re-equilibrium occurs between the free base and the cation form. The charged cation binds to the receptor site and is ultimately responsible for suppression of nerve transmission.

The sensory functions are lost in the following order and the return of sensation is in the reverse order:

- Pain
- Temperature
- Touch
- Proprioception
- Skeletal muscle tone

Classification of Local Anesthetics

1. Based on Source
   - Natural
     - Cocaine
   - Synthetic nitrogenous compounds
     - Ester Type
     - Amide Type
   - Synthetic non-nitrogenous compounds
     - Benzyl Alcohol
   - Miscellaneous drugs
     - Clove Oil
     - Phenol
2. Based on Chemical Group
   - Ester Group
     - Benzoic acid esters: Cocaine, Benzocaine
     - Para-amino benzoic acid esters: Procaine, 2-Chloroprocaine, Tetracaine, Propoxycaine
   - Non-ester group (Amide/Anilide Type): Lignocaine, Bupivacaine, Prilocaine, Dibucaine
   - Quinolones: Centbucridine
3. Based on site of Administration
   - Injectable anesthetics
     - Low potency (Short duration): Procaine, 2-Chloroprocaine
     - Intermediate potency (Medium duration): Lignocaine, Prilocaine
     - High potency (Long duration): Dibucaine, Tetracaine, Bupivacaine
   - Topical anesthetic
     - Water soluble: Cocaine, Lignocaine Hydrochloride, Tetracaine
     - Water insoluble: Benzocaine, Lignocaine Base, Butyl-amino Benzoate
4. Based on duration of action
   - Ultra short acting anesthetics (less than 30 minutes)
     - Procaine without a vasoconstrictor
     - 2-chloroprocaine without a vasoconstrictor
     - 2.0% Lignocaine without a vasoconstrictor
     - 4.0% Prilocaine without a vasoconstrictor for infiltration
   - Short acting anesthetics (45–75 minutes)
     - 2.0% Lignocaine with 1:1 lakh adrenaline
     - 2.0% Mepivacaine with 1:2 lakh adrenaline
     - 2.0% Procaine, 0.4% propoxycaine with a vasoconstrictor
     - 4.0% Prilocaine when used for nerve block
   - Medium acting anesthetics (90–150 minutes)
     - 2.0% Lignocaine and 2% Mepivacaine with a vasoconstrictor for pulpal anesthesia
     - 4.0% Prilocaine with 1:2 lakh adrenaline
   - Long acting anesthetics (more than 150 minutes)
     - 0.5% Bupivacaine with 1:2 lakh adrenaline
     - 0.5% or 1.5% Etidocaine with 1:2 lakh adrenaline
5. Based on biological site and mode of action
   - Class A: Acting at receptor site, located on external surface of nerve membrane
     - Tetrodotoxin, Saxitoxin
   - Class B: Acting at receptor site, located on internal surface of nerve membrane
     - Quaternary ammonium analogues of lidocaine, Scorpion venom
   - Class C: Acting by a receptor-independent physico-chemical mechanism
     - Benzocaine
   - Class D: Acting by combination of receptor-mediated and receptor-independent mechanisms
     - Lidocaine, Mepivacaine, Prilocaine (Most clinically useful local anesthetic)

Composition of an Injectable Local Anesthetic Solution

Each 1.0 ml of 2.0% Xylocaine with 1:2 lakh adrenaline consists of following:

1. ***Lignocaine hydrochloride (21.3 mg) (local anesthetic agent):*** *Lidocaine/Xylocaine/Octocaine* is used as hydrochloride salt which is readily water soluble and can withstand boiling and autoclaving.
   - *Pharmacology*: Diffuses readily through interstitial tissues and into the lipid rich nerves, giving a rapid onset of action. It is two times more potent and toxic as compared to procaine.
   - *Onset time*: 2–3 minutes
   - *Duration*: 30–75 minutes
   - *Dose*: 4.4 mg/kg (not to exceed 300 mg when not accompanied by a vasoconstrictor) and 7 mg/kg (not to exceed 500 mg when used with vasoconstrictor).
2. ***Adrenaline/epinephrine (vasoconstrictor) 0.005 mg***: It is the most potent vasoconstrictor used in dentistry. Concentrations from 1:50000 to 1:250000 are commonly used. Excessive doses may produce side effects primarily in cardiovascular, respiratory and central nervous system. Its addition in local anesthetic solution provides the following effects:
   - Prolongs duration of action of local anesthesia by decreasing their rate of removal from the local site into the circulation.
   - Enhances the intensity of nerve block.
   - Reduces systemic toxicity of local anesthesia by decreasing their absorption.
   - Provide hemostasis by vasoconstriction.
3. ***Sodium metabisulphite (preservative) (0.5 mg)***
   - Prevents oxidation when exposed to air.
4. ***Sodium chloride (6.0 mg)***
   - Makes the solution isotonic.
5. ***Methylparaben (1.0 mg)***
   - Used as preservative; however, it is primarily responsible for allergic reactions.
6. ***Distilled water (1.0 ml)***
   - Provides volume to solution (as diluent)
   - Thymol (fungicide) was present earlier as bacteriostatic agent; nowadays, it is not used.

TECHNIQUES OF REGIONAL ANESTHESIA

A. Anesthesia for Maxillary Nerve and its Subdivisions

32

1. Local Infiltration

Local infiltration anesthetizes terminal branches of the free nerve endings at that site. The area into which the local anesthesia is injected gets anesthetized. The anatomic landmarks are not much important.

It is indicated when only the mucous membrane and underlying connective tissues are to be anesthetized.

Technique

A long, 25 gauge needle is inserted beneath the mucous membrane into the connective tissue in the area to be anesthetized. The solution is injected slowly throughout the area (Fig. 32.1).

Probe or any other suitable instrument can be used to evaluate onset of anesthesia.

2. Block of Terminal Branches

Large terminal branches of any area are anesthetized. The anatomical landmarks depend on the areas to be anesthetized.

It is indicated for one or two maxillary teeth. Blocking the larger terminal branches in mandible is difficult because of its denseness. However, it may be used to block terminal branches of mandible in younger individuals.

Techniques

a. *Paraperiosteal technique*: The success of this technique depends on the diffusion of the solution through the periosteum and into the underlying bone to come in contact with the underlying nerves. The bone covering the deciduous maxillary teeth is thicker than the bone covering the maxillary permanent teeth. When one or two teeth are to be anesthetized, the 25 gauge needle is inserted into the mucobuccal fold so that it makes contact with the periosteum opposite and just above the apex of the tooth. 1.0–2.0 ml solution is deposited slowly. Sometimes, intraosseous (the solution is injected into the bone by creating a hole) or interseptal (the

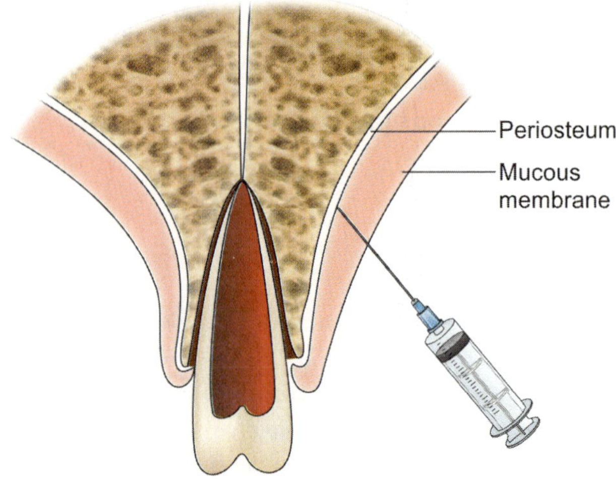

Fig. 32.1 Local infiltration (submucosal anesthesia)

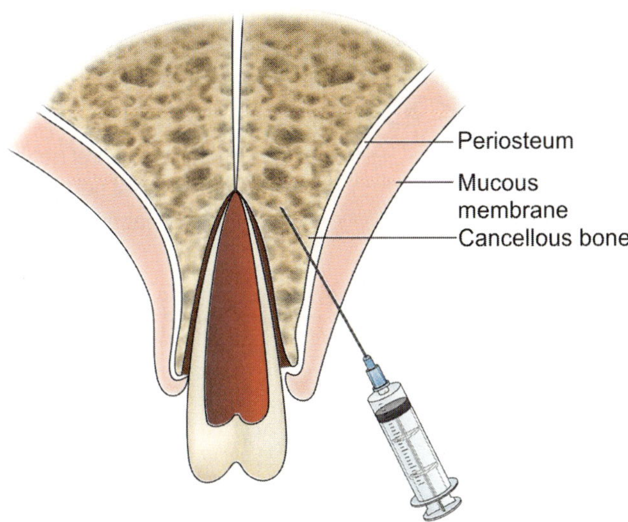

Fig. 32.2 Intraosseous anesthesia

solution is injected into the thin porous interseptal bone on either side of the tooth) techniques are also used (Fig. 32.2).

b. *Intraligamentary technique*: Special syringes have been developed to permit the solution to be injected under high pressure (Fig. 32.3a). The injection may also be given with conventional syringes. A 30 gauge needle is introduced through the gingival sulcus and into the periodontal ligament. The solution is injected with high pressure, forcing rather than diffusing the solution through periodontal ligament (Fig. 32.3b). It is advised that single rooted teeth be injected on the mesial/distal side or buccal/lingual side and the multirooted teeth be injected over each root.

It is documented that intraligamentary anesthesia produces immediate onset of anesthesia. When used as a primary injection, it is effective for 10–20 minutes; whereas, a supplemental injection with inferior alveolar nerve block, the effect is more pronounced.

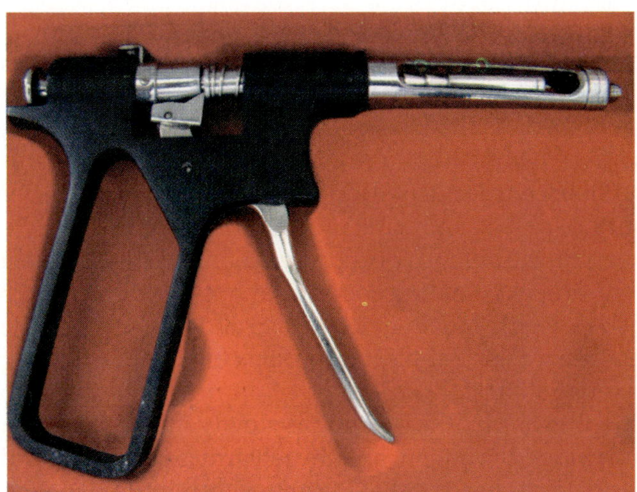
Fig. 32.3a Syringe for intraligamentary anesthesia

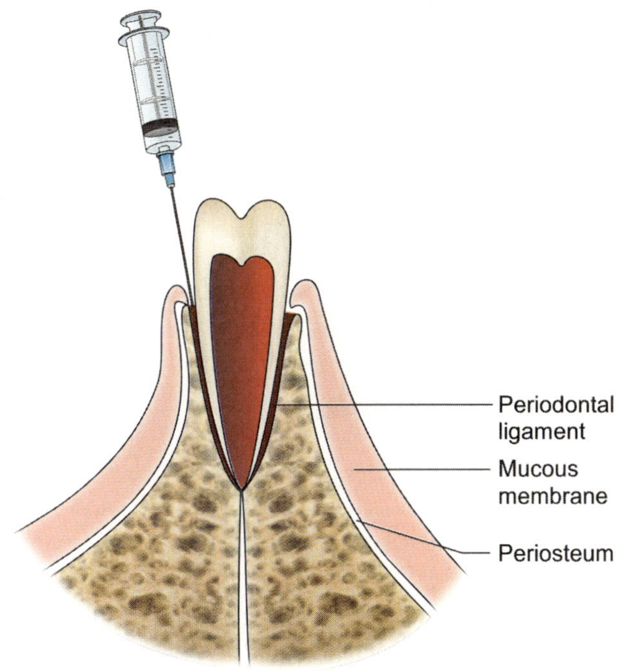

Fig. 32.3b Intraligamentary anesthesia

Complications

- *Postoperative discomfort*: The postoperative discomfort is related to the damage from the insertion of needle and not from the pressure of solution deposition. Initial discomfort mostly resolves within a day.
- *Avulsion*: Tooth avulsion, as hypothesized earlier, has not been documented adequately.
- *Occlusal disturbances*: Feeling of high in occlusion resolves within 24 hours.

c. *Intrapulpal*: Once the pulp chamber has been exposed, the needle may be introduced directly into the pulp (Fig. 32.4). The needle is wedged firmly into the pulp chamber or root canal and 0.1 to 0.2 ml solution is injected into canal. The anesthesia is achieved due to pressure and not by the amount of anesthetic solution injected into the canal.

3. Infraorbital Block (Anterior and Middle Superior Alveolar Nerves)

The infraorbital, anterior and middle superior alveolar, inferior palpebral, lateral nasal and superior labial nerves are anesthetized by this block. The incisors, cuspids, bicuspids and mesiobuccal root of first molar including the bony support and soft tissues, upper lip,

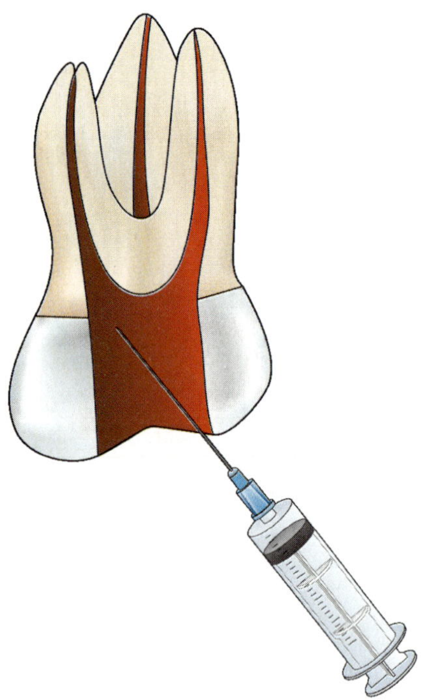

Fig. 32.4 Intrapulpal anesthesia

lower eyelid, portion of nose on the side of injection are the areas which get anesthetized.

The anatomical landmarks, viz. infraorbital ridge, infraorbital notch, anterior teeth and pupils of eyes are important for this block.

Technique

The supraorbital and infraorbital notches are palpated. An imaginary line is drawn passing through the pupils of the eye, the infraorbital foramen, bicuspid teeth and the mental foramen. The palpating finger is moved about 0.5 cm below infraorbital notch located on infraorbital rim where a shallow depression will be felt. This corresponds to infraorbital foramen. An appropriate long 25 gauge needle is inserted into the mucobuccal fold from either of the two techniques (directions) (Fig. 32.5). In the first technique the operator inserts in a line parallel with the supraorbital notch, the pupil of the eye, infraorbital notch, and the second bicuspid tooth. The needle should be inserted 5.0 mm buccal to the mucobuccal fold to pass over canine fossa. The thumb over the infraorbital foramen should be used to guide the needle into the position where it contacts the bone at the entrance of the infraorbital foramen.

The second technique of insertion bisects the crown of the central incisor from the mesioincisal angle to the disto-gingival angle of the same side. The needle is inserted towards the infraorbital foramen. In either approach, the needle should not penetrate more than three-fourth of an inch. This prevents the needle from

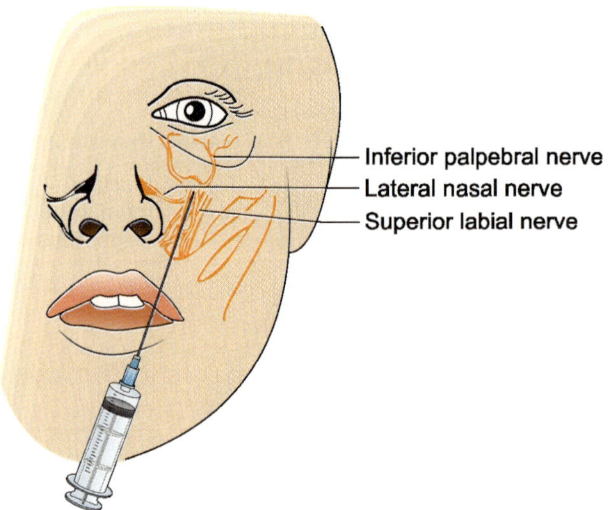

Fig. 32.5 Infraorbital nerve block

entering the orbital cavity. Approximately 2.0 ml of solution is injected in the area.

4. Posterior Superior Alveolar Block

The posterior superior alveolar nerve is anesthetized.

The maxillary molars, except the mesiobuccal root of first molar, buccal alveolar process of the maxillary molars including the overlying tissues are the areas which get anesthetized.

The anatomical landmarks viz. mucobuccal fold and its concavity, zygomatic process of the maxilla, infratemporal surface of maxilla, anterior border and coronoid process of the ramus of the mandible and tuberosity of the maxilla are important for this block.

This block is indicative for operative procedures of the maxillary molars and supporting structures.

Technique

For the right side block, the left forefinger is moved over the mucobuccal fold in a posterior direction from the bicuspid area until the zygomatic process of maxilla is reached. At this particular point the finger is rotated so that the fingernail is adjacent to the mucosa and its bulbous portion is still in contact with the posterior surface of the zygomatic process. The hand is lowered, keeping the bulbous portion of the finger still in contact with the zygomatic process. An appropriate long 25 gauge needle is held in pen grasp and inserted into the tissues in a line parallel to the index finger and bisecting the fingernail for a distance of approximately half to one-third inch. The solution is slowly injected. For left side block, the patient and the left arm is passed around the patients head so that the area may be palpated with the left forefinger.

5. Nasopalatine Nerve Block

Nasopalatine nerve is anesthetized. This nerve block is not commonly used in endodontics.

It is indicated for palatal anesthesia and also to complete the anesthesia of nasal septum.

The anterior portion of hard palate and overlying structures up to bicuspid area are anesthetized.

The anatomical landmarks, viz. central incisors and incisive papilla are important for this block.

6. Anterior Palatine Nerve Block (Greater Palatine Nerve Block)

Anterior palatine nerve is anesthetized. The posterior portion of hard palate and overlying structures up to first bicuspid are anesthetized.

It is indicated for palatal anesthesia to be used in conjunction with the posterior superior alveolar nerve block.

The anatomical landmarks, viz. second and third maxillary molars, palatal gingival margin of second and third maxillary molars, midline of palate, a line approximately 1.0 cm from the palatal-gingival margin towards the midline of the palate are important for this block.

Technique

The greater palatine foramen is approached from the opposite side with an appropriate long, 25 gauge needle, which is kept as near to right angle as possible with the curvature of the palatal bone. The needle is inserted till the palatal bone is encountered and then 0.25 to 0.5 ml of the solution is deposited very slowly.

B. Anesthesia for Mandibular Division and Subdivisions

1. Inferior Alveolar Nerves Block (Direct Conventional Inferior Alveolar Nerve Block): Open Mouth Approach

This is the most commonly used nerve block in endodontics.

The inferior alveolar nerve and its subdivisions, mental nerve, incisive nerve, and occasionally the lingual nerve and buccinator nerve are anesthetized.

The body of mandible and inferior portion of ramus, mandibular teeth, mucous membrane and underlying tissues anterior to the first mandibular molar are anesthetized.

It is indicated for procedures on the mandibular teeth and supporting structures, anterior to the first molar.

The anatomical landmarks, viz. mucobuccal fold, anterior border of the ramus of mandible, external oblique ridge, coronoid notch, retromolar triangle, internal oblique ridge, pterygomandibular ligament, buccal sucking pad, pterygomandibular space are important for this block.

Technique

The operator stands in front of the patient and with the left index finger or thumb palpates the mucobuccal fold. The finger is then moved posteriorly until contact is made with the external oblique ridge on the anterior border of ramus of mandible. When the finger or thumb contacts the ramus of mandible, it is moved up and down until the greatest depth of the anterior border of the ramus is identified. This is called the coronoid notch and is in direct line with the mandibular sulcus. The palpating finger is moved lingually across the retromolar triangle and onto the internal oblique ridge. The finger is then moved to the buccal side, taking with it the buccal sucking pad. An appropriate long, 25 gauge needle is then inserted parallel to the occlusal plane of the mandibular teeth from the opposite side (Fig. 32.6), at a level bisecting the finger nail. The depth of insertion is assessed by estimating when the needle tip has been advanced half the distance between the palpating index finger. Patient is asked to keep the mouth wide open. The needle is inserted gently, making contact with the internal surface of ramus. The needle is then withdrawn about 1.0 mm and 1.0–1.8 ml solution is injected. For left side, the operator stands slightly to the back and right side of the patient. The left arm is placed around the patients head so that the landmarks can be palpated with the left finger. The needle is slightly withdrawn and the lingual nerve is anesthetized.

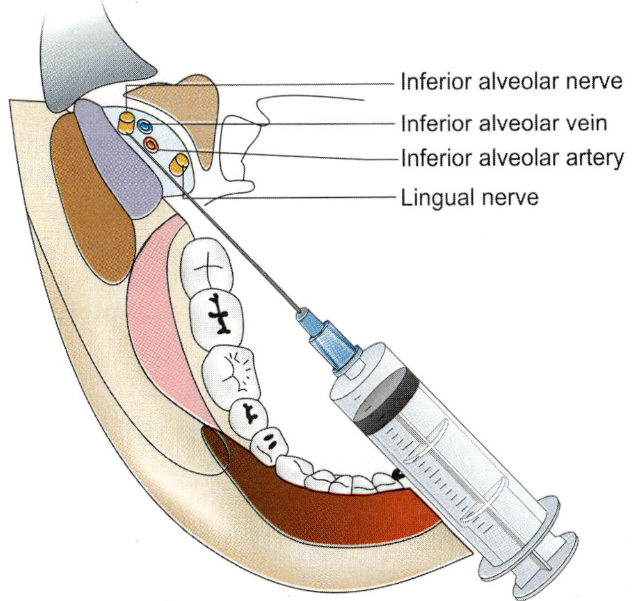

Fig. 32.6 Inferior alveolar nerve block

2. Vazirani-Akinosi Inferior Alveolar Nerve Block: Close-Mouth Approach

The inferior alveolar nerve and its subdivisions, mental and incisive nerves, lingual and buccinators nerves are anesthetized. The anesthetized area includes mandibular hard and soft tissue to the midline including the floor of mouth and anterior two-thirds of the tongue.

The anatomical landmarks are the occlusal plane of occluding teeth, mucogingival junction of the maxillary molar teeth and anterior border of ramus.

Technique

With the mouth closed, the needle is aligned parallel to the occlusal plane and positioned at the level of the muco-gingival junction of the maxillary molars. The operator retracts the patient's lip and the needle is penetrated about one and a half inches into the mucosa just medial to the ramus. After negative aspiration, the solution is slowly deposited.

Advantages

- Simple and easy to master technique.
- Three major nerves are anesthetized by single needle injection.
- Fear of injection into the throat does not exist.
- Useful in patients with limited mouth opening like trismus, space infection, etc.

Disadvantage

- Relies on minimum bony landmarks.

3. Inferior Alveolar Nerve Block (Gow-Gates Technique): True Mandibular Nerve Block

Inferior alveolar nerve and its subdivisions, mental nerve, incisive nerve, lingual nerve and buccinator, mylohyoid, auriculotemporal nerves are anesthetized by this technique.

All mandibular hard and soft tissues up to the midline including the floor of the mouth and anterior two-thirds of the tongue, the skin over the zygoma, the posterior portion of cheek, temporal region and a portion of external ear will be anesthetized.

It is indicated for operative and surgical procedure on the mandibular teeth.

Technique

The patient is placed in supine position and the operator stands to the right and slightly in front of the patient. Patient keeps the mouth wide open and remains in that position till injection is completed. An imaginary line is drawn from the corner of the mouth to the intertragic notch of the ear. The anterior border of the mandible is palpated, and the tendon of the temporal muscle is identified. Operator visually aligns the intraoral and extraoral landmarks, and the needle is introduced through the mucosa just medial to the temporal tendon and directed towards the target area on a line extending from the corner of the mouth to the intertragic notch. The degree of divergence of the external ear to the head is used as a guide to the lateral flare of the ramus. Needle insertion should be parallel to the flare of the ear. Needle is advanced till the fovea region of the condyle is contacted. Depth of insertion should not exceed 25–27 mm. If bone contact is not established, the needle should be withdrawn and redirected after checking the landmarks again. After injection, the patient is asked to keep the mouth open for 20–30 seconds to allow adequate bathing of the nerve trunk that has been straightened by open mouth. The onset of anesthesia takes five to seven minutes.

4. Lingual Nerve Block

Lingual nerve is anesthetized by this block leading to regional anesthesia of anterior two-thirds of the tongue and the floor of the mouth, mucosa and mucoperiosteum on the lingual side of the mandible.

It is indicated for procedure on the anterior two-thirds of the tongue, floor of the oral cavity and mucous membrane on the lingual side of the mandible.

Technique

Same as inferior alveolar nerve block.

5. Long Buccal Nerve Block

Long buccal nerve is anesthetized. The areas anesthetized are, buccal mucous membrane and mucoperiosteum of the mandibular molar.

The block is indicated for anesthesia of the mandibular buccal mucosa and to supplement the inferior alveolar nerve block.

The anatomical landmarks for block are external oblique ridge and retromolar triangle.

Technique

The needle is inserted in the buccal mucosa just distal to the third molar depositing 0.25–0.5 ml anesthetic solution in this area. An alternate technique is to insert the needle directly into the retromolar triangle.

Instrumentation is necessary for the demonstration of objective symptoms, since none of the subjective symptoms are present.

6. Mental Nerve Block

Mental nerve is anesthetized resulting in anesthesia of lower lip and mucous membrane in the mucobuccal fold anterior to the mental foramen.

It is indicated for the surgery of the lower lip or mucous membrane in the mucobuccal fold anterior to the mental foramen.

Technique

The apices of the bicuspid teeth should be estimated. The needle should be inserted into the mucobuccal fold after the cheek has been pulled to the buccal side. The tissues are penetrated till the periosteum of the mandible is contacted slightly anterior to the apex of the second bicuspid. 0.5–1.0 ml solution is injected.

Both subjective and objective symptoms are present. Subjective symptoms are tingling and numbness of lower lip; while for objective symptoms, instrumentation is necessary to demonstrate absence of pain sensation.

7. Incisive Nerve Block

Incisive nerve and mental nerve are anesthetized. Mandible and overlying labial structures anterior to the mental foramen, premolars, canines and incisors and lower lip are anesthetized.

It is indicated for anesthesia of the anterior mandible to the mental foramen and lower lip, when for some reason, the inferior alveolar nerve anesthesia is contraindicated or unnecessary.

Technique

It is same as that for mental nerve block, except that the needle point should penetrate into the mental foramen.

Subjective symptoms are numbness and tingling of lower lip; whereas, for objective symptoms, instrumentation is necessary to demonstrate absence of pain sensation.

8. Local Infiltration

Free nerve endings in the infiltrated area are anesthetized. Mucous membrane and mucoperiosteum in the infiltrated area are anesthetized.

It is indicated for soft tissue surgery in limited area.

Technique

The needle is inserted beneath the mucous membrane into the underlying tissues. More than one needle insertion may be necessary. The solution is deposited slowly and in minimal volumes.

Instrumentation is necessary for the demonstration of absence of pain, since none of the subjective symptoms are present.

Complications of Anesthesia

The complications of anesthesia are usually classified as:

1. Primary or secondary
2. Mild or severe
3. Transient or permanent

The complications can also be classified as:

1. Due to Solution Used

i. Toxicity
ii. Idiosyncrasy
iii. Allergy
iv. Anaphylactic reactions
v. Infections caused by infected solutions
vi. Local irritation or tissue reaction caused by the solution

2. Due to Insertion of Needle

i. Syncope
ii. Muscle trismus
iii. Pain or hyperalgesia
iv. Edema
v. Infections
vi. Broken needle
vii. Prolonged anesthesia other than from the anaesthetic solution
viii. Hematoma
ix. Sloughing
x. Bizarre neurological symptoms

Advances in Local Anesthesia

Various advances in local anesthesia are as follows.

a. Computerized Local Anesthetic Administration Device

A computerized local anesthetic delivery system has been developed as a possible means of eliminating pain due to injection. It consists of a conventional local anesthetic cartridge linked to a disposable Luer-lock needle.

The system delivers anesthesia at a constant pressure and controlled volume, regardless of the resistance in the tissues.

b. Electronic Dental Anesthesia

Transcutaneous electrical nerve stimulation (TENS) has been used for the management of acute and chronic pain.

In many instances, proper use of electronic nerve stimulation results in lack of need for local anesthetic. The patient controls the level of anesthesia needed, and once the unit is turned off, there is no numbness to recover from as with local anesthesia.

Patients with pacemakers, neurophysiological disorders (like epilepsy) and pregnant women should not be offered electronic anesthesia because of its harmful side effects.

c. EMLA (Eutectic Mixture of Local Anesthesia)

EMLA contains both lidocaine (2.5%) and prilocaine (2.5%). It significantly reduces pain experienced during needle insertion. It does not provide profound pulpal anesthesia for major endodontic procedures.

Lidocaine-prilocaine eutectic mixture is marketed as a cream base (EMLA cream) or a cellulose disk (EMLA patch). EMLA cream is used as a local anesthetic for topical application. EMLA is used to prevent pain associated with needle insertion, intravenous cannulation, laser hair removal and superficial surgery on skin.

EMLA patch (*DentiPatch*™) is an adhesive, which is absorbed by the mucosa. It is used as mild topical anesthesia for superficial dental procedures. It should be applied at least one hour or prior to local anesthetic injection.

Failure of Anesthesia in Endodontic Procedures

The failure of local anesthesia in endodontic procedures may be because of various reasons. The main reasons are:

a. Anatomic Causes

Accessory innervations to the mandibular teeth, especially molars, is the main cause of failure of local anesthesia. Various sources are: nerve to mylohyoid muscle, lingual nerve, upper cervical nerves and auriculotemporal nerve.

To overcome this problem, a nerve block given at a higher level (Gow-Gates or Vazirani-Akinosi nerve block technique) would predictably block the nerve impulses. Still, if pain persists, then the anesthetic solution is deposited at the apices of the teeth (intraligamentary or intraosseous route).

b. Effect of Inflammation on Local Tissue pH

As inflammation/infection produces acidosis, the low pH will result in a greater proportion of the local anesthetic being trapped in the changed acid form of the molecule and, therefore, unable to cross cell membranes. This is known as 'ion trapping'.

To overcome this problem, it is suggested that drugs like 3.0% mepivacaine should be used, which would increase the concentration of the molecules in the base form. The molecules can easily cross the cell membrane producing profound anesthesia even at low pH.

A few authors disagree with this hypothesis. Firstly, acidosis may be of minor magnitude, as extravasations of RBC's or protein products increases the buffering capacity of inflamed tissue. Secondly, change in pH is a localized event and should be concern for infiltration and not nerve block.

32

c. Increased Blood flow due to Vasodilation

In such cases, higher concentrations of vasoconstrictors may produce profound anesthesia, e.g. 1:100000 or 1:80000.

d. Effect of Inflammation on Nociceptors

Inflammatory mediators like Bradykinins, Prostaglandins, etc. activate or sensitize nociceptors. They also have a profound structural effect on these neurons. The Tetrodotoxin (TTX) resistant sodium channels are formed, which are less sensitive to lidocaine. To overcome this problem, the volume of anesthetic solution is increased (within the recommended maximum dose). It is helpful in two ways; first, it will expose a greater length of the nerve to be blocked and secondly, it will block the population of TTX resistant class of sodium channels.

e. Psychological Factors

Patients with the history of experiencing inadequate local anesthesia for dental procedures and those with high level of anxiety and apprehension may also contribute to local anesthetic failure. For managing such patients, a clinician should develop a positive and confident relationship with the patient. Also, drugs like alprazolam, midazolam, etc. can be administered.

PRINCIPLES OF SURGERY

The general principles involved in surgery are:

a. ***Painless surgery***: The assurance of painless surgery is important to avoid psychological and physical stress to the patient, which may predispose to shock, delay in recovery and make the surgery under local anesthesia more difficult.

Usually, most of the dental procedures can be carried out under local anesthesia; however, general anesthesia should also be the part of treatment option.

b. ***Asepsis***: Asepsis implies methods, which prevent contamination of wound by environment. Sterilization rather than disinfection is mandatory whenever tissue is penetrated or there is contact with blood or serum.

c. ***Minimal damage of vital tissues***: The damage of vital tissues during surgery should be minimum. Certain radical operations may require the sacrifice of vital structures; however, damage or loss of function should not be because of carelessness.

d. ***Adequate access***: The surgical incisions in the skin should be made along the 'Resting skin tension lines (RSTL)' or natural skin creases ensuring the scar to be more esthetic and less conspicuous.

Some commonly used skin incisions in the maxillofacial region are:
- Submandibular incision
- Retromandibular incision
- Preauricular incision
- Brows incision
- Infraorbital incision
- Coronal incision.

Principles of Surgical Incisions in Soft Tissues

The principles followed for surgical incisions in soft tissues are:

1. Incision must be made with a sharp blade. BP blade (15) is used in routine; however, during incision and drainage of an abscess, BP blade (11) is used. A sharp blade cleanly incises the tissues without damage. Such incisions heal without wound dehiscence.
2. Whenever an incision is made, blade should be held perpendicular to the epithelial surface and not obliquely.
3. The incision must be firm and stroke must be continuous and deep to the bone. Supraperiosteal incisions and multiple strokes result in tissue damage. The blood vessels are situated supraperiosteally; incising over the periosteum while reflecting flap protects supraperiosteal blood vessels. Short and interrupted incisions must be avoided. To reduce bleeding, injection of vasoconstrictor solution into the area can be given prior to making incision.
4. Incisions must be carefully planned in such a manner that vital structures are not damaged, e.g. incision parallel to the long-axis of vessels will not damage the vessels. When operating in vascular areas, the incision may be modified to reduce bleeding (electrosurgery may be used instead of scalpel).
5. The incisions should never be made over the operative site but rather in adjacent undisturbed areas so that flap will be supported by normal tissues and potential for revascularization is preserved.
6. Incisions should never be made in an area of thinned mucosa like that found over exostosis or other bony prominence because blood supply is reduced, suturing is difficult and rate of wound dehiscence is high.
7. Flap must be designed to provide adequate access to the surgical area.
8. Flap must have broad base and good vascular supply.
9. Length and breadth is an important factor. It is preferable that length of flap does not exceed the base.
10. When repositioned, it should rest on a healthy bone and not on a defect or hematoma.
11. Whenever incision is likely to involve free gingival margin, adequate care is taken not to disturb epithelial attachment, otherwise during wound healing there is distinct shift in epithelial reattachment exposing the cementum.
12. When the flap is raised, care should be taken to avoid perforation of flap. Such perforations may result in flap necrosis.
13. Flap is designed in such a way that there is no tension during retraction, surgery and suturing.
14. The flap should be handled gently. Gentle handling is preferred during retraction with appropriate retractors. Failure to do so will result in tissue laceration, postoperative edema and tissue damage.
15. Meticulous hemostasis during surgery is important. Excessive bleeding disturbs the fluid balance. It also results in poor visibility of the surgical field. Bleeding under the flap may result in subperiosteal hematoma, which interferes with healing of the flap.

Classification of Flaps

I. Based on bone exposure after reflection
- Full thickness flap (mucoperiosteal flap)
- Partial thickness flap (split thickness flap)
- Combination flap (full split type flap)

II. Based on presence/absence of vertical incisions
- Envelope flap (without vertical releasing incisions)
- Relaxed flap (with vertical releasing incisions)

III. Depending upon the shape of flap
- Two-sided/triangular flap
- Three-sided/trapezoidal flap
- Semilunar flap

IV. Based on the underlying specific blood vessel
- Pedicle flap
- Non-pedicle flap.

The routinely used flaps are:

Full Thickness Flap

The soft tissue including the periosteum is reflected to expose the underlying bone (Fig. 32.7a and b). A full thickness flap is performed by blunt dissection of the oral mucosa away from the teeth and alveolar bone. This is carried out with periosteal elevators or any other blunt instrument.

Indication

- Where access and visibility of the alveolar bone is required
- When primary wound healing is essential.

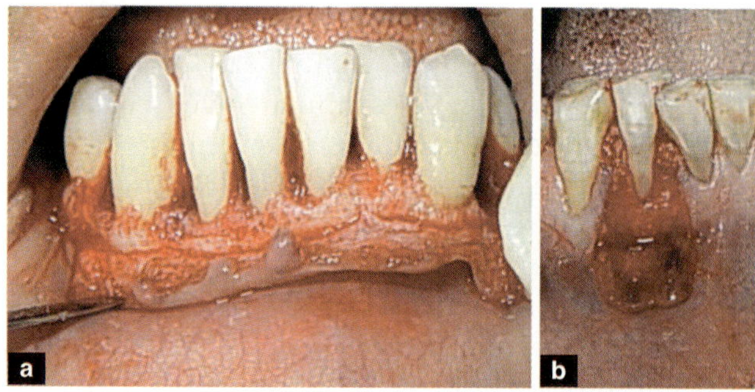
Fig. 32.7a and b Full thickness flap

Advantages
- Easy to perform than the split thickness flaps
- Improved visibility of the alveolar bone
- Generally associated with less bleeding and less post-operative pain.

Partial Thickness Flap

It includes only the epithelium and a layer of underlying connective tissue (Fig. 32.8a and b). Partial thickness flaps are accomplished by using a scalpel, which sharply dissect through the lamina propria of gingiva and alveolar mucosa.

Combination Flap

The combination of both complete thickness and partial thickness flap may be required to be used in certain procedures (Fig. 32.9).

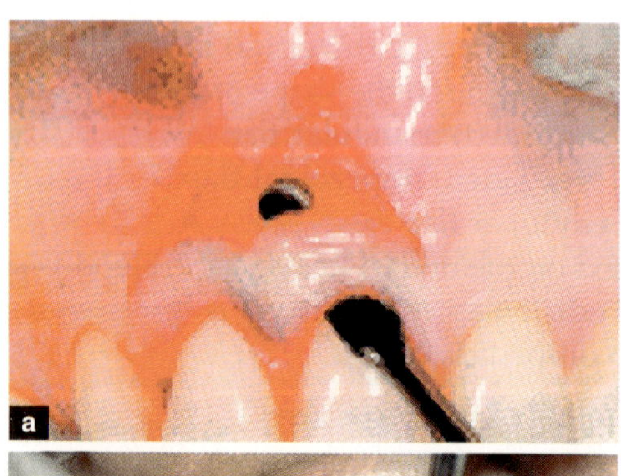
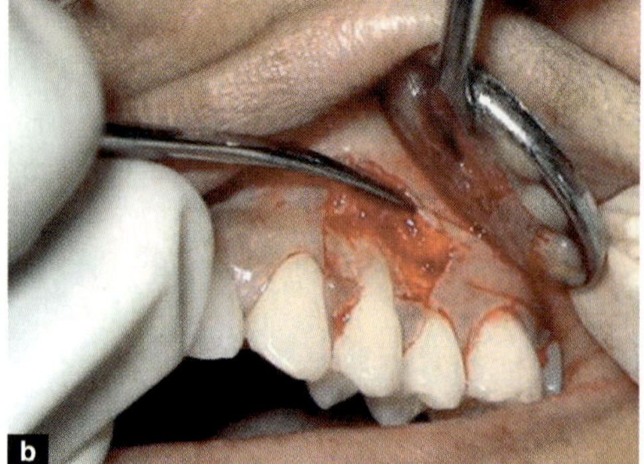
Fig. 32.8a and b Partial thickness flap

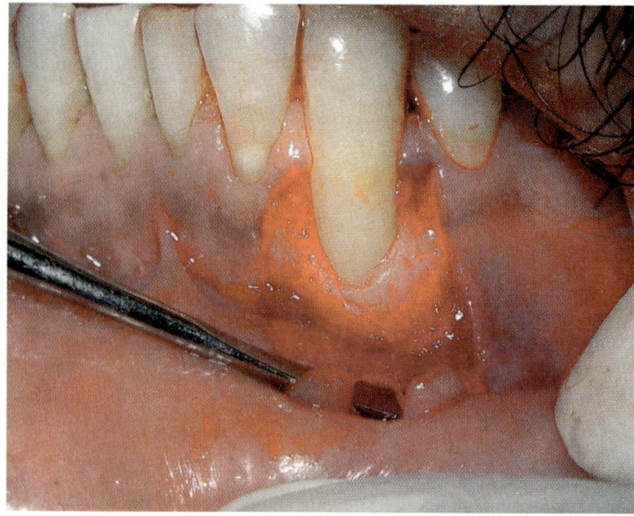
Fig. 32.9 Combination flap

Envelope Flap

No vertical incision is given and the flap begins and ends within the gingival sulcus of the contiguous teeth (Fig. 32.10).

Advantages
- Because envelope flaps have no vertical incisions, they are quicker to heal
- Less postoperative pain and bleeding.

Disadvantages
- Limit the access to the bony tissues
- Cannot be moved/repositioned to other locations.

Relaxed Flaps

These flaps have vertical releasing incisions and offer tremendous flexibility in terms of access and tissue control.

Advantages
- Better accessibility
- Can be repositioned to other locations.

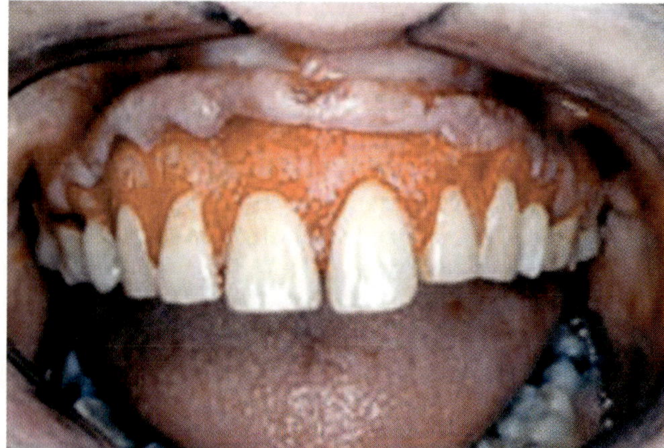
Fig. 32.10 Envelope flap

Disadvantages

- Vertical incisions delay healing as blood supply is compromised.
- Greater postoperative pain and bleeding.

Two-sided/Triangular Flap

Two-sided triangular flap is designed by making a releasing incision on the side of envelope flap that should be preferably divergent towards the vestibular sulcus forming an obtuse angle at the free gingival margin (Fig. 32.11a and b).

Three-sided/Trapezoidal Flap

Three-sided trapezoidal flap is a modification of two-sided triangular flap with addition of a second vertical incision towards vestibule to make better access (Fig. 32.12a and b). Care should be taken to keep the base of flap as broad as possible to ensure good blood supply (base to length ratio should be 2 : 1).

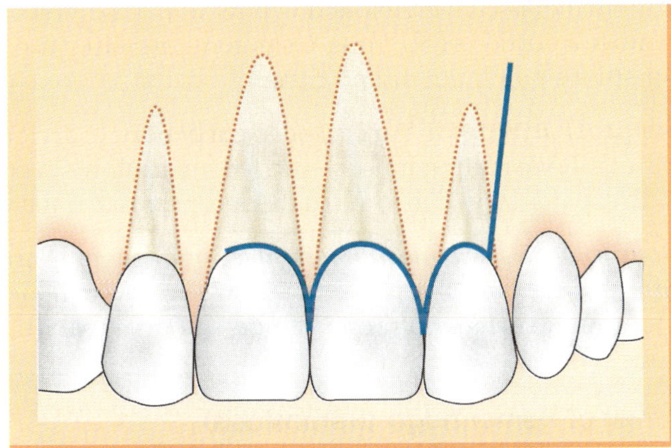

Fig. 32.11a Triangular flap (diagrammatic)

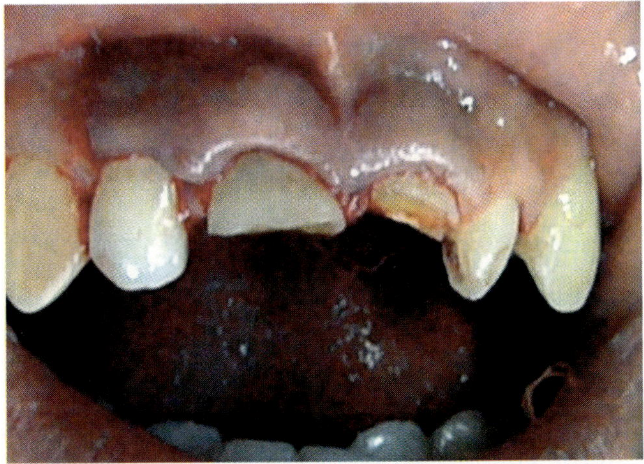

Fig. 32.11b Triangular (two-sided flap)

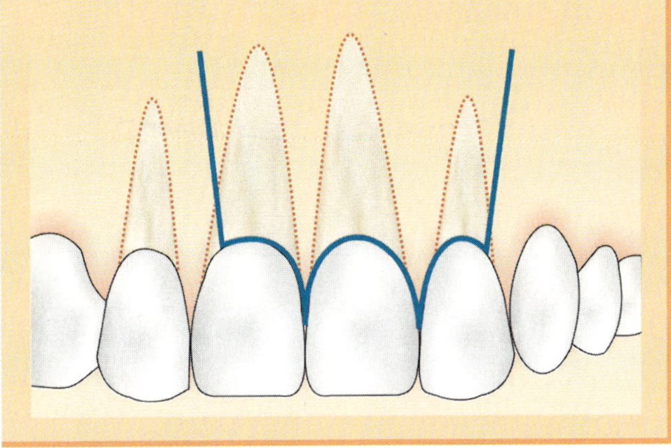

Fig. 32.12a Trapezoidal flap (diagrammatic)

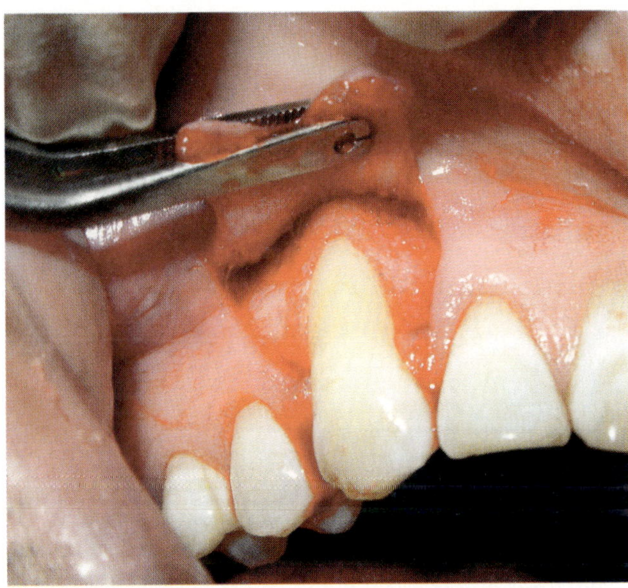

Fig. 32.12b Trapezoidal (three-sided flap)

Semilunar Flap

The semilunar flap is designed when periapical area is to be exposed. The height of incision is kept 5.0 mm away from the free gingival margin (Fig. 32.13a and b). This flap is preferred over the envelope flaps as there is no gingival retraction. The main disadvantage is that it leaves an unesthetic scar.

In edentulous case, horizontal incisions are placed on the alveolar crest and vertical incisions remain at the same place as in dentulous mouth.

Pedicle Flap

The flap based on specific blood vessel is known as pedicle flap, e.g. in palate, flap based on greater palatine vessels. If the flap is designed along the long-axis of the blood vessel, the base of the flap will be located around the maxillary third molar.

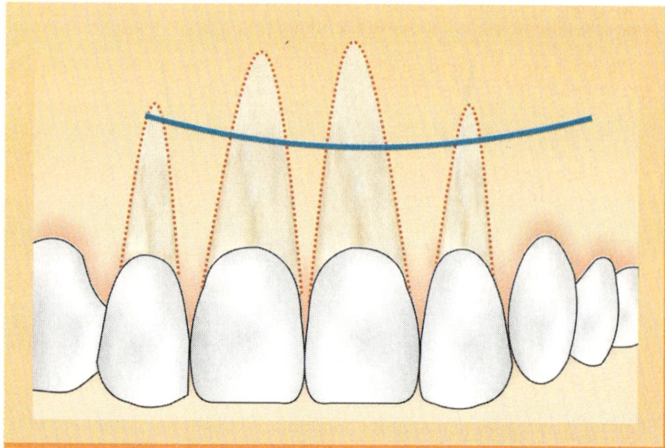

Fig. 32.13a Semilunar incision (diagrammatic)

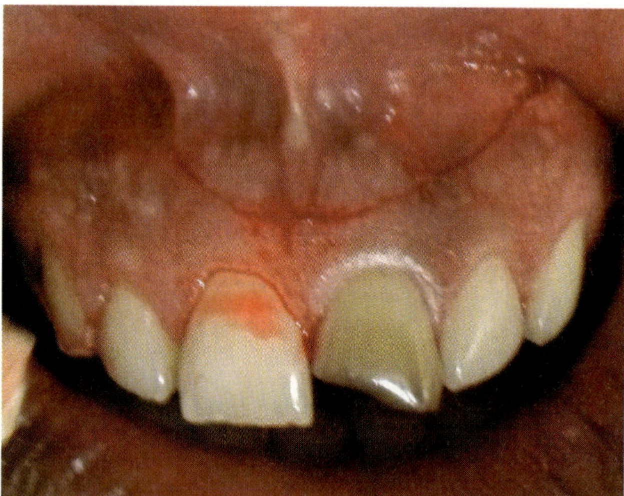

Fig. 32.13b Semilunar incision

Non-pedicle Flap

The flap not based on a specific blood vessel is termed non-pedicle flap.

Dissection and Reflection of Mucoperiosteal Flap

Adequate retraction is essential for surgical access. The retractor must rest on sound bone with light but firm pressure. The mucoperiosteal flap may be reflected with a periosteal elevator. The elevator is first inserted into the incision and starting in the buccal sulcus where periosteum is loosely attached, the first few millimeters at the edge of flap are gently freed along the periphery. Thereafter, it is reflected evenly along its periphery by a clear movement with the end pressed and firmly kept against bone. The reflective forces should be applied to the bone and periosteum with minimum force on the gingiva. Lifting movements are avoided as they tend to tear tissues. Bleeding tissue tags should not be removed during surgery as they help in healing.

The following features are important:

- When flap is reflected, care should be taken not to damage important anatomical structures like neurovascular bundles present around infraorbital and mental foramen
- Take care of muscular attachments during flap reflection
- Elevation of lingual mucoperiosteum near third molar carries risk of injury to lingual nerve
- Elevation of the mucoperiosteal flap in the palate needs careful consideration. Mucosa is tightly bound to midpalatine suture. The incision placed in the palate across the greater palatine vessels may results in brisk bleeding.

Bone Removal

Bone can be removed by chisel osteotome, surgical burs and bone rongeurs/files, etc.

***Chisel and osteotome*:** Chisel is a mono-bevelled instrument while osteotome is bi-bevelled. Chisel along with mallet is convenient and conventional method to remove a portion of the bone. Osteotome is mainly used for splitting of tooth or and bone.

***Surgical bur*:** Surgical bur is used to cut bone or to divide a tooth. Bone cutting must be carried out at slow speed with copious irrigation to avoid thermal necrosis of bone.

***Bone rongeurs or bone nibblers file*:** Bone rongeurs are useful in clipping sharp and irregular margins of bone. The rough surfaces of bone can be smoothened with bone file.

Arrest of Hemorrhage (Hemostasis)

The hemorrhage, if any, must be arrested before suturing the flap, otherwise accumulation of blood in the dead space becomes a nidus for growth of bacteria. Various methods used for hemostasis are:

- Digital pressure
- Hemostat or artery forceps
- Ligature
- Packing with gauge and hemostatic agents
- Electrocoagulation.

Débridement and Drainage

The debris and pathological tissues must be cleaned from the wound before closure. The bone cavity and flaps are trimmed off of all necrotic tissues or tags. Wound must be thoroughly irrigated with saline.

Dead space can be eliminated by adopting following features: Suturing tissue planes together to minimize the postoperative void, placing a pressure dressing over repaired wound, packing void until the bleeding has stopped and using drains, either alone or in addition to pressure dressing.

Wound Closure

Wound closure by suturing help obliterate dead spaces where accumulation of blood or other tissue fluids could prevent direct apposition of tissues and provide an environment favorable for bacterial growth. Sutures also distribute the tension of wound closure over a larger volume of tissues.

SUTURE MATERIALS

A suture is any thread or strand, which brings into apposition of surfaces or tissues, while a ligature is any thread or strands which obliterates the lumen of ductular structures. The suture material should be nonreactive, easy in handling and retain tensile strength till wound is completely healed.

Classification of Suture Materials

1. Absorbable
   a. Natural
      i. Catgut (plain and chromic)
      ii. Fascia lata
      iii. Kangaroo/beef tendon
   b. Synthetic
      i. Polyglactin 910 (vicryl)
         - Polyglycolic acid
         - Polydioxanone.
         - Polyglecaprone 25 (monocryl)
      ii. Irradiated Polyglactin 910 (vicryl rapid)
2. Nonabsorbable
   a. Natural
      - Silk
      - Cotton
      - Linen
   b. Synthetic.
      - Polyamide
      - Monofilament
      - Polyfilament (braided)
      - Polyester
      - Polyfilament
      - Uncoated
      - Coated (with polybutylate)
      - Polypropylene-monofilament (prolene)
      - Polybutester-novafil
      - Metals
      - Stainless steel
      - Platinum
      - Silver.

The commonly used sutures are:

Gut/Catgut

Gut/catgut is the most popular absorbable suture material. Plain catgut retains its tensile strength for approximately 10 days, while chromic catgut for 20 days. These are available in different sizes. Catgut is absorbed by proteolytic digestive enzymes released from inflammatory cells collected around the catgut (in the presence of infection catgut is rapidly absorbed).

Catgut is sterilized during preparation and kept in isopropyl alcohol. It should not be boiled or autoclaved as heat destroys the tensile strength. It should be wiped with saline prior to use.

Polyglactin 910 (Vicryl)

It is a synthetic absorbable suture material. It is braided to improve handling and is coated to reduce bacterial adherence and tissue drag. It is absorbed initially by hydrolysis and then phagocytosed by polymorphonuclear cells and other macrophages.

It is available in different sizes.

Advantages

- Minimum tissue reaction
- No fraying
- Excellent handling characteristics
- Distinct violet color is highly visible in the wound
- Unique molecular structure (retains its strength during the healing period and then get absorbed rapidly).

Disadvantage

Roughness.

Irradiated Polyglactin 910 (Vicryl Rapid)

It is braided synthetic absorbable, white color suture material, ideal for intraoral use.

It has a similar initial high tensile strength as that of the normal vicryl suture. It gives wound support up to 12 days. Its absorption is associated with minimal tissue reaction facilitating improved cosmetics and reduction of postoperative pain.

Silk

It is natural, nonabsorbable, polyfilament suture material, obtained from the cocoon of silkworm.

Advantages

- Does not soak fluids and never becomes brittle.
- Ties down smoothly and securely and its natural elasticity gives it an extensibility that signals when optimum knot placement has been achieved.

Disadvantage
- Infection rate is high as compared to synthetic materials.

Cotton

It is a natural, nonabsorbable (twisted polyfilament) suture, available in reels in an unsterile form. It can be sterilized by autoclaving.

Advantages
- Knot is secured
- Easy handling
- Cheap and freely available.

Disadvantages
- Absorbs fluids by capillary action (more chances of infection)
- Shows more tissue reaction
- Frays easily
- Low tensile strength.

Linen

It is a natural, nonabsorbable, polyfilament suture of natural linen color.

Advantages
- Knots slide down smoothly and tie securely
- Smooth and nonirritating.

Nylon

It is a synthetic, easily available nonabsorbable suture.

Advantages
- Smooth and nonirritating.
- High tensile strength, which is retained for a long-period.
- Cheaper.

Disadvantages
- Knot is slippery (may need 5–7 knots)
- Infection due to crevices in braided nylon.

Stainless Steel

Stainless steel wires are available in different sizes.

Disadvantages
- Knots are not firm and may break
- May excite tissue reaction.

Suture Selection

32

The selection of a suture material should be based on sound knowledge of the healing characteristics of the tissues to be approximated, physical and biological properties of the suture materials and condition of the wound to be closed.

- When a wound has reached maximal strength, sutures are no longer needed. Absorbable sutures are preferred in tissues that heal rapidly. Tissues that heal slowly are closed with nonabsorbable sutures.
- Multifilament sutures should be avoided in contaminated wounds as bacteria can linger within the suture.
- In case of cosmetic results, close and prolonged apposition of wound is achieved using inert monofilament suture (polyamide or prolene).
- Multifilament braided materials, such as black silk, or absorbable synthetic materials, such as polyglactin-910 are preferred for intraoral use.

SURGICAL NEEDLES

The surgical needles are sharp pointed instruments made of stainless steel or carbon steel. These are used for puncturing the tissue so as to guide the thread or wire to suture. The needles are available in a wide range of types, shapes, lengths and thickness.

Classification of Surgical Needles

- According to its eye
  - Eyeless needles (swaged)
  - Needles with eye
- According to shape
  - Straight needles
  - Curved needles
- According to cutting edge
  - Round body needles
  - Conventional cutting needles
  - Reverse cutting needles
- According to configuration tip
  - Triangular tipped needles
  - Round tipped needles
  - Blunt-point needles
  - Micro-point needles.

In endodontic surgery, the types of needles commonly used are:

i. *Eyeless needles*: One strand of suture material is attached to the swage of a needle during manufacturing.

Advantages
- Causes minimal tissue trauma as only a single swaged suture strand is drawn through the tissue.
- Each patient has the benefit of a new sharp needle. Reusable needles are potentially dull, blurred or tarnished.
- These needles do not unthread and can be easily recovered if accidentally dropped.
- Allows faster, more efficient surgery.

ii. ***Needles with eye***: These needles can be reused and are cheaper. The suture thread is changed with every surgery.

CLOSURE OF SURGICAL SITE (TECHNIQUES OF SUTURING)

The underside of reflected tissue, periradicular bone and the cavity should be inspected for any type of debris. The surgical site is repeatedly washed with normal saline. Gentle pressure is applied to reposition tissues to remove excess blood and to begin intimate attachment process. Reposition the flap and compress tissues against bone with moist sterilized gauze before suturing.

Principles of Suturing

- The needle holder should grasp the needle at approximately one-half to three-fourth of the distance from the point.
- The needle should enter the tissue perpendicular to the surface. If the needle pierces the tissue obliquely, a tear may develop.
- The needle should be passed through the tissue following the curve of the needle.
- The suture should be placed at an equal distance from the incision on both the sides and at an equal depth. This principle can be modified in case where the tissue edges are at different levels; then passing of the suture closer to the edge of the lower and farther from the edge of the higher side will tend to approximate the levels. Another method involves passing of the suture at an equal distance from the wound margins on both sides, but deeper into the tissues on the lower side and more superficially on the higher side.
- The needle should pass from the free tissue to the fixed side.
- If one tissue side is thinner than the other, the needle should pass from the thinner tissue to the thicker one.
- If one tissue plane is deeper than the other, then the needle should pass from the deeper to the superficial side.
- The distance that the needle is passed into the tissue should be greater than the distance from the tissue edge.
- The tissues should not be closed under tension, since they will tear or necrose around the suture. If tension is present, the tissues should be undermined to relieve it.
- The suture should be tied so that the tissue is merely approximated and the edges are everted.
- The knot should not be placed over the incision line.
- Sutures should be placed approximately 3.0–4.0 mm apart.
- If 'dog ear' occurs at the end of incisions, it should be eliminated.
- Apply firm pressure, at least for three to five minutes after suturing.

Knot Tying

The operator may use either the instrument tie or one or two hand tie. The instrument tie is more convenient in closed areas such as mouth, but can be used in open areas as well.

Surgeon's knot is formed by two throws of suture around the needle holder for first tie and one throw in opposite direction for second tie (Fig. 32.14).

Square knot: The basic knot is the square knot and requires at least three ties for surface knots. It is formed by wrapping ties around the needle holder once in opposite directions between ties (Fig. 32.15).

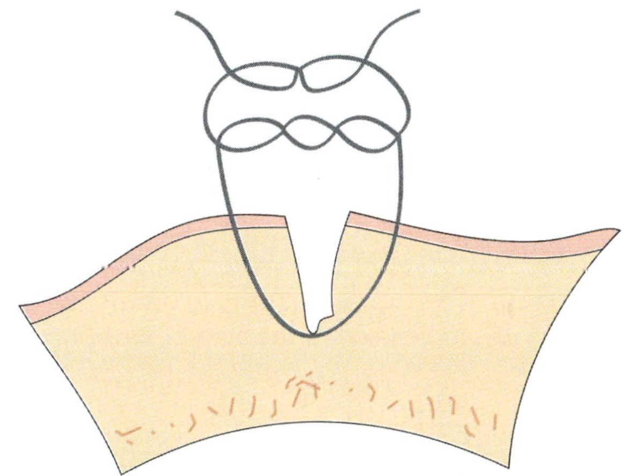

Fig. 32.14 Surgeon's knot

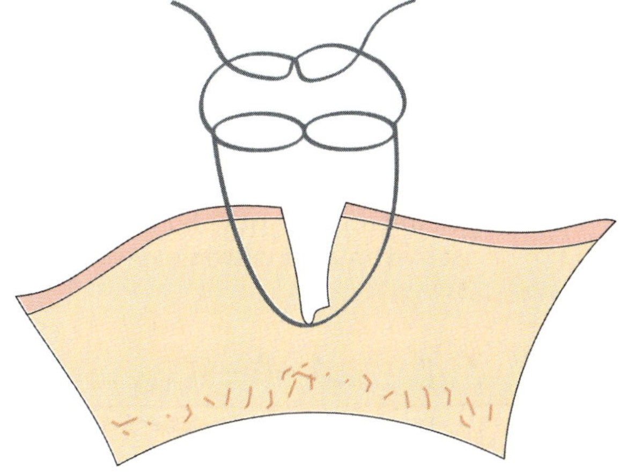

Fig. 32.15 Square knot

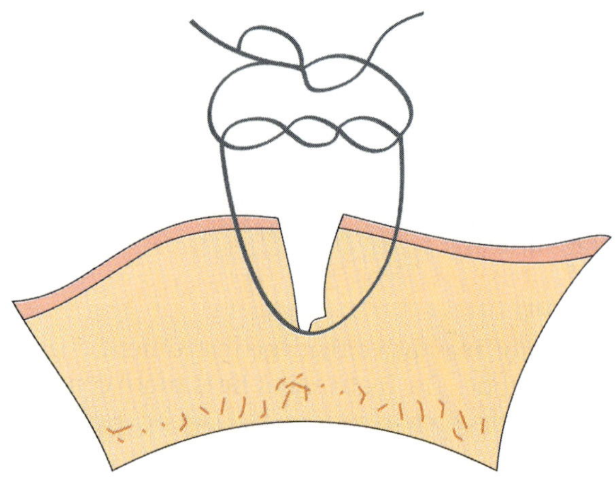

Fig. 32.16 Granny's knot

Granny's knot: This knot involves 1st tie in one direction followed by a 2nd tie in the same direction as the first. A 3rd tie is then squared in opposite direction on the second to hold the knot permanently (Fig. 32.16).

Methods of Suturing

The commonly used methods of suturing are:

- Interrupted suture
- Continuous suture
- Continuous locking suture
- Mattress suture
- Figure of '8' suture.

Interrupted Suture

The interrupted suture is the most commonly used (Fig. 32.17). It can be used in the area of tension.

Advantages

- Successive suture can be placed
- Each suture is independent of the next (loosening of one suture will not cause loosening of the others; and/or few sutures during reinfection can easily be removed).

Continuous Suture

The continuous suture provides a rapid technique for closure and even distribution of tension over the entire suture line. It provides water tight closure, which is especially important in intraoral bone grafting. It should not be used in areas of existing tension.

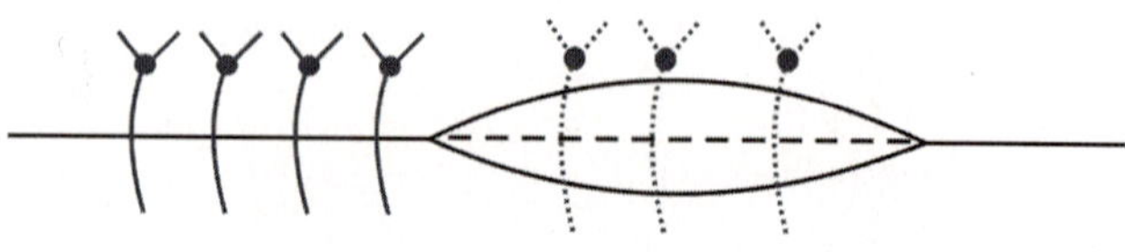

Fig. 32.17 Simple interrupted suture

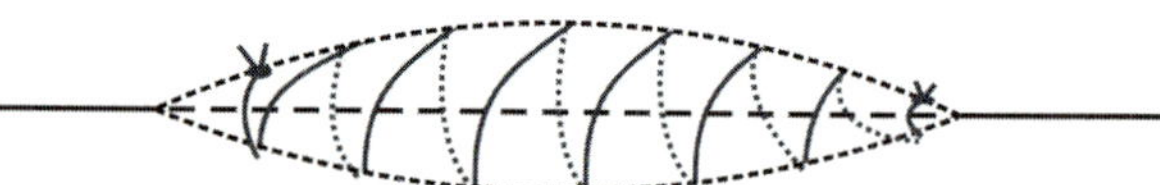

Fig. 32.18 Continuous suture

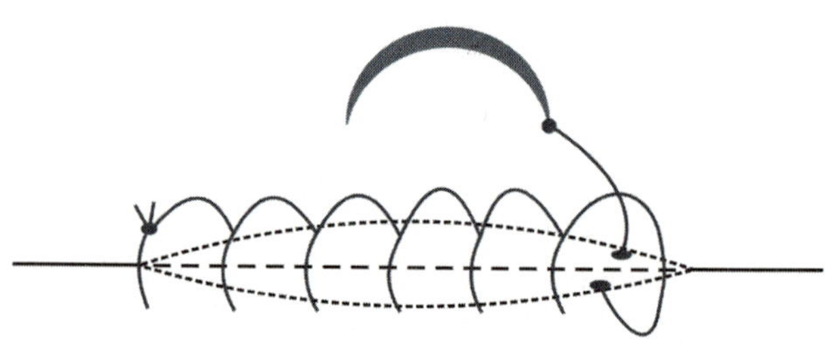

Fig. 32.19 Locking continuous suture

A simple interrupted suture is placed and needle is then inserted in continuous fashion (Fig. 32.18). The suture passes perpendicular to incision line underneath tissue and diagonally on surface and is ended by tying to last untightened loop of suture.

Continuous Locking Suture

The suture is passed perpendicular to incision line and degree of locking is provided by withdrawing suture through its own loop. The suture technique is begun and ended identical to continuous technique (Fig. 32.19).

Advantages

- The suture will align itself perpendicularly to the incision.
- The locking feature promotes continuous tightening of the suture as wound closure progresses. Care should be exercised not to tighten the individual lock excessively, since this can produce tissue necrosis.

Mattress Suture

Mattress sutures are of two types:

i. *Vertical*: The needle is passed close to incision line on both sides. When needle is brought back from second flap to first flap, the depth of penetration is more superficial (Fig. 32.20a).

   The vertical mattress suture is used to provide more tissue eversion and is used in areas where wound contraction could cause dehiscence and broad scar formation. The vertical mattress suture offers the advantage of running parallel to the blood supply of the edge of the flap and therefore not interfering with healing.

ii. *Horizontal*: The suture passes perpendicular to incision line underneath tissue and parallel to it on the surface; again perpendicular to incision line

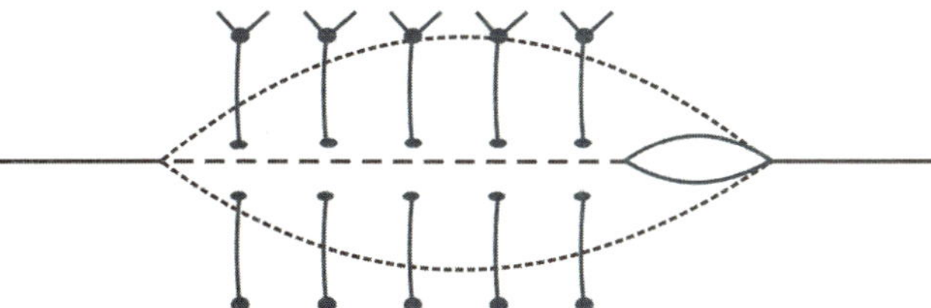

Fig. 32.20a Vertical mattress suturing

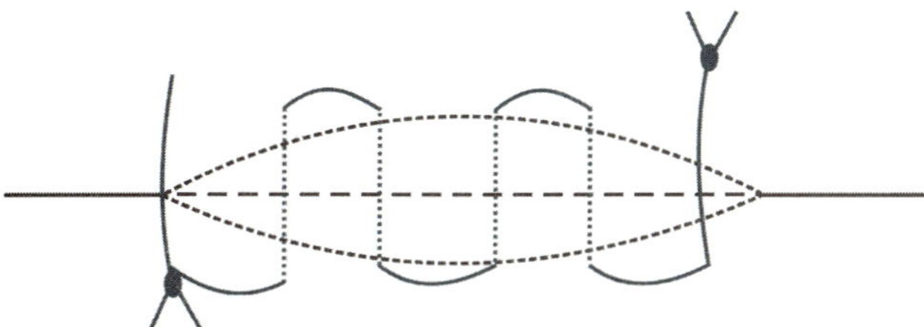

Fig. 32.20b Horizontal mattress suturing

underneath tissue to be knotted on that side (Fig. 32.20b).

The *interrupted horizontal mattress* suture produces broad contact of the wound margins and is useful where such a condition is needed. The disadvantage is the blood supply to the edges of the incision is constricted.

The *continuous horizontal mattress* suture is often used after intraoral bone grafting, as the eversion and continuity provide watertight closure.

Figure of '8' Suture

The figure of '8' suture is used over extraction sites where it provides protection to the socket and adaptation of the gingival papillae round the adjacent teeth (Fig. 32.21).

The only disadvantage is that the suture is difficult to remove after wound closure.

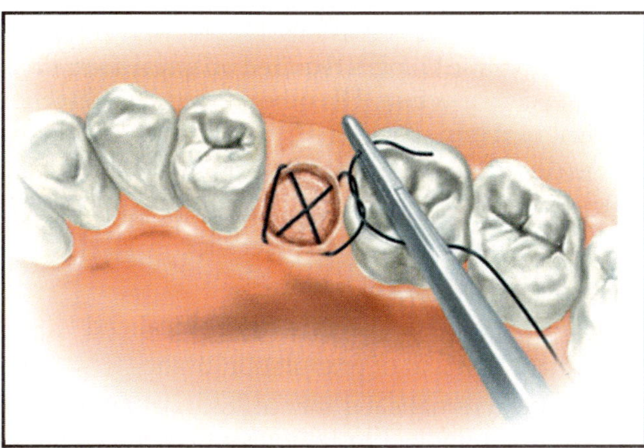

Fig. 32.21 Figure of '8' suture

Suture Removal

Suture should be grasped with an instrument and elevated above the epithelial surface during removal. A scissors should be used to transect side of the loop as close to the epithelial surface as possible. In this way a minimal portion of the suture laden with debris and bacteria (open to environment) will be dragged through the tissue.

Tissue Reaction to Sutures

The initial body response to sutures is almost identical in the first 4 to 7 days, regardless of the suture material. After one week the response is related to the type of suture material.

If the suture material leads through mucosal or skin surfaces, epithelial cells will begin tracking down the suture pathway. The longer the suture remains, the deeper is the epithelial invasion of the underlying tissue. When such sutures are removed, an epithelial tract remains. These cells may eventually disappear or remain to form keratin and epithelial inclusion cysts. A delay in sutures removal or excessive tension on the skin may also cause the site of the sutures to be visible and the typical 'railroad track' scar results.

The development of surgical infections is greatly enhanced by the presence of a suture in a contaminated wound. The use of monofilament sutures rather than braided sutures reduces the potential for infection as the multifilament sutures provide a heaven for bacteria, which can penetrate the interstices of the suture that are too small to allow granulocytes and macrophages. As a general rule, sutures should not be used in the presence of infections and should be removed if an infection becomes evident.

All sutures passing through the mucous membrane or skin provide a 'wick' down through which bacteria can gain access to the underlying tissues and may cause inflammation, subsequently granuloma or a stitch abscess. Because of this and the downward growth of the epithelial tissue, the sutures should be removed as early as possible consistent with adequate healing. Generally, sutures should be removed after 3 to 5 days on the skin of the head and neck, and 5 to 7 days intraorally. The sutures in case of cancer should be removed after two weeks.

SURGICAL ARMAMENTARIUM

The surgical armamentarium (Fig. 32.22) are:

For presurgical assessment

- Mirror and curved explorer
- Straight and curved periodontal probes.

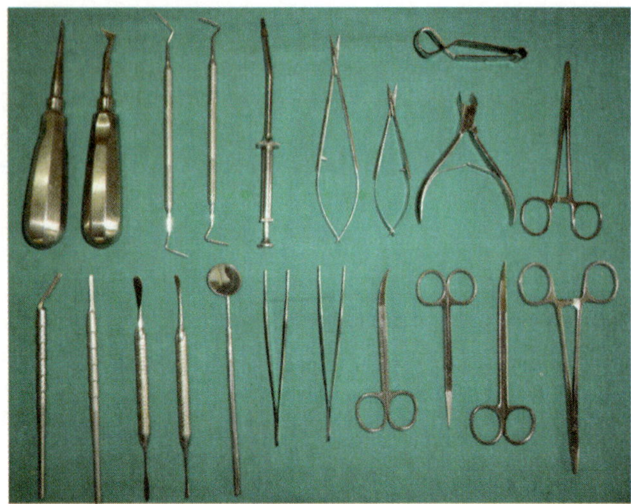

Fig. 32.22 Armamentarium for endodontic surgery

For soft tissue incision, elevation and reflection
- Scalpels
- Disposable blades (sizes 11, 12, 15)
- Mucoperiosteal elevator
- Mucoperiosteal retractor
- Tissue forceps
- Irrigating syringes and needles.

For periradicular curettage
- Spoon curette
- Periodontal curette
- Fine, curved mosquito forceps
- Small, curved surgical scissors.

For bone removal and root-end resection
- Surgical burs
- Bone curettes.

For root-end preparation and restoration
- Miniature contra-angle hand piece/ultrasonic hand piece
- Burs and ultrasonic tips
- Hemostatic agent
- Restorative carriers and condensers
- Small ball burnisher
- Small, fine explorer.

For suturing and soft tissue closure
- Surgical scissors
- Hemostat or fine needle holders
- Sutures (size 3-0 to 5-0)
- Sterile gauze for soft tissue compression.

SURGICAL PROCEDURES

Osseous Entry (Osteotomy)

32

The apical end of the root is identified. The bone surrounding the root tip may need to be removed to gain visual access to the surgical site. Bone removal is carried out with round and fissure burs under copious irrigation with normal saline. With the advent of ultrasonic tips and microsurgical gadgets, the diameter of an osteotomy is within 5.0 mm (exact position of root tip is identified prior to making small sized osteotomy). A periapical radiograph matches over the 'estimated' root tip. The area can be identified prior to use of surgical burs. A small sized osteotomy lead to reduced postoperative discomfort and faster healing.

Sometimes, a window is present in the bone due to growth of periapical granulation tissue. The window can be used as a starting point to cut bone round the apex. An appropriate size surgical curette is used to remove granulation tissue to improve visualization. The bony cavity can be modified for appropriate retrograde fillings.

Periradicular Curettage

Periradicular curettage is performed along with preparing bony cavity for better visualization of the root end. Sometimes, it is not possible to completely remove the granulation tissue without resecting root. Straight and angled bone curettes are usually used to excavate the diseased tissue. Injecting 0.5 ml of anesthetic solution in lesion decreases patient discomfort and also improves hemostasis. Curettes are used in a scrapping motion to detach soft tissue from bone. Loosened tissue is removed with the help of a tissue forceps. Caution must be taken to prevent damage to the vital structures when working in proximity to maxillary sinus, mental foramen or mandibular canal. The bony cavity is cleaned with sterilized gauge and checked for any residual bony spicules/diseased tissue. The cavity is then thoroughly washed with normal saline.

Apicoectomy (Root-end Resection)

The removal of apical portion of the root may or may not be necessary in all occasions. Usually, it is employed where retrograde filling is required or apical aberrations warrant such resection. The other reasons for resection of apical root are:

- Removal of iatrogenic mishaps, such as ledges, block, etc.
- Reduction of fenestrated apical root
- Evaluation of vertical fractures
- Achieving root canal access from apical end
- Facilitate removal of granulation tissues.

It has been established that at least 3.0 mm of root end must be removed to remove apical ramifications and to enhance visualisation of the periapical area.

The labial surface is beveled for better access and visibility. Earlier 30–45° bevel was recommended. Once the root has been exposed, the bur is placed at a desired angle and the root is shaved away. A couple of authors prefer cutting of root end without beveling. They are of the view that beveling exposes more surface area, which might lead to marginal leakage. It is established that 10° bevel is beneficial for manipulation at the root tip without leading to marginal leakage (Fig. 32.23). Extent of removal of root-end is dictated by following factors.

- Access and visibility to the surgical site
- Position of apical end of root within alveolar bone
- Presence of significant accessory canals
- Location of procedural error, if present
- Anatomical considerations, e.g. proximity of adjacent roots, level of remaining crestal bone, etc.

Stepwise procedure of apicoectomy of left maxillary central incisor tooth is depicted in Fig. 32.24. Apicoectomy of first mandibular molar is shown in Fig. 32.25.

Root-end Preparation

The root-end preparation is carried out to seal the apical opening of the root canal system. The preparation is made parallel to the anatomic outline of root. The depths of root end cavity depend upon the angle of beveling. 1.0–1.5 mm depth is sufficient if no bevel is given. Depth is more as the angle is increased (2.5 mm deep for 45° bevel). Root-end cavity can be prepared either with a bur used in a miniature handpiece or ultrasonics. Ultrasonic tips are used in light, sweeping motion (forward-backward). Interrupted strokes are more effective than the continuous ones. The prepared cavity is evaluated using micromirrors (Fig. 32.26). The ultrasonic tips allow good access to the root end and provide the requisite shape (Figs 32.27 and 32.28). The cavity should be free of debris including gutta-percha. The gutta-percha on the walls should be removed or packed down in the canal.

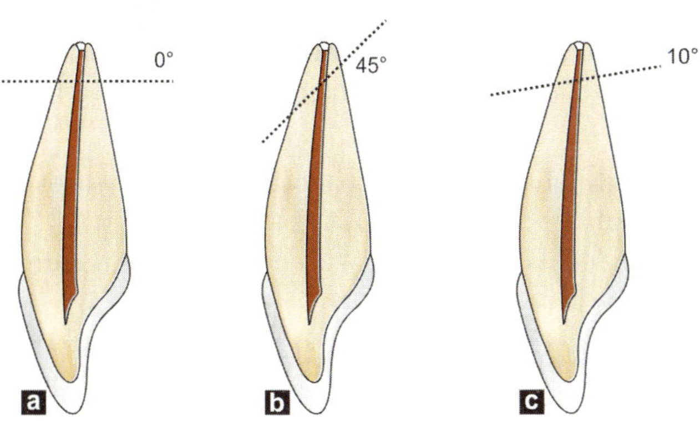

Fig. 32.23 (a) 0° bevel; (b) 45° bevel; (c) 10° bevel

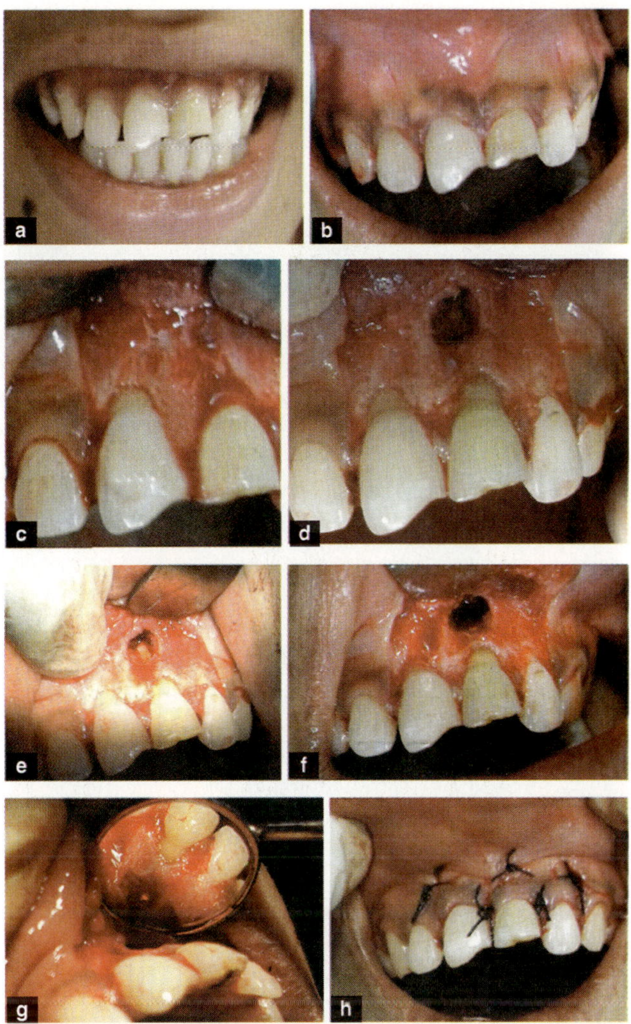

Fig. 32.24 Apicoectomy procedure (left maxillary central incisor): (a) Preoperative; (b) Incising the flap; (c) Flap raised; (d) Creating bony cavity; (e) Exposing root tip; (f) Root-end preparation; (g) Root-end filling; (h) Suture placed

Root-end Filling Materials

The root-end cavity is isolated. The hemostatic agent can be placed in the bony crypt. Manufacturer instructions should be followed while choosing the material for retrofilling and placing the same at the retrocavity prepared. The bony cavity should be cleaned thoroughly after the filling. The root-end filling material should have the following features:

- Potential to seal the root canal hermetically
- Biocompatible with no inflammatory reaction
- Radiopaque
- Nontoxic
- Should not promote or preferably inhibit the growth of pathogenic microorganisms
- Moisture friendly
- Dimensionally stable

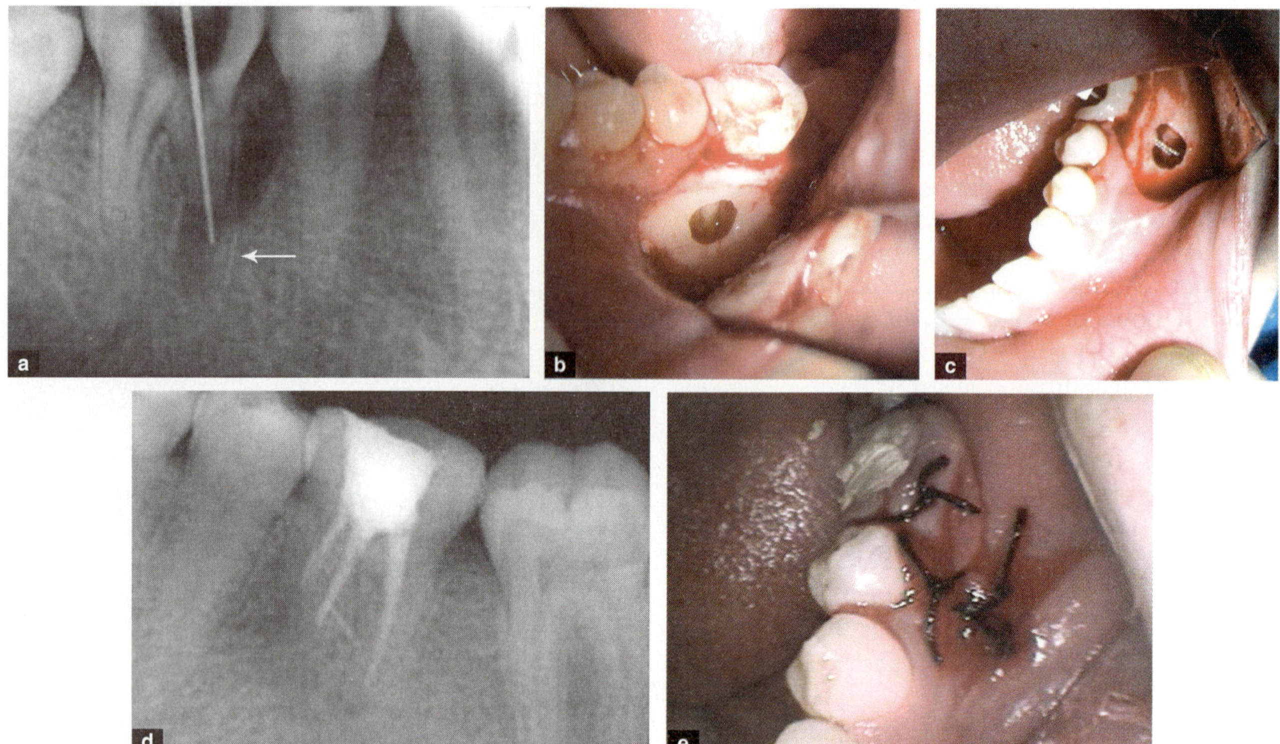

Fig. 32.25 Apicoectomy of first mandibular molar: (a) Fractured instrument lying in the periapical area (arrow); (b) Apicoectomy of mesial root of first mandibular molar; (c) Root canal files in mesial canal; (d) Postoperative radiograph; (e) Suture placed

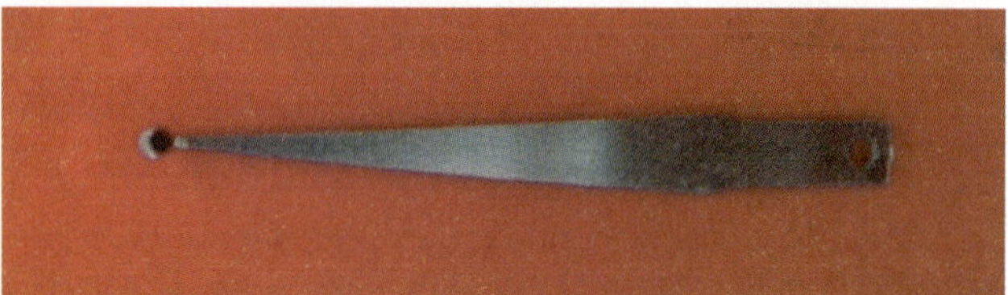

Fig. 32.26 Micro mirror

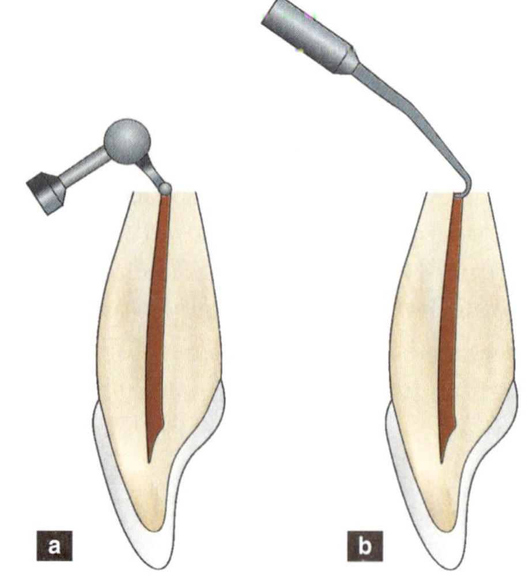

Fig. 32.27 Root-end cutting (a) Using round bur; (b) Using ultrasonic tip

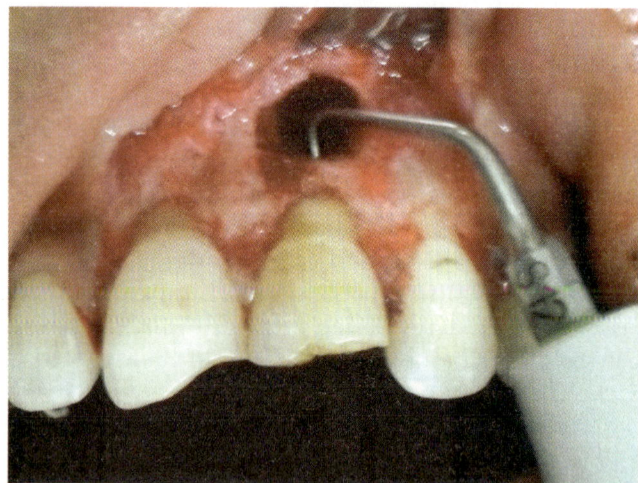

Fig. 32.28 Root-end preparation with ultrasonic tip

- Should not corrode or be electrochemically active
- Should not stain the tooth or tissues.

The details of commonly used retrofilling materials are described in Chapter 20.

Guided Tissue Regeneration (GTR)

The term regeneration implies reproduction or reconstruction of a lost or injured tissue. Guided tissue regeneration refers to regeneration of periodontal attachment (bone, periodontal ligament and cementum); whereas, guided bone regeneration refers to ridge augmentation and growth of bony tissue only.

Limited studies have been published using GTR techniques in endodontic surgeries. The most common lesion treated with GTR techniques are the endodontic–periodontic lesions, wherein considerable bone loss is evident. It has been established that GTR improves healing of transosseous defects as compared to endodontic surgery without using GTR.

Guided tissue regenerative technique can utilize bone grafts only or bone grafts with barrier membrane. The placement of barrier membrane (polytetrafluoroethylene, polyglactin, collagen, calcium sulfate, polylactic acid, etc.) prevents gingival epithelium and connective tissue from contacting the intended site of bone reformation and interfering with osteogenesis (bone formation) (Fig. 32.29a and b).

Advantages of using barrier membrane

- Membrane provides additional wound coverage and stability/protection of blood clot.
- Facilitates in-growth of cells and blood vessels from the base of the lesion.
- Maintain blood-clot area free of bacterial invasion.
- Prevent other tissues (connective tissue) entering the intended site of bone formation.

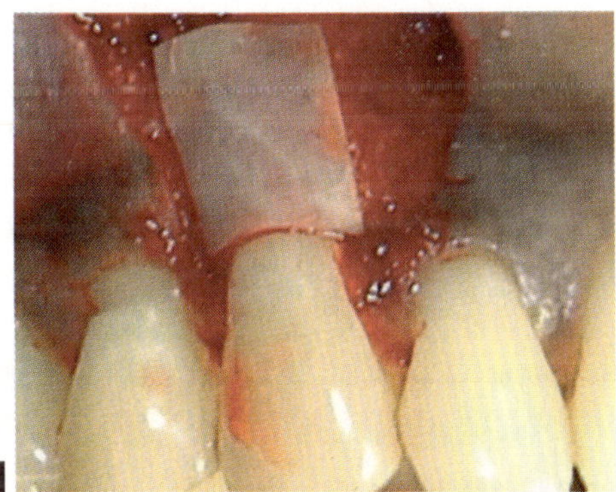

a

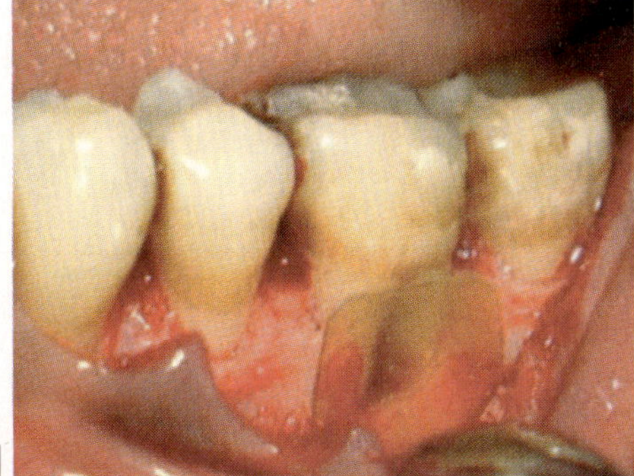

b

Fig. 32.29 Guided tissue regeneration: (a) Anterior tooth; (b) Posterior tooth

A classification is proposed (VonArx and Cochran-2001) for periradicular lesions suitable for GTR techniques (Table 32.1).

It has been shown that defects eroding both labial and palatal cortical plate normally do not heal completely; may fill with scar tissue (class Ib lesions). The use of membrane GTR technique has shown significant improvement in healing process. Class II lesions (endodontic–periodontal lesion) is always challenging. The loss of buccal bone compromises with the healing process. The operator must plan the placement of membrane and bone grafts with and without morphogenic scaffolds after assessing the bone loss configuration around each root. Lateral/furcation lesions (class III) have also been surgically treated using GTR approach. GTR therapy along with membrane placement is particularly indicated for treatment of furcation perforation lesions that communicate with the marginal periodontium.

It has been established that combination of graft and membrane is significantly better than barrier alone or control group of patients treated conventionally. However, a few authors have questioned the efficacy of GTR modality and opined that membrane might even prevent regeneration. It has also been questioned in case of root-end surgeries. The healing in root-end surgery without using any GTR modality is quite predictable.

It can be personal preference of the operator to use or not to use GTR techniques; however, using GTR along with bone grafting is always beneficial for long-term treatment outcome.

Although a substantial number of studies have preferred using GTR techniques; it should also be noted

Table 32.1	Periradicular lesions and guided tissue regeneration
Class I	Periapical bone defect without marginal lesion
Ia	Lingual/palatal cortex not eroded
Ib	Lingual/palatal cortex eroded (with a buccal surgical approach, this will result in a transosseous or through-and-through bone defect)
Class II	Periapical lesion (with or without lingual erosion) and concomitant marginal lesion)
IIa	No communication between the separate lesions
IIb	The two lesions are fused: endodontic–periodontal lesion
Class III	Lateral or furcation lesion (with or without marginal lesion)
IIIa	No communication to alveolar crest/marginal periodontium
IIIb	Communication to alveolar crest/marginal periodontium

that most of the studies did not evaluate the healing potential of GTR in control group, especially where the lesion was small.

Recently, bioabsorbable membrane instead of non-resorbable membrane, has been used in endodontic surgery. It is emphasized that GTR therapy, with or without grafts and barrier membrane, significantly improves healing, especially of large lesions.

Replantation/Intentional Replantation

Replantation implies planting avulsed tooth into the same socket (extraoral time varies, condition of tooth depends on patient); whereas, intentional replantation means extracting the tooth and replanting in the same socket (extraoral time depends on operator).

Indications

- Nonsurgical means are not feasible and the tooth would be extracted
- Patient unable to tolerate or not fit for lengthy endodontic surgery.

Contraindications

- Non-restorable tooth
- Severe periodontal disease
- Widely divergent/dilacerated roots or any abnormal morphology, which might lead to crown/root fracture.

Technique

- Root canal treatment should preferably be completed before extraction
- Minimize extraoral time (especially, if opt for root canal treatment after extraction)
- Restore access with amalgam or composites to prevent fracture
- Extraction should be atraumatic. Avoid injury to cementum
- Keep tooth moist after extraction, preferably with Hanks Balanced Salt Solution
- Do not curette walls of socket
- Replant (manually compress cortical plates over replant)
- Splint, if necessary
- Relieve occlusion
- Prescribe antibiotics to prevent inflammatory resorption.

Autotransplantation

32

Autotransplantation is the surgical repositioning of a tooth within the same patient (the socket will be different). The extracted tooth is implanted in a new, surgically prepared socket. The preservation and regeneration of periodontal ligament is the key to success of this treatment.

Indications

A chronically infected or severely fractured tooth or missing tooth requiring replacement (any non-functioning tooth, usually crowded tooth can be taken as donor). The third molar tooth replanting into first molar site is common. The teeth most commonly used as donor are premolars extracted because of orthodontic reasons.

Advantages

- The tooth continuously maintain alveolar bone and gingival margins
- Prosthesis is avoided
- No need to prepare adjacent tooth
- Cost-effective.

Disadvantages

- Possibility of resorption and loss of tooth
- May lead to ankylosis
- Need multidisciplinary approach for better results.

Decompression of Large Periradicular Lesions

The decompression is indicated in case of large lesion where surgery might devitalize the pulp of an adjacent tooth and nonsurgical treatment would lead to slow healing (Fig. 32.30).

Technique

- Fabricate tube with collar (section of intravenous tubing). A radiopaque nasogastric tube is preferred
- Aspirate lesion
- Small vertical incision is given into osseous fenestration

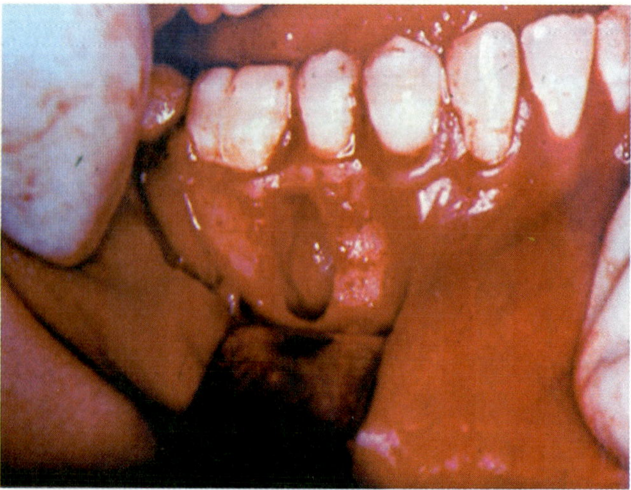

Fig. 32.30 Decompression of large periradicular lesion

- Trim tube to fit into depth of lesion without protruding
- Insert tube and irrigate with saline (10 ml three times a day)
- Monitor patient weekly and remove tube when no more debris is removed by flushing procedures
- Mucosal opening usually heal within one week
- Follow resolution of lesion with radiographs.

Perforation Repair

The perforation repair should preferably be carried out using nonsurgical modalities. In case surgery is mandatory; bone support of adjacent teeth is not to be sacrificed.

Access and visualization of the defect are essential for successful surgical repair (Fig. 32.31a to d). Usually only flaps are helpful in managing the perforation (up to furcation area). If perforation is deep rooted, bone cutting becomes necessary. The perforation site, once exposed, is washed thoroughly, excavated of any granulation tissue/debris and filled with an appropriate material. Intentional replantation can be considered if access is difficult.

Hemisection/Bicuspidization/Radisectomy

Hemisection refers to cutting the mandibular molar/ two rooted tooth to half and removing one half (used in case where one root cannot be treated endodontically). In bicuspidization, the mandibular molar/ two rooted tooth is cut into two and both the halves are preserved (used in case of un-managed furcation perforation). In case of maxillary molars, if only one or two roots need be extracted, the procedure is known as 'Radisectomy'.

The root canal of the healthy root(s) is prepared and obturated. The crown is bisected into two halves using fine bur, moving from lingual to buccal direction (prevents injury to tongue). The discs should be avoided. The diseased root is extracted slowly without disturbing the healthy one. The socket is curetted and sutured (Fig. 32.32a to f).

The treated and preserved root(s) is usually prone to fracture, especially if the occlusal forces are not in line with long-axis of the root. Do not restore the hemisected tooth as a cantilever.

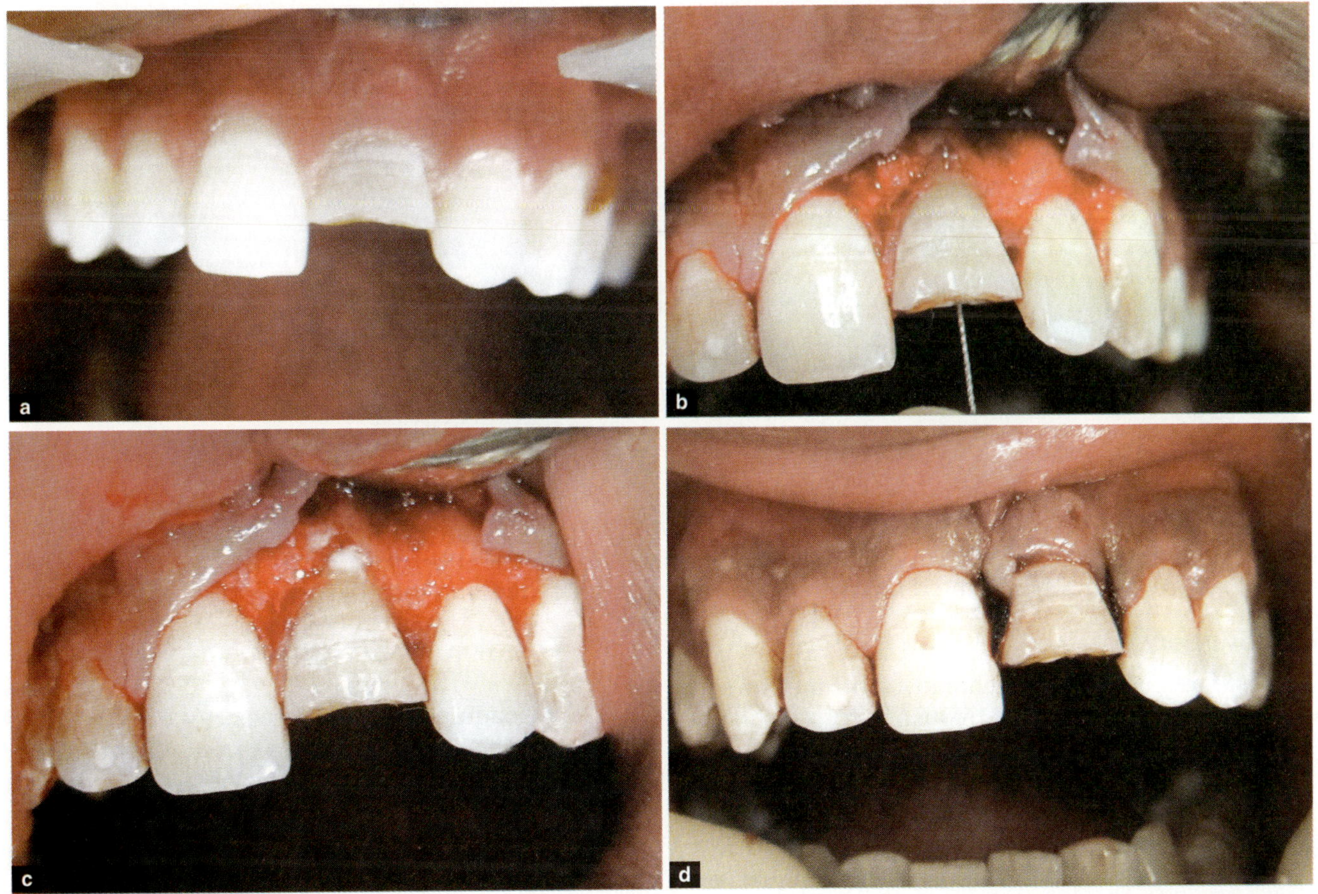

Fig. 32.31 Perforation repair (a) Preoperative; (b) File in perforation; (c) Sealing/filling of perforation; (d) Repositioning of flap and suturing

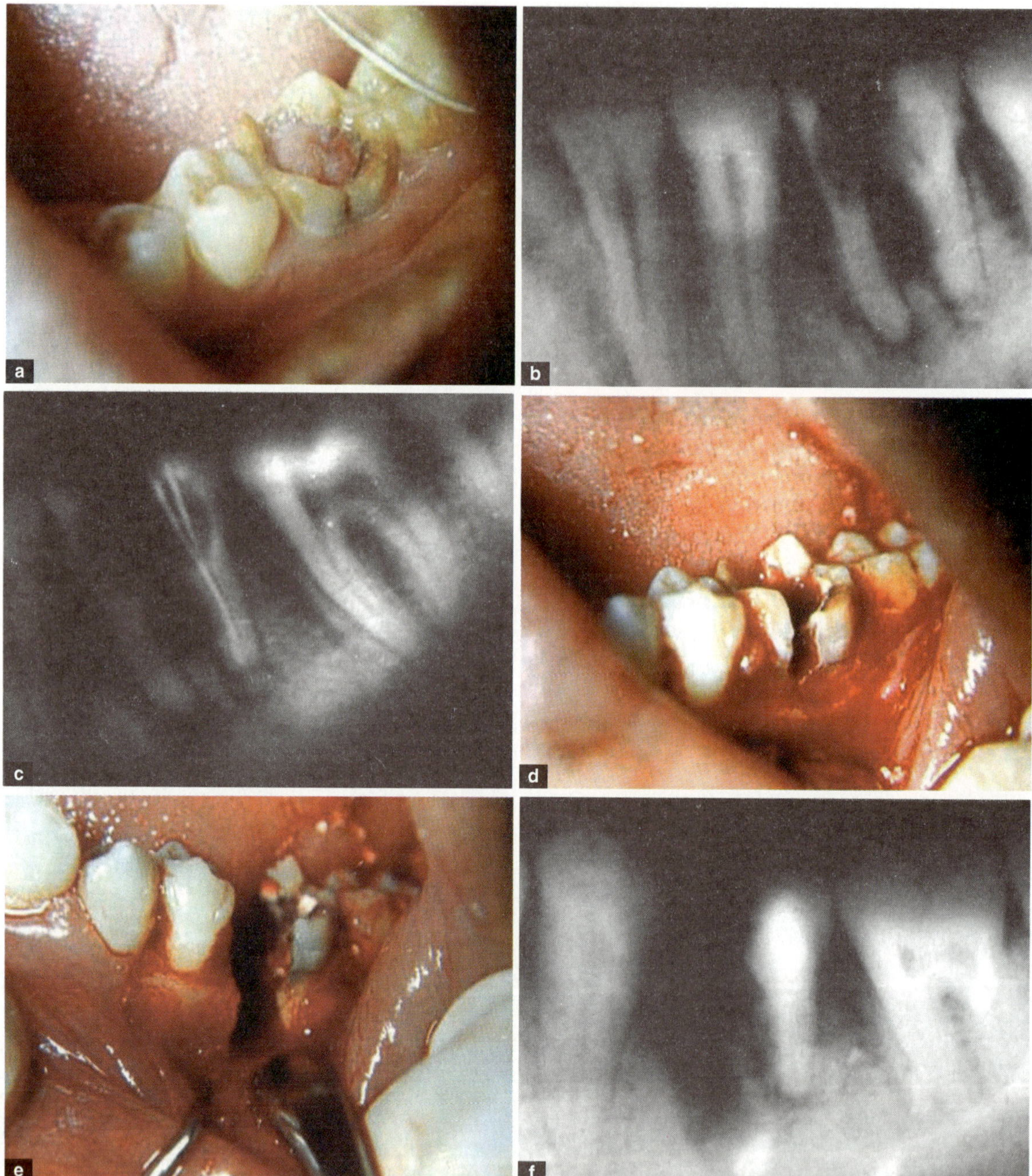

Fig. 32.32 Hemisection procedure: (a) Preoperative (clinical); (b) Preoperative (radiological); (c) Healthy root is prepared and obturated; (d) Crown is bisected into two halves; (e) Extraction of diseased root; (f) Postoperative radiograph

Electrosurgery

Electrosurgery is a surgical technique performed on soft tissues using controlled high frequency currents in the range of 1.5–7.5 million cycles per second or megahertz. The basic rule of electrosurgery is: always keep the tip moving. Prolonged/repeated application causes heat accumulation and tissue destruction.

The commonly used electrosurgical techniques are electrosection, electrocoagulation, electrofulguration and electrodesiccation.

- Electrosection is used for incision, excision and tissue planing.
- Electrocoagulation provides control of hemorrhage by using electrocoagulation current. (Electrosection and electrocoagulation are most commonly used in all areas of dentistry.)
- Electrofulguration and electrodesiccation are not used in dentistry.

The types of electrodes and their uses are tabulated in Table 32.2.

Table 32.2 Types of electrodes and their uses	
Type of electrode	*Use*
Needle electrode	• Removal of gingival enlargement and gingivoplasty • To make incision to establish drainage in treatment of acute periodontal abscess
Needle electrode supplemented by small ovoid loop or diamond-shaped electrodes	• Used for festooning • During reshaping, the electrode is activating and moved in a concise 'shaving' motion
Thin, bar-shaped electrode	• Control of bleeding points located interproximally • Electrosurgery is mainly helpful for the control of isolated bleeding points
Loop electrode	• Relocation of frenum and muscle attachments to facilitate pocket elimination • Removal of flap after the acute symptoms subside
Ball electrode	• Hemostasis

Disadvantages of electrosurgery

- Cannot be used in patients who have poorly shielded cardiac pacemakers
- Causes an unpleasant odor
- Electrosurgery point touching the bone may lead to irreparable damage
- Heat generated by injudicious use can cause tissue damage
- Electrode touching areas of cementum produces burns.

Cryosurgery

Cryosurgery involves the application of cold so as to freeze and destroy the tissues. Super-cooling of tissue is less destructive than slow freezing. Lower temperature is used to produce necrosis in vascular tissues than in epithelial tissues. Other factors that influence the amount of tissue damage are the rate of cooling, the final temperature reached, the time spent in frozen state, the rate of thawing and the medium in which these take place.

Cryosurgery has been used for a variety of clinical conditions, viz. premalignant lesions, mucous membrane tumors, neoplasm tumors, intraosseous tumors, ameloblastoma, giant cell lesions and certain bone cysts.

The depth of penetration is nonspecific in cryosurgery and has destructive effect on blood vessel, nerve, artery, etc.

Postoperative Care

Postoperative care is mandatory after every surgery. The patient should be informed of the complications/side effects of surgery. The patient is instructed to follow the following protocol (the instructions can be given verbally or in the written form).

- Use ice packs for first day in cycles of 20 minutes.
- Avoid alcohol, smoking and strenuous activity.
- Initial diet should consist of liquid supplements including fruit juices and vitamin supplements. Sticky food should be avoided.
- Do not tug or lift facial tissues.
- Oozing of blood from surgical site during first 24 hours is normal.
- Postsurgical discomfort may remain.
- Take analgesics/antibiotics as advised.
- Warm saline rinses are advised after 24 hours.

BIBLIOGRAPHY

1. Abella F, de Ribot J, Doria G, Duran-Sindreu F and Roig M. Applications of piezoelectric surgery in endodontic surgery: a literature review. J. Endod.: 2014; 40:325–332.
2. Arisu HD, Sakik B, Alimzhanova G and Turkoz E. Assessment of morphological changes and permeability of apical dentin surfaces induced by Nd:YAG laser irradiation through retrograde cavity surfaces. J. Contemp. Dent. Pract.: 2004; 15:102–113.
3. Artzi Z, Wasersprung N, Weinreb M, Steigmann M, Prasad HS and Tsesis I. Effect of guided tissue regeneration on newly formed bone and cementum in periapical tissue healing after endodontic surgery: An *in vivo* study in the cat. J. Endod.: 2012; 38:163–169.
4. Becker BD.: Intentional replantation techniques: a critical review. J. Endod.: 2018; 44:14–21.
5. Borisova-Papancheva T, Papanchev G, Peev S and Georgiev T. Posterior endodontic surgery—a case report. MedInform: 2016; 1:389–393.
6. Borisova-Papancheva T, Panov VI, Peev S and Papanchev G. Root-end filling materials-review. Scripta Sci. Med. Dent.: 2015; 1:9–15.
7. Bornstein MM, Lauber R, Sendi P and von Arx T. Comparison of periapical radiography and limited cone-beam computed tomography in mandibular molars for analysis of anatomical landmarks before apical surgery. J. Endod.: 2011; 37:151–157.
8. Clokie CM, Yau DM and Chano L. Autogenous tooth transplantation: an alternative to dental implant placement? J. Can. Dent. Assoc.: 2001; 67:92–96.
9. Corbella S, Taschieri S, Elkabbany A, Fabbro MD and von Arx T. Guided tissue regeneration using a barrier membrane in endodontic surgery. Swiss Dent. J.: 2016; 126:13–25.
10. Cotton TP, Geisler TM, Holden DT, Schwartz SA and Schindler WG. Endodontic applications of cone-beam volumetric tomography. J. Endod.: 2007; 33:1121–1132.

11. Day P and Littlewood SJ. Autotransplantation of teeth: An overview. Dent. Update: 2009; 36:102–104.
12. Eliyas S, Vere J, Ali Z and Harris I. Micro-surgical endodontics. Br. Dent. J.: 2014; 216:169–177.
13. El-Swiach, JM and Walker RT. Reasons for apicoectomies. A retrospective study. Endod. Dent. Traumatol.: 1996; 12: 185–191.
14. Floratos S and Kim S. Modern endodontic/Microsurgery concepts: A clinical update. Dent. Clin. N. Am.: 2017; 61: 81–91.
15. Freedman A and Horowitz I. Complications after apicoectomy in maxillary premolar and molar teeth. Int. J. Oral Maxillofacial Surg.: 1999; 28:192–194.
16. Gambruzzi JV and Marshall FJ. Molar endodontic surgery. J. Can. Dent. Assoc.: 1983; 1:61–66.
17. Garcia B, Martorell L, Marti E and Penarrocha, M.: Periapical surgery of maxillary posterior teeth. A review of the literature. Med. Oral Path. Oral Cin. Bucal.: 2006; 11:E146–150.
18. Garrett K, Kerr M, Hartwell G, O'Sullivan S and Mayer P. The effect of a bioresorbable matrix barrier in endodontic surgery on the rate of periapical healing: an *in vivo* study. J. Endod.: 2002; 28:503–506.
19. Gentile P, Chiono V, Tonda-Turo, Ferreira AM and Ciardelli G. Polymeric membranes for guided bone regeneration. Biotech. J.: 2011; 6:1187–1197.
20. Gouw-Soares S, Tanji E, Haypek P, Cardoso W and Esuardo CP. The use of Er:YAG, Nd:YAG and Ga-Al-As lasers in periapical surgery: a 3-year clinical study. J. Clin. Laser Med. Surg.: 2001; 19:193–198.
21. Gutmann JL and Gutmann MS. Historical perspectives on the evolution of surgical procedures in endodontics. J. Hist. Dent.: 2010; 58:1–42.
22. Gutmann JL. Is an apicoectomy ever successful? If so, under what conditions? A historic assessment with contemporary overtones. J. Hist. Dent.: 2013; 61:3–20.
23. Gutmann JL. Surgical endodontics: past, present and future. Endod. Topics: 2014; 30:29–43.
24. Gutmann JL and Pitford TR. Management of the resected root canal: a clinical review. Int. Endod. J. 1993; 26:273–283.
25. Guttmann JL and Harrison JW. Posterior endodontic surgery: anatomical considerations and clinical techniques. Int. Endod. J.: 1985; 18:8–34.
26. Hargreves KM and Khan A. Surgical preparation: anesthesia and hemostasis. Endod. Topics: 2005; 11:32–55.
27. Hauman CH, Chandler NP and Tong DC. Endodontic implications of the maxillary sinus: a review. Int. Endod. J.: 2002; 35:127–141.
28. Hoskinson AE. Hard tissue management: osseous access, curettage, biopsy and root isolation. Endod. Topics: 2005; 11:98–113.
29. Hsu YY and Kim S. The resected root surface. The issue of canal isthmuses. Dent. Clin. North Am.: 1997; 41:529–540.
30. Jacob SA and Amudha D. Guided tissue regeneration: a review. J. Dent. Health Oral Disor. Ther.: 2017; 6:1–7.
31. Khoury F and Hensher R. The bony lid approach for the apical root resection of lower molars. Int. J. Oral maxillofacial Surg. 1987; 16:166–170.
32. Kim S and Kratchman S. Modern endodontic surgery concepts and practice: a review. J. Endod.: 2006; 32:601–623.
33. Kim S and Rethnam S. Hemostatsis in endodontic microsurgery. Dent. Clin. North Am.: 1997; 41:499–511.
34. Kim S. Principles of endodontic microsurgery. Dent. Clin. North Am: 1997; 41:481–497.
35. Liu Z, Zhang D, Li Q and Xu Q. Evaluation of root-end preparation with a new ultrasonic tip. J. Endod.: 2013; 39:829–823.
36. Low KMT, Dula K, Burgin W and von Arx T. Comparison of periapical radiography and limited cone-beam tomography in posterior maxillary teeth referred for apical surgery. J. Endod.: 2008; 34:557–562.
37. Machado R, Vansan LP, da Cruz AM and da Silva EN. Surgical endodontic reintervention using a modern technique: 2 case reports. General Dent.: 2014:40–44.
38. Marques AM, Gerbi ME, dos Santos JN, Noia MP, Oliveria PC, Brugnera JA, Zanin FA and Pinheiro AL. Influence of the parameters of the Er:YAG laser on the apical sealing of apicoectomized teeth. Lasers Med. Sci.: 2011; 26:433–438.
39. Marx RE. Platelet-rich plasma (PRP): what is PRP and what is not PRP? Implant Dent.: 2001; 10:225–228.
40. Mendes RA and Rocha G. Mandibular third molar autotransplantation – literature review with clinical cases. J. Can. Dent. Assoc.: 2004; 70:761–766.
41. Naylor J, Mines P, Anderson A and Kwon D. The use of guided tissue regeneration techniques among endodontists: a web-based survey. J. Endod.: 2011; 37:1495–1498.
42. Niemczyk SP. Essentials of endodontic microsurgery. Dent. Clin. N. Am.: 2010; 54:375–399.
43. Park CH, Rios HE and Jin Q. Tissue engineering bone-ligament complexes using fiber-guiding scaffolds. Biomaterials: 2012; 33:137–145.
44. Park JH, Tai K and Hayashi D. Tooth autotransplantation as a treatment option: a review. J. Clin. Pediatr. Dent.: 2011; 35:129–135.
45. Payer M, Jakse N, Pertl C, Truschnegg A, Lechner E and Eskici A. The clinical effect of LLT in endodontic surgery: a prospective study of 72 cases. Oral Surg., Oral Med., Oral Pathol. Oral Radiol. Endod.: 2005; 100:375–379.
46. Pellegrini G, Pagni G and Rasperini G. Surgical approaches based on biological objectives: GTR versus GBR techniques. Int. J. Dent.: 2013; ID521547:1–13.
47. Peterson J and Gutmann JL. The outcome of endodontic surgery: a systematic review. Int. Endod. J.: 2001; 34:169–175.
48. Rahimi S, Yavari HR, Shahi S, Zand V, Shakour S, Reyhani MF and Pirzadeh A. Comparison of the effect of Er, Cr-YSGG laser and ultrasonic retrograde root-end cavity preparation on the integrity of root apices. J. Oral Sci.: 2010; 52:77–81.
49. Regan JD, Witherspoon DE and Foyle D. Surgical repair of root and tooth perforations. Endod. Topics: 2005; 11:152–178.
50. Reich PP. Autogenous transplantation of maxillary and mandibular molars. J. Oral Maxillofac. Surg.: 2008; 66:2314–2317.

51. Roy R, Chandler NP and Lin J. Peripheral dentin thickness after root-end cavity preparation. Oral Surg., Oral Med., Oral Pathol., Oral Radiol., Endod.: 2008; 105:263–266.

52. Scarano A, Artese L, Piattelli A, Carinci F, Mancion C and Iezzi G. Hemostasis control in endodontic surgery: a comparative study of calcium sulfate versus gauzes and versus ferric sulfate. J. Endod.: 2012; 38:20–23.

53. Stropko JJ, Doyon GE and Gutmann JJ. Root-end management: resection, cavity preparation, and material placement. Endod. Topics: 2005; 11:131–151.

54. Suebnukarn S, Rhienmora P and Haddawy P. The use of cone-beam computed tomography and virtual reality simulation for pre-surgical practice in endodontic microsurgery. Int. Endod. J.: 2012; 45:627–632.

55. Tang Y, Li X and Yin S. Outcome of MTA as root-end filling in endodontic surgery: a systematic review. Quint. Int.: 2010; 41:557–566.

56. Tanomaru-Filho M, Luis MR and Leonadro MR. Evaluation of periapical repair following retrograde filling with different root-end filling materials in dog teeth with periapical lesions. Oral Surg., Oral Med., Oral Pathol., Oral Radiol., Endod.: 2006; 102:127–132.

57. Taschieri S, delFabbro M and Testori T. Microscope versus endoscope in root-end management: a randomized controlled study. Int. J. Oral Maxillofac. Surg.: 2008; 37:1022–1026.

58. Taschieri S, delFabbro M, Testori T and Weinstein R. Efficacy of xenogenic bone grafting with guided tissue regeneration in the management of bone defects after surgical endodontics. J. Oral Maxillofac. Surg.: 2007; 65:1121–1127.

59. Tsesis I, Fuss Z, Lin S, Tilinger G and Peled M. Analysis of postoperative symptoms following surgical endodontic treatment. Quint. Int.: 2003; 34:756.

60. Tsesis I, Rosen E, Schwartz-Arad D and Fuss Z. Retrospective evaluation of surgical endodontic treatment: traditional versus modern techniques. J. Endod.: 2006; 32:412–416.

61. Tsurumachi T and Kakehashi Y. Autotransplantation of a maxillary third molar to replace a maxillary premolar with vertical root fracture. Int. Endod. J.: 2007; 40:970–978.

62. Velvart P and Peters CL. Soft tissue management in endodontic surgery. J. Endod.: 2005; 31:271–274.

63. Velvart P, Ebner-Zimmermann U and Ebner JP. Papilla haling following sulcular full thickness flap in endodontic surgery. Oral Surg., Oral Med., Oral Pathol., Oral Radiol. Endod.: 2004; 98:365–369.

64. Velvart P, Peters CI and Peters OA. Soft tissue management: flap design, incision, tissue elevation and tissue retraction. Endod. Topics: 2005; 11:78–97.

65. Velvart P. Papilla base incision: a new approach to recession-free healing of the interdental papilla after endodontic surgery. Int. Endod. J. 2002; 35:453–460.

66. vonArx T and AlSaeed M. The use of regenerative techniques in apical surgery: literature review. Saudi Dent. J.: 2011; 23:113–127.

67. vonArx T and Cochran DL. Rationale for the application of the GTR principle using a barrier membrane in endodontic surgery: A proposal of classification and literature review. Int. J. Periodont. Restor. Dent.: 2001; 21:127–139.

68. vonArx T and Salvi G. Incision techniques and flap designs for apical surgery in the anterior maxilla. Eur. J. Esthet. Dent.: 2008; 3:110–126.

69. vonArx T and Walker W. Microsrugical instruments for root-end cavity preparation following apicoectomy: a literature review. Endod. Dent. Traumatol. 2000; 16:47–62.

70. von Arx T, Friedli M, Sendi P, Lozanoff S and Bornstein MM. Location and dimensions of the mental foramen: a radiographic analysis by using cone-beam computer tomography. J. Endod.: 2013; 39:1522–1528.

71. vonArx T, Jensen SS, Hanni S and Schenk RK. Haemostatic agents used in periradicular surgery: an experimental study of their efficacy and tissue reactions. Int. Endod. J.: 2006; 39:800–808.

72. von Arx T, Salvi G, Janner S and Jensen SS. Gingival recession following apical surgery in the esthetic zone : a clinical study with 70 cases. Eur. J. Esthet. Dent.: 2009; 4:28–45.

73. vonArx T. Apical surgery : a review of current techniques and outcome. The Saudi Dent. J.: 2011; 23:9–15.

74. vonArx T. Failed root canals: the case for apicoectomy (periradicular surgery). J. Oral Maxillofac. Surg.: 2005; 63:832–837.

75. Von AT, Gerber G and Hardt P. Periradicular surgery of molars: a prospective clinical study with a 1-year follow-up. Int. Endod. J.: 2001, 34:520–525.

Chapter 33

Endodontic Implants

Preservation of natural dentition so as to achieve functional stomatognathic system is the main goal of restorative dentistry. Advanced caries and periodontal diseases may warrant the need of intrabone implant to stabilize the tooth and/or to improve the crown-root ratio. There are basically two types of implants; prosthetic implants that replace the missing tooth/root and endodontic implant that use the remaining tooth/root for anchorage.

An endodontic implant is a metallic extension of the root (Fig. 33.1), executed with the object of increasing the root-to-crown ratio so as to provide better stability to the tooth in the arch; subsequently maintaining the stomatognathic system (Fig. 33. 2).

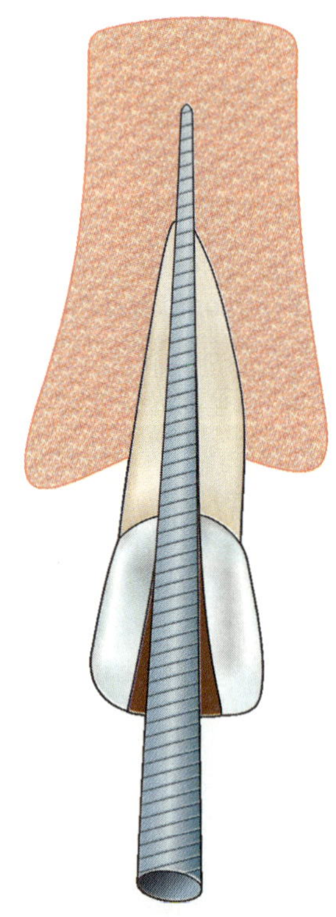

Fig. 33.1 Endodontic implant

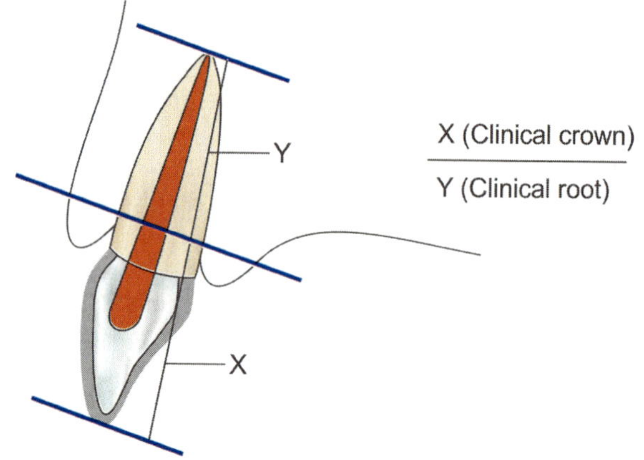

Fig. 33.2 Crown: Root ratio

Endodontic implants are also known as endodontic stabilizers, diodontic implants and endosseous endodontic implants. The endodontic implants increase the root anchorage in the bone by extension of the selected metal/material into the alveolar bone, stabilizing teeth with compromised alveolar support. As compared to prosthetic implants, endodontic implants are considered better since, these implants do not communicate with oral environment (separation from oral cavity reduces the complication of periodontal breakdown; one of the main cause of implant failure). Endodontic stabilizers have also been utilized in stabilizing two fractured root segments (Fig. 33.3).

Indications

The indications of endodontic implants are:

- Periodontally involved teeth requiring stabilization
- Transverse root fracture indicating removal of apical fragment, reducing the crown-root ratio
- Pathologic resorption of the root apex
- A pulpless tooth with an unusually short root
- Abutment teeth with inadequate root length
- A tooth in which additional root length is desired for improving its alveolar support

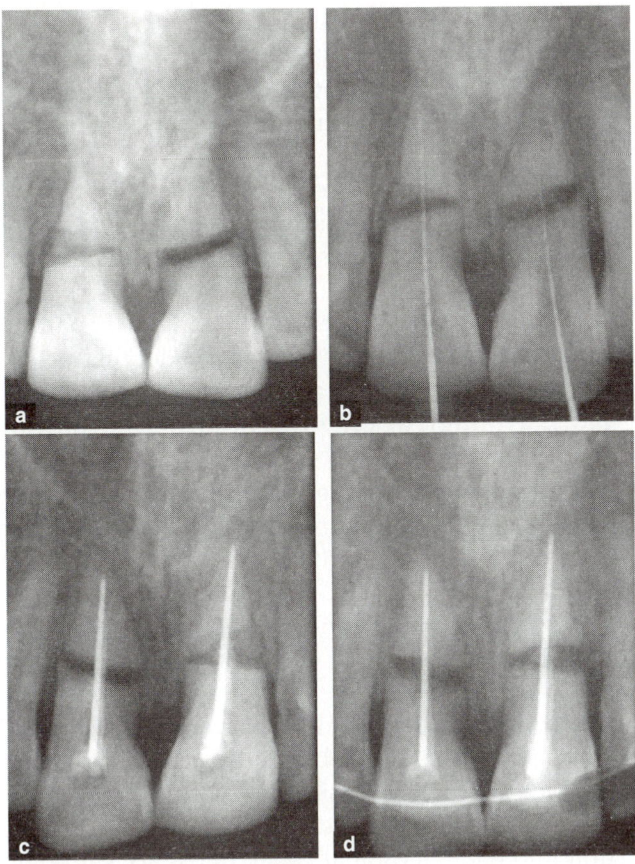

Fig. 33.3 Stabilizing two fractured root segments (a) Preoperative; (b) Assessing root canal; (c) Endodontic stabilization; (d) Postoperative (splinting)

- Apicoectomy where large portion of apical root is lost
- Primary molars with no permanent successors
- Grade II and III mobility
- Certain mobile reimplanted teeth
- Concomitant internal/external resorption leading to sacrificing apical portion of root.

Contraindications

The contraindications for the use of endodontic implants are:

- Periapical rarefaction/bone infection
- Previous radiation of the apical area
- Periodontal pockets communicating with the apical region
- Debilitating systemic conditions
- Roots with excessive curvatures
- Failed root canal treatment cases
- Inadequate vertical bone beyond the apex of tooth (minimum 6.0 mm bone required for implants)
- Anatomic structures approaching apex, such as maxillary sinus, inferior alveolar canal, mental foramen, etc. which are liable to be violated.

PATIENT SELECTION

The criteria used for patient selection requiring endodontic implants are:

i. ***Periodontal status of the tooth***: Aggressive periodontal problem with continuous loss of bone may lead to failure of endodontic implants. The periodontal therapy is to be instituted with or without grafting to ensure complete healing of periradicular bone. The active periodontal problem may also lead to soft tissue breakdown, facilitating communication of the implant with the oral cavity. This communication, if not managed at the initial stage may lead to failure of endodontic implant therapy.

ii. ***Anatomical considerations***: Anatomical structure, such as maxillary sinus, mental foramen, inferior alveolar canal may get violated during insertion of implant, especially when in near proximity to the apex of root. The inclination of root apex in the alveolar bone should also be evaluated before placing the endodontic implant.

iii. ***Patient's acceptance***: Patient selection is most important consideration for implant placement. Patient should be informed of all the implications involved during and after implant placement. The prognosis and longevity of the procedure should be clear to the patient prior to opting for implant therapy.

   (*Endodontic implants are not appropriate for all teeth that are mobile; and their placement may not resolve the advancing periodontal disease.*)

iv. ***Occlusal interference***: It is established that occlusal interferences affect treatment outcome in endodontic implants. Teeth in maximum occlusal interrelationships exhibit more mobility after placement of endodontic implants than those with no occlusion or at least minimum occlusal interference.

v. ***Clinician's skill***: The skill/competence of operator is also very important. The clinical information should be gathered and evaluated for each case in order to determine whether endodontic implant would be best and the last choice. And also the operator would be able to perform the treatment procedure with precision.

Implant Materials and Designs

The success of endodontic implant therapy mainly depends upon the material and the design of the implant.

Initially, vitallium (alloy of 65% cobalt, 30% chromium and 5% molybdenum) had been widely used as endodontic implant, considering it to be inert and non-corrosive. Later, investigators questioned the use of vitallium and also observed that it undergoes surface corrosion. These observations lead to discontinuation of vitallium as endodontic implant material.

Currently, two materials are being used as endodontic implants; Titanium and aluminium oxide, which is a single crystal sapphire. Titanium is biocompatible and exhibits superior physical properties. Stainless steel and Ni-Ti in the form of root canal files have also been used as endodontic implants.

The designs of endodontic implants currently in use are smooth-taper and threaded-taper. Another design of endodontic implant, the porous surface implant, is also under investigation (Fig. 33.4). The clinical success of smooth and threaded implants is almost same; both provide substantial fixation and adequate stress distribution to the surrounding tissues. Threaded implants displayed higher retention; however, the threads cutting into apical dentin may lead to high stresses and even microcracks in dentin, subsequently leading to root fracture and failure of implant therapy. Porous surface implant provides strong fixation by facilitating bony ingrowths. These implants also provide better retention in the root canal and better seal as well. Glass-ionomer and AH 26 cements provide better mechanical interlocking at cement-implant interface. Possibility of using aluminium, molybdenum with titanium for endodontic implant material is under investigation; porous surface design is showing promising results.

The efficacy of endodontic stabilizer depends upon following considerations:

- The implant/stabilizer should provide effective apical seal; seal at the apical zone area.
- The implant/stabilizer should remain retentive in the root canal.

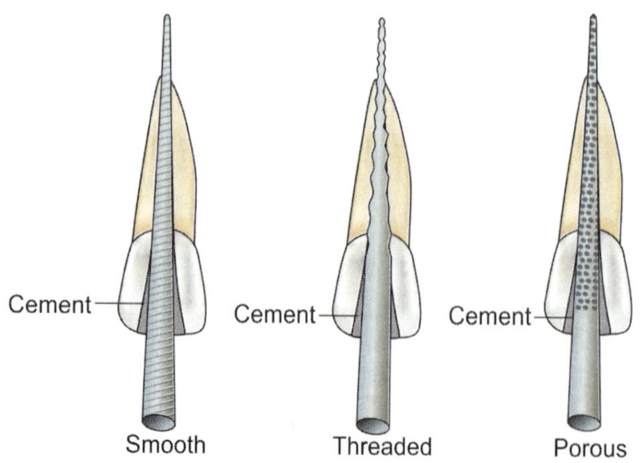

Fig. 33.4 Endodontic implants (surface variations)

33

- The implant/stabilizer should effectively fix into the jaw bone and get stabilized.
- The effective growth of bone around the implant provides necessary retention.

Clinical Criteria for a Successful Endodontic Implant

The success of endodontic implant therapy depends on various factors. The factors, which affect the long-term success of implants are:

- A radiographically normal attachment apparatus including the bone, cementum, and dentin.
- A stabilized functional, and symptomless tooth.
- Normal gingival crevice containing a normal epithelial attachment.
- The implant can be inserted through the prepared root canal up to the desired distance in the bone and remain there between the labial and lingual plates of bone.
- Sufficient alveolar bone should be available for retention and stability of both the tooth and the implant.
- Teeth with multiple canals, curved canals/curved root apices, calcified/obstructed canals should be avoided whenever possible.
- Caution must be exercised to avoid implant penetration into the mandibular canal, maxillary sinus, etc.
- Teeth with insufficient bone support and a hopeless periodontal prognosis are poor candidate for endodontic implant.

The ***limitations*** of endodontic implants, which can result in failure, are:

- Poor apical seal resulting in periapical rarefaction around the root apex.
- Extrusion of excessive sealer through the apical foramen into the periapical tissues; with resulting irritation.
- Limitation in the available length of the osseous portion of implants by local anatomic factors, such as the maxillary sinus, mandibular canal, etc. The labioversion/linguoversion of the tooth in the jaw also pose challenge.
- Perforation of the lateral root surface or perforation of a curved root near the root apex.
- A structurally weakened tooth, instrumented to a larger size than usual may fracture during function.

Three-dimensional apical seal is important feature for the success of implant therapy. In preparing a wide apical foramen, the root apex is ground away by the large endodontic instruments, which may lead to fracture the root tip or subsequently resorption of the root tip at a later stage. The result is an imperfect apical seal, which would lead to failure of the implant therapy.

IMPLANT PLACEMENT

The root canal is prepared following the conventional principles. In case the tooth is mobile (grade II mobility), the same should be splinted prior to root canal treatment. The access preparation should be larger and wider so as to accommodate the placement of a rigid implant that requires 'straight-line' insertion into the canal. The root canal must be enlarged to at least the size of a No. 60 instrument. The steps followed in implant placement are:

- Anesthetize the tooth and the surrounding areas.
- A marker is set on the 40 mm reamers at a level equivalent to the length of the tooth plus the number of millimetres the implant will extend beyond the root apex.
- The first 40 mm reamer used to perforate the root apex should be smaller than the last sized instrument, which was used to prepare root canal.
- The last 40 mm reamer should be of the size of last endodontic instrument; the bone is pierced to the desired length.
- Irrigate the root canal preferably with anesthetic solution, which débrides as well as controls hemorrhage within a few minutes.
- The canal is dried using sterile absorbent points.
- Select an implant of equivalent size to the last instrument used; the desired length is marked from the occlusal tip through the root canal to the exact length cut into the cancellous bone, and insert it into the bone through the root canal.
- The implant must penetrate into the bone up to the prepared length and should be tightly fit.
- If necessary, enlarge the root canal a little more to accommodate the implant, but the implant must fit snugly at the apical foramen.
- Insert a plugger into the canal opening until it binds, and measure the exact length; the implant can be inserted unimpeded into the canal.
- Using a diamond/carborundum disc, cut the butt end of the implant and adjust length equivalent to the measurement obtained by inserting the plugger into the root canal.
- This plugger is used to push the implant, because the butt end of the implant must be cut-off prior to insertion into the tooth.
- Glass-ionomer cement or AH 26 cement is preferred for cementation. Apply cement into the dried canal and try to avoid cement extrusion beyond the apical foramen.
- Using a hemostat, push the implant slowly into the canal and bone.
- Seat the implant by pressing the plugger firmly against the butt end of the implant, until it binds completely in the canal and the bone.

The rest of the space can be utilized for back-filling or postcore restoration depending on the remaining tooth structure, esthetics and the patient's expectations.

BIBLIOGRAPHY

1. Cardenas JE, Beltran EH and Ananos FH. Ni-Ti endodontic intraosseous implant. Dent. Press. Endod.: 2012; 2:38–41.
2. Chen H, Liu N, Xu X, Qu X and Lu E. Smoking, radiotherapy, diabetes and osteoporosis as risk factors for dental implant failure: a meta-analysis. PLoS ONE: 2013; 8:e71955.
3. Goldberg F. Endodontic implant: a scanning electron microscopic study. Int. Endod. J.: 1982; 15:17–78.
4. Konake VB and Patil SN. Management of grade III mobile anterior tooth in function using endostabilizer – a case report. J. Crit. And Diag. Res.: 2014; 8:6–7.
5. Larsen RM, Patten JR and Wayman BE. Endodontic endosseous implants: case report and update of materials. J. Endod.: 1989; 15:496–500.
6. Madison S and Bjorndal AM. Clinical application of endodontic implants. J. Prosthet. Dent.: 1988; 57:603–608.
7. Maniatopoulos C, Pilliar RM and Smith DC. Evaluation of the retention of endodontic implants. J. prosthet. Dent.: 1988; 59:438–446.
8. Marchand F, Raskin A and Dionnes-Hornes A. Dental implants and diabetes: conditions for success. Diabetes Metab.: 2012; 38:14–19.
9. Mittal S, Kumar T, Aggarwal V, Bansal R and Kaur D. Endodontic stabilizers for treating mid root fractures. J. Interdiscip. Dent.: 2011; 1:108–110.
10. Nivethithan T, Ramesh S and Raj JD. Endodontic stabilizers: A myth. Int. J. Pharma. Resch. Clin. Res.: 2015; 7:1–7.
11. Parmar G and Pramodkumar AV. Custom-fabricated endodontic implants: report of two cases. J. Endod.: 2000; 26:301–303.
12. Pereira FR, Brawuel JD, Roahen JO and Giambarresi L. Histological response to titanium endodontic endosseous implant in dogs. J. Endod.: 1996; 22:161–164.
13. Priyadarshini L and Narayan L. Endodontic miscellany: Use of an endodontic file as an endodontic implant. Endodontology: 2000; 12:37–39.
14. Sahelipour F. Endodontic stabilizers. J. Endod.: 2005; 18–21.
15. Sumi Y, Mitsudo K and Ueda M. Conservation of severely traumatized teeth using endodontic implants: A case report. J. Oral Maxillofac. Surg.: 1998; 56:240–242.
16. Sumi Y, Nakamura Y, Mitsudoh K and Ueda M. Application of titanium-alloy endodontic implants in conjunction with periradicular surgery. Oral Surg., Oral Med., Oral Pathol., Oral Radiol. Endod.: 1999; 88:484–7.
17. Sussman HI. Endodontic pathology leading to implant failure. A case report. J. Oral Implantol.: 1997; 23:112–116.
18. Torabinejad M and Goodacre CJ. Endodontic or dental implant therapy: the factor affecting treatment planning. JADA: 2006; 137:973–977.
19. Yadav RK, Tikku AP, Chandra A, Wadhwani KK, Kumar A and Singh M. Endodontic implants. Nat. J. Maxillofac. Surg.: 2014; 5:70–73.

Chapter 34

Endodontic–Periodontal Relationship

Each specialty of dentistry stands at a point where the patient care approach makes it mandatory to be involved with other specialties right from the phase of diagnosis to treatment planning and finally to that of maintenance. The specialties have been created for convenience to focus the knowledge on particular areas; however, for the benefit of patients, the interrelated areas should also be looked into and discussed.

Pulpal and periodontal problems are responsible for more than 50% of tooth mortality. The main pathways for communication between the dental pulp and periodontium are through lateral/accessory canals, apical foramen and also the dentinal tubules. The pathways of communications between pulp and periodontium often determine the progress of disease in these tissues.

Endodontic–periodontal (Endo–Perio) relationship implies the spread of inflammation and infection from one component to the other (spread of infection from endodontic lesion to periodontic tissues and from periodontic lesions to endodontic tissues). Thorough knowledge of Endo–perio relationship is crucial for proper diagnosis and treatment decision-making in diseases affecting these tissues.

PERIODONTAL PULPAL INTERRELATIONSHIP

The pulp is generally not affected by periodontal disease until the defect exposes accessory canal(s) to the oral environment. The pathogens may pass through these open accessory canals into the pulp and cause a localized inflammatory response, which may lead to pulpal necrosis. Certain procedures involved in root canal treatment, such as irrigants, intracanal medicaments, sealers, etc. if come in contact with periodontal tissues may lead to inflammatory response in the periodontium.

Periodontal defects may occur after procedural mishaps during root canal preparations, such as perforations of the floor of pulp chamber, strip perforations/root perforations, etc. Periodontal defects may also be caused by vertical root fractures, mostly associated with excessive force used during obturation of canal spaces.

The by-products of pulpal inflammation often lead to inflammation in the periodontal tissues. Inflammation in the infected pulp produces by-products that pass along the pathways of communications and elicit an inflammatory reaction in the periodontium. Similarly, the inflammatory by-products of the infected periodontal tissues can cause infection in the pulp. This is a vicious cycle that continues and often creates a dilemma for the clinician. A few authors are of view that periodontal disease would not cause pulpal disease because inflammation follows venous drainage and the venous blood flows outward from the pulp to the periodontium. Bacteria, viruses and fungi are the pathogens from diseased pulp that can cause periodontal lesions.

Bacteria

Bacteria play a critical role in both endodontic and periodontal diseases.

Initially proteolytic bacteria predominate in the root canals; later, anaerobic microbiota becomes prevalent. Spirochetes though associated with both endodontic and periodontal disease, are found more in subgingival plaque than in root canals. A large diversity of oral treponemas in subgingival biofilms of periodontal pocket has been identified; therefore, it was thought that the presence or absence of oral spirochetes can be used to differentiate between endodontic and periodontal lesions. However, the presence of spirochetes in the root canal has been well-documented by different identification techniques. The spirochete species most frequently found in root canals are *Treponema denticola* and *Treponema maltophilium*.

Bacteria associated with Pulp Diseases

- Spirochetes
- Eubacteria
- Peptostreptococci
- Fusobacterium
- Porphyromonas
- Prevotella
- Streptococci
- Lactobacillus
- Actinomyces.

Bacteria associated with Periodontal Lesions

- *Actinobacillus actinomycetemcomitans*
- *Porphyromonas gingivalis*
- *Bacteroides forsythus*
- *Prevotella intermedia*
- *Streptococcus intermedius*
- *Fusobacterium nucleatum*
- *Treponema denticola*
- *Eubacterium* spp.

Fungi

Candida albicans, Candida glabrata, Candida guillermondii, Candida incospicia and *Rodotorulamucilaginosa* are the common fungi species found in pulpal diseases.

The reduction of specific strains of bacteria in the root canal during endodontic treatment may allow fungal overgrowth in the remaining low nutrition environment. Fungi may gain access to the root canal from the oral cavity as a result of poor asepsis during endodontic treatment or postpreparation procedures. It has also been established that approximately 20% of periodontitis patients harbor subgingival yeasts.

Viruses

In patients with periodontal disease, herpes simplex virus was frequently detected in the gingival crevicular fluid and in the gingival biopsies of periodontal lesions. Human cytomegalovirus may be present in about 65% of the periodontal pocket samples and in about 85% of gingival tissue samples. Epstein-Barr virus Type 1 may be present in more than 40% of pocket samples and in about 80% of the gingival tissue samples. Active virus infection may give rise to production of an array of cytokines and chemokines with the potential to induce immunosuppression and tissue destruction.

Effect of Pulpal Disease on Periodontium

Pulpal tissue is enclosed in the pulp chamber and is separated from the periodontal tissue by dentin and cementum. The diseases of the pulp normally do not produce changes in the periodontal tissue; however, in some cases the pulpal inflammation may extend into the periodontium, e.g. a long-standing periapical abscess may drain through gingiva producing a periodontal pocket. This pocket formation is different from the common periodontal pocket and is termed *'retrograde periodontitis'*. The increased tension within the pulp chamber may facilitate passage of infected material into the periodontium along the pathways of communications, thereby spreading the disease.

Effect of Periodontal Disease on the Pulp

The pulpal diseases when initiated as a result of extension of infection from the periodontal tissue into the pulp, are termed *'retrograde pulpitis'*. During the root planing procedures, cementum may get exfoliated, exposing the dentinal tubules. The exposed dentinal tubules create direct pathway between the periodontium and the pulp. It is established that periodontal disease can produce atrophic changes like calcification and deposition of secondary dentin in the pulp.

CLASSIFICATION OF ENDODONTIC PERIODONTAL LESIONS

The endodontic-periodontal lesions have been classified by different authors. The accepted classifications are:

1. Simon's/Cohen's Classification

a. Primary endodontic lesions
b. Primary periodontal lesions
c. Combined lesions
  i. Primary endodontic disease with secondary periodontal involvement
  ii. Primary periodontal disease with secondary endodontic involvement
  iii. True combined diseases.

2. Grossman's Classification

a. Lesions that require endodontic treatment procedures only
  i. Periapical abscess
  ii. Root fractures
  iii. Root perforations
    - Teeth with incomplete root formation
    - Pulp exposures
b. Lesions that require periodontal treatment procedures only
  i. Occlusal trauma
  ii. Gingival inflammation
  iii. Periodontal pocket formation

c. Lesions that require combined endodontic periodontic treatment procedures
   i. Root resorption
   ii. Replants, transplants, etc.
      - Surgical intervention
      - Concomitant pulpal and periodontal involvement.

3. Weine's Classification

a. *Class I*: Tooth in which symptoms clinically and radiographically simulate periodontal disease; but are actually due to pulpal inflammation and/or necrosis.
b. *Class II*: Tooth that has concomitant pulpal/periapical and periodontal disease.
c. *Class III*: Tooth that has no pulpal problem but requires endodontic therapy (may need root amputation also) to achieve periodontal healing.
d. *Class IV*: Tooth that clinically and radiographically simulates pulpal/periapical disease; but actually has periodontal disease.

Simon's/Cohen's classification, based on pathology of origin of the lesion, is accepted and is described:

a. *Primary endodontic lesion*

Primary endodontic lesion is originally an endodontic lesion; the inflammatory by-products proceed from pulp spaces to the gingiva (Fig. 34.1a to c). Pulpal necrosis does not cause periodontal disease directly; however, it may form sinus tract, which allows passage of inflammatory products to the periodontal ligament. Osseous destruction is localized to the involved tooth.

b. *Primary periodontal lesions*

The periodontal lesions usually initiate in the sulcus and migrate apically (Fig. 34.2a to c). The plaque induced inflammation, lead to loss of surrounding alveolar bone and supporting periodontal soft tissues. The loss of clinical attachment of periodontal tissues initiates periodontal problems; subsequently, progression of periodontal disease leads to the formation of osseous defects along the lateral and furcation areas.

The affected tooth has vital pulp and responds normally on pulp testing.

c. *Combined lesions*

i. *Primary endodontic lesions with secondary periodontal involvement*: An untreated or poorly treated endodontic lesion usually lead to destruction of the periapical tissues; subsequently, this destruction progresses into the interradicular area. The persistent drainage from gingival sulcus coupled with accumulation of plaque/calculus results in periodontal disease and further apical migration of epithelial attachment (Fig. 34.3a to c).

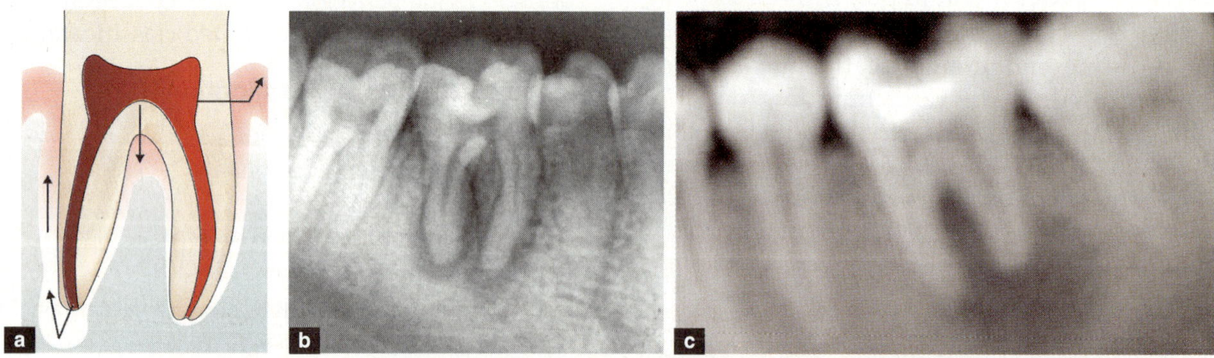

Fig. 34.1 Primary endodontic lesion: (a) Diagrammatic; (b) and (c) Radiographic

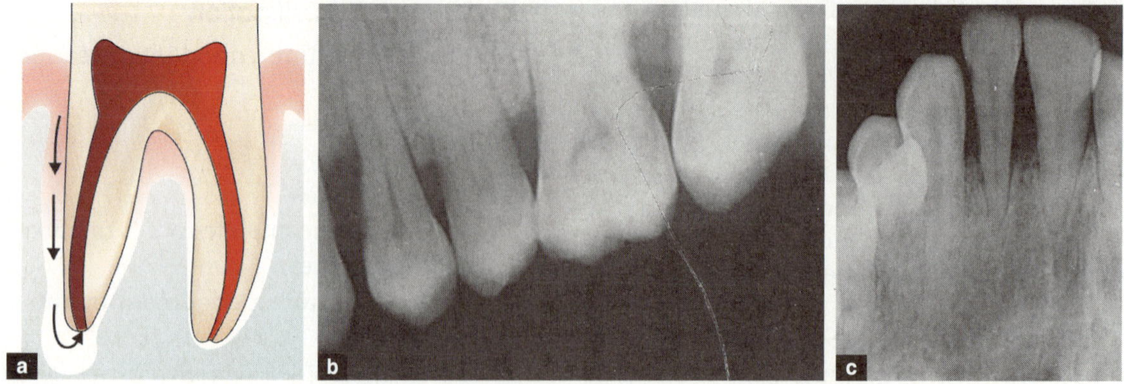

Fig. 34.2 Primary periodontal lesion (chronic periodontitis progresses apically along the root surface): (a) Diagrammatic; (b) Radiographic (premolars); (c) Radiographic (incisors)

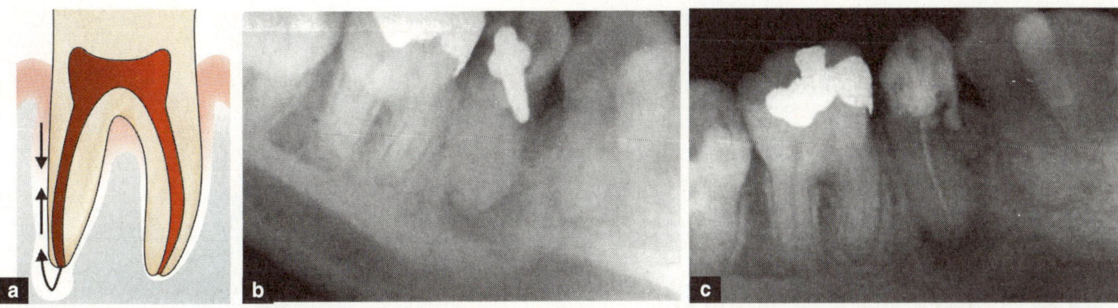

Fig. 34.3 Primary endodontic lesion with secondary periodontal involvement: (a) Diagrammatic; (b) Radiographic; (c) Case-treated with root canal therapy and bone grafting

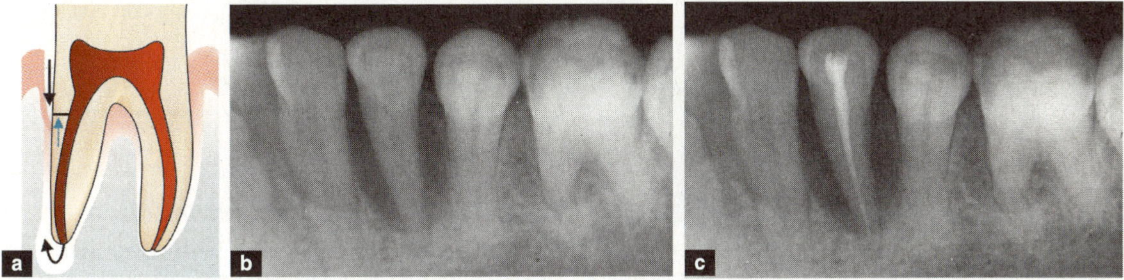

Fig. 34.4 Primary periodontal lesion with secondary endodontic involvement: (a) A periodontal pocket can infect the pulp through a lateral canal (blue arrow) and this in turn can result in a periapical lesion (diagrammatic); (b) Radiographic; (c) Case-treated with root canal therapy and curettage

These lesions usually have necrotic root canals and plaque/calculus accumulations can be seen clinically. Radiographs may show generalized periodontal defects at the initial site of endodontic involvement.

ii. *Primary periodontal lesions with secondary endodontic involvement*: Periodontal disease can have an effect on pulp through accessory/lateral canals or even through exposed dentinal tubules (Fig. 34.4a to c). Progressive osseous destruction due to periodontal disease can expose dentinal tubules, lateral accessory canals and the furcation area. Thus, a periodontal pocket can infect the pulp, subsequently resulting in a periapical lesion.

Primary periodontal lesions with secondary endodontic involvement usually exhibit pain and clinical signs of pulpal disease. This situation is evident when the periodontal disease progresses to expose the pulp to oral environment, generally leading to necrotic pulp.

The periodontally involved maxillary lateral incisor was treated with Fisiograft (Fig. 34.5) and root canal therapy (Fig. 34.6a to e).

iii. *True combined lesions*: Pulpal and periodontal disease may occur independently or concomitantly in and around the same tooth (Fig. 35.7a to c). Two independent periapical and periodontal lesions can coexist and may eventually fuse with each other. Once the separate endodontic and periodontal lesions coalesce, they are clinically indistinguishable and are known as *'True Combined lesions'*.

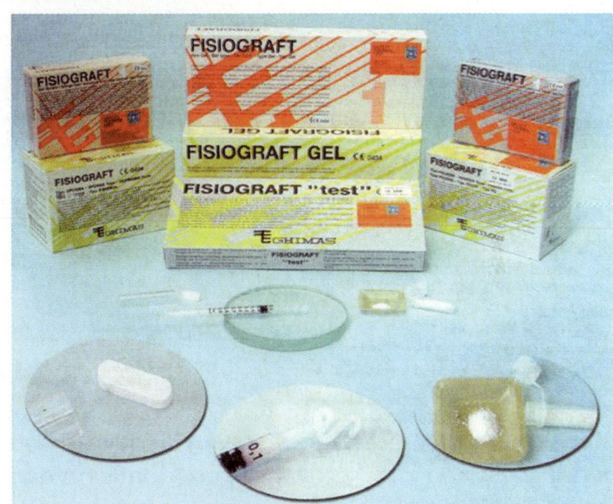

Fig. 34.5 Fisiograft

DIAGNOSIS

The pulp is vital and responsive to pulp testing in periodontal diseases; whereas, it is mostly infected and non-responsive in endodontic diseases. When the location is distinct and the lesion is discrete, the two can easily be differentiated. Once both the lesions progresses simultaneously or one affects the other, the diagnosis becomes challenging. Usually a similar

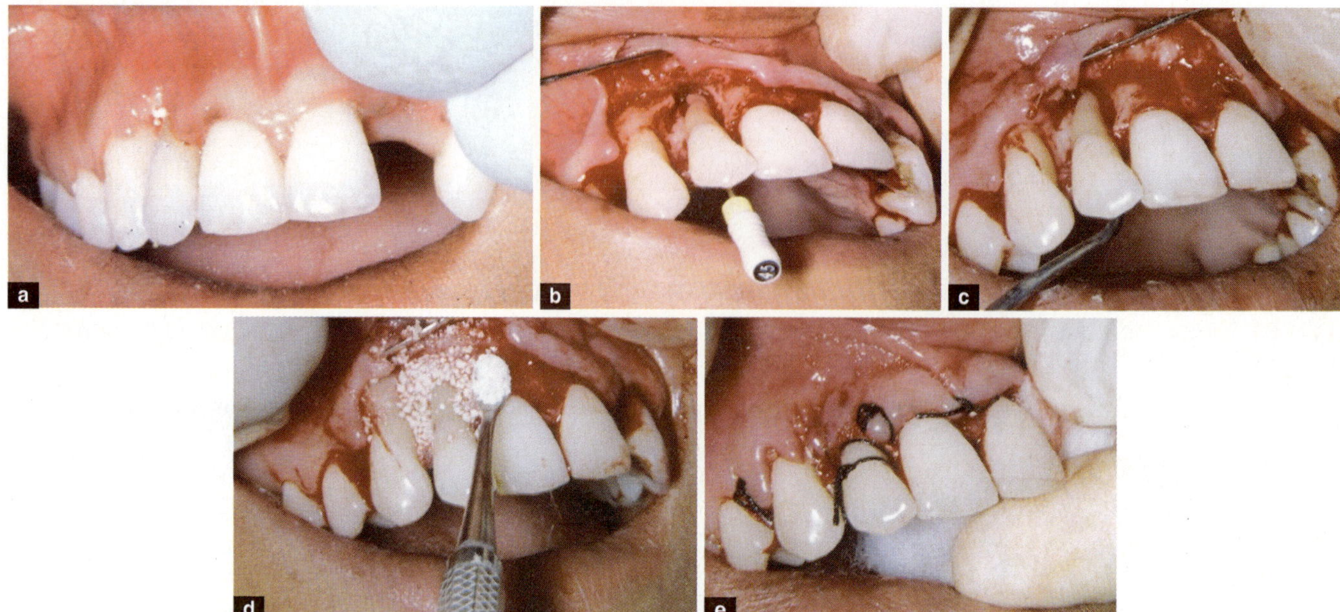

Fig. 34.6 Clinical management of maxillary lateral incisor (primary periodontal lesion with secondary endodontic involvement) (a) Preoperative; (b) Flap raised; root canal opened; (c) Curettage of bony defect; (d) Placement of fisiograft (after root canal completion); (e) Coapting the flap and suturing

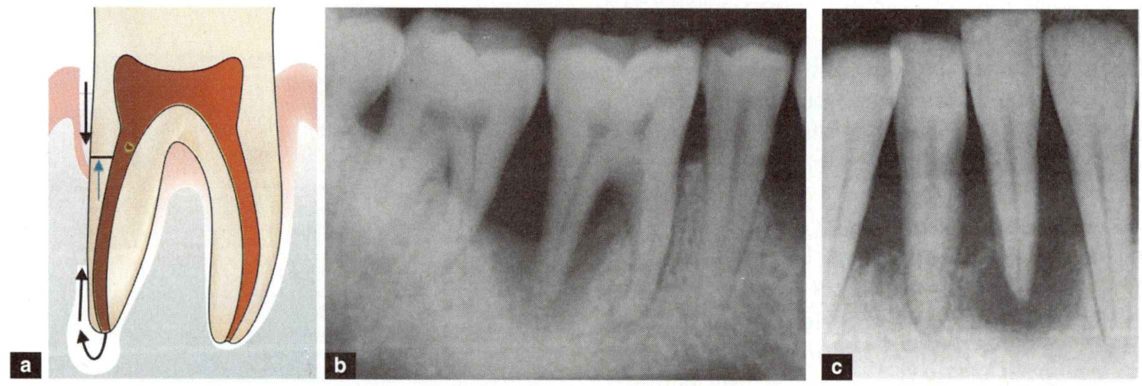

Fig. 34.7 True combined lesion: (a) Diagrammatic; (b) Radiographic (molar); (c) Radiographic (incisor)

clinical and radiological features are evident with both; a periapical lesion with secondary periodontal involvement and a periodontal lesion progressing to the apical area. The criteria of clinical identification of endodontic-periodontal lesions are tabulated in Table 34.1. The differentiation of sinus tract from an infrabony pocket is depicted in Table 34.2. The diagnostic features of both pulpal and periodontal lesions are given in Table 34.3.

In case diagnosis cannot be established, the lesion is considered to be of pulpal origin (an endodontic treatment can correct both lesions).

TREATMENT

The treatment decision-making depends on diagnosis of pulp vitality and extent of the periodontal defect. The suggestive treatment is described as per Simon's/Cohen's classification of Endodontic–Periodontal lesions.

Treatment: Key Features

- A few authors suggest that initial treatment be either endodontic or periodontal depending on origin of the initiating disease.
- Others recommend that endodontic treatment should be initiated followed by periodontal therapy; once a successful periodontal result has been achieved, the endodontic treatment is finalized.
- It is suggested that endodontic treatment should precede periodontal therapy, regardless of the cause of the disease; however, on exceptional occasions, the periodontal procedures should precede the endodontic treatment, such as when an unexpected need arises for radisectomy of a multi-rooted tooth, exposed during periodontal surgical procedure.

Table 34.1 Clinical identification of endodontic–periodontal lesions

Examination/diagnostic tests	*Primary endodontic lesion*	*Primary periodontal lesion*	*Primary endodontic lesions with secondary periodontal involvement*	*Primary periodontal lesions with secondary endodontic involvement*	*True combined lesion*
Visual examination	Presence of deep carious lesion/large-old restoration/ fractured restoration/ abrasion/cracks. Sinus opening may be present	Accumulation of plaque and subgingival calculus around multiple teeth/ inflamed gingiva. Presence of swelling around any tooth (indicating periodontal abscess)	Root perforation/fracture of root/post placed away from root canal. Seeping of exudate at the gingival margin of the affected tooth.	Presence of plaque/ sub gingival calculus around multiple teeth. Presence of generalized gingival recession Seeping of exudate from affected teeth.	Presence of varying degree of periodontitis. Presence of pus exudate along with chronic discolored (nonvital) tooth.
Pain	Sharp	Usually dull ache; abscess may present sharp pain	Usually sharp pain; chronic conditions present dull ache	Usually dull ache; Acute periodontal abscess present sharp pain	Usually dull ache (combined lesions are usually chronic)
Palpation	Usually no response (chronic periradicular inflammation may response positively)	Tender on palpation	Tender on palpation	Tender on palpation	Tender on palpation
Percussion	Tender on percussion	Usually not tender (acute case may response)	Tender on percussion	Tender on percussion	Tender on percussion
Tooth mobility	Fractured tooth/recently traumatized teeth show mobility	Presence of localized/ generalized mobility	Presence of localized mobility	Presence of generalized mobility	Presence of generalized mobility
Pulp vitality testing	A lingering response-irreversible pulpitis No response-necrotic pulp (nonvital)	The pulp is vital and responsive to testing	Pulp vitality tests negative	Pulp vitality may be positive in multirooted teeth	Usually negative because of nonvital pulp. Vitality tests may give positive response in multirooted teeth
Periodontal pocket evaluation	Presence of a solitary periodontal pocket in the absence of generalized periodontitis. (Such pocket may be seen in case of a vertical root fracture)	Multiple deep periodontal pockets	Presence of periodontal pocket along the affected tooth (teeth)	Presence of multiple deep periodontal pockets	Periodontal pockets in association with endodontically involved teeth
Radiographic sinus tracing using gutta-percha points	Gutta-percha point approaching apical area or furcation area in molars	Gutta-percha mainly depicted at the lateral aspect of the root	Gutta-percha mainly at the apical area or furcation area	Gutta-percha mainly depicted at the lateral aspect of the root	Sinus tract (gutta-percha) may not detect the lesion. Flap is to be raised to determine the exact etiology.
Conventional radiographic evaluation	Presence of deep carious lesions/extensive, old and defective restorations/poor root canal management/ root fractures. Periapical radiolucency may and may not be present.	Generalized vertical bone loss	Presence of deep carious lesions/extensive, old and defective restorations/poor root canal treatment/root fractures. Periapical radiolucency usually present.	Generalized angular bone loss	Generalized bone loss along with features of endodontic lesions.
Evaluating cracked tooth (teeth)	Painful response while chewing a wooden/ rubber platform; on releasing the biting pressure, pain increases.	No symptoms	Painful response while chewing a wooden/ rubber platform; on releasing the biting pressure, pain increases.	No symptoms	Painful response while chewing a wooden/rubber platform; on releasing the biting pressure, pain increases.

Table 34.2 Differentiation of a sinus tract from an infrabony pocket

	Sinus tract	*Infrabony pocket*
Origin	Originates from root canal and progresses occlusally from apical foramen or from a lateral canal	Originates from gingival crevice and progresses apically
Diagnosis	By means of gutta-percha cone or diagnostic wire	Periodontal probe
Treatment	Endodontic therapy	Periodontal therapy (endodontic therapy may be required)

Table 34.3 Differential diagnosis of pulpal and periodontal disease

	Pulpal	*Periodontal*
Clinical		
Cause	Pulpal infections	Periodontal infections
Vitality	Nonvital	Vital
Restoration	Deep or extensive	Not related
Plaque/calculus	Not related	Primary cause (must be present)
Inflammation	Usually acute, become chronic later	Usually chronic
Periodontal pockets	Not related	Deep/multiple
pH value	Often acidic	Often alkaline
Trauma	May lead to pulpal disease	Contributing factor
Flora	Few	Complex
Radiological		
Pattern	Localized	Generalized
Bone loss	Wider apically	Wider coronally
Periapical	Radiolucent	Not often related
Vertical bone loss	No	Yes
Histopathological		
Junctional epithelium	No apical migration	Apical migration
Granulation tissue	Minimal	larger
Gingiva	Normal	Usually recession

a. Primary Endodontic Lesions

Primary endodontic lesions usually heal following root canal treatment. Prognosis is always better in properly executed root canal treatment. The sinus tract extending into the gingival sulcus/furcation area, if present, disappears once the treatment is completed. Calcium hydroxide as an intracanal medicament, has been effective in the healing of large periapical lesion [Calcium hydroxide damages the microbial cytoplasmic membrane, suppresses enzyme activity, disrupts the cellular metabolism and inhibits deoxyribonucleic acid (DNA) replication by splitting DNA]. It also acts as a physical barrier that fills the space within the root canal walls and kills the remaining microorganisms by withholding substrates for their growth. In case of large periapical radiolucency, surgical intervention can be effective.

b. Primary Periodontal Lesions

34

Primary periodontal lesions are treated by appropriate periodontal therapy. The prognosis depends on the severity of the periodontal disease and the efficacy of periodontal therapy. Poor restorations and developmental grooves that are involved in the lesion must be removed. Periodontal surgery should be performed after the completion of hygiene phase of the treatment. The surgical periodontal procedures may remove cementum and expose dentinal tubules, (transporting irritants and causing pulpal inflammation); should be carried out judiciously. The clinicians should take precautions during periodontal therapy and avoid the use of irritating chemicals so as to minimize damage to cementum. Judicious use of periodontal surgical intervention can be effective.

Flowchart 34.1 summarizes the treatment of endodontic–periodontal lesions.

c. Combined Lesions

i. *Primary endodontic lesion with secondary periodontal involvement*

The prognosis for treatment of primary endodontic lesion with secondary periodontal involvement depends primarily on the severity of periodontal involvement. Such lesions should first be treated with

Flowchart 34.1: Stepwise treatment of endodontic–periodontal lesions

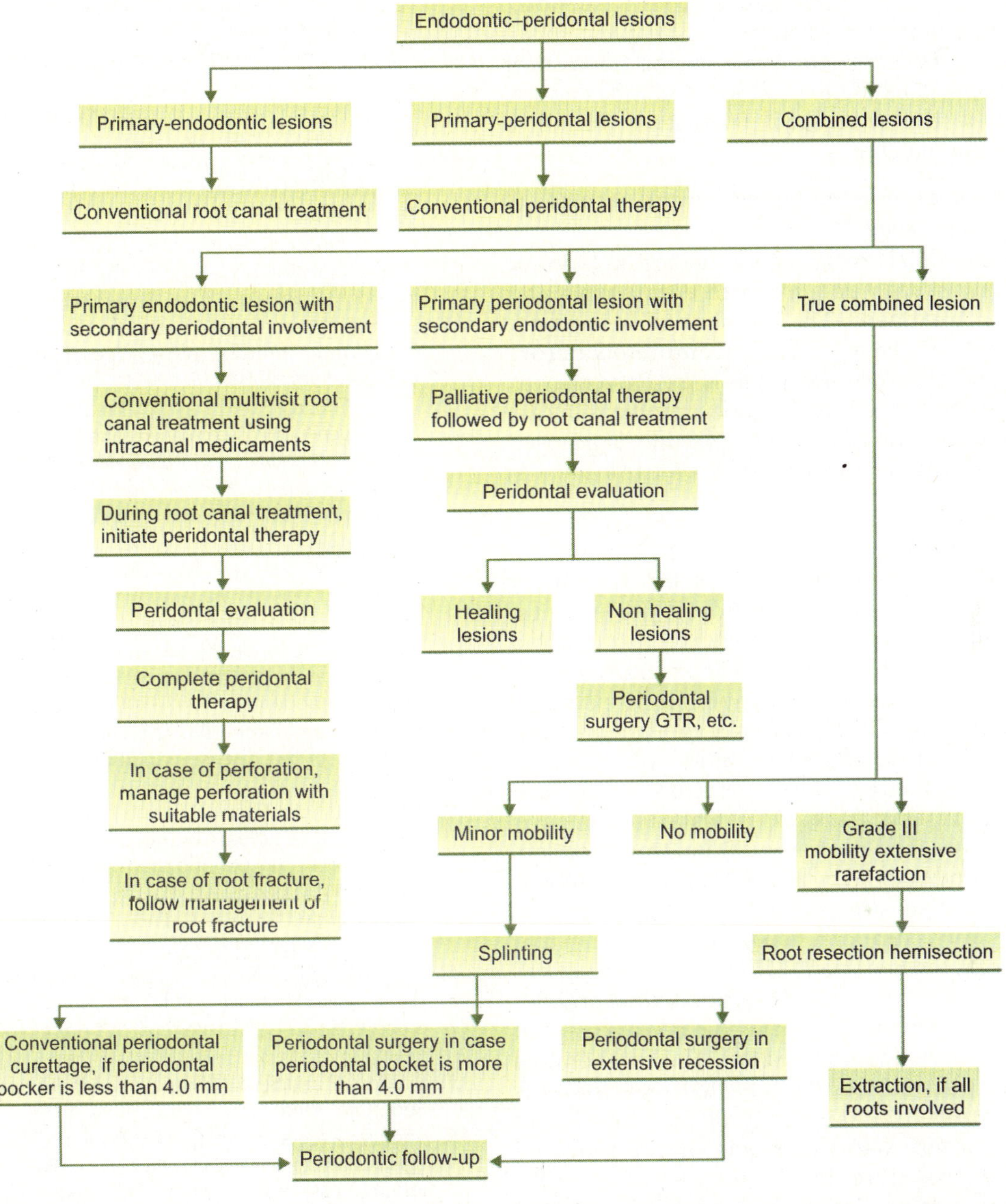

endodontic therapy followed by conventional periodontal treatment. Multivisit endodontics should be preferred placing intracanal medicament. The reduction in inflammation followed by repair should be evaluated periodically and then further periodontal treatment should be initiated. This way effect of pulpal inflammation on periodontal tissues can be evaluated. It is established that aggressive removal of the periodontal ligament and underlying cementum during initial endodontic therapy may adversely affect the periodontal healing. If the endodontic treatment is adequate, the prognosis depends on the severity of the periodontal tissue damage and the efficacy of periodontal treatment. Primary endodontic lesions with secondary periodontal involvement may also occur as a result of iatrogenic damage, such as root perforation or root fracture during root canal treatment. The outcome of the treatment of root perforations depends on the size, location, time of diagnosis and the degree of periodontal damage. It has been recognized that the success of the treatment depends mainly on immediate sealing of the perforation and appropriate infection control. Root fractures may also present as primary endodontic lesions with secondary periodontal involvement. Treatment depends on the tooth type, extent, duration and location of fracture, e.g. vertical root fracture of single rooted teeth has a poor prognosis, while molars can be managed by root resection/hemisection. Innovative techniques to treat and retain anterior teeth have been attempted using removal of the fractured segment followed by endodontic therapy or to bond the fractured fragments using a biocompatible material.

ii. *Primary periodontal lesions with secondary endodontic involvement*

Primary periodontal lesions with secondary endodontic involvement usually require both endodontic and periodontal treatment. The periodontal lesions are treated first (at least partially completed before initiating root canal treatment); may be by conventional, surgical and/or regenerative treatment protocol. In case of extensive periodontal lesion, splinting is advised for better results. The prognosis for such lesions is favorable.

iii. *True combined lesion*

True combined lesions should be treated as primary endodontic lesions with secondary periodontal involvement. Periodontal therapy should be completed followed by root canal treatment. The prognosis of true combined lesion is usually poor, especially in extensive periodontal lesions. The prognosis of combined lesions mainly rests with the efficacy of periodontal therapy. A tooth that requires a root to be resected always need root canal treatment; therefore, judicious planning is important as regard root amputation/hemisection. Ideally, the tooth should be root filled prior to surgery. The prognosis of an affected tooth can be improved by increasing bony support, using bone grafting and guided tissue regeneration (GTR). GTR therapy has been successfully carried out in the endodontic surgeries as a concomitant treatment during the management of the endodontic-periodontal lesions. The regenerative procedure is planned after verifying the nonvital status of the pulp, extent and severity of the periodontal destruction, and also prognosis of the planned regenerative procedure. In case the prognosis of the periodontal regenerative procedure is found to be favorable, then endodontic therapy should be initiated. A few authors suggest splinting of concerned tooth (teeth) before GTR procedure and root canal treatment. Root canal treatment does help reducing the mobility of tooth. Long-term follow-up is necessary to assess treatment success in such lesions.

BIBLIOGRAPHY

1. Bashutski JD and Wang HL. Periodontal and endodontic regeneration. J. Endod.: 2009; 35:321–328.
2. Chapple I and Lumley P: The periodontal-endodontic interface. Dent Update: 1999; 26:331.
3. Dahle UR, Tronstad L and Oslen I. Characterization of new periodontal and endodontic isolates of spirochetes. Eur. J. Oral Sci.: 1996; 104:41.
4. Goyal L. Clinical effectiveness of combining platelet rich fibrin with alloplastic bone substitute for the management of combined endodontic periodontal lesion. Restor. Dent. Endod.: 2014; 39:51–55.
5. Harrington GW, Steiner DR and Ammons WF. The periodontal-endodontic controversy. Periodontol2000.: 2002; 30:123–130.
6. Heijl L, Heden G, Svardstrom G and Frank AL. Enamel matrix derivative (EMDOGAIN) in the treatment of intrabony periodontal defects. J. Clin. Periodontol.: 1997; 24:705–714.
7. John V, Warner NA and Blanchard SB. Periodontic-Endodontic interdisciplinary treatment—A case report. Compendium: 2004; 25:179–185.
8. Oh SL, Fouad AF and Park SH. Treatment strategy for guided tissue regeneration in combined endodontic-periodontal lesions: Case report and review. J. Endod.: 2009; 35:1331–1336.
9. Parolia A, Gait TC, Porto IC and Mala K. Endo–perio lesion: A dilemma from 19th until 21st century. J. Interdisc. Dent.: 2013; 3:2–11.
10. Paul BF and Hutter JW. The endodontic–periodontal continuum revisited: new insights into etiology, diagnosis and treatment. J. Am. Dent. Assoc.: 1997; 128:1541.
11. Rostein I and Simon JH. Diagnosis, prognosis and decision-making in the treatment of combined periodontal-endodontic lesions. Periodontol.: 2002, 2004:34:165–203.
12. Rotstein I and Simon JH. The endo–perio lesion: A critical appraisal of the disease condition. Endod. Topics.: 2006; 13:34–56.
13. Rupf S, Kannengiesser S, Merte K, Pfister W, Sigusch B and Eschrich K. Comparison of profiles of key periodontal pathogens in the periodontium and endodontium. Endod. Dent. Traumatol.: 2000; 16:269.
14. Shenoy N and Shenoy A. Endo-perio lesion: diagnosis and clinical considerations. Ind. J. Dent. Res.: 2010; 21:579–585.
15. Simon JHS, Glick DH and Frank AL. The relationship of endo-dontic–periodontal lesions. J. Periodontal: 1972; 43:202–208.
16. Singh P. Endo–Perio Dilemma: A brief review. Dent. Res. J. (Isfahan): 2011; 8:39–47.
17. Siquiera JF and Sen BH. Fungi in endodontic infections. Oral Surg. Oral Med. Oral Pathol.: 2004; 97:632.
18. Somanath G, George G, Sinha JN and Gautam V. Inter-disciplinary approach in treatment of endodontic–periodontal lesion: A case report. J. Univ. Coll. Med. Sci.: 2013; 1:58–61.
19. Sunitha VR, Emmadi P, Namasivayam A, Thyegarajn R and Rajaraman V. The periodontal–endodontic continuum: A review. J. Conserv. Dent.: 2008; 11:54–62.
20. Taschieri S, Del Fabbro M, Testori T, Saita M and Weinstein R. Efficacy of guided tissue regeneration in the management of through-and-through lesions following surgical endodontics: A preliminary study. Int. J. Periodontics Restorative Dent.: 2008; 28:265–271.
21. Verma PK, Srivastava R, Gupta KK and Srivastava A. Combined endodontic–Periodontal lesion: A clinical dilemma. J. Interdis. Dent.: 2011; 1:119–124.
22. vonArx T and Cochran DL. Rationale for the application of the GTR principle using a barrier membrane in endodontic surgery: a proposal of classification and literature review. Int. J. Periodontics Restorative Dent.: 2001; 21:127–139.

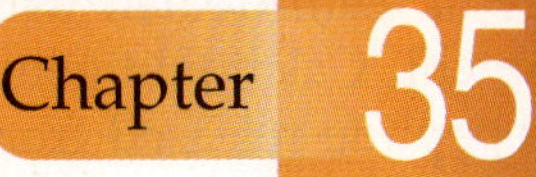

Chapter 35

Endodontic–Orthodontic Continuum

Almost all professional specialties of dentistry are interrelated. Endodontics is mainly interrelated to periodontics, orthodontics and restorative dentistry. The relation between orthodontics and endodontics has attracted less attention of the researchers. There might not be any definite guidelines on the subject, which make the treatment planning and execution difficult for the clinicians. The orthodontic movement inevitably causes biological reactions in periodontal and pulpal tissues. The clinician must be aware of the possible complications and also the management of such complications during orthodontic movement of teeth.

The combination of endodontics and orthodontics in majority of clinical situations present better results when treated both ways. The pulpal health, during orthodontic movement is to be analyzed periodically; in case of any indication of disease process, the same should be managed properly. These two specialties are intertwined theoretically and clinically; therefore, aptly referred to as *'Endodontic–orthodontic continuum'*.

Endodontic–orthodontic continuum is inseparable in the following situations:

- When orthodontic therapy warrants endodontic intervention (post-treatment resorption and loss of vitality of orthodontically treated teeth).
- When endodontic therapy warrants orthodontic intervention [loss of clinical crown due to advanced caries/resorption near alveolar crest/periodontal problems, requiring forced eruption (forced eruption is recommended in anterior teeth only)].
- When orthodontics requires endodontic intervention for better results (endodontic intervention to halt an ongoing resorption prior to starting of the orthodontic treatment).

IMPLICATIONS OF ORTHODONTIC TOOTH MOVEMENT

The force created by orthodontic tooth movement has definite effect on underlying tooth tissues. The clinical implications are:

a. Effect of Orthodontic Tooth Movement on Pulp

The magnitude of rapidity of orthodontic movement, which may cause pulpal damage has not been properly documented. The pulpal degeneration may occur after tipping forces or rapid tooth movement, owing to loss of collateral supply to the pulp. The 'tipping force' concept has been refuted, claiming successful rotation of 72–108° without any pulpal damage. The 'force', however, do affect pulpal vitality. The mechanisms which lead to changes in pulp vitality can be understood from the following factors:

i. Respiratory rate of the pulpal cells
ii. Blood flow to the pulp
iii. Neural response of the pulp.

i. Respiratory Rate of the Pulpal Cells

Respiration is a sign of vitality for any living tissue. Any change in the rate of respiration of any cell affects the state of its vitality. The pulp and its living components are no exception to it. Orthodontic movement depresses the respiratory rate by a mean value of 27.4%. A few authors have observed a significant correlation between amount of decrease in pulp tissue respiration rate and the age of the patient. This rate of respiratory depression is more in older patients due to the constriction of their apical foramina that decreases the blood flow. This also explains why younger teeth show less effect than the older ones. The changes in tissue respiration (possibly hypoxia), because of orthodontic movement of tooth, cause increase in aspartate aminotransferase (AST) activity level and affect pulp tissue, changing its neural response. It has also been opined that decrease of some protein expressions block the regeneration of pulp structure. Radiorespirometric methods have confirmed respiratory depression in pulp, which is under orthodontic tooth movement.

ii. Blood Flow to the Pulp

It is hypothesized that dynamic mechanisms exist in the control of blood flow in a tooth undergoing orthodontic movement. When an orthodontic force is applied, pulp tissue reacts with initial pulp hyperemia, subsequently proceeding to degranulation of mast cells characterized by cell damage and allied biochemical reactions. This is classical feature of acute inflammation. The initial stage of reactive hyperemia usually reverts back to normal in due course of time. When the pulp of teeth subjected to orthodontic forces was grown in culture, it showed sprouting of new vessels. Angiogenic changes have been observed after orthodontic movement (increase in number of microvessels), expressing rise of angiogenic growth factor in pulp. The factors responsible for such changes are platelet derived growth factor, vascular endothelial growth factor and transforming growth factor-β. Transforming growth factor β-1 (TGF-β1) and (TGF-β3) are responsible for stimulation of reactionary dentin and also reparative dentin after orthodontic tooth movement. Since dental pulp is limited in narrow area, the increase blood flow (dilatation of arterioles) cause increase in pulp pressure and compression of venous flow. It is established that most of the changes in pulpal blood are reversible (during tooth movement); only if pulp is not irritated earlier because of deep caries, trauma, etc. It is also asserted that fully developed (mature apex) teeth are sensitive to irreversible pulp inflammation and immature apex teeth are not sensitive. It is established that application of severe force for a longer period may affect pulpal blood flow than short-term application of same force (laser Doppler flowmetry evaluation). The two variables of decrease in pulpal respiration and an altered blood flow interplay to bring about dystrophic mineralization with deposition of reparative dentin in coronal and radicular portions of the tooth. It is established that such changes beginning at the periapex influence the odontoblasts in the formed teeth and Hertwig's Epithelial Root Sheath (HERS) in the developing teeth. Such changes, especially when accompanied with a history of previous trauma contribute to the mechanism of loss of pulp vitality after orthodontic movement.

iii. Neural Response of the Pulp

Neural response during orthodontic tooth movement has also been evaluated. A few authors examined pulp axon response to orthodontic tooth movement and observed no significant change in teeth treated with conservative orthodontic treatment. Calcitonin gene-related peptide (CGP), a neuropeptide released from C-type nerve fibers of pulp after injury, has the ability to initiate vasodilatation along with regulating inflammatory cells (macrophages, mast cells and lymphocytes). CGP has been shown to increase in teeth under orthodontic force as compared to normal neuropeptide values.

The decrease in the neural mediators causes a decreased sensation of pain. The partial to complete diminution of the pulp space may be evident on radiographs. A distinguishing feature is that such obliterations affect the apical third first followed by the coronal aspects of the canal. Any case presenting with altered sensation must be considered a manifestation of postorthodontic pulpal damage. The healing in such cases is believed to be normal. Orthodontic movement may not hinder periapical healing, but it certainly delays the process.

Clinical Management

- *After orthodontic treatment*: The resorption after orthodontic treatment may cause an insufficiency of the apical dentin matrix, which often leads to overfill. It is advocated to shorten the working length in such cases. The idea is to detect the most apical radio-dense point on the radiograph, which is usually 1.5–2.0 mm short of the apical end.
- *During orthodontic treatment*: Electrical pulp testing may not be possible due to placement of orthodontic bands. The electric pulp tester may also lead to inaccurate readings because of edema and local vascular damage. Also, the radiolucency due to orthodontic movement may often be confused with radiolucency of pulpal origin confounding the diagnosis. Isolation is also difficult in such cases as rubber dam placement becomes difficult. Calcifications, which may occur due to orthodontic treatment also make endodontic treatment challenging. In anterior teeth, the lingual brackets may force the endodontist to change the position of the access opening from the lingual to the incisal.

b. Orthodontic Force and Root Resorption

Root resorption due to application of orthodontic force on teeth is not uncommon. Resorption is generally described to be of three types: Surface resorption (occurring on cemental surfaces), inflammatory resorption (resorption reaches infected dentin and an inflammatory reaction follows) or replacement resorption (where part of resorbed area is replaced by bone causing ankylosis). Orthodontic forces cause surface or inflammatory resorption and rarely the replacement resorption. Apical resorption is four times

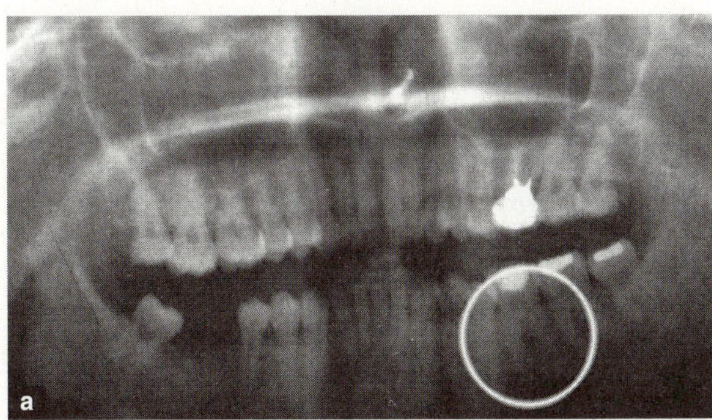

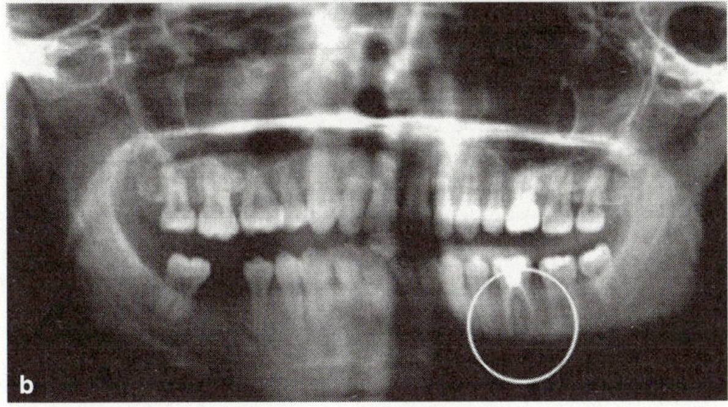

Fig. 35.1 Root resorption in mandibular first molar after Orthodontic treatment: (a) Preoperative (encircle); (b) Root canal treated (encircle)

more common than lateral resorption (Fig. 35.1a and b). This may be attributed to the use of excessive forces especially in case of extreme proclination. The incidence is increased further in the presence of existing defects like blunt rooted teeth and invaginations. It is established that adults are more prone to resorption because periodontal membrane becomes less vascularized and inflexible leading to difficulty in tooth movement with aging.

Mechanism

It is hypothesized that the pulp is responsible for resorptive changes as an after-effect of orthodontic treatment. The sympathetic neurons of the pulp (both Aδ and C fibers) release intraaxonal compounds like substance P, calcitonin, gene related peptide, neurokinin A, etc., which are neurogenic vasodilators that increase the blood supply of the pulp. The increased blood supply as caused by these mediators enhances the availability of osteoclast precursors, which are responsible for the resorption of roots.

Recently, specific genetic variables, IL-1β and 1L-1α have shown predisposition to root resorption, after orthodontic tooth movement. Root resorption in root filled teeth is significantly related to various intermediary genetic variations to inflammatory response.

A few authors studied predisposed factors associated with orthodontic tooth movement. They observed that increased age and prolonged pressure had significant effect on root resorption; whereas, morphology of roots and sex were not associated factors. CBCT evaluation also could not find any statistically significant difference in root resorption between root-filled and vital teeth.

Cervical root resorption, a destructive form of external resorption, characterized by osteoclastic cells adjacent to dentin, was also evaluated as an effect of orthodontic tooth movement. Authors were of view that orthodontic treatment was the most frequent predisposing factor in the development of cervical resorption (trauma and intracoronal bleaching are the other causes).

Routine periapical radiographs are generally effective in diagnosis of root resorption. CBCT, however, enables more accurate view of root resorption than traditional radiographs. CBCT provides even minute details of resorption without any distortion. Axial guided navigation, used to measure the axial length of teeth (from cups/incisal tip to root apex), has also been used to evaluate apical resorption.

c. Orthodontic Tooth Movement and Periapical Lesions

It is established that orthodontic tooth movement does not affect pathogenic and virulence of microbial biofilm and chronic inflammatory periapical lesions. The orthodontic forces can be applied 2–4 weeks later after completion of endodontic treatment (exudate and inflammatory leakage is absorbed within 2–4 weeks).

In case of teeth with apical periodontitis, the periapical environment is changed, having higher bacterial concentration and inflammatory bony changes. The existence of these factors may complicate healing process during orthodontic tooth movement. A few authors opined that orthodontic movement may delay the healing; however, did not prevent healing.

A few studies have evaluated the effect of orthodontic tooth movement on teeth subjected to periapical endodontic surgery. It is suggested that more apical resorption may develop as dentin is exposed at the apex coupled with irritation of root-end filling material (inflammation and leakage from the root end).

It has been established that persistence/partial regression of periapical lesions as a result of endodontic treatment is independent from orthodontic movement. Orthodontic movement is not a cause for endodontic failures.

d. Endodontic Surgery and Orthodontic Forces

The literature is deficient as regard orthodontic behavior of teeth after endodontic surgery. A healing period of three months to six months is recommended before attempting any forces on an endodontically treated tooth. Three months of healing period must be kept as a safety margin even for non-surgical cases with periapical radiolucency before attempting orthodontics.

ORTHODONTIC EXTRUSION (FORCED ORTHODONTIC ERUPTION)

Certain clinical situations may warrant forced orthodontic eruption of the affected tooth, such as caries causing loss of crown, resorption near alveolar crest, infrabony periodontal defects, etc.

Usually crown lengthening procedures utilizing periodontal surgery are followed to get access to tooth structure submerged under the gingival tissue. Orthodontic extrusion in such situations offers advantages as:

- No unnecessary bone cutting to maintain alveolar crest morphology
- Extrusion forces do not cause resorption (in fact they cause deposition)
- Eliminates periodontal defects without periodontal surgery
- Esthetically better than surgical intervention.

Guidelines

The following guidelines must be kept in mind for the health of periodontium and endodontium during orthodontic extrusion.

a. Periodontal Guidelines

The periodontal guidelines are:

i. ***Biological width***: The biological width (combined width of the connective tissue and junctional epithelium) should be taken care of during orthodontic extrusion. The crest of alveolar bone to cementoenamel junction is about 1.07 mm and to junctional epithelial attachment is about 0.71–1.35 mm. Thus additional 1.0–2.0 mm of sound tooth structure must be available coronal to the epithelial attachment. Distance from the alveolar crest to the coronal extent of remaining tooth structure should be minimum of 3.5–4.0 mm.

ii. ***Health of periodontal tissues***: Periodontal tissues must be maintained in a state of health. The entire periodontal apparatus moves alongside the tooth being extruded. In periodontal disease, the forces so exerted may cause deepening of the periodontal defect. Thus both, the biological width and the integrity of the periodontal apparatus, should be maintained.

b. Endodontic Guidelines

The endodontic guidelines are:

- The endodontic therapy is initiated in the beginning.
- During orthodontic movement, the canal is kept clean and temporarily sealed.
- The obturation may be delayed till orthodontic phase is over.
  (There is no contraindication to completion of treatment, except that the operator is at ease if the orthodontic appliances are not interfering).
- In case the root is filled with silver points or even in routine retreatment, the orthodontic extrusion is recommended first, followed by removal of silver points/gutta-percha (retreatment will be convenient).

c. Orthodontic Guidelines

The orthodontic guidelines are:

- Orthodontic movement should be initiated only in case of good periodontal health.
- Adequate anchorage must be considered (presence of two teeth on each side of tooth to be extruded) (Fig. 35.2b).
- Extrusion of anterior teeth is acceptable as it brings the conical portion of the root near the cemento-enamel junction of adjacent teeth. Thus, interdental environment is improved if root proximity is originally present (Fig. 35.2a).

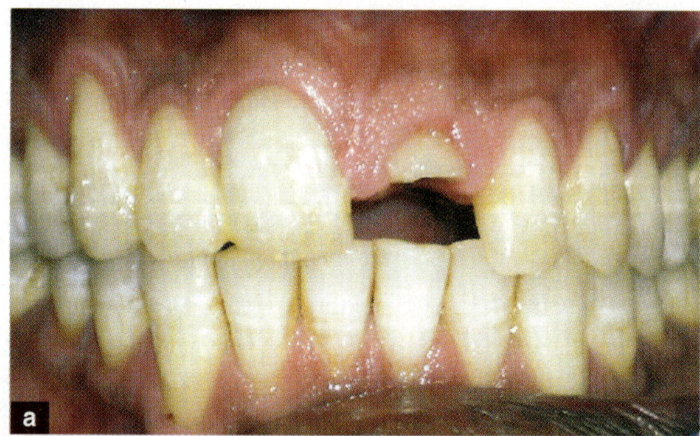

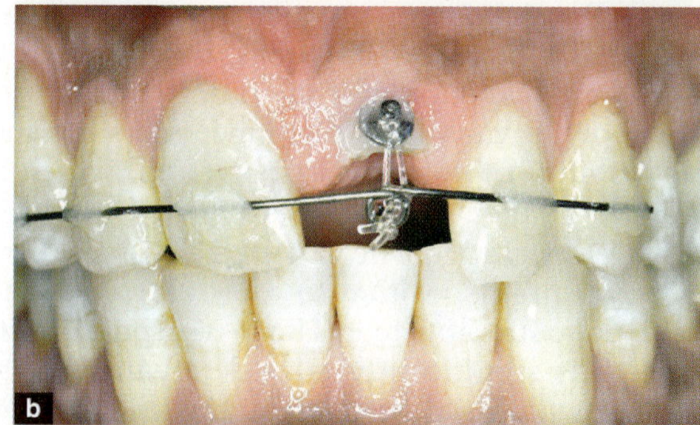

Fig. 35.2 Orthodontic extrusion: (a) Fractured central incisor; (b) Orthodontic extrusion (adequate anchorage from adjacent teeth)

- Extrusion of posterior teeth is not recommended as their access to forced extrusion is less and secondly, it brings the furcation close to the cementoenamel junction of the adjacent teeth. Thus, the chances of a furcation exposure increase. The problems of root proximity also increase especially in case of disto-buccal root of upper first molar and the mesiobuccal root of upper second molar.
- Prefer conventional fixed appliances. Removable appliances may offer greater anchorage, but are dependent on patient compliance and also do not stabilize the tooth after extrusion.
- Problems like accelerated mesial drift and unfavorable tipping must be corrected first.
- Adequate retention phase to prevent relapse (8–12 weeks with sign of apical bone fill).

Clinical Protocol

There is usually a time gap between the movement of the tooth and the movement of the attachment apparatus with it. The healthy attachment apparatus may move along with the tooth. Light force also reduces this gap time and the movement is nearly simultaneous. In case of heavy force, the attachment apparatus does not get adequate time for a simultaneous movement and only the tooth structure gets exposed.

Clinical protocol for forced extrusion depends upon whether the clinical crown is intact or not.

i. Tooth Lacking a Clinical Crown (Only Root)

An appropriate stainless steel wire with loop extension is cemented in the postspace. Semipermanent cement is used as this does not dislodge on pulling but does dislodge on rotation. The brackets are bonded to adjacent teeth. This is carried out as incisally as possible to increase distance between arch wire and loop. The arch wire must lie passively. Extrusion may take 4–6 weeks. After stabilization for 8–12 weeks, the root is restored with appropriate post and core restoration.

ii. Tooth with Intact Crown Portion

Place bracket as apical as possible on the tooth to be extruded and rest of the bonding procedures are followed as previously described. As the tooth approaches during extrusion, a flexible wire deflected 2.0–3.0 mm is used, which gives an extrusive force. The extruded tooth is stabilized for 8–12 weeks before permanent restoration.

Situations where Orthodontics Requires Endodontic Intervention for Better Results

The orthodontists do not sacrifice a key tooth as a part of the treatment plan. If such a tooth is pulpally involved, then a root canal treatment is the only way to achieve the treatment plan as originally intended. It is an essential prerequisite for an orthodontic treatment that all teeth be disease-free and endodontics plays a key role in achieving this requirement. Any tooth, which is marred by resorption before orthodontic treatment (resorption will be accentuated by the orthodontic forces), should be managed endodontically.

Orthodontic Behavior of Endodontically Treated Teeth

The entire orthodontic–endodontic continuum is based on the interaction of the endodontically treated tooth with the force applied by appliances. It has been questioned whether the endodontically treated teeth behave differently than those teeth, which have not undergone any such treatment.

It is hypothesized that an endodontically treated tooth (the neuropeptide influence is minimal) exhibits less resorption as the factors causing resorption are missing.

A few authors are of view that even though the teeth show the same movement but more resorption occurs in endodontically treated teeth.

It is established that endodontic treatment does not influence tooth movement. However, a fresh endodontically treated tooth in which the operator has inadvertently irritated the periapical tissues (slight overfill), can lead to complications. Such overfills can cause focal ankylosis which makes orthodontic movement very difficult. It is recommended that such teeth that need endodontic intervention during orthodontic treatment phase should be prepared and filled with calcium hydroxide initially and obturated only after the orthodontic movement is complete.

Fate of the Root Filling in Case of Resorption

The literature is deficient on the fate of the root fillings, once resorption sets in. The root filling may exfoliate along with the tooth; otherwise, it may be left behind in the bone after the tooth exfoliates and become encapsulated. The apical seal may or may not be lost by resorption depending on the nature of condensation of gutta-percha.

BIBLIOGRAPHY

1. Abuabara A. Biomechanical aspects of external root resorption in orthodontic therapy. Med. Oral Patol. Oral Cir. Bucal.: 2007; 12: E610–613.
2. Alomari FA, Al-Habahbeh R and Alsakarna BK. Responses to pulp sensibility tests during orthodontic therapy. Angle Orthod.: 2009; 79:166–171.

3. Aydin H and Er K. The effect of orthodontic tooth movement on endodontically treated teeth. J. Rest. Dent.: 2016; 4:31–41.
4. Beck VJ, Stacknik S, Chandler NP and Farella M. Orthodontic tooth movement of traumatized or root-canal-treated teeth: A clinical review. Nz. Dent. J.: 2013; 109:6–11.
5. Castro IO, Alencar AH, Valladares-Neto J and Estrela C. Apical root resorption due to orthodontic treatment detected by cone beam computed tomography. Angle Orthod.: 2013; 83:196–203.
6. Cave SG, Freer TJ and Podlich HM. Pulp-test responses in orthodontic patients. Aust. Orthod. J.: 2002; 18:27–34.
7. Caviedes-Bucheli J, Munoz HR, Azuero-Holguin MM and Ulate E. Neuropeptides in dental pulp: The silent protagonists. J. Endod.: 2008; 34:773–788.
8. Deepa D, Mehta DS, Puri VK and Shetty S. Combined periodontic–orthodontic–endodontic interdisciplinary approach in the treatment of periodontally compromised tooth. J. Ind. Soc. Periodontol.: 2010; 14:139–143.
9. Derringer KA and Linden RW. Vascular endothelial growth factor, fibroblast growth factor 2, platelet derived growth factor and transforming growth factor and transforming growth factor beta released in human dental pulp following orthodontic force. Arch. Oral Biol.: 2004; 49:631–641.
10. Durning P, Thomas M and McLaughlin W. Orthodontic extrusion: an interdisciplinary approach to patient management. Dent. Update: 2009; 36:212.
11. Esteves T, Ramos AL, Pereira CM and Hidalgo MM. Orthodontic root resorption of endodontically treated teeth. J. Endod.: 2007; 33:119–122.
12. Guevara MJ, McClugage SG and Clark JS. Response of the pulpal microvascular system to intrusive orthodontic forces. J. Dent. Res.: 1977; 56:243.
13. Hamilton RS and Gutmann JL. Endodontic–orthodontic relationships: A review of integrated treatment planning challenges. Int. Endod. J.: 1999; 32:343–360.
14. Ioannidou-Marathiotou I, Zafeiriadis AA and Papdopoulos MA. Root resorption of endodontically treated teeth following orthodontic treatment: A meta-analysis. Clin. Oral Investig.: 2013; 17:1733–1744.
15. Javed F, Al-Kheraif AA, Romanos EB and Romanos GE. Influence of orthodontic forces on human dental pulp: A systematic review. Arch. Oral Biol.: 2015; 60:347–356.
16. Lazzarett DN, Bortoluzzi GS, Torres Femandes LF, Rodriguez R, Grehs RA and Martins Hartmann MS. Histologic evaluation of human pulp tissue after orthodontic intrusion. J. Endod.: 2014; 40:1537–1540.
17. Popp TW, Artun J and Linge L. Pulpal response to orthodontic tooth movement in adolescents: A radiographic study. Am. J. Orthodont. Dentofacial Orthop: 1992; 101:228–233.
18. Sameshima GT and Sinclair PM. Predicting and preventing root resorption: Part I. Diagnostic factors. Am. J. Orthodont. Dentofacial Ortho.: 2001; 119:505–510.
19. Santamaria M Jr., Milagres D, Iyomasa MM, Stuani MB and Ruellas AC. Initial pulp changes during orthodontic movement: Histomorphological evaluation. Braz. Dent. J.: 2007; 18:34–39.
20. Veberiene R, Smailiene D, Baseviciene N, Toleikis A and Machiulskiene V. Change in dental pulp parameters in response to different modes of orthodontic force application. Angle Orthod.: 2010; 80:1018–1022.
21. von Bohl M, Ren Y, Fudalej PS and Kuijpers-Jagtman AM. Pulpal reactions to orthodontic force application in humans: A systematic review. J. Endod.: 2012; 38:1463–1469.
22. Walker SL, Tieu LD and Flores-Mir C. Radiographic comparison of the extent of orthodontically induced external apical root resorption in vital and root-filled teeth: A systematic review. Eur. J. Orthod.: 2013; 35:796–802.
23. Wang HL and Boyapati L. "PASS" principles for predictable bone regeneration. Implant Dent.: 2006; 15:8–17.

Chapter 36

Endodontic Failures and Retreatment

Endodontics undoubtedly is the most progressive branches of dentistry. The advancement in endodontic techniques and material has led to retaining significant number of teeth in older adults. Root canal treatment is effective in preventing and healing apical periodontitis with varying success. It is established that successful endodontics is based on the triad, i.e. correct diagnosis, adequate cleaning and shaping and three-dimensional obturation. The proper execution of these steps facilitates healing of the periapical lesion with the requisite osseous regeneration. Failure in root canal treatment is not uncommon. Root canal treatment usually fails when the standard protocol of 'triad' is not followed. Nevertheless, there are failures even after following the highest technical standards. Scientific evidences indicate that extraradicular and/or intraradicular infections, and intrinsic and/or extrinsic non-microbial factors are responsible for failure. A number of factors are considered responsible for the unsatisfactory outcome of well-treated cases. Regardless of the etiology, the main cause of failure is leakage and bacterial contamination. In a rough estimate, the percentage of success in endodontically treated teeth ranges from 10 to 50% globally.

Basis of Success

The definition of success has always been ambiguous. In endodontics, success implies clinical normalcy reinforced with normal radiographic and histopathological evidences. The percentage of success can vary if only clinical parameter is considered; histopathological and radiological parameters should also be recognized.

The goal of endodontic therapy is to heal the disease process and also prevent its recurrence. The treatment outcomes in reference to healing are:

i. *Healed*: Both the clinical and radiographic presentations are normal.

ii. *Healing*: Normal clinical presentation along with reducing radiolucency.

iii. *Diseased*: Radiolucency has emerged or persisted without change even when the clinical presentation is normal or clinical signs/symptoms are present even if the radiolucency is decreased.

The patient's perception of success is relief from acute symptoms, resolution of swelling or absence of pain and tenderness.

Basis of Failure

Failures can be classified as established failure and potential failure.

a. ***Established failure***: The failure is considered as 'established' when the patient and the operator are convinced of the clinical presentation, complaint and also the radiological assessment of the treated tooth.

b. ***Potential failure***: The failure is considered as 'potential' when one of the two (i.e. patient or the operator) is not convinced of the clinical and radiological assessments of the treated tooth.

The clinical and radiological features of established and potential failures are tabulated in Table 36.1.

Causes of Failure

The causes of endodontic failures are multifactorial; broadly classified as follows:

1. Biological factors
   a. Persistent intraradicular infection
   The intraradicular infection may persist because of: (i) Poor aseptic environment; (ii) use of incorrect irrigant/improper irrigation; (iii) inability to prepare till working length (Fig. 36.1a and b); (iv) missed canal(s)/hidden canal(s) (Fig. 36.2a and b); (v) procedural errors (Fig. 36.3a and b); (vi) poor obturation (Fig. 36.4a and b); (vii) coronal leakage; poor coronal filling (Fig. 36.5a and b); (viii) resistant microorganisms in the root canal intricacies
   b. Persistent extraradicular infection
2. Cystic lesions
3. Root fracture(s)
4. Incorrect diagnosis
5. Foreign body reaction
6. Neuropathic problem.

Table 36.1 Clinical and radiological features of failures

Types of failure	*Clinical features*	*Radiological features*
Potential failure	• Sporadic or vague symptoms, usually not reproducible. • Feeling of pressure or tightness. • Slight discomfort when chewing or pressing on tooth with finger or tongue. • Overlapping symptoms of sinusitis in the region of the treated teeth. • Occasional need of analgesics to alleviate discomfort.	• No change in periapical radiolucency or slight evidence of healing. • The periodontal ligament is not normal. • Evident space between filling and root canal walls. • Filling material/cement extending beyond the anatomic apex.
Established failure	• Persistent symptoms. • Recurrent sinus tract, swelling or pain. • Pain on percussion. • Unable to chew with the tooth. • Pain during functional movements.	• The periapical radiolucency has not changed or has enlarged. • The appearance of new periapical or lateral radiolucency. • Absence of formation of new lamina dura. • Evident space in the root canal that was not filled. • Excessive overfilling. • Evidence of progressive resorption.

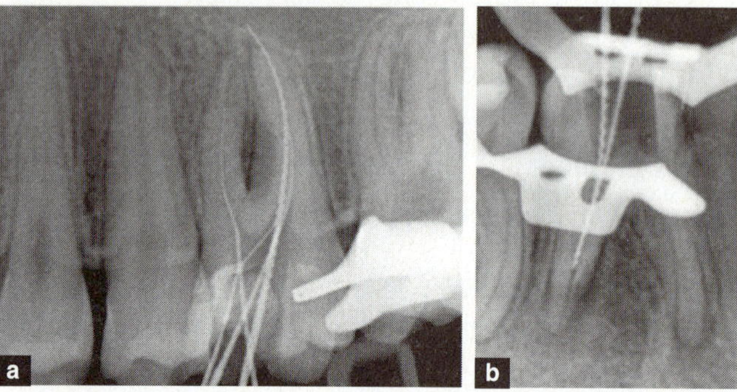

Fig. 36.1 Working length problem: (a) Short working length in mesial canal; (b) Improper working length

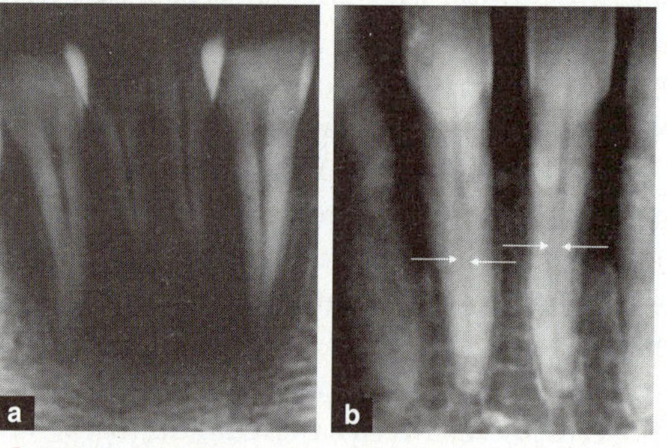

Fig. 36.2 Missed canals: (a) Missed canal in mandibular incisors; (b) Two root canals evident (arrows)

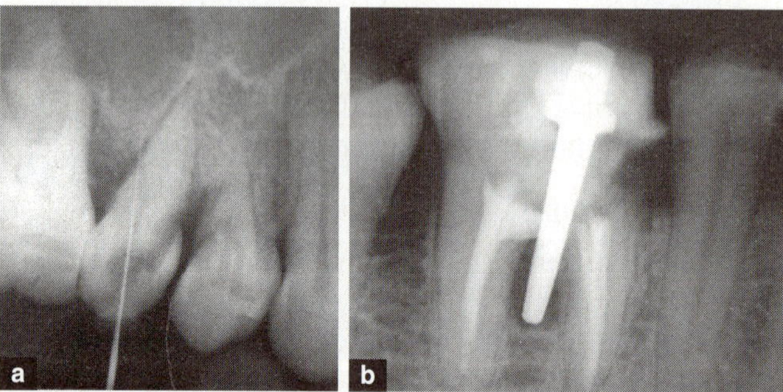

Fig. 36.3 Procedural errors: (a) Perforation during root canal preparation; (b) Perforation during postspace preparation

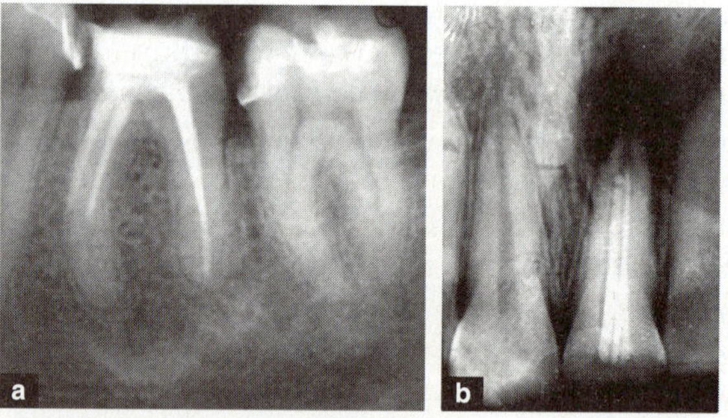

Fig. 36.4 Poor obturation: (a) Incomplete obturation (molar); (b) Poor condensation (incisor)

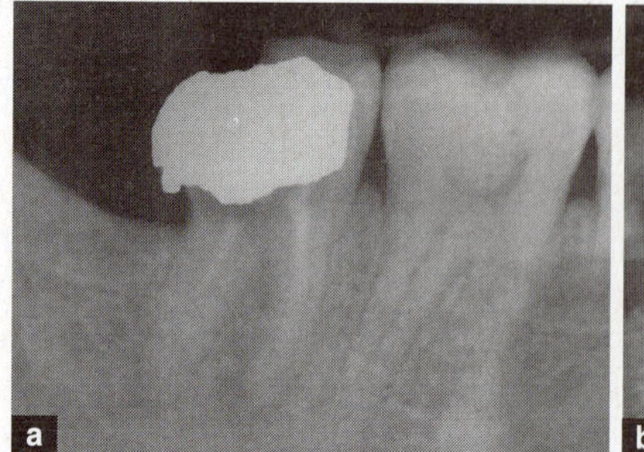

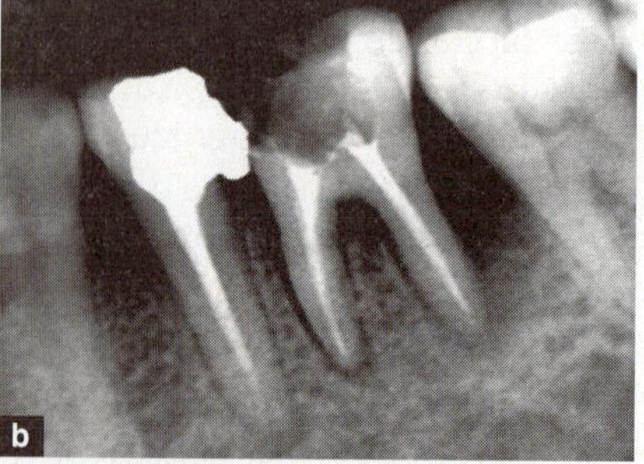

Fig. 36.5 Poor coronal restoration: (a) Leaky filling; (b) No coronal restoration since long

NONSURGICAL RETREATMENT

Retreatment in endodontics implies that procedures carried out on teeth that demonstrate incomplete endodontic treatment (showing signs of failure), to achieve successful results. Since, the causes of failure are summed up as leakage and bacterial contamination, the retreatment procedures are aimed at correcting the leakage and subsequently the bacterial contamination.

In order to control infection and its source, the root canals need to be reprepared and retreated. The process of renegotiating the canals can be carried out using either orthograde (nonsurgical retreatment) or a retrograde (surgical retreatment) methods. In a few cases, any of these methods are not feasible and the tooth is considered for extraction.

Surgical retreatment is preferred in cases of failure of nonsurgical methods, where root resection is indicated or the removal of post warrants fracture of root. Mostly nonsurgical retreatment procedures are carried out to overcome failures in root canal treatment.

Indications

The indications of nonsurgical retreatment are:

- Poorly sealed canals with a possibility to improve upon the quality of the previous instrumentation and obturation.
- Conventional root canal treatment failed; reasons conspicuous to the operator, where surgical intervention not required.

Contraindication

The conditions, which contraindicate nonsurgical retreatment are:

- Canal walls prone to perforation on further preparation due to thinness.
- Inability to débride the root canal system due to:
  - Failure in removal of post or broken instrument.
  - Sclerotic root canal, which cannot be negotiated.
- Root fracture, especially vertical fractures.
- Non-cooperative patient.

Objectives of Retreatment

The objectives of retreatment are the same as for the primary treatment of infected root canal system; to eliminate the substrate harboring microorganisms and hermetically sealing the space with biocompatible filling material. In retreatment cases, the operator may face root canals obstructed by posts, insoluble filling materials or separated instruments. Furthermore, during the previous treatment, a variety of procedural errors such as canal blockage, ledging, apical transportation and root perforation might have occurred. The rationale for retreatment is based on sound biological objectives of elimination and future exclusion of microorganisms from the root canal system, facilitating conducive environment for healing.

Treatment Planning

Patient's thorough history, clinical examination along with radiographs and other diagnostic tests should be performed to rule out non-odontogenic etiology. Inspection should always be carried out under dry condition, good illumination and magnification, which allows the clinician to identify significant conditions invisible to the naked eye, e.g. fracture, marginal leakage, etc. Dyes can also be a useful aid in diagnosing fracture lines, caries, marginal defects, etc.

Percussion test evaluates the status of periodontal tissues of previously root canal treated teeth. The electric pulp testing is usually of lesser value in root canal treated teeth. The positive result means that there may be remaining pulp tissue, but the negative result may not be correct for absence of pulp tissues. Such teeth, especially, if restored with full crowns, pose difficulties in evaluating status of pulp.

Intraoral periapical radiographs should be taken from various angulations; at least two radiographs, one conventional and the other one at mesial/distal angulation. The proximal caries and periodontal bone height can be evaluated using bite-wing radiographs. The origin and path of sinus tract is traced by inserting a suitable size gutta-percha point and getting a radiograph.

On the basis of clinical and radiological examination, a failure case can be categorized as a 'potential' or 'established' failure. For potential failure, the quality of the restoration and root canal obturation should be evaluated. If it is satisfactory, then it is better to wait and watch. If only coronal restoration looks compromised, then it is better to restore the coronal restoration; however, when the obturation is compromised and there is only a potential threat, one should wait and watch. When the failure is established, the access opening, without adversely affecting the tooth structure, should be carried out nonsurgically. In doubtful cases, resinifying therapy is the treatment of choice; however, non-accessible cases are preferably retreated with surgical means.

Patient's consent is extremely important in planning retreatment. Since, retreatment would involve a fair amount of time and expenses, the patient should be informed of the perceived prognosis and also other options, including extraction, etc.

The protocol for management of failure of root canal treatment is depicted in Flowchart 36.1.

Flowchart 36.1 Protocol for management of failure of root canal treatment

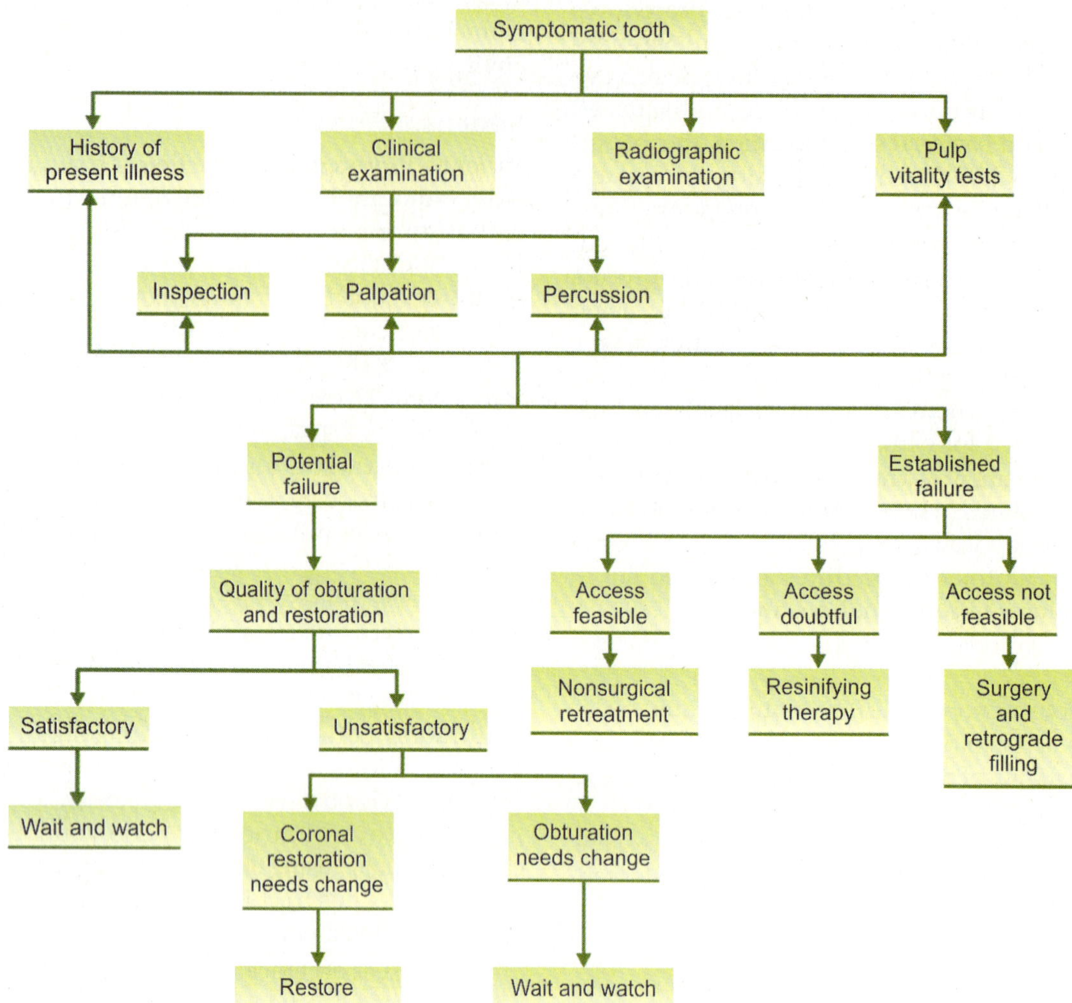

MANAGEMENT OF ENDODONTIC FAILURES

The features leading to endodontic failures and methods of retreatment are as follows.

1. Coronal Leakage

It has been established that poor coronal seal, even when the obturation is of good quality, affects the success of root canal treatment. The compromised coronal seal allows oral microorganism to invade the root canal system; subsequently, the failures. Both microorganisms and their endotoxins are capable to penetrate the obturated root canal; endotoxins may penetrate faster than microorganisms due to their smaller size. It has been hypothesized that *'hanging gutta-percha'* in the coronal aspect is one of the major cause of coronal leakage. It is important to restore the tooth with definite restorative material after removing the *'hanging gutta-percha'* points from the coronal chamber (Fig. 36.6a and b). When coronal leakage is the cause of failure, only rerestoration and/or revision of root canal treatment followed by coronal restoration (Fig. 36.6c) is the treatment of choice. Rerestoration of coronal filling should be avoided in chronic cases (where leakage continued for a sufficient long-time).

2. Inadequate Root Canal Treatment

Once the retreatment is planned, the first step is to identify the type of filling material present in the root canal(s) and also the anatomical variations. The method used to remove the root canal filling will depend on the type of material, the longevity of the treatment and the existing coronal restoration.

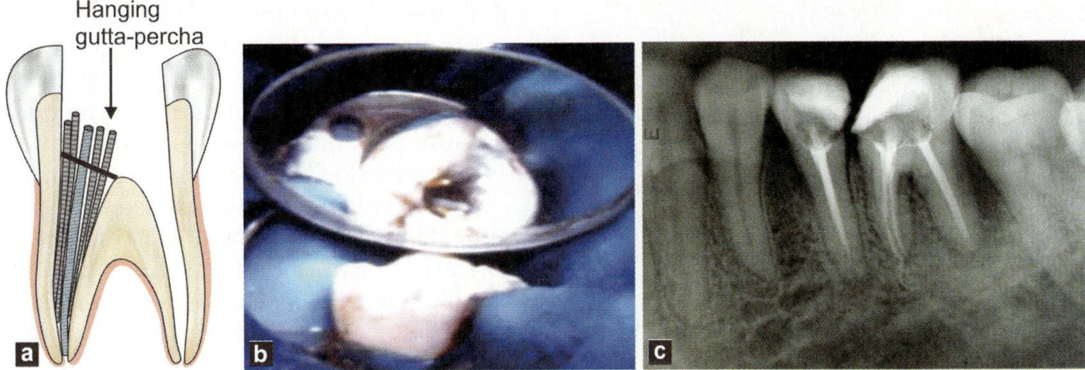

Fig. 36.6 Coronal leakage: (a) Hanging gutta-percha (diagrammatic); (b) Hanging gutta-percha (clinical); (c) Poor coronal restoration

a. Gaining Access through the Coronal Restoration

The coronal restorations, except for full crowns, is to be removed completely before starting the reaccess preparation. The coronal silver amalgam or cements, if not removed completely, can create problems in executing retreatment procedures (Fig. 36.7).

In case of well-fitting crown, which fulfills form, function and esthetics, the access can be gained through the crown (Fig. 36.8).

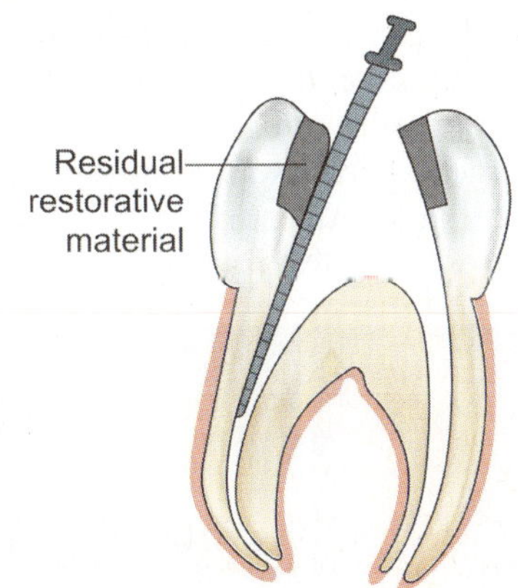

Fig. 36.7 Removal of coronal filling

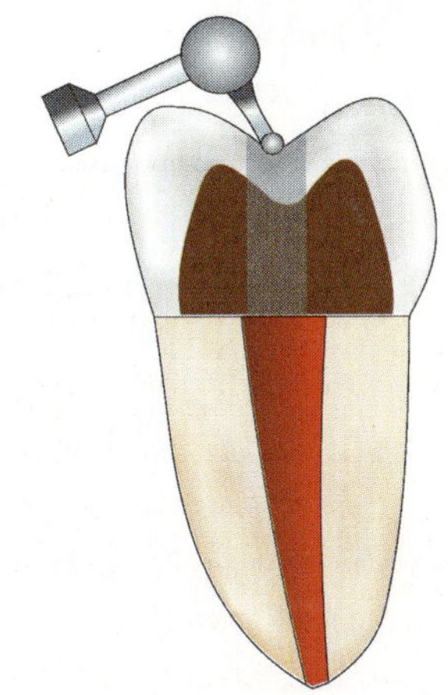

Fig. 36.8 Gaining access through crown

When the access is gained through the coronal restoration, care should be taken as the guidelines provided by the natural tooth are missing. Diamond points are usually preferred for access preparation in porcelain crowns (PFM or all-porcelain), while carbide burs are used for composite, amalgam alloy and the cast metal restorations. The size and shape of access opening should be such that the endodontic instruments should not scrape the cavity walls during instrumentation as it may shave off metal chips that might irreversibly block the canals, particularly in mandibular teeth. Use of copious irrigation during access preparation reduces the chances of microfractures and blockage of canal system by the remnants of these materials.

Advantages of retaining the restoration

The advantages of retaining the existing crown are that the isolation becomes easy, esthetics is not compromised and the occlusion is not disturbed. Retaining crown is also cost-effective.

Disadvantage of retaining the restoration

The disadvantages of retaining the crown are that it limits the visibility; subsequently, increasing the chances of iatrogenic mishaps. The decreased visibility also increases the chances of missing secondary caries, fracture lines, hidden canals, etc.

b. Gaining Access after Removal of Crown/and Bridges

The full veneer crowns usually make the retreatment difficult. Several techniques and methods are available, which facilitates easy and safe removal of such crowns. The removal of coronal restoration is known as 'coronal disassembly'.

Advantages

- Coronal disassembly allows better access to the actual axis of the tooth and the remaining coronal structure allows excavation of recurrent/hidden caries.
- Minor cracks and missed/additional canals can be negotiated easily.

Removal of Crown and Bridges

The restoration (crown and bridge or crown) is to be removed cautiously, not to fracture the teeth and/or the restoration. An effort is made to cement the same restoration after retreating the tooth. In case it is difficult to remove the restoration in one-piece without any damage, it is wise to cut the restoration in two or three pieces and removed. The safe removal of the restoration is important.

Safe removal depends upon many factors; such as the restorative material (porcelain crowns are difficult to remove than metal ones; porcelain fracture easily, especially at the margin), type of cement used during cementation (resin cement and glass-ionomer cements pose problem than zinc oxide and zinc phosphate cement). Experience of operator also affects safe removal of the crowns.

A variety of removal devices are available depending upon the principle on which they are based. Ultrasonics is useful to loosen the cement around the margins of a crown. Undermining the crown and opening up the margins allows placement of crown remover.

The routinely used devices are:

i. *Grasping instruments*: The instruments facilitate grasping of the restoration from two sides. The application of pressure on the handle increases the grip of instrument on the restoration. The pressure on the handle is adjusted so as not to damage the restoration and to avoid the slippage. These are coated with carborundum powder to prevent slipping. The instruments with rubber cup on the beaks are also available. Examples are KY Pliers (GC America); Wynman Crown Gripper (Miltex Instrument Company); and Trident Crown placer remover (Trident Dental Inc.) (Fig. 36.9).

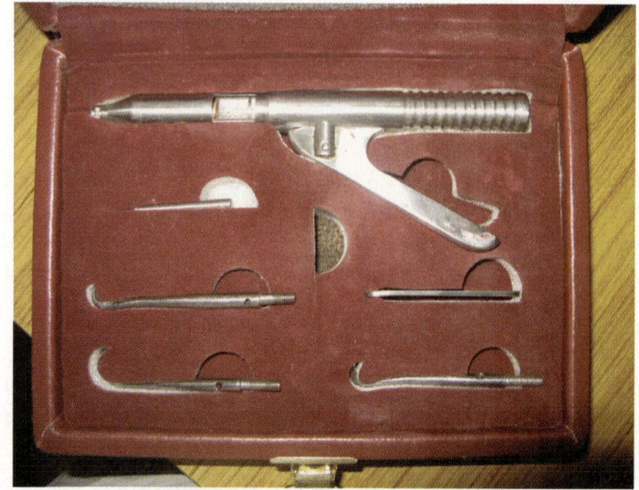

Fig. 36.9 Crown remover (conventional)

ii. *Percussive instruments*: These instruments apply percussive forces to the restoration, either directly or indirectly, in order to break the luting cement. However, this is an unpleasant technique, which may cause pain or fracture of crown and/or tooth. The SybronEndo Crown Splitter assists in safe and easy crown removal. Kavo Coronaflex works by delivering a pneumatic force. Pneumatic crown remover can be used with parachute technique (Fig. 36.10). Parachute technique uses metallic wires placed through two or more embrasures of the bridge in order to create loops acting as a rest for a metal rod. They are excellent device for removing intact restorations. Examples are Peerless Crown-a-Matic (Peerless International); and Coronaflex (Kavo, America).

iii. *Active instruments*: Active instruments work by first actively engaging the restoration to be dislodged and then applying the dislodging force. For actively engaging the restoration, these instruments need a small window, prepared on the restoration, which can later be restored. Examples are Metalift (Classic Practice Resources); Kline Crown Remover (Brasseler); Higa bridge Remover (Higa Manufacturing); and WamKey (Dentsply). For Metalift crown removal system, a tiny hole is created on occlusal surface of crown. A self-tapping instrument threads the metal on the occlusal surface, breaks the cement layer and subsequently loosening and removing the restoration. WamKeys need a small cut in the buccal or lingual surface of the crown and the crown is lifted using the appropriate keys (Fig. 36.11).

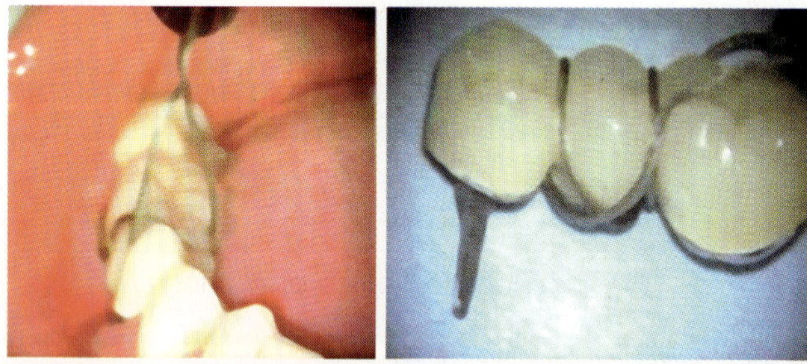

Fig. 36.10 Parachute technique

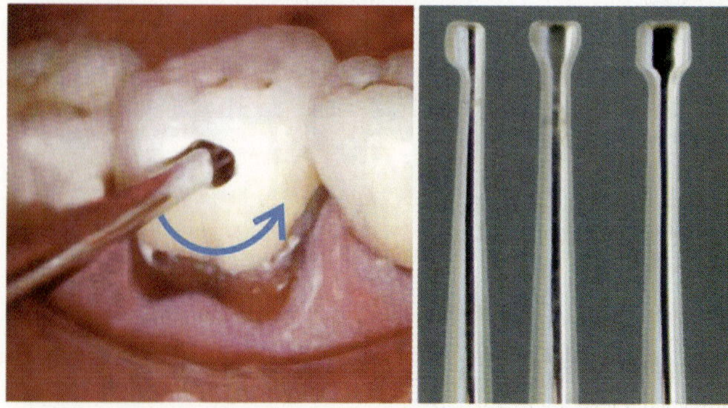

Fig. 36.11 WamKey system

Removal of Post and Cores

The removal of post in an endodontically treated teeth always present great difficulties because of risk of fracture/perforation of the root, especially when the remaining root dentin is less (Fig. 36.12a and b). However, with the recent technical advances, these sequelae have been minimized. The protocol of removal differs with the type of post and the material (whether metallic or fiber). The ultrasound and other mechanical post-removing devices, such as Post puller, Gonon post removal system, Masserann instrument, etc. have been tried to achieve postremoval.

The factors which influence removal of posts are:

- It is easier to remove tapering post than parallel. Similarly, passive post is easier to remove than active post.
- The resins cement and glass-ionomer cement, being more retentive, pose difficulty in removal than zinc phosphate cement and zinc oxide eugenol cement.
- It is easier to remove post when post's coronal end lies above the orifice of the root canal.
- Experience of the operator.

i. Removal of screw post

The screw post is removed using the wrench provided in the kit by the manufacturer (Fig. 36.13). Core material is carefully removed from around the coronal end of the post using a bur and ultrasonic tips. While removing the core, care should be taken not to damage the protruding head of the post in the pulp chamber.

Generally, the vibration created during drilling of core coupled with use of ultrasonic is sufficient to loosen the post. The ultrasonic tip is moved around the post in an anticlockwise direction to unscrew it. Ultrasonic vibrations need to be applied for sufficiently long-time to unscrew the post.

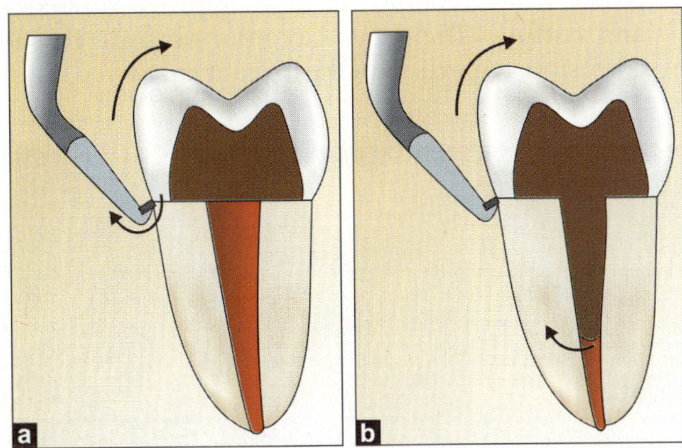

Fig. 36.12 Removal of post and core: (a) Removal of crown without post do not create stress in root; (b) Removal of crown with post creates stress (may lead to fracture of root)

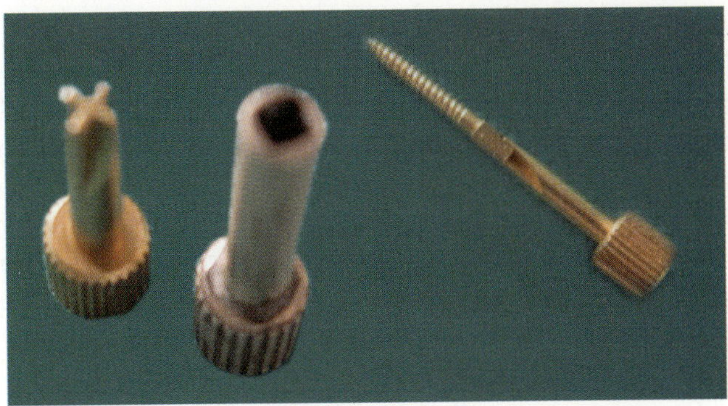

Fig. 36.13 Wrench for removing screw post

ii. Removal of fractured post

The post-fractured within the root canal pose difficulties in removal.

After getting excess to the post, the cement lute between the post and the root is to be broken. Ultrasonic vibrations along with certain devices (sword post puller, etc.) are used to loosen the post. Once the cement lute is separated, the post can be removed with the help of fine beaked forceps, e.g. Stieglitz forceps. When a post is broken deep inside the canal, the Masserann kit (Micro Mega) helps to remove post without damaging the root dentin.

The process of removal should be performed with great care to avoid undesirable complications, such as root fracture, canal perforation and extrusion of objects beyond root apex.

iii. Removal of fiber posts

The fiber posts are bonded to root dentin with bonding agents and are difficult to remove. It is hypothesized that in failed cases, coronal microleakage may disrupt the bond integrity facilitating removal of these posts.

Since fibers in fiber posts are tough materials and pose difficulty in removing, it is advised to use new removal drills. The fibers wear out the drills quickly and are susceptible to get separated inside the canal. Use of new removal drill is preferred in every case.

The sequence followed for removal of fiber posts is:

- The post is trimmed at the level of pulpal floor/canal orifice.
- A pilot drill is used to make a hole in the center of the post.
- The post is hollowed out by the successive drills available in the removal kits.
- The cement is softened using softening agents.
- The 'hollowed post' is screwed out, moving the appropriate peeso reamer/H-file, anticlockwise.
- The canal should be reprepared and reobturated before placing the new posts.

iv. Removal of core

It is difficult to remove cast cores as compared to composite and amalgam cores. A diamond point/ carbide bur can be used to remove core material. In certain cases, the core material is pushed 2.0 to 3.0 mm into the root canals. In such cases, after removing the coronal aspect of core material, an ultrasonic tip is used across the pulp floor and the coronal part of the root, removing the material slowly without risking perforation.

For cast post and core, attempt should be made to remove the post and core in one entity. If not possible, the core is separated, removed first and then the post can be loosened with the help of ultrasonics. The loosen post can be retrieved with the conventional gadgets.

Removal of Separated Instruments

The fracture of endodontic instruments (files, reamers, rotary instruments, pluggers, etc.) is quite common in clinical practice. The causes of fracture are:

- Improper handling
- Using instrument out of sequence
- Using excessive force, especially in rotary instrumentation
- Spending excessive time in root canal
- Lack of failure of inspection of the instrument prior to use
- Iatrogenic causes.

Factors affecting instrument removal

The factors, which favor easy removal of separated instruments are:

- Straighter the root canal easier the removal.
- Retrieval from coronal portion is easier than middle and apical portion of root canal. The separated instrument lying coronal to curvature is easier to remove than apical to curvature.
- Longer fragments are easier to remove.
- Hand instruments are easier to retrieve than rotary.
- Stainless steel instruments are easier to remove than Ni-Ti. Ni-Ti instruments may get straighten within a curvature in the root canal; posing difficulty in retrieval.

It is emphasized that all separated instruments need not be removed. The time and site of fracture are important. Time implies fracture of instrument prior to preparation, during preparation or after preparation of root canal. In case the instrument gets separated after the root canal preparation (during finishing stage), the same is left in the root canal, filling the rest of the root canal. The site implies fracture of instrument at coronal, middle or apical areas (Fig. 36.14a to c). Instrument fractured at apical area pose difficulties in removal; surgical interventions are only treatment of choice. In such cases, by-passing the fragmented instrument and engaging the same with other obturating material is preferred treatment modality.

There are three phases for removal of separated instruments.

i. In case the separated instrument is below orifice level, the coronal end of root canal is widened to get straight line access up to the coronal end of the separated instrument. The non-cutting tungsten carbide bur (Endo-Z) and diamond bur with non-cutting tip (LA Axxess) can be used to achieve the requisite straight line access (Fig. 36.15a to d).

ii. Once the separated instrument is visible, the ultrasonic energy is applied to the lateral surface of the fractured instrument to loosen the same. Ultrasonic energy is not applied at the coronal end. If the energy is applied to the coronal end, the instrument may get embedded deeper into the root canal. The ProUltra ENDO-3, 4, 5 ultrasonic tips are utilized for this purpose. Additionally, they are coated with zirconium nitride to improve durability and cutting efficiency. Zirconium nitride resists corrosion, regardless of the irrigant employed, does

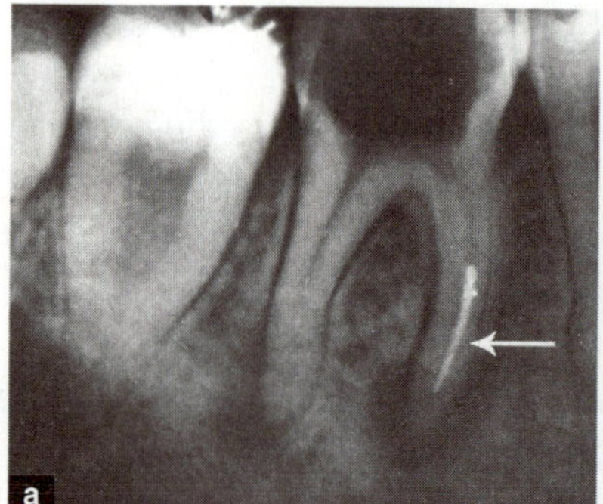

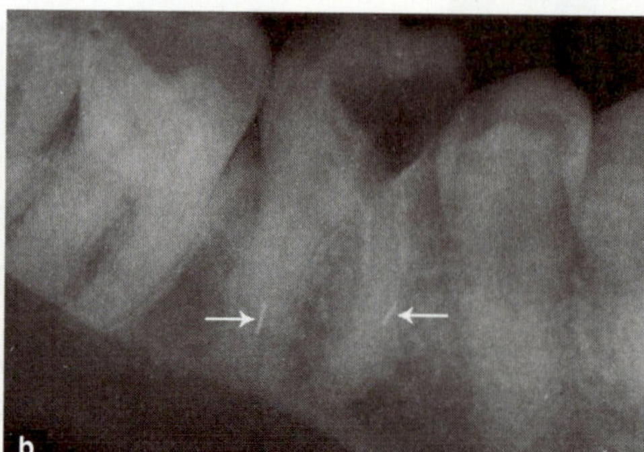

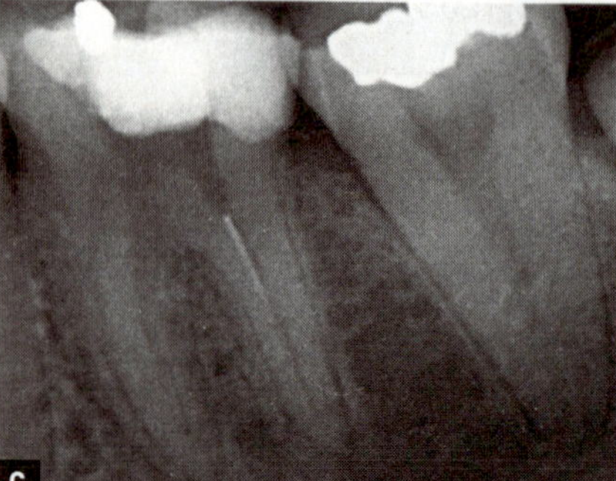

Fig. 36.14a to c Sites of separated instruments

36

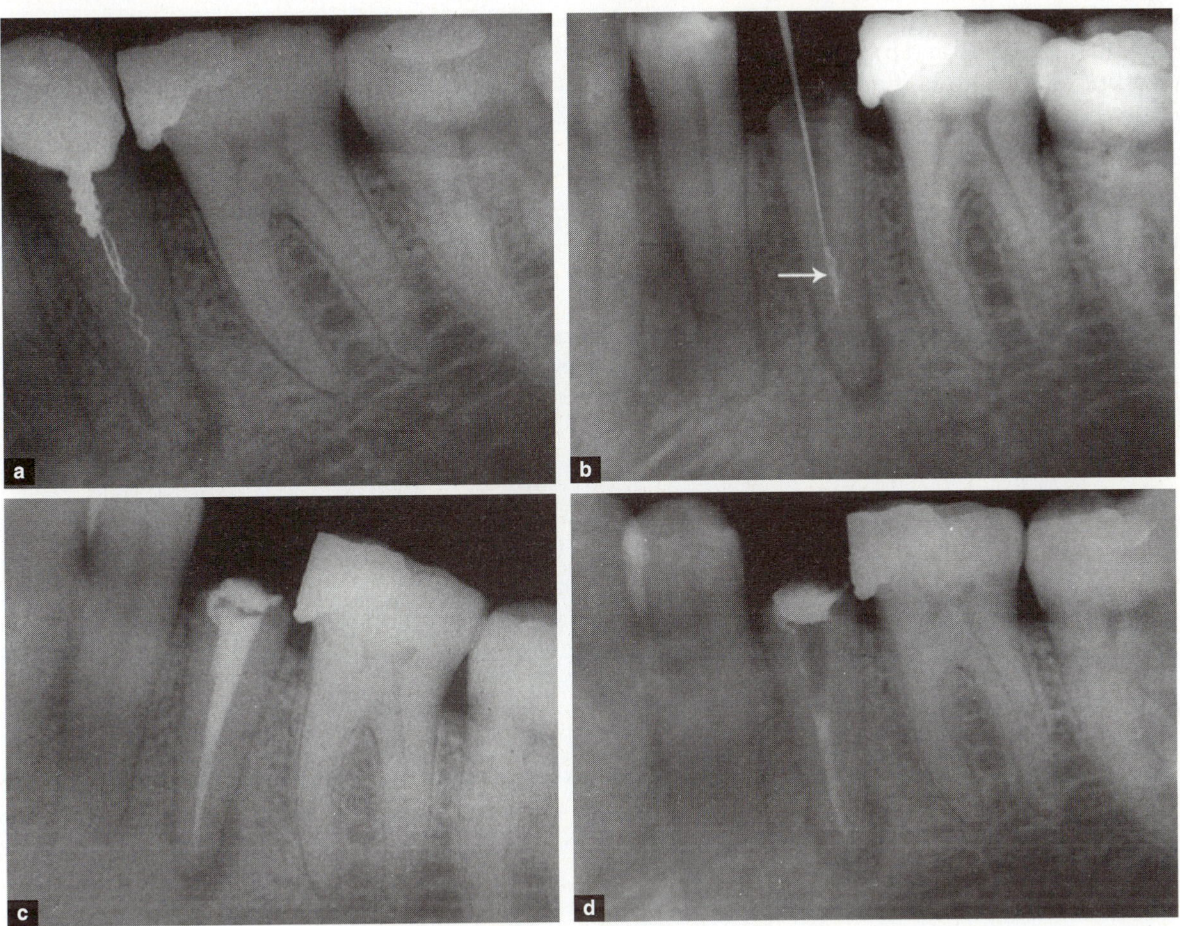

Fig. 36.15 Removal of separated instrument: (a) Preoperative (mandibular second premolar); (b) Separated instrument engaged and removed; (c) Root canal obturated; (d) Postspace preparation

not flake-off during use, and provides safety during intracanal procedures. The ENDO-6, 7 and 8 ultrasonic tips are made of titanium to provide clinicians with thinner diameters and longer lengths. These instruments are utilized in deeper spaces where access is more restrictive.

In case direct access is not feasible, by-passing the instrument is the treatment of choice. A drop of acid etch is trickled in the root canal where the instrument was broken. After a couple of minutes, by-passing the broken instrument is tried using small number file (Fig. 36.16). The residual acid etch

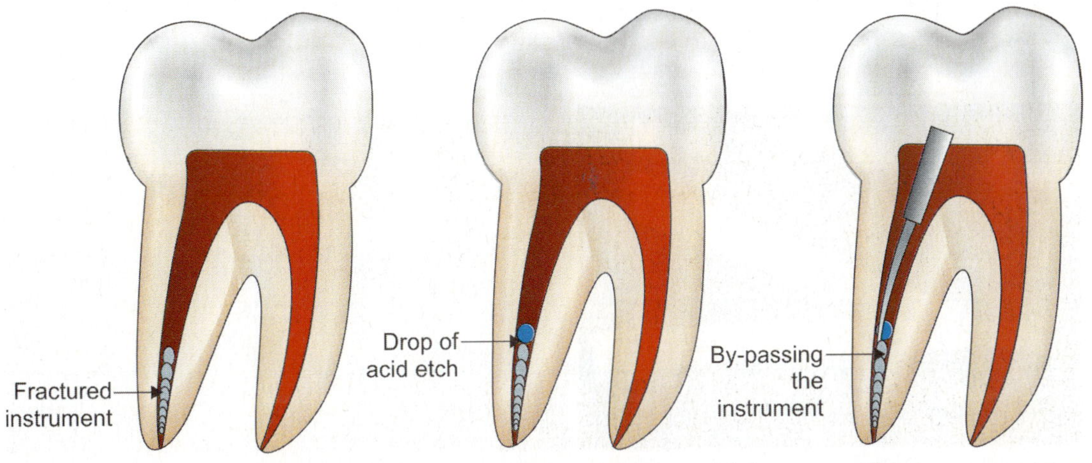

Fig. 36.16 By-passing the separated instrument (diagrammatic)

is washed out. The canal is prepared in routine and obturated (Fig. 36.17a and b). Alternatively, a small round bur is cut into half and reached up to the fractured site (Gary-Carr technique). It provides appropriate dentin for by-passing the fractured instrument (Fig. 36.18). The canal is prepared in routine and obturated.

iii. Another instrument (system) for removal of separated instruments has disposable tube to capture the separated file and lift it out. The disadvantage of these systems is that they require excessive removal of dentin for gaining direct access and engaging the separated instrument. The available systems are: Cancellier Extractor Kit, PRS System kit (Fig. 36.19a), Masserann kit, Spinal tap Needle, Endo extractor system (Fig. 36.19b), Meisinger Meitrac Instrument system, Instrument removal system, etc.

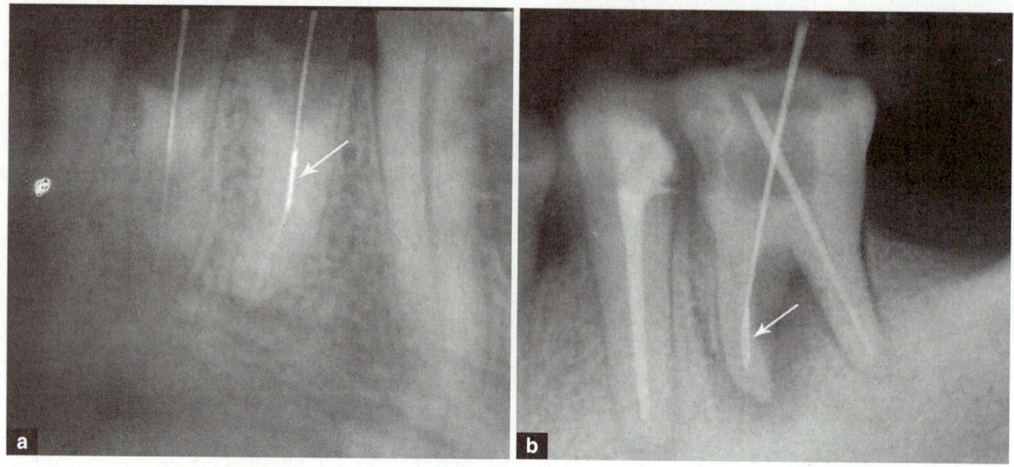

Fig. 36.17a and b By-passing the fractured instrument (arrow)

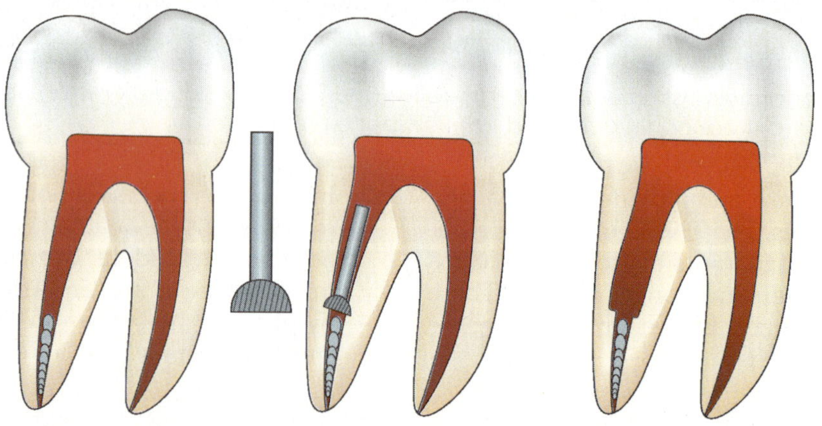

Fig. 36.18 Gary-Kerr technique

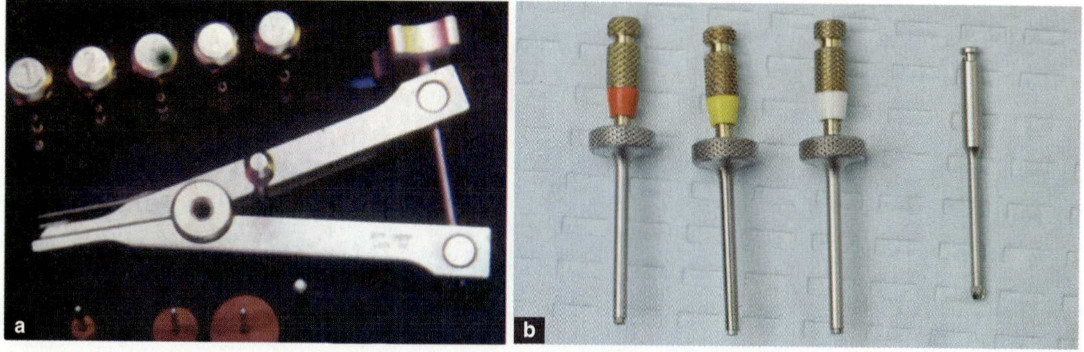

Fig. 36.19 Fractured instrument removal (kit): (a) PRS instrument removal system; (b) Endo extractor system

Instrument Removal System (IRS) is a two-component system, designed to mechanically engage separated instruments. Each microtube has a small-sized plastic handle to enhance vision during placement, a side window to improve mechanics, and a 45° beveled end to "scoop up" the coronal end of a broken instrument. Each screw wedge has a knurled metal handle, a left handed screw mechanism, and a solid cylinder that becomes tapered towards its distal end to facilitate engaging an instrument.

Removal of Obturating Materials

Various materials are being used, either alone or in combination, to obturate root canal. The complete removal of these materials may pose challenge in retreatment cases. The commonly used obturating materials and methods of their removal are:

i. *Removal of gutta-percha*

Gutta-percha has always been preferred as obturating material. In retreatment cases, removal of gutta-percha is comparatively easier than other obturating materials.

The methods employed for removing gutta-percha may differ according to obturating technique used.

- The single cone gutta-percha can be removed easily as the space around the gutta-percha cone is filled by the sealer. Similarly poorly condensed gutta-percha can be removed easily. A gap is created with an explorer and a suitable Hedstroem file is screwed into the space. A steady withdrawal force is exerted to remove the gutta-percha points. Gutta-percha is engaged on sides with a Hedstroem file and moving the file in pull-motion, gutta-percha is removed (Fig. 36.20). The endosonic file with irrigant can be used to break sealer layer. Heated instrument (plugger, file, etc.) can also be used to remove gutta-percha in pieces. Alternatively gutta-percha solvents can also be used (gutta-percha solvents should be used along with endodontic instrument). The over-extended gutta-percha points are difficult to retrieve as the gutta-percha extruded from the apical constriction tends to break from that point. A fine Hedstroem file is gently inserted extending 1.0–2.0 mm beyond the apical end of the root canal. The file is pulled gently retrieving the gutta-percha.
- When the gutta-percha is well-condensed, the mechanical means [gates glidden drills (No. 2 or 3)] are used to remove gutta-percha from coronal part. A rotary file of smaller size than the root canal is used to remove gutta-percha apical to the coronal area. Rotary files are also effective in generating heat, which further softens the gutta-percha. A heated instrument or heated plugger can also be used. The combination of solvent (xylene, eucalyptol, chloroform, methyl chloroform, halothane or rectified turpentine) and hedstroem file can then be used to remove the material from the remainder of the canals. In open apex cases, extra care must be taken to prevent the solvent or the softened gutta-percha from being forced out of apex. Chloroform is potential carcinogenic and mutagenic; however, it is unlikely that chloroform in small quantity (normally less than 1.0 ml) required in the endodontic retreatment would be hazardous. Specific gutta-percha removal instrument, as the GPX is also available. The C+ file (a stainless steel end-cutting hand file), with varying taper is effective to cut through well-condensed gutta-percha.

In curved root canals, there are increased chances of creating ledges, perforation and instrument fractures, etc. so extra care is exercised during removal of gutta-percha. Improper removal of gutta-percha and/or post-space preparation may lead to perforation (Fig. 36.21a and b).

ii. *Removal of carrier based obturating devices*

The carrier based obturating devices (e.g. Thermafil) usually consist of a metal or plastic carrier covered in alpha phase gutta-percha. The earlier Thermafil obturator had metallic carrier, which was later replaced by plastic carrier, facilitating easy retreatment. Once the carrier is exposed, the gutta-percha is removed slowly using H-file along the sides of carrier. Solvent

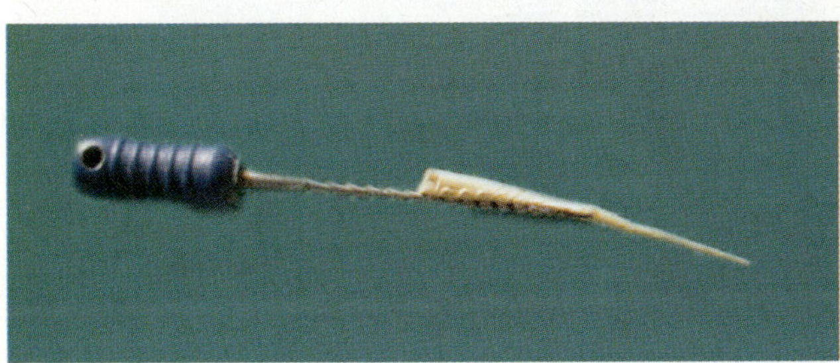

Fig. 36.20 Removal of gutta-percha with Hedstroem file

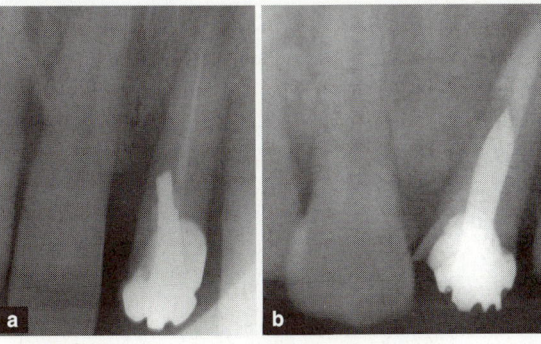

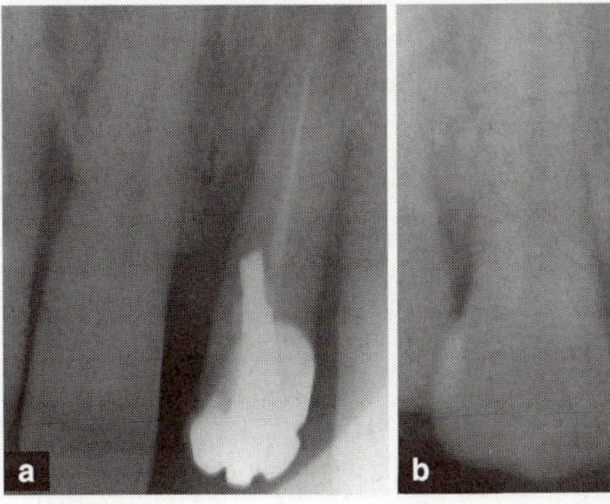

Fig. 36.21 Improper removal of gutta-percha: (a) Lateral perforation; (b) Labial perforation

can also be used along with H-file to facilitate softening and removal of gutta-percha. An appropriate file (usually 0.04 taper), depending upon the configuration of canal should be rotated in the groove of the carrier and advanced with light pressure. Frictional heat allows the instrument to advance apically and create a pilot channel. When resistance is felt, switch to greater taper (0.06 taper) file. Owing to the greater taper, the instrument will bind in the carrier, and the pulling force can take it out. Thermafil, if remain in place for a long, the gutta-percha usually become hard. Gutta-percha solvents can be useful in such cases (Fig. 36.22).

iii. *Removal of GuttaFlow*

GuttaFlow can be removed using similar techniques as used for removal of condensed gutta-percha. It is a cold gutta-percha filling system that utilizes a silicone matrix and shredded gutta-percha. The thermoplastic synthetic polymer (Resilon) when used as obturating material, can be softened with heat, or dissolved with solvents. Epiphany is a dual-cured resin sealer that is used with Resilon. It is claimed that it forms a monoblock with dentin. The removal is carried out by mechanical means.

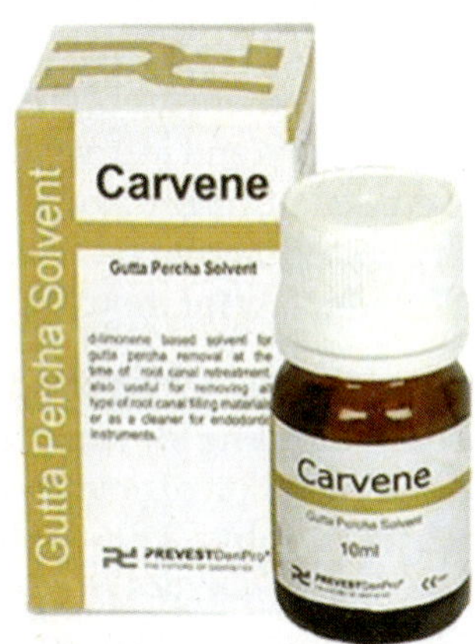

Fig. 36.22 Gutta-percha solvent

iv. *Removal of obturating pastes*

Various pastes are occasionally used as obturating material. Pastes normally have a soft consistency, but some materials can get hardened with time. The bacterial activity after microleakage may result in sludge-like consistency of the pastes.

The majority of material is removed by rotary instruments, the remaining tags can be removed by H-file/microdebrider along with endosonic irrigation. The vibrating file loosens the paste, which is flushed away by irrigant. Obturating pastes in the coronal and middle third are relatively easily removed; however, removal in apical third is difficult.

Certain cements may have radiopacity similar to that of dentin; hence, indistinguishable within the canal. The commonly encountered cements are AH 26, zinc phosphate and glass-ionomer, etc. The cements can be soluble and insoluble. Soluble cements can be softened by Endosolv E (for eugenol based cements) and Endosolv R (for resin based cements); whereas, insoluble cements are impervious to penetration by solvents. Long shank, fine sized carbide burs/diamond point can effectively remove insoluble cements. Fine filing should be carried out in slow motion, verifying the depth and direction of penetration. Good illumination along with use of magnification can allow the operator to distinguish between cement and the root dentin and can reduce the risk of perforation.

v. *Removal of silver points*

Silver points are no longer considered suitable for obturating root canals; however, operator may encounter previously obturated silver points for retreatment. Silver points are relatively easier to remove; the cement usually get dissolved by the time retreatment is planned. Generally, the root canal is not circular in cross-section but has an oval or fin-shaped morphology, leaving a space between dentin and silver point, which eases its removal (Fig. 36.23a to c).

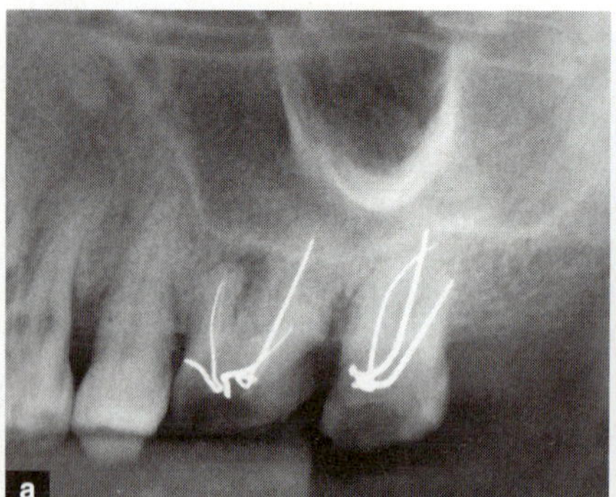

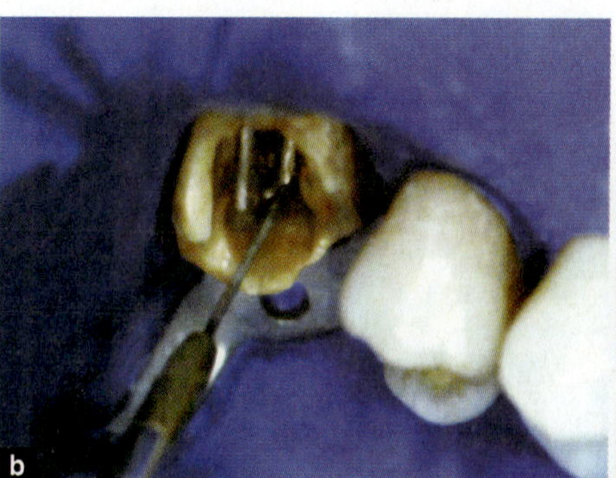

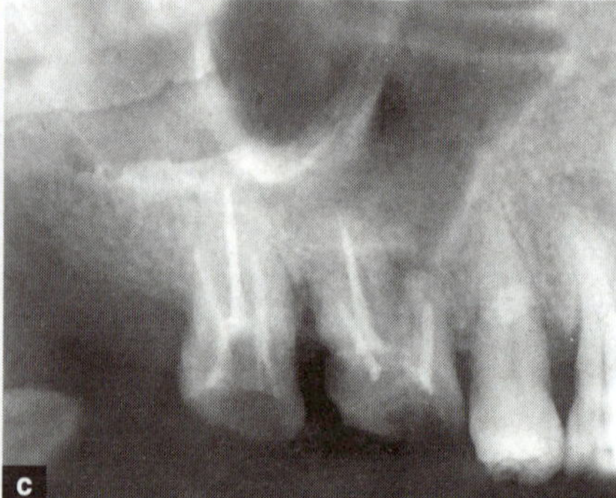

36

Fig. 36.23 Removal of silver points: (a) Maxillary molar restored with silver points; (b) Removal of silver points; (c) Tooth retreated with gutta-percha

The method of removing silver points varies as follows:

- *Removal of silver point extending in pulp chamber*: The silver points are easy to remove if they extend into the pulp chamber. The coronal end is grasped by either the Stieglitz forceps or narrow beaked artery forceps. Prior to this, the core material is removed using ultrasonic tips. Cement around the orifices of the silver cones can be removed using an endosonic tip. The point so loosen, can be gripped with Stieglitz forceps and withdrawn.
- *Removal of silver point lying in canal*: If the silver point lies in the straight portion of the root canal, the Masserann fragment remover kit will be useful. Removal of well-cemented silver points (newly obturated) can be challenging. The cement is carefully removed from pulp chamber using ultrasonics. An appropriate solvent is used to soften the cement. If the root is too slender to permit the use of the Masserann kit, attempts should be made to bypass and remove the points with Hedstroem files. If removal is not possible even after bypassing, the silver point should be incorporated with the new filling.
- *Removal of sectional silver point*: The sectional silver point, which is usually placed with a post, poses difficulty in removing. The root canal is enlarged coronally. After dissolving the cement lining, bypassing with H-files can be useful. Alternatively periapical surgery can be planned to expose and remove the silver point from the apical end.

3. Missed Canals

Missed canals have always been a source of failure in root canal treatment. Knowledge of possible deviations of root canal anatomy is mandatory for successful endodontics. In case of failure (persistent pain and infection), the possibility of extra canal should be explored before retreating the already obturated canals.

The features helpful in negotiating missed canals are:

i. Intraoral periapical radiographs taken at different horizontal angulations are helpful in locating missed canals. CBCT, providing three-dimensional view, is certainly beneficial.

ii. Proper illumination and working under magnification help visualize the internal anatomy of the pulp chamber much better than the naked eyes (Fig. 36.24). Magnification can be achieved by either loupes or surgical microscope. Surgical microscope provides magnified field as well as illumination.

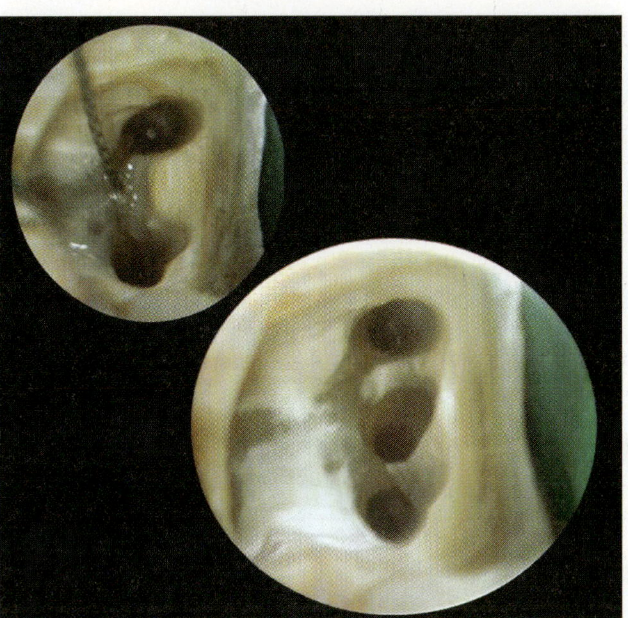

Fig. 36.24 Locating missed canal under microscope

iii. The access cavity is widened (diverging occlusally), involving the roof of pulp chamber. The floor of the pulp chamber is explored thoroughly with endodontic explorer for any catch, which may indicate orifice of missed canal.

iv. Location of canal orifice can also be negotiated by the use of dyes, ultrasonic tips, sodium hypochlorite, etc. Dyes, such as methylene blue is applied on the pulp chamber; upon rinsing and drying, the dye leaves the stains in orifices and isthmus areas indicating missed canals. The color of the dentin around the orifice is slightly darker than the surrounding dentin, which can be a good indication. Presence of pulpal remnants can cause bubbling with sodium hypochlorite; if flooded pulp chamber shows bubbling, it is also a good indicator for root canal orifice.

Once the orifice is located, the canal is negotiated with smaller files along with lubricants. Root canal preparation and obturation is carried out as in routine.

4. Canal Blockage

The dentinal mud is created during root canal preparation; and if not properly irrigated may block the root canal. Usually, the apical portion of the canal is blocked; however, any portion of root canal can be blocked (Fig. 36.25a and b). The residual cement after post-placement may also create block (Fig. 36.26a and b). The content of dentinal mud is frequently infected, thus may result in persistent disease. Blocks can be detected on radiographs as a short root filling. While managing blocks, the canal is widened using crown-

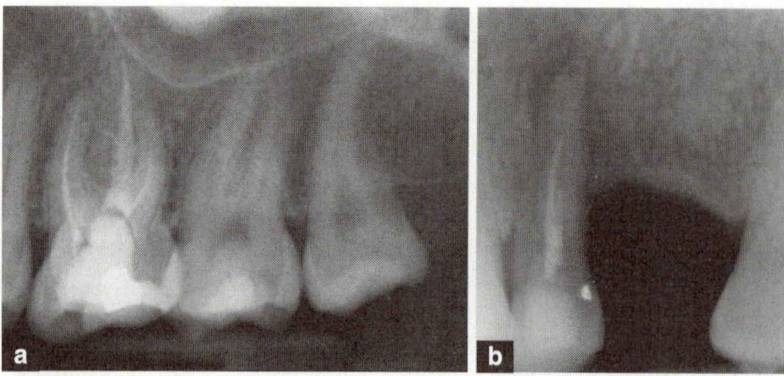
Fig. 36.25 Canal blockage: (a) Blockage in distobuccal root of maxillary first molar; (b) Blockage in maxillary premolar

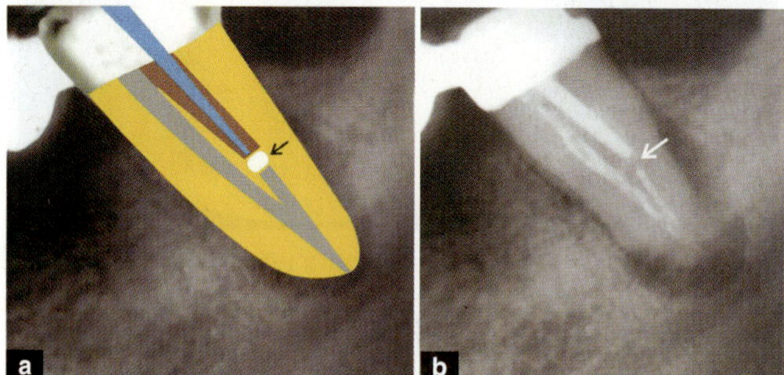
Fig. 36.26 Canal blockage: (a) Blockage due to residual cement (arrow)—diagrammatic; (b) Blockage due to residual cement (arrow)—radiographic

down technique up to the level of block. Copious irrigation is required to flush out the debris. The blockage is negotiated with precurved #8 or #10 file inserted slowly to crossover the debris. The chelating agents are used to soften the obstruction and facilitate the penetration of the file. Slowly, the file is pushed to the entire length of the canal. Once the length is negotiated, the blocked area is prepared using appropriate files. Ultrasonics can also be helpful to dislodge the blocked debris.

5. Ledges

The root canal instrumentation, if not properly gouged along the curvatures, may lead to creating a 'cut' in the dentin short of apical terminus; known as 'ledge' (Fig. 36.27a). It is usually created at the beginning of curvature when root canal instrument is used without precurving or using excessive amount of apical pressure. The radiograph suggests presence of ledge, when the apical extent of filling is not in the center of canal but on the outer side of the curve (Fig. 36.27b). The main problem with the ledge is that the instrument invariably lands at the ledge, while the original canal is not negotiated. As for management, non-end-cutting files are used up to the ledge to widen the canal (continuous irrigation is mandatory). Then a small file

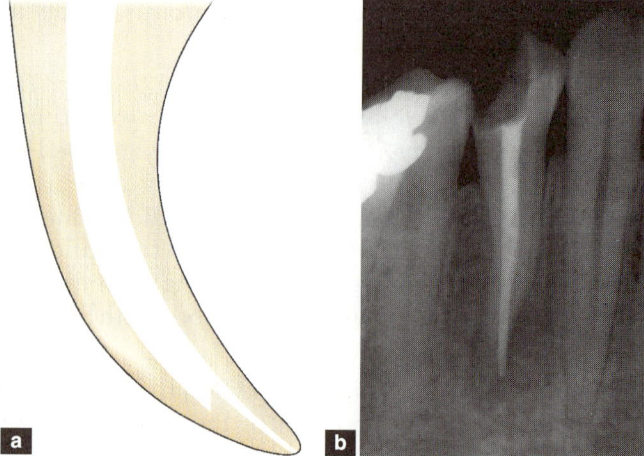
Fig. 36.27 Ledge: (a) Diagrammatic; (b) Radiographic (obturation follows this ledge)

(No. 8 or 10), precurved at 1.0–2.0 mm from the tip is inserted and rotated slowly to detect the original path of canal beyond the ledge. The file tip is slowly scraped along the internal wall of the canal curve slightly coronal to the level of ledge. A lubricant enhances the ability to place the file into the apical segment of the canal. Once the file reaches the estimated working length, a radiograph should be taken to verify its position. The filing is carried out circumferentially as in routine. Once the ledge has been bypassed and the canal can be negotiated with a conventional file, a non-end-cutting hand file with greater taper is tried to smoothen the ledge area. The anticurvature filing will enable the clinician to blend the ledge into canal preparation. Once the cleaning and shaping is completed, the canal is obturated (Fig. 36.28a and b). In rare instances, surgical intervention becomes necessary, if by passing the ledge is not feasible.

6. Canal Transportation

During root canal preparation, it is mandatory to maintain the shape of canal. The root canal instruments, if not properly used, especially at the apical area may

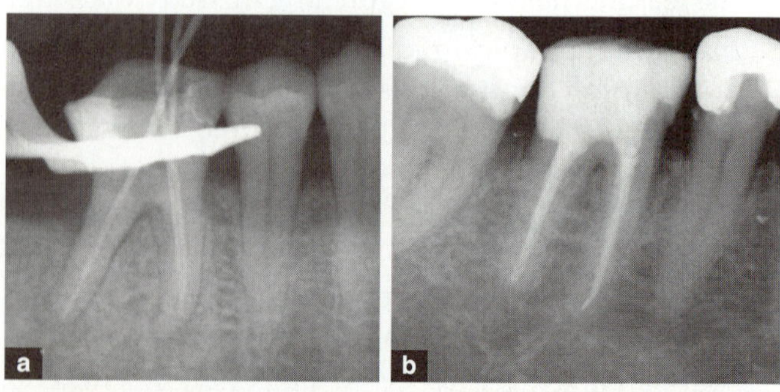
Fig. 36.28 Ledge: (a) Ledge in mesial canal of mandibular molar; (b) The retreated canals

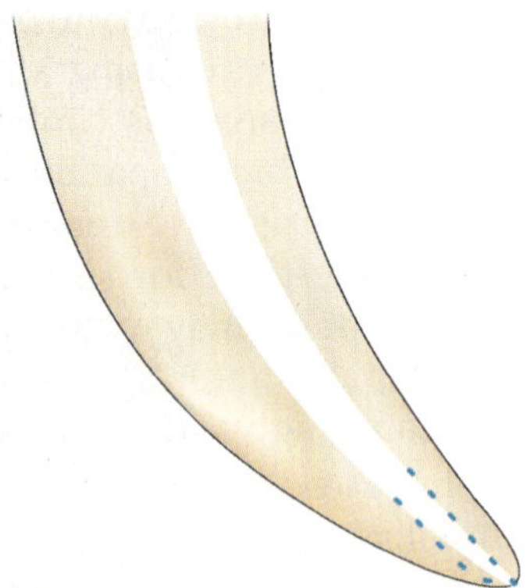

Fig. 36.29 Apical transportation (diagrammatic)

lead to deviated apical terminus. Such deviation from the actual terminus is referred to as *'canal transportation'* (Fig. 36.29). The degree of transportation can be minimal (less than 0.1 mm), moderate (0.1 mm) and severe (more than 0.1 mm). At the same time, that area does not provide resistance form to condense gutta-percha. Reverse architecture often lead to vertically overextended but actually underfilled canals.

The management of canal transportation varies according to the degree of transportation.

- When the change in location of apical terminus is 'minimal' the reverse architecture can be merged with the original path and obturated. Precaution should be taken to avoid strip perforation or weakening of dentinal walls.
- When the apical transportation is 'moderate' then it becomes difficult to correct the reverse architecture without weakening the residual apical dentin. Such cases need a barrier material, which provides hemostasis as well as a platform to condense gutta-percha. The commonly used barrier material, MTA (Fig. 36.30), sets within 4–6 hours and form cementum like barrier over it, thus allowing for a normal periodontal attachment (Fig. 36.31a and b).

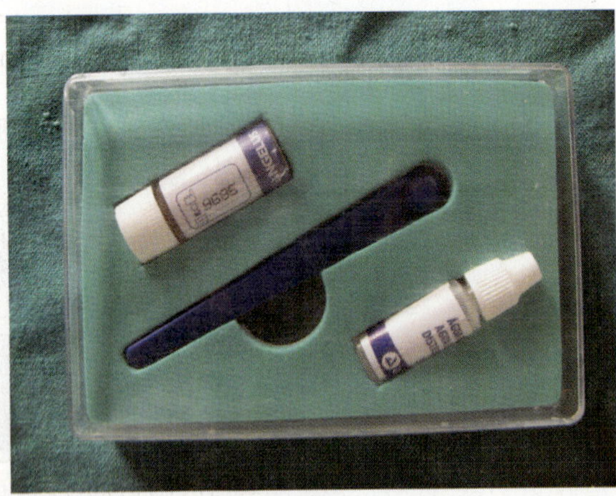

Fig. 36.30 MTA material

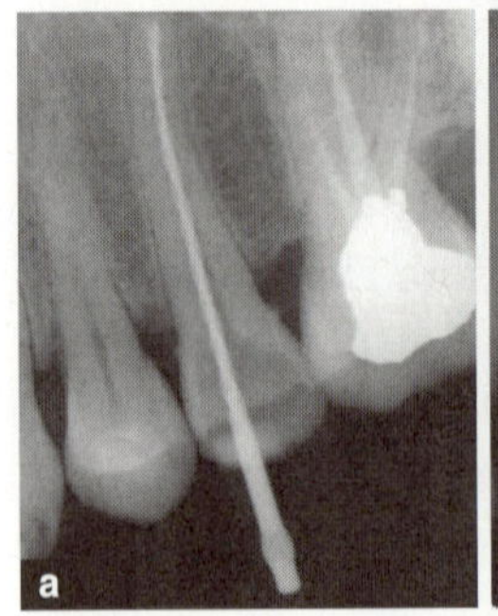

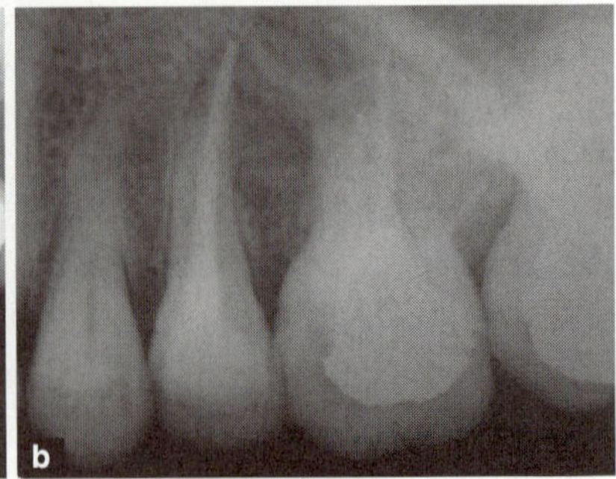

Fig. 36.31 Canal transportation in maxillary second premolar: (a) Preoperative; (b) Postoperative (treated with MTA)

- When the apical transportation is 'severe', the barrier material may not be effective; surgery is the only treatment of choice in such cases.

7. Perforation(s)

Perforation is the communication of root space with periodontal tissues. Perforation can occur during preparation of an access cavity (Fig. 36.32), cleaning and shaping of the root canal system (Fig. 36.33) and post-space preparation. The expansion of an inflammatory resorption defect may also lead to perforation.

Perforation can be classified as:

i. On the basis of size
   - Microperforation (less than 0.5 mm)
   - Macroperforation (more than 0.5 mm)

ii. On the basis of crestal level
   - Supracrestal
   - Crestal
   - Subcrestal

iii. On the basis of location
   - Coronal (at the pulpal floor)
   - Radicular (may be cervical, middle or apical).

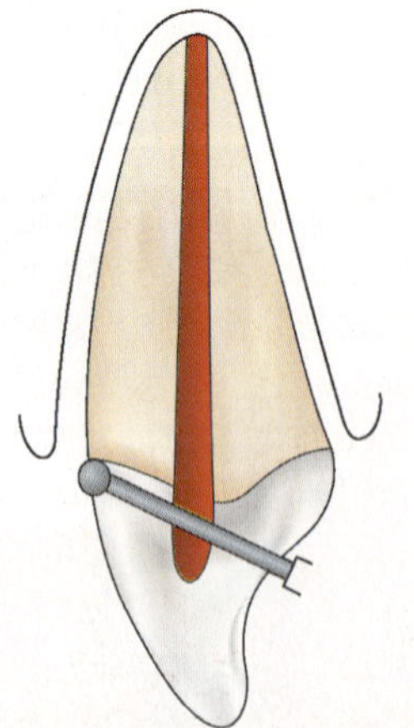

Fig. 36.32 Perforation during access cavity preparation

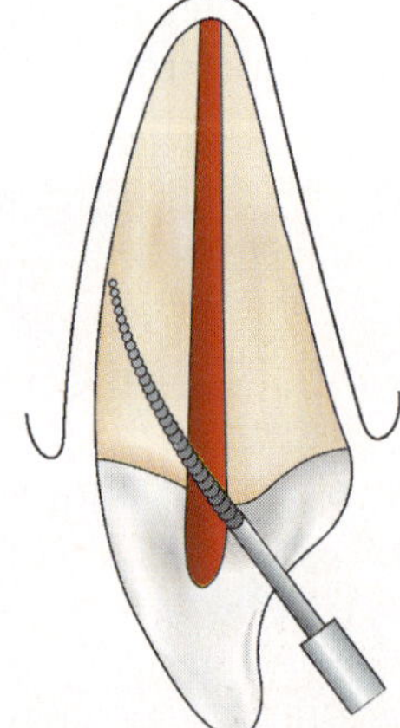

Fig. 36.33 Perforation during cleaning and shaping of root canal

The prognosis of management of perforation depends on its location, size and time elapsed since its occurrence. The perforation should preferably be sealed as soon as possible, since the delay leads to microleakage, infection and bone resorption. The radiographs taken at mesial/distal angulation are important in determining where a perforation exists and locating which surface(s) of the root have been perforated. Sometimes, the perforated area (usually very small) heals with time; evidences of healing in perforation need no treatment. However, in case perforation has led to inflammatory changes, surgical/nonsurgical treatment is initiated depending upon the size and site of perforation.

Advantages of nonsurgical approach

- Less destruction of periodontium in comparison to surgical approach
- Less chances of secondary infections.

Disadvantages of nonsurgical approach

- May be time consuming
- Prognosis remains doubtful.

Procedure

i. Microperforation when located coronally (pulpal floor) can be sealed using light cure composite or glass-ionomers. The site is disinfected before sealing (Fig. 36.34a to c).

ii. Macroperforations, particularly if associated with osseous defect, need a barrier or matrix, which serves as a hemostat. Hemostasis is achieved using collagen or calcium sulfate. Astringents, such as ferric sulfate, should be avoided because the coagulum they leave, may promote bacterial growth, subsequently compromising the seal. The barrier materials can be absorbable or non-absorbable. The absorbable are collagen materials and calcium sulfate. The non-absorbable are mineral trioxide aggregate and biodegradable ceramics. The *advantages* of using MTA are, it seals well even when the space is contaminated with blood and is highly biocompatible. The *disadvantages* are; it cannot be used for transgingival defects, as it requires long-time for setting; and direct contact with oral fluids may wash out the material. Fast setting repair material (e.g. Geristore) is preferred in transgingival defects.

   After control of bleeding and before placement of repair material, the root canals should be blocked with paper point or cotton, etc. so that the repair material should not enter the canal orifices.

iii. The furcation perforations are generally round; whereas, the lateral perforations are ovoid. The defect needs to be disinfected after isolation and prepared before receiving the restorative material. Ultrasonic instruments are employed to reshape the perforation site, if required. An appropriate barrier material and restorative material are selected; and the restoration is completed (Fig. 36.35a and b).

iv. The middle third area is usually perforated by misusing gates-glidden drills or misdirected post-preparations. For management, hemostasis and disinfection followed by restoration are carried out as for furcation perforations. In these cases, the defect lies deeper and further away from occlusal surface. To prevent obstructing the root canal space during repair procedure, any readily retrieval material is placed in the canal as space holders apical to the defect.

   In case the perforation is in the middle third of the root and sufficient access is available through the pulp chamber, the perforation can be repaired nonsurgically. The perforation site is cleaned and refined by Endo 4 ultrasonic tip to ensure an environment free of microbial contamination and necrotic tissue.

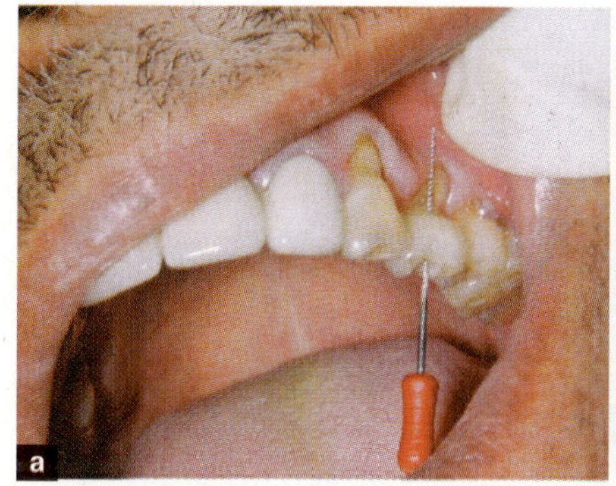

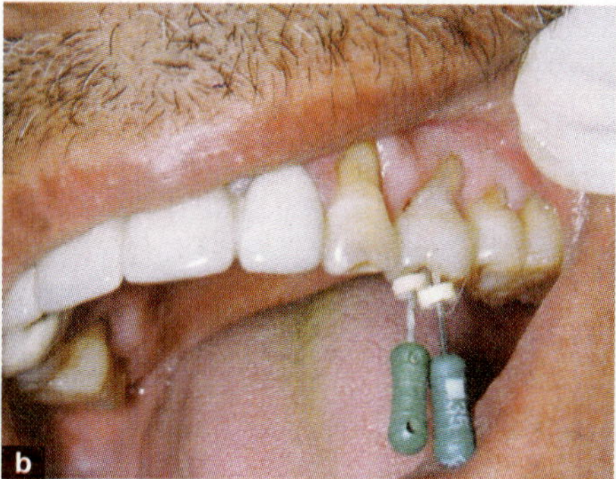

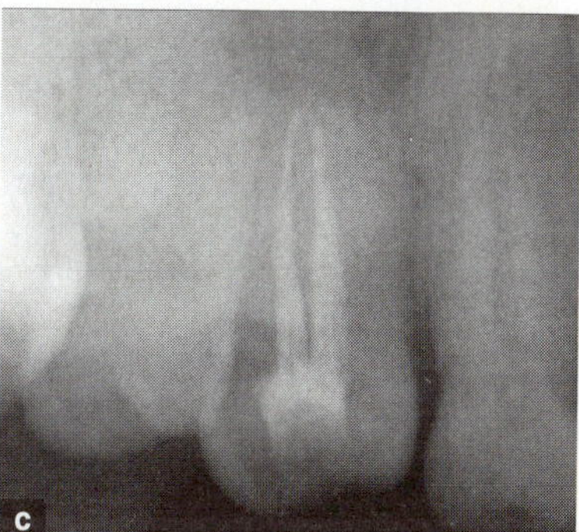

Fig. 36.34 Coronal perforation: (a) Cervical perforation of maxillary first premolar; (b) Perforation site filled and canals retreated; (c) Postoperative (radiograph)

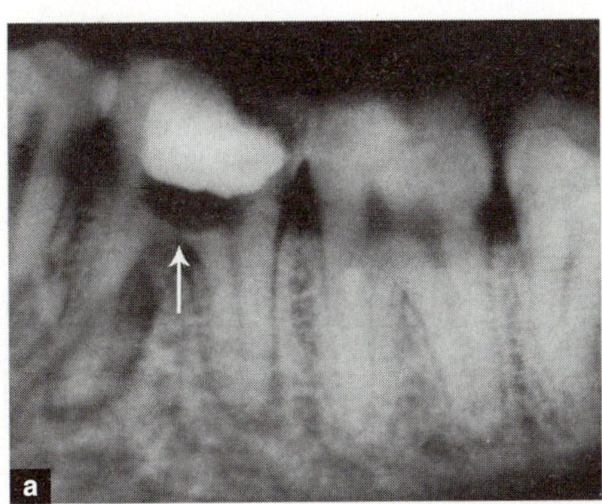

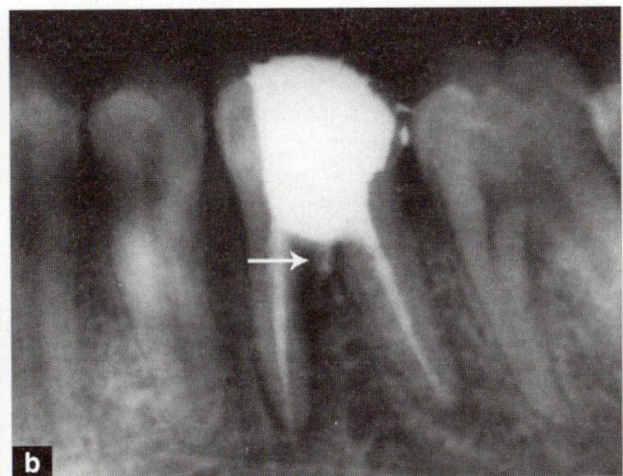

Fig. 36.35 Furcation perforation: (a) Preoperative (mandibular first molar); arrow showing perforation; (b) Postoperative (treated with MTA; arrow showing pushed out MTA)

A sterile, resorbable, and biocompatible collagen material is placed along the perforation site, to control hemostasis and prevent overfills; the material also acts as an internal matrix.

The Mineral Trioxide Aggregate forms a colloidal gel upon hydration, which solidifies in approximately four hours. Therefore, when used as a root repair material, moisture must be provided from the internal aspect of the root. The Mineral Trioxide Aggregate, because of its biocompatibility, is preferred as a material of choice to seal perforations. The location of the perforation is an important factor for its successful repair.

v. The perforation in the apical third of root canals is primarily due to faulty root canal preparation. A root canal perforated in apical area is usually blocked or ledged. The repair in apical portion of the canal is difficult because this involves negotiating, cleaning and filling the canal segment apical to perforation. The first attempt should be to negotiate the full length of the root canal. The precurved file is inserted and left in the canal so that during repair of the perforation, it can prevent blockage of the canal. To prevent the holding file from being cemented along with the repair material, the file is moved continually up and down. The canal is prepared and obturated using conventional means. Surgical intervention should be carried out, if need be.

BIBLIOGRAPHY

1. Ahonen M and Tjaderhane L. Endodontic-related paresthesia: A case report and literature review. J. Endod.: 2011; 37:1460–1464.
2. Akhavan H, Azdadi YK, Azimi S, Dadresanfar B and Ahmadi A. Comparing the efficacy of Mtwo and D-RaCe retreatment systems in removing residual gutta-percha and sealer in the root canal. Iran Endod. J.: 2012; 7:122–126.
3. Alhadainy HA and Abdalla AI. Artificial floor technique used for the repair of furcation perforations: a microleakage study. J. Endod.: 1998; 24:33–35.
4. Aqrabawi J. Management of endodontic failures: case selection and treatment modalities. Gen. Dent.: 2005; 53:63–65.
5. Aydemir S, Helvacioglu-Yigit D, Sinanoglu A and Emre O. Retreatment of a maxillary lateral incisor with two separate root canals confirmed with cone beam computed tomography. J. Clin. Med. Res.: 2015; 7:560–563.
6. Barrieshi-Nushair KM. Gutta-percha retreatment: effectiveness of nickel-titanium rotary instruments versus stainless steel hand files. J. Endod.: 2002; 28:454–456.
7. Bindal D. Endodontic non-surgical retreatment techniques – A review. SRM Univ. of Dent. Sci.: 2012; 3:32–40.
8. Bodrumlu E, Er O and Kayaoglu G. Solubility of root canal sealers with different organic solvents. Oral Surg., Oral Med., Oral Pathol., Oral Radiol. Endod.: 2008; 106: e67–69.
9. Cavenago BC, Ordinola-Zapata R and Duarte MA. Efficacy of xylene and passive ultrasonic irrigation on remaining root filling material during retreatment of anatomically complex teeth. Int. Endod. J.: 2014; 47:1078–1083.
10. Chong BS and Pitt Ford TR. Endodontic retreatment. 2: Methods. Dent. Update: 1996; 23:384.
11. Cicek E, Kocak MM, Kocak S and Saglam BC. Comparison of the amount of apical debris extrusion associated with different retreatment systems and supplementary file application during retreatment process. J. Cons. Dent.: 2016; 19:351–354.
12. DeDeus QD. Frequency, location and direction of the accessory canals. J. Endod.: 1975; 1:361–366.
13. Escoda-Francoli J, Canalda-Sahli C, Soler A, Figueiredo R and Gay-Escoda C. Inferior alveolar nerve damage because of over-extended endodontic material: A problem of sealer cement biocompatibility? J. Endod.: 2007; 33:1484–1489.
14. Farzaneh M, Abitbol S and Friedman S. Treatment outcome in endodontics: the Toronto Study. Phases I and II: Orthograde retreatment, J. Endod.: 2004; 30:627.
15. Fiedman S. Prognosis of initial endodontic therapy. Endodontic topics: 2002; 2:59–88.
16. Friedman S, Lost C, Zarraian M and Trope M. Evaluation of success and failure after endodontic therapy using glass-ionomer cement sealer. J. Endod.: 1995; 21:384.

17. Garrido AD, Oliviera AG, Osorio JE, Silva Sousa YT, Sousa NN. Evaluation of several protocols for the application of ultrasound during the removal of cast intraradicular posts cemented with zinc phosphate cement. Int. Endod. J.: 2009; 42:609–613.
18. Glick DH and Frank AL. Removal of silver points and fractured posts by ultrasonics. J. Prosth. Dent.: 1986; 55:212–215.
19. Iandolo A, Valletta A, Carratu P, Castiello G and Rengo S. Endodontic retreatment of maxillary first molar: the importance of the fourth canal. Giornale Italiano di Endod.: 2016; 30:27–32.
20. Karatas E, Kol E, Bayrakdar IS and Arslan H. The effect of chloroform, orange oil and eucalyptol on root canal transporation in endodontic retreatment. Aust. Soc. Endod.: 2016; 42, 37–40.
21. Keles A, Kamalak A, Keskin C, Akcay M and Uzun I. The efficacy of laser, ultrasound and self-adjustable file in removing smear layer debris from oval root canals following retreatment: A scanning electron microscopy study. Aust. Endod. J.: 2016; 1–8.
22. Kfir A, Blau-Venezia N, Tsesis I, Goldberger T and Metzger Z. Does root canal retreatment in necrotic pulp or retreatment cases with periapical lesions require anaesthesia? An *in vivo* clinical study. Int. Endod. J.: 2016:1–9.
23. Khedmat S, Azari A, Shamshiri AR, Fadae M and Fakhar HB. Efficacy of pro-taper and Mtwo retreatment files in removal of gutta-percha and guttaflow from root canals. Iran. Endod. J.: 2016; 11:184–187.
24. Kvist T and Reit C. Results of endodontic retreatment; a randomized clinical study comparing surgical and non surgical procedures. J. Endod.: 1999; 25:814.
25. Madani ZS, Simdar N, Moudi E and Bijani A. CBCT evaluation of the root canal filling removal using D-RaCe, Pro Taper retreatment kit and hand files in curved canals. Iran. Endod. J.: 2015; 10:69–74.
26. Muller GG, Schonhofen AP, Mora PM, Grecca FS, So MV and Bodanezi A. Efficacy of an organic solvent and ultrasound for filling material removal. Braz. Dent. J.: 2013; 24:585–590.
27. Nair PNR. Cholestrol as an aetiological agent in endodontic failures – a review. Aust. Endod. J.: 1999; 25:19–26.
28. Neskovic J, Slavolijub Z, Medojevic M and Maksimovic M. Outcome of orthograde endodontic treatment – A two-year follow-up. Srp. Arh. Celok. Lek.: 2016; 144:174–180.
29. Nudera WJ. Selective root retreatment: a novel approach. J. Endod.: 2015; 41, 1382–1388.
30. Ozyurek T, Demiryurek EO. Efficacy of different nickel-titanium instruments in removing gutta-percha during root canal retreatment. J. Endod.: 2016; 42:646–649.
31. Plotino G, Pameijer CH, Grande NM and Somma F. Ultrasonics in endodontics: a review of the literature. J. Endod.: 2007; 33:81–95.
32. Rehman K, Khan FR and Aman N. Comparison of orange oil and chloroform as gutta-percha solvents in endodontic retreatment. J. Contemp. Dent. Pract.: 2013; 14:478–482.
33. Riccuci D and Siqueira JF. Apical actinomycosis as a continuum of intraradicular and extraradicular infection: case report and critical review on its involvement with treatment failure. J. Endod.: 2008; 34:1124–1229.
34. Rodrigues RC, Antunes HS, Neves MA, Sequeira JE and Rocas IN. Infection control in retreatment cases: *In vivo* antibacterial effects of 2 instrumentation systems. J. Endod.: 2015; 41:1600–1605.
35. Rosa t P, Signoretti FG, Montagner F, Gomes BPF and Jacinto RC. Prevalence of *Treponema* spp. In endodontic retreatment-resistant periapical lesions. Braz Oral Res.: 2015; 29, 1–7.
36. Rubino GA, de Miranda Candeiro GT, Freire LG, Iglecias EF, de Mello Lemos E, Caldeira CL and Gavini G.: Micro-CT evaluation of gutta-percha removal by two retreatment systems. Iran. Endod. J.:2018; 13:221-227.
37. Ruddle CJ. Nonsurgical endodontic retreatment. CDA J.: 2004; 1–14.
38. Silva EJ. Brito ME, Ferreira VD, Belladonna FG, Neves AA, Senna PM and De-Deus G. Cytotoxic effect of the debris apically extruded during three different retreatment procedures. J. Oral Sci.: 2016; 58:211–217.
39. Siqueira JF and Rocas IN. Clinical implications and morphology of bacterial persistence after treatment procedures. J. Endod.: 2008; 34:1291–1301.
40. Siqueira JF. Aetilogy of root canal treatment failure. Why well treated teeth can fail. Int. Endod. J.: 2001; 34:1–10.
41. Stabholz A and Friedman S. Endodontic retreatment – case selection and technique. Part 2:treatment planning for retreatment. J. Endod.: 1988; 14:607–614.
42. Suter B, Lussi A and Sequiera P. Probability of removing fractured instruments from root canals. Int. Endod. J.: 2005; 38:112–123.
43. Topcuoglu HS, Demirbuga S and Tuncay O. The bond strength of endodontic sealers to root dentine exposed to different gutta-percha solvents. Int. Endod. J.: 2014; 47:1100–1106.
44. Ustun Y, Topcuoglu HS, Duzgun S and Kesim B. The effect of reciprocation versus rotational movement on the incidence of root defects during retreatment procedures. Int. Endod. J.: 2015; 48:952–958.
45. Vidal FT, Nunes E, Horta MC, Freitas M and Silveira FF. Evaluation of three different rotary systems during endodontic retreatment – Analysis by scanning electron microscopy. J. Clin. Exp. Dent.: 2016; 8:e125–129.
46. Ward JR, Parashos P and Messer HH. Evaluation of an ultrasonic technique to remove fractured rotary nickel titanium instruments from root canals. J. Endod.: 2003; 29:756.
47. Zmener O, Pameijer CH and Banegas G. Retreatment efficacy of hand versus automated instrumentation in oval-shaped root canals: an *ex vivo* study. Int. Endod. J.: 2006; 39: 521–526.

Chapter 37

Resinifying Therapy in Endodontics

The root canal treatment is becoming popular day by day. The world-wide dental surgeons are encouraged to provide better endodontic services by simplifying procedure, shortening the appointment times and maintaining original teeth in the arch. Different ways and means have been tried to save the teeth so as to maintain the stomatognathic system.

In certain cases, teeth with pulp involvement do not response to conventional root canal treatment. The reasons are multifactorial; however, complications pose difficulties in executing the treatment, so the success rate is compromised. Such cases and in other conditions where permanent treatment is to be delayed, resinifying therapy is the best choice.

Wang Manen (1957) initially suggested this treatment modality. In this therapy, the liquid phenol-aldehyde resin when inserted into root canal or poured over the tooth surface, becomes solid after polymerization. The microorganisms and associated debris get resinified. The resinifying agent has the potential to creep into tubules and set there, facilitating three-dimensional obturation of the root canal system. Even if the solution is pushed beyond the apex, it does not cause any major damage. After initial irritation, the healing progresses (the irritation and the healing has been documented in histopathological studies).

Sensitivity of resin resorcinol has been evaluated against eight commonly found microorganisms in the root canals, viz. *Enterococcus faecalis, Streptococcus haemolyticus, Streptococcus salivarius, Streptococcus mitis, Staphylococcus aureus, Escherichia coli, Lactobacilli and Actinomyces.* Zone of inhibition was observed both in *Staphylococcus aureus* and *Streptococci haemolyticus*, indicating that the resin has definite antibacterial effect both before and after polymerization.

Tsao (1984) recommended resinifying therapy of posterior teeth with larger periapical rarefied areas because of its simplicity and higher success rate.

Indications

- Necrosis of pulp
- Larger rarefied area at periapex
- Pulp exposure requiring pulp capping/pulpotomy
- Broken instruments/obstructions in the canal
- Lateral/accessory canal(s), which may cause problems during root canal procedures
- Vital dentin surface, as coating/temporization.

Contraindications

- Immature teeth with open apices
- Anterior teeth (resin may stain the teeth)
- Maxillary last molars are difficult; however, not contraindicated.

Advantages

- No need to remove the entire pulp
- Can be used as antimicrobial sealer
- No need for compaction or additional sealer
- Effective in retreatment cases, especially where the access is difficult.

Disadvantages

- Not radiopaque
- Delay in healing if leaks into periapical areas
- Staining of the treated teeth (reddish hue)

The differences between resinifying therapy and the conventional root canal treatment are summarized in Table 37.1.

Composition

Resinifying agent consists of three solutions (Fig. 37.1).

The composition of these solutions is as follows:

Solution I

Formaldehyde (38.48%)	62.0 ml
Cresol	12.0 ml
Alcohol (95%)	6.0 ml

Table 37.1 Differences between resinifying therapy and conventional root canal therapy

Procedure	*Conventional root canal therapy*	*Resinifying therapy*
Removal of pulp	Entirely removed	Not necessary
Preparation of canal	Mechanically enlarged	No need (many studies have shown better results with prepared root canals)
Disinfection of canal	Removal of infected dentinal wall, application of medication, sealing, etc.	No need
Use of sealer	Require appropriate sealer	No need
Root canal obturation	Require obturating material; gutta-percha, etc.	Resin sets in the canal and acts as obturator

Solution II

Resorcin	45.0 gm
Distilled water	55.0 ml

Solution III

Sodium hydroxide	1.0 gm
Distilled water	2.0 ml

The three solutions are mixed in a clean dappen dish/container (Fig. 37.2) in the ratio of 5 : 5 : 2. The solution is stirred prior to use. Solution III is a catalyst. The usual setting time of the mixed solution is four to five minute. In case, the operator requires early setting time, an extra drop of solution III can be added.

Fig. 37.1 Solutions used in resinifying therapy

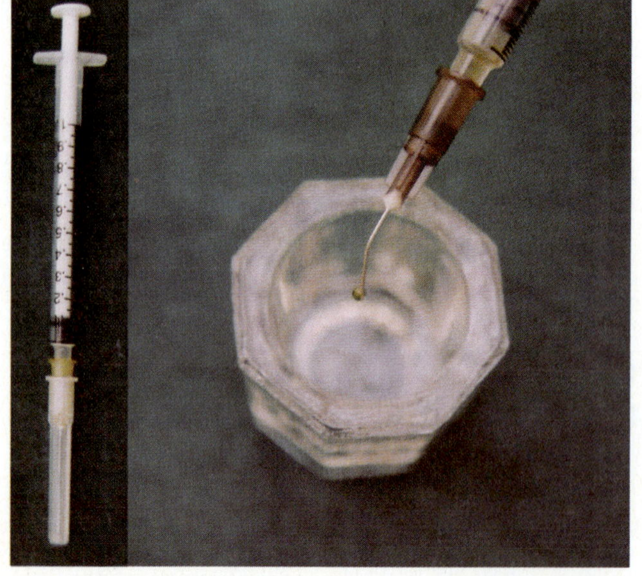

Fig. 37.2 Mixing of three solutions in the ratio of 5 : 5 : 2

UTILITY OF RESINIFYING THERAPY

Resinifying therapy can be used in variety of cases. The main are:

a. Resinifying agent as an Obturating Material

Isolate the selected tooth and open the root canals following standardized technique. In case of vital pulps, pulp residues in the apical end need not be removed. In necrotic pulps, root canals may not be prepared mechanically; however, a few authors recommend preparing the root canal with conventional methods, along with irrigation and dressing.

Procedure

Once the canal is ready for obturation, resinifying agent is introduced into the root canals. A small drop of resinifying agent is trickled over the coronal end of root canal. A small file is used with up-down motion to remove air and facilitate entry of the resinifying agent into the root canal(s). This process is repeated till the canal is filled. Leave the excess agent in the pulp chamber. Allow the liquid resin resorcinol solution to set in room environment (usual time of setting is 5–7 minutes). The coronal chamber is filled with interim restorative material.

The clinical and radiological observations strongly suggest that the resinifying agent has the capability to infiltrate into the root canals including the accessory canals. The resinifying agent has the potential to imbibe into the dentinal tubules up to 1/3rd or 1/4th of the total length (Fig. 37.3a and b). The residual pulp tissues and the irritants get resinified and retained in the canal without irritation to periapical areas. The root canals are obturated three dimensionally and the sealing of canals is maintained for a longer period. The clinical cases are exhibited in Figs 37.4a to d and 37.5a to d.

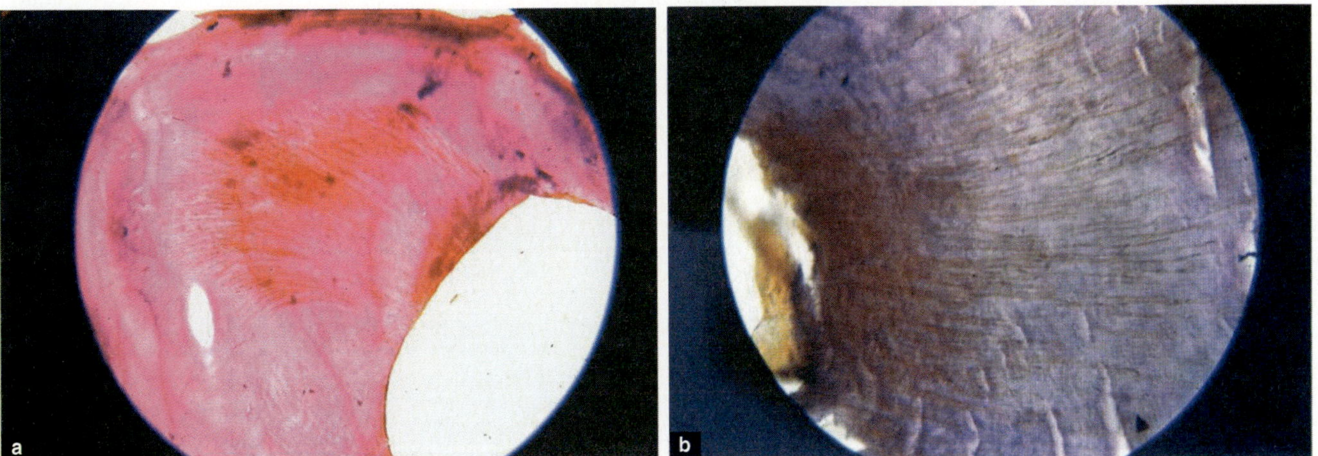

Fig. 37.3 Penetration of resinifying agent into dentinal tubules: (a) Low magnification; (b) High magnification

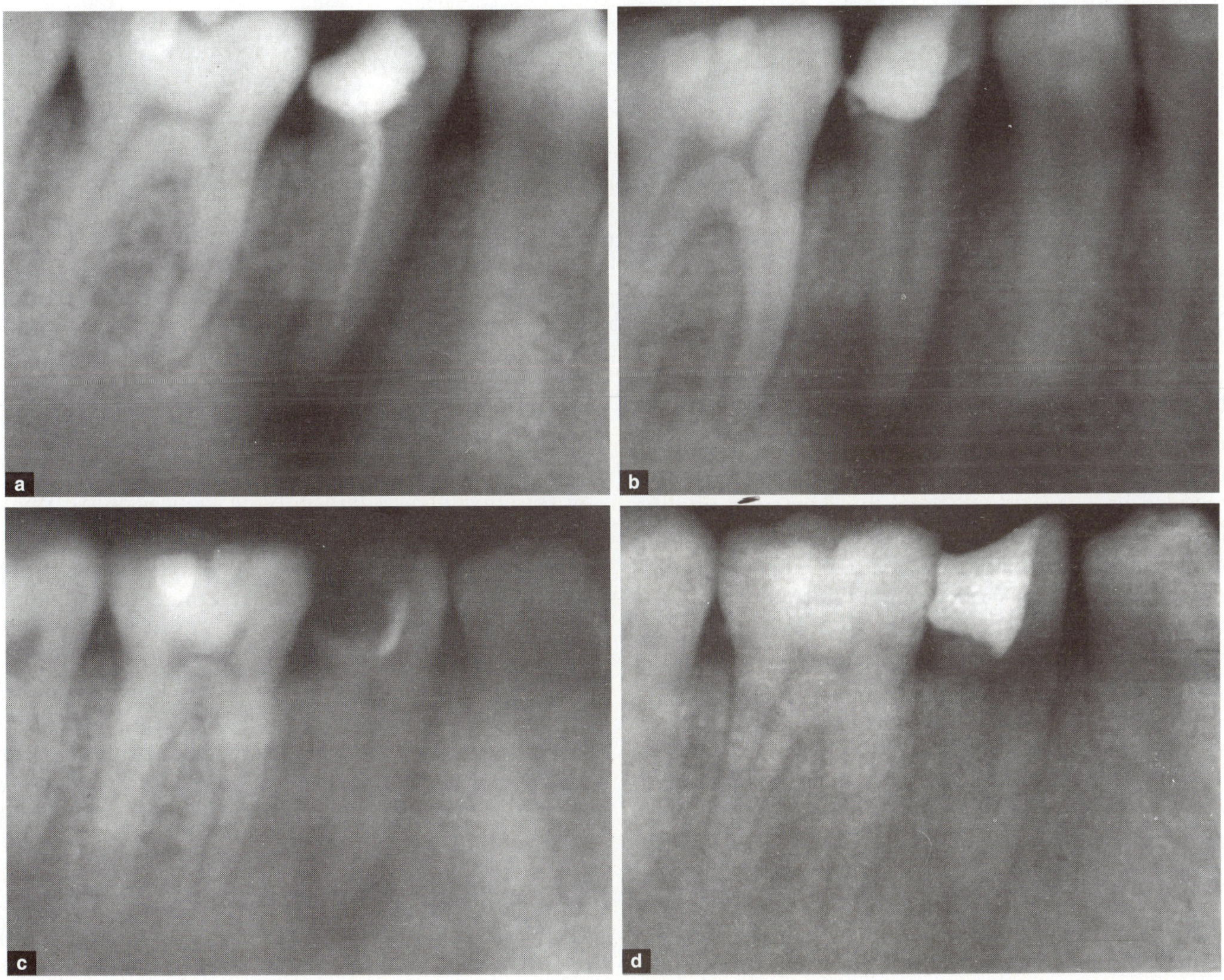

Fig. 37.4 Mandibular second premolar treated with resinifying therapy: (a) Preoperative (large rarefied area at periapex); (b) Tooth obturated with resinifying agent; (c) Postoperative (signs of healing at six month follow-up); (d) Postoperative (complete healing at one year follow-up)

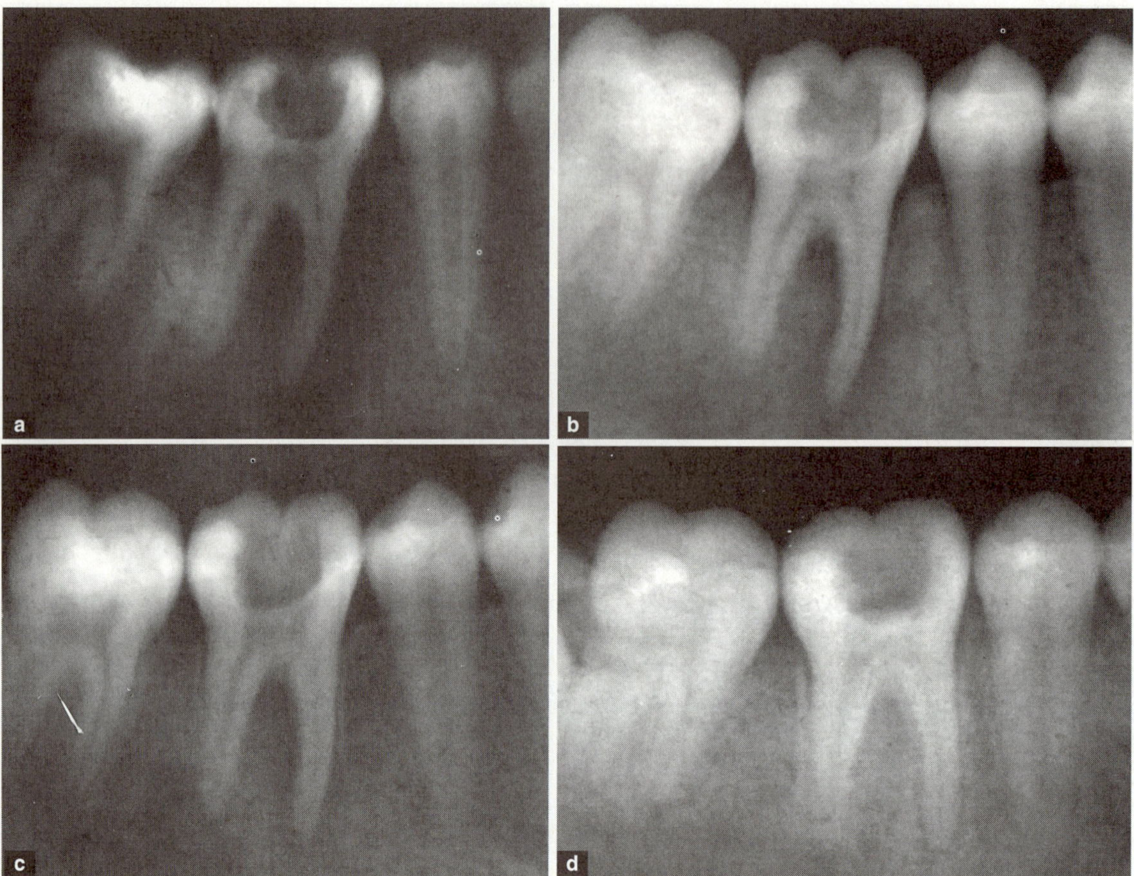

Fig. 37.5 Mandibular first molar treated with resinifying therapy: (a) Preoperative (large rarefied area around mesial root); (b) Tooth treated with resinifying therapy; (c) Postoperative (signs of healing at six month follow-up); (d) Postoperative (complete healing after one year follow-up)

b. Resinifying Agent as a Direct Pulp Capping Material

Direct pulp capping, though not so popular these days, is a treatment modality, whereby the exposed pulp is covered by a suitable material to retain pulp vitality. Direct pulp capping has always been controversial. Materials that have been tried as pulp capping agents range from pulp caps to tricalcium phosphate ceramics; the accepted one is calcium hydroxide. Earlier hypothesis that calcium of calcium hydroxide forms the dentin bridge has been disproved. The antibacterial environment created by calcium hydroxide, may however, be responsible for healing. The exposure site, if left bacteria free, may heal without any medicament. Resinifying agent has been successfully tried as direct pulp capping material (Fig. 37.6a and b).

Procedure

The exposure site is washed immediately with normal saline solution and isolated with sterilized cotton rolls. The exposure site and the rest of the cavity is wiped with cresophene. Two drops of freshly prepared resinifying solution is poured over the exposure site and let it set. The rest of the cavity is filled with Kalzinol, zinc phosphate cement or any other restorative material.

The effectiveness of resinifying agent as pulp capping material has been histologically proved.

Histological sections revealed areas of fibrosis and hyalinization in the pulp in the coronal area; however, in the middle and apical third of the sections, normal pulpal tissue was evident.

The fibroblastic activities present at the coronal sites are suggestive of the healing process. The normal pulp tissue, without any sign of necrosis, present in the middle and apical part of the root confirms that the resinifying agent can successfully be used in direct pulp capping.

c. Resinifying Agent as a Sealer

Resinifying agent has been tried as a sealer along with routinely used obturating materials. This sealer is antibacterial, but may shrink and leave a reddish hue on the outer tooth structure (hence the nickname 'Russian Red').

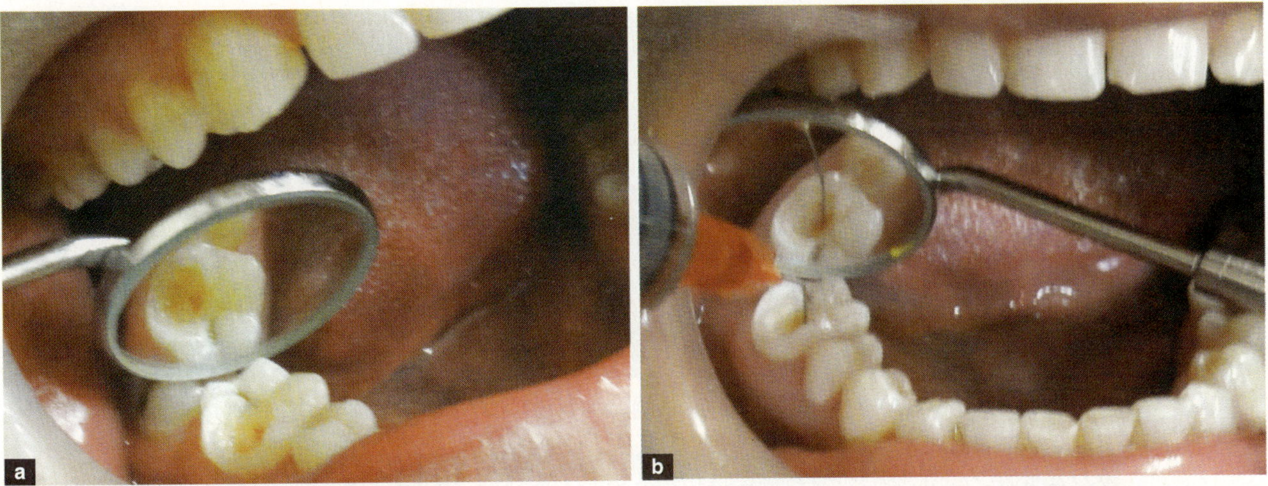

Fig. 37.6 Resinifying agent as direct pulp capping material: (a) Traumatic pulp exposure in mandibular first molar; (b) Application of resinifying agent at the exposure site

Procedure

When used as a sealer, once the resinifying agent is introduced to the root canals, single cone gutta-percha is pushed up to predetermined working length before the sealer sets. Once set, the excess gutta-percha is removed and the pulp chamber is filled with suitable materials (Fig. 37.7a and b).

d. Resinifying Agent as a Material for Temporization

Tooth preparation for full/partial veneer crowns needs immediate converge, especially in vital teeth. The laboratory procedures may take time, which may lead to hypersensitivity.

Procedure

Resinifying agent can be used to cover the prepared tooth prior to permanent restoration. The freshly prepared resinifying agent is applied to the tooth surface with the help of a camel brush. It will set within five minutes and form a resin coat over the tooth surface. The solution in the ratio of 5 : 5 : 3 can be used for fast setting (Fig. 37.8a and b).

e. Resinifying Agent in Complications

Resinifying agent has been used in complicated areas. Because of its liquid form, it can penetrate into inaccessible areas. It can be used in cases of:

- Broken instruments (Fig 37.9a to c)
- Obstructions/old filling materials in the canal, which are difficult to remove (Fig. 37.10)
- Ledges, where the root canal is not negotiated beyond ledge
- Teeth not responding to routine endodontic therapy.

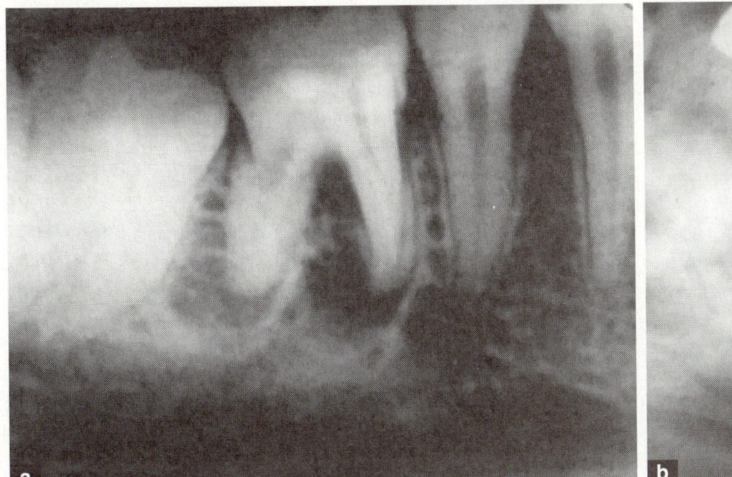

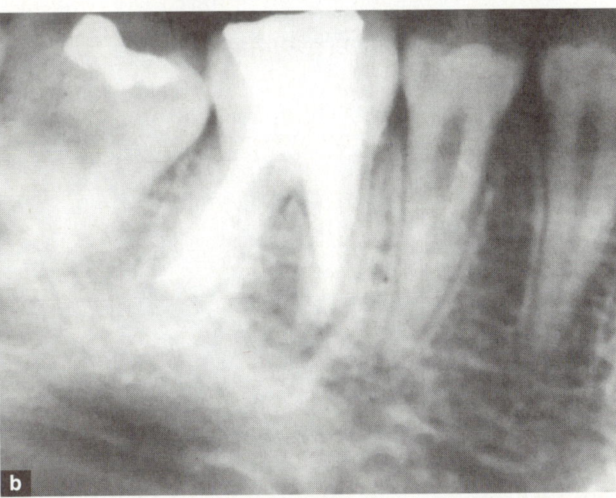

Fig. 37.7 Use of resinifying agent as sealer: (a) Preoperative (mandibular first molar); (b) Postoperative (signs of healing)

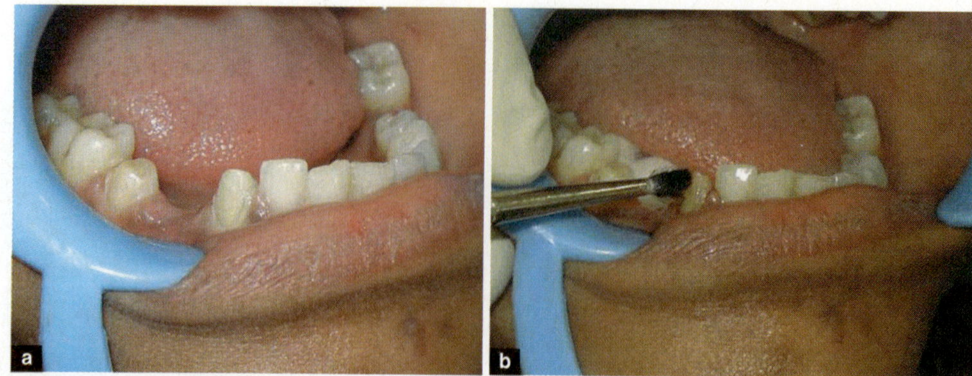

Fig. 37.8 Resinifying agent as interim restoration: (a) Crown preparation; (b) Application of resinifying agent

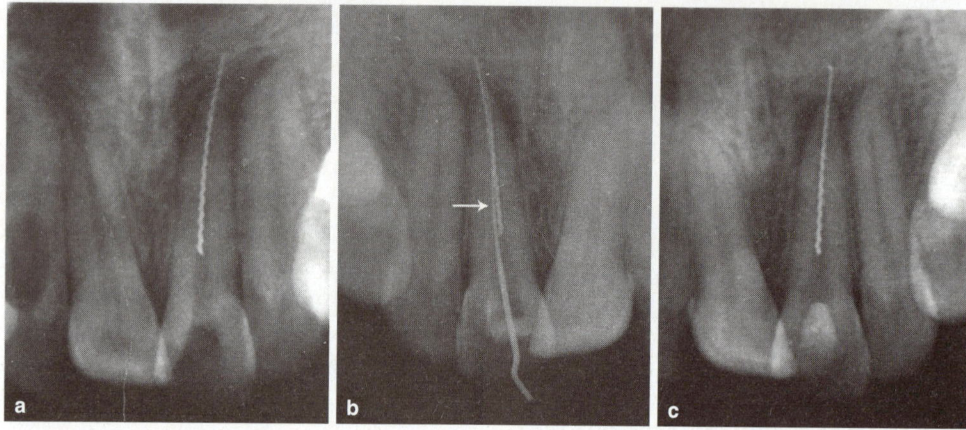

Fig. 37.9 Resinifying therapy in managing separated instruments: (a) Preoperative (broken instrument in maxillary central incisor); (b) Broken instrument by-passed (arrow) and treated with resinifying agent; (c) Postoperative (follow-up at six months; signs of healing)

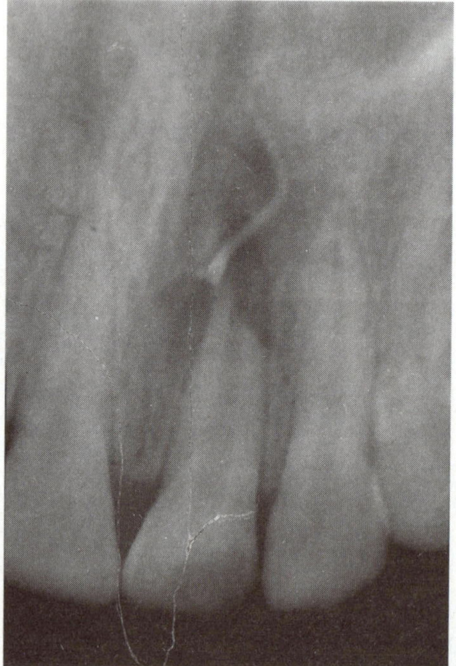

Fig. 37.10 Unretrievable gutta-percha treated with resinifying therapy

37

BIBLIOGRAPHY

1. Gound TG, Marx D and Schwandt NA. Incidence of flare-ups and evaluation of quality after retreatment of resorcinol-formaldehyde resin ("Russian Red Cement") endodontic therapy. J. Endod.: 2003; 29:624–626.
2. Lin KC and Kirk EEJ. Direct pulp capping: A review. Endod. and Dental Traumatol: 1987; 3:213–219.
3. Matthews JD. Pink teeth resulting from Russian endodontic therapy. JADA: 2000; 131:1598–1599.
4. Orstavik D. Materials used for toot canal obturation: technical, biological and clinical testing. Endodontic Topics: 2005;12:25–38.
5. Sikri V, Manjri M and Sikri P. Direct pulp capping with resorcinol: A clinical, radiological and histological evaluation. JCD: 1998; 1:90.
6. Sikri VK and Sikri P. Resinifying Therapy in Endodontics: A clinical and radiological evaluation. IJDR: 1995; 6:35–39.
7. Sikri VK, Sikri P, Singh J, Manjri M and Khanna S. Resinifying Therapy in Endodontics II. Histological and bacteriological evaluation. IJDR: 1996; 7:51–56.
8. Schwandt NW and Gound TG. Resorcinol-formaldehyde resin "Russian Red" endodontic therapy. J. Endod.: 2003; 29:435–437.
9. Tsao TF. Endodontic treatment in China. Int. Endod. J.: 1984; 17:163–175.
10. Wu Min-K. Clinical and experimental observations on Resinifying Therapy. O. Surg., O. Med., O. Path.: 1986; 62:441–448.

Chapter 38

Regenerative Endodontics

Regenerative endodontics is concerned with the development of biologically based treatment modalities that are used to replace diseased portion of the dental pulp or to allow complete formation of a dental pulp-like tissue that will act as the original dental pulp. A form of regenerative endodontics began many years ago with the development of direct and indirect pulp capping procedures. The need for scaffold, vascular supply, growth factors, signaling mechanisms, migration concept of cells differentiation are accepted regenerative procedures. Regenerative endodontic Procedures are defined as *'biologically based procedures designed to replace damaged tissues, including dentin, cementum and cells of the pulp-dentin complex as well'*. These procedures are also named *'revascularization'*, *'revitalization'*, and *'regenerative endodontics'*. An understanding of the processes and mechanisms to restore a vital, healthy tissue within a tooth is mandatory, which helps to gain greater knowledge of tissue engineering involving interactions at cellular and molecular levels.

The purpose of pulp treatment (maintaining the vitality of teeth damaged due to caries or trauma) is to maintain the tooth structure in order to preserve optimal function. Maintaining the pulp vitality is essential for continuous root development and apical closure, especially in case of immature permanent teeth.

If the pulp of immature permanent teeth is infected, traditional approach 'apexification' is followed, which includes removal of infected pulp and application of calcium hydroxide, MTA, etc. This treatment modality aids in closing the apical foramen; however, cannot maintain pulp vitality.

As the concept of regeneration endodontics is not new, various authors have tried regenerative treatment procedures with varying results. The important studies are tabulated below.

Author (Year)	*Procedure*
Hermann (1952)	First to carry out regenerative endodontic procedure; applied calcium hydroxide in vital pulp amputation.
Nygaard-Ostby (1961)	Established a blood clot to use as a scaffold to revascularize tissue within root canals of teeth.
Rule (1966)	Introduction of polyantibiotic paste; no bleeding in the canals was evoked; instrumentation short of what appeared to be the vital tissue.
Nygaard-Ostby (1971)	Use of antibiotics in the disinfection protocol and the intentional promotion of intracanal bleeding.
Hoshino (1993)	Use of triple antibiotic paste.
Iwaya and colleagues (2001)	Showed the revascularization potential of an immature permanent tooth without instrumentation and with the use of an antibiotic paste composed of ciprofloxacin and metronidazole (double antibiotic paste).
Banchs and Trope (2004)	Case reports on immature mandibular premolars (new protocol followed).
ADA (2011)	Adopted a new procedure code to allow clinicians to induce apical bleeding into the root canal in immature permanent teeth with necrotic pulps that have been extirpated.

Common Terms used in Regenerative Endodontics

Biomimetics: The science of reconstructing or mimicking natural process or tissue with the expectation that regeneration will follow.

Gene: Specific sequences of nucleotides along a molecule of DNA (or RNA in the case of some viruses) that represent the functional units of heredity.

Genetic engineering: Also called genetic modification, is the alteration of genetic make-up of an organism using techniques that introduce heritable material prepared outside the organism, either directly into the host or into the cell, that is then fused and hybridized with the host.

Gene therapy: The technique for the correction of defective genes that are responsible for the development of disease by the insertion, alteration or removal of genes within an individual's cells and biological tissues to treat disease.

Morphogens: They are extracellular secreted signals governing morphogenesis during epithelial-mesenchymal interactions. It is a biologic factor that regulates stem cells to form desirable cell type.

Repair: It is the restoration of tissue continuity without mimicking its original architecture or function.

Regenerative medicine: The engineering and growth of functional biological substitutes *in vitro* and/or the stimulus to the regeneration and remodeling of tissues *in vivo* for the purpose of repairing, replacing, maintaining or enhancing tissue and organ functions.

Regeneration: The restoration or new growth of organs, tissues, etc. that have been lost, removed or injured in an organism.

Scaffold: It provides a physiochemical and biological three-dimensional micro-environment for cell growth and differentiation, promoting cell adhesions and migration. The scaffold serves as a carrier for morphogens in protein therapy and for cells in cell therapy.

Stem cell: A cell that has the ability to continuously divide and produce progeny cells that differentiate into various other types of cells or tissues.

Stem cell plasticity: It refers to the phenomenon of generation of specialized cells of another generation by the adult stem cells of one generation.

Stem cell therapy: A technology in which persons own cells are triggered to revert to their primitive organic form, which then redifferentiate into mature cells of various organs.

Apexogenesis: A vital pulp therapy procedure performed to encourage continued development of root and physiological formation of its apical end.

Apexification: A method to induce a calcific barrier in root canal with an open apex; or continued development of root in teeth with necrotic pulp.

Revascularization: The methods involve in restoring vascularity of a tissue or organ.

Guided tissue regeneration: Induced/guided regeneration of the tissues.

Objectives of Regenerative Endodontic Treatment

The objective of regenerative treatment is to regenerate a fully functional pulp-dentin complex to aid in continued root development for immature teeth.

The goals of regenerative endodontic procedures are categorized as primary, secondary and tertiary; however, success of the treatment is confirmed by histological means. Histologic confirmation of dental pulp with an intact odontoblastic layer and restoration of a functional pulp is undoubtedly the prime goal.

- *Primary goal*: Elimination of symptoms along with evidence of bony healing.
- *Secondary goal*: (Desirable, may not be essential); increased root wall thickness and/or increased root length.
- *Tertiary goal*: (If achieved, indicates a high level of success); positive response to vitality testing.

TISSUE ENGINEERING

The application of the principles and methods of engineering and life sciences for the understanding of structure-function relationships in normal and pathological mammalian tissues; and the development of biological substitutes that restore, maintain, and/or improve tissue functions.

Tissue engineering is defined as *'an interdisciplinary field that integrates the principles of biology and engineering to develop biological substitutes that replace/regenerate human cells, tissues or organs in order to restore the normal function'*.

Regenerative procedures and tissue engineering hold the promise of a solution to a number of clinical problems in dentistry. The endodontists can adopt these scientific advances emerging from regenerative thereby developing regenerative endodontic procedures, subsequently improving patient care.

The ultimate goal of tissue engineering *vis-à-vis* regenerative endodontics is to develop therapies to restore lost, damaged or aging tissues using engineered or regenerated procedures derived from either donor or autologous cells.

The tissue of interest in regenerative endodontics includes dentin, pulp, cementum and periodontal tissues. Tissue engineering implies clinical approach for feeding more or less biodegradable scaffold with donor cells/growth factors, then culturing and implanting the scaffold to induce and direct the growth of new healthy tissues.

Triad of tissue engineering

The key elements of tissue engineering are stem cells, growth factors (morphogens) and an extracellular matrix scaffold; known as 'Triad of tissue engineering' (Fig. 38.1).

a. Stem cells

b. Growth factors

c. Scaffolds.

a. Stem Cells

Stem cells are unspecialized cells in the human body that are capable of becoming specialized cells, each with new specialized cell function.

A stem cell is defined as *'a cell that has the ability to continuously divide and produce progeny cells that differentiate (develop) into various other types of cells or tissues.'* "Stem cells are like little kids who, when they grow up, can enter a variety of professions," Dr Marc Hedrick of the UCLA School of Medicine says. "A child might become a fireman, a doctor or a plumber, depending on the influences in their life or environment. In the same way, the stem cells can become many tissues by making certain changes in their environment."

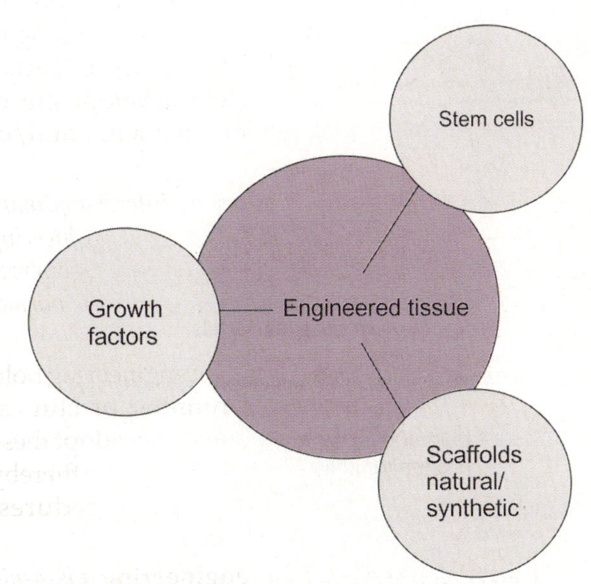

Fig. 38.1 Triad of regenerative procedure

William Sedgwick (1866) described certain cells for the regenerative properties of plants, the 'stem cells.' Stem cells are unprogrammed cells in the human body that can be described as 'shape shifters'.

Stem cells differ from other kinds of cells in the body. All stem cells regardless of their source have three general properties:

i. Capable of dividing and renewing themselves for long periods

ii. Unspecialized

iii. May give rise to specialized cell types

Isolation of stem cells involves enzymatic digestion of tissues followed by growth of isolated cells in a medium rich in growth factors. The differentiation of these cells involve: (i) Colony forming assays, (ii) Phenotypic assays and (iii) Flow cytometry.

These cells are stored in liquid nitrogen at –196°C (preservation in a liquid phase).

Culturing of Stem Cells

'Cell culture' is a term that refers to the growth and maintenance of cells in a controlled environment outside an organism. A successful stem cell culture is the one that keeps cells healthy, dividing and unspecialized.

Dental pulp stem cells can be cultured by following two methods:

1. ***Enzyme-digestion method*:** In this method, the pulp tissue is collected under sterile conditions and digested with appropriate enzyme; the resulting cell suspensions are incubated in culture dishes containing a special medium supplemented with necessary additives. Finally, the resulting colonies are subcultured before confluence and the cells are stimulated to differentiate.

2. ***Explant outgrowth method*:** In this method, the extruded pulp tissues are cut into 2.0 mm^3 cubes, shifted to a suitable substrate and are incubated directly in culture dishes containing essential medium. Ample time (up to 2 weeks) is needed to allow a sufficient number of migrants out of the tissues.

Classification of Stem Cells

i. Stem cells are classified as:

- *Embryonic/fetal*: Mostly cells are embryonic, so term embryonic is preferred.

- *Postnatal/adults*: Cells are similar at all age groups, so term postnatal is preferred.

Embryonic/fetal	*Postnatal/adults*
• Derived from inner cell mass of early embryo called blastocyst. • Capable of dividing and renewing themselves for long periods without differentiating whereas adult stem cells cannot • For example: Embryonic stem cells can differentiate into any type of specialized cells like Hematopoietic cells, Hepatic cells, osteoblasts, vascular endothelial cells, etc.	• Any stem cells taken from mature tissue. • They are lineage restricted and are referred to by their tissue of origin. • Play an important role in local tissue repair and regeneration. • For example: Dental pulp stem cells (DPSC), Stem cells from exfoliated deciduous teeth (SHED), etc.

ii. Stem cells are also classified according to their source and range of differentiation:

Type	*Source*
Totipotent	Cells from early (1–3 days) embryos (each cell can develop into a new individual)
Pluripotent	Some cells of blastocyst (5–14 days) [cells can form any (over 200) cell types]
Multipotent	Fetal tissue, cord blood, and postnatal stem cells including dental pulp stem cells (cells differentiated, but can form a number of other tissues)

iii. Stem cells have been classified, based on their source of genesis:

Allogenic	*Xenogenic*	*Isogenic*	*Autologous*
From same species (e.g. blood cells, bone marrow, cells of same species)	From individual of other species (blood cells, bone marrow cells of other species)	From genetically identical individual (twins) (any cell to be implanted)	From the same individual to whom required (any cell to be implanted)

Most stem cells found in the orofacial region are mesenchymal stem cells (Fig. 38.2). Flowchart 38.1 summarizes forms of dental stem cells.

The various postnatal mesenchymal cells can differentiate into odontoblast-like (dental) cells.

b. Growth Factors

Growth factors are proteins that bind to receptors on the cell and induce cellular proliferation and/or differentiation. Many growth factors are quite versatile, stimulating cellular division in numerous cell types, while others are more cell specific. Dentin contains many proteins capable of stimulating tissue responses. It is hypothesized that the therapeutic effect of calcium hydroxide may be because of its ability to extract growth factors from the dentin matrix. These growth factors play a key role in stimulating tertiary dentinogenesis, an accepted response of pulp-dentin repair.

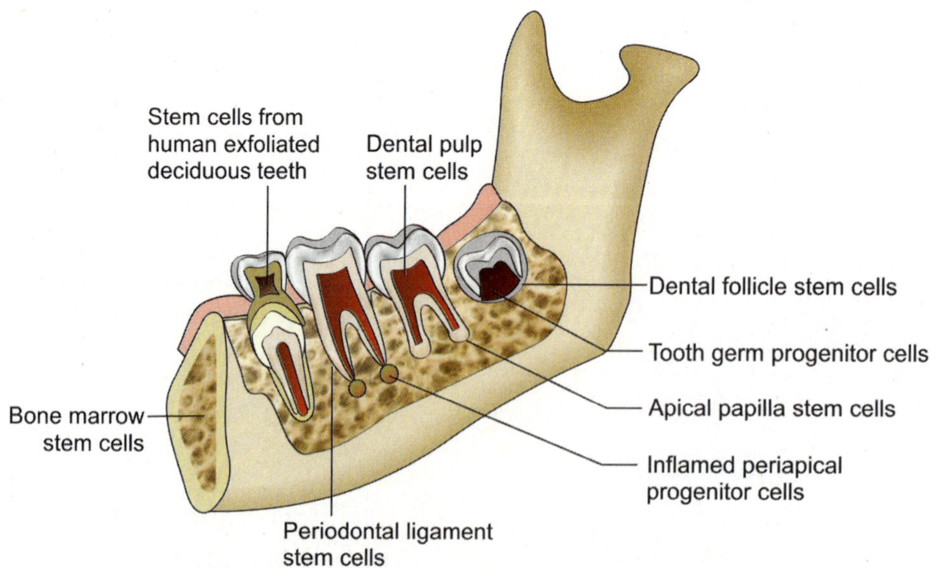

38

Fig. 38.2 Potential source of stem cells in oral environment (*Schematic representation: Adapted from* Hargreaves et al 2013)

Flowchart 38.1: Forms of dental stem cells

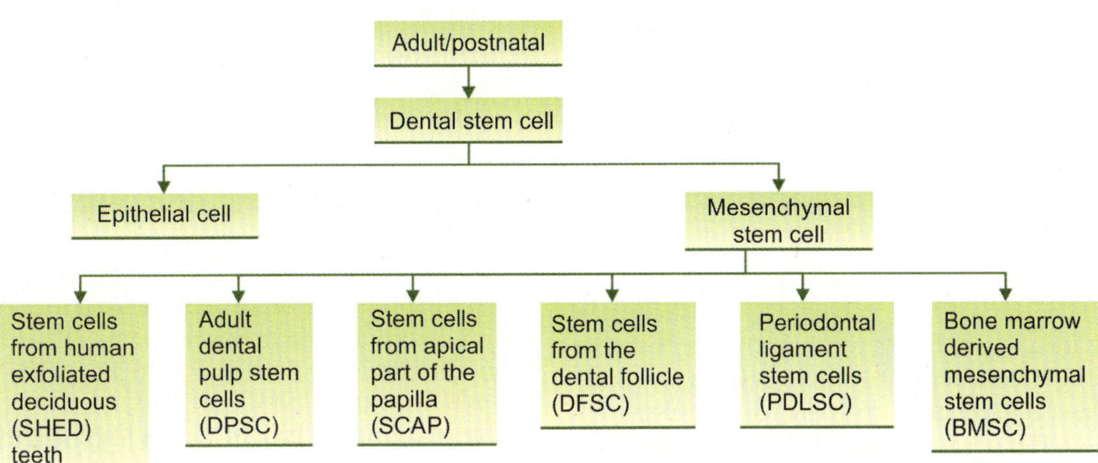

- Growth factors, especially transforming growth factor (β-TGF) are important for odontoblast differentiation and stimulation of dentin matrix secretion.
- Another important growth factors in regeneration is bone morphogenic proteins (BMPs). Recombinant human bone morphogenic protein (BMP) stimulates differentiation of osteoblasts; subsequently, bone mineralization.
- Fibroblast growth factors (FGF) are for general growth-promoting effects on most fibroblastic cells; it stimulates angiogenesis wound healing and cell migration *in vivo*.
- Platelet derived growth factor (PDGF) are derived from platelets and endothelial cells; promotes connective tissue cells.

The common growth factors, their source and cellular activity is tabulated in Table 38.1.

Table 38.1 Growth factors and cellular activity

Growth factor (source)	*Cellular activity*
Bone morphogenic protein (BMP) (bone matrix)	Induces differentiation of osteoblasts; stem cells synthesize secrete mineral matrix, subsequently bone mineralization
Epidermal growth factor (EGF) (submaxillary glands)	Promotes proliferation of mesenchymal and epithelial cells; increase stem cell numbers
Fibroblast growth factor (FGF) (a wide range of cells)	Promotes proliferation of many cells; increase stem cell numbers
Insulin-like growth factor I or II (IGF I or II; variety of cells)	Promotes proliferation of many cell types; increase stem cell numbers
Platelet-derived growth factor (PDGF) (platelets, endothelial cells, placenta)	Promotes proliferation of connective tissue; increase stem cell numbers
Transforming growth factor (β-TGF) (dentin matrix, activated T-helper cells	Anti-inflammatory, promotes wound healing, inhibits macrophage and lymphocyte proliferation; used to promote mineralization of pulp tissue
Nerve growth factor (NGF) (protein secreted by neuron's tissues)	Survival and maintenance of sympathetic and sensory neurons; promotes neuron outgrowth and neural cell survival

c. Scaffolds

A scaffold is an artificial three-dimensional frame structure that serves as a mimic of extracellular matrix for cellular adhesion, migration, proliferation, and tissue regeneration in three dimensions.

Ideal Requirements of a Scaffold

- Biocompatible
- Biodegradable
- Promote cell attachment, spreading and proliferation
- Strong enough to hold matrix
- Good transport properties
- Easy to connect to host's vascular system
- Conducive surface characteristics.

Types of Scaffold

a. *Biological/natural scaffolds*

These consist of natural polymers, such as collagen and glycosaminoglycan, which offer good biocompatibility and bioactivity. Collagen is the major component of the extracellular matrix and provides great tensile strength to tissues. As a scaffold, collagen allows easy placement of cells and growth factors and allows replacement and natural tissues after undergoing degradation. However, it has been reported that pulp cells in collagen matrices undergo marked contraction, which affects pulp tissue regeneration. For example;

- Collagen/dentin matrix
- Glycosaminoglycan
- Fibrin
- Platelet rich plasma (PRP).

Platelet rich plasma (PRP): An ideal scaffold

Platelet rich plasma (PRP) is being established as a potentially ideal scaffold for regenerative endodontic treatment regimen. An ideal scaffold selectively binds and localizes cells, contains growth factors and undergoes biodegradation over time. PRP contains growth factors, stimulates collagen production, recruits other cells to the site of injury, produces anti-inflammatory agents, initiates vascular ingrowth, induces cell differentiation, controls the local inflammatory response and improves soft and hard tissue wound healing.

It has increased concentration of growth factors that have the potential to attract stem cells present in the apical tissues (vital pulp cells, periodontal ligament, apical dental papilla, bone marrow) and even from periapical lesions.

Preparation of PRP involves taking—blood sample from the patient's arm (20 ml approximately); centrifuging the blood in the presence of an anticoagulant, removal of erythrocytes from the blood, and adding thrombin and calcium for coagulation of prepared PRP. It is then injected into the canal space up to the level of slightly short of coronal opening and allowed to clot for 5 minutes. Approximate 3.0 mm of grey MTA is placed directly over the PRP clot. The PRP clot provided an excellent matrix for placement of MTA. Subsequently permanent restoration is placed to prevent coronal leakage.

Advantages

- Relative ease of application
- Shorter time to induce vital tissues within the root canal system.

Disadvantages

- Need of special equipment and medications to prepare PRP in young patients.
- Increased cost of the treatment.

b. ***Artificial synthetic scaffolds***

These are synthetic polymers with controlled physicochemical features such as degradation rate, microstructure, and mechanical strength; for example:

- Polylactic acid (PLA), polyglycolic acid (PGA) and their copolymers–polylactic-co-glycolic acid (PLGA), etc.
- Synthetic hydrogels, including polyethylene glycol (PEG) based polymers.
- Scaffolds modified with cell surface adhesion peptides such as arginine, glycine and aspartic acid to improve cell adhesion and matrix synthesis within the three dimensional network.

c. Scaffolds containing inorganic compounds

Scaffolds containing inorganic compounds, such as hydroxyapatite (HA), tricalcium phosphate (TCP) and calcium polyphosphate (CPP) are used to enhance bone conductivity and have proved to be very effective for tissue engineering of dental pulp stem cells.

Clinical Applications of Tissue Engineering

Clinical techniques, whereby the tissues can be regenerated, include the surgical implantation of laboratory grown synthetic pulp and dentin tissues; implanting a mix of scaffold and growth factors and promoting endogenous recruitment of stem cells; or enhancing revascularization into root canals by encouraging stem cells to grow into natural fibrin clots.

On the basis of aforementioned principles of tissue engineering, the procedures for regenerating endodontium can be carried out following two approaches:

a. Creating an engineered tissue constructed in the laboratory and transplanting the same into the recipient tooth (pulp cavity).
b. Revascularization: Inducing host stem cells from the adjacent site to mobilize and inhabit the implanted/natural host matrix.

a. Implanting laboratory constructed tissue into the Pulp Cavity

The advancements in tissues engineering techniques facilitate stem cells be implanted onto a three dimensional conductive scaffold matrix rich in bioactive signaling molecules. The artificial pulp generated in the laboratory can be transplanted into the pulp cavity of the recipient tooth. However, construction of precise 3D models for each individual pulp cavity is difficult. Highly complex and variable internal anatomy amongst the teeth and also variations from tooth to tooth and individual to individual makes the task quite difficult.

Injecting a soft scaffold matrix impregnated with pulp stem cells and growth factors into the root canal system can overcome difficulties associated with implanting a rigid matrix. Scaffold material that can be injected includes synthetic hydrogels like polyethylene glycol polymers. Though delivery system is relatively easier with these polymers, problems of low cell survival and limited control over tissue formation exist.

Modifying hydrogel polymers with peptides like arginine, glycine or aspartic acid have helped in improving cell adhesion and matrix synthesis rendering them suitable for use. Making the hydrogels photo-polymerizable (injectable scaffold) so that they form a rigid framework after implantation into the receptor site is a better solution. Mineralizing genes have also been implanted into the pulp to promote tissue mineralization. Viruses have been genetically modified to hold human DNA. Therapeutic DNA can directly be inserted or transported to the membrane of the target cells through artificial lipid carrier. The ability to use this system *in vivo* need to be further evaluated. The conventional pulpotomy and regeneration of dentin-pulp organ is depicted in Figs 38.3a to c and 38.4a to d, respectively.

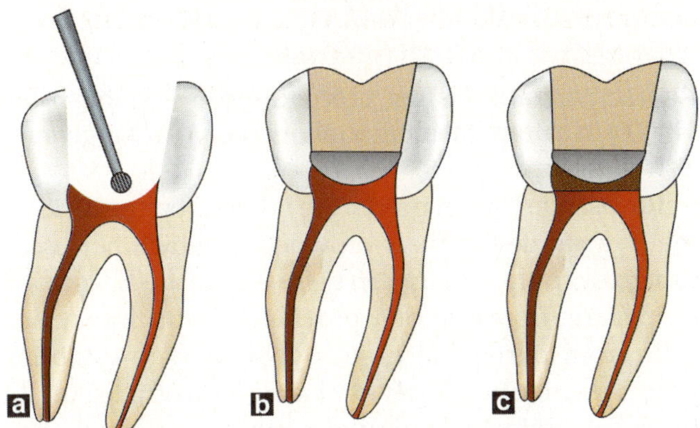

Fig. 38.3 Conventional vital pulpotomy: (a) Removal of coronal pulp; (b) Placement of MTA and restorative material; (c) Dentin bridge formation (no effect on dentin-pulp complex)

Cell Homing

Cell homing refers to two cellular processes; implanting and cell differentiation. The mesenchymal stem/progenitor cells having capacity to differentiate into various cell lineages forming dentin-pulp tissues are implanted into the root canal. Differentiation implies transformation of these stem/progenitor cells into odontoblasts, fibroblasts and also endothelial cells (Fig. 38.5 a to d).

Cell Homing is applicable to restoration of pulp vitality of both immature and mature permanent teeth. Cell Homing has the advantage wherein patient's own mesenchymal cells are implanted into endodontically prepared root canals and induce them to differentiate into pulp cells/odontoblastic lineage.

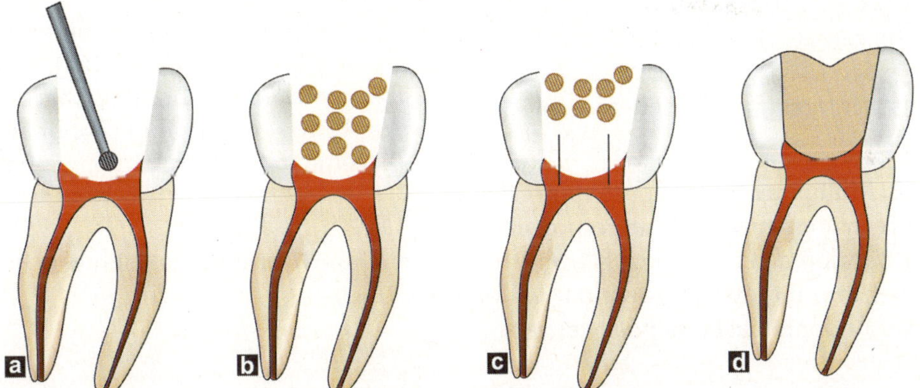

Fig. 38.4 Regeneration of dentin-pulp complex: (a) Residual pulp; (b) Implantation of growth factors and scaffolds; (c) Induced progenitor cells (stem cells) from pulp; (d) Regeneration of pulp-dentin complex

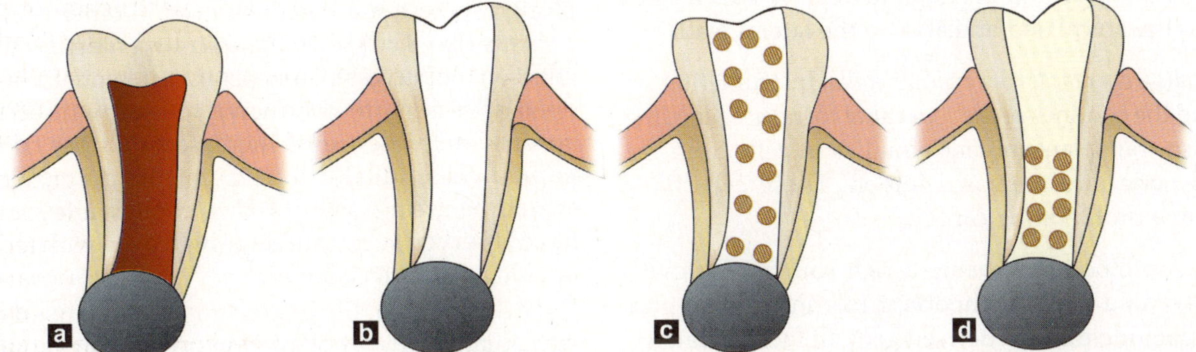

Fig. 38.5 Cell homing approach (diagrammatic): (a) Normal tooth with periapical lesion; (b) Root canal prepared; (c) Placement of scaffold into root canal; (d) Proliferation of stem cells

b. Revascularization (Inducing Endogenous Stem Cells Grow in Natural Fibrin Clot)

Revascularization is the procedure to re-establish the vitality in a nonvital tooth to allow repair and regeneration of tissues.

Revascularization procedure is based on the concept that if a sterile matrix is provided in which new cells can grow, pulp vitality can be re-established. Necrotic pulp, if free from infection, provides a matrix into which cells from periapical tissues grow and re-establish pulp vascularity, slowly replacing necrotic tissue. In immature infected nonvital teeth, an infection-free matrix is created by use of irrigants and/or tri-antibiotic pastes. This matrix acts as the scaffold for the regeneration of new pulp tissues.

Mechanism of revascularization: The possible mechanism of revascularization includes:

Vital apical pulp cells: It is speculated that a few vital pulp cells always remain at the apical end of the root canal. These cells might proliferate into the newly formed matrix and differentiate into odontoblast under the organizing influence of cells of Hertwig's epithelial root sheath, which are quite resistant to destruction, even in the presence of inflammation. The newly formed odontoblasts can lay down atubular dentin at the apical end (apexogenesis); also on lateral walls of the root canal, thus reinforcing and strengthening the root.

Multipotent stem cells: Multipotent dental pulp stem cells present in abundance in immature teeth are responsible for continued root development. These cells from the apical end might get into the existing dentinal walls and differentiate into odontoblasts; deposit tertiary/atubular dentin.

Stem cells in periodontal ligament: The stem cells present in the periodontal ligament can proliferate, grow into apical end and within the canal to deposit hard tissues both at the apical end and also on the lateral walls.

Stem cells from apical bone/apical papilla: Instrumentation beyond the confines of the root canal to induce bleeding can also transplant mesenchymal stem cells from the apical bone into the canal lumen. These cells have extensive proliferating capacity.

Blood clot: Blood clot, being a rich source of growth factors, could play an important role in regeneration. These include platelet-derived growth factor, platelet-derived epithelial growth factor, and tissue growth factor, which may stimulate differentiation and maturation of fibroblasts, odontoblasts, cementoblasts, etc. from the immature, undifferentiated mesenchymal cells in the newly formed tissue matrix.

Advantages

The advantages of revascularization are:

- Requires short treatment time: After control of infection, can be completed in a single visit
- Cost-effective; number of visits are reduced, and no additional material required
- Obturation of the canal is not required unlike in calcium hydroxide-induced apexification
- Continued root development (root lengthening) and strengthening of the root as a result of reinforcement of lateral dentinal walls with deposition of new dentin/hard tissues can be achieved successfully.

Limitations

The limitations of revascularization are:

- Long-term clinical results are yet to be documented.
- The entire canal might get calcified; potentially increasing the difficulty in future endodontic procedures, if required.
- Procedures are limited to the open apices, immature teeth.
- In case post and core are the final restorative treatment plan, revascularization is not the right treatment option because the vital tissue in apical two-thirds of the canal cannot be violated for post-placement.

Clinical Procedure

The clinical procedure followed in revascularization includes:

Case Selection

Necrotic pulp/immature pulp is a reasonable candidate of regenerative endodontic procedures.

Young patients (6–8 years of age) are preferred, though success has been observed in older age group patients also. The size of the apical opening has definite effect on the successful regenerative potential. Short and open root is more conducive to ingrowth of tissue, because of presence of increased number of apical papilla cells. Ideally the size of the apical opening should be greater than 1.0 mm, though a few authors have observed successful ingrowth even with an apical opening as less as 0.3 mm.

The cases to be excluded are: avulsed teeth immediately after replantation (revascularization may occur naturally in them), tooth cannot be adequately isolated, teeth with extensive loss of coronal tissue that require restoration with a post, medically compromised patients, patients on anticoagulants and with previous history of apical surgery.

Compliance of patient is essential. Patient should be informed of all the possible implications and make an informed consent.

Procedure

The **first stage** includes local anesthesia, rubber dam isolation and access preparation, followed by copious and gentle irrigation. No instrumentation is carried out during regenerative procedures (*use of instruments is limited to removal of loose/necrotic pulp tissue; no instrumentation of canal walls*). Hence, there is a need to rely heavily on chemical débridement and the use of intracanal medicaments to achieve disinfection and resolution of infection.

The selection of irrigant should not only be based on bactericidal property, but also ability to promote the survival and proliferative capacity of the patient's stem cells.

1.5% sodium hypochlorite is preferred, followed by normal saline; lower concentration of sodium hypochlorite minimizes cytotoxicity to stem cells in the apical tissue (Chlorhexidine is known cytotoxic to stem cells and should be avoided, especially in the second appointment). 5.0 ml of normal saline minimises the cytotoxic effect of sodium hypochlorite on vital tissues.

The **second stage** includes placement of antibiotic paste or calcium hydroxide after drying the canal.

i. Calcium hydroxide is effective as an antimicrobial, but it has certain limitations:
   - Calcium hydroxide limits the possibility of increasing the root canal wall thickness.
   - Effectiveness limited to the root canal only with inadequate dentin penetration.

ii. Triple antibiotic paste is very effective (1:1:1 by volume of ciprofloxacin/metronidazole/minocycline (0.1 mg/mL).

Note: *Undiluted slurry of antibiotics is cytotoxic to stem cells. Dilution of 1000 times (or g/ml) is necessary for stem cell survival and proliferation. Calcium hydroxide is still a preferred choice.*

Minocycline may stain dentin; however, staining can be avoided by:

- Sealing the pulp chamber with dentin bonding agent or flowable composite
- Elimination of minocycline from the composition and use as double antibiotic paste
- Cefaclor is used in place of minocycline.

The canal is sealed with appropriate temporary material.

The **third stage** includes stimulating bleeding and placing scaffold.

The initial treatment is assessed thoroughly to ensure no sensitivity to palpation and percussion. If signs/symptoms of infection persist, additional treatment time with antimicrobial or use of alternative antimicrobial is recommended.

The area is anesthetized (epinephrine should be avoided as it prevents blood flow to create a scaffold) and isolated with rubber dam.

Antibiotic paste/calcium hydroxide is removed by copious irrigation using EDTA. (EDTA removes smear layer and exposes dentinal tubules. It also stimulates and conditions the dentin to release growth factors).

Bleeding is created into canal system by over instrumenting (blood clot consists of a network of fibrin platelets, red blood cells and white blood cells).

The canal is finally irrigated with 5.0 ml normal saline. After drying the canal, a sterilized pre-bent H-file is used to cause mechanical irritation of the periapical tissues. The canal is allowed to be filled with blood; wait for 15 minutes for the blood to clot.

Clinical Tips

- Place a small bend in the file, dip the file in EDTA and over instrument to achieve blood clot just below the cemento-enamel junction (coronal openings).
- In canals where a blood clot cannot be evoked, blood from adjacent canals can be placed in the canal under treatment to create a clot.

Autologous fibrin matrix (AFM) can be preferred as a 3D scaffold than a blood clot with increased concentration of growth factors. Use of AFM is advantageous, being easy to collect, provides a 3D scaffold and supplies a concentrated source of growth factor.

Platelet rich fibrin (PRF) is commonly used autologous fibrin matrix. It is rich in pre-existing growth factors like PDGF, TGF-β, etc., which helps in migration of fibroblasts and endothelial cells. Platelet rich fibrin is prepared by collecting venous blood from the patient without anticoagulant. It employs a centrifuge kit and a collection kit. The blood is immediately centrifuged at a speed of 2700 rpm for 12 minutes. The resultant product consists of PRF clot in the middle and RBC at the bottom.

Once bleeding has been evoked or AFM has been injected, place a collagen matrix, such as Collaplug or Collacote at the orifice (prevents over extension of restorative material). A case, achieving revascularization in deciduous first molar, is depicted in Fig. 38.6a to d.

Place 3.0–4.0 mm of MTA over the collagen matrix to provide a seal (white MTA may stains dentin, GIC can be used as an alternate in esthetic areas).

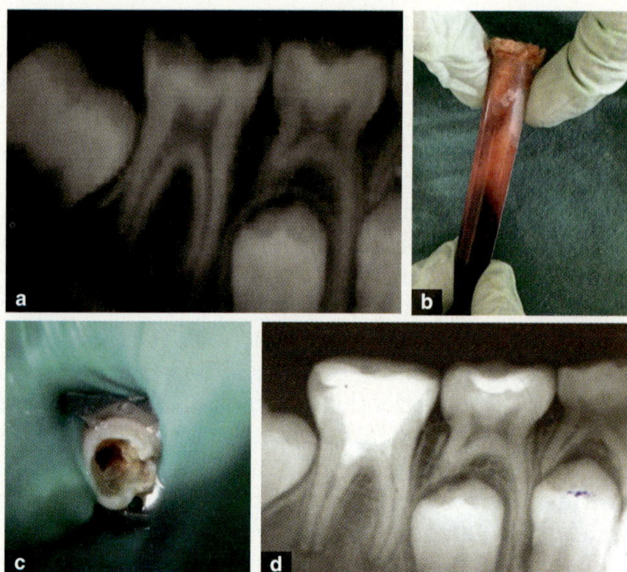

Fig. 38.6 Revascularization using plasma rich fibrin (PRF) in deciduous first molar: (a) Immature apex and periapical radiolucency in relation to mandibular first molar; (b) Plasma rich fibrin (PRF) prepared; upper layer of plasma, fibrin clot and RBC's below; (c) Placing PRF in canals; (d) Post-operative radiograph showing closure of apex and root development (at six month follow-up)

Materials used for Sealing

The materials currently available for sealing the teeth intended for revascularization are Mineral Trioxide Aggregate (MTA), Bioceramics, Glass-ionomer cement and Calcium enriched mixture (CEM).

Mineral Trioxide Aggregate (MTA)

MTA has been successfully used as a sealing agent along with glass-ionomer cement in the revascularization process. It is biocompatible and osseoconductive and sets in the presence of moisture. However, it does not strengthen the remaining tooth structure (Fig. 38.7a to h).

A clinical case of revascularization with MTA is shown in Fig. 38.8a and b.

Bioceramics

Bioceramics have also been successfully tried for sealing of root canals and as root repair materials. Their aluminium free composition makes them more biocompatible as compared to MTA. The ability to form hydroxyapatite while setting and then easy availability makes them the choice of materials for the apexification procedures.

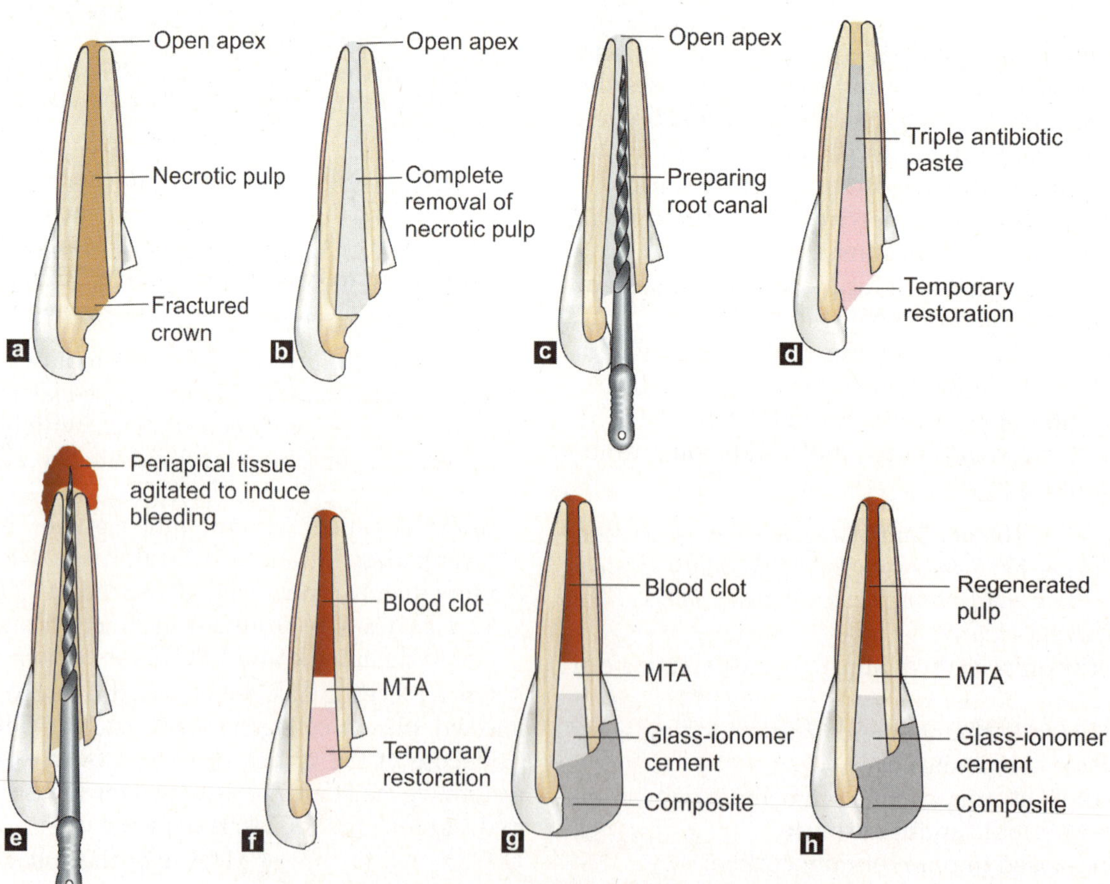

Fig. 38.7a to h Revascularization using MTA as sealing agent

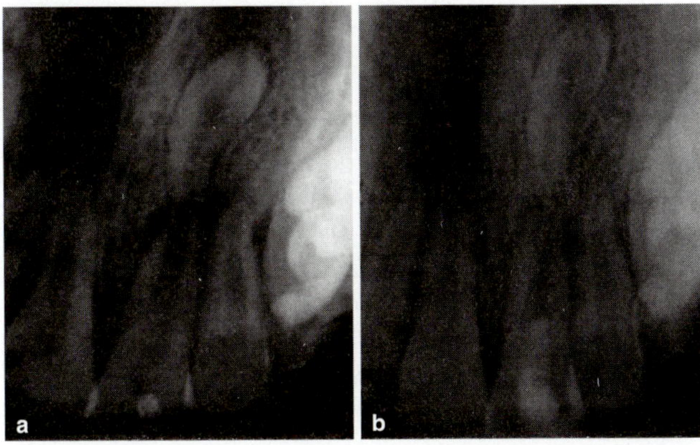

Fig. 38.8 Revascularization using MTA in maxillary left central incisor: (a) Incomplete root formation; (b) Recall at six months showing root apex formation

Glass-Ionomer Cement

It is also used as a sealing agent in revascularization.

Calcium Enriched Mixture (CEM)

Calcium enriched mixture (CEM) is a new biomaterial, which can be used for regenerative endodontic therapy. It is established that CEM is biocompatible material in vital pulp therapies and its sealing ability, biocompatibility and cementogenic properties are identical to those of MTA. CEM is also an antibacterial biomaterial (an appropriate sealing biomaterial over blood clot in revascularization). Unlike MTA, CEM has the advantage of being tooth colored and prevent discoloration caused by presence of MTA. Moreover, the surface characteristics of set CEM cement as well as distribution pattern of calcium phosphorous and oxygen ions are similar to human tooth dentin, which can promote differentiation process of stem cells.

Follow-up

The final stage is the follow-up procedure, which include both clinical and radiographic evaluation. The success pattern should depict as:

- Radiographic evidence of bony healing (6–8 months)
- Radiographic evidence of root development (12–16 months)
- Increased root length
- Responsive pulp vitality tests.

Limitations of Regenerative Procedures

Regenerative procedures are being followed with varying success. The possible limitations are:

- Current procedures are directed to stimulate repair rather than regeneration of new tissues
- Hard tissue development in root canals may hinder future endodontic procedures
- Control over growth factors is mandatory to get desired quality results
- Appropriate biodegradable scaffolds are required for formation of engineered tissues
- Isolation and organization of dental stem cells for regeneration procedures is practically challenging
- Procedural problems, such as discoloration, insufficient bleeding, etc. should also be taken care of.

There is a need for biologically based endodontic procedures that offer the potential to replace tissues lost due to trauma or disease. Regenerative endodontic procedure of future will involve cell biologist and also the concept of tissue engineering so as to achieve successful results.

BIBLIOGRAPHY

1. Albuquerque MT, Valera MC, Moreira CS, Bresciani E, De Melo RM and Bottino MC. Effects of ciprofloxacin-containing scaffolds on *Enterococcus faecalis* biofilms. J. Endod.: 2015; 41, 710–714.
2. Bottino MC, Kamocki K, Yassen GH, Platt JA, Vail MM and Ehrlich Y. Bioactive nanofibrous scaffolds for regenerative endodontics. J. Dent. Res.: 2013; 92:963–969.
3. Chrepa V, Henry MA and Daniel BJ. Delivery of apical mesenchymal stem cells into root canals of mature teeth. J. Dent. Res.: 2015; 94:1653–1659.
4. Chueh LH and Huang GT. Immature teeth with periradicular periodontitis or abscess undergoing apexogenesis: a paradigm shift. J. Endod.: 2006; 32:1205–1213.
5. Chueh LH, Ho YC, Kuo TC, Lai WH, Chen YH and Chiang CP. Regenerative endodontic treatment for necrotic immature permanent teeth. J. Endod.: 2009; 35:160–164.
6. Cordeiro MM, Dong Z and Kaneko T. Dental pulp tissue engineering with stem cells from exfoliated deciduous teeth. J. Endod.: 2008; 34:962–969.
7. Deepak BS and Nandini DB. Stem cell: challenges in endodontics. J. Pharma. And Bioallied Sci.: 2012; 4:84.
8. Diogenes A, Ruparel NB and Teixeira FB. Translational science in disinfection for regenerative endodontics. J. Endod.: 2014; 40:S52–57.
9. Diogenes A and Ruparel NB. Regenerative endodontic procedures: clinical outcomes. Dent. Clin. N. Am.: 2017; 61:111–125.
10. Dissanayaka WL, Hargreaves KM, Jin L, Samaranayake LP and Zhang C. The interplay of dental pulp stem cells and endothelial cells in an injectable peptide hydrogel on angiogenesis and pulp regeneration *in vivo*. Tissue Engg.: 2015, 21:550–563.
11. Fawzy El-Sayed KM, Jakusz K, Jochens A, Dorfer C and Schwendicke F. Stem cell transplantation for pulpal regeneration: a systematic review. Tissue Eng. Part B Rev.: 2015; 21:451–460.

12. Fouad AF. The microbial challenge to pulp regeneration. Adv. Dent. Res.: 2011; 23:285–289.
13. Freymiller EG, Aghaloo TL. Platelet rich plasma: ready or not? J Oral Maxillofac. Surg. 2004, 62; 484.
14. Garcia-Goday F and Murray PE. Recommendations for using regenerative endodontic procedures in permanent immature traumatized teeth. Dent. Traumatol.: 2012; 28:33–41.
15. Gong T, Heng BC, Lo EC and Zhang C. Current advance and future prospects of tissue engineering approach to dentin/pulp regenerative therapy. Stem Cells Int.: 2016; ID9204574.
16. Hargreaves K, Geisler T, Henry M, Wang Y: Regeneration potential of the young permanent tooth: what does the future hold? J. Endod.: 2008, 34; 51.
17. He L, Zhong J, Gong Q, Cheng B, Kim SG, Ling J and *Mao JJ*. Regenerative endodontics by cell homing. Dent. Clin N. Am.:2017; 61:143–159.
18. Hotwani K and Sharma K. Platelet rich fibrin - a novel acumen into regenerative endodontic therapy. Restor. Dent. Endod.: 2014; 39:1–6.
19. Huang GJ. Apexification: the beginning of its end. Int. Endod. J.: 2009; 42:855–866.
20. Huang GT and Garcia-Godoy F. Missing concepts in *de Novo* Pulp Regeneration. J. Dent. Res.: 2014; 93:717–724.
21. Huang GT. A paradigm shift in endodontic management of immature teeth: conservation of stem cells for regeneration. J. Dent.: 2008; 36:379–386.
22. Huang GTJ, Gronthos S and Shi S. Mesenchymal stem cells derived from dental tissues vs. those from other sources: their biology and role in regenerative medicine. J. Dent. Res.: 2009; 88:792–806.
23. Iohara K, Murakami M and Takeuchi N. A novel combinatorial therapy with pulp stem cells and granulocyte colony-stimulating factor for total pulp regeneration. Stem Cells Translational Medicine: 2013; 2:521–533.
24. Ishizaka R, Hayashi Y, Iohara K, Sugiyama M, Murakami M. and Yamamoto T. Stimulation of angiogenesis, neurogenesis and regeneration by side population cells from dental pulp. Biomaterials: 2013; 34:1888–1897.
25. Ishizaka R, Iohara K and Murakami M. Regeneration of dental pulp following pulpectomy by fractioned stem/progenitor cells from bone marrow and adipose tissue. Biomaterials: 2012; 33:2109–2118.
26. Kamocki K, Nor JE and Bottino MC. Dental pulp stem cell responses to novel antibiotic-containing scaffolds for regenerative endodontics. Int. Endod. J.: 2015; 48:1147–1156.
27. Kim JH, Kim Y, Shin SJ, Park JW and Jung IY. Tooth discoloration of immature permanent incisor associated with triple antibiotic therapy: a case report. J. Endod.: 2010; 36:1086–1091.
28. Kim S, Zheng Y, Zhou J, Chen M, Embree MC and Song K. Dentin and dental pulp regeneration by the patient's endogenous cells. Endod. Topics: 2013; 28:106–117.
29. Laurent P, Camps J and About I. Biodentine ™ induces TGF-beta1 release from human pulp cells and early dental pulp mineralization. Int. Endod. J.: 2012; 45:439–448.
30. Laureys WG, Cuvelier CA, Dermaut LR and De Paw GA. The critical apical diameter to obtain regeneration of the pulp tissue after tooth transplantation, replantation, or regenerative endodontic treatment. J. Endod.: 2013; 39:759–763.
31. Law AS. Considerations for regeneration procedures. J. Endod.: 2013; 39:S44–56.
32. Lee BN, Moon JW, Chang HS, Hwang IN, Oh WM and Hwang YC. A review of the regenerative endodontic treatment. Restor. Dent. Endodo.: 2015; 40:179–187.
33. Leong DJX, Setzer FC, Trope M and Karabucak B. Biocompatibility of two experimental scaffolds for regenerative endodontics. Restor. Dent. Endod.: 2016; 41:98–105.
34. Liu J, Yu F, Sun Y, Jiang B, Zhang W, Yang J, Xu GT, Liang A and Liu S. Concise reviews: characteristics and potential applications of human dental tissue-derived mesenchymal stem cells. Stem Cells: 2015; 33:627–638.
35. Mari-Beffa M, Segura-Egea JJ and Diaz-Cuenca A. Regenerative endodontic procedures: a perspective from stem cell niche biology. J. Endod.: 2017; 43:52–62.
36. Miran S, Mitisiadis TA and Pagella P. Innovative dental stem cell-based research approaches: The future of dentistry. Stem Cells Int.: 2016; Article. ID7231038: 1–7.
37. Mitisiadis TA and Harada H. Regenerated teeth: the future of tooth replacement. An Update. Regenerative Medicine: 2015; 10:5–8.
38. Mitisiadis TA, Feki A, Papaccio G and Caton J. Dental pulp stem cells, niches and notch signaling in tooth injury. Adv. Dent. Res.: 2011; 23:275–279.
39. Mitisiadis TA, Orsini G and Jimenez-Rojo L. Stem cell-based approaches in dentistry. Eur. Cells and Mater.: 2015; 30: 248–257.
40. Mjor IA, Smith MR, Ferrari M and Mannoci F. The structure of dentin in the apical region of human teeth. Int. Endod J.: 2001, 34; 346–353.
41. Murray PE, Garcia-Goday F and Hargreaves KM. Regenerative endodontics: a review of current status and a call for action. J. Endod.: 2007; 33:377–390.
42. Nakashima M and Iohara K. Regeneration of dental pulp by stem cells. Adv. Dent. Res.: 2011; 23:313–319.
43. Nosrat A, Seifi A, Asgary S. Regenerative endodontic treatment (revascularization) for necrotic immature permanent molars: a review and report of two cases with a new biomaterial. J. Endod.: 2011, 37; 562.
44. Pan S, Dangaria S, Gopinathan G, Yan X, Lu X and Kotokythas A. SCF promotes dental pulp progenitor migration, neurovascularization, and collagen remodeling-potential applications as a homing factor in dental pulp regeneration. Stem Cell Rev.: 2013; 29:655–667.
45. Peters OA. Translational opportunities in stem cell-based endodontic therapy: where are we and what are we missing? J. Endod.: 2014; 40:S82–S85.
46. Petrino JA, Boda KK, Shambarger S, Bowles WR and McClanahan SB. Challenges in regenerative endodontics: a case series. J. Endod. 2010, 36; 536.

47. Potdar PD and Jethmalani YD. Human dental pulp stem cells: applications in future regenerative medicine. Word J. Stem Cells: 2015; 7:839–851.
48. Rafter M. Apexification: a review. Dent. Traumatol.: 2005;21:1–8.
49. Saito MT, Silverio KG, Casati MZ, Sallum EA and Nociti FH. Tooth-derived stem cells: update and perspectives. World J. Stem Cells: 2015; 7:399–407.
50. Scheller EL, Krebsbach PH and Kohn DH. Tissue engineering: state of the art in oral rehabilitation. Journal of oral rehabilitation.: 2009, 6; 358.
51. Shah N, Logani A, Bhaskar U, Aggarwal V. Efficacy of revascularisation to induce apexification/apexogenesis in infected, non-vital, immature teeth: a pilot clinical study. J. Endod: 2008, 34; 919.
52. Simon SR, Tomson PL and Berdal A. Regenerative endodontics: regeneration or repair? J. Endod.:2014; 40:S70–75.
53. Smith AJ, Duncan HE, Diogenes A, Simon S and Cooper PR. Exploiting the bioactive properties of the dentin-pulp complex in regenerative endodontics. J. Endod.: 2016; 42:47–56.
54. Sonoyama W, Liu Y, Yamaza T, Tuan RS, Wang S, Shi S and Huang GT. Characterization of the apical papilla and its residing stem cells from human immature permanent teeth: a pilot study. J. Endod.: 2008; 34:166–171.
55. Suzuki T, Lee CH, Chen M, Zhao W, Fu SY and Qi JJ. Induced migration of dental pulp stem cells for *in vivo* pulp regeneration. J. Dent. Res.: 2011; 90:1013–1018.
56. Thibodeau B. and Trope M: Pulp revascularization of a necrotic infected immature permanent tooth: case report and review of the literature. Pediat. Dent 29, 47, 2010.
57. Thomson A and Kahler B. Regenerative endodontics—biologically-based treatment for immature permanent teeth: a case report and review of the literature. Aust. Dent. J.: 2010; 55:446–452.
58. Torabinejad M, Parirokh M. Mineral trioxide aggregate: a comprehensive literature review: part II – leakage and biocompatibility investigations. J. Endod. 36,190, 2010.
59. Torabinejad M, Turman M. Revitalization of tooth with necrotic pulp and open apex by using platelet rich plasma: a case report. J. Endod.: 37, 265 , 2011.
60. Tziafas D. Dentinogenic potential of the dental pulp: facts and hypotheses. Endod. Topics: 2010; 17:42–64.
61. Vijayaraghavan R, Mathia VM, Sundaram AM, Karunakaran R and Vinodh S. Triple antibiotic paste in root canal therapy. J. Pharm. Bioallied Sci.: 2012; 4:S230–S233.
62. Volponi AA, Pang Y and Sharpe PT. Stem cell-based biological tooth repair and regeneration. Trends in Cell Biol.: 2010; 20:715–722.
63. Widbiller M, Driesen RB, Eidt A, Lambrichts I, Hiller KA, Buchalla W, Schmalz G and Galler KM.: Cell homing for pulp tissue engineering with endogenous dentin matrix proteins. J. Endod.: 2018; 1–7.
64. Wiggler R, Kaufman AY, Lin S, Steinbock N, Hazan-Molina H and Torneck CD. Revascularization: a treatment for permanent teeth with necrotic pulp and incomplete root development. J. Endod.: 2013; 39:319–326.
65. Yang J, Yuan G and Chen Z. Pulp regeneration: current approaches and future challenges. Frontiers in Physiology: 2016; 7:1–8.
66. Zheng Y, Wang XY and Wang YM. Dentin regeneration using deciduous pulp stem/progenitor cells. J. Dent. Res.: 2012, 91, 676–682.
67. Zhou J, Shi S, Shi Y, Xie H, Chen L and He Y. Role of bone marrow-derived progenitor cells in the maintenance and regeneration of dental mesenchymal tissues. J. Cell. Physiol.: 2011; 226:2081–2090.

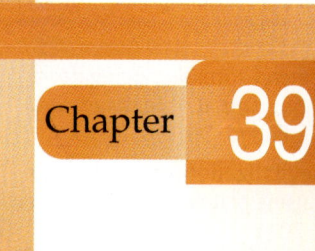

Chapter 39

Ethics in Endodontics

The word ethics is derived from a Greek word *'ethos'* meaning 'conduct' or 'character'. It is the philosophy of human conduct, a way of stating and evaluating principles by which problems of behavior can be solved. In simple terms 'Ethics' is the ability to know the difference between what you consider as a right to do and what is right to do. Ethics is the philosophy of human conduct or the science of what is morally right. The conduct is a voluntary action carried out without any compulsion and the ethics is concerned with evaluating the human conduct and judging whether the action is right or wrong. Ethics is interchangeably used with the word 'moral' (latin word *mores*: meaning conduct or habits). Collectively ethics are only moral obligations, not imposed by any law. A few professions may have written ethical codes; however, basic principle should be followed by one and all. Dental ethics implies moral duties and obligations of the dental professionals towards patients, colleagues and the society at large.

A few authors have notified ETHICS alphabets as, E: Expertise, T: Truthful, H: Honesty, I: Integrity, C: Compassion and S: Sagacity.

Ethics and society are interrelated and influence each other. Individuals following ethics make better society. The gap between general and professional ethics is marginal. There is difference of degree only and not of quality. For example, 'do not steal', a principle in general ethics is equally applicable to the professional ethics.

The code of dental ethics, created by American Dental Association, serve as a standard to which all dental professionals should adhere with sincerity. Each member of dental fraternity is responsible for maintaining the ethical standards of the profession.

Ethics is one of the three branches of philosophy (other two are metaphysics and epistemology) that is concerned with study of those concepts that are used to evaluate human activities; especially, the concepts of goodness and obligation. Ethics may be defined as *'a normative study that deals with the conduct of human beings in private or in public'*. Ethics is thus, a normative science, not a descriptive one. The descriptive science deals with the factual truths; whereas, moral values are evaluated in a normative science. Ethics does not teach us what to do; rather it seeks to find out what should be the base for our actions. It is a search for principles that guide our conduct and moral perceptions in the society.

Other two branches of philosophy, i.e. metaphysics and epistemology also have a bearing on ethics. *Metaphysics* is concerned with our perception of ultimate nature of reality. *Epistemology* deals with the conditions under which our claims to knowledge and belief are either valid or invalid. The relation between ethics and epistemology is well-described by forensic science, which defines the ethicolegal status of an action on the basis of evidence of facts.

The nucleus of ethics is moral behavior, which develops in following three stages:

Stage 1: Person decides what is 'right' or 'wrong' on the basis of inborn/innate feelings.

Stage 2: Those forms of conduct is considered 'right' which were approved by customary modes of behavior in the society.

Stage 3: It is the individual's conscience with his capacity to judge what is 'right' and what is 'wrong'.

Usually our moral judgments are not decided on the basis of instincts or customs. The transition from customary to conscience/reflective morality makes the individual responsible for his/her choice of action.

The ethical postulates to be followed are:

- To differentiate between right and wrong actions (know the difference between right and wrong).
- Knowledge of morality make a genuine impact on human behavior.

- Despite certain constraints, one has the capacity to exercise one's rationality to make moral decisions.
- Individual's capacity to fix priority of decisions.

History of Ethics

The 'Hippocratic oath' has been regarded as a standard of professional ethics. Descriptive theories define the meaning of good; may be moral or non-moral characteristics. Prescriptive theories define ethical terms as carrying mandatory force, e.g. 'ethical rules for dentists' framed by Dental Council of India. Various theories have been put forward regarding ethics:

1. *Theory of utilitarian ethics*: Focuses on utility.
2. *Theory of deontologic ethics*: Focuses on morality of act rather than its consequences; emphasis on action irrespective of the consequence and do not compromise with duty.
3. *Theory of virtue ethics*: Focuses on what a virtuous person would have reacted in a particular circumstance.

Modern Version of the Hippocratic Oath (Revised in 1964 by Louis Lasagna)

In India, The Dentist Act was amended via section 17A (amendment in August 1988) empowering the Dental Council of India to prescribe standards of professional conduct and etiquettes.

The famous 'Hippocratic Oath' written in 4th Century BC, is still the nucleus of professional ethics. The initial version 'do no harm' has been modified and considered as the nucleus of modern version of the Hippocratic Oath.

I swear to fulfil, to the best of my ability and judgment, this covenant:

- I will respect the hard-won scientific gains of those physicians in whose steps I walk, and gladly share such knowledge as is mine with those who are to follow.
- I will apply, for the benefit of the sick, all measures which are required, avoiding those twin traps of overtreatment and therapeutic nihilism.
- I will remember that there is art to medicine as well as science, and that warmth, sympathy, and understanding may outweigh the surgeon's knife or the chemist's drug.
- I will not be ashamed to say "I know not," nor will I fail to call in my colleagues when the skills of another are needed for a patient's recovery.
- I will respect the privacy of my patients, for their problems are not disclosed to me that the world may know. Most especially, must I treat with care in matters of life and death. If it is given me to save a life, all thanks. But it may also be within my power to take a life; this awesome responsibility must be faced with great humbleness and awareness of my own frailty. Above all, I must not play at God.
- I will remember that I do not treat a fever chart, a cancerous growth, but a sick human being, whose illness may affect the person's family and economic stability. My responsibility includes these related problems, if I am to care adequately for the sick.
- I will prevent disease whenever I can, for prevention is preferable to cure.
- I will remember that I remain a member of society, with special obligations to all my fellow human beings, those sound of mind and body as well as the infirm.
- If I do not violate this oath, may I enjoy life and art, respected while I live and remembered with affection thereafter. May I always act so as to preserve the finest traditions of my duties and may I long experience the joy of healing those who seek my help.

Ethical Dilemmas

The specific problems and moral issues emerged due to changed modern circumstances for dealing with patients are called Ethical Dilemmas. A branch of normative ethics, which deals with these specific ethical problems is called *'Applied Ethics'*. It includes (a) medical ethics, (b) business ethics, (c) media ethics, (d) legal ethics and (e) environment ethics.

The *principles* followed for making decisions in the *ethical dilemmas* are:

1. *Analyzing:* Dividing a problem into its leading alternatives.
2. *Weighing:* Assessing the strength and weakness of alternatives by balancing one against the other.
3. *Justifying:* Providing a compelling and sufficient moral reason that appeal to an established moral principle such as to tell the truth.
4. *Choosing:* Selecting alternatives for which some justification can be made.
5. *Evaluating:* Re-examining the choice and the justification based on one's exposure to other similar moral issues.

Code of Dental Ethics

A profession consists of a limited group of persons who have acquired some special skill and are able to perform that function in society better than an average normal person. A professional person is expected to have respect for human beings, competence in his chosen field, integrity and primary concern with service rather than with prestige and profit. A systematic set of rules is needed that upholds the dignity and honor of any profession upgrading its standards and sphere of usefulness. The members of the concerned association should understand their duties and obligations, not only to their fellow beings but also to the society. Ethical codes are the result of an attempt to direct moral consciousness of members of the profession to a peculiar problem. Hippocrates wrote first voluntary code of regulations for medical profession, protecting the rights of patients and appealing to finer instincts of physicians. Standards for protection of human subjects were created in 1947 and called *'Nuremberg Code'.*

In dentistry, the American Dental Association's (ADA) principles of ethics are followed in routine, labelled as a code of ethics and conduct. This code contains five major sections:

1. Service to public and quality of care
2. Education
3. Governing the profession
4. Research and development
5. Professional announcement.

Ethical Principles

The fundamental duty of a dental surgeon is to achieve proper ethical conduct in a dental setting; the patient's interest and needs should be balanced. For maintaining the balance, the following principles of ethics are prescribed.

1. To Do No Harm (Non-maleficence)

This is the foundation of social morality, which states that dental surgeon should not cause any unnecessary harm to the patients specifically.

'Conservative Dentistry' literally embodies the principle, which implies that preservation of what remains is more important than the meticulous replacement of what is lost. Newer methods of cavity preparation and recent advances in material technology are already providing attractive minimal invasive options for treatments that once required extensive unnecessary removal of tooth structure.

Endodontists must explain alternatives to patients as regard restorative aspects. Implants are an enticing lucrative business currently in vogue; however ethically speaking, if the damaged tooth can be salvaged, all measures must be taken to preserve it by endodontic treatment and an adequate postendodontic restorations.

In case where pain cannot be avoided, all appropriate measures must be attempted to minimize the pain during treatment. The aim should be to provide 'painless endodontics' to all the patients. It is imperative that the dental surgeons must update their knowledge regularly, and under all constraints, can perform the procedure in the best interest of the patients.

39

2. To Do Good (Beneficence)

Doctors are generally equated to God and it is our moral duty not to abuse this power.

The healthcare professionals are expected to initiate beneficial actions for their patients honoring an unspoken agreement between the doctor and the patient that some good will result.

The dental professionals must realize that it is not enough to feel satisfied that the treatment will not cause any harm to the patient. Make sure that endodontic therapy/restorative treatment or re-evaluation at a later date will definitely be for the benefit to the patient and relieve them of their discomfort.

This principle can be explained as 'there are two types of bad people—those who do bad things; and those who see bad things and do not make any attempt to rectify them'.

If the patient's previous treatment is unsatisfactory (say partial endodontic treatment or an overhanging restoration) causing pain or discomfort, it is the duty of the operating doctor to do his/her level best without undermining and abusing the other doctor. Your work will convey the clear message of your supremacy of the subject.

3. Respect for Persons

One of the most important principles, respect for persons, incorporate two fundamental ethical considerations, namely:

a. *Autonomy*: Autonomy implies that healthcare professionals respect the patient's capacity for self-determination in making decision concerning their treatment.

Patients should be explained the pros and cons of their decision and should be allowed to abide by their decision, whether or not the operator believe that these choices are wise or beneficial (in case of discontentment the patient is referred to another dental surgeon for opinion).

During planning the treatment, the patient should be an active participant and not as a mere by stander.

More often we, the dental surgeons, are guilty of withholding information, restricting choices or making choices for the patient without their consent, even if we believe that the decision is in 'best interests of the patient'.

Restoring some adjoining teeth when patient ask for a specific restoration, or propagating the use of a particular material insisting it is the best option, must be avoided as misleading the patients is always unethical and may lead to legal hassles.

b. *Informed consent*: *'Informed Consent'* is an essential component of respecting a person under ethical norms. The attributes of informed consent (Nuremberg code) are:

- It should be voluntarily given by the patient.
- It should be legally valid.
- It should be informed.
- It should be comprehending.

In certain populations, the concept of individual autonomy may be comprehended. In such situations, informed consent is negotiated with a leader. This can also be followed in cases where persons because of illiteracy or otherwise cannot participate actively. The ethical principles require special justification before treatment is carried out on vulnerable individuals. Vulnerable population also includes women who might be subservient to their spouses. Women may or may not be literate, but should participate in discussion. Illiteracy may not create any problem because informed consent can be taken by talking rather than reading. This empowers even women to protect their own interests.

The *'Consent Form'* is an instrument designed to protect the interests of the investigators and their institutions; and also to defend them against any civil or criminal liability. The informed consent actually consists of two steps. In first step, the investigator/operator presents whole of the information regarding the procedure to the subject/patient and in second step, his queries about that procedure are cleared.

Step 1: Information is presented to the patient regarding the procedure to be undertaken, advantages, disadvantages, associated risks, need for treatment as well as the future prognosis to some extent.

Step 2: Patient understand the process (may be by reading the document or by narrating the same in his/her language) and based upon this understanding either agrees or refuses to undergo treatment.

A list of information conveyed to the perspective patient/subject includes:

i. A statement that the study involves research coupled with explanation of the purpose of research and expected duration of subjects' involvement. A description of the procedure followed should also be identified.
ii. A description of any benefit to the subjects.
iii. A description of any reasonably foreseeable risks or discomforts to the patient.
iv. Whether any medical treatment available during risk.
v. Availability of alternative procedure, if any.
vi. A statement highlighting how the confidentiality of records will be maintained.
vii. Availability of person(s) for answer to pertinent questions about ongoing research.
viii. A statement that participation is voluntary and refusal to participate will involve no penalty or loss of benefits to which the subject is otherwise entitled and the subject may discontinue participation at any time.

These eight features are known as 'Elements of Information' in the informed consent.

Informed consent must be recorded in every case along with date and must be duly signed by the patient.

Informed Consent of Endodontic Treatment

In case not opting for endodontic treatment, the options may be:

- Extracting the tooth
- Endodontic surgery

In case opting for endodontic treatment (endodontic treatment may have 5–10% failure rate); the possible risks and complications may be:

- Pre-existing gum disease requiring additional treatment
- Problems due to local anesthesia
- Instrument separation
- Perforation of the canal
- Infection, discomfort, numbness
- Allergic/adverse reaction of the materials used
- Tooth fracture
- Incomplete healing

After endodontic therapy, it is important to restore the tooth as early as possible (say within two weeks).

I understand that endodontic therapy may have 5–10% failure rate under optimal conditions. I agree to face the problems, if any. I have had the opportunity to ask questions and all my questions have been answered to my satisfaction. I trust the operative capabilities of my doctor and I hereby offer my consent to have root canal treatment for tooth ....

Diagnosis: ....

Clinical/Radiological findings: ....

Name of patient/guardian   Signature   Date

4. Justice

Justice is described as fairness and equal acceptance given to other individuals. The principal of justice, emphasising on equality, calls for an obligation to protect the weaker section of the society and to ensure equality in their rights and benefits.

It is the society which determines what is just and unjust; therefore, it is imperative that dental surgeons should be in touch with society for ethical compliance of justice.

The dental professional in general and endodontist in particular can offer discount services to needy or spare some time in clinics for low income patients.

They can support local or state level program that seek to extend oral healthcare to the needy people in society.

5. Truthfulness (Veracity)

Veracity implies being truthful and respecting the trust that is essential in patient–doctor relationship. The patient–doctor relation being based on trust, lying of any kind may jeopardize the relations.

It is unethical to recommend any unnecessary treatment to the patients and also charging for the treatment procedures which was never carried onto the patients (doctor may charge for two restorations when only one tooth was restored). Unnecessary referral is also considered unethical. Advertisements based on partial truths are also sort of lying to patients. Another area of veracity (truthfulness) is the credential of the dental surgeon. Any fake degree or specialization as shown by the doctor lead to 'lying'; subsequently, guilty of diluting this ethical principle.

6. Confidentiality

Patients have the right to expect that all communications and records pertaining to their case will be treated as confidential. The relationship of patient and the doctor is based on the understanding that any information revealed by the patient will not be divulged without the patient's consent.

In the field of conservative dentistry, which pertains largely to esthetics as well, the operator may advertise/display the pre- and post-treatment photographs; however, in doing so without the consent of the patient, would undeniably break a bond of trust between the dental professional and the patient. In case the dental surgeon has some personal relations with the patient, it is important to understand that in professional dealing, the personal and professional relationship will have to be dealt separately.

Advertising in Dentistry

Advertising has traditionally been seen as a controversial issue especially for health professionals. The use of advertising media to promote a professional practice is relatively new in medical field. However, advertising by healthcare professionals in India has increased dramatically during the past decade, and this trend in all probability is to continue.

Three types of advertising commonly used amongst dental professional are:

a. Comparable advertising
b. Competitive advertising
c. Informational advertising.

a. *Comparable advertising* is the use of comparisons between the advertiser and others in the same market. An example of 'comparable' type of advertisement, which states that Dr X is the 'only dental surgeon recognized as a Master'. These are usually seen as statements of superiority. Such advertisements can easily be misinterpreted by the public; so considered false and misleading. A few professionals claim that advertising one's achievements is informational and not a statement of superiority. Explanation may and may not be convincing; however, such advertisements must not mislead the patients and therefore should be used with caution. Advertisements regarding superiority are comparative and not information, since they promote the impression that the particular dental surgeon is superior to or better than others in the field.

b. *Competitive advertising* implies offering discounts on dental procedures or offering of the same product or service for less cost than others in the same market. A few dental surgeons have seen offering discounted services, such as 'fillings free with ortho treatment', or 'one child will be treated free if parents are also patients', or 'free treatment for first five patients' and so on.

c. *Informational advertising* is the most acceptable mode of advertisement in medical field. It is the use of information that only pertains to the advertiser and does not refer to any other service providers. This type of advertisement informs the selected population of the person (advertiser), the advertiser's location, and the services available from the advertiser. It also communicates general information regarding the services to educate the target audience. These types of advertisements generally comply with various state ethical codes and the ADA Code of Professional Conduct.

In some countries, dental surgeons have the right to advertise their practice within legal limits; however, in India the rules do not permit advertisements. In the Dentists (Code of Ethics) Regulations 1976, advertising, 'whether directly or indirectly, for the purpose of obtaining patients or promoting their own professional advantage', or acquiescing in the publication of notice directing attention to the operator's skills, knowledge or qualifications, is considered as unethical, equal to conniving at or aiding in any kind of illegal practice. Under the code of ethics, any advertisements by dental professionals should be limited to the announcement of the opening of a practice, a change of address, a change of ownership, or the introduction of a new partner. Despite these rules, a number of practitioners ignore the code of ethics to advertise their services. Many dental surgeons feel that advertising is a necessary part of running a business, and a few also argue that it has the potential to be beneficial. Supporters of advertising claim that information advertising can empower consumers to make good decisions regarding their oral health; increase the community's awareness of dental healthcare; encourage better quality dental services; and help consumers choose their dental surgeon. However, there are also those who defend the traditional view that dentistry is primarily a health profession and not a business; and that the ethical considerations of a profession should be given priority. It is also a fact that industry competition has allowed commercialization of medical profession in general, which risks undermining the ethical standing of the profession. The concept of commercialization is considered inappropriate and misleading. The opponents object to the increased emphasis on fee structure, viz. discounts and 'treatment packages' etc. The dental surgeons are encouraged to regard patients as customers, rather than patients in need of help. A few professionals believe that advertising could have an adverse effect on the image of the profession in general and no impact on competitive price reduction. The dichotomy between the dual role of dental surgeons as a healthcare provider and as a business entity is the main impinging factor. Commercial goals are one side of the coin; whereas, professional goals are other side of the coin. However, business itself is not unethical, and the reality is: if the practice fails as a business, the practitioner fails as a professional.

The issue of poorly designed advertisements is also of concern of the ethical principles. Many dental advertisements can be seen with poor design that lead to discredit to the profession. Some of these advertisements may well be within the guidelines of state dental council acts but convey a non-professional message to the society. Such advertisements, being unethical damage the professionalism of dentistry and insult the social contract that dentistry enjoys by being a profession and not a business.

In spite of the ban on advertising by dental professionals, there are few who keep on resorting to advertising to promote their professional services. Unethical advertising is neither appreciated nor condoned, but there is a demand for relaxation in the restrictions, which would be beneficial for the budding dental professionals. The majority of young and budding dental surgeons approve of advertising, while their seniors reject it. This may be a reflection of industry competition, a drop in ethical standards, or a greater familiarity with the world of advertising and media among younger age groups. The ethical objections to advertising by healthcare professionals, including dental professionals, persist with good cause. The rise of new technologies and media is another challenge, but the ethical issue remain the same.

Standard of Care

The standard of care in dental profession is defined as the degree of care that a concerned dental surgeon would exercise under similar circumstances. The standard has been expressed as the capability/expertise of the operator as compared to other dental surgeons in the community with similar education and experience. The dental surgeon should be aware of their responsibilities and commitment towards their patients.

Any conduct failing to conform to the standard of care constitutes a breach of duty and an element of negligence.

The dental surgeon practicing general dentistry are expected to execute standard of care under any circumstances.

Endodontists are expected to set a higher standard of care as compared to general dental practitioner.

The element of negligence on the part of the dental surgeon is looked into by the attorneys (judges), who analyse whether standard of care was followed or not. The evidence and justification of standard of care presented to the patient at that given time and circumstances are to be explained to the judge by the dental surgeon.

It is important to comply with the following basic criteria:

- Complete dental and medical history is to be recorded.
- The affected teeth along with other oral tissues should be thoroughly examined.

- Do not rely on old radiograph, take a new good quality radiograph; may be more than one at different angulations.
- Analyze the previous treatment plan and never hesitate to suggest more conservative/feasible options; do not straight away disregard the earlier plan.
- Inform the patient about prognosis of the affected tooth and also possible time span.
- Refer the patient whenever treatment protocol is beyond your control and expertise.

Advances in technology continue to make dentistry a truly dynamic profession. The standard of care in each and every ailment is improving over the years.

For example, the standard of care in the direct placement of Class II restoration in early eighties differs from the present standard of care. It requires a commitment to continuous learning to offer standard of care of the level prevalent at any given time. Participating in continuing education courses, and professional meetings help updating the knowledge on periodic basis.

The dental surgeons should strive to use current technology, materials and knowledge to offer the requisite standard of care to their patients.

Refer or Not to Refer

The concept of 'referral' has never been properly understood and followed in our country. Patients keep on moving from one dental surgeon to another; may not get satisfaction of their choice. By and large, patients are not aware of their problems; and also who is the perfect person to solve that problem. The ethics and the concept of referral implies certain objectives.

The common objective is that no patient shall move from one practitioner to another without someone in command. Every patient should learn and understand the importance of the first dental surgeon visited (patient has the right to choose and select the initial doctor).

In case of referral, the basic 'headquarter' remains with the first operator; the patient is to be sent back after the requisite consultation/treatment. General practitioner refer the patient to a specialist for treatment; whereas, one specialist can refer the patient to another for seeking opinion. The referred operator, after sincerely analysing, inform his/her opinion to the first operator (the relevant fee can be charged).

The decision to make a referral is personal, based on the individual's own experience, an honest assessment of one's abilities in particular areas and the comfort level, drawing the line as to where one's expertise ends.

Guidelines for Referral

- Is the treatment technically beyond my capability?
- Is there a high-risk of complications for the indicated procedure?
- Will the patient feel comfortable if I perform the procedure?
- My experience and confidence with the said procedure.

The accepted principle is 'When in doubt, refer to some experienced operator'. The dental surgeon should follow certain duties (guidelines) while referring his/her patient to a consultant. The duties are:

Duties towards the patients

The duties towards the patients are:

- Dental surgeon has the ethical obligation to furnish record of the patient to the referral doctor, either free or accepting nominal fee.
- A reasonable arrangement for emergency care of a patient, (may be direct or referred) should be available in every dental clinic.
- Dental surgeon shall be obliged to seek consultation, if need be; the referred consultant upon completion of the treatment shall return the patient to the referring dental surgeon.
- Dental surgeons have an obligation to use their knowledge and experience for overall improvement of dental health of the society.

Duties towards the referral doctor (consultant)

The duties towards the referral dental surgeon are:

a. The dental surgeon should exercise control in making comments on oral health of the patient, e.g. for example, a difference of opinion as regard disease or treatment should not be communicated to patient in a manner which may offend him.
b. One should never criticize the fellow dental surgeon, especially in front of other patients.

The following features are considered unethical towards professional colleagues:

- Paying or accepting commissions of referrals.
- Undercutting of charges in order to solicit patients for future.
- If planned treatment is beyond the competence of the initial dental surgeon; even then the patient is not referred to a consultant.
- The patient is not sent back to the previous doctor after the requisite service of the consultant completes.
- The consultant should charge as per advice of the referred dental surgeon.

Endodontic Referrals

A. Referred from

Doctor's Name: ____________________ Contact: __________

Clinic Address: ____________________

Patient Name: ____________________

a. Signs and Symptoms
- Pain in tooth
- Swelling

b. Radiological findings
- Apical Radiolucency
- Periodontal condition
- Status of pulp spaces
- Any abnormal findings

c. Any specific complaint
- Trauma or fracture

Treatment already performed
- Prescribed medicines (also report any allergy/sensitivity to drugs)
- Caries excavation
- Root canal opened (report all root canal separately)
- Incision/drainage
- Mishaps (if any)

B. Referred to

Doctor's Name: ____________________ Contact: __________

Clinic Address: ____________________

Patient Name: ____________________

Referred For
- Diagnostic consultation
- Root canal treatment
- Endodontic surgery
- Managing root canal mishaps
- Any specific problem

Referred to Dr. ....

Referred by Dr. .... Signature and Date

Negligence and Malpractice

Dental negligence is a violation of the standard of care during dental treatment; an injury caused to the patient as a result of negligent dental treatment. The dental surgeon is liable to face criminal charges for such negligence.

Any kind of negligence or poor quality dental treatment is considered as dental malpractice.

Substandard dental care resulting in the above can be due to (i) Clinician not possessing a required qualification (ii) Qualified persons perform carelessly without professional responsibility.

Endodontic treatment procedure is the second highest number of malpractice reported in India. Teeth to be treated endodontically should be evaluated for any aberrant morphology/anatomy such as curved roots, calcified canals, and any other potential complicating factors. Good preoperative X-rays and use of a rubber dam are mandatory. Infections due to endodontic procedures can be 'deadly'; mainly because of their anaerobic nature. If the operator breaks any root canal instrument in a canal, which cannot be retrieved, the patient should be advised and referred appropriately.

The endodontic negligence, is mainly because of failure to carry out proper preoperative assessments or devise inappropriate treatment plans, substandard operative procedures and inadequate information to the patient as regard postoperative maintenance phase.

In case of legal implications, the lawyer will take a detailed statement from the dental surgeon to find out exactly what happened during treatment. The lawyers usually seek an independent expert opinion as to whether that particular dental practice was acceptable and whether it caused any harm to the patient. Depending on that opinion, the lawyers tries to settle the claim off the court's jurisdiction.

Traditionally, dental cases do not get into the courts, probably because the sums claimed might be less than the expenses of the courts. There have been a few exceptions in recent years; most of the cases related to cosmetic dentistry.

The dental surgeons should put sincere efforts to diffuse patient dissatisfaction; mostly the patients are not heard properly and need psychological motivation. Dental surgeon's conduct and practice, usually solve most of the problems. The nucleus is how to deal with the complaint, rather to involve lawyers, etc.

Failure to provide the standard care to the patients may have many parameters; main are as follows:

a. Failure to Provide Adequate Isolation

Failure to use rubber dam while performing an endodontic procedure is considered as negligence. Use of rubber dam is mandatory as it provides appropriate safety measures during root canal procedures.

It prevents the aspiration, inhalation or ingestion of endodontic instruments and irrigants like sodium hypochlorite, etc. It also reduces microbial contamination and reinfection.

In case the instrument is ingested/aspirated, the dental surgeon should:

- Inform the patient
- Reassure the patient
- Refer patient to medical care
- Pay all the bills of patient.

The barrier technique such as sterilized gloves, face mask, protective eye shields and disposal of waste, etc. should also be followed during endodontic treatment.

b. Failure to record Quality Radiographs

Good quality radiographs are mandatory; if not recorded properly, will be considered as negligence. Avoid excessive radiation exposure to patient at all expenses.

Whenever possible, take digital radiographs, so as to incorporate all the affected teeth in least number of radiographs, coupled with minimum exposing the patient.

X-ray units and other related armamentarium should be checked before use.

c. Negligence related to Pain Management

Pain management is mainly carried out by using local anesthesia in dental set up. Injecting local anesthesia may lead to problems such as:

- Syncope
- Fracture of needle in site
- Hematoma
- Trismus
- Drug allergy
- Infection (postoperative).

In few cases, patients have moved consumer courts with allegations of negligence by the operator.

d. Injuries Leading to Burns

Burns can be because of thermal or chemical reasons.

i. *Thermal burns*: Thermal burns can occur due to:

- Over used burs; especially at high speeds
- Curing lights and few lasers (less chances)
- Insufficiently cooled instruments after sterilization
- Heated instruments especially during sealing off gutta-percha during obturation.

Care should be taken to avoid these mishaps, such as:

- Handpiece should be regularly oiled and maintained.
- New and sharp burs should be used.
- Soft tissues should be properly managed during endodontic procedures.
- Continuous irrigation should be carried out during root canal treatment.

ii. *Chemical burns*: Many strong chemicals, medicaments and irrigants can cause chemical burns in the oral cavity, which can be avoided by:

- Proper training of assistants
- Avoid overuse of chemicals
- Alternate between strong irrigants/acids with normal saline
- Avoid carrying chemicals over patient's face.

e. Negligence in use of Sodium Hypochlorite

Sodium hypochlorite, when extruded beyond tooth apex, manifest as combination of severe pain, swelling and profuse bleeding both through tooth and interstitially.

Such accidents are managed by aspiration, ice packs, analgesics, wound débridement and warm compress (after 24 hours).

Following principles help in preventing such accidents:

- Using needles with closed end and lateral vents
- The tip of the needle be 1.0–2.0 mm short of apex if open on top
- Do not allow binding of needle in root canal
- Do not force irrigants in root canals.

f. Iatrogenic Negligence

i. *Tissue emphysema*: Collection of gas or air in the tissue space of facial planes leads to tissue emphysema. While using air pressure, blast of air should be directed at horizontal direction against the walls of tooth and not periapically.

ii. *Overlooking periodontal concerns*: In case the affected tooth has caries progressing subgingivally or into the furcation area, or if the periradicular area shows signs of bone loss/inflammation; the dental surgeon should seek opinion of a periodontist or other specialist before proceeding to endodontic treatment.

iii. *Instrument separation*: Instrument separation usually occurs in routine endodontic practice. A sincere effort to retrieve the instrument or to bypass the separated instrument to negotiate rest of canal is mandatory. If unable to manage the separated instruments, the guidelines are:

- Explain the patient about the incident.
- Show the remaining part of the instrument and assure that the tooth will remain asymptomatic.
- Record the methods tried to retrieve or bypass the separated instrument.
- Refer the case to someone expert and follow till satisfaction of the patient.
- Keep the records for any medicolegal reference.

iv. *Perforations*: Perforation is a common procedural accident, mainly due to unpredictable anatomy. The endodontists are usually competent enough to tackle the situation. In case the perforation is unmanageable, the case can be referred to the expert operator for management. The patients should also be explained of the implications of perforations.

v. *Overextensions*: Overextensions is a rare procedural error; endodontists are mostly aware of the precautions to be taken to avoid such mishap.

There is a controversy regarding what actually constitutes as an 'overextended obturation'. It is fine if the filling is within the tip of the apex; 1.0–2.0 mm beyond the apex constitute overextension (patient may be asymptomatic). Sealer causing paresthesia are usually not used these days; the problem caused by obturating materials is usual transient and get resolved within one week. The case should be followed up properly.

ETHICS IN ENDODONTIC RESEARCH

Research in the dental profession is moving forward expeditiously. A fairly large amount of research articles are being published by Indian authors. Apart from institutional trust, the authors should adhere to the Code of Ethics in every aspect of research and publications. This is fundamental professional responsibility and commitment to an ethical pursuit of knowledge.

All of us, especially the budding researchers are expected to cooperate in the implementation of this Code. Misconduct casts doubt on the integrity of individuals and may lead to complications at any stage of life.

The prevention of misconduct in research is best achieved by properly educating all individuals involved in research. It is suggested that researchers should participate in appropriate educational activities, keeping abreast with the latest knowledge. Constant review of current literature in various national and international journals pertaining to our own branch as well as parallel branches of dentistry should be carried out in routine to be able to innovate ideas for the betterment of the concerned subject.

All participating investigators and their colleagues conducting any research should follow ethical practice, with due consideration of any local legislation and regulations. Ethical committee approval must be obtained along with written informed consent by the participants in their own language.

Where the population is vulnerable to exploitation, it is important to respect their human rights and ensure that the research has relevance and potential benefit to their well-being.

Human Research

The declaration of Helsinki is a statement of ethical principles for research involving human participants; a subject of ethical standards that promote respect for all human participants and protect their health and rights.

Research must adhere to the fundamental principles: respect the needs for autonomy, beneficence, justice, veracity, fidelity, anonymity and nonmaleficence. Human research comprises, investigative clinical research, clinical trials and studies using tissue samples. Biogenetics, using stem cells and utilizing tissue banks require complete transparency in all aspects of consenting and confidentiality.

Animal Research

An investigator using animals in research should understand basic principles of ethics and also contribute to the improvement of animal health and welfare. Researchers should sincerely make efforts to protect misuse of animals.

Every effort must be made to:

- Preferably replace the use of live animals by non-animal alternatives
- Reduce the number of animals used in research to the minimum mandatory requirement
- Refine the procedures so that the animal's suffering is kept to a minimum during research.

Conflicts of Interest

Each individual is expected to follow ethical ways to avoid conflict in terms of decision-making and publication of data. The appearance of a conflict of interest, such as the potential for financial and personal gain, can be as damaging as an actual act of conflict of interest. Full disclosure of any potential conflict of interest must be made to the investigator's institution or to the association as applicable.

The intellectual property rights of all participating researchers should be protected (intellectual property rights apply to any potential commercial gain, and must be agreed at the outset of the project by the investigators, their institutions and/or any other external body, such as a sponsoring company).

Dissemination of Information

Most scientific journals ask authors to make declarations at submission about the integrity of their research. Many journals have experienced plagiarism; the editors need to develop policies to minimize the publication of articles containing evidence of scientific misconduct. It is expected that authors, representing a body of research in a process of publication should:

- not inappropriately fragment data into several different publications
- inform sources of funding
- adhere to predetermined guidelines regarding order of authorship
- agree to its submission for review and publication.

Appropriate written permission must be obtained to publish any type of image, which should not identify the participant.

Misconduct is the fabrication, falsification, plagiarism, or any other deviation from accepted practices in proposing, carrying out, or reporting results from research. It is the failure to comply with international, national, local and institutional requirements for the protection of researchers, human participants, laboratory animals and the public at large. It is also the failure to meet other legal requirements governing research.

Misconduct includes:

- Submission of the same article simultaneously to more than one journal without informing the editors concerned.
- Lack of consent by coauthors (coauthorship of an article indicates that all individuals who have genuinely participated in research, have full knowledge of, and are in total agreement with, the content of the article).
- Lack of acknowledgment of financial support.
- Premature release of scientific data prior to presentation or publication in a peer-reviewed forum.

Any individual, who is involved in any form of misconduct or misuse of ethical principles is expected to report the matter to the concerned authorities. Only then the profession will adapt to a state of satisfaction in any field of research, precisely Endodontics.

Ethics and Esthetics

The term 'esthetic dentistry' has been used to refer to the application of tooth colored restoration in either anterior or posterior regions. Such restorations should function properly maintaining the stomatognathic system.

Cosmetic dentistry implies application of restorative techniques purely to remove the appearance while not necessarily improving function. These type of restorative protocol should not be at the cost of unnecessary tooth reduction.

It is important to note that we must resist the provocative call of cosmetic gurus to limit your practice to esthetics. Cosmetic dentistry should be undertaken keeping in view the need and analyzing each aspect of the procedure.

The dental surgeons are usually attuned to their patient's esthetic desires and aspirations. Many of them have added the requisite know-how of the subject and are willing to help improving patient's dental appearance by using biologically sound and minimally destructive means following ethical principles.

Esthetic problems are generally managed ethically following detailed discussions and careful evaluation of the various options available (including the ones that other disciplines or skills could possibly provide) coupled with appropriate training and skills.

Cosmetic dentistry is regarded as just one aspect of decent restorative dentistry. Restorative dentistry has always been about managing dental disease; maintaining function and improving looks as well. However, in seeking to do so, the 'risk-to-reward ratio' must be considered and enough time must be taken to ethically weigh up the real potential esthetics benefits against the many risks involved; (risks include long-term biologic damage of the tooth tissue or stability, that might be involved in performing such procedures).

Laws in Dentistry

The laws applicable to dental practice are same as those applicable to anyone who provides personal services. As a private practitioner, the dental surgeons are governed by *tax laws*, *employment laws* and *law of contract*. The dental profession is also subject to a special statue, commonly referred to as *dental law or dental practice act*.

The laws that are applicable under the act are as follows:

- The name under which a dental surgeon conducts his practice should not be false or misleading in any respect.
- The name of the dental surgeon no longer actively associated with the practice may not be used for more than one year.
- A dental surgeon, who by any means of communication, announces that he/she is certified or a diplomate in an area of dentistry not recognized by Dental Council of India, amounts to making a false or misleading representation to the public.

Laws that are related to third party payment are:

- A dental surgeon who accepts third party payment under a co-payment plan, as payment without disclosing details to the third party is unethical.
- It is unethical for a dental surgeon to increase the fee to a patient solely because the patient is insured.
- Payments received under a government funded program or constituent dental society sponsored program should not be overbilled.
- A dental surgeon who submits a claim form to a third party reporting arbitrary treatment dates so as to assist a patient in obtaining benefits under a dental plan is unethical.
- A dental surgeon who incorrectly describes a dental procedure in order to receive a greater payment or reimbursement is unethical.
- A dental surgeon who performs unnecessary dental procedures is also unethical.

We, the dental professionals, should strive to do what is 'right'. Usually, it is tempting to do what is easy. Simeroth's words clearly explain 'Science takes us to the next level, but it is ethics that keeps us there'. Ethical codes tries to direct the moral consciousness of the members of the profession to a particular situation and are important in developing standards of moral conduct. It is imperative to concentrate doing the right thing in the right perspective rather than repenting why you did that wrong.

BIBLIOGRAPHY

1. Angell E, Sutton AJ, Windridge K and Dixon-Woods M. Consistency in decision making by research ethics committees: a controlled comparison. J. Med. Ethics: 2006; 32:662–664.
2. Castledine G. The importance of keeping patient records secure and confidential. Br. J. Nurs.: 2006; 15:466.
3. Chamber DW. The ethics of experimenting in dental practice. Dent. Clin. North Am.: 2002; 46:29–44.
4. Chambers DW. A primer on dental ethics: Part I. Knowing about ethics. J. Am. College of Dentists: 2006; 73:38–46.
5. Chambers DW. A primer on dental ethics: Part II. Moral Behaviour. J. Am. College of Dentists: 2007; 74:38–49.
6. Ellen P and Singleton R. Human rights and ethical considerations in oral health research. JCDA: 2008; 74:439–439e.
7. Garbin CA, Garbin AJ, Saliba N, de Lima DC and Macedo AP. Analysis of the ethical aspects of professional confidentiality in dental practice. J. Appl. Oral Sci.: 2008; 16:75–80.
8. Grady C. Enduring and emerging challenges of informed consent. N. Engl. J. Med.: 2015; 372:855–862.
9. Hayden JE. Digital manipulation in scientific images: some ethical considerations. J. Biocommun.: 2000; 27:11–19.
10. Jeffocoat MK. A well-founded trust: a sever-tier defence against scientific misconduct. J. Am. Dent. Assoc.: 2002; 133:804, 806.
11. Kegley JA. Challenges to informed consent. EMBO Rep.: 2004; 5:832–836.
12. Macklin R. Understanding informed consent. Acta. Oncol.: 1999; 38:83–87.
13. Main BG and Adair SR. The changing face of informed consent. Br. Dent. J.: 2015; 219:325–327.
14. Nicholl J. The ethics of research ethics committees. BMJ: 2000; 320:1217.
15. Nichols PS and Winslow GR. How strict is confidence? Gen. Dent.: 2004; 52:15–17.
16. Nicol TE. Confidentiality versus disclosure of a patient's infectious status. Gen. Dent.: 1997; 45:78–80.
17. O'Neill O. Some limits of informed consent. J. Med. Ethics: 2003; 29:4–7.
18. Phaosavasdi S, Thaneepanichskul S, Tannirandorn Y, Pupong V, Uerpairojkit B, Pruksapongs C and Kajanapitak A. The idealistic ethical doctor. J. Med. Assoc. Thai.: 2007; 90: 201–202.
19. Renson CE. Ethical dilemmas in dentistry. Dent. Update: 1994; 21:225–226.
20. Shaw D. Ethics, professionalism and fitness to practice: three concepts, not one. BDJ: 2009; 207:59–62.
21. Sikri V and Sikri P. Ethics and endodontic intervention. JIDA: 1990; 2:31–33.
22. Skene L. Undertaking research in other countries: national ethico-legal barometers and international ethical consensus statements. PLoS Med.: 2007; 4:e10.
23. Smith AJ. Human embryonic stem cell research and its regulation. J. Dent. Res.: 2007; 86:197.
24. Smith D. Five principles for research ethics. Am Psychological association: 2003; 34:56.
25. Sotelo J. Regulation of clinical research sponsored by pharmaceutical companies: a proposal. PloS Med.: 2006; 3:e306.
26. Trathen A and Gullaghor JF. Dental professionalism: definitions and debate. BDJ: 2009; 206:249–253.
27. Zabala-Blanco J, Alconero-Camarero AR, Casaus-Perez M, Gutierrez-Torre E and Saiz-Fernandez G. Evaluation of bioethical aspects in health professionals. Enferm Clin.: 2007; 17:56–62.

Index

D

E

U

V

W

X

Z